Basic
Neurochemistry

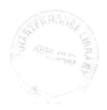

Basic
Neurochemistry

Molecular, Cellular and Medical Aspects
Sixth Edition

Editor-in-Chief

George J. Siegel, M.D.
Chief, Neurology Service
Edward Hines Jr. Veterans Affairs Hospital
Hines, Illinois and
Professor of Neurology and Cellular and Molecular Biochemistry
Loyola University Chicago Stritch School of Medicine
Maywood, Illinois

Editors

Bernard W. Agranoff, M.D.
Ralph Waldo Gerard Professor of
Neurosciences
Department of Psychiatry and
Professor, Department of Biological Chemistry
University of Michigan
Ann Arbor, Michigan

R. Wayne Albers, Ph.D.
Chief, Section on Enzyme Chemistry
Laboratory of Neurochemistry
National Institute of Neurological Disorders
and Stroke
National Institutes of Health
Bethesda, Maryland

Stephen K. Fisher, Ph.D.
Professor, Department of Pharmacology
Senior Research Scientist
Mental Health Research Institute
University of Michigan
Ann Arbor, Michigan

Michael D. Uhler, Ph.D.
Associate Professor, Department of
Biological Chemistry
Research Scientist
Mental Health Research Institute
University of Michigan
Ann Arbor, Michigan

Illustrations by Lorie M. Gavulic, M.F.A.

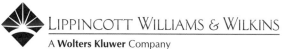

LIPPINCOTT WILLIAMS & WILKINS
A **Wolters Kluwer** Company
Philadelphia · Baltimore · New York · London
Buenos Aires · Hong Kong · Sydney · Tokyo

Acquisitions Editor: Mark Placito
Developmental Editor: Anne M. Sydor
Manufacturing Manager: Tim Reynolds
Production Manager: Kathleen Bubbeo
Cover Designer: Karen Quigley
Indexer: Phyllis Manner
Compositor: Maryland Composition
Printer: World Color

Cover figures: The background electron micrograph is Figure 1-9, showing synaptic vesicles in two axodendritic synapses. Atop the electron micrograph is a model of the crystal structure of the potassium channel. (Reprinted with permission from Doyle, D.A., Cabral, J.M., Pfuetzner R. A., et al. The structure of the potassium channel: Molecular basis of K^+ conduction and selectivity. *Science* 280:69–81, 1998. Copyright 1998 American Association for the Advancement of Science.)

Printed in the United States of America

9 8 7 6 5 4 3 2

Library of Congress Cataloging-in-Publication Data

Basic neurochemistry : molecular, cellular and medical aspects /
editor-in-chief, George J. Siegel ; editors, Bernard W. Agranoff...
[et al.] ; illustrations by Lorie M. Gavulic. — 6th ed.
    p.   cm.
  Includes bibliographical references and index.
  ISBN 0-397-51820-X
  1. Neurochemistry.   I. Siegel, George J.
  [DNLM: 1. Neurochemistry.   2. Nervous System Physiology.
3. Nervous System Diseases.   WL 104 B311 1998]
QP356.3.B27   1998
612.8′ 042—dc21
DNLM/DLC
for Library of Congress   98-21392
                                                                  CIP

Care has been taken to confirm the accuracy of the information presented and to describe generally accepted practices. However, the authors, editors, and publisher are not responsible for errors or omissions or for any consequences from application of the information in this book and make no warranty, express or implied, with respect to the contents of the publication.

The authors, editors, and publisher have exerted every effort to ensure that drug selection and dosage set forth in this text are in accordance with current recommendations and practice at the time of publication. However, in view of ongoing research, changes in government regulations, and the constant flow of information relating to drug therapy and drug reactions, the reader is urged to check the package insert for each drug for any change in indications and dosage and for added warnings and precautions. This is particularly important when the recommended agent is a new or infrequently employed drug.

Some drugs and medical devices presented in this publication have Food and Drug Administration (FDA) clearance for limited use in restricted research settings. It is the responsibility of the health care provider to ascertain the FDA status of each drug or device planned for use in their clinical practice.

Contents

Boxes

Contributors

Bernard W. Agranoff, M.D.
Ralph Waldo Gerard Professor of Neurosciences
Professor, Department of Biological Chemistry
Senior Research Scientist
Mental Health Research Institute
University of Michigan
1103 East Huron Street
Ann Arbor, Michigan 48104-1687

R. Wayne Albers, Ph.D.
Chief, Section on Enzyme Chemistry
Laboratory of Neurochemistry
National Institutes of Health
National Institute of Neurological Disorders
*   and Stroke*
9000 Rockville Pike
Bethesda, Maryland 20892

Margaret Altemus, M.D.
Assistant Professor
Department of Psychiatry
Cornell University Medical College
525 East 68th Street
New York, New York 10021

Jack D. Barchas, M.D.
Professor and Chairman
Department of Psychiatry
Cornell University Medical College
525 East 68th Street, Box 171
New York, New York 10021

Robert L. Barchi, M.D., Ph.D.
David Mahoney Professor and Chair
Department of Neurology
University of Pennsylvania School of Medicine
3400 Spruce Street
Philadelphia, Pennsylvania 19104

Nicolas G. Bazan, M.D., Ph.D.
Boyd and Villere Professor of Ophthalmology,
*   Biochemistry and Molecular Biology, and*
*   Neurology*
Louisiana State University Medical Center
Director, Neuroscience Center of Excellence
2020 Gravier Street, Suite D
New Orleans, Louisiana 70112

Joyce A. Benjamins, Ph.D.
Professor, Associate Chair for Research
Department of Neurology
Wayne State University School of Medicine
421 East Canfield Avenue
Detroit, Michigan 48201-1908

A. Lorris Betz, M.D., Ph.D.
Crosby-Kahn Professor of Neurosurgery and
*   Neuroanatomy*
Professor of Pediatrics, Surgery and Neurology
University of Michigan
D2337 Medical Professional Building
Ann Arbor, Michigan 48109-0532

John P. Blass, M.D., Ph.D.
Professor of Neurology, Medicine and
*   Neuroscience*
Cornell University Medical College at the Burke
*   Medical Research Institute*
785 Mamaroneck Avenue
White Plains, New York 10605

Scott T. Brady, Ph.D.
Associate Professor
Department of Cell Biology and Neuroscience
University of Texas Southwestern Medical Center
5323 Harry Hines Boulevard
Dallas, Texas 75235-9111

Joan Heller Brown, Ph.D.
Professor
Department of Pharmacology
School of Medicine
University of California, San Diego
La Jolla, California 92093-0636

Roger F. Butterworth, Ph.D., D.Sc.
Professor of Medicine
University of Montreal, Campus Saint-Luc
1058 Rue Saint-Denis Street
Montreal, Quebec H2X 3J4
Canada

Ellen Carpenter, Ph.D.
UCLA Mental Retardation Research Center
760 Westwood Plaza, 68-177 NPI
Los Angeles, California 90024

William A. Catterall, Ph.D.
Professor and Chairman
Department of Pharmacology
University of Washington
Seattle, Washington 98195

Astrid Chapman, Ph.D.
Senior Lecturer
Department of Neurosciences
Institute of Psychiatry
De Crespigny Park
Denmark Hill
London SE5 8AF
United Kingdom

Dennis W. Choi, M.D., Ph.D.
Professor and Head
Department of Neurology
Washington University School of Medicine
660 South Euclid Avenue, Box 8111
St. Louis, Missouri 63110

Donald D. Clarke, Ph.D.
Professor, Department of Chemistry
Fordham University
441 East Fordham Road
Bronx, New York 10458

David R. Colman, Ph.D.
Professor
Brookdale Center for Molecular Biology
Mount Sinai School of Medicine
One Gustave L. Levy Place
New York, New York 10029

Pastor R. Couceyro, Ph.D.
Research Associate
Division of Neuroscience
Yerkes Primate Research Center
Emory University
954 Gatewood Road NE
Atlanta, Georgia 30329

Carl W. Cotman, Ph.D.
Professor of Neurology and Psychobiology
Institute for Brain Aging & Dementia
University of California, Irvine
Irvine, California 92697-4540

Timothy M. DeLorey, Ph.D.
Staff Scientist
Molecular Research Institute
854 Page Mill Road
Palo Alto, California 94304

Ariel Y. Deutch, Ph.D.
Professor
Departments of Psychiatry and Pharmacology
*   and Center for Molecular Research*
Vanderbilt University School of Medicine
1601 23rd Avenue South
Nashville, Tennessee 37212

Jean de Vellis, Ph.D.
Professor of Neurobiology
Director, Mental Retardation Research Center
760 Westwood Plaza, 68-177 NPI
Los Angeles, California 90024-1759

Darryl C. De Vivo, M.D.
Sidney Carter Professor of
*   Neurobiology*
Department of Neurology
Columbia University
710 West 168th Street
New York, New York 10032

Salvatore diMauro, M.D.
Lucy G. Moses Professor of Neurology
Department of Neurology
Columbia University
710 West 168th Street
New York, New York 10032

Raymond Dingledine, Ph.D.
Professor and Chairman
Department of Pharmacology
Emory University School of Medicine
5001 Rollins Research Center
1510 Clifton Road
Atlanta, Georgia 30322-3090

Laura L. Dugan, M.D.
Assistant Professor
Departments of Neurology and Medicine
Washington University School of Medicine
660 South Euclid Avenue
St. Louis, Missouri 63110

Ronald S. Duman, Ph.D.
Associate Professor
Department of Psychiatry
Yale University School of Medicine
Connecticut Mental Health Center
34 Park Street
New Haven, Connecticut 06508

James Eberwine, Ph.D.
Professor
Departments of Pharmacology and
  Psychiatry
University of Pennsylvania Medical School
36th Street and Hamilton Walk
Philadelphia, Pennsylvania 19104

Betty A. Eipper, Ph.D.
Professor
Departments of Neuroscience and
  Physiology
Johns Hopkins University School of Medicine
725 North Wolfe Street
Baltimore, Maryland 21205-2185

Marie T. Filbin, Ph.D.
Professor
Department of Biology, HN 927
Hunter College
695 Park Avenue
New York, New York 10021

Caleb E. Finch, Ph.D.
ARCO and William F. Kieschnick Professor in the
  Neurobiology of Aging
Neurogerontology Division
Andrus Gerontology Center and Department of
  Biological Sciences
University of Southern California
3715 McClintock Avenue
Los Angeles, California 90089-0191

Stuart J. Firestein, Ph.D.
Associate Professor
Department of Biological Sciences
Columbia University
New York, New York 10027

Stephen K. Fisher, Ph.D.
Professor, Department of Pharmacology
Senior Research Scientist, Mental Health
  Research Institute
University of Michigan
1103 East Huron Street
Ann Arbor, Michigan 48104-1687

Alan Frazer, Ph.D.
Chairman, Department of Pharmacology
University of Texas Health Science Center
7703 Floyd Curl Drive
San Antonio, Texas 78284-7764

Kirk A. Frey, M.D., Ph.D.
Professor, Division of Nuclear Medicine
Senior Researcher
Mental Health Research Institute
1103 East Huron Street
Ann Arbor, Michigan 48104-1687

M. Gerlach, M.D.
Department of Psychiatry
University of Würzburg
Füchsleinestrasse 15
D-97080 Würzburg
Germany

Gary E. Gibson, Ph.D.
Professor of Neuroscience
Department of Neuroscience and Neurology
Cornell University Medical College
Burke Medical Research Institute
785 Mamaroneck Avenue
White Plains, New York 10605

Peter Gillespie, Ph.D.
Associate Professor of Physiology and Neuroscience
Department of Physiology
Johns Hopkins University School of Medicine
725 North Wolfe Street
Baltimore, Maryland 21205

Gary W. Goldstein, M.D.
Professor of Neurology and Pediatrics
Johns Hopkins University School of Medicine
President, Kennedy Krieger Research Institute
707 North Broadway
Baltimore, Maryland 21205

Paul Greengard, Ph.D.
Vincent Astor Professor
Head, Laboratory of Molecular and Cellular
*   Neuroscience*
The Rockefeller University
1230 York Avenue
New York, New York 10021

Amiya K. Hajra, Ph.D.
Professor of Biological Chemistry and Senior
*   Research Scientist*
Mental Health Research Institute
University of Michigan
1103 East Huron Street
Ann Arbor, Michigan 48104

Julie G. Hensler, Ph.D.
Assistant Professor
Department of Pharmacology
University of Texas Health Science Center
7703 Floyd Curl Drive
San Antonio, Texas 78284-7764

Bertil Hille, Ph.D.
Professor
Department of Physiology and Biophysics
University of Washington School of Medicine
Seattle, Washington 98195-7290

Ronald W. Holz, M.D., Ph.D.
Professor
Department of Pharmacology
Medical Research Sciences Building 3, Room 1301
University of Michigan
Ann Arbor, Michigan 48109

Lindsay B. Hough, Ph.D.
Professor
Department of Pharmacology and Neuroscience
Albany Medical College
Albany, New York 12208

Richard L. Huganir, Ph.D.
Investigator, Howard Hughes Medical Institute
Professor, Department of Neuroscience
Johns Hopkins University School of Medicine
725 North Wolfe Street
Baltimore, Maryland 21205

Richard F. Keep, Ph.D.
Senior Associate Research Scientist
Department of Surgery (Neurosurgery)
University of Michigan
R5605 Kresge I
Ann Arbor, Michigan 48109-0532

Sue Kinnamon, Ph.D.
Associate Professor
Departments of Anatomy and Neuroscience
Colorado State University
Fort Collins, Colorado 80523

Laura L. Kirkpatrick, Ph.D.
Department of Cell Biology and Neuroscience
University of Texas Southwestern Medical
*   Center*
5323 Harry Hines Boulevard
Dallas, Texas 91115-7523

Michael J. Kuhar, Ph.D.
Charles Howard Candler Professor and Chief
Division of Neuroscience
Yerkes Primate Research Center
Emory University
954 Gatewood Northeast
Atlanta, Georgia 30329

Philip D. Lambert, Ph.D.
Research Associate
Division of Neuroscience
Yerkes Primate Research Center
Emory University
954 Gatewood Road Northeast
Atlanta, Georgia 30329

Gary E. Landreth, Ph.D.
Professor of Neurology and Neurosciences
Case Western Reserve University School of
  Medicine
Alzheimer's Research Lab, Room E504
10900 Euclid Avenue
Cleveland, Ohio 44106

Peter J. Lansbury, Jr., M.D.
Associate Professor of Neurology and
  Neuroscience
Harvard Medical School
Center for Neurologic Diseases
Brigham and Women's Hospital
75 Francis Street
Boston, Massachusetts 02115

John Laterra, M.D., Ph.D.
Associate Professor
Neurology, Oncology and Neurosciences
Johns Hopkins University School of Medicine
Kennedy Krieger Research Institute
707 North Broadway
Baltimore, Maryland 21205

Lit-fui Lau, Ph.D.
Postdoctoral Fellow
Department of Neuroscience
Johns Hopkins University School of Medicine
725 North Wolfe Street
Baltimore, Maryland 21205

Joel M. Linden, Ph.D.
Professor of Medicine and Molecular Physiology
  and Biological Physics
University of Virginia Health Sciences Center
Charlottesville, Virginia 22902

Richard E. Mains, Ph.D.
Professor of Neuroscience and Physiology
Johns Hopkins University School of Medicine
725 North Wolfe Street
Baltimore, Maryland 21205

Robert L. Macdonald, M.D.
Professor of Neurology and Physiology
Department of Physiology
University of Michigan
1103 East Huron Street
Ann Arbor, Michigan 48104

Robert F. Margolskee, M.D., Ph.D.
Associate Investigator
Howard Hughes Medical Institute
Associate Professor
Mount Sinai School of Medicine
1425 Madison Avenue
New York, New York 10029

Chris J. McBain, Ph.D.
Chief, Unit of Cellular and Synaptic Plasticity
National Institutes of Health
NICHD/LCMN
Building 49, Room 5A78
Bethesda, Maryland 20892

Bruce S. McEwen, Ph.D.
Professor and Head
Margaret Milliken Laboratory of
  Neuroendocrinology
The Rockefeller University
66th and York Avenue
New York, New York 10021

Henry F. McFarland, M.D.
Chief, Neuroimmunology Branch
National Institutes of Health
National Institute of Neurological Disorders and
  Stroke
Building 10, Room 5B16
MSC-1400
Bethesda, Maryland 20892-1400

Brian Meldrum, M.B., Ph.D.
Professor
Department of Clinical Neurosciences
Institute of Psychiatry
De Crespigny Park
Denmark Hill
London SE5 8AF
United Kingdom

Herbert Y. Meltzer, M.D.
Professor of Psychiatry and Pharmacology
Director, Psychopharmacology Division
Psychiatric Hospital at Vanderbilt
1601 23rd Avenue South, Suite 306
Nashville, Tennessee 37212

Pierre Morell, Ph.D.
Professor of Biochemistry and Neurobiology
University of North Carolina Neuroscience
Center
Chapel Hill, North Carolina 27599

Torben R. Neelands, B.S.
Department of Neurology
University of Michigan
1103 East Huron Street
Ann Arbor, Michigan 48104

Eric J. Nestler, M.D., Ph.D.
Elizabeth Means and House Jameson Professor
Departments of Psychiatry and Neurobiology
Yale University School of Medicine
Connecticut Mental Health Center
34 Park Street
New Haven, Connecticut 06508

Richard W. Olsen, Ph.D.
Professor
Department of Molecular and Medical
Pharmacology
University of California at Los Angeles School of
Medicine
Center for Health Sciences, Room 23-120
Los Angeles, California 90095

David E. Pleasure, M.D.
Loeb Neuroscience Chair and Director
Department of Neurology
The Children's Hospital of Philadelphia
Abramson Research Building, Room 516H
3517 Civic Center Boulevard
Philadelphia, Pennsylvania 19104

James W. Putney, Jr., Ph.D.
Chief, Calcium Regulation Section
National Institute of Environmental Health
Sciences
National Institutes of Health
P.O. Box 12233
Research Triangle Park, North Carolina
27709-2233

Richard H. Quarles, Ph.D.
Chief, Laboratory of Molecular and Cellular
Neurobiology
National Institutes of Health
National Institute of Neurological Disorders and
Stroke
Building 49, Room 2A28
49 Covent Drive, MSC 4440
Bethesda, Maryland 20892-4440

Cedric S. Raine, Ph.D.
Professor of Pathology, Neurology and Neuroscience
Albert Einstein College of Medicine
1300 Morris Park Avenue
Bronx, New York 10461

P. Riederer, Ph.D.
Professor of Clinical Neurochemistry
Department of Psychiatry
University of Würzburg
D-97080 Würzburg
Germany

George S. Roth, Ph.D.
Chief, Molecular Physiology and Genetics Section
Laboratory of Cellular and Molecular Biology
National Institute of Aging
5600 Nathan Shock Drive
Baltimore, Maryland 21224

Dennis J. Selkoe, M.D.
Professor of Neurology and Neuroscience
Harvard Medical School
Co-director, Center for Neurologic Diseases
Brigham and Women's Hospital
77 Avenue Louis Pasteur
Harvard Institutes of Medicine 730
Boston, Massachusetts 02115

Hitoshi Shichi, Ph.D.
Professor of Ophthalmology
Wayne State University School of Medicine
Kresge Eye Institute
4717 Saint Antoine
Detroit, Michigan 48210

J. Sian, Ph.D.
Postdoctoral Research Fellow
University of Würzburg
Füchschleinestrasse 15
D-97080 Würzburg
Germany

George J. Siegel, M.D.
Chief, Neurology Service
Edward Hines Jr. Veterans Affairs Hospital
Hines, Illinois 60141
Professor of Neurology and Cellular and
   Molecular Biochemistry, and
Vice-Chairman, Department of Neurology
Loyola University of Chicago Stritch School of
   Medicine
Maywood, Illinois 60153

Louis Sokoloff, M.D.
Chief, Laboratory of Cerebral Metabolism
National Institutes of Health
National Institute of Mental Health
Building 36, Room 1A-05
36 Covent Drive, MSC 4030
Bethesda, Maryland 20892

David L. Stenoien, Ph.D.
Department of Cell Biology and Neuroscience
University of Texas Southwestern Medical Center
5323 Harry Hines Boulevard
Dallas, Texas 91115-7523

Thomas C. Südhof, M.D.
Professor of Molecular Genetics
Director, Center for Basic Neuroscience
Investigator, Howard Hughes Medical Institute
5323 Harry Hines Boulevard
Dallas, Texas 75235

Kunihiko Suzuki, M.D.
Director, Neuroscience Center
Professor of Neurology and Psychiatry
University of North Carolina School of Medicine
Chapel Hill, North Carolina 27599-7250

Palmer Taylor, Ph.D.
Sandra and Monroe Trout Professor and
   Chairman of Pharmacology
Department of Pharmacology
School of Medicine
University of California, San Diego
La Jolla, California 92093-0636

George R. Uhl, M.D., Ph.D.
Chief, Molecular Neurobiology
National Institute on Drug Abuse
P.O. Box 5180
Baltimore, Maryland 21224

Michael D. Uhler, Ph.D.
Associate Professor
Department of Biological Chemistry
Research Scientist
Mental Health Research Institute
1103 East Huron Street
Ann Arbor, Michigan 48104-1687

Marie T. Vanier, M.D., Ph.D.
Biochémie, INSERM U189
Faculté de Médecine Lyon-Sud
F 69921 Oullins Cedex
France

Moussa B. H. Youdim, Ph.D.
Professor of Pharmacology
Finkelstein Professor of Life Sciences
Department of Pharmacology
Technion—Faculty of Medicine
Efron Street 2
P.O. Box 9697
31096 Haifa
Israel

Marc Yudkoff, M.D.
Professor of Pediatrics
Division of Child Development
Children's Hospital of Pennsylvania
1 Children's Center
Philadelphia, Pennsylvania 19104

Acknowledgments

We express our debt to all the former authors for their contributions that have made this book so useful over the years, some of which we have carried forward into this sixth edition. In particular, we note with thanks the earlier work of former co-editors, Dr. Robert Katzman in the first three editions and Dr. Perry Molinoff in the fourth and fifth editions. We express our gratitude to the many investigators whose important research made this new edition necessary and possible. Much important work cannot be specifically referenced in a textbook. These are given more explicit acknowledgment in the expanded bibliographies contained in the accompanying CD-ROM version of the book. We are indebted to artist Lorie (Manzardo) Gavulic for preparing the illustrations throughout the book. We also thank Roderick MacKinnon, Ph.D. and the AAAS for their kind permission to re-use their figure of the potassium channel on our front cover.

We are particularly grateful to Anne M. Sydor, Ph.D., Developmental Editor, Lippincott Williams & Wilkins, for her knowledge of neuroscience and her dedication and diligence throughout guiding all aspects of the production of this edition and in keeping us all on track to ensure its timely and successful completion. Finally, we thank Mark Placito, Senior Editor; Kathey Alexander, Editor-in-Chief; and the staff of Lippincott Williams & Wilkins for their support and fostering of this project.

George J. Siegel
Bernard W. Agranoff
R. Wayne Albers
Stephen K. Fisher

Excerpts from the Preface to the Fourth Edition

The addition of the phrase, "Molecular, Cellular and Medical Aspects" to the title of this Fourth Edition of *Basic Neurochemistry* emphasizes our belief that the flourishing of neurochemistry derives from correlations among phenomena that are observed at multiple levels. As discussed in the Preface to the First Edition in 1972, integrating hypotheses are being developed to account for the functioning of the nervous system in terms of molecular events. The current growth of correlative power stems not only from increases in sensitivity and resolution of analytical biochemistry—more data from smaller samples—but equally from technology that permits observing and quantitating molecular events in functioning, complex and relatively intact biological structures. Examples range from recording the conductance of single ion channels in patches of membrane, to measuring processes in transfected cells or transgenic animals, to imaging receptor-ligand binding, metabolism and blood flow in brains of awake functioning humans.

Advances in molecular genetics have generated an enthusiastic sense of anticipation among neurobiologists over the past decades. The derivative applications are, on the one hand, revealing more about molecular structures and, on the other, elucidating nervous system development and the bases of genetic diseases affecting human behavior. We are encouraged to believe that increased knowledge of the molecular basis of neurobiology will ultimately lead to an understanding of the coding of experiences that comprise memory and are the substrate of behavior and mind.

Basic Neurochemistry had its origin in the Conference on Neurochemistry Curriculum initiated and organized by R. Wayne Albers, Robert Katzman and George J. Siegel under the sponsorship of the National Institute for Neurological Diseases and Stroke, June 19 and 20, 1969, Bronx, New York. At this conference, a group of 30 neuroscientists constructed a syllabus outline delineating the scope of a neurochemistry curriculum appropriate for medical, graduate and postgraduate neuroscience students. Out of this outline grew the first edition, edited by R. Wayne Albers, George J. Siegel, Robert Katzman and Bernard W. Agranoff. It was anticipated that the book would evolve with the emergence of the field and would stimulate continuing reappraisal of the scientific and educational aspects of neurochemistry. The Editors elected to assign the copyright and all royalties to the American Society for Neurochemistry, the royalties to be used for educational purposes. These funds have been used to sponsor the Annual Basic Neurochemistry Lectureship.

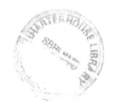

Preface

We have tried to make this sixth edition both current and comprehensive with respect to the dynamic field of neurochemistry, while maintaining a single volume text. Our initial task, to determine how the field has evolved, was accomplished with advice from many of the contributors to previous editions and from numerous colleagues with whom we consulted prior to and during our initial planning meeting in March, 1996. Consistent with our previous editions, these revisions have involved identifying new topics and, in some cases, recruitment of new chapter authors and reassignment of subjects to new chapters. We particularly wish to thank again all of the contributors to the fifth and earlier editions, much of whose work remains an essential part of this book.

Completely new chapters by new authors represent about one-third of the sixth edition. These include such subjects as cell-cell interactions, adhesion molecules and extracellular matrix, intracellular trafficking, cytosol-nuclear communication, nerve growth and regeneration, excitotoxicity, apoptosis, drug addiction and prion diseases. Many previous chapters were extensively revised. Although the nearly three years that have elapsed from initial planning to publication is consistent with previous editions, the increasing pace of research makes this a greater concern. Our response to this has been to introduce three devices: separate "boxes" on specific topics that came up during the editing process were inserted into pertinent chapters; authors were encouraged to add significant new references at a late stage of editing; and, perhaps the ultimate in "currency," a CD-ROM version of the entire book was produced, including abstracts of key references and an integral function for searching the Medline database, thus making the entire on-line biomedical literature available while reading the book.

As in all previous editions, the copyright and all royalties for *Basic Neurochemistry: Molecular, Cellular and Medical Aspects* are assigned to the American Society for Neurochemistry for use in neuroscience education, including the support of the annual Basic Neurochemistry Lectureship. Information about these lectureships and a continuing forum on basic neurochemistry may be found at the American Society for Neurochemistry website, currently to be found at http://www.tmc.edu/asn/asn.html.

George J. Siegel
Bernard W. Agranoff
R. Wayne Albers
Stephen K. Fisher
Michael D. Uhler

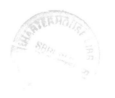

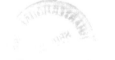

Cellular Neurochemistry and Neural Membranes

1

Neurocellular Anatomy

Cedric S. Raine

UNDERSTANDING NEUROANATOMY IS NECESSARY TO STUDY NEUROCHEMISTRY

Despite the advent of molecular genetics in neurobiology, our understanding of the functional relationships of the components of the central nervous system (CNS) remains in its infancy, particularly in the areas of cellular interaction and synaptic modulation. Nevertheless, the fine structural relationships of most elements of nervous system tissue have been described well [1–5]. The excellent neuroanatomical atlases of Peters et al. [3] and Palay and Chan-Palay [1]

Basic Neurochemistry: Molecular, Cellular and Medical Aspects, 6th Ed., edited by G. J. Siegel et al. Published by Lippincott–Raven Publishers, Philadelphia, 1999. Correspondence to Cedric S. Raine, Department of Pathology, Albert Einstein College of Medicine, 1300 Morris Park Avenue, Bronx, New York 10461.

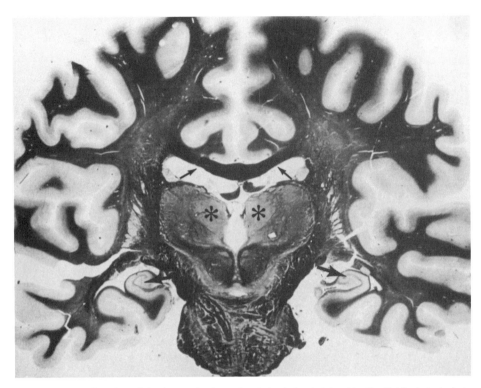

FIGURE 1-1. Coronal section of the human brain at the thalamic level stained by the Heidenhain technique for myelin. Gray matter stains faintly; all myelinated regions are black. The thalamus (*) lies beneath the lateral ventricles and is separated at this level by the beginning of the third ventricle. The roof of the lateral ventricles is formed by the corpus callosum *(small arrows)*. Ammon's horns are shown by the *large arrows*. Note the outline of gyri and sulci at the surface of the cerebral hemispheres, sectioned here near the junction of the frontal and parietal cortices.

should be consulted for detailed ultrastructural analyses of specific cell types, particularly of neurons with their diverse forms and connections. This chapter provides a concise description of the major cytoarchitectural features of the nervous system and an entrance into the relevant literature. Although the fine structure of the organelles of the CNS and peripheral nervous system (PNS) is not peculiar to these tissues, the interactions between cell types, such as synaptic contacts between neurons and myelin sheaths around axons, are unique. These specializations and those that allow for the sequestration of the CNS from the outside world, namely, the blood–brain barrier (BBB) and the absence of lymphatics, become major issues in considerations of normal and disease processes in the nervous system. For the sake of simplicity, the present section is subdivided into a section on general organization and a section regarding major cell types.

Diverse cell types are organized into assemblies and patterns such that specialized components are integrated into a physiology of the whole organ

The CNS parenchyma is made up of nerve cells and their afferent and efferent extensions, dendrites and axons, all closely enveloped by glial cells. Coronal section of the cerebral hemispheres of the brain reveals an outer convoluted rim of gray matter overlying the white matter (Fig. 1-1). Gray matter, which also exists as islands within the white matter, contains mainly nerve cell bodies and glia and lacks significant amounts of myelin, the lipid component responsible for the whiteness of white matter. More distally along the neuraxis in the spinal cord, the cerebral situation is reversed: white matter surrounds gray matter, which is arranged in a characteristic H formation (Fig. 1-2).

A highly diagrammatic representation of

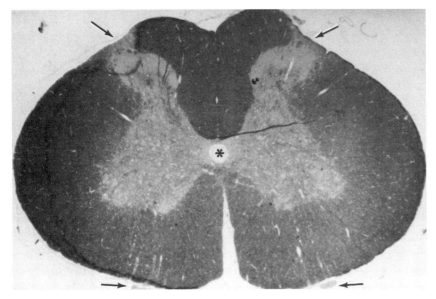

FIGURE 1-2. Transverse section of a rabbit lumbar spinal cord at L-1. Gray matter is seen as a paler staining area in an H configuration formed by the dorsal and ventral horns with the central canal in the center (*). The dorsal horns would meet the incoming dorsal spine nerve roots at the *upper arrows*. The anterior roots can be seen below *(lower arrows)*, opposite the ventral horns, from which they received their fibers. The white matter occupies a major part of the spinal cord and stains darker. Epon section, 1 μm, stained with toluidine blue.

the major CNS elements is shown in Figure 1-3. The entire CNS is bathed both internally and externally by cerebrospinal fluid (CSF), which circulates throughout the ventricular and leptomeningeal spaces. This fluid, a type of plasma ultrafiltrate, plays a significant role in protecting the CNS from mechanical trauma, balancing electrolytes and protein and maintaining ventricular pressure (see Chap. 32). The outer surface of the CNS is invested by the triple-membrane system of the meninges. The outermost is the dura mater, derived from the mesoderm, which is tightly adherent to the inner surfaces of the calvaria. The arachnoid membrane is closely applied to the inner surface of the dura mater. The innermost of the meninges, the pia mater, loosely covers the CNS surface. The pia and arachnoid together, derived from the ectoderm, are called the leptomeninges. CSF occupies the subarachnoid space, between the arachnoid and the pia, and the ventricles. The CNS parenchyma is overlaid by a layer of subpial astrocytes, which in turn is covered on its leptomeningeal aspect by a basal lamina (see Fig. 1-3). On the inner, or ventricular, surface, the CNS parenchyma is separated from the CSF by a layer of ciliated ependymal cells,

which are thought to facilitate the movement of CSF. The production and circulation of CSF are maintained by the choroid plexus, grape-like collections of vascular tissue and cells that protrude into the ventricles. Resorption of CSF is effected by vascular structures known as arachnoid villi, located in the leptomeninges over the surface of the brain (see Chap. 32).

Ependymal cells abut layers of astrocytes, which in turn envelop neurons, neurites and vascular components. In addition to neurons and glial cells, such as astrocytes and oligodendrocytes, the CNS parenchyma contains blood vessels, macrophages and microglial cells.

The PNS and the autonomic nervous system consist of bundles of myelinated and nonmyelinated axons enveloped by Schwann cells, the PNS counterpart of oligodendrocytes. Nerve bundles are enclosed by the perineurium and the epineurium, which are tough, fibrous, elastic sheaths. Between individual nerve fibers are isolated connective tissue, or endoneurial cells, and blood vessels. The ganglia, such as dorsal root and sympathetic ganglia, are located peripherally to the CNS and are made up of large neurons, usually unipolar or bipolar, surrounded by satellite cells, which

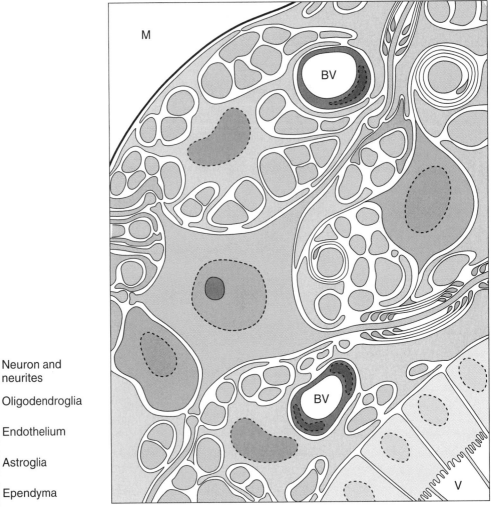

FIGURE 1-3.   The major components of the CNS and their interrelationships. Microglia are not depicted. In this simplified schema, the CNS extends from its meningeal surface *(M)* through the basal lamina *(solid black line)* overlying the subpial astrocyte layer of the CNS parenchyma and across the CNS parenchyma proper (containing neurons and glia) and subependymal astrocytes, to ciliated ependymal cells lining the ventricular space *(V)*. Note how the astrocyte also invests blood vessels *(BV)*, neurons and cell processes. The pia-astroglia (glia limitans) provides the barrier between the exterior (dura and blood vessels) and the CNS parenchyma. One neuron is seen **(center),** with synaptic contacts on its soma and dendrites. Its axon emerges to the right and is myelinated by an oligodendrocyte **(above).** Other axons are shown in transverse section, some of which are myelinated. The oligodendrocyte to the lower left of the neuron is of the nonmyelinating satellite type. The ventricles *(V)* and the subarachnoid space of the meninges *(M)* contain cerebrospinal fluid.

are specialized Schwann cells. A dendrite and an axon, both of which can be up to several feet in length, arise from each neuron.

CHARACTERISTICS OF THE NEURON

From a historical standpoint, no other cell type has attracted as much attention or caused as much controversy as the nerve cell. It is impossible in a single chapter to delineate comprehensively the extensive structural, topographical and functional variation achieved by this cell type. Consequently, despite an enormous literature, the neuron still defies precise definition, particularly with regard to function. It is known that the neuronal population usually is established shortly after birth, that mature neurons do not divide and that in humans there is a daily dropout of neurons amounting to approximately 20,000 cells. These facts alone make the neuron unique.

Neurons can be excitatory, inhibitory or modulatory in their effect and motor, sensory or secretory in their function [6]. They can be influenced by a large repertoire of neurotransmitters and hormones (see Chap. 10). This enormous repertoire of functions, associated with different developmental influences on different neurons, is largely reflected in the variation of dendritic and axonal outgrowth. Specialization also occurs at axonal terminals, where a variety of junctional complexes, known as synapses, exist. The subtle synaptic modifications are best visualized ultrastructurally, although immunohistochemical staining also permits distinction among synapses on the basis of transmitter type.

General structural features of neurons are the perikarya, dendrites and axons

The stereotypical image of a neuron is that of a stellate cell body, the perikaryon or soma, with broad dendrites emerging from one pole and a fine axon emerging from the opposite pole. This impression stems from the older work of Purkinje, who first described the nerve cell in 1839, and of Deiters, Ramón y Cajal and Golgi (see [3]) at the end of the nineteenth century and the early twentieth century. However, this picture does not hold true for many neurons. The neuron is the most polymorphic cell in the body and defies formal classification on the basis of shape, location, function, fine structure or transmitter substance. Although early workers described the neuron as a globular mass suspended between nerve fibers, the teased preparations of Deiters and his contemporaries soon proved this not to be the case. Later work, using impregnation staining and culture techniques, elaborated on Deiters' findings. Before the work of Deiters and Ramón y Cajal, both neurons and neuroglia were believed to form syncytia, with no intervening membranes. Today, of course, we are familiar with the specialized membranes and the enormous variety of nerve cell shapes and sizes. They range from the small, globular cerebellar gran-

ule cells, with a perikaryal diameter of approximately 6 to 8 μm, to the pear-shaped Purkinje cells and star-shaped anterior horn cells, both of which may reach diameters of 60 to 80 μm in humans. Perikaryal size is generally a poor index of total cell volume, however, and it is a general rule in neuroanatomy that neurites occupy a greater percentage of the cell surface area than does the soma. For example, the pyramidal cell of the somatosensory cortex has a cell body that accounts for only 4% of the total surface area, whereas from its dendritic tree the dendritic spines alone claim 43% (Mungai, quoted by Peters et al. [3]). Hyden [2] quotes Scholl (1956), who calculated that the perikaryon of a "cortical cell" represents 10% of the neuronal surface area. In the feline reticular formation, some giant cells possess ratios between soma and dendrites of about 1:5. A single axon is the usual rule, but some cells, like the Golgi cells of the cerebellum, are endowed with several axons, some of which may show branching.

The extent of the branching displayed by the dendrites is a useful index of their functional importance. Dendritic trees represent the expression of the receptive fields, and large fields can receive inputs from multiple origins. A cell with a less developed dendritic ramification, such as the cerebellar granule cell, has synapses with a more homogeneous population of afferent sources.

The axon emerges from a neuron as a slender thread and frequently does not branch until it nears its target. In contrast to the dendrite and the soma, the axon is myelinated frequently, thus increasing its efficiency as a conducting unit. Myelin, a spirally wrapped membrane (see Chap. 4), is laid down in segments, or internodes, by oligodendrocytes in the CNS and by Schwann cells in the PNS. The naked regions of axon between adjacent myelin internodes are known as nodes of Ranvier (see below).

Neurons contain the same intracellular components as do other cells

No unique cytoplasmic inclusions of the neuron distinguish it from any other cell. Neurons have all the morphological counterparts of other cell types, the structures are similarly distributed and

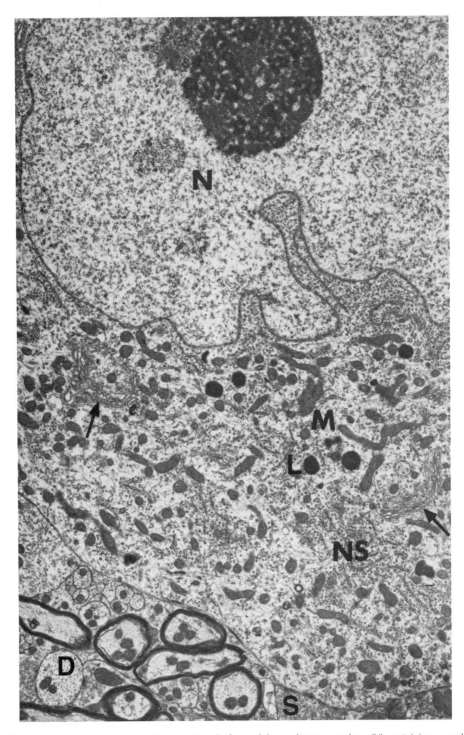

FIGURE 1-4. A motor neuron from the spinal cord of an adult rat shows a nucleus *(N)* containing a nucleolus, clearly divisible into a pars fibrosa and a pars granulosa, and a perikaryon filled with organelles. Among these, Golgi apparatus *(arrows)*, Nissl substance *(NS)*, mitochondria *(M)* and lysosomes *(L)* can be seen. An axosomatic synapse *(S)* occurs below, and two axodendritic synapses abut a dendrite *(D)*. ×8,000.

some of the most common, the Golgi apparatus and mitochondria, for example, were described first in neurons (Fig. 1-4).

The nucleus is large and usually spherical, containing a prominent nucleolus. The nucleochromatin is invariably pale, with little dense heterochromatin. In some neurons, such as the cerebellar granule cells, the nucleoplasm may show more differentiation and dense heterochromatin. The nucleolus is vesiculated and clearly delineated from the rest of the nucleoplasm. It usually contains two textures: the pars fibrosa, which are fine bundles of filaments, and the pars granulosa, in which dense granules predominate. An additional juxtaposed structure, found in neurons of the female of some species, is the nucleolar satellite, or sex chromatin, which consists of dense but loosely packed, coiled filaments. The nucleus is enclosed by the nuclear envelope, made up on the cytoplasmic side by the perikaryon inner membrane, which sometimes is seen in continuity with the endoplasmic reticulum (Fig. 1-5), and a more regular membrane on the inner, or nuclear, aspect of the envelope. Between the two is a clear channel of between 20 and 40 nm. Periodically, the inner and outer membranes of the envelope come together to form a single diaphragm, a nuclear pore (Fig. 1-5). In tangential section, nuclear pores are seen as empty vesicular structures, approximately 70 nm in diameter. In some neurons, as in Purkinje cells, that segment of the nuclear envelope which faces the dendritic pole is deeply invaginated.

The perikaryon, or body of the neuron, is rich in organelles (Fig. 1-4). It often stands out poorly from a homogeneous background neuropil, most of which is composed of nonmyelinated axons and dendrites, synaptic complexes and glial cell processes. Closer inspection shows that, like all cells, the neuron is delineated by a typical triple-layered unit membrane approximately 7.5 nm wide. Among the most prominent features of the perikaryal cytoplasm is a system of membranous cisternae, divisible into rough or granular endoplasmic reticulum (ER), which forms part of the Nissl substance; smooth or agranular ER; subsurface cisternae; and the Golgi apparatus. Although these various components are interconnected structurally, each possesses distinct enzymological properties. Also present within the cytoplasm are abundant lysosomes; lipofuscin granules, which also are termed *aging pigment*; mitochondria; multivesicular bodies; neurotubules; neurofilaments; and ribosomes.

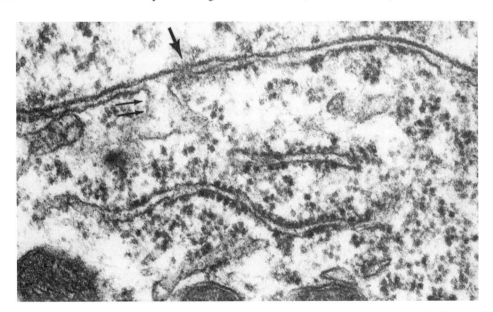

FIGURE 1-5.   Detail of the nuclear envelope showing a nuclear pore *(single arrow)* and the outer leaflet connected to the smooth endoplasmic reticulum (ER) *(double arrows)*. Two cisternae of the rough ER with associated ribosomes are also present. ×80,000.

Nissl substance consists of the intracytoplasmic basophilic masses that ramify loosely throughout the cytoplasm and is typical of most neurons (Figs. 1-4 and 1-5). The distribution of Nissl substance in certain neurons is characteristic and can be used as a criterion for identification. By electron microscopy (EM), this substance is seen to comprise regular arrays or scattered portions of flattened cisternae of the rough ER surrounded by clouds of free polyribosomes. The membranes of the rough ER are studded with rows of ribosomes, which produce the granular appearance of the rough ER. A space of 20 to 40 nm is maintained within cisternae. Sometimes, cisternal walls meet at fenestrations. Unlike the rough ER of glandular cells or other protein-secreting cells, such as plasma cells, the rough ER of neurons probably produces most of its proteins for use within that neuron, a feature imposed by the extraordinary functional demands placed on the cell. Nissl substance does not penetrate axons but does extend along dendrites.

Smooth endoplasmic reticulum is present in most neurons, although it is sometimes difficult to differentiate it from the rough ER owing to the disorderly arrangement of ribosomes. Ribosomes are not associated with these membranes, and the cisternae usually assume a meandering, branching course throughout the cytoplasm. In some neurons, the smooth ER is quite prominent, for example, in Purkinje cells. Individual cisternae of the smooth ER extend along axons and dendrites (see Chaps. 8 and 9).

Subsurface cisternae are a system of smooth, membrane-bound, flattened cisternae that can be found in many neurons. These structures, referred to as hypolemmal cisternae by Palay and Chan-Palay [1], abut the plasmalemma of the neuron and constitute a secondary membranous boundary within the cell. The distance between these cisternae and the plasmalemma is usually 10 to 12 nm, and in some neurons, such as the Purkinje cells, a mitochondrion may be found in close association with the innermost leaflet. Similar cisternae have been described beneath synaptic complexes, but their functional significance is not known. Some authors have suggested that such a system may play a role in the uptake of metabolites. Membrane structures are described in Chapter 2.

The *Golgi apparatus* is a highly specialized form of agranular reticulum and is visualized best using the metal impregnation techniques of Golgi. Ultrastructurally, the Golgi apparatus consists of aggregates of smooth-walled cisternae and a variety of vesicles. It is surrounded by a heterogeneous assemblage of organelles, including mitochondria, lysosomes and multivesicular bodies. In most neurons, the Golgi apparatus encompasses the nucleus and extends into dendrites but is absent from axons. A three-dimensional analysis of the system reveals that the stacks of cisternae are pierced periodically by fenestrations. Tangential sections of these fenestrations show them to be circular profiles. A multitude of vesicles is associated with each segment of the Golgi apparatus, particularly "coated" vesicles, which proliferate from the lateral margins of flattened cisternae (Fig. 1-6) (see Chap. 9). Such structures have been variously named, but the term *alveolate vesicle* seems to be generally accepted. Histochemical staining reveals that these bodies are rich in acid hydrolases, and they are believed to represent primary lysosomes [7]. Acid phosphatase also is found elsewhere in the cisternae but in lesser amounts than in alveolate vesicles.

The *lysosome* is the principal organelle responsible for the degradation of cellular waste. It is a common constituent of all cell types of the nervous system and is particularly prominent in neurons, where it can be seen at various stages of development (Fig. 1-4). It ranges in size from 0.1 to 2 μm in diameter. The primary lysosome is elaborated from Golgi saccules as a small, vesicular structure (Fig. 1-6). Its function is to fuse with the membrane of waste-containing vacuoles, termed *phagosomes*, into which it releases hydrolytic enzymes (see Chap. 41). The sequestered material is then degraded within the vacuole, and the organelle becomes a secondary lysosome; it is usually electron-dense and large. The matrix of this organelle will give a positive reaction when tested histochemically for acid phosphatase. Residual bodies containing nondegradable material are considered to be tertiary lysosomes, and in the neuron some are represented by lipofuscin granules (Fig. 1-7). These granules contain brown pigment and lamellar stacks of membrane material and are more common in the aged brain [7].

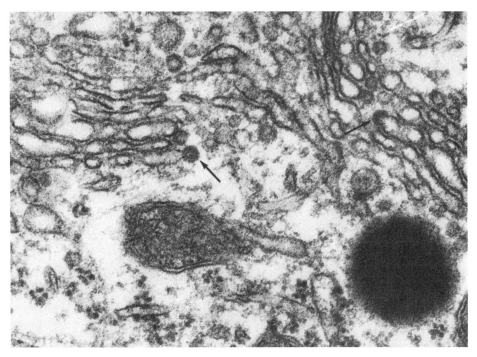

FIGURE 1-6.   A portion of a Golgi apparatus. The smooth-membraned cisternae appear beaded. The many circular profiles represent tangentially sectioned fenestrations and alveolate vesicles (primary lysosomes). Two of the latter can be seen budding from Golgi saccules *(arrows)*. Mitochondria and a dense body (secondary lysosomes) are also present. ×60,000.

Multivesicular bodies usually are found in association with the Golgi apparatus and are visualized by EM as small, single membrane-bound sacs approximately 0.5 μm in diameter. They contain several minute, spherical profiles, sometimes arranged about the periphery. They are believed to belong to the lysosome series prior to secondary lysosomes because they contain acid hydrolases and apparently are derived from primary lysosomes.

Neurotubules have been the subject of intense research [8]. They usually are arranged haphazardly throughout the perikaryon of neurons but are aligned longitudinally in axons and dendrites. Each neurotubule consists of a dense-walled structure enclosing a clear lumen, in the middle of which may be found an electron-dense dot. Axonal neurotubules display 5-nm filamentous interconnecting side-arms known to be involved in axoplasmic transport in association with the proteins dynein and kinesin (see Chap. 28). The diameter of neurotubules varies between 22 and 24 nm. High-resolution studies indicate that each neurotubule wall consists of 13 filamentous subunits arranged helically around a lumen (see also Chaps. 8 and 28).

Neurofilaments belong to the family of intermediate filaments and usually are found in association with neurotubules. The function of these two organelles has been debated for some time [8,9], and current views of their roles in the maintenance of form and in axoplasmic transport are discussed in Chapters 8 and 28. Neurofilaments have a diameter of approximately 10 nm, are of indeterminate length and frequently occur in bundles. They are constant components of axons but are rarer in dendrites. In the axon, individual filaments possess a minute lumen and interconnect by proteinaceous side-arms, thereby forming a meshwork. Because of these cross-bridges, they do not form tightly packed bundles in the normal axon, in contrast to filaments within astrocytic processes (see Fig. 1-14), which lack cross-bridges. Neurofilaments within neuronal somata usually do not display cross-bridges and can be found in tight bundles. A form of filamentous structure

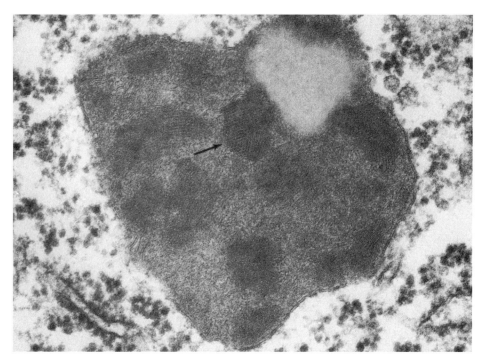

FIGURE 1-7. A lipofuscin granule from a cortical neuron shows membrane-bound lipid (dense) and a soluble component (gray). The denser component is lamellated. The lamellae appear as paracrystalline arrays of tubular profiles when sectioned transversely *(arrow)*. The granule is surrounded by a single-unit membrane. Free ribosomes also can be seen. ×96,000.

finer than neurofilaments is seen at the tips of growing neurites, particularly in the growth cones of developing axons. These structures, known as microfilaments, are 5 nm in size and are composed of actin. They facilitate movement and growth since it has been shown that axonal extension can be arrested pharmacologically by treatment with compounds that depolymerize these structures. The biochemistry of neurotubules and neurofilaments is dealt with in more detail in Chapter 8 and in Soifer [8] and Wang et al. [9].

Mitochondria are the centers for oxidative phosphorylation. These organelles occur ubiquitously in the neuron and its processes (Figs. 1-4 and 1-6). Their overall shape may change from one type of neuron to another, but their basic morphology is identical to that in other cell types. Mitochondria consist morphologically of double-membraned sacs surrounded by protuberances, or cristae, extending from the inner membrane into the matrix space [7].

The axon becomes physiologically and structurally divisible into the following distinct regions as it egresses: the axon hillock, the initial segment, the axon proper and the axonal termination [3]. The segments differ ultrastructurally in membrane morphology and the content of the rough and smooth ER. The axon hillock may contain fragments of Nissl substance, including abundant ribosomes, which diminish as the hillock continues into the initial segment. Here, the various axoplasmic components begin to align longitudinally. A few ribosomes and the smooth ER persist, and some axoaxonic synapses occur. More interesting, however, is the axolemma of the initial segment, the region for the generation of the action potential, which is underlaid by a dense granular layer similar to that seen at the nodes of Ranvier. Also present in this region are neurotubules, neurofilaments and mitochondria. The arrangement of the neurotubules in the initial segment, unlike their scattered pattern in the distal axon, is in fascicles; they are interconnected by side-arms [3,9]. Beyond the initial segment, the axon maintains a relatively uniform morphology. It contains the axolemma without any structural modification, except at nodes and the termination, where submembranous densities are seen; microtubules, sometimes cross-linked; neurofilaments, connected by side-arms; mitochondria; and tubulovesicular profiles, probably derived from the smooth ER. Myelinated axons show granular densifications beneath the axolemma at the nodes of Ranvier [6,10], and synaptic complexes may occur in the same regions. In myelinated fibers, there is a concentration of sodium channels at the nodal axon, a feature underlying the rapid, saltatory conduction of such fibers [11] (see Chaps. 6 and 10). The terminal portion of the axon arborizes and enlarges at its synaptic regions, where it might contain synaptic vesicles beneath the specialized presynaptic junction.

The dendrites are the afferent components of neurons and frequently are arranged around the neuronal soma in stellate fashion. In some neurons, they may arise from a single trunk, from which they branch into a dendritic tree. Unlike axons, they generally lack neurofilaments, although they may contain fragments of Nissl substance; however, large branches of dendrites in close proximity to neurons may contain small bundles of neurofilaments. Some difficulty may be encountered in distinguishing small unmyelinated axons or terminal segments of axons from small dendrites. In the absence of synaptic data, they often can be assessed by the content of neurofilaments. The synaptic regions of dendrites occur either along the main stems (Fig. 1-8) or at small protuberances known as dendritic spines or thorns. Axon terminals abut these structures.

The synapse is a specialized junctional complex by which axons and dendrites emerging from different neurons intercommunicate [12]. This was proposed first by Sherrington in 1897, who also proposed the term synapse. The existence of synapses was immediately demonstrable by EM and can be recognized today in a dynamic fashion by Nomarski and confocal optics, light microscopy and scanning EM. With the development of neurochemical approaches to neurobiology, an un-

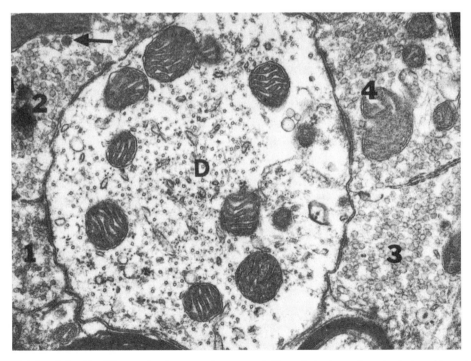

FIGURE 1-8. A dendrite *(D)* emerging from a motor neuron in the anterior horn of a rat spinal cord is contacted by four axonal terminals: terminal *1* contains clear, spherical synaptic vesicles; terminals *2* and *3* contain both clear, spherical and dense-core vesicles *(arrow)*; and terminal *4* contains many clear, flattened (inhibitory) synaptic vesicles. Note also the synaptic thickenings and, within the dendrite, the mitochondria, neurofilaments and neurotubules. ×33,000.

derstanding of synaptic form and function becomes of fundamental importance. As was noted in the first ultrastructural study on synapses (Palade and Palay in 1954, quoted in [4]), synapses display interface specialization and frequently are polarized or asymmetrical. The asymmetry is due to the unequal distribution of electron-dense material, or thickening, applied to the apposing membranes of the junctional complex and the heavier accumulation of organelles within the presynaptic component. The closely applied membranes constituting the synaptic site are overlaid on the presynaptic and postsynaptic aspects by an electron-dense material similar to that seen in desmosomes and separated by a gap or cleft of 15 to 20 nm. The presynaptic component usually contains a collection of clear, 40- to 50-nm synaptic vesicles. These synaptic vesicles are important in packaging, transport and release of neurotransmitters and after their discharge into the synaptic cleft, they are recycled with the axon terminal [6,13]. Also present are small mitochondria approximately 0.2 to 0.5 μm in diameter (Figs. 1-8–1-10). Occasionally, 24-nm microtubules, coated vesicles and cisternae of the smooth ER are found in this region. On the postsynaptic side is a density referred to as the subsynaptic web, but apart from

an infrequent, closely applied packet of smooth ER or subsurface cisternae belonging to the hypolemmal system, there are no aggregations of organelles in the dendrite. At the neuromuscular junction, the morphological organization is somewhat different. Here, the axon terminal is greatly enlarged and ensheathed by Schwann cells; the postsynaptic or sarcolemmal membrane displays less density and is infolded extensively.

Before elaborating further on synaptic diversity, it might be helpful to outline briefly other ways in which synapses have been classified in the past. Using the light microscope, Ramón y Cajal (see [14]) was able to identify 11 distinct groups of synapses. Today, most neuroanatomists apply a more fundamental classification schema to synapses, depending on the profiles between which the synapse is formed, such as axodendritic, axosomatic, axoaxonic, dendrodendritic, somatosomatic and somatodendritic synapses. Unfortunately, such a list disregards whether the transmission is chemical or electrical, and in the case of chemical synapses, this classification does not address the neurotransmitter involved.

In terms of physiological typing, three groups of synapses are recognized: excitatory,

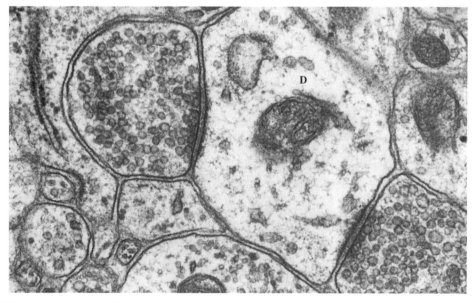

FIGURE 1-9. A dendrite *(D)* is flanked by two axon terminals packed with clear, spherical synaptic vesicles. Details of the synaptic region are clearly shown. ×75,000.

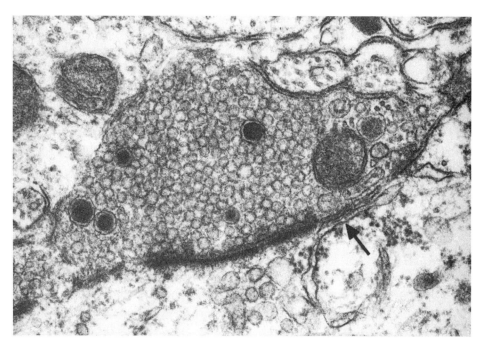

FIGURE 1-10.   An axonal terminal at the surface of a neuron from the dorsal horn of a rabbit spinal cord contains both dense-core and clear, spherical synaptic vesicles lying above the membrane thickenings. A subsurface cisterna *(arrow)* is also seen. ×68,000.

inhibitory and modulatory. Some neuroanatomical studies [14] have claimed that excitatory synapses possess spherical synaptic vesicles, whereas inhibitory synapses contain a predominance of flattened vesicles (Fig. 1-8). Other studies [15] have correlated this synaptic vesicular diversity with physiological data. In his study on the cerebellum, Gray [15] showed that neurons, with a known predominance of excitatory input on dendrites and an inhibitory input on the cell body, possessed two corresponding types of synapses; however, although this interpretation fits well in some loci of the CNS, it does not hold true for all regions. Furthermore, some workers consider that the differences between flat and spherical vesicles may reflect an artifact of aldehyde fixation or a difference in physiological state at the time of sampling. In light of these criticisms, it is clear that confirmation of the correlation between flattened vesicles and inhibitory synapses is required.

Another criterion for the classification of synapses by EM was introduced in 1959 by Gray [15]. Briefly, certain synapses in the cerebral cortex can be grouped into two types, depending on the length of the contact area between synaptic membranes and the amount of postsynaptic thickening. Relationships have been found between type 1 synapses, which have closely apposed membranes over long distances and a large amount of associated postsynaptic thickening, and excitatory axodendritic synapses. Type 2 synapses, which show less close apposition and thickening at the junction, are mainly axosomatic and believed to be inhibitory. This broad grouping has been confirmed in the cerebral cortex by a number of workers, but it does not hold true for all regions of the CNS.

Most of the data from studies on synapses *in situ* or on synaptosomes have been on cholinergic transmission. There is a vast family of chemical synapses that utilize biogenic amines (see Chap. 12) as neurotransmitter substances. Morphologically, catecholaminergic synapses are similar but possess, in addition to clear vesicles, slightly larger dense-core or granular vesicles of variable dimension (Figs. 1-8 and 1-10). These vesicles were identified first as synaptic vesicles by Grillo and Palay (see Bloom [16]), who segregated classes of granular vesicles based on vesicle and core size, but no relationship was made between granular vesicles and transmitter substances. About the same time, EM autoradiographic techniques were being employed and, using tritiated norepinephrine, Wolfe and coworkers [17] labeled granular vesicles within axonal terminals. Catecholaminergic vesicles generally are classified on a size basis, and not all have dense cores. Another, still unclassified, category of synapses may be the so-called silent synapses observed in CNS tissue both *in vitro* and *in vivo*. These synapses are morphologically identical to functional synapses but are physiologically dormant.

Finally, with regard to synaptic type, there is the well-characterized electrical synapse [18], where current can pass from cell to cell across regions of membrane apposition that essentially lack the associated collections of organelles present at the chemical synapse. In the electrical synapse (Fig. 1-11), the unit membranes are closely apposed, and indeed, the outer leaflets sometimes fuse to form a pentalaminar structure; however, in most places, a gap of approximately 20 nm exists, producing a so-called gap junction. Not infrequently, such gap junctions are separated by desmosome-like regions [3]. Sometimes, electrical synapses exist at terminals that also display typical chemical synapses; in such cases, the structure is referred to as a mixed synapse. The comparative morphology of electrical and chemical synapses has been reviewed by Pappas and Waxman [18].

Molecular markers can be used to identify neurons

Characterization of the vast array of neuron-specific cytoskeletal elements, such as intermediate filaments, microtubules and their associated proteins [19,20], and the neurotransmitters and their receptors [6,21] has led to the development of correspondingly large numbers of molecular and immunological probes, which now are applied routinely in neuroanatomical analyses. The neuron is incapable of participating in T-cell interactions via the expression of major histocompatibility complex (MHC) antigens or the production of soluble mediators, such as cytokines. However, neurons do possess unique proteins, some of which are antigenic, that normally are sequestered by the BBB from the circulating

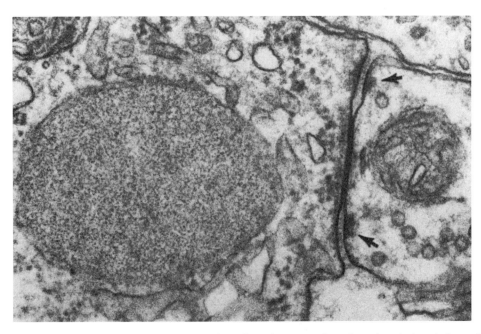

FIGURE 1-11. An electrotonic synapse is seen at the surface of a motor neuron from the spinal cord of a toadfish. Between the neuronal soma **(left)** and the axonal termination **(right),** a gap junction flanked by desmosomes *(arrows)* is visible. (Photograph courtesy of Drs. G. D. Pappas and J. S. Keeter.) ×80,000.

immune system. This theoretically renders the CNS vulnerable to immune-mediated damage should the BBB be breached.

CHARACTERISTICS OF NEUROGLIA

In 1846, Virchow (see [3]) first recognized the existence in the CNS of a fragile, non-nervous, interstitial component made up of stellate or spindle-shaped cells, morphologically distinct from neurons, which he named neuroglia, or "nerve glue." It was not until the early part of the twentieth century that this interstitial element was classified as consisting of distinct cell types [3,4]. Today, we recognize three broad groups of glial cells: (i) true glial cells or macroglia, such as astrocytes and oligodendrocytes, of ectodermal origin, the stem cell of which is the spongioblast; (ii) microglia, of mesodermal origin; and (iii) ependymal cells, also of ectodermal origin and sharing the same stem cell as true glia. Microglia invade the CNS at the time of vascularization via the pia mater, the walls of blood vessels and the tela choroidea. Glial cells differ from neurons in that they possess no synaptic contacts and retain the ability to divide throughout life, particularly in response to injury. The rough schema represented in Figure 1-3 demonstrates the interrelationships between the macroglia and other CNS components.

Virtually nothing can enter or leave the central nervous system parenchyma without passing through an astrocytic interphase

The complex packing achieved by the processes and cell bodies of astrocytes underscores their involvement in brain metabolism. Although astrocytes traditionally have been subdivided into protoplasmic and fibrous astrocytes [4], these two forms probably represent the opposite ends of a spectrum of the same cell type. However, Raff et al. [22] have suggested that the two groups might derive from different progenitors and that the progenitor of the fibrous astrocyte is the same as that of the oligodendrocyte. The structural components of fibrous and protoplasmic astrocytes are identical; the differences are

quantitative. In the early days of EM, differences between the two variants were more apparent owing to imprecise techniques, but with the development of better procedures, the differences became less apparent.

Protoplasmic astrocytes range in size from 10 to 40 μm, frequently are located in gray matter in relation to capillaries and have a clearer cytoplasm than do fibrous astrocytes (Fig. 1-12). Within the perikaryon of both types of astrocyte are scattered 9-nm filaments and 24-nm microtubules (Fig. 1-13); glycogen granules; lysosomes and lipofuscin-like bodies; isolated cisternae of the rough ER; a small Golgi apparatus opposite one pole of the nucleus; and small, elongated mitochondria, often extending together with loose bundles of filaments along cell processes. A centriole is not uncommon. Characteristically, the nucleus is ovoid and the nucleochromatin homogeneous, except for a narrow, continuous rim of dense chromatin and one or two poorly defined nucleoli. The fibrous astrocyte occurs in white matter (Fig. 1-13). Its processes are twig-like, being composed of large numbers of 9-nm glial filaments arranged in tight bundles. The filaments within these cell processes can be distinguished from neurofilaments by their close packing and the absence of side-arms (Figs. 1-13 and 1-14). Desmosomes and gap junctions occur between adjacent astrocytic processes.

In addition to protoplasmic and fibrous forms, regional specialization occurs among astrocytes. The outer membranes of astrocytes located in subpial zones and adjacent to blood vessels possess a specialized thickening. Desmosomes and gap junctions are very common in these regions between astrocytic processes. In the cerebellar cortex, protoplasmic astrocytes can be segregated into three classes, each ultrastructurally distinct: the Golgi epithelial cell, the lamellar or velate astrocyte and the smooth astrocyte [1].

Astrocyte functions have long been debated. Their major role is related to a connective tissue or skeletal function since they invest, possibly sustain and provide a packing for other CNS components. In the case of astrocytic ensheathment around synaptic complexes and the bodies of some neurons, such as Purkinje cells, it has

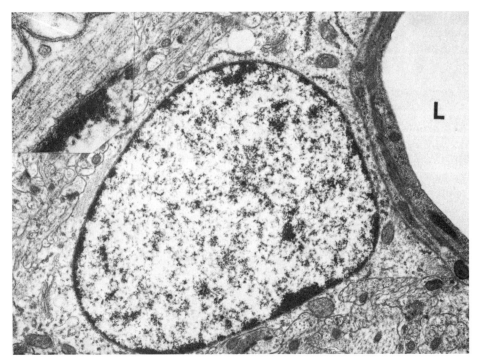

FIGURE 1-12. A protoplasmic astrocyte abuts a blood vessel (lumen at *L*) in rat cerebral cortex. The nucleus shows a rim of denser chromatin, and the cytoplasm contains many organelles, including Golgi and rough endoplasmic reticulum. ×10,000. **Inset:** Detail of perinuclear cytoplasm showing filaments. ×44,000.

been speculated that the astrocyte isolates these structures.

One well-known function of the astrocyte is concerned with repair. Subsequent to trauma, astrocytes invariably proliferate, swell, accumulate glycogen and undergo fibrosis by the accumulation of filaments, expressed neurochemically as an increase in glial fibrillary acidic protein (GFAP). This state of gliosis may be total, in which case all other elements are lost, leaving a glial scar, or it may be a generalized response occurring against a background of regenerated or normal CNS parenchyma. Fibrous astrocytosis can occur in both the gray and white matter, thereby indicating common links between protoplasmic and fibrous astrocytes. With age, both fibrous and protoplasmic astrocytes accumulate filaments. In some diseases, astrocytes become macrophages. It is interesting to note that the astrocyte is probably the most disease-resistant component in the CNS because very few diseases, other than alcoholism, cause depletion of astrocytes.

Another putative role of the astrocyte is its involvement in transport mechanisms (see Chap. 5) and in the BBB system (see Chap. 32). Astrocytes interact with neurons in various metabolic and transport processes. It was believed for some time that transport of water and electrolytes was effected by the astrocyte, a fact never definitively demonstrated and largely inferred from pathological or experimental evidence. It is known, for example, that damage to the brain vasculature, local injury due to heat or cold and inflammatory changes produce focal swelling of astrocytes, presumably owing to disturbances in fluid transport. The astrocytic investment of blood vessels suggests a role in the BBB system, but the studies of Reese and Karnovsky [23] and Brightman [24] indicate that the astrocytic end-feet provide little resistance to the movement of molecules and that blockage of the passage of material into the brain occurs at the endothelial cell-lining blood vessels (see Chap. 32). CNS endothelial cells display selective transport by transcytosis. During inflammation, these mechanisms are disrupted and there are alterations in permeability of endothe-

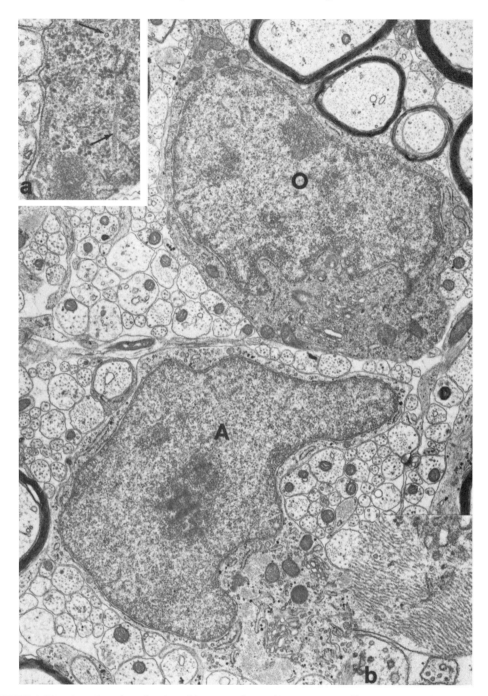

FIGURE 1-13.   A section of myelinating white matter from a kitten contains a fibrous astrocyte *(A)* and an oligodendrocyte *(O)*. The nucleus of the astrocyte *(A)* has homogeneous chromatin with a denser rim and a central nucleolus. That of the oligodendrocyte *(O)* is denser and more heterogeneous. Note the denser oligodendrocytic cytoplasm and the prominent filaments within the astrocyte. ×15,000. **Inset a:** Detail of the oligodendrocyte, showing microtubules *(arrows)* and absence of filaments. ×45,000. **Inset b:** Detail of astrocytic cytoplasm showing filaments, glycogen, rough endoplasmic reticulum and Golgi apparatus. ×45,000.

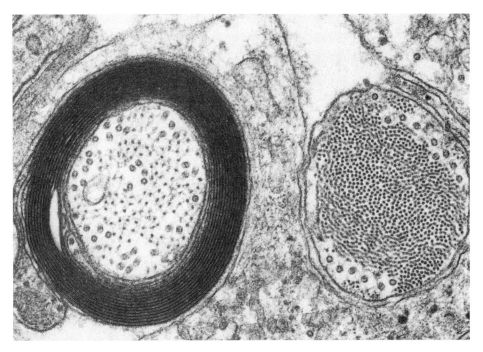

FIGURE 1-14.   Transverse sections of a myelinated axon **(left)** and the process of a fibrous astrocyte **(right)** in dog spinal cord. The axon contains scattered neurotubules and loosely packed neurofilaments interconnected by side-arm material. The astrocytic process contains a bundle of closely packed filaments with no cross-bridges, flanked by several microtubules. Sometimes, a lumen can be seen within a filament. ×60,000.

lial tight junctions and formation of edema. Astrocytes also are involved in reuptake of the neurotransmitter glutamate (see Chaps. 5 and 15). Finally, it is believed that astrocytes are responsible for the regulation of local pH levels and local ionic balances.

Molecular markers of astrocytes. Although antigenically distinct from other cell types by virtue of its expressing GFAP [17], there is no documented evidence of astrocytic disease related to an immunological response to GFAP on any astroglial molecule. GFAP remains singularly the most used cytoplasmic marker of astrocytes. A reliable marker for astrocytic membranes remains to be described. Interestingly, there is increasing evidence demonstrating the ability of astrocytes to serve as accessory cells of the immune system in a number of immune-mediated conditions [27,28]. In this regard, astrocytes are known for their ability to express class II MHC antigens *in vitro*, which are molecules essential for the presentation of antigen to helper/inducer CD4[+] T cells, as well as their ability to synthesize a number of cytokines,

such as interleukin-1, tumor necrosis factor and interferon γ (see Chaps. 35 and 39). It appears, therefore, that in circumstances in which the BBB is interrupted, the astrocyte is a facultative phagocyte with the potential to interact with lymphocytes.

Oligodendrocytes are myelin-producing cells in the central nervous system

The ultrastructural studies of Schultz and co-workers (1957) and Farquhar and Hartman (1957) (discussed in [4]) were among the first to contrast the EM features of oligodendrocytes with astrocytes (Fig. 1-12). The study of Mugnaini and Walberg [4] more explicitly laid down the morphological criteria for identifying these cells, and apart from subsequent technical improvements, our EM understanding of these cells has changed little since that time [5,29].

As with astrocytes, oligodendrocytes are highly variable, differing in location, morphology and function, but definable by some morphological criteria. The cell soma ranges from 10 to 20 μm and is roughly globular and more dense than that of an astrocyte. The margin of the cell is irregular and compressed against the adjacent neuropil. Few cell processes are seen, in contrast to the astrocyte. Within the cytoplasm, many organelles are found. Parallel cisternae of the rough ER and a widely dispersed Golgi apparatus are common. Free ribosomes occur, scattered amid occasional multivesicular bodies, mitochondria and coated vesicles. Distinguishing the oligodendrocyte from the astrocyte are the apparent absence of glial filaments and the constant presence of 24-nm microtubules (Fig. 1-13). Microtubules are most common at the margins of the cell, in the occasional cell process and in the cytoplasmic loops around myelin sheaths. Lamellar dense bodies, typical of oligodendrocytes, are also present [5]. The nucleus is usually ovoid, but slight lobation is not uncommon. The nucleochromatin stains heavily and contains clumps of denser heterochromatin; the whole structure is sometimes difficult to discern from the background cytoplasm. Desmosomes and gap junctions occur between interfascicular oligodendrocytes [5].

Ultrastructural and labeling studies on the developing nervous system (see Chap. 27) have demonstrated variability in oligodendrocyte morphology and activity. Mori and Leblond (see [5]) separated oligodendrocytes into three groups based on location, stainability and DNA turnover. Their three classes correspond to satellite, intermediate and interfascicular, or myelinating, oligodendrocytes. Satellite oligodendrocytes are small (~10 μm), restricted to gray matter and closely applied to the surface of neurons. They are assumed to play a role in the maintenance of the neuron and are potential myelinating cells. Interfascicular oligodendrocytes are large (~20 μm) during myelination but, in the adult, range from 10 to 15 μm, with the nucleus occupying a large percentage of the cell volume. Intermediate oligodendrocytes are regarded as satellite or potential myelinating forms. The nucleus of these cells is small, the cytoplasm occupying the greater area of the soma.

Myelinating oligodendrocytes have been studied extensively [5,30] (see Chap. 4). Examination of the CNS during myelinogenesis (Fig. 1-15) reveals connections between the cell body and the myelin sheath [31]; however, connections between these elements have never been demonstrated in a normal adult animal, unlike the PNS counterpart, the Schwann cell. In contrast to the Schwann cell (see below), the oligodendrocyte is capable of producing many internodes of myelin simultaneously. It is estimated that oligodendrocytes in the optic nerve produce between 30 and 50 internodes of myelin [5]. In addition to this heavy structural commitment, the oligodendrocyte possesses a slow mitotic rate and a poor regenerative capacity. Damage to only a few oligodendrocytes, therefore, can be expected to produce an appreciable area of primary demyelination. In most CNS diseases in which myelin is a target, oligodendrocytes are among the most vulnerable elements and the first to degenerate (see Chap. 39).

Somewhat analogous to the neuron, the relatively small oligodendrocyte soma produces and supports many more times its own volume of membrane and cytoplasm. For example, consider an average 12-μm oligodendrocyte producing 20 internodes of myelin [5]. Each axon has a diameter of 3 μm and is covered by at least six lamellae of myelin, each lamella representing two fused layers of unit membrane. By statistical analysis, taking into account the length of the myelin internode, which is possibly 500 μm, and the length of the membranes of the cell processes connecting the sheaths to the cell body (~12 μm), the ratio between the surface area of the cell soma and the myelin it sustains is approximately 1:620. In most cases, however, this ratio is probably in the region of 1:3,000. In rare instances, oligodendrocytes elaborate myelin around structures other than axons in that myelin has been documented around neuronal somata and nonaxonal profiles.

Molecular markers of oligodendrocytes. The oligodendrocyte is potentially highly vulnerable to immune-mediated damage since it shares with the myelin sheath many molecules with known affinities to elicit specific T- and B-cell responses, which lead to its destruction. Chapter 39 describes the immune process in demyelination. Many of these molecules, such as myelin basic protein, proteolipid protein, myelin-associated glycoprotein, myelin/oligodendrocyte protein, galactocerebroside, myelin oligodendrocyte glycoprotein (MOG) and others, have been used to generate specific antibodies, which are routinely applied to anatomical analyses of oligodendro-

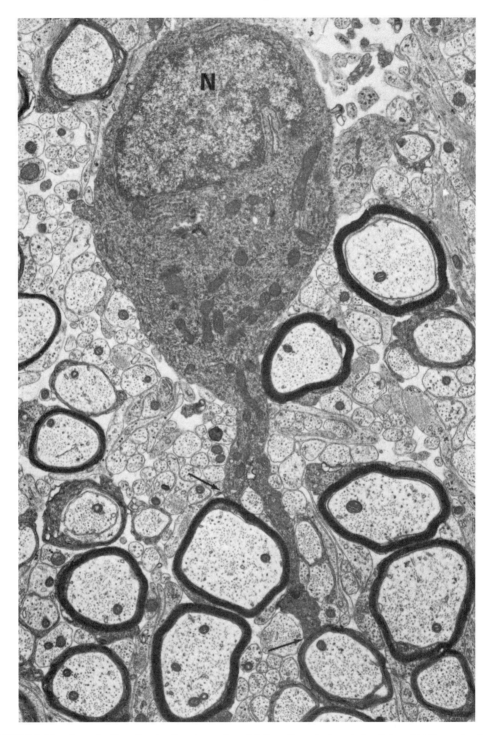

FIGURE 1-15.   A myelinating oligodendrocyte, nucleus *(N),* from the spinal cord of a 2-day-old kitten extends cytoplasmic connections to at least two myelin sheaths *(arrows).* Other myelinated and unmyelinated fibers at various stages of development, as well as glial processes, are seen in the surrounding neuropil. ×12,750.

cytes *in vivo* and *in vitro*. However, unlike the astrocyte, the oligodendrocyte expresses no class I or II MHC molecules suggestive of interactions with the immune system [32].

The microglial cell plays a role in phagocytosis and inflammatory responses

Of the few remaining types of CNS cells, the most interesting, and probably the most enigmatic, is the microglial cell, a cell of mesodermal origin, located in the normal brain in a resting state and purported to become a very mobile, active macrophage during disease (see Chap. 35). Microglia can be stained selectively and demonstrated by light microscopy using Hortega's silver carbonate method, but no comparable technique exists for their ultrastructural demonstration. The cells have spindle-shaped bodies and a thin rim of densely staining cytoplasm difficult to distinguish from the nucleus. The nucleochromatin is homogeneously dense, and the cytoplasm does not contain an abundance of organelles, although representatives of the usual components can be found. During normal wear and tear, some CNS elements degenerate and microglia phagocytose the debris (Fig. 1-16). Their identification and numbers, as determined by light microscopy, differ from species to species. The CNS of rabbit is richly endowed. In a number of disease instances, such as trauma, microglia are

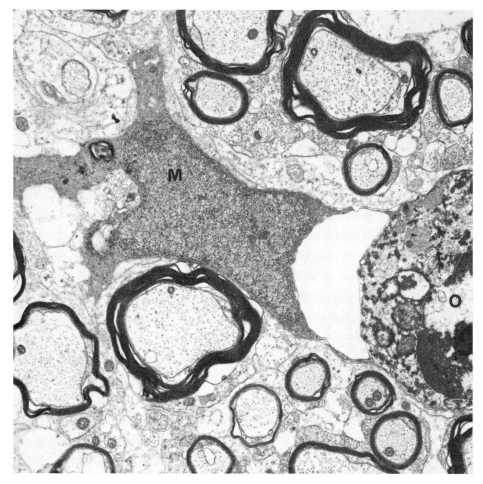

FIGURE 1-16.   A microglial cell *(M)* has elaborated two cytoplasmic arms to encompass a degenerating apoptotic oligodendrocyte *(O)* in the spinal cord of a 3-day-old kitten. The microglial cell nucleus is difficult to distinguish from the narrow rim of densely staining cytoplasm, which also contains some membranous debris. ×10,000.

stimulated and migrate to the area of injury, where they phagocytose debris. The relatively brief mention of this cell type in the major EM textbooks [3] and the conflicting EM descriptions [33] are indicative of the uncertainty attached to their identification. Pericytes are believed by some to be a resting form of microglial cell. Perivascular macrophages, which are of bone marrow origin and are distinct from parenchymal microglia, also have been described.

Molecular markers of microglial cells. There has been a veritable explosion of activity in the field of microglial cell biology with the realization that this cell type is capable of functioning as a highly efficient accessory cell of the immune system. While no particularly microglia-specific molecule has been identified, a number of antibodies raised against monocytic markers and complement receptor molecules stain microglial cells *in situ* and *in vitro*. There is strong evidence that microglia express class II MHC upon activation [34–37], frequently in the absence of a T-cell response. This suggests that class II MHC ex-

pression may represent a marker of activation or in some way elevate the cells to a state of immunological awareness. Microglia are also producers of a number of proinflammatory cytokines with known effects upon T cells. Taken in concert, the increasing evidence of an immunological role for microglia in a wide spectrum of conditions probably supports the putative monocytic origin of this cell type.

Ependymal cells line the brain ventricles and the spinal cord central canal

Ependymal cells are arranged in single-palisade arrays and line the ventricles of the brain and central canal of the spinal cord. They are usually ciliated, their cilia extending into the ventricular cavity. Their fine structure has been elucidated by Brightman and Palay [38]. They possess several features that clearly differentiate them from any other CNS cell. The cilia emerge from the apical pole of the cell, where they are attached to a blepharoplast, the basal body (Fig. 1-17), which is anchored in the cytoplasm by means of ciliary rootlets and a basal

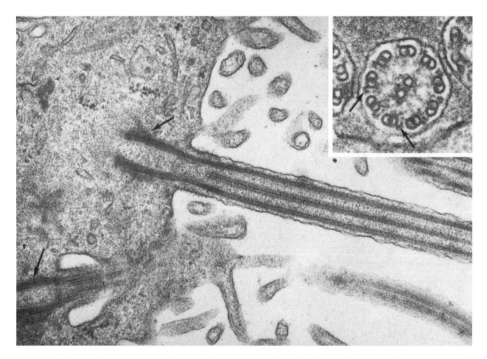

FIGURE 1-17.   The surface of an ependymal cell contains basal bodies *(arrows)* connected to the microtubules of cilia, seen here in longitudinal section. Several microvilli are also present. ×37,000. **Inset:** Ependymal cilia in transverse section possess a central doublet of microtubules surrounded by nine pairs, one of each pair having a characteristic hook-like appendage *(arrows).* ×100,000.

foot. The basal foot is the contractile component that determines the direction of the ciliary beat. Like all flagellar structures, the cilium contains the common microtubule arrangement of nine peripheral pairs around a central doublet (Fig. 1-17). In the vicinity of the basal body, the arrangement is one of nine triplets; at the tip of each cilium, the pattern is one of haphazardly organized single tubules. Also, extending from the free surface of the cell are numerous microvilli containing actin microfilaments (Fig. 1-17). The cytoplasm stains intensely, having an electron density about equal to that of the oligodendrocyte, whereas the nucleus has a similar density to that of the astrocyte. Microtubules; large whorls of filaments; coated vesicles; rough ER; Golgi apparatus; lysosomes; and abundant small, dense mitochondria are also present. The base of the cell is composed of involuted processes that interdigitate with the underlying neuropil. The lateral margins of each cell characteristically display long, compound, junctional complexes (Fig. 1-18) made up of desmosomes, termed *zonula adherentes*, and gap junctions [3]. Overlying specialized secretory zones around the ventricles, the so-called subventricle organs and choroid plexus, the ependymal lining is different and the cells are connected at their apical poles by tight junctions called *zonula occludentes*. Desmosomes and gap junctions are also present at the lateral aspects of the cells [39].

The biochemical properties of these structures are known. Desmosomes display protease sensitivity, divalent cation dependency and osmotic insensitivity; and their membranes are mainly of the smooth type. In direct contrast to desmosomes, the tight junctions as well as gap junctions and synapses display no protease sensitivity, divalent cation dependency or osmotic sensitivity, while their membranes are complex. These facts have been used in the development of techniques to isolate purified preparations of junctional complexes.

The Schwann cell is the myelin-producing cell of the peripheral nervous system

When axons leave the CNS, they lose their neuroglial interrelationships and traverse a short transitional zone, where they are invested by an

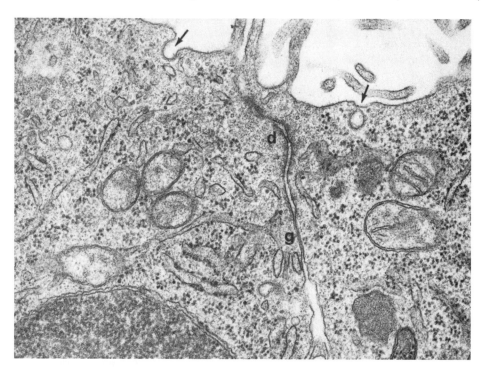

FIGURE 1-18. A typical desmosome *(d)* and gap junction *(g)* between two ependymal cells. Microvilli and coated pits *(arrows)* are seen along the cell surface. ×35,000.

astroglial sheath enclosed in the basal lamina of the glia limitans. The basal lamina then becomes continuous with that of axon-investing Schwann cells, at which point the astroglial covering terminates. Schwann cells, therefore, are the axon-ensheathing cells of the PNS, equivalent functionally to the oligodendrocyte of the CNS (see Chap. 4). Along the myelinated fibers of the PNS, each internode of myelin is elaborated by one Schwann cell and each Schwann cell elaborates one internode [30]. This ratio of one internode of myelin to one Schwann cell is a fun-

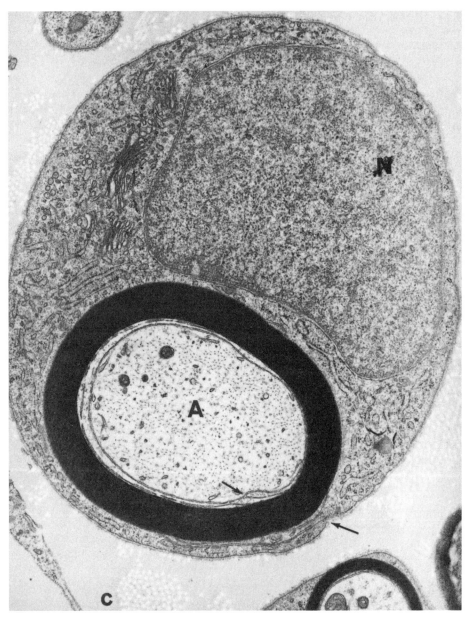

FIGURE 1-19. A myelinated PNS axon *(A)* is surrounded by a Schwann cell, nucleus *(N)*. Note the fuzzy basal lamina around the cell, the rich cytoplasm, the inner and outer mesaxons *(arrows)*, the close proximity of the cell to its myelin sheath and the 1:1 (cell:myelin internode) relationship. A process of an endoneurial cell is seen **(lower left)**, and unstained collagen *(c)* lies in the endoneurial space *(white dots)*. ×20,000.

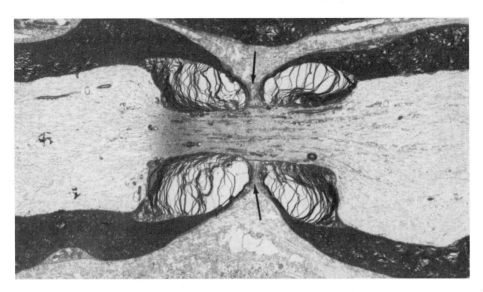

FIGURE 1-20. Low-power electron micrograph of a node of Ranvier in longitudinal section. Note the abrupt decrease in axon diameter and the attendant condensation of axoplasmic constituents in the paranodal and nodal regions of the axon. Paranodal myelin is distorted artifactually, a common phenomenon in large-diameter fibers. The nodal gap substance *(arrows)* contains Schwann cell fingers; the nodal axon is bulbous; and lysosomes lie beneath the axolemma within the bulge. Beaded smooth endoplasmic reticulum sacs are also seen. ×5,000.

damental distinction between this cell type and its CNS analog, the oligodendrocyte, which is able to proliferate internodes in the ratio of 1:30 or greater. Another distinction is that the Schwann cell body always remains in intimate contact with its myelin internode (Fig. 1-19), whereas the oligodendrocyte extends processes toward its internodes. Periodically, myelin lamellae open up into ridges of Schwann cell cytoplasm, producing bands of cytoplasm around the fiber, Schmidt-Lanterman incisures, reputed to be the stretch points along PNS fibers. These incisures usually are not present in the CNS. The PNS myelin period is 11.9 nm in preserved specimens, which is some 30% less than in the fresh state, in contrast to the 10.6 nm of central myelin. In addition to these structural differences, PNS myelin differs biochemically and antigenically from that of the CNS (see Chap. 4). Not all PNS fibers are myelinated, but in contrast to nonmyelinated fibers in the CNS, nonmyelinated fibers in the PNS are suspended in groups within the Schwann cell cytoplasm, each axon connected to the extracellular space by a short channel, the mesaxon, formed by the invaginated Schwann cell plasmalemma.

Ultrastructurally, the Schwann cell is unique and distinct from the oligodendrocyte. Each Schwann cell is surrounded by a basal lamina made up of a mucopolysaccharide approximately 20 to 30 nm thick that does not extend into the mesaxon (Fig. 1-19). The basal laminae of adjacent myelinating Schwann cells at the nodes of Ranvier are continuous, and Schwann cell processes interdigitate so that the PNS myelinated axon is never in direct contact with the extracellular space. These nodal Schwann cell fingers display intimate relationships with the axolemma (Figs. 1-20 and 1-21), suggesting that the entire nodal complex might serve as an electrogenic pump for the recycling of ions [10]. A similar arrangement between the nodal axon and the fingers of astroglial cells is seen in the CNS. The Schwann cells of nonmyelinated PNS fibers overlap, and there are no nodes of Ranvier.

The cytoplasm of the Schwann cell is rich in organelles. A Golgi apparatus is located near the nucleus, and cisternae of the rough ER occur throughout the cell. Lysosomes, multivesicular bodies, glycogen granules and lipid granules, also termed pi granules, also can be seen. The cell is rich in microtubules and filaments, in contrast

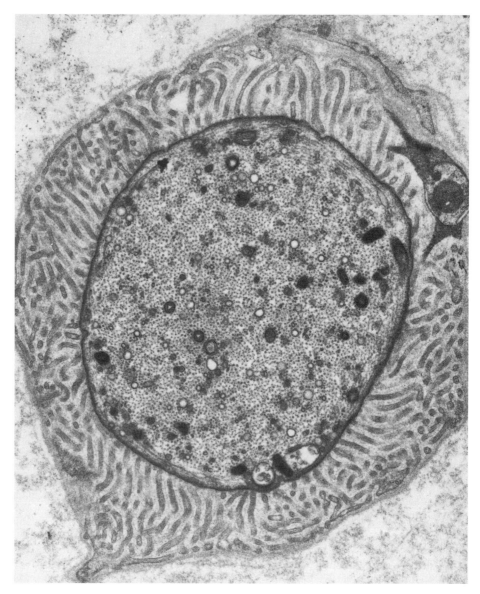

FIGURE 1-21.   A transverse section of the node of Ranvier (7 to 8 μm across) of a large fiber shows a prominent complex of Schwann cell fingers around an axon highlighted by its subaxolemmal densification and closely packed organelles. The Schwann cell fingers arise from an outer collar of flattened cytoplasm and abut the axon at regular intervals of approximately 80 nm. The basal lamina of the nerve fiber encircles the entire complex. The nodal gap substance is granular and sometimes linear. Within the axoplasm, note the transversely sectioned sacs of beaded smooth endoplasmic reticulum (ER); mitochondria; dense lamellar bodies, which appear to maintain a peripheral location; flattened smooth ER sacs; dense-core vesicles; cross-bridged neurofilaments; and microtubules, which in places run parallel to the circumference of the axon **(above left** and **lower right),** perhaps in a spiral fashion. ×16,000.

to the oligodendrocyte. The plasmalemma frequently shows pinocytic vesicles. Small, round mitochondria are scattered throughout the soma. The nucleus, which stains intensely, is flattened and oriented longitudinally along the nerve fiber. Aggregates of dense heterochromatin are arranged peripherally [3].

In sharp contrast to the oligodendrocyte, the Schwann cell responds vigorously to most forms of injury (see Chap. 39). An active phase of mitosis occurs following traumatic insult, and the cells are capable of local migration. Studies on their behavior after primary demyelination have shown that they are able to phagocytose damaged myelin. They possess remarkable reparatory properties and begin to lay down new myelin approximately 1 week after a fiber loses its myelin sheath. Studies on PNS and CNS re-myelination [40] have shown that by 3 months after primary demyelination, PNS fibers are well remyelinated, whereas similarly affected areas in the CNS show relatively little proliferation of new myelin (see Chap. 29). Under circumstances of severe injury, such as transection, axons degenerate and the Schwann cells form tubes, termed *Büngner bands*, containing cell bodies and processes surrounded by a single basal lamina. These structures provide channels along which regenerating axons might later grow. The presence and integrity of the Schwann cell basal lamina is essential for reinnervation.

The extracellular space between peripheral nerve fibers is occupied by bundles of collagen fibrils, blood vessels and endoneurial cells

Endoneurial cells are elongated, spindle-shaped cells with tenuous processes relatively poor in organelles except for large cisternae of the rough ER. There is some evidence that these cells proliferate collagen fibrils. Sometimes mast cells, the histamine producers of connective tissue, can be seen. Bundles of nerve fibers are arranged in fascicles emarginated by flattened connective tissue cells forming the perineurium, an essential component in the blood–nerve barrier system. Fascicles of nerve fibers are aggregated into nerves and invested by a tough elastic sheath of cells known as the epineurium [41].

ACKNOWLEDGMENTS

The excellent technical assistance of Everett Swanson, Howard Finch and Miriam Pakingan is appreciated. The work represented by this chapter was supported in part by USPHS Grants NS 08952 and NS 11920 and by Grant NMSS RG 1001-I-9 from the National Multiple Sclerosis Society.

REFERENCES

1. Palay, S. L., and Chan-Palay, V. *Cerebellar Cortex: Cytology and Organization.* New York: Springer, 1974.
2. Hyden, H. The neuron. In J. Brachet and A. E. Mirsky (eds.), *The Cell.* New York: Academic, 1960, Vol. 5, pp. 215–323.
3. Peters, A., Palay, S. L., and Webster, H. de F. *The Fine Structure of the Nervous System: The Cells and Their Processes.* New York: Oxford University Press, 1991.
4. Mugnaini, E., and Walberg, F. Ultrastructure of neuroglia. *Ergeb. Anat. Entwicklungsgesch.* 37:194–236, 1964.
5. Raine, C. S. Oligodendrocytes and central nervous system myelin. In R. L. Davis and D. M. Robertson (eds.), *Textbook of Neuropathology,* 3rd ed. Baltimore: Williams & Wilkins, 1997, pp. 137–164.
6. Kandel, E. R., Schwarz, J. H., and Jessell, T. M. (eds.), *Principles of Neural Science.* Amsterdam: Elsevier, 1991.
7. Novikoff, A. B., and Holtzman, E. *Cells and Organelles.* New York: Holt, Rinehart and Winston, 1976.
8. Soifer, D. (ed.), Dynamic aspects of microtubule biology. *Ann. N. Y. Acad. Sci.* 466, 1986.
9. Wang, E., Fischman, B., Liem, R. L., and Sun, T.-T. (eds.), Intermediate filaments. *Ann. N. Y. Acad. Sci.* 455, 1985.
10. Raine, C. S. Differences in the nodes of Ranvier of large and small diameter fibres in the PNS. *J. Neurocytol.* 11:935–947, 1982.
11. Ritchie, J. M. Physiological basis of conduction in myelinated nerve fibers. In P. Morell (ed.), *Myelin.* New York: Plenum, 1984, pp. 117–146.
12. Peters, A., and Palay, S. L. The morphology of synapses. *J. Neurocytol.* 25:687–700, 1996.
13. Bauerfeind, R., Galli, T., and DeCamilli, P. Molecular mechanisms in synaptic vesicle recycling. *J. Neurocytol.* 25:701–716, 1996.
14. Bodian, D. Synaptic diversity and characterization by electron microscopy. In G. D. Pappas and D. P. Purpura (eds.), *Structure and Function of Synapses.* New York: Raven, 1972, pp. 45–65.
15. Gray, E. G. Electron microscopy of excitatory and inhibitory synapses: A brief review. *Prog. Brain Res.* 31:141, 1969.
16. Bloom, F. E. Localization of neurotransmitters by electron microscopy. In *Neurotransmitters (Proc. ARNMD).* Baltimore: Williams & Wilkins, 1972, Vol. 50, pp. 25–57.
17. Wolfe, D. E., Potter, L. T., Richardson, K. C., and

Axelrod, J. Localizing tritiated norepinephrine in sympathetic axons by electron microscopic autoradiography. *Science* 138:440–442, 1962.

18. Pappas, G. D., and Waxman, S. Synaptic fine structure: Morphological correlates of chemical and electronic transmission. In G. D. Pappas and D. P. Purpura (eds.), *Structure and Function of Synapses.* New York: Raven, 1972, pp. 1–43.

19. Liem, R. K. H. Neuronal intermediate filaments. *Curr. Opin. Cell Biol.* 2:86–90, 1990.

20. Cleveland, D. W., and Hoffman, P. N. Neuronal and glial cytoskeletons. *Curr. Opin. Neurobiol.* 1:346–353, 1991.

21. McGeer, P. L., Eccles, J. C., and McGeer, E. G. (eds.), *Molecular Neurobiology of the Mammalian Brain.* New York: Plenum, 1987.

22. Raff, M. C., Miller, R. H., and Noble, M. A. Glial progenitor cell that develops in vitro into an astrocyte or an oligodendrocyte depending on culture medium. *Nature* 303:390–396, 1983.

23. Reese, T. S., and Karnovsky, M. J. Fine structural localization of a blood–brain barrier to exogenous peroxidase. *J. Cell Biol.* 34:207–217, 1967.

24. Brightman, M. The distribution within the brain of ferritin injected into cerebrospinal fluid compartments. II. Parenchymal distribution. *Am. J. Anat.* 117:193–220, 1965.

25. Brosnan, C. F., Claudio, L., and Martinez, J. A. The blood brain barrier during immune responses. *Semin. Neurosci.* 4:193–206, 1992.

26. Claudio, L., Raine, C. S., and Brosnan, C. F. Evidence of generalized blood–brain barrier abnormalities in chronic progressive multiple sclerosis. *Acta Neuropathol.* (Berlin) 90:228–238, 1995.

27. Yong, V. W., and Antel, J. P. Major histocompatibility complex molecules on glial cells. *Semin. Neurosci.* 4:231–240, 1992.

28. Benveniste, E. N. Cytokine expression in the nervous system. In R. W. Keane and W. F. Hickey (eds.), *Immunology of the Nervous System.* New York: Oxford University Press, 1997, pp. 419–459.

29. Norton, W. T. (ed.), *Oligodendroglia. Advances in Neurochemistry,* Vol. 5. New York: Plenum, 1984.

30. Raine, C. S. Morphology of myelin and myelination. In P. Morell (ed.), *Myelin,* 2nd ed. New York: Plenum, 1984, pp. 1–50.

31. Bunge, R. P. Glial cells and the central myelin sheath. *Physiol. Rev.* 48:197–248, 1968.

32. Raine, C. S. The Dale E. McFarlin Memorial Lecture: The immunology of the multiple sclerosis lesion. *Ann. Neurol.* 36:561–572, 1994.

33. Fujita, S., and Kitamura, T. Origin of brain macrophages and the nature of the microglia. In H. Zimmerman (ed.), *Progress in Neuropathology.* New York: Grune and Stratton, 1976, Vol. 2, pp. 1–50.

34. Dickson, D. W., Mattiace, L. A., Kure, K., et al. Biology of disease. Microglia in human disease, with an emphasis on acquired immune deficiency syndrome. *Lab. Invest.* 64:135–156, 1991.

35. Matsumoto, Y., Ohmori, K., and Fujiwara, M. Microglial and astroglial reactions to inflammatory lesions of experimental autoimmune encephalomyelitis in the rat central nervous system. *J. Neuroimmunol.* 37:23–33, 1992.

36. Ling, E. A., and Wong, W. C. The origin and nature of ramified and amoeboid microglia: an historical review and current concepts. *Glia* 7:84–92, 1993.

37. Perry, V. H., and Gordon, S. Microglia and macrophages. In R. W. Keane and W. F. Hickey (eds.), *Immunology of the Nervous System.* New York: Oxford University Press, 1997, pp. 155–172.

38. Brightman, M., and Palay, S. L. The fine structure of ependyma in the brain of the rat. *J. Cell Biol.* 19:415–440, 1963.

39. Milhorat, T. H. (ed.), *Cerebrospinal Fluid and the Brain Edemas.* New York: Neuroscience Society of New York, 1987.

40. Raine, C. S., Wisniewski, H., and Prineas, J. An ultrastructural study of experimental demyelination and remyelination. II. Chronic experimental allergic encephalomyelitis in the peripheral nervous system. *Lab. Invest.* 21:316–327, 1969.

41. Babel, J., Bischoff, A., and Spoendlin, H. Ultrastructure of the peripheral nervous system and sense organs. In *Atlas of Normal and Pathologic Anatomy.* St. Louis: Mosby, 1970, pp. 1–171.

2

Cell Membrane Structures and Functions

R. Wayne Albers

Basic Neurochemistry: Molecular, Cellular and Medical Aspects, 6th Ed., edited by G. J. Siegel et al. Published by Lippincott–Raven Publishers, Philadelphia, 1999. Correspondence to R. Wayne Albers, Laboratory of Neurochemistry, National Institute of Neurological Diseases and Stroke, National Institutes of Health, Bethesda, Maryland 20892.

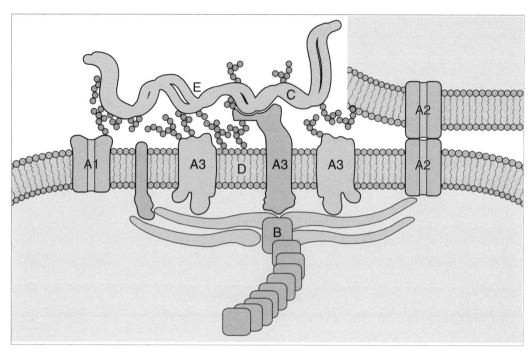

FIGURE 2-1. Overview of plasma membrane structure. Plasma membranes are distinguishable from other cellular membranes by the presence of both glycolipids and glycoproteins on their outer surfaces and the attachment of cytoskeletal proteins to their cytoplasmic surfaces. Interrelations among typical membrane components are depicted. Proteins that are inserted through the lipid bilayer *(A1–A3)*, termed "integral" membrane proteins, are often glycosylated *(dark orange circles)*, as are some bilayer lipids *(D)* and many components of the extracellular matrix *(E)*. Many interactions at the extracellular surface are stabilized by hydrogen bonding among these glycosyl residues. Certain integral membrane proteins can interact by virtue of specific receptor sites with intracellular proteins *(B)*, with extracellular components *(C)* and to form specific junctions with other cells *(A2)*. A host of integral membrane proteins mediates different signal-transduction and active-transport pathways.

Neurons are specialized to integrate environmental stimuli, both spatially and temporally. The processes of integration generate signals that are rapidly transmitted along axonal plasma membranes to other cells. This chapter begins with a discussion of the physical chemistry underlying the structure of cell membranes. Subsequent sections describe the general organization of membranes and examples of different classes of membrane proteins (Fig. 2-1). Finally, the biochemical processes that produce and maintain plasma membranes are summarized with attention to those that are important for neural functions.

PHOSPHOLIPID BILAYERS

Cells are separated from their environment by lipid bilayers

The fundamental importance of lipids in membrane structure was established early in this century by demonstrations that positive correlations exist between cell membrane permeabilities to small nonelectrolytes and the oil/water partition coefficients of these molecules. Contemporary measurements of the electrical impedance of cell suspensions suggested that cells are surrounded by a hydrocarbon barrier, which was first estimated to be about 3.3 nm thick. It was originally thought that a membrane containing a lipid monolayer could account for these data. However, subsequent experiments established that the ratio of the area of a monolayer formed from erythrocyte membrane lipids to the surface area of these cells is nearly 2. These and other studies of the physical chemistry of lipids fortified the concept that a continuous lipid bilayer is a major component of cell membranes. This concept has received support from many other studies, including the interpretation of X-ray diffraction data obtained from intact cell membranes.

Forces acting between lipids and between lipids and between proteins are primarily noncovalent, consisting of electrostatic, hydrogen-bonding and van der Waals' interactions. Although these are weak interactions relative to covalent bonds, their sum can produce very stable associations. Ionic and polar parts of molecules exposed to water will become hydrated. Substances dissolve in a solvent only if their molecules interact with the solvent more strongly than with each other. Complex molecules may have two or more surface domains that differ in polarity. In aqueous solution their apolar surfaces form an internal hydrophobic phase that minimizes their exposure to water and their more polar surfaces form an external hydrated phase. Molecules with segregated polar and nonpolar surfaces are termed amphipathic. These include most biological lipids and many proteins.

Amphipathic molecules form bilayered lamellar structures spontaneously if they have an appropriate geometry

Most of the major cell membrane lipids have a polar head, commonly a glycerophosphorylester moiety and a hydrocarbon tail, usually consisting of two esterified fatty acids (Chap. 3). The head groups can interact with water and aqueous phase solutes, whereas the nonpolar tails aggregate to form an internal phase.

Three principal phases with different structures are formed by phospholipids in the presence of water [1] (Fig. 2-2). Although the lamellar, or bilayer, structure is generally found in cell membranes, the two hexagonal phases probably occur during some membrane transformations. The importance of molecular geometry for bilayer stability is illustrated by the effects of the phospholipase A$_2$ component of many venoms: they remove one fatty acid from a phospholipid to produce lysophosphatides, which ultimately destabilize bilayers relative to hexagonal phase structures. In sufficient amounts, lysophosphatides disrupt cell membranes and lyse cells. Detergents are amphipathic molecules with similar abilities to transform lipid bilayers into water-soluble micelles. In contrast to the destabilizing effects of lysophosphatides and other detergents, cholesterol stabilizes bilayers by in-

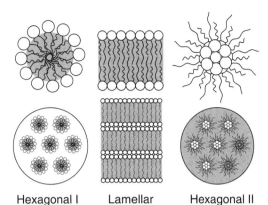

Hexagonal I   Lamellar   Hexagonal II

FIGURE 2-2. Complex lipids interact with water and with each other to form different states of aggregation, or "phases," shown here schematically. *Open circles* or *ellipses* represent the more polar head groups, and *dark lines and areas* represent nonpolar hydrocarbon chains. The phase structures are generally classified as illustrated in the **lower row** of the figure. The hexagonal I and lamellar phases can be dispersed in aqueous media to form the micellar structures shown in the **top row.** Hexagonal II phase lipids will form "reverse micelles" in nonpolar solvents. The stability of lamellar structures relative to hexagonal structures depends upon fatty acid chain length, presence of double bonds, relative sizes of polar head and hydrocarbon tail groups and temperature.

tercalating at the interface between head and tail regions of phospholipid so as to satisfy the bulk requirements for a planar geometry.

Multilamellar bilayer structures (Fig. 2-2) form spontaneously if small amounts of water are added to solid or liquid phase phospholipids. These can be dispersed in water to form vesicular structures called *liposomes*. These are often employed in studies of bilayer properties and may be combined with membrane proteins to reconstitute functional membrane systems. A valuable technique for studying the properties of proteins inserted into bilayers employs a single bilayer lamella, also termed a *black lipid membrane*, formed across a small aperture in a thin partition between two aqueous compartments. Because pristine lipid bilayers have very low ion conductivities, the modifications of ion-conducting properties produced by membrane proteins can be measured with great sensitivity (Chap. 6).

In aqueous systems, phospholipid structures may manifest either gel, that is, rigid, or liquid-crystalline, that is, two-dimensionally fluid, properties. In the case of pure phospholipids, these states interconvert at a well-defined transition temperature, T_c, that increases with alkyl chain length and decreases with introduction of unsaturation. In cell membranes, there is marked heterogeneity in both the polar and nonpolar domains of the bilayer. Alkyl chain heterogeneity and the presence of cholesterol maintain cell membrane bilayers in the fluid state over a broad temperature range. Bilayer fluidity causes membrane lipids and proteins to diffuse rapidly within the plane of the bilayer.

Functional importance of bilayer asymmetry. Although there is rapid diffusion within the plane of a bilayer, spontaneous transverse migration of phospholipids from one bilayer leaflet to another is rare. This allows the two leaflets of a cell membrane bilayer to have very different compositions (Chap. 3). Aminophospholipids are normally confined almost exclusively to the cytoplasmic leaflet, whereas most glycolipids and sphingolipids are in the extracytoplasmic leaflet. This is accomplished by an ATP-dependent process that "pumps" the head groups of aminophospholipids toward the cytoplasmic surface. A second ATP-dependent pumping process may be involved in maintaining the extracytoplasmic orientation of phosphatidylcholine (Chap. 5). High intracellular Ca^{2+}, which can arise from any condition that depletes intracellular ATP, activates a "scramblase" protein, which catalyses random transverse lipid movements. The appearance of substantial amounts of phosphatidylserine on outer cell surfaces can initiate apoptosis and phagocytosis [2].

Insertion of lipids into bilayers. Most biosynthesis of membrane lipids occurs in the endoplasmic reticulum (ER) (Chap. 3). Glycosphingolipids can segregate laterally in the bilayer to form microdomains, or "rafts," with cholesterol [3]. In apical membranes of epithelial cells, these domains are associated with the sites of formation of small vesicles, called "caveolae" (see below), which transport cholesterol and, perhaps, other lipids to plasma membranes [4].

Most bilayer phospholipids are physically constrained by association with integral membrane proteins

In addition to interacting with each other to form the bilayer, membrane lipids may interact to varying degrees with membrane proteins [5]. Some physical measurements, such as electron spin resonance, have indicated that the acyl moieties of lipids immediately surrounding integral membrane proteins are motionally restricted and reoriented relative to the bilayer. This "annulus" fraction can comprise 20 to 90% of the total membrane phospholipid. Because the annulus lipids appear to equilibrate rapidly, within microseconds, with the bulk membrane lipids in comparison with the time scale of most enzyme-catalyzed reactions, which occur in milliseconds, the significance of such interactions has been questioned. However, phosphatidylethanolamine is now known to be a component of the crystalline structure of the membrane protein, cytochrome oxidase [6]. Some proteins, including certain integral membrane proteins, contain domains that can interact directly and strongly with phospholipids (see below).

Diffusional flow of water directly through lipid bilayers largely accounts for the water permeability of most cell membranes

The water permeability of ion channels is estimated to account for only about 1% of the total cell water permeability. Measurements of water permeability of bilayers of varying lipid composition have ranged from 2 to 1,000 $\times$ 10^{-5} cm²/sec [7]. Measurements of cell membrane water permeabilities are in the same range for many cell types. Erythrocytes are a known exception, with a water permeability of about 2 $\times$ 10^{-2} cm². The high water permeability of the plasma membranes of erythrocytes, kidney epithelia, certain glia and other cells results from the presence of specific membrane proteins, designated *aquaporins*. These are the eukaryotic members of a large and widespread family of membrane channel proteins that select water and, in some cases, admit small neutral molecules such as urea and glycerol [8]. Aquaporin-2 mediates vasopressin-sensitive water transport [9]. Aquaporin-4 is expressed in high levels in certain glial and ependymal cells [10].

The head–group regions of phospholipid monolayers facilitate lateral diffusion of protons and possibly of other ions

In model systems, pH changes have been shown to be transmitted more rapidly along these interfaces than in bulk solution. This may have particular importance in mitochondrial ATP synthesis and other processes that depend on transmembrane proton gradients [11]. This high mobility may not be restricted to protons: nuclear magnetic resonance studies have shown that the exchange of metal cations among phospholipid head groups can also be more rapid than in free solution.

MEMBRANE PROTEINS

Integral proteins have transmembrane domains that insert directly into the lipid bilayer

These transmembrane domains consist predominantly of nonpolar amino acid residues and may traverse the bilayer once or several times. High-resolution structural information is available for only a few integral membrane proteins, primarily because it is difficult to obtain membrane protein crystals that are adequate for X-ray diffraction measurements. Consequently, much of our knowledge of integral membrane protein structure derives from the application of various topographical mapping techniques.

Transmembrane domains are usually α helices

The peptide bond is intrinsically polar and can form internal hydrogen bonds between carbonyl oxygens and amide nitrogens, or either of these may hydrate. Within the lipid bilayer, where water is essentially excluded, peptides usually adopt the configuration that maximizes their internal hydrogen bonding, which is an α helix. A length of α helix sufficient to span the usual width of a lipid bi-

layer requires 18 to 21 amino acid residues (Fig. 2-3). Because the surface properties of an α helix are determined by its side chains, a single helical segment that anchors a protein by insertion into the bilayer consists largely of hydrophobic residues. Integral membrane proteins with multiple transmembrane helices may have amphipathic amino

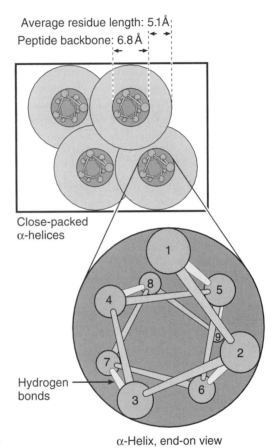

Average residue length: 5.1 Å
Peptide backbone: 6.8 Å

Close-packed α-helices

Hydrogen bonds

α-Helix, end-on view

FIGURE 2-3.   The transmembrane domains of integral membrane proteins are predominantly α helices. This structure causes the amino acid side chains to project radially. When several parallel α helices are closely packed, their side chains may intermesh as shown, or steric constraints may cause the formation of interchain channels. The outwardly directed residues must be predominantly hydrophobic to interact with the fatty acid chains of lipid bilayers. The bilayer is about 3 nm thick. Each peptide residue extends an α helix by 1.5 Å. Thus, although local modifications of the bilayer or interactions with other membrane polypeptides may alter this requirement, transmembrane segments usually require about 20 residues to span the bilayer. Integral membrane proteins are characterized by the presence of hydrophobic segments approximating this length.

acid sequences, with the more polar residues involved in helix–helix interactions, intramembrane channel formation and other interactions. Derivation of "hydrophobicity profiles" from protein sequence data often provides major insights about transmembrane protein topography.

Proteins with one transmembrane domain may have soluble domains at either or both surfaces

Cytochrome b5 has a single hydrophobic segment that forms a hairpin loop, which acts as an anchor to the cytoplasmic surface but is thought not to penetrate the bilayer totally. It is an example of a monotopic protein. Bitopic proteins are more common, having a single transmembrane helix, which, if oriented with the N-terminus on the extracytoplasmic surface, is classified as type I or, if on the cytoplasmic surface, as type II [12] (Fig. 2-4).

Bitopic membrane proteins are often involved in signal transduction. For example, some of the receptor-activated tyrosine kinases are bitopic (Chap. 25). Agonist occupation of an extracytoplasmic receptor domain can transmit structural changes via a single transmembrane segment to activate latent kinase activity in its cytoplasmic domain.

Ion channels, transport pumps and many receptor–effector complexes are polytopic. Their predominantly hydrophobic transmembrane segments are commonly interspersed with polar and helix-destabilizing residues. Such proteins that perform tasks within the bilayer frequently have amphipathic helices that interact to form the requisite functional structures.

Transmembrane helices are usually closely packed

Two examples of this are bacteriorhodopsin and the sarcoplasmic Ca^{2+} pump. Peptide bonds have substantial dipole moments that are transmitted to the ends of α helices. This circumstance would be expected to favor close packing of antiparallel helices and is, in fact, consistent with the observed disposition of helices in bacteriorhodopsin [13]. However, intersubunit packing in oligomeric proteins can involve interactions of extramembranous protein domains and may encompass some bilayer lipids.

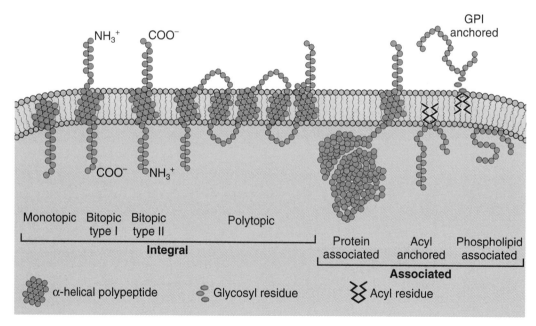

FIGURE 2-4. **Left:** Integral membrane proteins can be classified with respect to the orientation and complexity of their transmembrane segments. **Right:** Proteins may associate with membranes through several types of interactions with the bilayer lipids and by interacting with integral membrane proteins. *GPI,* glycosylphosphatidylinositol.

The fluidity of the lipid bilayer permits dynamic interactions among membrane proteins

For example, the interactions of a neurotransmitter or hormone with its receptor can dissociate a "transducer" protein, which in turn will diffuse to interact with other effector proteins (Chap. 20). A given effector protein, such as adenylyl cyclase, may respond differently to different receptors because of mediation by different transducers. These dynamic interactions require rapid protein diffusion within the plane of the membrane bilayer. Receptor occupation can initiate extensive redistribution of membrane proteins, as exemplified by the clustering of membrane antigens consequent to binding bivalent antibodies [14].

In contrast to these examples of lateral mobility, the surface distribution of integral membrane proteins can be fixed by interactions with other proteins. Membranes may also be partitioned into local spatial domains by networks of cytoskeletal proteins. This partitioning may restrict the transla-tional motion of enmeshed proteins and yet allow rapid rotational diffusion. Examples of such spatial localization include restriction of Na^+ pumps to the basolateral domains of most epithelial cells, Na^+ channels to nodes of Ranvier and nicotinic acetylcholine receptors to the postsynaptic membranes of neuromuscular junctions.

Mechanical functions of cells require interactions between integral membrane proteins and the cytoskeleton

These functions include cell motility, endo- and exocytosis, formation of cell junctions and regulation of cell shape. Several different families of membrane-associated proteins mediate specific interactions among integral membrane proteins, cytoskeletal proteins and contractile proteins. Many of these *linker proteins* consist largely of various combinations of conserved protein-association domains, which often occur in multiple variant copies (Table 2-1).

TABLE 2-1. **SOME PROTEIN–PROTEIN INTERACTION DOMAINS THAT OCCUR IN MEMBRANE-ASSOCIATED PROTEINS**[a]

Domain (proteins)	Residues per domain	Domains per molecule	Target proteins	Reference
Spectrin (spectrins, dystrophins)	100–120	17–26	Ankyrin	[44]
Ankyrin (ankyrin)	33	24	Anion transporter, sodium pump, sodium channels	[45]
Armadillo (β-catenin plakoglobin, SMAP)	42	11–13	Cadherins, α-catenin, EGFR	—
PH (pleckstrin homology)	100	1–2	$G_{\beta\gamma}$, PIP_2	[46,47]
SH2 (src homology 2)	100	1–2	Phosphotyrosine	[47]
SH3 (src homology 3)	60	1–2	Proline-rich	[47]
PDZ	90	1–5	Variable short consensus sequences	[48]
GUK (guanylyl kinase homology)	190	1	SAPAPs, GKAPs	[49,50]
Actin-binding (β-spectrin, actinin, dystrophin, dystonin)	240–275	1–3	F-actin	—

[a]SMAP, small G protein regulator associated protein; EGFR, epidermal growth factor receptor; PIP_2, phosphatidylinositol 4,5-bisphosphate; SAP, synapse associated protein; SAPAP, SAP associated protein; GKAP, guanylyl kinase associated protein.

The spectrin–ankyrin network. In erythrocytes and most other cells, the major structural link of plasma membranes to the cytoskeleton is mediated by interactions between ankyrin and various integral membrane proteins, including Cl^-/HCO_3^- antiporters, sodium ion pumps and voltage-dependent sodium ion channels (Table 2-1). Ankyrin also binds to the ~100-nm, rod-shaped, antiparallel $\alpha\beta$ heterodimers of spectrin and, thus, secures the cytoskeleton to the plasma membrane. Spectrin dimers self-associate to form tetramers and further to form a polygonal network parallel to the plasma membrane (Fig. 2-5D). Neurons contain both spectrin I, also termed erythroid, and spectrin II, also termed fodrin. Spectrin II is found throughout neurons, including axons, whereas spectrin I occurs only in the soma and dendrites. This spectrin network further binds to actin microfilaments and to numerous other ligands. These associations are probably dynamic. For example, phosphorylation of ankyrin can alter its affinity for spectrin. Spectrin II has binding sites for microtubules. The functions of the multiple protein-interaction domains of both spectrin and ankyrin have been as yet only partially defined (see Chap. 8).

Membrane structural specializations. The spectrin–ankyrin network comprises a general form of membrane-organizing cytoskeleton within which a variety of membrane-cytoskeletal specializations are interspersed. Many of these are concerned with cell–cell or cell–matrix interactions (Chap. 7). The several morphological types of cell–cell junctions are associated with junction-specific structural and linking proteins. For example, tight junctions, also termed *zona occludens,* are constructed of the integral membrane protein occludin, which binds the linking proteins ZO-1 and ZO-2 [15]. These linking proteins are members of a large family, termed membrane-associated guanylyl kinase homologs (MAGUKs). The general structure of this family has, distributed from the N- to C-terminus, one or more PDZ-binding domains, a src homology 3 (SH3) domain (see Chap. 25) and a guanylyl kinase homolog domain (Table 2-1). Other members of the PDZ family are expressed in neurons at postsynaptic densities. One of these, PSD-95, contains two N-terminal PDZ domains

that can bind to a motif, –E–S/T–D–V–, that occurs in *N*-methyl-D-aspartate (NMDA) receptors and in certain types of K^+ channel. Multimeric clusters of these receptors or channels can be formed through disulfide cross-linking between cysteines of the N-terminal domains of PSD-95 molecules [16]. Different PDZ domains within a single linker protein can display different peptide motif selectivities. Accordingly, it has been suggested that a given linker protein may simultaneously bind to multiple different channels and receptors to produce complex clusters at various postsynaptic sites.

Certain transmembrane glycoproteins can mediate interactions between the cytoskeleton and the extracellular matrix

Many glycoproteins link sites on extracellular matrix proteins or on other cell surfaces with cytoskeletal proteins (Chap. 7). In some cases, the extracellular binding specificity is for sites found on matrix proteins, while the intracellular specificity is for a cytoskeletal protein, such as talin, which may further interact with an intermediate filament protein (Fig. 2-4) (see Chap. 8). Integrins are a major family of transmembrane receptors with these properties [17]. Their adhesion to extracellular ligands can be up- or downregulated by cytoplasmic signals and, thus, function in cell migration, cell aggregation and other intercellular interactions. Conversely, their interactions with cytoskeletal components and protein kinases can be modulated by extracellular ligands [18].

Neural cell adhesion molecules (NCAMs) belong to a widely distributed family of cell-surface glycoproteins that have extracellular domains structurally related to the immunoglobulins (see Chap. 7). They can be homotypic; that is, they can bind to each other, but they can also interact with heparin in the matrix. Differential splicing of their mRNAs can result in the expression of different polypeptides from a single NCAM gene. Two of these are transmembrane glycoproteins with identical extracellular domains and differing cytoplasmic domains. A third NCAM is not a transmembrane protein and does not participate in transmembrane sig-

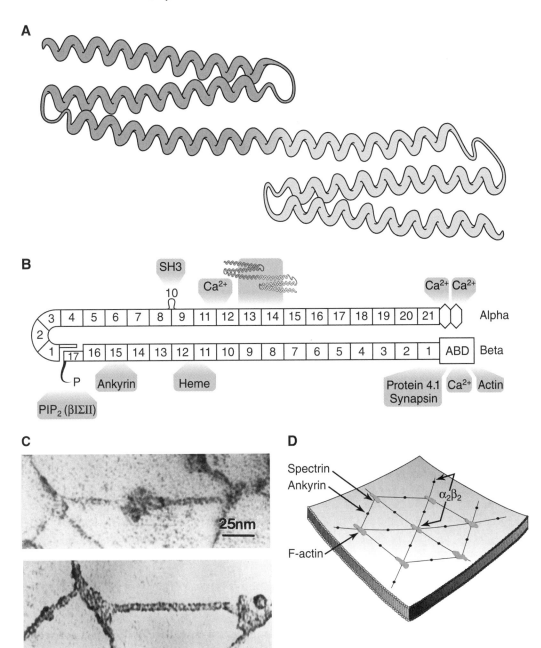

FIGURE 2-5. The ankyrin–spectrin lattice. **A:** Structural model of a spectrin repeat unit based on the crystal structure of a dimer of the fourteenth repeat unit of *Drosophila* spectrin. (Adapted from [39], with permission.) **B:** Cartoon of the domain structure of a spectrin dimer. Many of the repeat units of spectrin constitute binding domains with different specificities. Some of these have been identified and are labeled here. ABD, actin binding domain; PIP$_2$, phosphatidylinositol-4,5-bisphosphate domain occurs only on the βIΣII isoform; SH3, src homology 3 domain. See Table 2-1 for references. (Adapted from [40] with permission). **C:** Electron micrographs of rotary-shadowed spectrin tetramers (courtesy of J. Ursitti). Note the periodic substructure of spectrin filaments and the putative site of a complex with an ankyrin molecule **(top, center)**. **D:** Schematic organization of the spectrin–ankyrin cytoskeleton on the cytoplasmic surface of neurons. (Redrawn from [41], with permission.)

naling because it is wholly extracellular and anchored to the membrane only through a covalent attachment involving glycosylphosphatidylinositol (Fig. 2-4) (Chap. 3). The N-terminal extracellular domains of NCAMs are heavily glycosylated, and their adhesive properties can be suppressed by further addition of long polysialic acid chains (Chaps. 7 and 28).

Cadherins are Ca^{2+}-dependent, homotypic adhesion proteins that may be largely responsible for the preferential adhesion of similar cell types [19]. They associate intracellularly with actin microfilaments at adherens junctions by means of linker proteins called catenins and to the intermediate filaments α-actinin and vinculin at desmosomes by means of other linker proteins called desmoplakins.

Covalently attached lipids often participate in binding proteins to membranes

Myristate can be added cotranslationally to the N-terminal glycine of a number of peripheral proteins, thus participating in binding them to the cytoplasmic membrane surface. The catalytic subunit of cAMP-dependent protein kinase, calcineurin B and NADH-cytochrome b5 reductase are myristoylated proteins [20] (Fig. 2-4).

Fatty acids, most commonly palmitate, can link as thioesters to a cysteine residue that is usually located near a membrane-binding domain. Both integral membrane proteins, such as rhodopsin and transferrin receptor, and membrane-associated proteins, such as ankyrin and vinculin, may be acylated. A number of proteins can be post-translationally prenylated [21]. One synthetic pathway for prenyl anchors involves precursor proteins with a C-terminal sequence, CXXX. A C_{20} acyl group from geranylgeranyl pyrophosphate is transferred to the cysteine sulfhydryl. The three terminal amino acids are then cleaved, and finally, a methyl group is added to the newly exposed cysteine α-carboxyl. Prenylated proteins include many signal transducers of the small G protein class and γ subunits of heterotrimeric G proteins (see Chap. 20). Proteins can be anchored to the external bilayer leaflet by covalent linkage to complex glycosylated phosphoinositides [22]. Glycosylphos-phatidylinositol (GPI)-anchored proteins include alkaline phosphatase, 5′-nucleotidase, one form of acetylcholinesterase and one form of NCAM.

Membrane associations can occur by selective protein binding to lipid head groups

One example is spectrin, which binds to cytoplasmically oriented phosphatidylinositol-4,5-bisphosphate by means of a pleckstrin-homology (PH) domain [23] (Table 2-1) (Chap. 25). Several enzymes and structural proteins become membrane-bound in response to Ca^{2+} activation. These include protein kinase C (PKC), phospholipase A_2 and synaptotagmin.

Allosteric regulation of the hydrophobicity of protein-binding surfaces frequently occurs. One of the best known cases is the Ca^{2+}-dependent binding of calmodulin to other proteins (Chap. 23). Annexins are a family of proteins that exhibit Ca^{2+}-dependent associations with cell membranes through direct interaction with phospholipids, and conversely, interactions with phospholipids increase their affinities for Ca^{2+} [24].

MEMBRANE DYNAMICS

Nascent membrane proteins must be inserted through the bilayer and transported to their destinations

The information that targets a polypeptide to the ER membrane is contained in a segment near the N-terminus called a *signal sequence*. These sequences are highly variable but include a hydrophobic segment of nine or more residues bracketed by basic residues at the N-terminus and a mixture of acidic and basic residues at the C-terminus. Membrane proteins possess additional, predominantly hydrophobic segments, termed "topogenic sequences," that determine their primary membrane topologies, that is, the number of times they traverse the bilayer [25].

The predominant pathway for targeting proteins to the ER in animals begins with interaction of a signal-recognition particle (SRP) with the nascent signal sequence as it emerges from the mRNA–ribosome complex (Fig. 2-6). SRP is an 11S ribonucleoprotein consisting of six different peptides and one 7S RNA. Translation is arrested if SRP binds to the complex in the absence of ER membranes. Elongation of the nascent peptide can proceed after the ribosome-bound SRP interacts with the SRP receptor or docking protein, a component of the ER membrane. This is followed by SRP dissociation from the ribosome and insertion of the signal sequence into the ER membrane, permitting the mRNA translation to continue. GTP binding and hydrolysis are required at this step. Both SRP and the SRP receptor have GTP-binding domains, but present evidence implicates binding to the receptor at this stage [26]. Once a conjunction of the ribosomal complex with the ER membrane is effected, the growing peptide passes through the membrane. This mechanism is called *cotranslational insertion.*

Secreted proteins are synthesized as "proproteins" with amino-terminal signal sequences. After the rest of the peptide has been exported, the signal sequence is cleaved from the secreted product by a signal peptidase, itself a membrane protein with its active site within the ER lumen (see Chap. 18). Membrane proteins that have a single anchoring segment near the NH_2-terminus may insert by a similar mechanism involving an uncleaved signal sequence (Fig. 2-6). Membrane proteins that have a single anchor near their COOH-terminus require a stop-transfer sequence to form a permanent transmembrane segment and, finally, cleavage of the initial signal peptide.

Many membrane proteins contain two or more topogenic sequences. An example is opsin, which traverses the membrane seven times (Chap. 47). Since it has four intralumenal domains, as many as four stop-transfer sequences may be required. By the use of selectively deleted cDNA and subsequent translation of the corresponding RNA transcripts, the experimental indications are that, in fact, the first and sixth transmembrane segments of opsin contain the stop-transfer sequences hypothesized to be necessary for proper membrane insertion [27].

Not all cases of membrane protein insertion seem to conform to this cotranslational

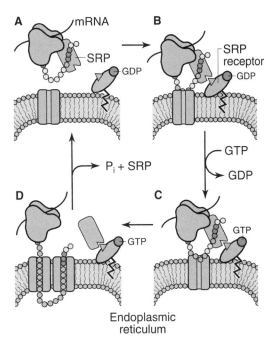

FIGURE 2-6. Initiation of membrane protein insertion into the endoplasmic reticulum (ER). **A:** Signal-recognition particles (, *SRP*) associate with ribosomes (), and the signal sequences () of nascent membrane proteins. **B:** These complexes associate with SRP receptors in the ER membrane. The SRP receptors contain bound GDP. **C:** Bound GDP is exchanged for cytoplasmic GTP, and **D:** translocation of peptides occurs as GTP is hydrolyzed. The peptides are oriented N⇒C outward as they insert through a membrane. (Adapted from [42], with permission.)

model. Ribosomal synthesis of some integral membrane proteins does not require formation of an SRP–membrane complex. For example, the Ca^{2+} pump ATPase contains stop-transfer sequences, and although SRP is required for membrane insertion, the absence of membranes containing the docking protein does not arrest its synthesis [28]. Other integral membrane proteins, such as cytochrome b5, can be synthesized on free ribosomes and subsequently insert into membranes in the absence of SRP.

To account for all possible configurations of integral membrane proteins, it was postulated that translocator proteins in the ER membrane interact with topogenic sequences to form channels that allow hydrophilic protein segments to traverse the bilayer. Combinations of stop-transfer sequences, cleaved signal sequences and

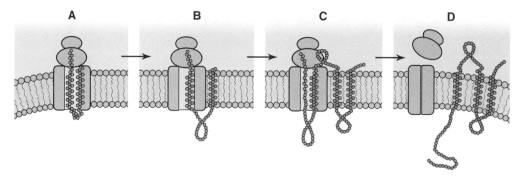

FIGURE 2-7. Throughout the synthesis of polytopic membrane proteins, including **A:** the transmembrane segments, **B:** lumenal domains and **C:** even cytoplasmic domains, the ribosome seals the lumen of the translocator channel. As transmembrane domains are completed, they move laterally into the lipid bilayer. **D:** When translation is complete, the ribosome detaches and the channel closes. (Adapted from [26], with permission.)

appropriate responses by the translocator proteins to these signals account for most of the observed transmembrane dispositions of polypeptide segments [29].

Channel-forming proteins with the requisite properties have been detected in rough ER: 250 pS conductance events are induced in these membranes when protein synthesis is aborted with puromycin [30]. Because puromycin causes nascent peptides to dissociate from ribosomes, ribosomes lacking such peptides can combine with translocator proteins to form and open channels in the ER. These channels remain closed in the absence of ribosomes and do not conduct ions while they are occupied by ribosomes that are generating nascent peptides (Fig. 2-7). The peptide translocator channels are formed from a heterotrimeric complex [31].

"Molecular chaperones" are frequently required to mediate correct protein folding

It was long held that nascent polypeptides assume their "native" conformations spontaneously as they emerge from the ribosome. In its strict form, this model implied that the genetic information that specifies a primary sequence completely defines the native protein conformation. This concept has been revised because of the discovery of auxiliary proteins, "molecular chaperones," that regulate polypeptide folding [32]. The SRP and other proteins that recognize topogenic sequences are examples of this functional class.

Numerous chaperones are resident within the ER lumen. For example, calnexin is an ER-resident chaperone that complexes selectively with certain partially glycosylated proteins, including the GLUT-I glucose transporter and the α and β subunits of the nicotinic acetylcholine receptor. BiP is another ER-resident chaperone. BiP interacts with newly synthesized γ subunits of nicotinic acetylcholine receptors [33] and binds ATP. Mature nicotinic receptors are pentamers of four different subunits, $\alpha_2\beta\gamma\delta$, in which the two α subunits are not adjacent (Chap. 11). BiP will bind to $\alpha\gamma$ and $\alpha\delta$ complexes but not to the mature receptor. This binding apparently assists in the correct assembly of this and probably many other oligomeric membrane proteins. The peptide-binding site of BiP involves seven adjacent residues. The site specificity is rather broad and similar to the composition of the interior of folded proteins, the composition of which is not very different from that of many transmembrane segments. Peptide binding causes hydrolysis of bound ATP, which causes release of the peptide.

Newly synthesized plasma membrane proteins travel from the endoplasmic reticulum through a succession of Golgi compartments

During this time they may undergo post-translational modifications such as glycosylation, finally fusing with pre-existing plasma membrane from the trans-Golgi network [34] (Fig. 2-8).

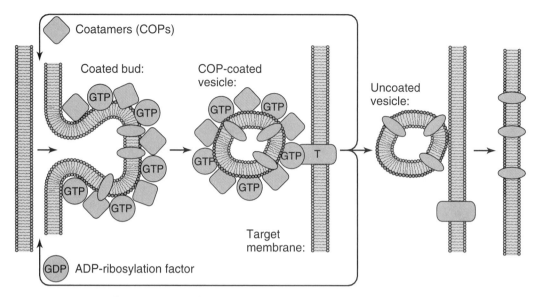

FIGURE 2-8.   Model for the transport of membrane components from one Golgi compartment to the next. **Left:** Area of a Golgi membrane containing the transiting proteins *(dark orange)* that bind resident proteins, including coat proteins *(COPs)* and the ADP-ribosylation factor. This initiates the formation of a coated vesicle. The detached vesicle binds to an unknown component, *T,* of the target membrane, which may be another Golgi compartment, the plasma membrane or an intracellular organelle. Coat proteins are released and recycled as the vesicle and the transiting proteins fuse with the target membrane **(right)**. (Adapted from [43], with permission.)

Each transit event appears to be initiated by a set of "coat proteins," also termed "COPs" or "coatomers," which bind to a patch of the cytoplasmic surface of a Golgi membrane to form a "coated pit." Coated pits transform into vesicles. Scission of the vesicles from one Golgi compartment is followed by their fusion with the membrane of the next compartment.

Subunits of the intra-Golgi vesicle coat complex, termed α-, β-, γ- and δ-COP, have been identified. Among these, α-COP has similarities to clathrin heavy chain (see below) and β-COP has similarities to the clathrin-associated adaptins. One hypothesis is that the process mediated by this complex consists of a nonselective "bulk flow" of most of the membrane proteins and soluble components through successive Golgi compartments. These proteins are progressively subjected to various covalent modifications by enzymes that reside in different Golgi compartments. Thus, both the ER and the various Golgi compartments contain characteristic resident proteins. Although the "default" mechanism of vesicular traffic outward from the ER is nonselective, there are "active" and selective

mechanisms for retaining the resident proteins, such as retrograde, or "salvage," transport from Golgi to ER. A C-terminal signature sequence, Lys-Asp-Glu-Leu or "KDEL," occurs in ER-resident proteins and is recognized by the salvage mechanism.

A different set of coat proteins, the clathrin complexes, function between the trans-Golgi network and its target membranes [35] (Fig. 2-9). Clathrin complexes consist of three molecules of clathrin heavy chain, which form a "triskelion" by joining together near their C-termini. Clathrin light chains associate with the proximal domains of the heavy chains. Each heavy chain is divided into proximal and distal domains by a hinge region. The clathrin triskelions self-assemble into extensive lattices by interacting at their heavy-chain N-termini. However, the interaction of these lattices with membrane proteins is mediated by another set of proteins, the adaptins. The combination of lattice forming by clathrin and protein selection by adaptins produces a concentration of targeted integral membranes within "coated pits" in both trans-Golgi and plasma membranes. Different

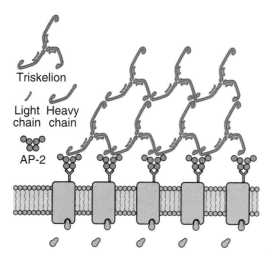

Triskelion

Light   Heavy
chain   chain

AP-2

FIGURE 2-9. Endocytosis of membrane components. The scheme shown here is derived from studies of the recycling of membrane receptors for ligands such as transferrin and insulin. Recycling of synaptic vesicle membranes occurs by a similar process. Ligand binding to the receptor appears to induce a conformational change that permits a tyrosine-containing β turn in the cytoplasmic domain to interact with one of the adaptins *(AP-2)*. Clathrin binding to the adaptins then produces the "coated pits" that develop into endocytotic vesicles. Clathrin consists of three heavy chains (~190 kDa each) that join near their C-termini to form a triskelion. Three light chains, of undetermined function, associate with the proximal segments of the heavy chains, possibly via an amphipathic α helix (heptad repeats) found in their central domains.

adaptins reside in different membranes. For example, the adaptin AP-2 is involved in the assembly of coated pits on the plasma membrane that occurs during endocytosis, whereas AP-1 participates in the corresponding assembly on the trans-Golgi network that occurs during secretion.

Fusion of vesicles with their target membranes involves disassembly of the coat proteins. In the case of clathrin, this is mediated by an "uncoating ATPase," identical to hsp70, a constitutive member of the heat-shock protein family, which includes several molecular chaperones. Each step of vesicular transit from the Golgi to the target membrane appears to involve both ATPase and GTPase activities.

Little is known about the mechanisms that direct membrane proteins to their ultimate targets. In both epithelial cells and neurons, membrane proteins with GPI anchors move almost exclusively to the apical plasma membrane, the neuronal analog of which is the axon [36]. Some proteins that are retained in the basolateral membranes of epithelial cells and, equivalently, in the soma and dendrites of neurons contain a cytoplasmic tyrosine-containing β-turn similar to the endocytotic signal sequence for coated vesicles (Fig. 2-9).

In addition to the clathrin-coated vesicle pathway of secretion and endocytosis, there is another pathway involving uncoated vesicles, or *caveolae*, that contain high concentrations of sphingolipids, gangliosides, cholesterol and the cholesterol-binding protein caveolin. Other proteins that are reported to occur in caveolae include heterotrimeric and monomeric G proteins, inositol 1,4,5-trisphosphate (IP$_3$) receptors and tyrosine kinases. GPI-anchored proteins, originally considered to be associated with caveolae [3], have been shown in several instances to reside in distinct membrane domains and to be internalized via conventional endosomes [37].

Neurons have special forms of vesicular transport. Some of the vesicles that bud from the trans-Golgi network are carried by *fast axoplasmic transport* (Chap. 28) to targets in nerve processes. Voltage-dependent exocytosis of neurotransmitters, triggered by the presynaptic influx of Ca^{2+}, may occur within 200 μsec of the stimulus. Maintenance of adequate supplies of the membrane constituents that package these rapidly secreted neurotransmitters is facilitated by recycling synaptic vesicle components from the presynaptic plasma membranes (Chap. 9).

Some membrane proteins can be selectively tagged by ubiquitin for recycling or degradation

Ubiquitin (Ub) is a 76-residue polypeptide that can be covalently linked via its C-terminal carboxyl to lysines on various proteins to target them for further processing. In certain cases, the Ub tags are elongated by esterification of additional Ub molecules.

Many normal membrane proteins are subject to regulatory downregulation. For example, some receptors are endocytosed following ligand binding. A pathway for some of these proteins involves ubiquitination followed by endocytosis and lysosomal degradation (see Chap. 46). However, endocytosed membrane proteins may also be de-ubiquitinated and recycled to the plasma membrane. Various forms of stress can also initiate selective ubiquitination, leading to rapid endocytosis and degradation of certain membrane proteins. Defective membrane proteins, such as the cystic fibrosis transmembrane conductance regulator (CFTR) protein, are ubiquitinated and degraded by the proteosome pathway within the ER. It is likely that proteins enter this pathway because of improper folding. Three enzymes involved in ubiquitination occur in several differentially expressed isoforms. Different isoforms may direct molecules to different pathways. There is indirect evidence for this from studies of yeast in which the tag directing proteins to proteosomes involves poly-Ub with linkage to lys-46 of the proximal Ub. In contrast, the activation of endocytosis of a membrane protein, maltose permease, is via either a single Ub or, more effectively, poly-Ub with linkage to lys-63 of the proximal Ub [38].

REFERENCES

1. Tanford, C. *The Hydrophobic Effect: Formation of Micelles and Biological Membranes*, 2nd ed. New York: Wiley Interscience, 1980.
2. Martin, S., Reutelingsperger, C., McGahon, A., et al. Early redistribution of plasma membrane phosphatidylserine is a general feature of apoptosis regardless of the initiating stimulus: Inhibition by overexpression of Bcl-2 and Abl. *J. Exp. Med.* 182:1545–1556, 1995.
3. Simons, K., and Ikonen, E. Functional rafts in cell membranes. *Nature* 387:569–572, 1997.
4. Smart, E., Ying, Y., Donzell, W., and Anderson, R. A role for caveolin in transport of cholesterol from endoplasmic reticulum to plasma membrane. *J. Biol. Chem.* 271:29427–29435, 1996.
5. Jost, P. C., and Griffith, O. H. The lipid–protein interface in biological membranes. *Ann. N.Y. Acad. Sci.* 348:391–407, 1980.
6. Tsukihara, T., Aoyama, H., Yamashita, E., et al. The whole structure of the 13-subunit oxidized cytochrome c oxidase at 2.8 Å. *Science* 272:1136–1144, 1996.
7. Finkelstein, A. Water movement through membrane channels. *Curr. Top. Membr. Transp.* 21:298–308, 1984.
8. Park, J., and Saier, M. J. Phylogenetic characterization of the MIP family of transmembrane channel proteins. *J. Membr. Biol.* 153:171–180, 1996.
9. Fushimi, K., Sasaki, S., and Marumo, F. Phosphorylation of serine 256 is required for cAMP-dependent regulatory exocytosis of the aquaporin-2 water channel. *J. Biol. Chem.* 272:14800–14804, 1997.
10. Nielsen, S., Nagelhus, E., Amiry-Moghaddam, M., Bourque, C., Agre, P., and Ottersen, O. Specialized membrane domains for water transport in glial cells: High-resolution immunogold cytochemistry of aquaporin-4 in rat brain. *J. Neurosci.* 17:171–180, 1997.
11. Heberle, J., Riesle, J., Thiedemann, G., Oesterhelt, D., Dencher, N. A. Proton migration along the membrane surface and retarded surface to bulk transfer. *Nature* 370:379–382, 1994.
12. Jennings, M. L. Topography of membrane proteins. *Annu. Rev. Biochem.* 58:999–1027, 1989.
13. Kimura, Y., Vassylyev, D., Miyazawa, A., et al. Surface of bacteriorhodopsin revealed by high-resolution electron crystallography. *Nature* 389:206–211, 1997.
14. Poo, M. Mobility and localization of proteins in excitable membranes. *Annu. Rev. Neurosci.* 8:369–406, 1985.
15. Tsukamoto, T., and Nigam, S. Tight junction proteins form large complexes and associate with the cytoskeleton in an ATP depletion model for reversible junction assembly. *J. Biol. Chem.* 272:16133–16139, 1997.
16. Hsueh, Y., Kim, E., and Sheng, M. Disulfide-linked head-to-head multimerization in the mechanism of ion channel clustering by PSD-95. *Neuron* 18:803–814, 1997.
17. Chothia, C., and Jones, E. The molecular structure of cell adhesion molecules. *Annu. Rev. Biochem.* 66:823–862, 1997.
18. Dedhar, S., and Hannigan, G. Integrin cytoplasmic interactions and bidirectional transmembrane signalling. *Curr. Opin. Cell. Biol.* 8:657–669, 1996.
19. Hynes, R. O., and Lander, A. D. Contact and adhesive specificities in the associations, migrations, and targeting of cells and axons. *Cell* 68:303–322, 1992.
20. Casey, P. Protein lipidation in cell signaling. *Science* 268:221–225, 1995.
21. Gelb, M. Protein prenylation, et cetera: signal transduction in two dimensions. *Science* 275:1750–1751, 1997.
22. Udenfriend, S., and Kodukula, K. How glycosylphosphatidylinositol-anchored membrane proteins are made. *Annu. Rev. Biochem.* 64:563–591, 1995.

23. Wang, D., and Shaw, G. The association of the C-terminal region of βIΣII spectrin to brain membranes is mediated by a PH domain, does not require membrane proteins, and coincides with a inositol-1,4,5 triphosphate binding site. *Biochem. Biophys. Res. Commun.* 217:608–615, 1995.

24. Mollenhauer, J. Annexins: What are they good for? *Cell. Mol. Life Sci.* 53:506–507, 1997.

25. von Heijne, G. Membrane protein assembly: Rules of the game. *Bioessays* 17:25–30, 1995.

26. Mothes, W., Heinrich, S., von Heijne, G., Brunner, J., and Rapoport, T. Molecular mechanism of membrane protein integration into the endoplasmic reticulum. *Cell* 89:523–533, 1997.

27. Friedlander, M., and Blobel, G. Bovine opsin has more than one signal sequence. *Nature* 318:338, 1985.

28. Anderson, D. J., Mostov, K. E., and Blobel, G. Mechanisms of integration of *de novo*-synthesized polypeptides into membranes. *Proc. Natl. Acad. Sci. USA* 80:7249–7253, 1983.

29. Singer, S. J., Maher, P. A. A., and Yaffe, M. P. On the translocation of proteins across membranes. *Proc. Natl. Acad. Sci. USA* 84:1015–1019, 1987.

30. Simon, S. M., and Blobel, G. A protein-conducting channel in the endoplasmic reticulum. *Cell* 65:371–380, 1991.

31. Rapoport, T., Jungnickel, B., and Kutay, U. Protein transport across the eukaryotic endoplasmic reticulum and bacterial inner membranes. *Annu. Rev. Biochem.* 65:271–303, 1996.

32. Burston, S., and Clarke, A. Molecular chaperones: Physical and mechanistic properties. *Essays Biochem.* 29:125–136, 1995.

33. Blount, P., and Merlie, J. BIP associates with newly synthesized subunits of the mouse muscle nicotinic receptor. *J. Cell Biol.* 113:1125–1132, 1991.

34. Rothman, J., and Orci, L. Budding vesicles in living cells. *Sci. Am.* 274:70–75, 1996.

35. Schekman, R., and Orci, L. Coat proteins and vesicle budding. *Science* 271:1526–1533, 1996.

36. Dotti, C., Parton, R., and Simons, K. Polarized sorting of glypiated proteins in hippocampal neurons. *Nature* 349:158–161, 1991.

37. Henke, R., Hancox, K., and Jeffrey, P. Characterization of two distinct populations of detergent resistant membrane complexes isolated from chick brain tissues. *J. Neurosci. Res.* 45:617–630, 1996.

38. Galan, J., and Haguenauer-Tsapis, R. Ubiquitin Lys63 is involved in ubiquitination of a yeast plasma membrane protein. *EMBO J.* 16:5847–5854, 1997.

39. Yan, Y., Winograd, E., Viel, A., Cronin, T., Harrison, S., and Branton, D. Crystal structure of the repetitive segments of spectrin. *Science* 262:2027–2030, 1993.

40. Ursitti, J., Kotula, L., DeSilva, T., Curtis, P., and Speicher, D. Mapping the human erythrocyte β-spectrin dimer initiation site using recombinant peptides and correlation of its phasing with the α-actinin dimer site. *J. Biol. Chem.* 271:6636–6644, 1996.

41. Goodman, S., Zimmer, W., Clark, M., Zagon, I., Barker, J., and Bloom, M. Brain spectrin: Of mice and men. *Brain Res. Bull.* 36:593–606, 1995.

42. Rapoport, T. A. Protein transport across the ER membrane. *Trends Biochem. Sci.* 15:355–358, 1990.

43. Rothman, J., and Orci, L. Molecular dissection of the secretory pathway. *Nature* 355:409–415, 1992.

44. Viel, A., and Branton, D. Spectrin: On the path from structure to function. *Curr. Opin. Cell Biol.* 8:49–55, 1996.

45. Michaely, P., and Bennett, V. Mechanism for binding site diversity on ankyrin. Comparison of binding sites on ankyrin for neurofascin and the Cl^-/HCO_3^- anion exchanger. *J. Biol. Chem.* 270:31298–31302, 1995.

46. Ma, A., Brass, L., and Abrams, C. Pleckstrin associates with plasma membranes and induces the formation of membrane projections: Requirements for phosphorylation and the NH2-terminal PH domain. *J. Cell. Biol.* 136:1071–1079, 1997.

47. Shaw, G. The pleckstrin homology domain: An intriguing multifunctional protein module. *Bioessays* 18:35–46, 1996.

48. Sheng, M. PDZs and receptor/channel clustering. *Neuron* 17:575–578, 1996.

49. Tsunoda, S., Sierralta, J., Sun, Y., et al. A multivalent PDZ-domain protein assembles signalling complexes in a G-protein-coupled cascade. *Nature* 388:243–249, 1997.

50. Naisbitt, S., Kim, E., Weinberg, R. J., et al. Characterization of guanylate kinase-associated protein, a postsynaptic density protein at excitatory synapses that interacts directly with postsynaptic density-95/synapse-associated protein 90. *J. Neurosci.* 17:5687–5696, 1997.

3

Lipids

Bernard W. Agranoff, Joyce A. Benjamins and Amiya K. Hajra

Since lipids constitute about one-half of brain tissue dry weight, it is not surprising that lipid biochemistry and neurochemistry have evolved together. The brain contains many complex lipids, including gangliosides, cerebrosides, sulfatides and phosphoinositides, that were first discovered in

Basic Neurochemistry: Molecular, Cellular and Medical Aspects, 6th Ed., edited by G. J. Siegel et al. Published by Lippincott–Raven Publishers, Philadelphia, 1999. Correspondence to Bernard W. Agranoff, Neuroscience Laboratory, University of Michigan, 1103 E. Huron, Ann Arbor, Michigan 48104-1687.

brain, where they are highly enriched compared to other tissues. Phospholipids account for the high total phosphorus content of brain, which led to an alchemical mystique in the nineteenth century that associated phosphorescence with thought and to the apocryphal claim that fish are good "brain food" since fish, too, are rich in phosphorus.

PROPERTIES OF BRAIN LIPIDS

Lipids have multiple functions in brain

They have two principal functions in the body: as repositories of chemical energy in storage fat, primarily triglycerides, and as structural components of cell membranes. The brain contains virtually no triglyceride, so it is in their role as membrane components that brain lipids initially commanded the attention of neurochemists. Later, some biomessenger functions of non-membrane lipids, such as steroid hormones and eicosanoids, became evident. Some membrane lipids, such as inositides and phosphatidylcholine, which were previously believed to have only a structural role, also have important functions in signal transduction across biological membranes. In addition, lipids covalently coupled to proteins play a major role in anchoring marker proteins within biomembranes (see below). These discoveries established that lipids participate in both the function and the structure of neural membranes.

Membrane lipids are amphiphilic molecules

All membrane lipids have a small polar, or hydrophilic, and a large nonpolar, or hydrophobic, component. The hydrophilic regions of lipid molecules associate with water and water-soluble ionic compounds by hydrogen and electrostatic bonding. The hydrophobic regions cannot form such bonds and, thus, associate with each other outside the aqueous phase. Depending on the relative dominance of the hydrophobic and hydrophilic regions of a given lipid molecule, the amphiphiles will form either aggregates, also termed micelles, or bilayers. Lipid molecules containing comparatively large polar groups,

such as lysolipids, gangliosides and natural or synthetic detergents which are fairly soluble in water, tend to form micelles once the solubility limit, or critical micellar concentration, is reached. Most membrane lipids tend to associate in a hydrophobic "tail-to-tail" fashion to form bilayers (see Chap. 2).

The hydrophobic components of many lipids consist of either isoprenoids or fatty acids and their derivatives

Lipids were originally defined operationally, on the basis of their extractability from tissues with organic solvents such as a chloroform/methanol mixture, but this is no longer the sole criterion. For example, the protein component of myelin proteolipid is extractable into lipid solvents but, nevertheless, is not considered to be a lipid since its structure is that of a highly hydrophobic polypeptide. In fact, many integral membrane proteins contain "hydrophobic" membrane-spanning regions (see Chap. 2). Conversely, gangliosides are considered to be lipids on the basis of their structure, even though they are water-soluble. It is apparent, then, that lipids are defined not only by their physical properties but also on the basis of their chemical structure. Chemically, lipids can be defined as compounds containing long-chain fatty acids and their derivatives or linked isoprenoid units. Fatty acids in lipids are either esterified to the trihydroxy alcohol glycerol, or are present as amides of sphingosine, a long-chain dihydroxyamine. The isoprenoids are made up of branched-chain units and include sterols, such as cholesterol.

Isoprenoids have the unit structure of a five-carbon branched chain

Isoprenoid units have the formula C_5H_8 and the structure

$$\begin{array}{c} CH_3 \\ H | H H \\ -C-C=C-C- \\ H H \end{array}$$

The most abundant of these in brain is cholesterol. Unlike other tissues, normal adult brain contains virtually no cholesterol esters. Desmo-

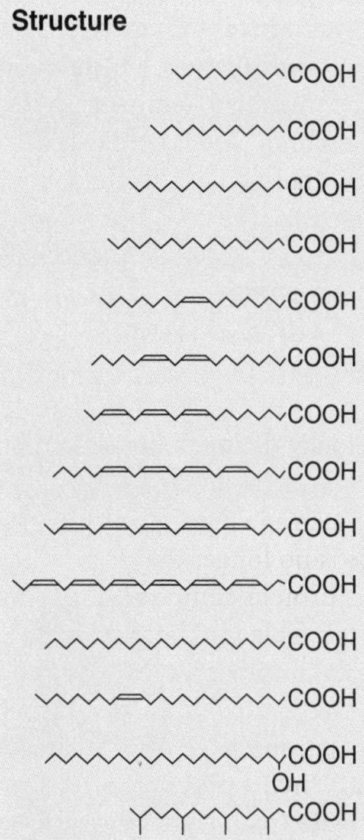

Structure	Chemical name	Trivial name	Abv.
⌇⌇⌇⌇COOH	Dodecanoic acid	Lauric acid	12:0
⌇⌇⌇⌇COOH	Tetradecanoic acid	Myristic acid	14:0
⌇⌇⌇⌇COOH	Hexadecanoic acid	Palmitic acid	16:0
⌇⌇⌇⌇COOH	Octadecanoic acid	Stearic acid	18:0
⌇⌇⌇⌇COOH	9-Octadeceanoic acid	Oleic acid	18:1(n-9)
⌇⌇⌇⌇COOH	9,12-Octadecadienoic acid	Linoleic acid	18:2(n-6)
⌇⌇⌇⌇COOH	9,12,15-Octadecatrienoic acid	Linolenic acid	18:3(n-3)
⌇⌇⌇⌇COOH	5,8,11,14-Eicosatetraenoic acid	Arachidonic acid	20:4(n-6)
⌇⌇⌇⌇COOH	5,8,11,14,17-Eicosapentenoic acid	EPA	20:5(n-3)
⌇⌇⌇⌇COOH	4,7,10,13,16,19-Docosahexenoic acid		22:6(n-3)
⌇⌇⌇⌇COOH	Tetracosanoic acid	Lignoceric acid	24:0
⌇⌇⌇⌇COOH	15-Tetracoseanoic acid	Nervonic acid	24:1(n-9)
⌇⌇⌇⌇COOH OH	2-Hydroxytetracosanoic acid	Cerebronic acid	24h:0
⌇⌇⌇⌇COOH	3,7,11,15-Tetramethylhexadecanoic acid	Phytanic acid	

FIGURE 3-1. Structures of some fatty acids of neurochemical interest (see also Fig. 3-7 and text). The "n minus" nomenclature for the position of the double bond(s) is given here. Note that the position of the double bond from the carboxyl end can be indicated by the symbol Δ, so that linoleic acid may be also be designated as $18:2\Delta^{9,12}$. The linolenic acid shown is the α isomer.

sterol, the immediate biosynthetic precursor of cholesterol, is found in developing brain and in some brain tumors but not in normal adult brain. Other isoprenoid substances present in brain are the dolichols, very long (up to C_{100}) branched-chain alcohols which are cofactors for glycoprotein biosynthesis; squalene, which is the linear C_{30} precursor of all steroids; and the carotenoids, including retinal and retinoic acid. Some isoprene units, such as farnesyl (C_{15}) and geranyl-geranyl (C_{20}), have been shown to be covalently linked via thioether bonds to membrane proteins (see Fig. 3-6 for structures of some of these compounds and for the numbering system for cholesterol).

Brain fatty acids are long-chain carboxylic acids which may contain one or more double bonds

The brain contains a variety of straight-chain monocarboxylic acids, usually with an even number of carbon atoms ranging from C_{12} to C_{26}. The hydrocarbon chain may be saturated or may contain one or more double bonds, all in *cis* (Z) configuration. When multiple double bonds are present, they are nonconjugated and almost always three carbons apart. The unsaturated fatty acids are classified by the location of the double bond most distal from the carboxyl end. The most prevalent series, n being the number of carbon atoms in the fatty acid, are n − 3 (n minus 3) n − 6 and n − 9. Thus, linoleic acid, which has 18 carbons (Fig. 3-1), is a member of the n − 6 family because the double bond most distal from the carboxyl end is at 18 − 6, or the C-12 position. Since the next double bond is separated by three carbon atoms, it is between C_9 and C_{10}. A similar, widely used but nonstandard nomenclature employs the omega (ω) designation, indicating the position of the first double bond counting from the methyl (ω-carbon) end. These nomenclature conventions are convenient from both the biochemical and the nutritional points of view since fatty acids are elongated or degraded *in vivo* by two carbon units from the carboxyl end and animals need certain polyunsaturated fatty acids, termed essential fatty acids, in their diet, as discussed below and in Chapter 33. The complete shorthand notation for fatty acids consists of the number of carbon atoms followed by the number of double bonds and the position of the first double bond. Linoleic acid is thus 18:2 (n − 6) or, alternatively, 18:2ω6. The brain contains some unusual fatty acids, such as very long (20 to 26 carbons), odd-numbered and 2-hydroxy fatty acids, prevalent in the cerebrosides. A list of major brain fatty acids with their common names and structures is given in Figure 3-1.

COMPLEX LIPIDS

Glycerolipids are derivatives of glycerol and fatty acids

Most brain glycerolipids are derivatives of phosphatidic acid (PtdOH), which is diacylated *sn*-glycerol-3-phosphate. The notation *sn* refers to stereochemical numbering, with the secondary hydroxyl group of glycerol at C-2 shown on the left, that is, the L-configuration of Fischer's projection, and the phosphate at C-3. This special nomenclature is employed because, unlike the trioses or other carbohydrates, glycerol does not have a reporter carbonyl group to assign an absolute D- or L-configuration. As shown in Figure 3-2, the

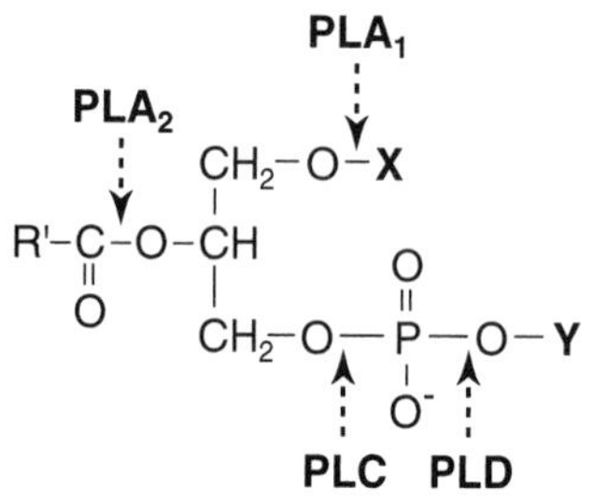

Y	Lipid	Abv.
H	Phosphatidate	PtdOH
$CH_2\text{-}CH_2\text{-}\overset{+}{N}H_3$	Phosphatidylethanolamine	PtdEtn
$CH_2\text{-}CH_2\text{-}\overset{+}{N}(CH_3)_3$	Phosphatidylcholine	PtdCho
$CH_2 - \underset{H}{\overset{NH_3^+}{C}} - COO^-$	Phosphatidylserine	PtdSer
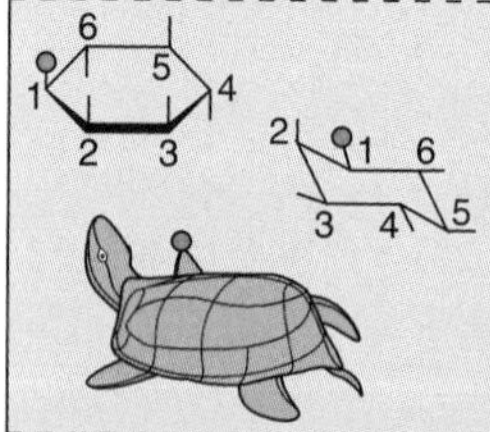	Phosphatidylinositol	PtdIns
$CH_2\text{-}CH(OH)\text{-}CH_2HO$	Phosphatidylglycerol	PtdGro
Phosphatidylglycerol	Cardiolipin	PtdGroPtd

FIGURE 3-2. The structure of phosphoglycerides. In most lipids, X is acyl, that is, R—(C═O). In alkyl ethers, present mainly in brain ethanolamine phosphoglycerides (2 to 3%), X is a long-chain hydrocarbon (C_{16}, C_{18}). For plasmalogens, which constitute about 60% of adult human brain PtdEtn, X is 1-alk-1′enyl (that is, —CH═CH—R). *Arrows* indicate sites of enzymatic hydrolysis of the phosphoglycerides. *PLA₁*, phospholipase A_1; *PLA₂*, phospholipase A_2; *PLC*, phospholipase C; *PLD*, phospholipase D. Note that *myo*-inositol is written in the D-configuration, where the 1′ position is linked to the PtdOH moiety. For polyphosphoinositides, additional phosphate groups are present in the 3, 4 or 5 positions. See Chapter 21 for further detail regarding the stereochemistry of inositol and the use of the turtle representation.

hydroxyl groups on C-1 and C-2 of glycerolipids are esterified with fatty acids. The substituent at *sn*-1 is usually saturated, whereas that at *sn*-2 is unsaturated. In addition, there are lipid species in which *sn*-1 is ether-linked either to an aliphatic alcohol, termed an alkyl, or to an α,β-unsaturated alcohol, alk-1′-enyl. The latter lipids are referred to as plasmalogens (Fig. 3-2). While diacylglycerophospholipids are saponifiable, that is, they contain alkali-labile ester bonds, and are acid-stable, the alkenyl ethers are alkali-stable and acid-labile. Alkyl ethers are stable to both acids and bases. A useful general term that includes all of these various aliphatic substituents, acyl, alkenyl and alkyl, is "radyl," for example, 1,2-diradyl-*sn*-glycerol-3-phosphorylethanolamine is a term that includes phosphatidylethanolamine (PtdEtn) as well as its plasmalogen analogs.

If positions 1 and 2 are acylated and the *sn*-3 hydroxyl group is free, the lipid is 1,2-diacyl-*sn*-glycerol (DAG). The DAGs play both a biosynthetic (see later) and a cellular regulating role in that they activate protein kinase C (PKC) (see Chaps. 21 and 24). In addition, DAGs can be fusogenic and have been proposed to play a role in altering cell morphology, for example, in fusion of synaptic vesicles (see Chap. 9). Other nonphosphorus-containing glycerides of interest are DAG-galactoside and its sulfate. These minor glycolipids are found primarily in white matter and appear to be analogous to their sphingosine-containing counterparts, the cerebrosides, described below.

Glycerophospholipid classes are defined on the basis of the substituent base at *sn*-3 of the diacylglycerophosphoryl (phosphatidyl) function (Fig. 3-2). The bases are short-chain, polar alcohols phosphodiester-linked to PtdOH. The amount and distribution of these lipids vary with brain regions and with age [1,2]. In quantitatively decreasing order in adult human brain, they are PtdEtn, including plasmalogens; phosphatidylcholine (PtdCho, "lecithin"); and phosphatidylserine (PtdSer). The phosphoinositides include phosphatidylinositol (PtdIns), phosphatidylinositol-4-phosphate (PtdIns-4-P), and phosphatidylinositol 4,5-bisphosphate (PtdIns(4,5)P_2); they are quantitatively minor phospholipids but play an important role in signal transduction. They are also abbreviated as PI, PIP and PIP_2 respectively, and are discussed in more detail, as are the phosphatidylinositide-3-phosphate (PI3P) family of inositides, in Chapter 21. The phosphatidylglycerols in brain, as in other tissues, are present in mitochondrial membranes. Of these, cardiolipin (bisphosphatidylglycerol) is the most prevalent.

Each phospholipid class in a given tissue has a characteristic fatty acid composition. Though the same fatty acid may be present in a number of lipids, the quantitative fatty acid composition is different for each class of lipids and remains fairly constant during the growth and development of the brain. The molecular species composition of different lipids in adult rat brain is shown in Table 3-1, which illustrates the varieties of lipid present in neural membranes. Not only do they differ in the structure of the polar head groups, or phospholipid classes, but within each class there are a variety of combinations of pairs of fatty acids, giving rise to molecular species which differ in the nature and positional distribution of fatty acids esterified to the glycerol backbone. From Table 3-1, we see, for example, that the 1-stearoyl, 2-arachidonyl (18:0–20:4) species is predominant in inositides, while 22:6 acids are enriched in PtdEtn and PtdSer. While the values in Table 3-1 are for whole brain, it should be noted that the fatty acid substituents for a given phospholipid class isolated from white and gray matter may differ dramatically. For example, white matter PtdEtn contains 42% 18:1 and 3% 22:6, while gray matter PtdEtn contains only 12% 18:1 and 24% 22:6 [4]. As noted below, brain lipids contain some unusually long and polyunsaturated fatty acids from both the ω3 and ω6 families of essential fatty acids, which cannot be biosynthesized in the animal body *de novo* (see also Chap. 33). This implies the existence of a mechanism for transporting essential fatty acids across the blood–brain barrier. There is considerable interest in the role of the polyunsaturated fatty acids and their metabolites in brain after breakdown of their parent phospholipids in conditions such as ischemia and anoxia (see Chaps. 34 and 35).

TABLE 3-1. **DISTRIBUTION PROFILE OF THE MAJOR INDIVIDUAL MOLECULAR SPECIES IN THE DIACYLGLYCEROL MOIETIES OF RAT BRAIN PHOSPHOGLYCERIDES**[a]

Fatty acid		PtdIns	PtdIns4,5P$_2$	PtdCho	PtdEtn	PtdSer
C-1	C-2	(mol %)	(mol %)	(mol %)	(mol %)	(mol %)
16:0	22:6	1.4	0.1	3.3	4.8	0.8
16:0	20:4	7.8	9.5	4.4	2.3	0.6
18:1	20:3	4.1	1.1	Tr	Tr	Tr
18:0	22:6	Tr	1.0	2.5	17.6	42.4
14:0	16:0	0.6	0.4	3.1	1.5	0.8
18:0	22:5	1.0	0.7	0.4	0.2	5.3
18:0	20:4	49.5	66.1	3.8	22.5	3.8
18:1	18:1	1.7	2.1	3.4	11.1	7.0
16:0	18:1	12.7	6.5	36.2	15.8	9.1
16:0	16:0	6.9	1.4	19.2	0.7	Tr
18:0	18:1	7.0	4.6	14.1	14.8	23.7

[a]Adapted from [3]. PtdIns, phosphatidylinositol; PtdIns(4,5)P$_2$, phosphatidylinositol-4,5-*bis*phosphate; PtdCho, phosphatidylcholine; PtdEtn, phosphatidylethanolamine; PtdSer, phosphatidylserine.

In sphingolipids, the long-chain aminodiol sphingosine serves as the lipid backbone

Sphingosine resembles a monoradyl glycerol but has asymmetric carbons at both C-2 and C-3. The chiral configuration is like that of the tetrose D-erythrose. That is, the amino group at C-2 and hydroxyl group at C-3 are in *cis* configuration (2S, 3R). Unlike unsaturated fatty acids, the double bond between C-4 and C-5 in sphingosine is in the *trans* (E) configuration. In the IU-

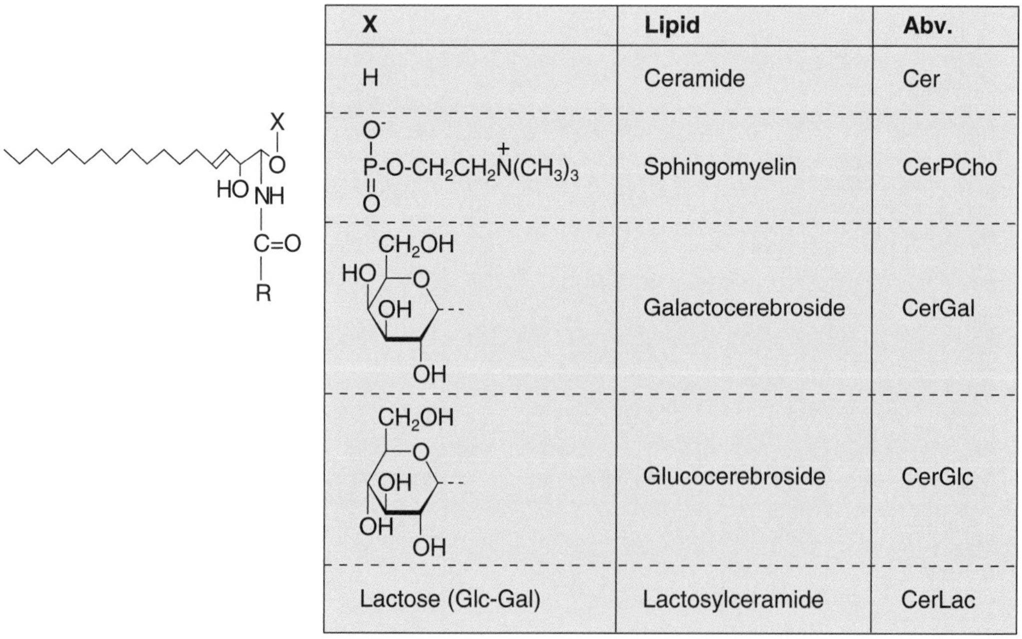

FIGURE 3-3. Structure of some simple sphingolipids. X may be a complex polysaccharide either containing sialic acid (gangliosides) or not (globosides). See also Figures 3-4 and 3-9 for the nomenclature and structure of some of the complex brain sphingolipids.

PAC-IUB nomenclature, the saturated analog of sphingosine, dihydrosphingosine or D-erythro-2-amino-1,3-octadecanediol, is termed sphinganine and sphingosine is (E-4) sphingenine. While in most sphingolipids the sphingosine is 18 carbons long, in brain gangliosides, there is a significant representation of the C_{20} homolog.

In sphingolipids, the amino group of sphingosine is acylated with long-chain fatty acids and the N-acylated product is termed a ceramide (Fig. 3-3). C-1 of ceramide is linked to different head groups to form various membrane lipids. For example, sphingomyelin is the phosphodiester of ceramide and choline. The fatty acids in sphingomyelin have a bimodal distribution: in white matter they are mostly 24 carbons long (lignoceric and nervonic, see Fig. 3-1), while in gray matter, stearic acid (18:0) predominates. Most of the glycolipids in brain consist of ceramide glycosidically linked at C-1 with different mono- or polysaccharides. The major glycolipid of mammalian brain is galactocerebroside, in which galactose is β-glycosidically linked to ceramide; it constitutes about 16% of total adult human brain lipid. Sulfatide is galactocerebroside esterified to sulfate at the 3′ position of galactose and constitutes about 6% of brain lipid. Cerebrosides are present mainly in brain white matter, especially in myelin, and generally contain very-long-chain normal (lignoceric and nervonic), α-hydroxy (cerebronic) and odd-numbered fatty acids, such as 23:0 and 23h:0. Myelin is a specialized plasma membrane that surrounds nerve processes and is elaborated by oligodendroglial cells in the CNS and by Schwann cells in the PNS (see Chaps. 1 and 4). A number of neurological disorders appear to involve selectively myelin (Chap. 39). Brain also contains many other glycolipids that are polysaccharide derivatives of glucocerebroside (Cer-Glc). Many monosaccharides, such as galactose (Gal), glucose (Glc), N-acetylglucosamine (GlcNAc), N-acetylgalactosamine (GalNAc), fucose and others, are present in various linkages in these carbohydrate head groups. One important carbohydrate is sialic acid, or N-acetyl (or N-glycolyl)-neuraminic acid (NANA), an N-acylated, nine-carbon amino sugar (Fig. 3-4B) containing a free carboxyl group. NANA is

enzymatically formed by condensation of N-acetyl (or N-glycolyl)-manosamine with phosphoenolpyruvate. The sialic acid-containing glycolipids are acidic in nature because of the presence of the free carboxylic group and are termed gangliosides. Many gangliosides have been identified in neural and other tissues, making their classification and nomenclature somewhat complex. One popular nomenclature system is that of Svennerholm, who classified the

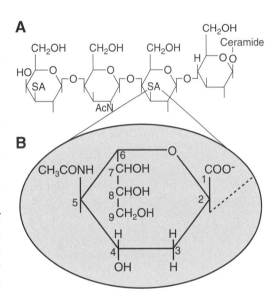

FIGURE 3-4. **A:** The structure of a major brain ganglioside, which is termed GD1a according to the nomenclature of Svennerholm. G denotes ganglioside, D indicates disialo, 1 refers to the tetrasaccharide (Gal-GalNac-GalGlc-) backbone and a distinguishes positional isomers in terms of the location of the sialic acid residues (see also Fig. 3-9). In IUPAC-IUB nomenclature, this ganglioside is termed IV^3NeuAc,II^3NeuAc-Gg_4Cer, where the roman numerals indicate the sugar moiety (from ceramide) to which the sialic acids (NeuAC) are attached and the arabic numeral superscript denotes the position in the sugar moiety where NeuAC are attached; Gg refers to the ganglio (Gal-GalNAC-Gal-Glc) series and the subscript 4 to the four-carbohydrate backbone for the "ganglio" series. **B:** The structure of sialic acid, also called N-acetyl neuraminic acid (NeuAc or NANA). Human brain gangliosides are all N-acetyl derivatives; however, some other mammalian, such as bovine, brain may contain the N-glycolyl derivatives. The metabolic biosynthetic precursor for sialylation of glycoconjugates is CMP-sialic acid, forming the phosphodiester of the 5′OH of cytidine and the 2-position of neuraminic acid.

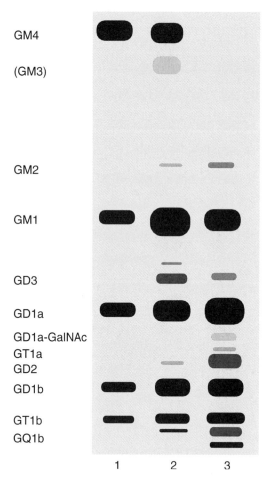

GM4

(GM3)

GM2

GM1

GD3

GD1a

GD1a-GalNAc
GT1a
GD2

GD1b

GT1b
GQ1b

1   2   3

FIGURE 3-5. Diagrammatic representation of thin-layer chromatograms of gangliosides from normal human white matter *(lane 2)* and gray matter *(lane 3)*. Lane 1 contains a mixture of isolated standards. Each lane contains about 7 μg sialic acid. Merck precoated HPTLC plates (silica gel 60, 200 μm thick) were used. The plate was developed with chloroform–methanol–water, 60:40:9 (containing 0.02% $CaCl_2 \cdot 2H_2O$). The bands were visualized with resorcinol–hydrochloric acid reagent. (Courtesy of R. K. Yu, see also Yu and Ando [5].) See legend to Figures 3-4 and 3-9 for nomenclature.

ANALYSIS OF BRAIN LIPIDS

Chromatographic methods are employed to analyze and classify brain lipids

The lipids from brain are generally extracted by a mixture of chloroform and methanol, by methods that are variations of one originally described by Folch and coworkers. In most procedures, the tissue or homogenate is treated with 19 volumes of a 2:1 (v/v) mixture of chloroform–methanol. A single liquid phase is formed, leaving behind a residue of macromolecular material, primarily protein, with lesser amounts of DNA, RNA and polysaccharides. The subsequent addition of a small amount of water to the $CHCl_3$–methanol extract leads to separation into chloroform-rich and aqueous methanol phases; the lower chloroform phase contains the lipids, whereas low-molecular-weight metabolites and polar lipids, such as gangliosides, are in the upper phase. If the lower phase is evaporated to dryness and taken back up in a lipid solvent such as chloroform, proteolipid protein remains undissolved and can be removed at this point. Gangliosides can be extracted from the aqueous phase by repartitioning into an apolar solvent. Acidic phospholipids such as the polyphosphoinositides are poorly extracted at neutral pH, so it is necessary to acidify the initial chloroform–methanol mixture for their recovery [6]. Unfortunately, the acidity leads to cleavage of plasmalogens, primarily alkenyl-acyl PtdEtn. There is thus no single procedure that results in quantitative recovery of all brain lipids. Lipid classes are separated from a lipid extract by thin-layer chromatography (TLC), ion-exchange chromatography or high-performance liquid chromatography (HPLC) using silicic acid as the stationary phase. To analyze individual fatty acids in a given lipid class, methyl esters can be prepared directly by alkaline methanolysis of extracted lipid bands scraped from TLC plates following visualization, usually with a fluorescent spray. The amide-bound fatty acids of the sphingolipids require more vigorous conditions of methanolysis, such as treatment with hot HCl–methanol. The

gangliosides according to the number of sialic acid residues present in the molecule and its relative migration rate on thin-layer chromatograms (Fig. 3-5). IUPAC-IUB has proposed a different systematic nomenclature for both gangliosides and neutral glycolipids, or globosides. The structure and nomenclature of a major brain ganglioside are given in Figure 3-4A (see Fig. 3-9 below for other gangliosides).

TABLE 3-2. **LIPID COMPOSITION OF NORMAL ADULT HUMAN BRAIN**[a]

Constituent	Gray matter (%)			White matter (%)		
	Fresh wt.	Dry wt.	Lipid	Fresh wt.	Dry wt.	Lipid
Water	81.9	—	—	71.6	—	—
Chloroform–methanol—insoluble residue	9.5	52.6	—	8.7	30.6	—
Proteolipid protein	0.5	2.7	—	2.4	8.4	—
Total lipid	5.9	32.7	100	15.6	54.9	100
Upper-phase solids	2.2	12.1	—	1.7	6.0	—
Cholesterol	1.3	7.2	22.0	4.3	15.1	27.5
Phospholipid, total	4.1	22.7	69.5	7.2	25.2	45.9
PtdEtn	1.7	9.2	27.1	3.7	13.2	23.9
PtdCho	1.9	10.7	30.1	2.4	8.4	15.0
Sphingomyelin	0.4	2.3	6.9	1.2	4.2	7.7
Phosphoinositides	0.16	0.9	2.7	0.14	0.5	0.9
PtdSer	0.5	2.8	8.7	1.2	4.3	7.9
Galactocerebroside	0.3	1.8	5.4	3.1	10.9	19.8
Galactocerebroside sulfate	0.1	0.6	1.7	0.9	3.0	5.4
Ganglioside, total[b]	0.3	1.7	—	0.05	0.18	—

[a]Modified from Suzuki [7].
[b]Phospholipid fractions include plasmalogen, assuming that all plasmalogen is present as PtdEtn. Ratios of PtdEtn to PtdCho are 4:1 in white matter and 1:1 in gray matter. In intact brain (based on analysis of rapidly microwaved rat brain), phosphoinositides are present in both white and gray matter in the ratio of 5:0.3:1 for phosphatidylinositol (Pt-dIns) phosphatidylinositol-4-phosphate (PtdIns4P$_2$), phosphatidylinositol-4,5-bisphosphate (PtdIns4,5P$_2$). Gangliosides are calculated on the basis of total sialic acid, assuming that sialic acid constitutes 30% of the weight of a typical ganglioside; GD$_{1a}$ is the major ganglioside of both gray and white matter. PtdEtn, phosphatidylethanolamine; PtdCho, phosphatidylcholine; PtdSer, phosphatidylserine.

methyl esters are then separated by gas-liquid chromatography (GLC). It is sometimes possible to separate subclasses of intact phospholipids on the basis of the number of fatty acid double bonds if Ag$^+$ is present in the silica gel of the TLC plates. This separation is based on the bonding of Ag$^+$ with the π-electrons of the fatty acid double bonds. The molecular species can also be separated by reverse-phase HPLC. For this purpose, a reporter group, such as the UV-absorbing benzoyl group, can be attached either directly to the lipids in the carbohydrate portion of glycolipids or to the DAG backbone of lipid after hydrolysis of the polar head group [3]. In this method, separation of the derivatized DAGs is achieved on the basis of their differences in hydrophobicity. Gangliosides are separated from each other by HPTLC, as shown in Figure 3-5.

The lipid composition of mammalian brain analyzed by these methods is found to change with age and is different from one region to another [1]. A typical lipid composition of gray and white matter in adult human brain is given in Table 3-2.

BRAIN LIPID BIOSYNTHESIS

Acetyl coenzyme A is the precursor of both cholesterol and fatty acids

The hydrophobic chains of lipids, that is, fatty acids and isoprenoids, are biosynthesized from the same two-carbon donor, acetyl-CoA, with differences in condensation leading to different products. In cholesterol biosynthesis, two acetyl-CoAs are condensed to form acetoacetyl-CoA, which can be further condensed with a third acetyl-CoA to form a C$_6$ branched-chain dicarboxylic acyl-CoA, termed β-hydroxy-β-methylglutaryl (HMG)-CoA. HMGCoA is reduced by 2NADPH$^+$ to form mevalonic acid, and this reduction is catalyzed by the enzyme HMGCoA reductase, the principal regulatory enzyme for the biosynthesis of isoprenoids [8]. Mevalonic acid undergoes pyrophosphorylation by two consecutive reactions with ATP, and the product is decarboxylated to form isopentenyl pyrophosphate. This C$_5$H$_8$ isoprene unit is the building

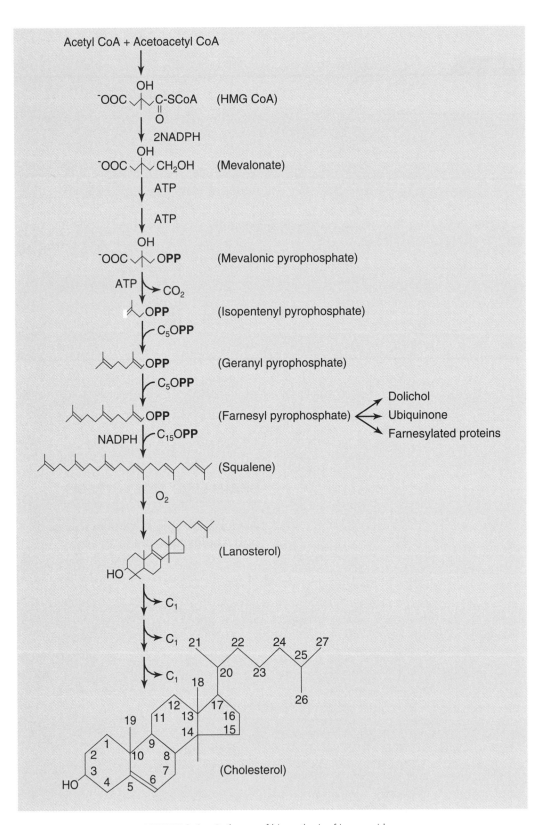

FIGURE 3-6. Pathways of biosynthesis of isoprenoids.

block of all isoprenoids. Two isoprene units, isopentenyl pyrophosphate and dimethyl allyl pyrophosphate, condense to form geranyl pyrophosphate (C_{10}), which then condenses with another C_5 unit to form farnesyl pyrophosphate (C_{15}), the precursor of many different isoprenoids, such as dolichol, a very-long-chain (up to C_{100}) alcohol; a redox coenzyme, ubiquinone; and cholesterol. Polyisoprenyl pyrophosphates also alkylate some proteins via a thioether bond, which attaches them to biomembranes (see below). During cholesterol biosynthesis, two farnesyl pyrophosphate molecules reductively condense in a head-to-head manner to form squalene, a C_{30} hydrocarbon. Squalene is oxidatively cyclized to form lanosterol, a C_{30} hydroxysteroid. After three demethylations, lanosterol is converted to cholesterol (C_{27}). An outline of the pathway of biosynthesis of cholesterol is shown in Figure 3-6. Once formed, brain cholesterol turns over very slowly, and there is both metabolic and analytic evidence to indicate an accretion of brain cholesterol with age.

Fatty acids are biosynthesized via elongation by C_2 units. Here, acetyl-CoA is carboxylated by bicarbonate to form malonyl-CoA, which then condenses with an acyl-CoA to form a β-ketoacyl-CoA and CO_2. This release of CO_2 (HCO_3^-) drives the reaction forward and elongates the chain by acetyl units. The ketone group is then enzymatically reduced, dehydrated and hydrogenated, resulting in an acyl-CoA that is two carbons longer than the parent acyl-CoA. NADPH acts as the reducing agent for the reduction of both the ketone group and the double bond. All four reactions, condensation, reduction, dehydration and hydrogenation, are carried out by fatty acid synthase, a large, multifunctional, dimeric enzyme. This cycle is repeated until the proper chain length ($>C_{12}$) is attained, after which the fatty acid is hydrolyzed from its thioester link with the enzyme. Preformed or exogenous fatty acids are extended by a similar mechanism and catalyzed by enzyme(s) present in the endoplasmic reticulum [9]. There is also a minor mitochondrial chain-elongation system in which acetyl-CoA rather than malonyl-CoA is utilized to lengthen the fatty acid chain. Fatty acids are converted to unsaturated fatty acids mainly in the endoplasmic reticulum. Fatty acyl-

CoA desaturases, of which Δ^9-desaturase is most active in all organisms, remove two hydrogens from the $-CH_2-CH_2$ groups of long-chain intermediates, such as octadecanoyl-CoA, by oxidizing them with molecular oxygen. In brain, this enzyme is responsible for the conversion of stearic acid (18:0) to oleic acid (18:1ω9) and palmitic acid (16:0) to palmitoleic acid (16:1ω7) (see Fig. 3-1). The electrons are transferred via cytochrome b_5 which in turn is reduced to NADH via cytochrome b_5 reductase. In brain, polyunsaturated fatty acids, such as arachidonic (20:4ω6) and decosahexenoic acids (22:6ω3), are major phospholipid components. They are formed by chain elongation and desaturation of shorter-chain fatty acids (Fig. 3-7). In animals, additional double bonds can be introduced only between an existing double bond and the fatty acid carboxyl group. For example, stearic acid (18:0) is converted to oleic acid (18:1ω9) in brain but cannot be further converted to linoleic acid (18:2ω6). This means that the fatty acids of the ω3 and ω6 series can be obtained only via dietary sources, mainly from plants, and so are termed "essential fatty acids" (see also Chap. 33) and have important physiological roles. If the ω3 and ω6 precursors are not available in the diet, then ω9 fatty acids are further chain-elongated and desaturated to form abnormal fatty acids, as a compensatory response of the brain. One of these is 20:3ω9 (Fig. 3-7), termed "Mead acid" because it was discovered by James Mead in the tissues of animals fed a fat-free diet over extended periods. Mead acid substitutes for arachidonic acid and, like arachidonic acid in normal animals, is enriched in the inosites of essential fatty acid-deficient animals.

Fatty acids are degraded by two-carbon units in a manner similar to their biosynthesis. The acyl-CoAs are first dehydrogenated to α,β-unsaturated acyl-CoA, and then hydrated to β-hydroxyacyl-CoA, followed by oxidation to β-ketoacyl-CoA. The C–C bond between C-2 and C-3 of the latter compound is broken by a free CoA molecule via thiolysis to form an acyl-CoA that is two carbons shorter and acetyl-CoA. Unlike fatty acid biosynthesis, each step of the β oxidation of fatty acids is catalyzed by a distinct enzyme. These are present both in mitochondria and in peroxisomes. Though the biochemical

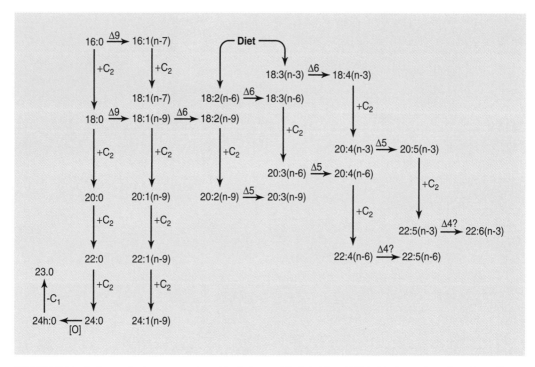

FIGURE 3-7.   Pathways for interconversion of brain fatty acids. Palmitic acid (16:0) is the main end product of brain fatty acid synthase. It may then be elongated, desaturated and/or β-oxidized to form different long-chain fatty acids. The monoenes ($18:1\Delta^9$, $18:1\Delta^7$, $24:1\Delta^{15}$) are the main unsaturated fatty acids formed *de novo* by Δ^9 desaturation and chain elongation. As shown, the very-long-chain fatty acids are α-oxidized to form α-hydroxy and odd-numbered fatty acids. The polyunsaturated fatty acids are formed mainly from exogenous dietary fatty acids, such as linoleic (ω6) and α-linolenic (ω3) acids, by chain elongation and desaturation (Δ^5, Δ^6), as shown. It is doubtful whether there is a Δ^4 desaturase in brain; the apparent Δ^4 desaturation is probably effected by first chain elongation (+C_2), then Δ^6 desaturation in microsomes, followed by peroxisomal β oxidation (C_2), that is, by "retroconversion." In severe essential fatty acid deficiency, the abnormal polyenes, such as 20:3, ω9, are also biosynthesized *de novo*.

steps are similar in the two cellular compartments, there are some differences between peroxisomal and mitochondrial β-oxidation pathways. In mitochondria, the first dehydrogenation is carried out by an FAD-containing enzyme, which is coupled to oxidative phosphorylation, thus generating ATP. In peroxisomes, however, this dehydrogenation is carried out by a flavin-containing oxidase, which reacts directly with molecular oxygen to form H_2O_2, which is further decomposed by peroxisomal catalase to H_2O and O_2, thus wasting the chemical energy. Two separate mitochondrial enzymes, enoyl-CoA hydratase and β-hydroxy acyl-CoA dehydrogenase, catalyze the next two reaction steps, while in peroxisomes both the reactions are catalyzed by a single multifunctional enzyme protein. The peroxisomal β-oxidation pathway is probably responsible for the oxidation of very-long-chain

fatty acids ($>C_{22}$), which are enriched in brain. Evidence for this is provided by a number of genetic diseases involving peroxisomal disorders, such as Zellweger's cerebrohepatorenal syndrome and adrenoleukodystrophy, in which there is an accumulation of such very-long-chain fatty acids [10], especially in neural tissues (see Chap. 41).

In addition to the classical β oxidation of fatty acids, known to occur in all tissues, significant α oxidation, especially of the fatty acids of galactocerebroside, occurs in brain. In this reaction, carbon 2, termed the α carbon, of a long-chain fatty acid is hydroxylated, then oxidized and decarboxylated to form a fatty acid one carbon shorter than the parent fatty acid. This quantitatively minor α-hydroxylation pathway may explain the origins of both the comparatively large amounts of odd carbon fatty acids and of 2-hydroxy fatty acids in brain galactocerebrosides. Another α-oxidation pathway normally present in liver and other tissues is defective in the genetic disorder Refsum's disease. This results in the failure to metabolize the dietary branched-chain fatty acid phytanic acid (see Fig. 3-1), which can be initially metabolized only by ω oxidation in these patients [11]. In Refsum's disease, this branched-chain fatty acid accumulates in nervous tissues, resulting in severe neuropathy (see Chap. 41).

Phosphatidic acid is the precursor of all glycerolipids

sn-Glycerol-3-phosphate (G-3-P), formed from the reduction of dihydroxyacetone phosphate (DHAP) by NADH catalyzed by glycerophosphate dehydrogenase, is consecutively acylated with two acyl-CoAs to form PtdOH. Alternatively, DHAP may be first acylated then reduced by NADPH to lysophosphatidate, or 1-acyl-GP, which is further acylated to form PtdOH. Acyl DHAP is also the precursor of ether lipids. The ether bond is formed in a reaction where the acyl group of acyl DHAP is substituted by a long-chain alcohol to form 1-*O*-alkyl DHAP, which is then reduced and converted to 1-alkyl,2-acyl-*sn*-G-3-P, and which is in turn converted to the alkyl ether analog of PtdEtn, the precursor of PtdEtn plasmalogen (Fig. 3-8).

Phosphatidate may be hydrolyzed to 1,2-diacyl-*sn*-glycerol (DAG), which is the precursor of the zwitterionic membrane lipids; PtdCho; PtdEtn; and PtdSer. PtdCho is formed by the transfer of the phosphocholine group from CDP-choline to DAG, and PtdEtn is formed by a corresponding transfer of the head group from CDP-ethanolamine. The enzymes catalyzing the synthesis of CDP-choline and CDP-ethanolamine regulate the overall biosynthesis of PtdCho and PtdEtn. In a minor alternative pathway, PtdEtn is converted to PtdCho by sequential methylations, the methyl donor being *S*-adenosylmethionine. In animals, there is no direct pathway for the formation of PtdSer. PtdSer is formed in brain by a base-exchange reaction between PtdEtn, or PtdCho, and serine. PtdSer is in turn decarboxylated in mitochondria to form PtdEtn [12].

The acidic phospholipids are synthesized by a completely different pathway, in which the phosphate group in PtdOH is retained in the product. In this scheme, PtdOH is converted to the liponucleotide CMP-PtdOH (CDP-DAG) (Fig. 3-8). CDP-DAG reacts with inositol to form PI or with *sn*-glycerol-3-phosphate (Gro3-P) to form phosphatidyl glycerophosphate, which is then converted to cardiolipin (bisphosphatidylglycerol), a mitochondria-specific phospholipid. PI is phosphorylated in the inositol moiety to form PIP, which is an intermediate in a pathway that mediates signal transduction across membranes (see Chap. 21). The pathways from brain phospholipid biosynthesis, including the enzymes that catalyze each step, are summarized in Figure 3-8.

The newly biosynthesized phosphoglycerides undergo deacylation to the corresponding lysolipids, which can be further degraded or reconverted to the parent lipids by reacylation often with a different fatty acyl substitute. The reacylation of lysolipids occurs by transferring acyl groups from acyl-CoAs or from other phospholipids either by CoA-dependent or CoA-independent acyltransferase. The acyltransferase(s) catalyzing the reacylation reactions is very specific toward the acyl donor and lysolipid substrates. It is thought that the specific distribution of fatty acids in each individual class of membrane phosphoglycerides is regulated by these "deacylation–reacylation" mechanisms. Thus, the initial fatty acid composition of a biosynthesized lipid may not reflect its ultimate composition.

Most of the enzymes catalyzing the biosynthesis of glycerolipids are bound to endoplasmic reticular membranes, although those catalyzing the biosynthesis of cardiolipin are mitochondrial. The acyl-DHAP pathway enzymes, obligatory for the synthesis of ether lipids, are in peroxisomes, a finding that explains the deficiency of ether lipids in patients suffering from genetic peroxisomal disorders, as noted above [13].

The phosphoglycerides are hydrolyzed by specific phospholipases, as indicated in Figure 3-2. The acyl groups at C-1 and C-2 are hydrolyzed by phospholipases A_1 and A_2 (PLA$_1$, PLA$_2$), respectively. The presence of PLA$_1$ in brain is inferential. The head groups are hydrolyzed by

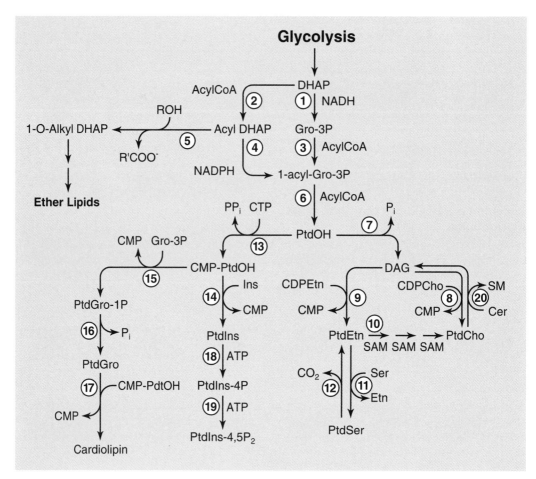

FIGURE 3-8. Schematic representation of glycerophospholipid biosynthesis. Note that dihydroxyacetone phosphate *(DHAP)* may be reduced to glycerophosphate or may be first acylated and then serve as a precursor of ether lipid. The alkyl analog of phosphatidic acid (that is, 1-*O*-alkyl,2-acyl-*sn*-glycerol-3-P) is converted to the alkyl analog of phosphatidylethanolamine *(PtdEtn)* by the same diacylglycerol *(DAG)* pathway as shown for the diacyl lipids, and the alkyl analog of PtdEtn is dehydrogenated to form the 1-alk-1′enyl analog of PtdEtn, plasmalogen (not shown). As mentioned in the text, phosphatidic acid *(PtdOH)* is converted to DAG, which is converted to the major brain lipids phosphatidylcholine *(PtdCho)* and PtdEtn. The acidic lipids are formed via the conversion of PtdOH to CDP-DAG (CMP-PtdOH). PtdCho and PtdEtn are interconverted either via methylation or via base-exchange reactions to phosphatidylserine *(PtdSer)*. Not only PtdEtn (as shown) but also PtdCho is converted to PtdSer by base-exchange reaction. Exchange of the head group of PtdCho with ceramide to form sphingomyelin is also shown. The enzymes catalyzing lipid biosynthesis are as follows: *1*, glycerophosphate dehydrogenase; *2*, dihydroxyacetone phosphate acyltransferase; *3*, *sn*-glycerol-3-phosphate acyltransferase; *4*, acyl/alkyl dihydroxyacetone phosphate reductase; *5*, alkyl dihydroxyacetone phosphate synthase; *6*, 1-acyl glycerol-3-phosphate acyltransferase; *7*, phosphatidate phosphohydrolase; *8*, diacylglycerol cholinephosphotransferase; *9*, diacylglycerol ethanolaminephosphotransferase; *10*, phosphatidylethanolamine *N*-methyl transferase and phosphatidyl-*N*-methylethanolamine *N*-methyl transferase; *11*, phosphatidylethanolamine:serine transferase; *12*, phosphatidylserine decarboxylase; *13*, phosphatidate cytidyltransferase; *14*, phosphatidylinositol synthase; *15*, CDP-DAG:glycerol-3-phosphate phosphatidyltransferase; *16*, phosphatidylglycerol phosphatase; *17*, cardiolipin synthase; *18*, phosphatidylinositol-4-kinase; *19*, phosphatidylinositol-4-phosphate 5-kinase; *20*, phosphatidylcholine:ceramide cholinephosphotransferase.

class-specific phospholipases. Thus, PtdCho and PI are cleaved by different phospholipases. The bond between DAG and phosphate is hydrolyzed by PLC, whereas that between the phosphate and the polar alcohol is hydrolyzed by phospholipase D. These enzymes can be important not only for the catabolism of these lipids but also for the generation of biological signal-transduction-messenger lipid products, such as DAG or arachidonic acid (see Chap. 21). Many of these enzymes are regulated, indirectly or directly, by cell-surface receptors. The brain also contains specific hydrolases, plasmalogenase and lysoplasmalogenase, which catalyze the hydrolysis of the alkenyl ether bond to form long-chain aldehydes and lysolipids or glycerophosphorylethanolamine, respectively.

Sphingolipids are biosynthesized by adding head groups to the ceramide moiety

Sphinganine, also termed dihydrosphingosine, is biosynthesized by a decarboxylating condensation of serine with palmitoyl-CoA to form a keto intermediate, which is then reduced by NADPH (Fig. 3-9). Sphinganine is acylated, then dehydrogenated to form ceramide. Free sphingosine, also termed sphingenine, "salvaged" from sphingolipid breakdown can be enzymatically acylated with acyl-CoA to form ceramide.

Ceramide is the precursor of all sphingolipids; sphingomyelin is formed by a reaction that transfers the head group of PtdCho to ceramide to form sphingomyelin and DAG (Figs. 3-8 and 3-9), while sphingosine-containing glycolipids are formed from consecutive glycosylation of ceramide by various nucleotide–carbohydrate derivatives. For example, galactocerebroside is formed by glycosylation of ceramide with UDPGal, whereas glucocerebroside is formed by glycosylation of ceramide with UDPGlc [14]. The latter, Cer-Glc, is the precursor of neutral glycolipids, also termed globosides, and acidic glycolipids, also termed gangliosides. The CMP derivative of the *N*-acetyl (or *N*-glycolyl) neuraminic acid NANA, or NeuAc, is the donor of this moiety to form gangliosides. Some of the reactions forming these complex glycolipids are shown in Figure 3-9. These reactions occur in Golgi bodies, and it is the specificity of these membrane-bound glycosyl transferases toward the lipid substrate and to the water-soluble nucleotide derivatives that determines the structures of the products.

These same glycolipids are broken down by specific hydrolases present in lysosomes and stimulated by noncatalytic lysosomal proteins. A congenital deficiency of either one of the hydrolases or in the helper proteins results in the accumulation of lipid intermediates in lysosomes, leading to a lysosomal storage disease. For example, in Gaucher's disease, Cer-Glc accumulates because of a defect in its hydrolysis, whereas in Tay-Sachs disease, the GM2-ganglioside concentration is increased because of a deficiency in the hydrolase releasing *N*-acetylgalactosamine (see Chap. 41). Because of interest in these genetic diseases, genes coding for a number of these hydrolytic enzymes have been identified and cloned. Progress has also been made in the elucidation of genes coding for biosynthetic enzymes, including several transferases in the pathway for ganglioside formation and the UDP-galactosyltransferase that leads to cerebroside formation (see Chap. 4). In pathways for phospholipid synthesis, the cDNA coding for the enzyme CDP-DAG synthase has been cloned from a human cell line [15].

LIPIDS IN THE CELLULAR MILIEU

Lipids are transported between membranes

As indicated above, lipids are often biosynthesized in one intracellular membrane and must be transported to other intracellular compartments for membrane biogenesis. Because lipids are insoluble in water, special mechanisms must exist for the inter- and intracellular transport of membrane lipids. The best understood of such mechanisms is vesicular transport, wherein the lipid particles are enclosed in membrane vesicles which bud out from the donor membrane and travel to and then fuse with the recepient membrane. The well-characterized transport of plasma cholesterol into cells via receptor-medi-

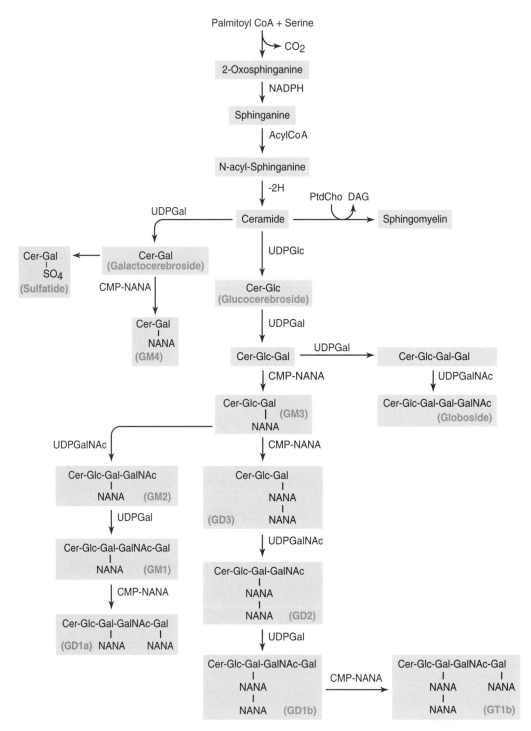

FIGURE 3-9. Pathways for biosynthesis of sphingolipids. Ceramide *(Cer)* is the precursor of all sphingolipids. Ceramide is converted to cerebroside *(Cer-Gal)*, the main brain glycolipid, which is further converted to cerebroside sulfate (sulfatide) as shown. Cer-Gal is also converted to ganglioside *(GM4)*, which is present in brain myelin. Most other gangliosides originate from Cer-Glc, and the main pathways for formation of these lipids are shown. The abbreviations using Svennerholm's nomenclature are shown in parentheses. (See Figs. 3-4 and 3-5.) The first letter, G, is for ganglioside. The second letter, M, D, T or Q, represents the number of sialic acid residues. Isomeric configurations of NANAs are distinguished by a and b. The main gangliosides of adult human brain are GM1, GD1a, GD1b and GT1b.

ated endocytosis is a useful model of this type of lipid transport. It is believed that transport of cholesterol from the endoplasmic reticulum to other membranes and of glycolipids from the Golgi bodies to the plasma membrane is mediated by similar mechanisms. The transport of phosphoglycerides is less clearly understood but is believed to occur via a carrier-mediated mechanism; that is, the lipids are complexed with a specific water-soluble protein carrier, which picks up lipids from one membrane and delivers them to another. A number of cellular proteins which catalyze a rapid exchange of lipids from one membrane to another have been identified. Some of these proteins are specific for particular lipids, such as PtdCho or PI, whereas others are nonspecific. Such lipid-exchange proteins have been identified in brain. Since they thus far have been shown only to exchange lipids, however, it is not clear how they can effect net transport of lipids from one membrane to another.

Membrane lipids may be asymmetrically oriented

In the "fluid-mosaic" model of biomembranes, the lipids form a bimolecular leaflet in which proteins are embedded (see Chap. 2). This model, with some modifications, is useful in explaining a number of membrane phenomena, but it does not take into account the complex arrangement and function of various polar head groups and different fatty acids present in biomembrane lipids. In some biomembranes, such as those of red blood cells, the choline-containing phospholipids PtdCho and sphingomyelin are known to be enriched in the outer leaflet, while the amino lipids PtdEtn and PtdSer are concentrated in the inner leaflet of the plasma membrane. This arrangement probably also exists in the plasma membrane of most other cells. Studies with the serine-binding protein annexin V indicate that PtdSer appears in the plasma membrane outer leaflet in apoptosis [16]. The glycolipids, especially the gangliosides, are enriched in the extracellular side of the plasma membrane, where they may function in intercellular communication and act as receptors for certain ligands; for example, GM1 acts as a receptor for cholera toxin and GD1b for tetanus toxin. It is not clear how this asymmetric distribution of lipids in biomembranes originates. Lipids can move freely within the same plane of the bilayer but their movement from one leaflet of the bilayer to another is thermodynamically restricted. It is postulated that membrane may contain some proteins which catalyze a "flip-flop" transbilayer movement of lipids. Specificity of such "flippase" activity may be responsible for the asymmetric distribution of lipids between the inner and outer leaflets of the membrane bilayer. In support of this hypothesis, it has been shown that plasma membrane contains an ATP-dependent phospholipid translocase that selectively catalyzes the transport of the aminophospholipids PtdSer and PtdEtn but not of PtdCho from the outer to the inner lipid layer of the membrane [17] (see Chaps. 2 and 5).

Some proteins are bound to membranes by covalently linked lipids

In recent years, a number of membrane-bound proteins have been shown to be covalently linked with various lipids, which anchor the protein to the lipid bilayer. PI-anchored proteins constitute a major family of membrane-tethered proteins (see Box 3-1). In brain proteolipid protein, fatty acids (14:0, 16:0) are attached to the protein via ester to a serine or threonine moiety or a thioester to a cysteine moiety linkage. A number of cellular proteins are also acylated with myristic acid (14:0) to the free amino group of N-terminal amino acids. A class of proteins, including Ras, a proto-oncogene product, has been shown to form covalent links with farnesyl (C_{15}) or C_{20} isoprenes via a thioether linkage to cysteine [18]. The lipid anchor in Ras, which occupies a central position in intracellular signal transduction, is required for its activity. Cholesterol may also be linked covalently to membrane protein. Hedgehog, a family of developmental signaling proteins, contains cholesterol covalently linked to the amino terminal signaling domain [19].

Lipids have multiple roles in cells

Recent discoveries show that the same lipid may have both structural and regulatory roles in the cell. For example, while arachidonic acid

---

Box 3-1

GLYCOSYLPHOSPHATIDYLINOSITOL-ANCHORED PROTEINS

A bacterial phosphatidylinositol specific phospholipase C (PI-PLC) had been available for many years before it was demonstrated to strip a number of membrane-bound proteins from eukaryotic cell surfaces [1]. Such proteins are anchored by a PI moiety in which the 6 position of inositol is glycosidically linked to glucosamine, which in turn is bonded to a polymannan backbone (see Figure). The polysaccharide chain is joined to the carboxyl terminal of the anchored protein via amide linkage to ethanolamine phosphate.

A

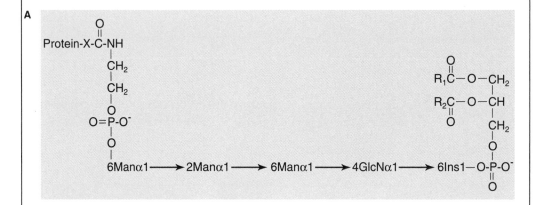

B

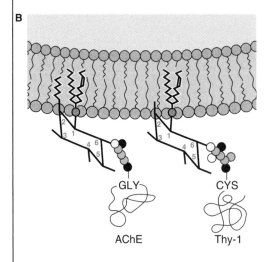

FIGURE.   Structure of phosphatidylinositol anchors. **A:** The backbone structure of a glycosylphosphatidylinositol (GPI) anchor. Additional phosphoethanolamine or galactose may be attached to one of the mannose moieties. **B:** The structure of two mammalian GPI anchors, Thy-1 antigen and erythrocyte acetylcholinesterase *(AChE)*. AChE has an additional fatty acid moiety (16:0) attached to the 2 position of inositol. Phosphorylethanolamine, ●; mannose, (●); galactose, (○); GlcN, (●). See Chapter 21 for other inositol lipids.

(20:4ω6) is a major constituent of brain inositides and PtdEtn, the free acid is also a precursor of a number of important biomessengers, the eicosanoids, such as prostaglandins, prostacyclins, leukotrienes and thromboxanes (see Chap. 35). Arachidonic acid itself acts as a biomessenger by activating certain isoforms of PKC. It may also be found in a derivatized form. It has been identified in amide linkage with ethanolamine as anandamide or esterified to the 2-position of glycerol, and both have been proposed as possible endogenous ligands for brain cannabinoid

---

Box 3-1 (Continued)

The presence of a free NH_2 group in the glucosamine residue makes the structure labile to nitrous acid. Bacterial PI-PLC hydrolyzes the bond between DAG and phosphatidylinositols, releasing the water-soluble protein polysaccharide-inositol phosphate moiety. These proteins are said to be tethered by glycosylphosphatidylinositol (GPI) anchors. They occur widely in nature, from trypanosome cell-surface antigens to placental alkaline phosphatase. In yeast and protozoa, cell-surface proteins appear to be ceramide- or GPI-anchored. The concept of a hydrophilic cell-surface protein tethered by a membrane lipid may be misleading since some GPI-anchored proteins appear to fulfill roles generally served by membrane-spanning proteins in higher animal cells, such as signal-transducing receptor proteins, ion channels and transporters. GPI-anchored proteins of neurobiological interest include rat Thy-1 antigen, neural cell adhesion molecules (NCAMs) and prion protein (see Chaps. 7 and 46). Interest in the GPI-anchored protein complex also stems from indications that they may be linked to trophic proteins that mediate chemical affinity gradients during development. The inositol–glycan complex of GPI may also have messenger-like properties in growth factor actions. A defect in GPI-anchor formation gives rise to the blood disorder paroxysmal nocturnal hemoglobinuria. For some GPI anchors, the PI moiety may contain alkyl ethers at C-1 of the glycerol, generally not found in free PI, and the 2-position of inositol can be esterified with a fatty acid, which renders the molecule resistant to PLC action. The lipid polysaccharide backbone is biosynthesized by sequential addition of the carbohydrate moiety to PtdIns, which initially reacts with UDPGlcNAc to form PI-6-1Glc NAc, and is then deacetylated. D-Mannose moieties are next transferred from dolichol-P-mannose to make the polysaccharide backbone, which then undergoes phosphodiesteratic linkage with phosphoethanolamine derived from phosphatidylethanolamine [2,3]. The GPI is anchored via amide linkage of the ethanolamine amino group and the C-terminal amino acid of a protein, and the complex is then transported to the outer surface of the plasma membrane. While the sequence of carboxy-terminal amino acids that signal GPI linkage is complex, it has been possible to splice nucleotide sequences coding for such sequences to mRNAs and to transfect cells which then produce novel cell-surface proteins. Proteins released by phospholipase have been shown to be reincorporated and GPI-anchored, even into other cell types. This has led to the concept of "painting" cell surfaces for potential therapeutic uses, such as prevention of transplant rejection [4].

—*Bernard W. Agranoff*

REFERENCES

1. Low, M. G. The glycosyl-phosphatidylinositol anchor of membrane proteins. *Biochim. Biophys. Acta.* 988:427–454, 1989.
2. Udenfriend, S., and Kodukula, K. How glycosylphosphatidylinositol-anchored membrane proteins are made. *Annu. Rev. Biochem.* 64:563–591, 1995.
3. Takeda, J., and Kinoshita, K. GPI-anchor biosynthesis. *Trends Biochem. Sci.* 20:367–370, 1995.
4. Medof, M. E., Nagargian, S., and Tykocinski, M. L. Cell-surface engineering with GPI-anchored proteins. *FASEB J.* 10:574–586, 1996.

---

receptors [20]. Oleic acid amide has been reported to be an endogenous sleep-promoting factor [21], as has the prostanoid prostaglandin D_2 [22].

DAG is an important precursor for lipid biosynthesis in the endoplasmic reticulum, but in the plasma membrane it acts as a second messenger, activating PKC. Major structural lipids, such as PI and PtdCho, are also intimately involved in the signal-transduction process (see Chap. 21). The ether lipid 1-*O*-hexadecyl-2-acetyl-*sn*-glycero-3-phosphocholine, termed platelet activating factor, commonly referred to as PAF, has potent biomessenger activity in aggregating platelets and releasing eicosanoids [23] (see Chap. 35). Sphingolipids, including ceramide, sphingosine and sphingosine-1-phosphate, have been implicated in cell regulatory processes, such as cell-cycle arrest, apoptosis and stress-activated protein kinase actions [24,25]. For example, tumor necrosis factor, the cytokine interleukin-1β and nerve growth factor act through their receptors to induce sphingomyelin hydrolysis to ceramide, which then activates a number of downstream activities, including protein kinases and phosphatases, triggering cell-cycle arrest, proliferation, differentiation or cell death (see also Chaps. 19 and 27).

REFERENCES

1. Sastry, P. S. Lipids of nervous tissue: Composition and metabolism. *Prog. Lipid Res.* 24:69–176, 1985.
2. Wells, M. A., and Dittmer, J. C. A comprehensive study of the postnatal changes in the concentration of the lipids of developing rat brain. *Biochemistry* 10:3169–3175, 1967.
3. Lee, C., and Hajra, A. K. Molecular species of diacylglycerols and phosphoglycerides and the postmortem changes in the molecular species of diacylglycerols in rat brain. *J. Neurochem.* 56: 370–379, 1991.
4. O'Brien, J. S., and Sampson, E. L. Lipid composition of the normal human brain: Gray matter, white matter, and myelin. *J. Lipid Res.* 6:537–544, 1965.
5. Yu, R. K., and Ando, S. Structures of some new complex gangliosides. In L. Svennerholm, P. Mandel, H. Dreyfus, and P.-F. Urban (eds.), *Structure and Function of Gangliosides.* New York: Plenum, 1980, pp. 33–45.
6. Hajra, A. K., Fisher, S. K., and Agranoff, B. W. Isolation, separation and analysis of phosphoinositides from biological sources. In A. A. Boulton, G. B. Baker and L. A. Horrocks (eds.), *Neuromethods (Neurochemistry). Lipids and Related Compounds,* Vol. 8. Clifton, NJ: Humana Press, 1987.
7. Suzuki, K. Chemistry and metabolism of brain lipids. In G. J. Siegel, R. W. Albers, B. W. Agranoff, and R. Katzman (eds.). *Basic Neurochemistry,* 3rd ed. Boston: Little, Brown, 1981, pp. 355–370.
8. Brown, M. S., and Goldstein, J. L. A receptor-mediated pathway for cholesterol homeostasis. *Science* 232:34–47, 1986.
9. Cinti, D. L., Cook, L., Nagi, M. N., and Suneja, S. K. The fatty acid chain elongation system of mammalian endoplasmic reticulum. *Prog. Lipid Res.* 31:1–51, 1992.
10. Moser, H. W., and Moser, A. B. Adrenoleukodystrophy (X-linked). In C. R. Scriver, A. L. Beaudet, W. S. Sly, and D. Valle (eds.), *The Metabolic and Molecular Basis of Inherited Disease,* 7th ed. New York: McGraw-Hill, 1997, pp. 1511–1532.
11. Steinberg, D. Refsum disease. In C. R. Scriver, A. L. Beaudet, W. S. Sly, and D. Valle (eds.), *The Metabolic and Molecular Basis of Inherited Disease,* 7th ed. New York: McGraw-Hill, 1997, pp. 2351–2369.
12. Kennedy, E. P. The biosynthesis of phospholipids. In J. A. F. Op den Kamp, B. Roelofsen, and K. W. A. Wirtz (eds.), *Lipids and Membranes: Past, Present and Future.* Amsterdam: Elsevier, 1986, pp. 171–206.
13. Hajra, A. K. Glycerolipid biosynthesis in peroxisomes (microbodies). *Prog. Lipid Res.* 34 343–364, 1995.
14. Radin, N. S. Biosynthesis of the sphingoid bases: A provocation. *J. Lipid Res.* 25:1536–1560, 1984.
15. Heacock, A. M., Uhler, M. D., and Agranoff, B. W. Cloning of CDP-diacylglycerol synthase from a human neuronal line. *J. Neurochem.* 67: 2200–2203, 1996.
16. Martin, S. J., Reutelingsberger, C. P., McGahon, A. J., vanSchie, R. C., LaFace, D. M. and Green, D. R. Early redistribution of plasma membrane phosphatidylserine is a general feature of apoptosis regardless of the initiating stimulus: Inhibition by overexpression of Bcl-2 and Abl. *J. Exp. Med.* 182:1545–1556, 1995.
17. Devaux, P. F. Protein involvement in transmembrane lipid asymmetry. *Annu. Rev. Biophys. Biomol. Struct.* 21:417–439, 1992.
18. Glomset, J. A., Gebb, M. H., and Farnsworth, C. C. Prenyl proteins in eukaryotic cells: A new type of membrane anchor. *Trends Biochem. Sci.* 15: 139–142, 1990.
19. Porter, J. A., Young, K. E., and Beachy, P. A. Cholesterol modification of hedgehog signaling proteins in animal development. *Science* 274: 255–357, 1996.
20. Sheskin, T., Hanus, L., Slager, J., Vogel, Z., and Mechoulam, R. Structural requirements for binding of anandamide-type compounds to the brain cannabinoid receptor. *J. Med. Chem.* 40:659–667, 1997.
21. Cravatt, B. F., Prospero-Garcia, O., Siuzdak, G., et al. Chemical characterization of a family of brain

lipids that induce sleep. *Science* 268:1506–1509, 1995.

22. Satoh, S., Matsumura, H., Suzuki, F., and Hayaishi, O. Promotion of sleep mediated by the A_{2a}-adenosine receptor and possible involvement of this receptor in the sleep induced by prostaglandin D_2 in rats. *Proc. Natl. Acad. Sci. USA* 93: 5980–5984, 1996.

23. Bazan, N. G., and Allan, G. Platelet-activating factor in the modulation of excitatory amino acid neurotransmitter release and of gene expression. *J. Lipid Mediat. Cell Signal.* 3:321–330, 1996.

24. Hannun, Y. A. Functions of ceramide in coordinating cellular responses to stress. *Science* 274: 1855–1859, 1996.

25. Kolesnick, R., and Golde, D. W. The sphingo-myelin pathway in tumor necrosis factor and interleukin-1 signaling. *Cell* 77:325–328, 1994.

GENERAL REFERENCES

Prescott, M. P. (ed.) A thematic series on phospholipases. *Journal of Biological Chemistry 1997 Mini-review Compendium.* Am. Soc. for Biochem. and Mol. Biol., Bethesda, Maryland, 1997.

Vance, D. E., and Vance, J. (eds.) *Biochemistry of Lipids, Lipoproteins and Membranes. New Comprehensive Biochemistry,* Vol. 31. Amsterdam: Elsevier Science, 1996.

4

Myelin Formation, Structure and Biochemistry

Pierre Morell and Richard H. Quarles

Basic Neurochemistry: Molecular, Cellular and Medical Aspects, 6th Ed., edited by G. J. Siegel et al. Published by Lippincott–Raven Publishers, Philadelphia, 1999. Correspondence to Pierre Morell, Neuroscience Center, University of North Carolina at Chapel Hill, Chapel Hill, North Carolina 27599-7250.

The morphological distinction between white matter and gray matter is one that is useful for the neurochemist. White matter, named for its glistening white appearance, is composed of myelinated axons, glial cells and blood vessels. Gray matter contains the nerve cell bodies with their extensive dendritic arborizations. The predominant element of white matter is the myelin sheath, which comprises about 50% of the total dry weight and is responsible for the gross chemical differences between white and gray matter.

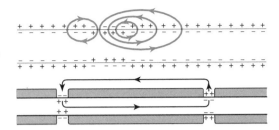

FIGURE 4-1. Impulse conduction in unmyelinated **(top)** and myelinated **(bottom)** fibers. Arrows show the flow of action currents in local circuits into the active region of the membrane. In unmyelinated fibers, the circuits flow through the adjacent piece of membrane, but in myelinated fibers the circuit flow jumps to the next node.

THE MYELIN SHEATH

The myelin sheath is a greatly extended and modified plasma membrane wrapped around the nerve axon in a spiral fashion [1]. The myelin membranes originate from and are a part of the Schwann cells in the peripheral nervous system (PNS) and the oligodendroglial cells in the central nervous system (CNS) (see Chap. 1). Each myelin-generating cell furnishes myelin for only one segment of any given axon. The periodic interruptions where short portions of the axon are left uncovered by myelin are the nodes of Ranvier, and they are critical to the functioning of myelin.

Myelin facilitates conduction

Myelin is an electrical insulator; however, its function of facilitating conduction in axons has no exact analogy in electrical circuitry. In unmyelinated fibers, impulse conduction is propagated by local circuits of ion current that flow into the active region of the axonal membrane, through the axon and out through adjacent sections of the membrane (Fig. 4-1). These local circuits depolarize the adjacent piece of membrane in a continuous, sequential fashion. In myelinated axons, the excitable axonal membrane is exposed to the extracellular space only at the nodes of Ranvier; this is the location of sodium channels [2]. When the membrane at the node is excited, the local circuit generated cannot flow through the high-resistance sheath and, therefore, flows out through and depolarizes the membrane at the next node, which might be 1 mm or farther away (Fig. 4-1). The

low capacitance of the sheath means that little energy is required to depolarize the remaining membrane between the nodes, which results in local circuit spreading at an increased speed. Active excitation of the axonal membrane jumps from node to node; this form of impulse propagation is called saltatory conduction (Latin *saltare*, "to jump"). Such movement of the wave of depolarization is much more rapid than in unmyelinated fibers. Furthermore, because only the nodes of Ranvier are excited during conduction in myelinated fibers, Na^+ flux into the nerve is much less than in unmyelinated fibers, where the entire membrane is involved. An example of the advantage of myelination is obtained by comparison of two different nerve fibers, both of which conduct at 25 m/sec at 20°C. The 500-mm diameter unmyelinated giant axon of the squid requires 5,000 times as much energy and occupies about 1,500 times as much space as the 12-mm diameter myelinated nerve in the frog.

Conduction velocity in myelinated fibers is proportional to the diameter, while in unmyelinated fibers it is proportional to the square root of the diameter. Thus, differences in energy and space requirements between the two types of fiber are exaggerated at higher conduction velocities. If nerves were not myelinated and equivalent conduction velocities were maintained, the human spinal cord would need to be as large as a good-sized tree trunk. Myelin, then, facilitates conduction while conserving space and energy [3].

Myelin has a characteristic ultrastructure

Myelin, as well as many of its morphological features, such as nodes of Ranvier and Schmidt-Lantermann clefts, can be seen readily with light microscopy (Fig. 4-2). Further insight comes from biophysical studies of structures with parallel axons: sciatic nerve as representative of the PNS and optic nerve or tract as representative of the CNS. Myelin, when examined by polarized light, exhibits both a lipid-dependent and a protein-dependent birefringence. Low-angle X-ray diffraction studies of myelin provide electron-density plots of the repeating unit that show three peaks which correspond to protein plus lipid polar groups and two troughs which correspond to lipid hydrocarbon chains. The repeat distance varies somewhat depending on the species and whether the sample is from the CNS or the PNS. Thus, the results from these two techniques are consistent with a protein–lipid–protein–lipid–protein structure, in which the lipid portion is a bimolecular leaflet

and adjacent protein layers are different in some way. Data for mammalian optic nerve show a repeat distance of 80 Å (Fig. 4-3). This spacing can accommodate one bimolecular layer of lipid (about 50 Å) and two protein layers (about 15 Å each). The main repeating unit of two such fused unit membranes is twice this figure, or 160 Å [5]. Although it is useful to think of myelin in terms of alternating protein and lipid layers, this concept has been modified somewhat to be compatible with the "fluid mosaic" model of membrane structure, which includes intrinsic transmembrane proteins as well as extrinsic proteins.

Information concerning myelin structure is also available from electron-microscopic studies, which visualize myelin as a series of protein layers appearing as alternating dark and less dark lines separated by lipid hydrocarbon chains which appear as unstained zones (Figs. 4-4–4-7). There is asymmetry in the staining of the protein layers. The less dark, or intraperiod, line represents the closely apposed outer protein coats of the original cell membrane; the membranes are

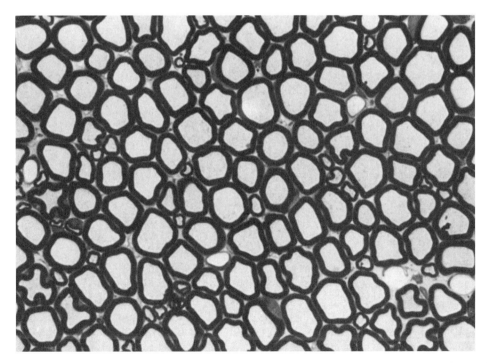

FIGURE 4-2.   Light micrograph of a 1-μm Epon section of rabbit peripheral nerve (anterior root) stained with toluidine blue. The myelin sheath appears as a thick black ring around the pale axon. ×600, before 30% reduction. (Courtesy of Dr. Cedric Raine.)

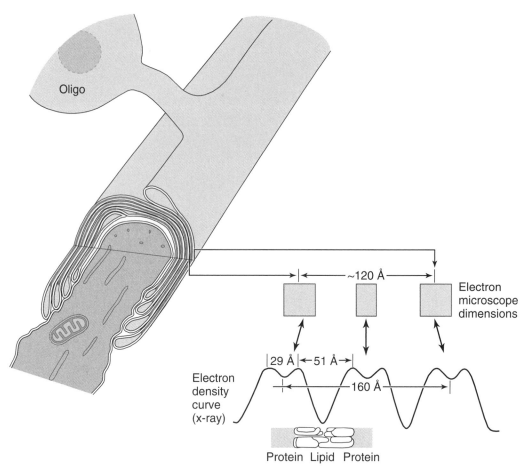

FIGURE 4-3.   A composite diagram summarizing some of the ultrastructural data on CNS myelin. At the top, an oligodendroglial cell is shown connected to the sheath by a process. The cutaway view of the myelin and axon illustrates the relationship of these two structures at the nodal and paranodal regions. Only a few myelin layers have been drawn for the sake of clarity. At the internodal region, the cross-section reveals the inner and outer mesaxons and their relationship to the inner cytoplasmic wedges and the outer loop of cytoplasm. Note that, in contrast to PNS myelin, there is no full ring of cytoplasm surrounding the outside of the sheath. The lower part of the figure shows roughly the dimensions and appearance of one myelin-repeating unit as seen with fixed and embedded preparations in the electron microscope. This is contrasted with the dimensions of the electron-density curve of CNS myelin obtained by X-ray diffraction studies in fresh nerve. The components responsible for the peaks and troughs of the curve are sketched below. (Modified from [4], with permission of Lea & Febiger, publishers.)

not actually fused since they can be resolved as a double line at high resolution (Figs. 4-6 and 4-7). The dark, or major period, line is the fused, inner protein coat of the cell membrane. The repeat distances observed by electron microscopy are less than those calculated from the low-angle X-ray diffraction data, a consequence of the considerable shrinkage that takes place after fixation and dehydration. However, the difference in pe-

riodicity between PNS and CNS myelin is maintained; peripheral myelin has an average repeat distance of 119 Å and central myelin, 107 Å.

Nodes of Ranvier.   Two adjacent segments of myelin on one axon are separated by a node of Ranvier. In this region, the axon is not covered by myelin. At the paranodal region and the Schmidt-Lantermann clefts, the cytoplasmic

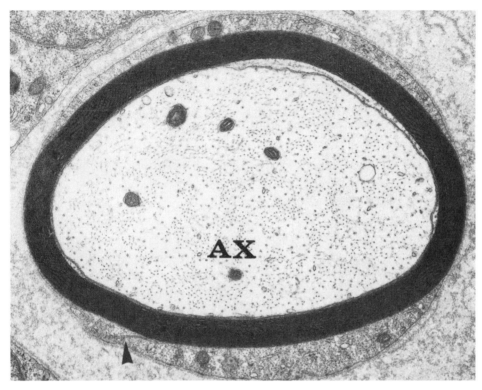

FIGURE 4-4.   Electron micrograph of a single peripheral nerve fiber from rabbit. Note that the myelin sheath has a lamellated structure and is surrounded by Schwann cell cytoplasm. The outer mesaxon *(arrowhead)* can be seen at the lower left. *AX,* axon. ×18,000. (Courtesy of Dr. Cedric Raine.)

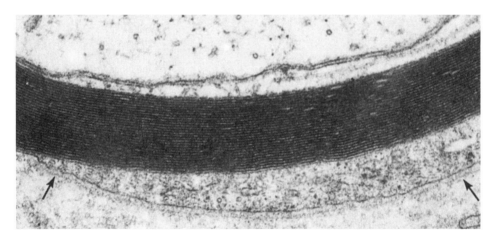

FIGURE 4-5.   Higher magnification of Figure 4-4 to show the Schwann cell cytoplasm covered by basal lamina *(arrows).* ×50,000.

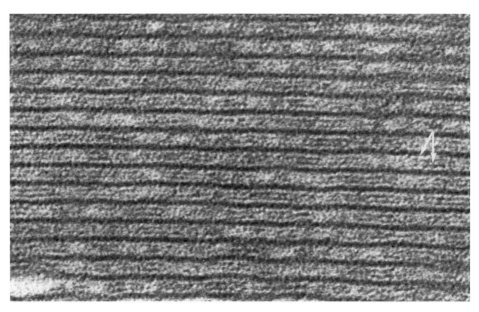

FIGURE 4-6.   Magnification of the myelin sheath of Figure 4-4. Note that the intraperiod line *(arrows)* at this high resolution is a double structure. ×350,000. (Courtesy of Dr. Cedric Raine.)

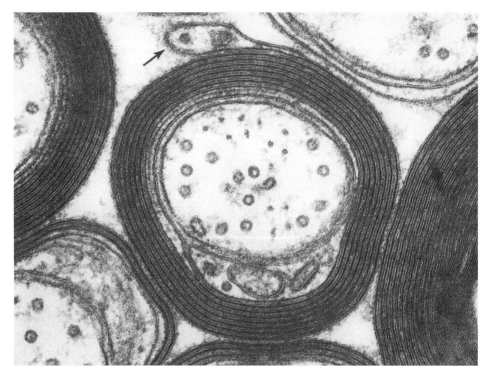

FIGURE 4-7.   A typical CNS myelinated fiber from the spinal cord of an adult dog. Contrast this figure with the PNS fiber in Figure 4-3. The course of the flattened oligodendrocytic process, beginning at the outer tongue *(arrow),* can be traced. Note that the fiber lacks investing cell cytoplasm and a basal lamina, as is the case in the PNS. The major dense line and the paler, double intraperiod line of the myelin sheath can be discerned. The axon contains neurotubules and neurofilaments. ×135,000.

surfaces of myelin are not compacted and
Schwann or glial cell cytoplasm is included
within the sheath. To visualize these structures,
one may refer to Figures 4-8 and 4-9, which
show that if myelin were unrolled from the axon,
it would be a flat, spade-shaped sheet surrounded by a tube of cytoplasm. Thus, as shown
in electron micrographs of longitudinal sections
of axon paranodal regions, the major dense line
formed by apposition of the cytoplasmic faces
opens up at the edges of the sheet, enclosing cytoplasm within a loop (see Figs. 4-3 and 4-9).
These loop-shaped terminations of the sheath at
the node are called *lateral loops*. The loops form
membrane complexes with the axolemma called
transverse bands, whereas myelin in the internodal region is separated from the axon by a gap
of *periaxonal* space. The transverse bands are helical structures that seal the myelin to the axolemma but provide, by spaces between them, a
tortuous path from the extracellular space to the
periaxonal space.

Schmidt-Lantermann clefts are structures
where the cytoplasmic surfaces of the myelin
sheath have not compacted to form the major
dense line and, instead, contain Schwann or
glial cell cytoplasm (Fig. 4-9). These regions
are common in peripheral myelinated axons
but rare in the CNS. These inclusions of cytoplasm are present in each layer of myelin. The
clefts can be visualized in the unrolled myelin
sheet as tubes of cytoplasm similar to the tubes
making up the lateral loops but in the middle
regions of the sheet, rather than at the edges
(Fig. 4-9).

Myelin is an extension of a cell membrane

In the PNS, myelination is preceded by invasion
of the nerve bundle by Schwann cells, rapid multiplication of these cells and segregation of the
individual axons by Schwann cell processes.
Smaller axons (≤1 μm), which will remain unmyelinated, are segregated; several may be enclosed in one cell, each within its own pocket,
similar to the structure shown in Figure 4-10A.
Large axons (≥1 μm) destined for myelination
are enclosed singly, one cell per axon per inter-

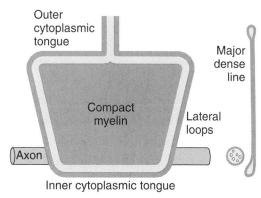

FIGURE 4-8.   A diagram showing the appearance of
CNS myelin if it were unrolled from the axon. One can visualize this structure arising from Figure 4-3 if the glial
cell process were pulled straight up and the myelin layers
separated at the intermediate period line. The whole
myelin internode forms a spade-shaped sheet surrounded by a continuous tube of oligodendroglial cell cytoplasm. This diagram shows that the lateral loops and
inner and outer cytoplasmic tongues are parts of the
same cytoplasmic tube. The drawing on the right shows
the appearance of this sheet if it were sectioned along
the vertical line, indicating that the compact myelin region is formed of two unit membranes fused at the cytoplasmic surfaces. The drawing is not necessarily to scale.
(Adapted from [6].)

node. These cells line up along the axons with intervals between them; the intervals become the
nodes of Ranvier.

Before myelination, the axon lies in an in-
vagination of the Schwann cell (Fig. 4-10A).
The plasmalemma of the cell then surrounds
the axon and joins to form a double-mem-
brane structure that communicates with the
cell surface. This structure, called the *mesaxon*,
elongates around the axon in a spiral fashion
(Fig. 4-10). Thus, formation of myelin topo-
logically resembles rolling up a sleeping bag;
the mesaxon winds about the axon, and the cytoplasmic surfaces condense into a compact
myelin sheath and form the major dense line.
The two external surfaces form the myelin intraperiod line.

In the CNS, the structures of myelin are
formed by the oligodendroglial cell [7]. This
has many similarities but also points of difference with respect to myelination in the PNS.
CNS nerve fibers are not separated by connective tissue, nor are they surrounded by cell cytoplasm, and specific glial nuclei are not obvi-

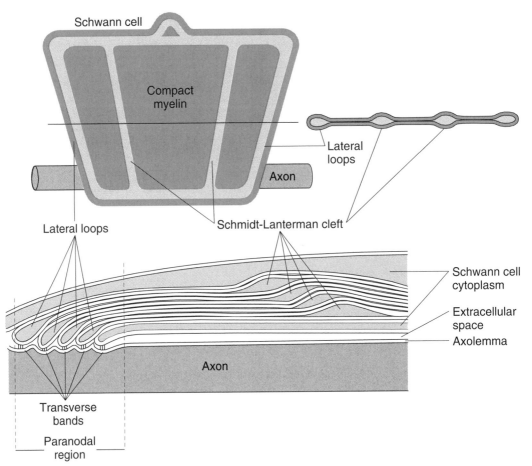

FIGURE 4-9.   A diagram similar to Figure 4-8 but showing one Schwann cell and its myelin sheath unrolled from a peripheral axon. The sheet of PNS myelin is, like CNS myelin, surrounded by a tube of cytoplasm and has additional tubes of cytoplasm, which make up the Schmidt-Lantermann clefts, running through the internodal regions. The horizontal section **(top right)** shows that these additional tubes of cytoplasm arise from regions where the cytoplasmic membrane surfaces have not fused. Diagram at **bottom** is an enlarged view of a portion of **top left,** with the Schwann cell and its membrane wrapped around the axon. The tube forming the lateral loops seals to the axolemma at the paranodal region, and the cytoplasmic tubes in the internodal region form the Schmidt-Lantermann clefts. These drawings are not to scale. (Adapted from [6].)

ously associated with particular myelinated fibers. CNS myelin is a spiral structure similar to PNS myelin; it has an inner mesaxon and an outer mesaxon that ends in a loop, or tongue, of glial cytoplasm (Fig. 4-3). Unlike the peripheral nerve, where the sheath is surrounded by Schwann cell cytoplasm, the cytoplasmic tongue in the CNS is restricted to a small portion of the sheath. This glial tongue is continuous with the plasma membrane of the oligodendroglial cell through slender processes. One glial cell can myelinate 40 or more separate axons [8].

Myelin deposition in the PNS may result in a single axon having up to 100 myelin layers; therefore, it is improbable that myelin is laid down by a simple rotation of the Schwann cell nucleus around the axon. In the CNS, such a postulate is precluded by the fact that one glial cell can myelinate several axons. During myelination, there are increases in the length of the internode, the diameter of the axon and the number of myelin layers. Myelin, therefore, expands in all planes at once. Any mechanism to account for this growth must assume that the membrane system is able to expand and contract and that layers slip over each other.

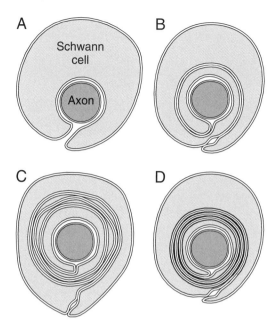

FIGURE 4-10. Myelin formation in the peripheral nervous system. **A:** The Schwann cell has surrounded the axon, but the external surfaces of the plasma membrane have not yet fused in the mesaxon. **B:** The mesaxon has fused into a five-layered structure and spiraled once around the axon. **C:** A few layers of myelin have formed but are not compacted completely. Note the cytoplasm trapped in zones where the cytoplasmic membrane surfaces have not yet fused. **D:** Compact myelin showing only a few layers for the sake of clarity. Note that Schwann cell cytoplasm forms a ring both inside and outside of the sheath. (Modified from [4]. With permission of Lea & Febiger, publishers.)

Myelin can be isolated in high yield and purity by conventional methods of subcellular fractionation

If CNS tissue is homogenized in media of low ionic strength, myelin peels off the axons and reforms in vesicles of the size range of nuclei and mitochondria. Because of their high lipid content, these myelin vesicles have the lowest intrinsic density of any membrane fraction of the nervous system. Procedures for isolation of myelin take advantage of both the large vesicle size and the low density [9].

In a widely used method, a homogenate of rodent nervous tissue, or dissected white matter in the case of larger animals, in isotonic sucrose (0.3 M) is layered directly onto 0.85 M sucrose and centrifuged at high speed. Mitochondria and synaptosomes sediment through the denser sucrose, and many of the smaller membrane fragments from other organelles remain in the 0.3 M sucrose layer. A crude myelin layer collects at the interface. The major impurities, microsomes and axoplasm trapped in the vesicles during the homogenization procedure are released by subjecting the myelin to osmotic shock in distilled water. The larger myelin particles can then be separated from the smaller, membranous material by low-speed centrifugation or by repeating the density gradient centrifugation on continuous or discontinuous gradients, usually of sucrose. Preparations of purified myelin can be subdivided further and arbitrarily into fractions of different densities by centrifugation on expanded continuous or discontinuous density gradients. These fractions differ somewhat in composition.

Demonstration of purity for a myelin preparation includes electron-microscopic appearance; however, the difficulty of identifying small membrane vesicles of microsomes in a field of myelin membranes and the well-known sampling problems inherent in electron microscopy make this characterization unreliable after a certain purity level has been reached.

Markers characteristic of myelin include certain proteins, lipids and enzymes described in the following sections. Although such assays are useful, like electron microscopy they are not sensitive to small amounts of impurities. If purity of a myelin preparation is an issue, it is important to assay contamination of myelin by other subcellular fractions using markers such as succinic dehydrogenase for mitochondria; Na,K-ATPase and 5′-nucleotidase for plasma membranes; NADH-cytochrome-C reductase for microsomes; DNA for nuclei; RNA for nuclei, ribosomes and microsomes; lactate dehydrogenase for cytosol; β-glucosidase for lysosomes; and acetylcholinesterase for neuronal fragments. Although all of these markers are low in purified myelin and set an outside limit for levels of contamination by other membranes, the actual contamination may be less than calculated by such methods since low levels of many different enzymes appear to be intrinsic to myelin.

Peripheral nerve myelin can be isolated by similar techniques, but especially vigorous homogenization conditions are required because of the large amounts of connective tissue and, sometimes, adipose tissue present in the nerve. The slightly lesser density of PNS myelin requires some adjustment of gradient composition to prevent loss of myelin.

CHARACTERISTIC COMPOSITION OF MYELIN

Myelin *in situ* has a water content of about 40%. The dry mass of both CNS and PNS myelin is characterized by a high proportion of lipid (70 to 85%) and, consequently, a low proportion of protein (15 to 30%). In contrast, most biological membranes have a higher ratio of proteins to lipids.

Central nervous system myelin is enriched in certain lipids

Table 4-1 lists the composition of bovine, rat and human myelin compared to bovine and human white matter, human gray matter and rat whole brain (see Chap. 3). All of the lipids assayed in whole brain are also present in myelin; that is, there are no lipids localized exclusively in some nonmyelin compartment, with the exception of

the mitochondria-specific lipid diphosphatidyl-glycerol, not included in the table. We also know that the reverse is true; that is, there are no myelin lipids that are not also found in other subcellular fractions of the brain.

Even though there are no absolutely "myelin-specific" lipids, cerebroside, also known as galactosylceramide, is the most typical of myelin. With the exception of early development, the concentration of cerebroside in brain is directly proportional to the amount of myelin present. As much as one-fifth of the total galactolipid in myelin occurs in the form of sulfatide, in which the 3-hydroxyl moiety on the galactose of cerebroside is sulfated. Because of the specificity and quantitative significance of galactocerebroside in oligodendrocytes and myelin, it has been assumed for decades that it is essential for oligodendroglial differentiation and the specialized structure and function of myelin. This dogma was overthrown by the creation of a knockout mouse lesioned in UDP-galactose:ceramide galactosyltransferase, the obligate terminal step in cerebroside biosynthesis, also required for sulfatide formation [10]. Surprisingly, the myelin formed appears relatively normal, although subtle differences in structure and

TABLE 4-1.   COMPOSITION OF CNS MYELIN AND BRAIN

Substance[a]	Myelin			White matter		Gray matter (human)	Whole brain (rat)
	Human	Bovine	Rat	Human	Bovine		
Protein	30.0	24.7	29.5	39.0	39.5	55.3	56.9
Lipid	70.0	75.3	70.5	54.9	55.0	32.7	37.0
Cholesterol	27.7	28.1	27.3	27.5	23.6	22.0	23.0
Cerebroside	22.7	24.0	23.7	19.8	22.5	5.4	14.6
Sulfatide	3.8	3.6	7.1	5.4	5.0	1.7	4.8
Total galactolipid	27.5	29.3	31.5	26.4	28.6	7.3	21.3
Ethanolamine phosphatides	15.6	17.4	16.7	14.9	13.6	22.7	19.8
Lecithin	11.2	10.9	11.3	12.8	12.9	26.7	22.0
Sphingomyelin	7.9	7.1	3.2	7.7	6.7	6.9	3.8
Phosphatidylserine	4.8	6.5	7.0	7.9	11.4	8.7	7.2
Phosphatidylinositol	0.6	0.8	1.2	0.9	0.9	2.7	2.4
Plasmalogens[b]	12.3	14.1	14.1	11.2	12.2	8.8	11.6
Total phospholipid	43.1	43.0	44.0	45.9	46.3	69.5	57.6

[a]Protein and lipid figures in percent dry weight; all others in percent total lipid weight.
[b]Plasmalogens are primarily ethanolamine phosphatides.

changes in axon conduction velocity can be demonstrated. With age, animals develop a progressive hindlimb paralysis and extensive vacuolation of myelin in the spinal cord. These findings indicate that cerebroside and/or sulfatide are not required for myelin formation but play important roles in its insulating capacity and stability.

In addition to cerebroside, the major lipids of myelin are cholesterol and ethanolamine-containing plasmalogens (see Chap. 3). Lecithin is also a major myelin constituent, and sphingomyelin is a relatively minor one. Not only is the lipid composition of myelin highly characteristic of this membrane, the fatty acid composition of many of the individual lipids is distinctive.

The data in Table 4-1 suggest that myelin accounts for much of the total lipid of white matter and that the lipid composition of gray matter is quite different from that of myelin. The composition of brain myelin from all mammalian species studied is very much the same. There are, however, some species differences; for example, myelin of rat has less sphingomyelin than bovine or human myelin (Table 4-1). Although not shown in the table, there are also regional variations; for example, myelin isolated from the spinal cord has a higher lipid-to-protein ratio than brain myelin from the same species.

Besides the lipids listed in Table 4-1, there are several others of importance. If myelin is not extracted with acidified organic solvents, the polyphosphoinositides (see Chap. 3) remain tightly bound to the myelin protein and, therefore, are not included in the lipid analysis. Triphosphoinositide accounts for between 4 and 6% of the total myelin phosphorus and diphosphoinositide for 1 to 1.5%.

Minor components of myelin include at least three fatty acid esters of cerebroside and two glycerol-based lipids, diacylglyceryl-galactoside and monoalkylmonoacylglycerylgalactoside, collectively called galactosyldiglyceride. Some long chain alkanes also appear to be present. Myelin from mammals contains 0.1 to 0.3% gangliosides, which are complex sialic acid-containing glycosphingolipids. The proportion of the different gangliosides to each other is different in myelin, which is greatly enriched in monosialoganglioside GM1 relative to other brain membranes, which are enriched in the polysialo species. Myelin from certain species, including human, contains an additional unique ganglioside as a major component, sialosylgalactosylceramide, GM4.

Peripheral and central nervous system myelin lipids are qualitatively similar

There are quantitative differences. PNS myelin has less cerebroside and sulfatide and considerably more sphingomyelin than CNS myelin. Of interest is the presence of ganglioside LM1, also termed sialosyl-lactoneotetraosylceramide, as a characteristic component of myelin in the PNS of some species. These differences in lipid composition between CNS and PNS myelin are not, however, as dramatic as the differences in protein composition discussed below.

Central nervous system myelin contains some unique proteins

The protein composition of CNS myelin is simpler than that of other brain membranes, with the proteolipid protein and basic protein(s) making up 60 to 80% of the total in most species. Many other proteins and glycoproteins are present to lesser extents. With the exception of the basic proteins, myelin proteins are neither easily extractable nor soluble in aqueous media. However, like other membrane proteins, they may be solubilized in sodium dodecylsulfate (SDS) solutions and, in this condition, separated readily by electrophoresis in polyacrylamide gels. This technique separates proteins primarily according to molecular weight. The presence of bound carbohydrates or unusual structural features somewhat disrupts the relationship between migration and molecular weight so that terminology for location of a protein in such a gel is taken to mean apparent molecular weight, which sometimes is written M_r for relative molecular mass. Protein compositions of human and rat brain myelin are illustrated in Figure 4-11B and D, respectively. The quantitative predominance of two proteins, the positively charged myelin

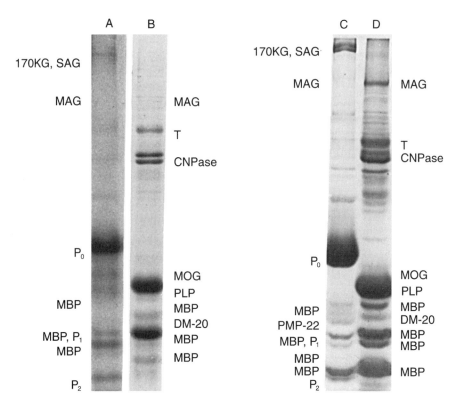

FIGURE 4-11. Polyacrylamide gel electrophoresis of myelin proteins in the presence of sodium dodecyl sulfate (SDS). The proteins of **A:** human PNS myelin, **B:** human CNS myelin, **C:** rat PNS myelin and **D:** rat CNS myelin were solubilized with the detergent SDS, electrophoresed and stained with Coomassie brilliant blue. The electrophoretic system separates proteins primarily according to their molecular size, with the smallest proteins migrating the farthest toward the bottom of the gel. The three myelin basic protein *(MBP)* bands in lanes **A** and **B** are the 17.2-, 18.5- and 21.5-kDa isoforms generated by alternative splicing of the mRNA in humans, and the four MBP bands in lanes **C** and **D** are the 14.0-, 17.0-, 18.5- and 21.5-kDa isoforms generated in rats (see Fig. 4-12). The 18.5-kDa MBP also is called P_1 in the terminology for the PNS. The 26-kDa myelin-oligodendrocyte glycoprotein *(MOG)* is probably the faint band just above proteolipid protein *(PLP)*, which is most apparent in lane **D.** 2':3'-Cyclic nucleotide-3'-phosphodiesterase *(CNPase)* electrophoresis is a tight doublet, and the lower and upper bands are sometimes referred to as CNP1 and CNP2, respectively. *T,* tubulin; PMP-22, peripheral-myelin-protein-22. Note that the location shown for myelin-associated glycoprotein *(MAG)*, which stains too faintly to be seen well on the gels, is just above a discrete Coomassie blue-stained band in lane **D,** which is probably the 96-kDa subunit of Na$^+$, K$^+$-ATPase. The 170-kDa glycoprotein in PNS myelin is labeled both as 170KG and SAG for the name of Schwann cell membrane glycoprotein (see text).

basic protein (MBP) and proteolipid protein (PLP), in the gel pattern of human CNS myelin is clear. These proteins are major constituents of all mammalian CNS myelins, and similar proteins are present in myelins of many lower species.

Proteolipid protein. Myelin PLP, also known as the Folch-Lees protein [11], has the unusual physical property of solubility in organic solvents. The molecular weight of PLP from sequence analysis is about 30,000, although it migrates anomalously fast on SDS gels. The amino acid sequence, strongly conserved during evolution, contains several membrane-spanning domains. PLP contains about 3 moles of fatty acids, primarily palmitate, oleate or stearate, per mole protein in ester linkage to hydroxy amino acids. There is rapid turnover of the fatty acids independent of the peptide backbone [12].

In addition to PLP, myelin of the CNS has lesser quantities of a related protein, DM-20, named for its M_r of 20,000. This protein is coded by an alternative splicing of the RNA, which gives rise to the major PLP. Both DNA and protein-sequencing data indicate that the structure of DM-20 is related to that of PLP by a deletion of 35 amino acids [13,14]. DM-20-related message appears earlier than PLP during development, even before myelin formation in some cases; and it might have a role in oligodendrocyte differentiation in addition to a structural role in myelin. The PLP and DM-20 proteins may be evolved from an ancestral gene encoding a pore-forming polypeptide [15], lending support to the hypothesis that myelin may be involved in ion movement. Although PLP and DM-20 serve important functions, they are not essential. Contrary to the general expectation that PLP would be needed for formation of compact, multilamellar myelin, a knockout mouse for PLP/DM-20 [16] is relatively normal with respect to myelin formation, although there is a difference at the level of the intraperiod line. In this knockout mouse, life span and sophisticated motor performance also are affected. In contrast, a variety of naturally occurring mutations in PLP (see Chap. 39) or overexpression of normal PLP [17] have severe functional consequences, apparently due to cellular toxicity of mutated forms of the protein or even just excess amounts of normal PLP. A curiosity is that, although significant amounts of PLP and DM-20 are restricted to the CNS, mRNA for PLP is expressed in the PNS and small amounts of protein are synthesized but not incorporated into myelin in appreciable amounts.

Myelin basic protein has long been of interest because it is the antigen that, when injected into an animal, elicits a cellular immune response that produces the CNS autoimmune disease *experimental allergic encephalomyelitis* (EAE) (see Chap. 39). MBP can be extracted from myelin as well as from white matter with either dilute acid or salt solutions; once extracted, it is very soluble in water. The amino acid sequence of the major basic protein is similar in a number of species [11]. These proteins have molecular weights of around 18,500; they are highly unfolded, with essentially no tertiary structure in solution. This basic protein shows microheterogeneity upon electrophoresis in alkaline conditions, due to a combination of phosphorylation, loss of the C-terminal arginine and deamidation. There is also heterogeneity in the degree of methylation of an arginine at residue 106. MBP is located on the cytoplasmic face of the myelin membranes corresponding to the major dense line. The rapid turnover of the phosphate groups present on many of the MBP molecules [18,19] suggests this post-translational modification might influence the close apposition of the cytoplasmic faces of the membrane. It also has been speculated that phosphorylation may modify this process in a dynamic manner. Of interest is that mRNA coding for MBP is preferentially localized far from the cell perikaryon, in the region where myelin compaction is taking place [20].

In addition to the major MBP, most species of mammals that have been studied contain various amounts of other basic proteins related to it in sequence. Mice and rats have a second smaller MBP of 14-kDa. The small MBP has the same N- and C-terminal sequences as the larger MBP but differs by a deletion of 40 residues. The ratio of these two basic proteins to each other changes during development: mature rats and mice have more of the 14-kDa protein than of the 18-kDa protein. Two other MBPs seen in many species have molecular weights of 21,500 and 17,000, respectively. These two proteins are related structurally to the large and small basic proteins, respectively, by the addition of a polypeptide sequence of M_r ~3,000 near the amino-terminal end of the protein. Another basic protein, present to some extent in humans, has a molecular weight of 17,200 and is now known to be slightly different from the 17-kDa protein in other species. The different MBPs arise from alternative splicing of a common mRNA precursor. A diagrammatic representation of some of these alternative splicing schemes is presented in Figure 4-12. The physiological significance of the heterogeneity of MBPs is an open question. It is relevant that the exons which can be combined to make the various myelin basic proteins are also part of a larger set of exons of a gene, *GOLLI*. Transcripts of this gene are expressed as Golli proteins, which contain MBP sequences as well as unique peptide sequences, during early development and in various neural cell types, including neurons [22].

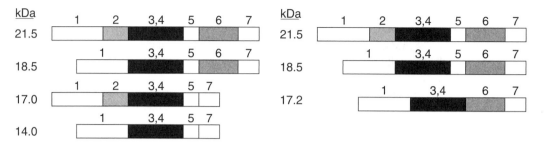

FIGURE 4-12. The amino acid sequences corresponding to the various mouse myelin basic proteins (MBPs) are encoded in a gene containing at least seven exons (separated by introns, DNA regions whose base sequence does not code directly for proteins). The precursor RNA transcribed from this gene can be spliced to give a message containing all seven exons; this message codes for the 21.5-kDa MBP. Alternative splicings result in messenger RNA species with deletions of exons 2 and/or 6, which code for the other MBPs. The exons forming the various mouse messenger species are indicated **above, left.** The corresponding gene in humans also contains seven exons, which have minor base changes relative to the corresponding mouse sequences. Messenger RNA species derived from the human genome are indicated **above, right.** Messengers for the 21.5kDa and 18.5-kDa MBPs are formed in a manner analogous to that of the corresponding mouse proteins. Note, however, that the 17-kDa human protein contains a slightly different exon complement from the 17-kDa mouse MBP. (Adapted from Kamholz et al. [21].)

2′:3′-Cyclic nucleotide-3′-phosphodiesterase. There are many higher molecular weight proteins present in the gel-electrophoretic pattern of myelin. These vary in amount depending on species; for example, mouse and rat may have as much as 30% of the total myelin protein in this category. These proteins also vary depending on the degree of maturity, such that the younger the animal, the less myelin but the greater the proportion of higher molecular weight proteins. A double band with M_r ~50,000 is present in myelin from most species. It has been identified with an enzyme activity, 2′:3′-cyclic nucleotide-3′-phosphodiesterase (CNP), which comprises several percent of myelin protein [23]. Although there are low levels of this enzymatic activity associated with the surface membrane of many different types of cell, it is much enriched in myelin and in cells committed to the formation of myelin. The enzyme is extremely active against 2′,3′-cAMP, as well as the cGMP, cyclic cytidine monophosphate (cCMP) and cyclic uridine monophosphate (cUMP) analogs, all of which are hydrolyzed to the corresponding 2′-isomer. This is probably an artifactual activity; recall that the biologically active cyclic nucleotides are those with a 3′:5′ structure. The amino acid sequence is relatively conserved in different species. In mice, the two CNP polypeptides are generated by alternative splicing of the mRNA,

with the larger polypeptide having an extra 20 amino acids at the N-terminus.

CNP is not a major component of compact myelin but is concentrated in specific regions of the myelin sheaths associated with cytoplasm, such as the oligodendroglial processes, inner and outer tongue processes and lateral loops. The biological function of CNP is not known, but it is of interest that it contains a consensus sequence found in G proteins. It also has been proposed, in part because of its isoprenylation, that CNP plays a role in events involving the cytoskeletal network of myelin [24]. Examination of aberrant myelination occurring in transgenic mice overexpressing CNP suggests that it is an early regulator of cellular events that culminate in CNS myelination [25].

Myelin-associated glycoprotein and other glycoproteins of CNS myelin. The myelin-associated glycoprotein (MAG) is a quantitatively minor, 100-kDa glycoprotein in purified myelin [26] that electrophoreses at the position shown in Figure 4-11. However, because it is less than 1% of total protein and stains weakly with Coomassie blue, it does not correspond to one of the discrete protein bands visible in the figure. MAG has a single transmembrane domain that separates a heavily glycosylated extracellular part of the molecule, composed of five immunoglobulin-like domains and eight or nine sites for *N*-linked glycosylation,

from an intracellular carboxy-terminal domain. Its overall structure is similar to that of neural cell adhesion molecule (NCAM). MAG in rodents occurs in two developmentally regulated isoforms, which differ in their cytoplasmic domains and are generated by alternative splicing of mRNA. The isoform with a longer C-terminal tail (L-MAG) is predominant early in development during active myelination of the CNS, whereas the isoform with a shorter cytoplasmic tail (S-MAG) increases during development to become prominent in adult rodents. These cytoplasmic domains are phosphorylated on serine and threonine residues by protein kinase C, and L-MAG is phosphorylated also on tyrosine-620.

MAG is not present in compact, multilamellar myelin but is located exclusively in the periaxonal oligodendroglial membranes of CNS myelin sheaths. Both its location next to the axon and its membership in the immunoglobulin superfamily (see Chap. 7) suggest that it functions in adhesion and signaling between myelin-forming oligodendrocytes and the axolemma. MAG is a member of the I-type lectin subfamily of the immunoglobulin superfamily and binds to glycoproteins and gangliosides with terminal 2–3-linked sialic acid moieties. Thus, the axolemmal ligand(s) for MAG is probably a sialoglycoconjugate, but the identity of its physiological receptor is unknown. Furthermore, MAG may bind to other components on the axolemma by different mechanisms. A relationship of MAG to other adhesion proteins also is demonstrated by the presence in most species of a sulfate-containing carbohydrate HNK-1 epitope, which is expressed on a large number of neural adhesion proteins, including NCAM and MAG, and functions in cell–cell interactions. As with other proteins in the immunoglobulin superfamily, it is likely that the interaction of MAG with its ligand(s) on the axolemma mediates cell–cell signaling by mechanisms involving phosphorylation [19,26]. For example, the cytoplasmic domain of MAG interacts with *fyn* tyrosine kinase and phospholipase Cγ by mechanisms that appear to involve phosphorylated amino acids on MAG.

Although MAG is presumed to function in important signaling mechanisms between axons and oligodendrocytes during myelin formation, there may be some redundancy involved since young MAG knockout mice myelinate relatively normally and exhibit only subtle periaxonal structural abnormalities. However, as the null mutants age to 8 to 10 months, they develop a dying-back oligodendrogliopathy [27] and a peripheral neuropathy affecting both myelin and axons, suggesting that the most critical functions of MAG may be for maintenance of axon–myelin complexes. Also, although MAG generally has been thought to function in axon-to-glia signaling, the neuronal abnormalities found in aging MAG-null mutants suggest that it may also function in glia-to-axon signaling [26]. Furthermore, MAG is one of the factors in CNS white matter that inhibits neurite outgrowth in tissue culture [26]. Whatever the possible physiological implications of this for neuronal regeneration *in vivo* following injury, the findings are consistent with a MAG-mediated signaling mechanism from glia to axons that can affect the properties of neurons.

There are a large number of other glycoproteins associated with white matter and myelin, many of which have not yet been studied well. However, in addition to MAG, a few have been cloned and partially characterized. One of these is a minor protein of 26 kDa called the myelin-oligodendrocyte glycoprotein (MOG) [28]. MOG also is a transmembrane glycoprotein, contains a single immunoglobulin-like domain and one site for N-linked glycosylation and expresses the adhesion-related HNK-1 epitope. Unlike MAG, which is sequestered at the interior of myelin sheaths, MOG is localized on the surface of myelin sheaths and oligodendrocytes. Because of its surface location, it may function in transmitting extracellular information to the interior of oligodendrocytes and has been implicated as a target antigen in autoimmune aspects of demyelinating diseases of the CNS (see Chap. 39).

There is also a 120-kDa glycosylated protein in white matter called the oligodendrocyte-myelin glycoprotein [29]. This glycoprotein is membrane-bound through a phosphatidylinositol linkage and characterized by a cysteine-rich motif at the N-terminus and a series of tandem leucine-rich repeats. Unlike MAG and MOG, it is not a member of the immunoglobulin superfamily but does express the HNK-1 carbohydrate epitope. The leucine-rich repeats and adhesion-related HNK-1 epitope suggest that it also may function in cell–cell interactions.

Small amounts of proteins characteristic of membranes in general can be identified on gels of myelin proteins. Noted in Figure 4-11 is tubulin; although this may be present because of contamination of myelin preparation by other membranes, there is evidence suggesting that it is an authentic myelin component. High-resolution electrophoretic techniques demonstrate the presence of other minor protein bands; these may relate to the presence of numerous enzyme activities associated with the myelin sheath (see below).

Peripheral myelin contains some unique proteins and some shared with central nervous system myelin

P_0 is the major PNS myelin protein. Gel-electrophoretic analysis (Fig. 4-11A,C) shows that a single protein, of 30 kDa, P_0 accounts for more than half of the PNS myelin protein. The cloning and sequencing of the message for this protein [30,31] led to derivation of amino acid sequences from several species. From this, it has been deduced that the protein has about 220 amino acids with an intracellular domain, a hydrophobic transmembrane domain and a single extracellular immunoglobulin-like domain. The amino-terminal extracellular domain includes a signal sequence for insertion of protein into the membrane and a glycosylation site. In addition to the well-characterized carbohydrate chain, other post-translational modifications include sulfation, phosphorylation and acylation.

It is interesting to note that PLP and P_0 protein, although different in sequence, post-translational modifications and structure, may have similar roles in the formation of structures as closely related as myelins of the CNS and PNS. These proteins are not mutually exclusive; they are coexpressed in certain fish and amphibians [32]. Transfection of non-neural cells with the P_0 gene results in cell–cell interaction, which can be demonstrated to be due to homophilic interactions of the extracellular domains of P_0 [33,34]. Elucidation of the crystal structure of the extracellular domain of P_0 shows tetrameric

packing of P_0 molecules, suggesting that the extracellular domains of P_0 project from the myelin membrane surface as tetramers [35]. The complete knockout of P_0 has profound consequences on myelin structure and function [36], in contradistinction to the previously noted, relatively benign consequences for CNS in animals with a deletion of the PLP gene.

Myelin basic protein content in the PNS varies from approximately 5 to 18% of total protein, in contrast to the CNS, where it is on the order of 30%. In rodents, the same four MBPs found in the CNS are present in the PNS, with molecular weights of 21,000, 18,500, 17,000 and 14,000 respectively. In adult rodents, the 14-kDa MBP is the most prominent component and is termed "P_r" in the PNS nomenclature. The 18-kDa component is present and often is referred to as the P_1 protein in the nomenclature of peripheral myelin proteins. Another species-specific variation occurs in humans. In human PNS, the major basic protein is not the 18.5-kDa form, which is most prominent in the CNS, but rather the 17.2-kDa form [11]. MBP may not play as critical a role in myelin structure in the PNS as it does in the CNS. The murine mutant *Shiverer* is lesioned with respect to MBP synthesis. CNS myelin has no dense line structure; this contrasts to the PNS, which has almost normal myelin amount and structure but lacks MBP.

PNS myelin contains another positively charged protein, referred to as P_2, with M_r ~15,000. It is unrelated in sequence to either P_1 or P_r but shows strong homology to a family of cytoplasmic lipid-binding proteins that are present in a variety of cell types [37]. This suggests the possibility of P_2 protein involvement in lipid assembly or turnover within the myelin sheath. The amount of P_2 protein is highly variable from species to species, accounting for about 15% of total protein in bovine PNS myelin, 5% in humans and less than 1% in rodents. Within a species, P_2 is more prominent in the thicker myelin sheaths. P_2 protein generally is considered in the context of PNS myelin proteins, but it is expressed in small amounts of CNS myelin sheaths of some species. P_2 is an antigen for experimental allergic neuritis (EAN), the PNS counterpart of EAE (see Chap. 39). P_2 appears to be present in the major dense line of myelin sheaths, where it may play a structural role similar to MBP, and there appears to be substantially more P_2 in large sheaths than small ones. The large variation in the amount and distribution of the protein from species to species and sheath to sheath raises questions about its function. Its similarities to cytoplasmic proteins, whose functions appear to involve solubilization and transport of fatty acids and retinoids, suggest that it might function similarly in myelination; but there is currently no experimental evidence to support this hypothesis.

Other glycoproteins of PNS myelin. In addition to the major P_0 glycoprotein, compact PNS myelin contains a 22-kDa glycoprotein called peripheral myelin protein-22 (PMP-22) [38], which accounts for less than 5% of the total protein (Fig. 4-11C). PMP-22 has four potential transmembrane domains and a single site for *N*-linked glycosylation. It is referred to as a *growth arrest protein* because its cDNA was cloned from nondividing fibroblasts and the synthesis of PMP-22 and other myelin proteins ceases when Schwann cells begin to proliferate following nerve transection. Since it is quantitatively a rather minor component, it may perform some unknown dynamic function in myelin assembly or maintenance rather than a major structural role. Its putative tetraspan structure is similar to that of PLP, suggesting that its role might be one of the functions of PLP in CNS myelin. Also, as is the case with PLP, any significant deviation in gene dosage for PMP-22 or disruption caused by point mutations has severe functional consequences [39]. Abnormalities of the PMP-22 gene are responsible for the *trembler* murine mutant and several inherited human neuropathies (see Chap. 39).

Similarly to the CNS, MAG is present in the periaxonal membranes of the myelin-forming Schwann cells, but it is also present in the Schwann cell membranes constituting the Schmidt-Lentermann incisures, paranodal loops and outer mesaxon [26]. All of these locations are characterized by 12- to 14-nm spacing between the extracellular surfaces of adjacent membranes and the presence of cytoplasm on the inner side of the membranes. Therefore, in addition to a role in Schwann cell–axon interactions in the PNS, MAG may function in interactions between adjacent Schwann cell membranes at the other locations. Both isoforms of MAG are present in the PNS of rodents, although S-MAG is the predominant isoform at all ages. As mentioned earlier, the peripheral neuropathy affecting both myelin and axons that develop in aging MAG knockout mice suggests that MAG-mediated signaling from axons to Schwann cells, and *vice versa* may be important for the maintenance of myelin–axon complexes. Clinical interest in PNS MAG derives from the demonstration that human IgM monoclonal antibodies in patients with neuropathy in association with gammopathy react with a carbohydrate structure in MAG that is very similar to the adhesion-related HNK-1 carbohydrate epitope (see Chap. 39).

PNS myelin also contains a glycoprotein of 170 kDa that accounts for about 5% of the total myelin protein and appears to be the same as a protein that was characterized further and called the Schwann cell membrane glycoprotein (SAG) [40]. It appears to be expressed in locations distinct from compact myelin by both myelinating and nonmyelinating Schwann cells, but very little is known about its structure and function at this time. In addition, avian Schwann cells contain a glycoprotein with relatively high amino acid sequence homology to MAG, the Schwann cell myelin protein (SMP) [26]. Although it is not thought to be the avian homolog of MAG because of differences in its pattern of expression and less than expected sequence homology, the structural and functional relationships between SMP and MAG remain to be established.

Myelin contains enzymes that function in metabolism and possibly ion transport

Several decades ago, it was generally believed that myelin was an inert membrane that did not carry out any biochemical functions. More recently, however, a large number of enzymes have been discovered in myelin [41]. These findings imply that myelin is metabolically active in synthesis, processing and metabolic turnover of some of its own components. Additionally, it may play an active role in ion transport with respect to not only maintenance of its own structure but also participation in buffering of ion levels in the vicinity of the axon.

A few enzymes, such as the previously mentioned CNP, are believed to be fairly myelin-specific, although they are probably also present in oligodendroglial membranes. CNP is very low in peripheral nerve and PNS myelin, suggesting some function more specialized to the CNS. A pH 7.2 cholesterol ester hydrolase also may be relatively myelin-specific, although the enzyme is prominent in myelin. N-Acetyl-L-aspartate aminohydroxylase, an enzyme operating on a substrate of unknown metabolic significance, also is enriched in myelin.

There are many enzymes that are not myelin-specific but appear to be intrinsic to myelin and not contaminants. Several proteolytic activities have been identified in purified myelin; the presence of neutral protease activity is well documented. The presence in myelin of cAMP-stimulated kinase, calcium/calmodulin-dependent kinase and protein kinase C activities has been reported. Phosphoprotein phosphatases are also present. Protein kinase C and phosphatase activities are presumed to be responsible for the rapid turnover of phosphate groups of MBP. Enzyme activity for acylation of PLP is also intrinsic to myelin.

Enzymes involved in the metabolism of structural lipids include a number of steroid-modifying and cholesterol-esterifying enzymes, UDP-galactose:ceramide galactosyltransferase and many enzymes of glycerophospholipid metabolism (see Chap. 3). The latter grouping includes all of the enzymes necessary for phosphatidyl ethanolamine synthesis from diradyl-*sn*-glycerol and ethanolamine; it is likely that phosphatidylcholine also can be synthesized within myelin. Perhaps even more elemental building blocks can be assembled into lipids by myelin enzymes. Acyl-CoA synthetase is present in myelin, suggesting the capacity to integrate free fatty acids into myelin lipids. The extent of the contribution of these enzymes in myelin, relative to enzymes within the oligodendroglial perikaryon, to metabolism of myelin lipids is not known.

Other enzymes present in myelin include those involved in phosphoinositide metabolism: phosphatidylinositol kinase, diphosphoinositide kinase, the corresponding phosphatases and diglyceride kinases. These are of interest because of the high concentration of polyphosphoinositides of myelin and the rapid turnover of their phosphate groups. This area of research has expanded toward characterization of a signal-transduction system(s). There is evidence for the presence in myelin of muscarinic cholinergic receptors, G proteins, phospholipases C and D and protein kinase C.

Certain enzymes present in myelin could be involved in ion transport. Carbonic anhydrase generally has been considered a soluble enzyme and a glial marker, but myelin accounts for a large part of the membrane-bound form in brain. This enzyme may play a role in removal of carbonic acid from metabolically active axons. The enzymes 5′-nucleotidase and Na,K-ATPase have long been considered specific markers for plasma membranes and are found in myelin at low concentrations. The 5′-nucleotidase activity may be related to a transport mechanism for adenosine, and Na,K-ATPase could function in transport of monovalent cations. The presence of these enzymes suggests that myelin may have an active role in transport of material in and out of the axon. In connection with this hypothesis, it is of interest that the PLP gene family may have evolved from a pore-forming polypeptide [15]. K^+ channels in myelin vesicles also have been described [42]. An isoform of glutathione-S-transferase is present in myelin and may be involved in transport of certain larger molecules.

DEVELOPMENTAL BIOLOGY OF MYELIN

Myelination follows the order of phylogenetic development

As the nervous system matures, portions of the PNS myelinate first, then the spinal cord and the brain last. In all parts of the nervous system, there are many small fibers that never myelinate. Even within the brain, different areas myelinate at different rates, the intracortical association areas being the last to do so. In humans, the motor roots begin to myelinate in the fifth fetal month, and the brain is almost completely myelinated by the end of the second year of life.

It is generally true that pathways in the nervous system become myelinated before they become completely functional. A relevant observation is that the CNS of rats and other nest-building animals myelinates largely postnatally, and the animals are quite helpless at birth. Grazing animals, such as horses, cows and sheep, have considerably more myelin in the CNS at birth and correspondingly a much higher level of complex activity immediately postnatally. Despite the attractiveness of the hypothesis that myelination is the terminal step in preparing a nervous system pathway for function, it should be noted that the period of maximal myelination coincides with many other changes in the nervous system.

Although it is easy to ascertain when myelination begins, it is difficult to determine when the process of accumulation stops. In the rat, myelin is still being deposited in the brain well past one year of age and possibly longer. The rat, however, continues to grow in body size and brain weight for most of its life span, and such a prolonged period of myelination may not occur in all species. Even in the human, myelination continues in the neocortex at least through the end of the second decade.

The composition of myelin changes during development

Nervous system development is marked by several overlapping periods, each defined by one major event in brain growth and structural maturation. In the rat CNS, there is considerable development postnatally and the maximal rate of cellular proliferation, much of which involves oligodendroglial precursor cells, occurs at 10 days. The rat brain begins to form myelin postnatally at about 10 to 12 days. Although the maximal rate of accumulation of myelin in the rat is at about 20 days of age, myelin accumulation continues at a decreasing rate throughout adulthood. At 6 months of age, 60 mg of myelin can be isolated from one brain. This represents an increase of about 1,500% over the 4 mg of myelin content of the brains of 15-day-old animals. During the same 5.5-month period, the brain weight increases by only 50 to 60%.

The myelin that is deposited first has a different composition from that of the adult [9]. As the rat matures, myelin galactolipids increase by about 50% and lecithin decreases by a similar amount. Similar changes are seen in human myelin. The very small amount of desmosterol declines, but the other lipids remain relatively constant. In addition, the polysialogangliosides decrease and the monosialoganglioside GM1 increases to become the predominant ganglioside. These changes are not complete until the rat is about 2 months old. Both basic protein and PLP increase in the myelin sheath during development, whereas the amount of higher molecular weight protein decreases.

Myelin subfractions may represent transitional forms of myelin

The studies summarized above on the composition of myelin from immature brains are consistent with the idea that myelin first laid down by the oligodendroglial cell may represent a transitional form with properties intermediate between those of mature compact myelin and the oligodendroglial cell membrane. As mentioned earlier, in the section on isolation, myelin can be separated into subfractions of different densities; in young animals depositing myelin, the dense fractions are prominent. The lighter fractions are enriched in multilamellar myelin, whereas the denser fractions contain a large proportion of single-membrane vesicles that resemble microsomes or plasma membrane fragments. Generally speaking, as one goes from light myelin fractions to heavier, the lipid-to-protein ratio decreases; the amount of basic protein decreases; the amount of MAG and of unidentified high-molecular-weight proteins increases; CNP, carbonic anhydrase and other enzymes increase; and the amount of PLP stays relatively constant. Metabolic studies described later lend support to the view that the dense fractions represent transitional forms.

SYNTHESIS AND METABOLISM OF MYELIN

Synthesis of myelin components is rapid during deposition of myelin

A remarkable amount of synthetic work is done by the oligodendroglial cell during the period of maximal myelination. Myelin accumulates in a 20-day-old rat brain at a rate of about 3.5 mg per day. Rough calculations show that there are about 20×10^6 oligodendroglia in such a brain, with each cell body having a dry weight of about 50×10^{-9} mg. Thus, on average, each cell makes about 175×10^{-9} mg of myelin per day, more than three times the weight of the perikaryon. Rates of myelin accumulation increase rapidly prior to this peak and decrease considerably afterward.

Myelin synthesis can be measured by studying the activity *in vitro* of enzymes involved in the synthesis of specific myelin components, by measuring incorporation *in vivo* of labeled precursors into myelin components and by carrying out similar studies using tissue slices. For example, the activity of UDP-galactose:ceramide galactosyltransferase, which is the enzyme that catalyzes the last step of cerebroside synthesis, in mouse brain microsomes increases fourfold from 10 days to a peak activity at 20 days, just preceding the age of maximal rate of myelin accumulation. It then gradually declines, paralleling the declining rate of myelination. The synthesis of glucocerebroside, which is not a myelin lipid, follows a completely different developmental pattern. Many other enzymes involved in the synthesis of lipids represented in myelin show increases during the period of rapid myelination.

In vivo studies using radioactive precursors generally furnish results similar to those of the enzyme assays *in vitro*. Incorporation of precursor into myelin-specific lipids is greatest if the injection of precursor is at the time of the greatest myelin accumulation, which is around 20 days in the rat, and decreases at earlier or later ages. Similar results are obtained when radioactive precursors, such as acetate for lipids or leucine for proteins, are presented to brain and spinal cord slices. Incorporation of radioactive precursors into myelin is greatest when slices are obtained from rats at about 20 days of age.

Sorting and transport of lipids and proteins take place during myelin assembly

After myelin components have been synthesized, they have to be assembled to form the membrane. Following intracranial injection of a radioactive amino acid or application of a labeled precursor to tissue slices, radioactive basic protein is synthesized and integrated into myelin very rapidly, with a lag time of only a few minutes [43]. In contrast, substantial amounts of radioactive PLPs are not found in myelin until after about 45 min. Thus, following synthesis, PLP enters a pool that is on its way to being integrated into myelin; in contrast, basic protein is incorporated into myelin as soon as it is made. This interpretation is compatible with the demonstration that PLP is synthesized on bound polysomes in the perikaryon. Presumably, the pool of PLP consists of membranous vesicles, including those involving the endoplasmic reticulum and Golgi membrane, on their way to the myelin being formed at the end of the oligodendroglial cell processes. In contrast, MBP is synthesized on free polysomes, which are associated with or in very close proximity to the myelin sheath [20]. Another difference in the processing of the two proteins during myelin assembly is that, following a pulse of incorporation of radioactive amino acids into newly synthesized protein, radioactive MBP appears more or less simultaneously in myelin subfractions of different densities. In contrast, PLP appears first in the densest myelin fractions and later in lighter, or more mature, myelin fractions in a manner which suggests a precursor–product relationship. Metabolic experiments suggest that MAG resembles PLP, while other high-molecular-weight proteins resemble basic protein, with respect to the kinetics of entry into myelin. Different classes of lipid show similar heterogeneity with respect to processing on the way to form myelin. The large and small MAG isoforms also sort differentially, possibly related to performance of different functions [44].

The available information is not yet sufficient to provide a detailed model of membrane assembly, but a general picture emerges. Many high-molecular-weight proteins are present in a lipid-poor precursor oligodendroglial cell membrane, with all of the PLP and some basic protein added during the early stages of myelin formation. More of the basic protein and other high-molecular-weight proteins are added at later states of transition. Addition of PLP might be a rate-limiting step in myelin formation. The bulk of the lipids are added at later stages of myelin assembly, and their entry is directed by the proteins already present.

Myelin components exhibit great heterogeneity of metabolic turnover

A standard type of experiment to determine lipid turnover is to inject a radioactive metabolic precursor into rat brains and then, after sufficient time to allow for incorporation, to follow loss of radioactivity from individual lipids as a function of time. Structural lipid components of myelin, notably cholesterol, cerebroside and sulfatide, are relatively stable metabolically, with half-lives on the order of many months. Phospholipids of myelin are more metabolically active, but even so, any given phospholipid turns over more slowly in myelin than in total membrane fraction or microsomes from whole brain.

For many lipids, the relationship between loss of radioactivity, usually referred to as apparent half-life, and the real rate of degradation is complicated by reutilization. For example, radioactive acetate is incorporated into fatty acids, which are processed further to become part of glycerolipid molecules. At some future time, when these lipids are degraded, the fatty acid can, to a large extent, be reutilized for synthesis of new lipids. In contrast, radioactive glycerol also is incorporated into glycerolipids, but upon degradation, the glycerol moiety is metabolized preferentially rather than being reutilized for biosynthesis. The apparent half-life of phosphatidylcholine varies depending on whether the molecule is labeled with radioactive phosphate, acetate, choline or glycerol, the latter precursor yielding the shortest and presumably most accurate estimate. Even within a phospholipid class, turnover of the glycerol backbone is influenced greatly by the fatty acid composition of the lipid [45].

A further complication is that the metabolic turnover of individual myelin components is multiphasic; that is, at least two turnover rates can be measured. When young animals incorporate radioactive precursors, a significant percentage of the total incorporated label is still present in phospholipids some months later. One of several possible interpretations of these data is on the basis of morphology, the more stable metabolic pool consisting of deeper layers of myelin that may be less accessible for metabolic turnover. Much of the myelin deposited in young animals during the period of rapid myelin accumulation is transferred rapidly to the metabolically stable pool. Some of the newly formed myelin may remain in outer layers and stay accessible for whatever mechanisms are involved in catabolism, thus accounting for the rapid turnover of this pool. In contrast, in older animals, radioactive precursors are incorporated less efficiently because myelin accumulates less rapidly and the label incorporated into phospholipids turns over rapidly; because of the slow rate of myelin accumulation, newly synthesized phospholipid remains for a longer time in the metabolically active compartment.

The overall picture appears to be that myelin glycerophospholipids have metabolic half-lives on the order of one week or less for the fast phase of turnover and on the order of one month for the slower phase of turnover. If radioactive precursors other than glycerol are utilized, the apparent half-life of a given lipid is longer and in the case of precursors which label fatty acyl moieties up to several times longer. Plasmalogens are unusual in their metabolism in that the hydrophilic moieties, that is, the acyl chain and vinyl ether chain, are reutilized so efficiently that when these chains are labeled *in vivo* with acetate or glucose the plasmalogens appear metabolically stable.

Myelin proteins show the same type of biphasic turnover as lipids. Whereas in the fast phase, both basic protein and PLP show half-lives on the order of 2 to 3 weeks, several studies show that both of these proteins are metabolically stable in the slow phase, showing half-lives too long to be calculated accurately. Again, as with the lipids, myelin protein decay curves vary with the precursor used and the age of the animals injected. Shorter half-lives are seen if adult animals are labeled.

Although the discussion above indicates a half-life on the order of days to months for most myelin components, some aspects of myelin metabolism have a half-life on the order of minutes. The phosphate group of MBPs is in this category. Measurements of half-life are limited by the time taken for injected [^{32}P] phosphate to equilibrate with ATP, but it is clear that much of the phosphate cycles on and off the peptide backbone, with a half-life which is on the order of minutes or faster [18,19]. Also, the monoesterified phosphate groups of polyphosphatidylinositol at positions 3 and 4 are labeled very quickly even in mature animals and presumably have a rapid half-life. There is evidence that a significant portion of the phosphatidylinositol of myelin rapidly incorporates phosphate, suggesting degradation to the extent of phospholipase C cleavage and subsequent resynthesis of at least some phosphatidylinositol of myelin. Finally, evidence for the presence in myelin of signal-transduction systems suggests that myelin metabolism includes many rapid events.

MOLECULAR ARCHITECTURE OF MYELIN

The currently accepted view of membrane structure is that of a lipid bilayer with some integral membrane proteins embedded and other extrinsic proteins attached to one surface or the other by weaker linkages. Both proteins and lipids are distributed asymmetrically with the asymmetry of lipids being partial. The molecular architecture of the layered membranes of compact myelin appears to be determined by similar principles. Molecular models of compact myelin are hypothesized based on data from electron microscopy, immunostaining, X-ray diffraction, surface probe studies, structural abnormalities in mutant mice, correlations between structure and composition in various species and predictions of protein structure from sequencing information [5].

Presumably, the glycolipids in myelin, as in other membranes, are preferentially at the extracellular surfaces in the intraperiod line. Based on a finding referred to earlier in mice unable to synthesize galactocerebroside and sulfatide [10], one or both of these major glycolipids may contribute to the stability of the intraperiod line. Diffraction studies demonstrate that cholesterol also is enriched in the extracellular face of the myelin membrane, whereas ethanolamine plasmalogen is localized asymmetrically to the cytoplasmic half of the bilayer.

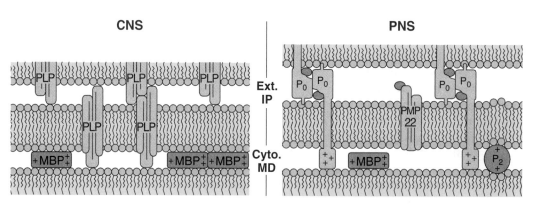

FIGURE 4-13. Diagrammatic representation of current concepts of the molecular organization of compact CNS and PNS myelin. Apposition of the extracellular *(Ext.)* surfaces of the oligodendrocyte or Schwann cell membranes to form the intraperiod *(IP)* line is shown in the upper part of the figure. Apposition of the cytoplasmic *(Cyto.)* surfaces of the membranes of the myelin-forming cells to form the major dense *(MD)* line is shown in the lower part of the figure. See the text for a detailed description of this model. The dark orange structures on P_0 and peripheral myelin protein-22 *(PMP-22)* represent the single oligosaccharide moieties on each protein. The blip at the apex of P_0 represents the tryptophan residue, which X-ray analysis suggests may interact with the apposing bilayer; but the expected tetramerization of P_0 is not shown for diagramatic simplification. Although proteolipid protein *(PLP)* molecules may exhibit homophilic interactions, as suggested at one position in the figure, there is no strong experimental evidence to support this, as in the case of P_0. This figure does not include 2':3'-cyclic nucleotide-3'-phosphodiesterase (CNP), myelin-associated glycoprotein (MAG) or other quantitatively minor proteins of isolated myelin because they probably do not play a major structural role in most of the compact myelin. In fact, many of them are localized selectively in regions of myelin sheaths distinct from the compact myelin. MBP, myelin basic protein.

A diagrammatic representation of current ideas about the molecular organization of proteins in compact myelin of the CNS and PNS is shown in Figure 4-13. Although several models for the orientation of PLP in the membrane have been proposed, it is now widely believed that all four hydrophobic domains pass entirely through the membrane with both the N- and C-termini on the cytoplasmic side, as shown in Figure 4-13. By contrast, MBP is an extrinsic protein localized exclusively at the cytoplasmic surface in the major dense line, a conclusion based on its amino acid sequence, inaccessibility to surface probes and direct localization at the electron-microscope level by immunocytochemistry. MBP may form dimers and may be the principal protein stabilizing the major dense line of CNS myelin, possibly by interacting with negatively charged lipids. Failure of compaction of the major dense line in MBP-deficient mutants supports this hypothesis (see Chap. 39). An important role for PLP in stabilizing the intraperiod line generally has been assumed, based largely on the extracellular loops of this protein being present at this location. The intraperiod line is condensed abnormally both in the PLP/DM-20 knockout mouse [16] and in spontaneously occurring PLP-deficient mutants (see Chap. 39), confirming a structural role for PLP in determining the architecture of the intraperiod line. Because myelin formation is relatively normal in PLP knockout mice this major protein is not required for spiraling of the membrane or compaction of extracellular surfaces. This suggests that other proteins or lipids of myelin may contribute to the adherence of extracellular faces during compaction. However, myelin in the PLP-null mutant is extrasensitive to osmotic shock during fixation, suggesting that PLP does enhance the stability of myelin, possibly by forming a zipper-like structure after it is compacted.

In the PNS, the major P_0 protein transverses the bilayer once and is believed to stabilize the intraperiod line by homophilic binding between extracellular domains on adjacent layers (Fig. 4-13). The relatively large, glycosylated, extracellular, immunoglobulin-like domain of P_0 probably accounts for the greater separation of extracellular surfaces in PNS myelin in comparison to CNS myelin, where closer apposition of these surfaces is possible in the presence of the smaller extracellular domains of PLP. This hypothesis is supported by findings in fish, the species in which compact myelin first appeared during evolution, which have P_0 in both PNS and CNS myelin and no PLP in CNS myelin [5]. The spacing of the intraperiod line in fish CNS myelin is greater than that in higher vertebrates and comparable to that of P_0-containing PNS myelin in other species. Homophilic interactions between P_0 molecules may involve both protein–protein and protein–carbohydrate interactions [26]. Furthermore, the crystal structure of the extracellular domain of P_0 [35] suggests that P_0 molecules emanate from each apposing membrane surface as tetramers. A tryptophan residue at the apex of its extracellular domain may interact directly with the lipid bilayer of the apposing membrane. A more detailed description of the function of P_0 as an adhesion molecule is provided in Chapter 7. P_0 protein also has a relatively large positively charged domain on the cytoplasmic side of the membrane, which contributes significantly to stabilization of the major dense line in the PNS. As a result, MBP is not as important for stability of the major dense line as in the CNS, where there is more of it. Comparison of animals doubly deficient in the genes for P_0 and MBP to animals deficient in one or the other indicates that both contribute to compaction of the cytoplasmic surfaces in PNS myelin [46]. The P_2 protein also may contribute to the stability of the major dense line, although its amount varies drastically from species to species. Interestingly, larger amounts of P_2 protein in myelin of various species correlate with larger widths of the major dense lines as determined by X-ray diffraction [5]. Although the tetraspan PMP-22 is localized in compact PNS myelin, as shown in Figure 4-13, it is not known if its extracellular or cytoplasmic domains play an important structural role. The relatively small amount of PMP-22 suggests a dynamic function.

Although the above model is a static representation, the relatively rapid metabolism of certain myelin components suggests that there may be some dynamic aspect of myelin structure, such as occasional separation of the cytoplasmic faces of the membranes. More detailed analysis of both the static structural aspect and the dynamic properties of the myelin sheath awaits conceptual and analytical advances.

ACKNOWLEDGMENTS

We thank Dr. Cedric Raine for the elegant photomicrographs that illustrate this chapter. We note with much appreciation that the organization and much of the information included in this chapter reflect those presented by Dr. William T. Norton in the first three editions of this book.

REFERENCES

1. Raine, C. S. Morphology of myelin and myelination. In P. Morell (ed.), *Myelin,* 2nd ed. New York: Plenum, 1984, pp. 1–41.
2. Waxman, S. G., and Ritchie, J. M. Molecular dissection of the myelinated axon. *Ann. Neurol.* 33:121–136, 1993.
3. Ritchie, J. M. Physiological basis of conduction in myelinated nerve fibers. In P. Morell (ed.), *Myelin,* 2nd ed. New York: Plenum, 1984, pp. 117–141.
4. Norton, W. T. The myelin sheath. In E. S. Goldensohn and S. H. Appel (eds.), *Scientific Approaches to Clinical Neurology.* Philadelphia: Lea & Febinger, 1977, pp. 259–298.
5. Kirschner, D. A., and Blaurock, A. E. Organization, phylogenetic variations and dynamic transitions of myelin. In R. E. Martenson (ed.), *Myelin: Biology and Chemistry.* Boca Raton, FL: CRC Press, 1991, pp. 413–448.
6. Hirano, A., and Dembitzer, H. M. A structural analysis of the myelin sheath in the central nervous system. *J. Cell Biol.* 34:555–567, 1967.
7. Bunge, R. P. Glial cells and the central myelin sheath. *Physiol. Rev.* 48:197–248, 1968.
8. Davison, A. N., and Peters, A. Myelination. Springfield, IL: Charles C. Thomas, 1970.
9. Norton, W. T., and Cammer, W. Isolation and characterization of myelin. In P. Morell (ed.), *Myelin,* 2nd ed. New York: Plenum 1984, pp. 147–180.
10. Coetzee, T., Fujita, N., Dupree, J., et al. Myelination in the absence of galactocerebroside and sulfatide: Normal structure with abnormal function and regional instability. *Cell* 86:209–219, 1996.

11. Lees, M. B., and Brostoff, S. W. Proteins of myelin. In P. Morell (ed.), *Myelin,* 2nd ed. New York: Plenum, 1984, pp. 197–217.
12. Lees, M. B., and Bizzozero, O. A. Structure and acylation of proteolipid protein. In R. E. Martenson (ed.), *Myelin: Biology and Chemistry.* Boca Raton, FL: CRC Press, 1991, pp. 413–448.
13. Griffiths, I. R., Montague, P., and Dickinson, P. The proteolipid protein gene [Review]. *Neuropathol. Appl. Neurobiol.* 21:85–96, 1995.
14. Mikoshiba, K., Okano, H., Tamura, T., and Ikenaka, K. Structure and function of myelin protein genes. *Annu. Rev. Neurosci.* 140:201–217, 1991.
15. Kitagawa, K., Sinoway, M. P., Yang, C., Gould, R. M., and Colman, D. R. A proteolipid protein gene family: Expression in sharks and rays and possible evolution from an ancestral gene encoding a pore-forming polypeptide. *Neuron* 11:433–448, 1993.
16. Klugmann, M., Schwab, M. H., Pühlhofer, A., et al. Assembly of CNS myelin in the absence of proteolipid protein. *Neuron* 18:59–70, 1997.
17. Readhead, C., Schneider, A., Griffiths, I., and Nave, K. A. Premature arrest of myelin formation in transgenic mice with increased proteolipid protein gene dosage. *Neuron* 12:583–595, 1994.
18. DesJardins, K. C., and Morell, P. The phosphate groups modifying myelin basic proteins are metabolically labile; the methyl groups are stable. *J. Cell Biol.* 97:438–446, 1983.
19. Eichberg, J., and Iver, S. Phosphorylation of myelin protein: Recent advances. *Neurochem. Res.* 21:527–535, 1996.
20. Brophy, P. J., Boccaccio, G. L., and Colman, D. R. The distribution of myelin basic protein mRNAs within myelinating oligodendrocytes. *Trends Nat. Sci.* 16:515–521, 1993.
21. Kamholz, J., de Ferra, F., Puckett, C., and Lazzarini, R. Identification of three forms of human myelin basic protein by cDNA cloning. *Proc. Natl. Acad. Sci. USA* 83:4962–4966, 1986.
22. Landry, C. F., Ellison, J. A., Pribyl, T. M., Campagnoni, E., Kampf, K., and Campagnoni, A. T. Myelin basic protein gene expression in neurons: Developmental and regional changes in protein targeting within neuronal nuclei, cell bodies, and processes. *J. Neurosci.* 16:2452–2462, 1996.
23. Tsukada, Y., and Kurihara, T. 2′,3′-Cyclic nucleotide 3′-phosphodiesterase: Molecular characterization and possible functional significance. In R. E. Martenson (ed.), *Myelin: Biology and Chemistry.* Boca Raton, FL: CRC Press, 1992, pp. 449–480.
24. DeAngelis, D. A., and Braun, P. E. 2′,3′-Cyclic nu-

cleotide 3′-phosphodiesterase binds to actin-based cytoskeletal elements in an isoprenylation-independent manner. *J. Neurochem.* 67:943–951, 1996.

25. Gravel, M., Peterson, J., Yong, V. W., Koittis, V., Trapp, B. and Braun P. E. Overexpression of 2′,3′ cyclic nucleotide-3′-phosphodiesterase in transgenic mice alters oligodendrocyte development and produces aberrant myelination. *Mol. Cell. Neurosci.* 7:453–466, 1996.

26. Quarles, R. H. Glycoproteins of myelin sheaths. *J. Mol. Neurosci.* 8:1–12, 1997.

27. Lassmann, H., Bartsch, U., Montag, D., and Schachner, M. C. Dying back oligodendrogliopathy: A late sequel of myelin-associated glycoprotein deficiency. *Glia* 19:104–110, 1997.

28. Gardinier, M. V., Amiguet, P., Linington, C., and Matthieu, J. M. Myelin/oligodendrocyte glycoprotein is a unique member of the immunoglobulin superfamily. *J. Neurosci Res.* 33:177–187, 1992.

29. Mikol, D. D., Gulcher, J. R., and Stefansson, K. The oligodendrocyte-myelin glycoprotein belongs to a distinct family of proteins and contains the HNK-1 carbohydrate. *J. Cell. Biol.* 110:471–479, 1990.

30. Lemke, G. The molecular genetics of myelination: An update. *Glia* 7:263–271, 1993.

31. Uyemura, K., Asou, H., and Takeda, Y. Structure and function of peripheral nerve myelin proteins. *Prog. Brain Res.* 105:311–318, 1993.

32. Yoshida, M., and Coleman, D. R. Parallel evolution and coexpression of the proteolipid proteins and protein zero in vertebrate myelin. *Neuron* 16:1115–1126, 1996.

33. D'Urso, D., Brophy, P. J., Staugatis, S. M., et al. Protein zero of peripheral nerve myelin: Biosynthesis, membrane insertion, and evidence for homotypic interaction. *Neuron* 2:449–460, 1990.

34. Filbin, M. T., Walsh, F. S., Trapp, B. D., Pizzey, J. A., and Tennenkoon, G. I. Role of myelin P_0 protein as a homophilic adhesion molecule. *Nature* 344:871–872, 1990.

35. Shapiro, L., Doyle, J. P., Hensley, P., Colman, D. R., and Hendrickson, W. A. Crystal structure of the extracellular domain from P_0, the major structural protein of peripheral nerve myelin. *Neuron* 17:435–449, 1996.

36. Martini, R., Zielasek, J., Toyka, K. V., Giese, K. P., and Schachner, M. Protein zero (P_0)-deficient mice show myelin degeneration in peripheral nerves characteristic of inherited human neuropathies. *Nat. Genet.* 11:281–286, 1995.

37. Martenson, R. E., and Uyemura, K. Myelin P2, a neuritogenic member of the family of cytoplasmic lipid-binding proteins. In R. E. Martenson (ed.), *Myelin: Biology and Chemistry.* Boca Raton, FL: CRC Press, 1992, pp. 509–528.

38. Suter, U., and Snipes, G. J. Peripheral myelin protein-22: Facts and hypotheses. *J. Neurosci. Res.* 40:145–151, 1995.

39. Magyar, J. P., Martini, R., Ruelicke, T., et al. Impaired differentiation of Schwann cells in transgenic mice with increased PMP22 gene dosage. *J. Neurosci.* 16:5351–5360, 1996.

40. Dieperink, M. K., O'Neill, A., Magnoni, G., et al. SAG: A Schwann cell membrane glycoprotein. *J. Neurosci.* 12:2177–2185, 1992.

41. Ledeen, R. W. Enzymes and receptors of myelin. In R. E. Martenson (ed.), *Myelin: Biology and Chemistry.* Boca Raton, FL: CRC Press, 1992, pp. 531–570.

42. Morell, P., Roberson, M. D., Meissner, G., and Toews, A. Myelin: From electrical insulator to ion channels. In G. Hashim (ed.), *Dynamic Interactions of Myelin Proteins,* New York: Wiley-Liss, 1989, pp. 1–23.

43. Benjamins, J. A., and Smith, M. E. Metabolism of myelin. In P. Morell (ed.), *Myelin,* 2nd ed. New York: Plenum, 1984, pp. 225–249.

44. Minuk, J., and Braun, P. E. Differential intracellular sorting of the myelin-associated glycoprotein isoforms. *J. Neurosci. Res.* 44:411–420, 1996.

45. Ousley, A. H., and Morell, P. Individual molecular species of phosphatidylcholine and phosphatidylethanolamine in myelin turn over at different rates. *J. Biol. Chem.* 267:10362–10369, 1992.

46. Martini, R., Mohajeri, M. H., Kasper, S., Giese, K. P., and Schachner, M. Mice doubly deficient in the genes for both P_0 and myelin basic protein show that both proteins contribute to formation of the major dense line in peripheral nerve myelin. *J. Neurosci.* 15:4488–4495, 1995.

5

Membrane Transport

R. Wayne Albers and George J. Siegel

Basic Neurochemistry: Molecular, Cellular and Medical Aspects, 6th Ed., edited by G. J. Siegel et al. Published by
Lippincott–Raven Publishers, Philadelphia, 1999. Correspondence to R. Wayne Albers, Laboratory of Neurochemistry, National Institute of Neurological Diseases and Stroke, National Institutes of Health, Bethesda, Maryland 20892.

TRANSPORT PROCESSES

Ion gradients are generated across cell membranes by transport proteins and are required for some of the most basic neural functions

These ion gradients produce the voltages across plasma membranes that drive the propagated signaling functions of neurons. Other uses of the potential energy of ion gradients include the synthesis of ATP in mitochondria; the concentrative acquisition or recovery of nutrients, metabolites and neurotransmitters; and the regulation of intracellular ionic concentrations.

Some transporters are electrogenic; that is, their operation can move electrical charge across membranes [1]. Well-characterized examples of transport proteins in each category are discussed. These are now sufficiently numerous to inspire analyses of their structural and evolutionary interrelations. One generalization permitted from present evidence is that most of the major families of transport proteins arose early in evolution, prior to the divergence of eukaryocytes from prokaryocytes [1].

Concentration gradients across membranes result from two opposing processes: diffusion and active transport

The Gibbs equation describes the free energy (ΔG) released by the diffusion of a solute or required for its transport in the opposite direction:

$$\Delta G_{\text{diff}} = RT \ln(C_2/C_1) \qquad (1)$$

where $R = 1.99$ cal/deg Kelvin, T is degrees Kelvin and C_1 and C_2 are concentrations of the solute on opposite sides of a permeable membrane.

Because cell membranes are selective in their ion permeabilities, the active transport of charged solutes produces electrical as well as chemical potentials (Chap. 6). The energy stored as electrical potential is given by the following:

$$\Delta G_{\text{emf}} = ZFV \qquad (2)$$

where Z is valence, F is the Faraday constant (23,500 cal/volt/mol) and V is the transmembrane potential difference in volts. The free energy change related to movement of 1 mol of a solute with respect to the combined electrochemical gradient is described by the sum of equations 1 and 2:

$$\Delta G_{\text{total}} = RT \ln(C_2/C_1) + ZFV \qquad (3)$$

The chemical and electrical diffusion components are equal and opposite only in an equilibrium state. When work occurs, ΔG is not equal to zero and a steady state can be maintained only if sufficient energy is supplied by some exergonic process.

In the case of neurons and certain other cells in which the ionic currents are carried primarily by Na$^+$ and K$^+$, the energy input to maintain a steady-state electrochemical gradient can be approximated by the application of equation 3 to just these species:

$$\begin{aligned}
\Delta G_{\text{total}} &= RT \ln([\text{Na}_e^+/[\text{Na}^+]_i) + ZFV \\
&\quad + RT \ln([\text{K}^+]_i/[\text{K}^+]_e) - ZFV \qquad (4) \\
&= RT \ln([\text{Na}^+]_e[\text{K}^+]_i/[\text{Na}^+]_i[\text{K}^+]_e)
\end{aligned}$$

Assuming typical values for Na$^+$ and K$^+$ concentration gradients, that is, $[\text{Na}^+]_e/[\text{Na}^+]_i = 12$ and $[\text{K}^+]_i/[\text{K}^+]_e = 50$, then ΔG is about 3.8 kcal per mole of Na$^+$ exchanged for K$^+$. The hydrolysis of a high-energy phosphate bond of ATP may yield about 12 kcal per mole, thus permitting the exchange of about three equivalents of cation for each mole of ATP hydrolyzed. This ratio of Na^+ transported per mole of ATP has been confirmed by measurements in several tissue preparations.

Membrane-transport processes store energy, whereas channel-mediated processes dissipate energy

The direction and rate of diffusion of ions or molecules across membranes through channels is determined by prevailing electrochemical gradients. Channels achieve adequate selectivity without strong interactions with ions. This allows typical ion channels to conduct several thousand ions per millisecond (Chap. 6). In contrast, transport proteins form highly specific and relatively strong complexes with their substrates. These interactions initiate conformational transitions of the transport proteins, culminating in release of the substrate ions on the opposite face of the membrane. Because of these strong interactions, transport processes typically require several milliseconds per ion. The relationships between solute concentration and rate of transport can be described by saturation kinetics, as is the case for the relationship of enzyme reaction rate and substrate concentration.

Selective transport of molecules or ions through membranes may occur without coupling to any other substrate. Such a process is termed facilitative, or uncoupled, transport. An example is the stereoselective entrance of D-glucose into neurons. In this case, binding of a transport substrate is sufficient to initiate an uncoupled transport cycle, in which the substrate is conveyed across the membrane and the unoccupied transport-binding site is restored to its original orientation (Fig. 5-1).

Secondary or flux-coupled transport processes obligatorily couple the transport of one molecular or ionic species to the transport of another. The coupled processes are termed symport or antiport according to the relative directions of the two transport events (Fig. 5-1). Many essential nutrients are accumulated by symport systems coupled to Na^+ or proton gradients. Neurotransmitter reuptake systems are similarly coupled symporters and are described below. In coupled transport, both substrates must be available, either simultaneously or sequentially, on the same side of the membrane in the case of a symporter and on opposite sides in the case of an antiporter. The kinetic behavior of these systems can be described by substrate–velocity functions analogous to those of multisubstrate enzymes. More than two substrates are involved in some secondary transport systems, as exemplified by the bumetanide-sensitive (Na^+, K^+, $2Cl^-$)-symporter (see below).

Primary active transport processes comprise those in which one or more substrates are transported in concert with a chemical reaction that provides the free energy for concentrative substrate accumulation (Fig. 5-1). All of the known primary processes transport cations: H^+, Na^+, K^+ and Ca^{2+}. The principal function of primary Na^+ and K^+ transport in most cells is to store energy. In contrast, H^+ and Ca^{2+} pumps act as regulators of intracellular or intraorganellar concentrations of these ions, which in turn control the rates of other cell functions (see below).

Energy transduction. Biochemical terminology is curiously inadequate to describe proteins that have energy-transducing functions. Members of this group include, in addition to proteins that implement primary active transport, proteins that produce contractile forces, such as myosins and dyneins (see Chaps. 8, 28 and 43); those that transport macromolecules and organelles intracellularly, such as kinesins (Chaps. 8 and 28); those that transform the shapes or relative positions of other macromolecules, such as peptidyl transferases, DNA helicases and topoisomerases; and those that transform physical stimuli into chemical messages, such as in phototransduction (Chap. 47). Most of these proteins catalyze ATP or GTP hydrolysis. However, such enzyme activities are only a byproduct of their primary energy-transducing functions, which are to produce various forms of local ordering of the cell structure or environment. These functions transcend the usual definition of an enzyme as a cat-

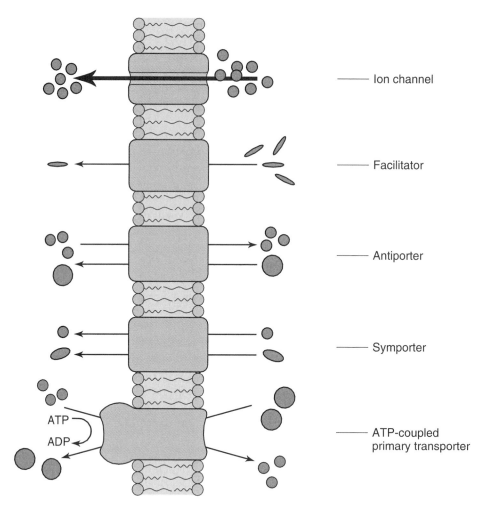

FIGURE 5-1. Types of membrane transport proteins. *Ion channels* provide gated diffusion paths across cell membranes that are regulated by membrane voltage, interactions with ligands and/or phosphorylation (see Chap. 6). *Facilitators,* or *uncoupled transporters,* provide highly selective pathways, such as for D-glucose, but are not coupled to energy sources and, therefore, cannot concentrate their substrates. Transporters that are coupled to energy sources can alter the steady-state distribution of their substrate ions and/or molecules. *Secondary transporters* derive energy from existing ion gradients to transport a second ion or molecule in a direction that is either the same as *(symport)* or opposite to *(antiport)* that of the energizing ion. *Primary transporters* couple a chemical reaction to protein conformational transitions, which supply energy to generate concentration gradients of one or more substrates across cell membranes.

alyst because they are "uphill" reactions that move the system away from chemical equilibrium and reduce the local entropy of the system. For this reason, primary active-transport proteins are preferably called "pumps" rather than enzymes. Another problem in terminology is the use of the term "substrate," which, in enzymology, is restricted to molecules that are chemically transformed as a result of interactions with enzymes. However, in the case of membrane

pumps, the molecules or ions that are transported are not chemically altered. Their interactions with transporters are similar to enzyme–substrate interactions, and they will frequently be called substrates in the following discussions.

The principal generators of transmembrane, cation gradients are members of a family of proteins designated "P-type" ATPases because their transport mechanisms involve phosphorylation of the catalytic-site aspartyl residue. Until recently, the known functions of these pumps were confined to cation transport across plasma and endoplasmic reticulum membranes. However, one member of this family has now been shown to transport aminophospholipids across membranes [2]. The general structural features of the P-type cation-transport ATPases are highly conserved in this family (Fig. 5-2). The transport mechanisms are also highly conserved and analogous to that described in Figure 5-3.

THE ATP-DEPENDENT NA$^+$,K$^+$ PUMP

The principal primary active-transport system in neurons, as in most other animal cells, is a P-type pump that concurrently extrudes Na$^+$ and accumulates K$^+$. For brevity, we will refer to it as the Na,K-ATPase. Depending on their functions, different tissues have vastly different requirements for pumping Na$^+$ and K$^+$. Transport by Na,K-ATPases is specifically inhibited by cardiac glycosides, such as ouabain. The Na$^+$ pump consists of two protein subunits. The α subunit contains the catalytic and ionophoric domains. It is polytopic, with ten probable transmembrane domains (Fig. 5-2A). The large cytoplasmic structure probably consists of the B and C domains and perhaps includes the N-terminal domain (compare Fig. 5-2A and B). It is connected to the major transmembrane domain by a stalk, probably consisting of the regions labeled S1–6 in Figure 5-2A. Anionic and hydrogen-bonding residues that are critical for cation binding occur in M4, M5, M6 and M8. These segments are likely components of the ionophoric domain, which may have the form of a doubly gated channel. The β subunit is a monotopic glycoprotein with a large extracellular domain that exhibits some of the characteristics of adhesion molecules (Chap. 7). The α subunit is not functional and remains within the endoplasmic reticulum if it is expressed in the absence of the β subunit.

The minimum oligomeric size required for a functional Na$^+$ pump has not been established. An αβ heterodimer exhibits most of the ATPase and cation-binding properties of the functional pump, but its kinetic behavior is different from that of a membrane-bound pump. It is known that $(\alpha\beta)_2$ and higher oligomers exist in cell membranes, and it is likely that oligomeric interactions are important for efficient energy transduction.

Three different α-subunit isoforms are specified by three different genes in mammals

Although in kidney and most other tissues the major expressed isoform is α1, all three isoforms are expressed in mammalian brains. The three isoforms show about 85% sequence similarity, with the most substantial differences occurring in their N-terminal regions. When expressed in HeLa cells, the isoforms differ substantially in their responses to $[Na^+]_i$: half-maximal activations, $[Na^+]_{0.5V}$, of α1 < α2 < α3 in one study [3] and in another, $[K^+]_{0.5V}$ of α3 < α2 = α1 [4].

Three β-subunit genes have also been identified, the β1 isoform being most generally expressed [5]. In embryonic brain, the β2 isoform was first identified as adhesion molecule on glia (AMOG) that is transiently expressed on the surface of cerebellar Bergman glia during the differentiation of granule cells. As the brain matures, β2 becomes widely expressed on astrocytes and disappears from most neurons. The specific β-subunit isoform that pairs with an α subunit appears to have little effect on pump parameters, and no preferential association of particular α and β isoforms is demonstrable in cerebellum [6]. A major function of β subunits is to target the Na$^+$ pump to the plasma membrane [7]. Different β isoforms may determine different cellular and subcellular localizations [8].

A major fraction of cerebral energy production is required for extrusion of intracellular Na$^+$ that enters during excitation and secondary transport

Cation flux during action potentials is two to three orders of magnitude greater than in the resting state. For example, Na$^+$ entry and K$^+$ efflux from a squid giant axon during a single ac-

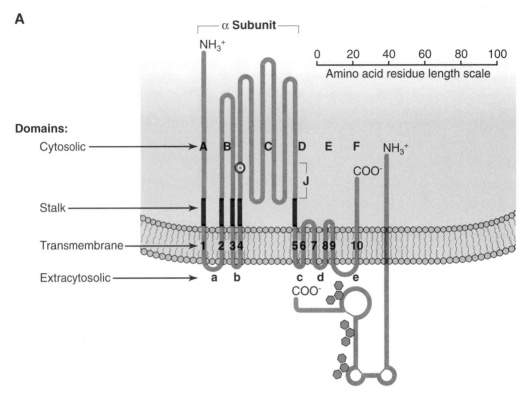

FIGURE 5-2. A: Topological map of the P-type cation pumps. The catalytic subunit, α, contains a consensus sequence (indicated by ⊙ in the large cytoplasmic loop, *C*) that defines this family of transport proteins. All members of this family contain an aspartyl residue at this site, which is alternately phosphorylated and dephosphorylated during each transport cycle. Conformational energy is transmitted from the catalytic site to the ionophoric domains to drive ion transport. Region *J*, near the other end of domain *C*, is highly conserved and may participate in energy transduction to the ionophoric domains. Most P-type cation pumps appear to have ten transmembrane segments. There is evidence that the ionophoric domains that mediate cation binding and transport involve transmembrane segments *4, 5, 6* and probably *8*. A β subunit has not been identified for all of the P-type transporters. When present, it is characterized by a cytosolic N-terminal domain, a single transmembrane domain and a C-terminal domain that is heavily glycosylated (indicated by ⬡) and has several disulfide-stabilized loops. The tight association of α and β subunits involves the extracytoplasmic domain of the β subunit near its C-terminus and the *d* loop of the α subunit.

tion potential, which has a duration of ~1 msec, is about 3×10^{-12} mol · cm^{-2} membrane. The resting membrane flux in this tissue is 12×10^{-12} mol · cm^{-2} · sec^{-1} (Chap. 6). Therefore, it would take the pump about 0.25 sec to regenerate the flux of one spike at the resting membrane-pump rate. Based on these estimates, in order to maintain a steady state at conduction frequencies ranging from 10 to 100 impulses/sec, the Na$^+$ pump rate would have to increase by 2.5 to 25 times its resting level.

It is estimated that 25 to 40% of brain energy utilization may be related to Na,K-ATPase activity. The energy expenditure for biosynthetic processes in mature brain, including osmotic work, protein and lipid synthesis and turnover of neurotransmitters, is relatively small, probably less than 10% of total ATP utilization. Other energy-utilizing processes include axoplasmic transport, Ca^{2+} transport, vesicle recycling and aminophospholipid translocation. While all of these are significant, Na$^+$ transport accounts for the largest share of energy flux.

Coupled active transport of Na$^+$ and K$^+$ results from a cycle of conformational transitions of the transport protein

The ATPase activity that is associated with the Na$^+$ pump is actually the sum of Na$^+$-dependent

B

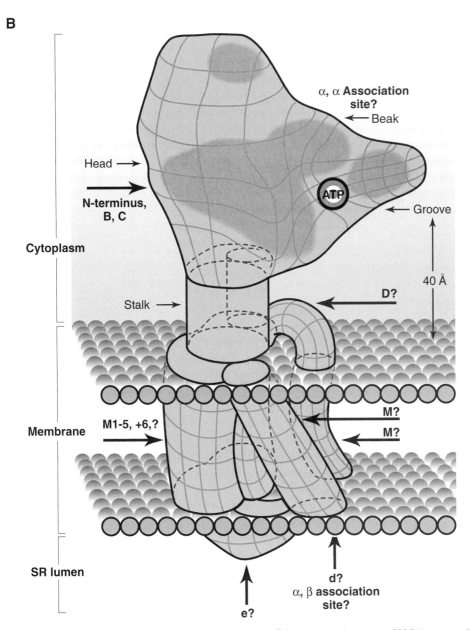

FIGURE 5-2. *(Continued.)* **B:** Three-dimensional cartoon of the P-type cation pump, SERCA, or smooth endoplasmic reticulum Ca^{2+} antiporter. The general shape of the molecule is derived from cryoelectron microscopy at about 14 Å resolution from tubular crystals of the calcium pump from rabbit muscle. The location of the ATP-binding site was determined by comparing the electron-diffraction images of crystals prepared with and without chromium-ATP. Correlations of other parts of the molecule with the primary structure is speculative and based mostly on sequence analysis and the results of a variety of studies on effects of point mutations and of site-specific reagents on pump functions. Structural information about the Na^+ pump and other P-type transporters is generally consistent with this model. (Modified from [51], with additional data from [52].) The resolution of this structure has been improved to 8 Å [52a].

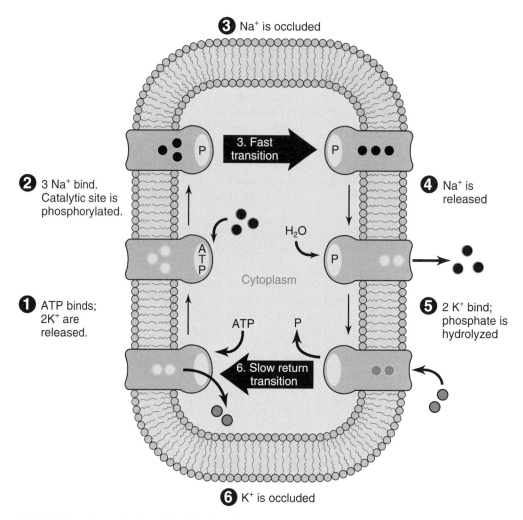

FIGURE 5-3.   The mechanism of the ATP-dependent Na^+ pump. The sequence of reaction steps is indicated by the *large arrows.* **Left:** Pump molecules are in the E_1 conformation, which has high affinity for Na^+ and ATP and low affinity for K^+. Ionophoric sites are accessible only from the cytoplasmic side. *Step 1:* K^+ is discharged as metabolic energy is added to the system by ATP binding. *Step 2:* Three Na^+ bind and the enzyme is reversibly phosphorylated. *Step 3:* The conformational transition from $E_1{\sim}P$ to E_2-P, shown at the top, is the "power stroke" of the pump, during which the ionophoric sites with their three bound Na^+ become accessible to the extracellular side and decrease their affinity for Na^+. Part of the free energy of the enzyme acylphosphate has been dissipated in this process. **Right:** Pump molecules are in the E_2 conformation. *Step 4:* Three Na^+ dissociate from E_2-P. *Step 5:* Two K^+ bind and more free energy is dissipated as the enzyme acylphosphate is hydrolyzed. At this point, the two K^+ become tightly bound ("occluded"). *Step 6:* E_2 reverts to E_1 carrying the K^+ to the cytoplasmic side.

phosphorylation of an aspartyl residue at the catalytic site of the pump protein and subsequent K^+-dependent hydrolysis of the enzyme acylphosphate (Fig. 5-3). These molecular events channel metabolic energy into the pumping process. The initial catalytic-site phosphorylation occurs only after three Na^+ have bound to ionophoric sites from the cytoplasmic side. In

this "E1$\sim$P" conformation, the phosphorylation by ATP is readily reversible; that is, the energy state of the protein acylphosphate is comparable to that of the ATP phosphate bond. However, phosphorylation initiates a rapid conformational transition to the E2-P state, from which the Na^+ is discharged extracellularly. K^+ then binds to E2-P, initiating hydrolysis of the acylphosphate.

This causes E2 to spontaneously revert to E1, carrying two K^+ into the cell. The cycle is completed as the K^+ dissociates in concert with initiation of the next cycle by binding ATP.

The Na^+,K^+ pump and the cell-membrane potential interact with each other

A stoichiometry of three Na^+ exchanged for two K^+ as one ATP is hydrolyzed has been observed in nearly all of the numerous cell types and reconstituted systems that thus far have been studied. Because there is a net outward flow of positive charge, the membrane tends to hyperpolarize. Therefore, the Na^+ pump is termed *electrogenic*. The membrane electrical potential contributed by Na^+ pumping is usually less than 10 mV. This can be sufficient to shorten the duration of the action potential and to contribute to negative afterpotentials. In heart muscle, hyperpolarization due to increased Na^+ pumping can be observed after sustained increases in firing rate and may be a factor in cardiac arrhythmias. Conversely, the membrane potential modifies the pump rate. Hyperpolarization appears to slow Na^+ dissociation from the pump [9].

Phosphorylation of the catalytic subunit by cAMP-dependent protein kinase reduces pump activity

This occurs at the serine of the consensus sequence RRNSVF in the C-terminal cytoplasmic loop (*e* in Fig. 5-2A). This sequence occurs in all three isoforms as well as in the gastric H^+,K^+-exchange pump and is highly conserved across species. Inhibitory phosphorylation of Na,K-ATPase appears to occur in some neurons. The $\alpha1$ isoform can also be phosphorylated by protein kinase C (PKC), but the functional consequences of this are uncertain.

The isoforms of the α-subunit genes differ with respect to regulatory DNA base sequences in their 5′-flanking regions

These may enhance or obstruct the assembly of the preinitiation complex of RNA polymerase and relevant transcription factors [10]. The neuron specificity of $\alpha3$ expression appears to be related to a neural-restrictive silencer element and a positively acting *cis* element [11].

The "basal promoter," required for constitutive expression of the $\alpha1$ gene, is a positive regulatory element termed ARE [12] and contains binding sites for several transcription factors, including the cAMP-responsive element (CRE). CRE occurs within promoters of many cAMP-inducible genes and can interact with CRE-binding (CREB) and -modulatory (CREM) proteins and activating transcription factor 1 (ATF-1), which are a subgroup within the leucine zipper family defined by their amino acid-sequence similarity and ability to heterodimerize with each other. The CRE site is subject to regulation by several pathways, including some involving cAMP, Ca^{2+} and transforming growth factor β (TGFβ). Phosphorylation of ATF-1 and CREB by either cAMP-dependent protein kinase (PKA) or PKC can enhance their binding to the ATF/CRE site and may be required for transcription of the ATPase $\alpha1$ gene [13].

Regulation by hormones. In the rat hippocampus, the dentate granular cells express the $\alpha1$ and $\alpha3$ isoforms (Fig. 5-4). In adrenalectomized rats, aldosterone selectively regulates $\alpha3$ in these cells. In other cortical neurons which express both mRNAs, however, aldosterone has no effect on either [14]. In the kidney, aldosterone regulates the level of expression of $\alpha1$. Regulation by aldosterone is evidently determined by local factors, such as cell type and location, in addition to the presence of the corticoid receptor. These local factors in gene regulation, which may be positive or negative, have been termed the "cell context."

During postnatal development days 1 to 20, $\alpha3$ mRNA is the isoform predominantly expressed in rat brain and is the one most decreased by thyroidectomy [15]. The genes for the $\beta1$ and $\beta2$ subunits also contain numerous consensus sequences for transcription factors, including, in the case of $\beta1$, potential binding sites for thyroid and glucocorticoid receptors [16].

Na^+-dependent regulation of Na^+-pump expression. Alterations in the local ionic environment, probably mainly through changes in cyto-

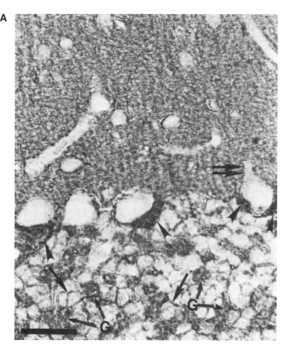

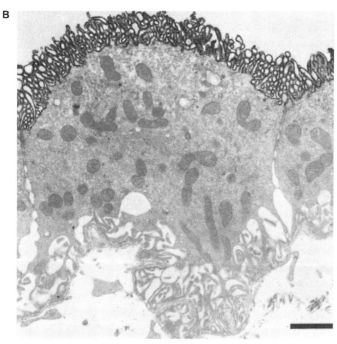

FIGURE 5-4. **A:** Immunocytochemical localization of the Na,K pump in cerebellum. Cerebellar cortex has intensely stained basket regions adjacent to Purkinje cells and little staining along the apical dendrites *(double arrows)* of Purkinje cells. While the reaction product is dense over glomeruli *(G)*, a fine deposition outlines the plasmalemma of granule cell bodies *(arrows)*. Original magnification: ×620; bar = 50 μm. (From [53].) **B:** Immunocytochemical localization of the Na,K pump in choroid plexus. Choroid plexus contains epithelial cells with intensely stained microvillar and intermicrovillar plasma membranes. The basal and lateral plasma membrane surfaces are not stained. Original magnification ×8000; bar = 2.0 μm. (From [54].)

FIGURE 5-4. *(Continued.)* **C:** *In situ* hybridization for α1 and α3 mRNAs of Na,K-ATPase in 3-month-old rat cerebellum. **Left,** α 1. **Right,** α3. Note the prominent clusters of α3 mRNA over Purkinje cells *(long arrow)*, basket cells *(short arrow)*, stellate cells *(black arrowhead)* and Golgi cells *(white arrowheads)*. In contrast, α1 mRNA is diffusely distributed, with higher concentrations in the granular layer *(GL)* and white matter *(WM)* than in the molecular layer *(ML)* and lowest concentrations in the Purkinje cell layer *(PCL)*. (From [55], see also [56].)

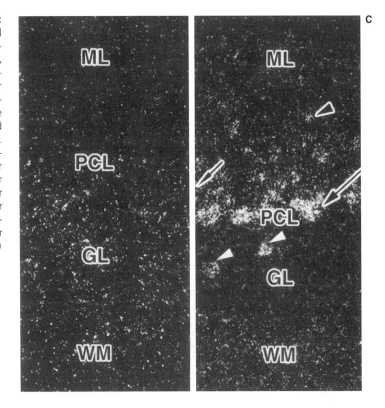

plasmic Ca^{2+} and Na^+, can affect expression of the Na^+ pump and of early-response genes [17]. There is evidence for a Na^+-responsive element in the 5′-flanking regions of each of the α-subunit genes [18].

Differential localization of isoforms. The activity of rat brain Na,K-ATPase per milligram of protein increases about ten times during the developmental stage just prior to rapid myelination, which occurs 2 to 12 days postnatally and corresponds to the time of glial proliferation, elaboration of neuronal and glial processes and increasing neuronal excitability. In the nervous system, Na^+ pumps are concentrated in membrane regions associated with high ionic flux. These include neuronal axon terminals, synapses, perikarya and dendritic processes, as well as glial processes that occur in the neuropil of gray matter (see cerebellum, Fig. 5-4A). Na,K-ATPase is demonstrable in neuritic extensions in cell cultures and at the node of Ranvier but not in myelin wrappings of adult rat optic nerve. Within the retina, heavy concentrations are found in photoreceptor inner segments. In reti-

nal pigment epithelium and choroid plexus ependyma, the Na^+ pump is concentrated on apical or luminal surfaces (Fig. 5-4B). In contrast, almost all epithelial cells adapted for secretion or reabsorption, such as kidney tubules and exocrine glands, express the Na^+ pump asymmetrically, on the basolateral or antiluminal surfaces but not on the apical surface.

All three α-subunit isoforms are expressed in the CNS but to varying extents in different regions and cell types. The α1 isoform appears in glia, Schwann cells, choroid plexus epithelium and some neurons. The α2 isoform is found diffusely throughout the CNS in glia, although some neuronal localization is not excluded. The α3 isoform is found only in neurons. In the rat nervous system, α3 mRNA is most abundant within the perikarya of retinal ganglion cells, cortical and hippocampal pyramidal cells, certain interneurons, Purkinje cells, brainstem nuclei, subcortical nuclei and anterior and posterior spinal cord gray columns. The α1 mRNA is most abundant in rat hippocampal and cerebellar granule cell layers, sparse in Purkinje cells and diffusely distributed in neuropil and white matter (Fig. 5-4C). In the spinal cord, α1 expression is restricted to a set of laterally situated anterior horn cells and to intermediolateral thoracic cord cells. Different dorsal root ganglion cells express α3 alone or together with α1 but do not express α1 alone. In contrast to the rat, one study of human cerebellum shows that α1 mRNA is about equal in granule and Purkinje cell layers. Aging-related changes in α-isoform gene expression are discussed in Chapter 30.

In human cerebral cortex (Fig. 5-5), as in rat, α3 mRNA is clustered over pyramidal and other neurons while α1 mRNA is distributed diffusely through the neuropil. In nondemented, aged humans, there are slight increases in α1 mRNA, not reaching statistical significance, while there are significant but small reductions in the neuronal perikaryal content of α3 mRNA. In contrast, in dementing Alzheimer's disease (Chap. 46), the neuronal perikaryal and total neuropil α3 mRNA contents diminish markedly prior to neuronal dystrophic changes, reflecting changes in neuronal function early in the neurodegenerative process (Fig. 5-5).

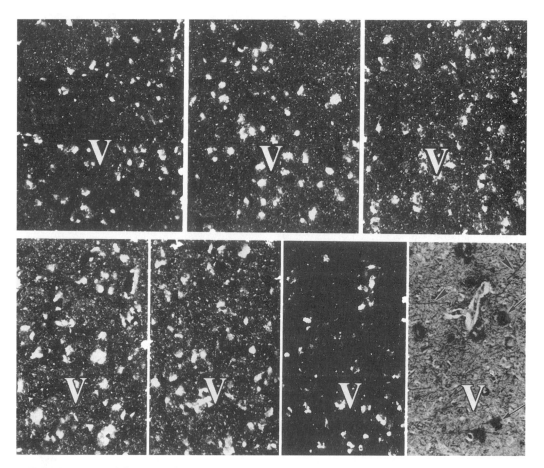

FIGURE 5-5. *In situ* hybridization for α1 and α3 mRNAs of Na,K-ATPase in postmortem human superior frontal cortex (layers IV, V). **Top row, α1; left to right:** 39-year-old normal, 78-year-old normal and 78-year-old Alzheimer's disease (AD). Note the mildly increased hybridization signal for α1 mRNA in the normal age-matched and AD brains compared to the young control brain. **Bottom row, α3; left to right:** adjacent sections to those in top row. **Far right,** Bielschowsky stain of adjacent AD cortex. Note the small decrease in α3 mRNA hybridization signal over neurons in the aged normal relative to the young control and the large decrease in total α3 mRNA signal over neurons and neuropil in AD relative to young and age-matched control brains. The Bielschowsky silver stain shows dark-appearing amyloid plaques *(arrows)* and neuropil fibers *(arrowheads)* in the AD brain. (From [57].)

ATP-DEPENDENT CA^{2+} PUMPS

ATP-dependent Ca^{2+} pumps and Na$^+$,Ca^{2+} antiporters act in concert to maintain a low concentration of free cytosolic Ca^{2+}

The concentration of cytosolic free calcium ion, $[Ca^{2+}]_i$, in unstimulated cells is between 10^{-8} and 10^{-7} M, which is several orders of magni-tude lower than that of extracellular free Ca^{2+}. Cells also maintain Ca^{2+} stores in the endoplas-mic reticulum (Fig. 5-6). Regulation of $[Ca^{2+}]_i$ is particularly important in the regulation of in-traneuronal signals. Cytosolic free Ca^{2+} regu-lates certain plasma membrane cation channels (Chap. 6), acts in second-messenger systems (Chaps. 21–23) and participates in neurotrans-mitter release (Chap. 9). Impairment of Ca^{2+} regulation can be catastrophic to the cell

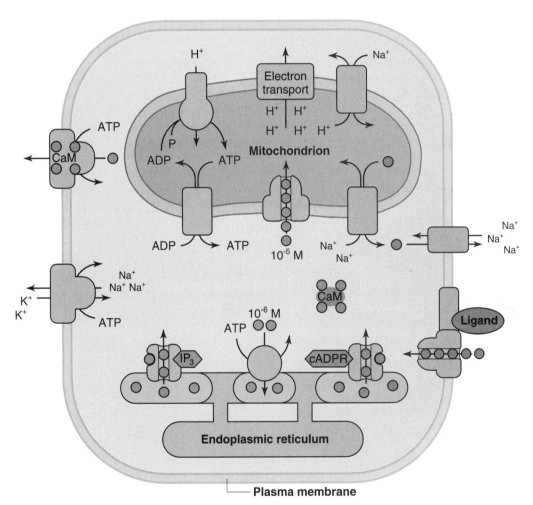

FIGURE 5-6. Calcium homeostasis. Ca^{2+} enters cells through a variety of ligand- and voltage-regulated channels, but intracellular free Ca^{2+} is normally maintained at less than micromolar concentrations. Intracellular Ca^{2+} is proba-bly regulated coordinately by a Na$^+$, Ca^{2+} antiporter in plasma membranes and by several different Ca-ATPases in plasma membranes and endoplasmic reticulum. The driving force for Na$^+$, Ca^{2+} antiporter exchange is the inwardly directed Na$^+$ gradient, which is maintained by the Na,K-ATPase. Mitochondria may participate transiently in Ca^{2+} homeostasis if the capacities of these other systems are exceeded. Internal stores of Ca^{2+} may be released from en-doplasmic reticulum through the action of second messengers, such as inositol 1,4,5-trisphosphate (*IP$_3$*) or Ca^{2+} it-self, in response to various receptor systems. In the figure, Ca^{2+} is represented by ●. *CaM*, calmodulin; *cADPR*, cADP receptor.

(Chaps. 23 and 34). Ca^{2+} enters the cytosol through both voltage- and ligand-gated channels in the plasma membrane (Chap. 6) and lig-and-gated channels in the endoplasmic reticulum (Chap. 23).

Plasma membranes contain two types of Ca^{2+} transporter. The first is a low-affinity, high-transport-capacity Na^+, Ca^{2+} exchanger, or antiporter. It is energetically driven by the Na^+ gradient (see below). The second is a P-type, plasma-membrane Ca^{2+} pump (PMCA) with high affinity for Ca^{2+} ($K_m = 100$ to 200 nM) but relatively low transport capacity [19]. The stoichiometry of PMCA is one Ca^{2+} transported for each ATP hydrolyzed. These pumps probably do not carry out bulk movements of Ca^{2+} but are most effective in maintaining very low concentrations of cytosolic Ca^{2+} in resting cells. A distinguishing characteristic of the PMCAs is that, in addition to binding Ca^{2+} as a substrate, they are further activated by binding Ca^{2+}/calmodulin. The effect of calmodulin binding is to increase the affinity of the substrate Ca^{2+} site by 20- to 30-fold. This highly cooperative activation mechanism makes the PMCAs very sensitive to small changes in $[Ca^{2+}]_i$.

A group including at least five PMCAs forms a multigene family. Three isoforms that occur in brain are designated PMCA1–3, and each has a distinct distribution in brain [20]. For example, PMCA1 mRNA is widely distributed, with highest concentrations in CA1 pyramidal cells of hippocampus, whereas that of PMCA2 is highest in cerebellar Purkinje neurons and that of PMCA3 is highest in habenula and choroid plexus.

The smooth endoplasmic reticulum Ca^{2+} antiporter (SERCA) found in brain is the same as the sarcoplasmic reticulum pump expressed in high concentrations in skeletal muscle, where it brings about muscle relaxation by rapidly sequestering cytoplasmic Ca^{2+} into the sarcoplasmic reticulum (Chap. 43). There are at least three separate genes for SERCA. Of these, SERCA-2 is the major form expressed in brain. It is widely distributed and expressed at relatively high levels in cerebellar Purkinje cells, hippocampus, cerebral cortex, thalamus and other areas. SERCA-type Ca^{2+} pumps interact with phospholamban, a regulatory protein which increases pump activity when phosphorylated by PKA [19].

OTHER P-TYPE CATION TRANSPORTERS

Copper-transport defects underlie two genetic diseases, Wilson's and Menke's, with major neurological components (Chap. 45). The Wilson's disease gene codes for a transport protein, expressed chiefly in liver, that probably functions in Cu^{2+} excretion. The Menke's disease gene codes for a closely related protein that may function in intestinal Cu^{2+} absorption. From structural considerations, both of these pumps belong to a rather divergent subclass of the P-type cation pumps [21].

An ATP-dependent aminophospholipid translocase creates the asymmetric distribution of phosphatidylserine and phosphatidylethanolamine across cell membranes (Chaps. 2 and 3). The aminophospholipid translocase is a member of a subfamily of the P-type pumps [2].

MITOCHONDRIAL AND VACUOLAR ATPases

F-type ATPases occur as part of the F_1F_0 ATP synthase of mitochondria, chloroplasts and prokaryocyte plasma membranes

ATP synthesis utilizes energy derived from a proton gradient generated by electron-coupled proton pumps, such as cytochrome oxidase. ATP synthesis involves binding ADP and orthophosphate in close proximity on the surface of the β subunits. The $\alpha\beta$ dimers form a trimeric, wheel-like structure centrally attached to the F_0 transmembrane proton channel. Rotation of an asymmetric, rod-like γ subunit within this channel is driven by the proton flow. The γ-subunit rotation within the $(\alpha\beta)_3$ wheel causes the dimers to assume three successively different conformations. Thus, at any instant, each $\alpha\beta$ dimer is in a different conformational state. These conformational transitions evidently drive the dehydration of the bound substrates and effect dissociation of the nascent ATP molecules [22]. Dissipation of the proton gradient by various means will convert the synthase into an ATPase. The F_1 complex also incorporates δ and ϵ subunits of uncertain function.

Vacuolar ATP-dependent proton transporters occur in Golgi-derived membranes

These include Golgi cisternae, lysosomes, endosomes, endocrine secretory vesicles and the presynaptic vesicles that store neurotransmitters and peptide hormones. The vacuolar, ATP-dependent proton transporters (V-type ATPases) pump H^+ from the cytoplasm to acidify the vesicular or cisternal lumen. Transport of neurotransmitters into presynaptic vesicles is energized by the proton gradient so created (see below). The sequences and subunit structures of vacuolar proton pumps are very similar to those of the F-type ATPases.

ATP-BINDING CASSETTE PROTEINS

The ATP-binding cassette proteins are members of a superfamily with functions that encompass transport, ion conductance and regulation

Their structural unit is a "cassette," comprising six transmembrane segments and a cytoplasmic nucleotide-binding domain [23].

It has been proposed that a subfamily, the multidrug-resistance proteins (MDR, also called P-glycoproteins), may function to "flip" amphipathic molecules from the inner to the outer leaflet of plasma membranes [24]. One member, MDR3, selectively transports phosphatidylcholine [25]. MDR1 and MDR2 are the classic *multidrug-resistance proteins* (MRP), consisting of two cassettes within a single peptide chain. Their elevated expression during chemotherapy can produce decreased chemosensitivity of cancer cells by pumping the drugs out of the cells. They can also flip a broad range of amphipathic molecules, including membrane phospholipids and sphingolipids [25]. One or more P-glycoproteins appears to be expressed at high concentrations in the lumenal membranes of brain capillaries ([26], but see [27]) and probably accounts for many drug-exclusion functions of the blood–brain barrier (Chap. 32). Another subfamily of MRP can transport a variety of amphipathic organic anions from cells but has not been reported in brain.

According to one proposed mechanism for energizing transport by ATP-binding cassette (ABC) proteins, both nucleotide-binding domains may participate in an ATPase cycle that drives the transport: substrate binding permits ATP hydrolysis at one domain, which generates an activated conformation; transport results from a subsequent relaxation upon ATP binding at the other domain [28].

MDR apparently can function in some contexts as a volume-activated, ATP-dependent Cl^- channel [29]. Two other important ABC proteins, the cystic fibrosis gene product (CFTR) and the sulfonylurea receptor (SUR), are also ATP-regulated Cl^- and K^+ channels, respectively, with complex properties but possibly no transport functions.

In *Drosophila,* tryptophan and guanine transport are both mediated by ABC proteins that are dimers of three different gene products. The *white* gene protein dimerizes with the *scarlet* gene protein to form a tryptophan transporter and with the *brown* gene protein to form a guanine transporter. Each subunit consists of a single cassette. Human and mouse homologs of the *white* gene have been cloned and are expressed in several tissues including brain, but their function is unknown [30].

Adrenoleukodystrophy and the Zellweger's syndrome (Chap. 41) result from defects in two different genes that specify "single cassette" proteins targeted to peroxisomes. Both of these genes have homologs in yeast, where there is evidence that their proteins occur in the same heterodimers [31]. Because the defect in adrenoleukodystrophy involves β oxidation of the CoA derivatives of very-long-chain fatty acids, this transporter may function to move very-long-chain fatty acids into peroxisomes (Chap. 41).

Other members of the ABC superfamily participate in transmembrane peptide transport. One example is the presentation of class I major histocompatibility antigens on cell surfaces. This has led to the suggestion that similar transporters may function as peptide hormone transporters [32].

SECONDARY TRANSPORT SYSTEMS

Secondary active-transport systems mediate diverse neural functions

A variety of molecules and ions are regulated by specific symporters or antiporters linked to the Na^+ gradient (Fig. 5-1). Examples are discussed in the following sections.

The clearance of amine and amino acid neurotransmitters from the synaptic cleft and their storage in cytoplasmic vesicles is accomplished by the tandem action of plasma-membrane and vesicular-transport systems. Symporters in the plasma membranes of neurons and glia mediate neurotransmitter reuptake from synaptic clefts, whereas antiporters function in neurons to concentrate neurotransmitters from neuronal cytoplasm into synaptic vesicles (Fig. 5-7).

Neurotransmitter symporters. All neurotransmitter reuptake is driven by the Na^+ gradient created by the Na^+, K^+ pump. Symporters have been identified and partially characterized for the major neurotransmitters. While their demands on cerebral energy metabolism are unknown, it has been proposed that they could contribute substantially to the increased metabolism associated with neuronal activity (Chap. 31).

There are two distinct subfamilies of Na^+-dependent symporters that function in plasma membranes. One subfamily includes the $(Na^+ + Cl^-)$-dependent transporters for GABA, glycine, norepinephrine, dopamine and serotonin. Their topology includes 12 traverses of the plasma membrane. The other subfamily includes the $(Na^+ + Cl^- + K^+)$-dependent glutamate transporters, which traverse the plasma membrane ten times.

Five glutamate-symporter isoforms have been identified in human brain. Two of these

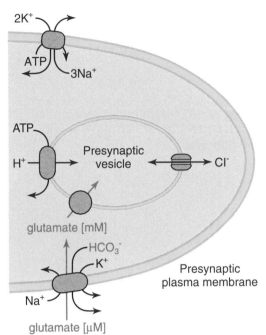

FIGURE 5-7. Processes involved in neurotransmitter uptake at nerve endings. Concentration into the cytoplasm is achieved by means of a Na^+ symporter with high affinity for the neurotransmitter. Synaptic vesicle membranes contain an ATP-dependent H^+ pump and Cl^- channels which acidify their internal space. These membranes also contain transporters that are selective for the neurotransmitter. Whether these operate as proton antiporters or as potential-driven facilitators has not been determined.

isoforms, glutamate–aspartate transporter (GLAST) and glutamate transporter-1 (GLT-1) (Chap. 15), are selectively expressed in astrocytes, while others display selective localization in certain neuronal cell types. The different isoforms probably have different regulatory interactions. For example, two of them have been shown to respond oppositely to exposure to arachidonic acid [33]. Astrocytes appear to play an important role in glutamate clearance from synaptic clefts. Rendering mice [34] and rats [35] deficient in GLAST or GLT-1 produces elevated extracellular glutamate concentrations and leads, in the case of mice, to lethal seizures.

Glutamate symporters have a relatively complex ion requirement, which has been investigated in a study of glutamate uptake by salamander retinal glia: one glutamate and two Na^+ are taken into the cell in exchange for the extrusion of one K^+, HCO_3^- or OH^-. Another study has concluded that three Na^+ enter with each glutamate [36]. In either case, there will be a net depolarizing influx of positive charge. The anion efflux produces intracellular acidification and extracellular alkalinization. The regulation of glutamate concentration is of special interest because the accumulation of extracellular glutamate is a probable factor in various pathologies (Chap. 34). While brain glutamate concentration is about 10 mM, "extracellular" glutamate as measured by *in vivo* microdialysis is normally only 3 to 4 μM. Glutamate within the synaptic cleft must be maintained at still lower concentrations in the resting state. With "normal" membrane potentials and ion concentrations, the glutamate transporter can theoretically reduce this value to 0.6 μM or less. However, under depolarizing or anoxic conditions, the membrane potential and the Na^+ and K^+ gradients can be reduced to levels that cause the symporter to fail or to operate in reverse to produce 100- to 1,000-fold increases in extracellular glutamate. Glutamate accumulated by astrocytes is converted to glutamine, which is, at least partly, shunted back into neurons.

Studies on the mechanisms of secondary transport. Voltage-clamp techniques (Chap. 6) can provide some insights into the mechanisms of ion-coupled secondary transport. Charge movements that are direct reflections of transport events can be detected in voltage-clamped membranes containing transport proteins. For example, capacitative currents occur in *Xenopus* oocyte membranes containing GABA transporters when the external medium is rapidly changed between Na^+-containing and Na^+-free Ringer's solutions. These currents can be related to transport because they are suppressed by specific GABA transport-blocking agents. Several deductions regarding the transport mechanism are inferred from such measurements: the apparent affinity of the transport sites for Na^+ is voltage-dependent; the amount of charge movement is a cooperative function of $[Na^+]$, indicative of two Na^+-binding sites per transporter; external Cl^- increases Na^+ affinity without changing the capacitative current. These are all events that involve the extracellularly available

transporter domains when measured in the absence of external GABA. Accordingly, they are considered to be "priming reactions" that prepare the transporter to rapidly bind and remove GABA as it appears in a synaptic cleft [37].

Ionic currents through transporters have been observed in the presence of neurotransmitters but in the absence of energizing ion gradients. Voltage-clamp recordings of several of the neurotransmitter symporters have exhibited brief, 2 to 3 msec, electrical events that are comparable to discrete ion-channel openings. For example, serotonin symporters exhibit Na^+ conductances of 6 to 13 pS, whereas glutamate symporters exhibit Cl^- conductances of ~0.7 pS. In both cases, these channel-like events can be blocked by selective transport inhibitors and they occur at much lower frequencies than the turnover rates of the symporters. Although their physiological relevance is unknown, they are undoubtedly associated with these ion-coupled symporters [38].

Vesicle neurotransmitter antiporters. As discussed above, proton-dependent antiporters concentrate neurotransmitters into presynaptic vesicles (Fig. 5-7). Protons are transported into the vesicles by a vacuolar-type ATPase, as discussed above.

Two closely related vesicular membrane antiporters (VMAT), VMAT1 and VMAT2 (Chap. 12), are broadly selective for the monoamine neurotransmitters dopamine, norepinephrine and serotonin. VMAT1 is expressed in peripheral neuroendocrine cells, VMAT2 in neurons and both in adrenal chromaffin cells [39]. VMAT2 expression is restricted to the membranes of dense-core vesicles. It also transports histamine and is expressed in histamine-storing cells. Selective inhibitors of both VMAT1 and VMAT2 include reserpine and ketanserin, whereas tetrabenazine inhibits only VMAT2. The related vesicular acetylcholine transporter (VAChT) is present in small cholinergic synaptic vesicles of the CNS. The membrane topology of all of these synaptic vesicle antiporters seems to consists of 12 transmembrane segments, beginning and ending on the cytoplasmic side.

Uptake of neurotransmitters into synaptic vesicles can be blocked by nigericin, by proton ionophores or by other agents which dissipate the proton gradient and by *N*-ethylmaleimide, which inhibits V-type ATPases. Uptake into synaptic vesicles is not affected by agents that act on other transport systems, such as Na^+, Ca^{2+}, ouabain, vanadate or oligomycin. A low concentration of extravesicular Cl^- stimulates the uptake of glutamate and catecholamines into their respective vesicles but does not affect glycine or GABA vesicular uptake.

Na^+, H^+ antiporters. Five isoforms of mammalian Na^+, H^+ antiporters (NHE) have been identified that catalyze an electroneutral exchange of protons for Na^+. The membrane topology is similar in all isoforms and includes ten to twelve putative transmembrane segments within the first 500 N-terminal residues. This fragment has been shown to be sufficient to mediate exchange of protons for Na^+. The more variable C-terminal cytoplasmic segment of about 300 residues appears to contain isoform-dependent regulatory domains. NHE1 is the most widely distributed and intensively studied isoform. It can be activated by a variety of stimuli, including neurotransmitters, hormones, growth factors and cell volume decrease. These factors act through second messengers to increase the affinity for protons, resulting in cytoplasmic alkalinization. Functions ascribed to Na^+, H^+ antiporters include roles in pH and volume regulation, cell adhesion, cell proliferation and ion and water transport. The NHE1 and NHE3 isoforms are expressed in the basolateral and apical membranes, respectively, of epithelia. The NHE5 isoform is primarily expressed in brain, spleen and testes.

Na^+, Ca^{2+} antiporters are present in plasma membranes and endoplasmic reticulum and act in concert with ATP-coupled Ca^{2+} pumps. The exchange process is electrogenic since the stoichiometry is three Na^+ per Ca^{2+}. The antiporters have lower affinities for Ca^{2+} than the P-type pumps, but because in some tissues the antiporter pumping capacity may be up to ten times that of the Ca^{2+}-ATPases, they may be important for rapidly lowering high cytoplasmic Ca^{2+}.

Anion Antiporters. Because CNS energy production derives almost entirely from aerobic glycolysis, the rate of metabolic CO_2 production is essentially equal to the rate of oxygen consumption. In adult human brain, this is about 2.5 mM per minute (Chap. 31). Most neurons express only low concentrations of carbonic anhydrase, and most carbonic anhydrase in brain is nonneuronal. Thus, most CO_2 diffuses unhydrated out of neurons and is rapidly converted to HCO_3^- before it enters the blood. A major component of erythrocytes is a Cl^-/HCO_3^- antiporter, known as band 3 protein, which mediates rapid uptake of HCO_3^- in exchange for Cl^- in peripheral tissues and releases HCO_3^- in exchange for Cl^- in the lungs. A neuron-specific isoform of the Cl^-/HCO_3^- antiporter has been identified, which suggests that significant anion exchange may occur across neuronal and/or glial membranes. Since some neurons express significant concentrations of cytoplasmic carbonic anhydrase, Cl^-/HCO_3^- exchange may have unrecognized functions. Its operation in neurons could influence both Cl^- potentials and cytoplasmic pH.

Rapid clearance of K^+ from the extracellular space is critical because high extracellular K^+ depolarizes neurons

Neural activity discharges K^+ into the extraneuronal space. If not rapidly removed, this K^+ lowers the membrane potential of adjacent cells. Normal neuronal activity can lead to elevations of 1 to 3 mM in extracellular K^+ ($[K^+]_e$), and during epileptogenesis, concentrations can be three to four times higher. Usually, the upper limit of axonal impulse-conduction frequency is set by a conduction block that occurs when extracellular K^+ accumulates to a concentration of 25 to 30 mM (Chap. 37). Both neurons and astroglia are involved in K^+ uptake, and both active and passive transport are probably important. The relative contributions of the two cell types and of the two cell processes remain controversial. It is clear that neurons accumulate K^+ almost exclusively by means of active transport, but the Na^+,K^+ pump is slow relative to the channel-mediated K^+ release from neurons and to the rates of K^+ increase in the extracellular space. Moreover, the neuronal Na^+,K^+ pump is saturated at low $[K^+]_e$, making it an ineffective regulator for this purpose.

Glial processes invest nearly all extrasynaptic neuronal surfaces (Chap. 1), and one of their principal functions is to regulate $[K^+]_e$. The extracellular space of the brain consists primarily of the 150 to 250 Å clefts separating glia and neurons. Astrocytes have higher K^+ permeability than most neurons, and they are extensively interconnected by gap junctions (Chap. 2). K^+ efflux from a neuron can diffuse into the local glial cytoplasm, and compensatory K^+ efflux can occur from more distal reaches of the glial syncytium, where the $[K^+]_e$ is lower (Fig. 5-8A). It should be noted that this "spatial buffering" is a diffusion process that requires no energy input. Measurements on retinal Müller cells have provided relevant data. These cells are specialized forms of astrocytes which do not form syncytia. Rather, they extend from the deep layers of the retina to form endfeet at the retinal interface with the vitreous body (see Fig. 47-1). The K^+ conductance of these cells is about 30 times higher at the endfeet in contact with the vitreous fluid than elsewhere. Moreover, K^+ currents through the plasma membranes other than endfeet are carried by inward-rectifying channels, whereas the K^+ channels at the endfeet are high-conductance and non-rectifying [40]. This seems designed to facilitate diffusive currents of K^+ from the retina into the Müller cell, which are balanced by K^+ efflux into the vitreous space and constitute a relatively "infinite" sink, equivalent to the syncytium of the generalized astrocytes.

Although spatial buffering can effectively prevent accumulation of moderate concentrations of extracellular K^+, this diffusion process may be inadequate at very low and very high rates of neuronal K^+ efflux. Several K^+ transporters occur in astrocytes and probably broaden the range of effective $[K^+]_e$ regulation. Glial swelling accompanies neural activity. This reflects the operation of a $(Na^+,K^+,2Cl^-)$ symporter in response to the volume-regulation mechanism discussed below. This symporter is driven by the Na^+ gradient generated by the Na^+ pump and may clear extracellular K^+ when an adequate K^+ sink is not present.

An outwardly directed Cl^- pump is necessary for the inhibitory, that is, hyperpolarizing, functions of GABA- and glycine-gated ion channels

The principal inhibitory neurotransmitters, GABA and glycine, hyperpolarize mature neurons by opening Cl^- channels (Chap. 16). This occurs because their internal Cl^- concentration is maintained at less than its equilibrium value and Cl^- flows inward. The most likely mechanism for reducing internal Cl^- involves a KCl symporter, a neuron-specific isoform of which occurs in brain [41]. Although indirect evidence for ATP-dependent primary Cl^- transport has been reported, a corresponding ATPase protein has not been identified [42]. The importance of an outward Cl^- pump for the inhibitory function of GABA-gated channels is made evident by observations that at early developmental stages GABA-gated channels in cortical neurons are depolarizing. They become hyperpolarizing only with maturation as a Cl^- transport system appears and the internal Cl^- concentration decreases [43].

Intracellular pH in brain is regulated by Na^+,H^+ antiporters, anion antiporters and Na^+, HCO_3^- symporters

The products of cerebral energy metabolism, primarily water and CO_2, could in principle leave the brain and enter the circulation without disturbing the ionic balance. However, to the extent that oxidation is incomplete, that is, to the extent that lactate or ketoacids are produced (Chap. 31), or that CO_2 equilibrates to $H^+ + HCO_3^-$, local pH will decrease. Other processes, such as local influx of Ca^{2+}, can also produce local pH changes. The cerebral metabolic rate is sensitive to such changes and decreases with decreasing pH. Without adequate pH control, local metabolic deficits can be intensified and propagated [44]. In addition to the increase of $[K^+]_e$ discussed above, intracellular acidification and extracellular alkalinization accompany neuronal activity [45]. The pH response of astrocytes to membrane depolarization is opposite to the neuronal pH response: intracellular alkalinization and extracellular acidification occur [46]. The neuronal acidification appears to involve the anion antiporter exchange of HCO_3^- for Cl^-, whereas astrocytic alkalinization is probably mediated by a Na^+, HCO_3^- symporter. This is an oversimplification of CNS pH regulation in view of the fact that additional secondary transporters are involved in various aspects of local pH regulation.

Na^+, H^+ antiporters occur in synaptosomes, glia and neuroblastoma cells (Fig. 5-8B). They are relatively inactive at neutral pH, but with a decrease in intracellular pH they produce an efflux of protons at the expense of the Na^+ gradient. The Na^+, H^+ transport stoichiometry is 1:1. Activation by an internal pH decrement apparently results from protonation of a cytoplasmic site, which allosterically increases the affinity of the proton ionophoric site. In some cells, the Na^+, H^+ antiporter is under additional control by receptor mechanisms. Several growth factors and hormones produce transient cytoplasmic alkalinization, probably by mediating a protein kinase phosphorylation of the antiporter, which increases its internal proton affinity.

Cell-volume regulation involves control of the content of osmotically active impermeant molecules and ions

Cell volume will change because of an altered internal solute content, termed isotonic response, or because of altered extracellular solute concentration, termed hyper- or hypotonic responses (Fig. 5-8B). Impairment of brain energy metabolism, such as may ensue from ischemia, anoxia or trauma, produces an isotonic cellular swelling called "cytotoxic edema" and further effects by the coincident release of glutamate (Chaps. 34 and 38). Cellular swelling is also produced by extracellular hypotonicity. This is most often caused by hyponatremia, which can result acutely from postsurgical fluid therapies.

Chronic hyponatremia can arise from congestive heart failure, Addison's disease or a "syndrome of inappropriate vasopressin release." A general reduction in brain size resulting from acute extracellular hypertonicity may produce neurological disturbances. This condition may be a component of pathology originating outside the brain, such as kidney disease (uremia) and diabetes mellitus (hyperglycemia). Central pontine myelinolysis, which is produced experimentally by acute infusion of hypertonic saline, can occur as a complication of liver transplantation.

Cells have short-term mechanisms that tend to restore their volume toward "normal" primarily by shifting the distributions of Na^+, K^+ and Cl^-. The details of the mechanisms appear to vary with cell type. Subsequent to cell swelling, regulatory volume decrease usually involves opening ion channels. Subsequent to hyperosmotic shrinking, regulatory volume increase frequently involves activation of Na^+, H^+ antiporters and Na^+, K^+, $2Cl^-$ symporters. The primary detectors of volume and osmotic changes are presently unknown. Although cell membranes can readily change shape, they do not stretch significantly. However, cytoskeletal proteins attached to membrane proteins could form tensile elements that could mediate volume changes (Fig. 5-8B). Cell shape is determined by interactions of cytoskeletal elements, membranes and components of the extracellular matrix (Chaps. 2 and 8). Stretch-activated cation channels have been detected both in neuroblastoma cells and in cultured astrocytes (see Box 47-1). Activation of Cl^- channels by cellular swelling is an identified characteristic of both the MDR and CFTR proteins [47], at least one of which occurs in astrocytes.

Altered extracellular tonicity can induce compensatory changes in the concentrations of certain intracellular osmolytes through mecha-

FIGURE 5-8. **A:** Spatial buffering by astrocytes. This conceptual diagram indicates the pathways available for potassium ions to diffuse through the glial syncytium *(light orange)* subsequent to their release from neuronal membranes *(dark orange)* during neural activity. **B:** Regulation of cell volume. The mechanisms of osmotic activation of ion pathways vary with cell type. Detection of volume changes may involve cytoskeletal proteins which interact with channels and/or transporters. Regulatory volume decrease *(RVD)* may be initiated by stretch-activated channels that permit efflux of KCl. Acute regulatory volume increase *(RVI)* produces NaCl influx, with or without coupling to K^+ influx. Chronic exposure to hypertonic media initiates adaptation mechanisms that include transcriptional activation of osmolyte symporters.

A

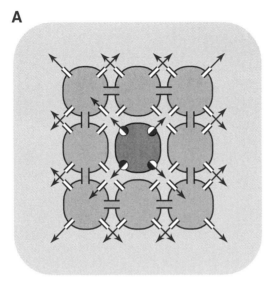

◐ Voltage gated
  potassium channels

∥ Inward-rectifying
  potassium channels

▬ Gap junctions

B

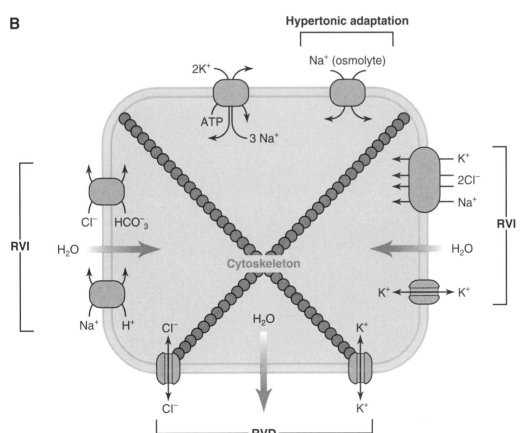

nisms involving gene regulation. Glioma cells in culture have been shown to respond after a few hours of exposure to hypertonic medium by transcribing high levels of the Na^+, inositol symporter. In brain, active osmolytes include taurine, glutamine, glutamate, myo-inositol, creatine, glycerophosphorylcholine and choline. Na^+-dependent symporters for most of these compounds have been identified [48].

Unclassified energy-requiring pumps. Three different but closely related mammalian proteins, called ZnT-1, -2 and -3, have been related to Zn^{2+} transport. The best evidence indicates that ZnT-1 mediates Zn^{2+} efflux across cell membranes, whereas ZnT-2 mediates vesicular sequestration of Zn^{2+}. ZnT-3 is selectively expressed in brain and testes. In brain it may be associated with presynaptic vesicles in certain glutamatergic neurons [49]. The ZnT proteins are structurally related to a family of yeast proteins that confer resistance to Zn^{2+} and Co^{2+} toxicity. At present, there is no information about the energy source for Zn^{2+} transport in eukaryotes. An *E. coli* Zn^{2+}-resistance gene has been shown to encode a P-type ATPase.

UNCOUPLED TRANSPORTERS

Glucose crosses the cells that constitute the blood–brain barrier and the plasma membranes of neurons and glia by means of uncoupled transporters that facilitate diffusion (Fig. 5-1). It is noteworthy that, despite the vital dependence of brain on an adequate supply of glucose (Chap. 31), there appears to be no mechanism for active transport of glucose into brain. Instead, local blood flow must be closely regulated to maintain the highly variable local metabolic requirements (Chaps. 31 and 54).

Seven different isoforms of uncoupled glucose transporters (GLUT-1–7) have been identified in mammalian cells. They seem to vary chiefly in their responses to regulatory influences: GLUT-1 is negatively regulated by glucose; GLUT-4 can be held in an extracellular reserve of endocytotic vesicles that respond to insulin by fusion with the plasma membrane. Although regulation of the other forms has not

been defined, all are differentially expressed. GLUT-3 is expressed by glia and certain neurons, whereas GLUT-1 is expressed in the epithelial and endothelial cells that comprise the blood–brain barrier and in glia, Schwann cells and the perineurium of peripheral nerves. GLUT-5 occurs in microglia; GLUT-2, GLUT-4 and GLUT-7 have been detected in brain at lower levels of expression and are confined to more discrete regions [50].

REFERENCES

1. Laüger, P. *Electrogenic Ion Pumps.* Sunderland, MA: Sinauer Associates, 1991.
2. Tang, X., Halleck, M. S., Schlegel, R. A., and Williamson, P. A subfamily of P-type ATPases with aminophospholipid transporting activity. *Science* 272:1495–1497, 1996.
3. Zahler, R., Zhang, Z. T., Manor, M., and Boron, W. F. Sodium kinetics of Na,K-ATPase α isoforms in intact transfected HeLa cells. *J. Gen. Physiol.* 119:201–213, 1997.
4. Munzer, J. S., Daly, S. E., Jewell-Motz, E. A., Lingrel, J. B., and Blostein, R. Tissue- and isoform-specific kinetic behavior of the Na,K-ATPase. *J. Biol. Chem.* 269:16668–16676, 1994.
5. Besirli, C. G., Gong, T. W., and Lomax, M. I. Novel β3 isoform of the Na,K-ATPase β subunit from mouse retina. *Biochim. Biophys. Acta* 1350:21–26, 1997.
6. Peng, L., Martin-Vasallo, P., and Sweadner, K. J. Isoforms of Na,K-ATPase α and β subunits in the rat cerebellum and in granule cell cultures. *J. Neurosci.* 17:3488–3502, 1997.
7. Geering, K., Beggah, A., Good, P., et al. Oligomerization and maturation of Na,K-ATPase: Functional interaction of the cytoplasmic NH2 terminus of the β subunit with the α subunit. *J. Cell Biol.* 133:1193–1204, 1996.
8. Lecuona, E., Luquin, S., Avila, J., Garcia-Segura, L. M., and Martin-Vasallo, P. Expression of the β1 and β2 (AMOG) subunits of the Na,K-ATPase in neural tissues: Cellular and developmental distribution patterns. *Brain Res. Bull.* 40:167–174, 1996.
9. Fendler, K., Froehlich, J., Jaruschewski, S., et al. Correlation of charge translocation with the reaction cycle of the Na,K-ATPase. In J. Kaplan and P. De Weer (eds.), *The Sodium Pump: Recent Developments.* New York: Rockefeller University Press, 1991, pp. 525–530.

10. Potaman, V. N., Ussery, D. W., and Sinden, R. R. Formation of a combined H-DNA/open TATA box structure in the promoter sequence of the human Na,K-ATPase α2 gene. *J. Biol. Chem.* 271:13441–13447, 1996.

11. Pathak, B. G., Neumann, J. C., Croyle, M. L., and Lingrel, J. B. The presence of both negative and positive elements in the 5′-flanking sequence of the rat Na,K-ATPase α3 subunit gene are required for brain expression in transgenic mice. *Nucleic Acids Res.* 22:4748–4755, 1994.

12. Nomoto, M., Gonzalez, F. J., Mita, T., Inoue, N., and Kawamura, M. Analysis of cis-acting regions upstream of the rat Na^+/K^+-ATPase α1 subunit gene by *in vivo* footprinting. *Biochim. Biophys. Acta* 1995:35–69, 1995.

13. Kobayashi, M., Shimomura, A., Hagiwara, M., and Kawakami, K. Phosphorylation of ATF-1 enhances its DNA binding and transcription of the Na,K-ATPase α1 subunit gene promoter. *Nucleic Acids Res.* 25:877–882, 1997.

14. Farman, N., Bonvalet, J. P., and Seckl, J. R. Aldosterone selectively increases Na^+-K^+-ATPase α3-subunit mRNA expression in rat hippocampus. *Am. J. Physiol.* 266:C423–C428, 1994.

15. Chaudhury, S., Bajpai, M., and Bhattacharya, S. Differential effects of hypothyroidism on Na-K-ATPase mRNA α isoforms in the developing rat brain. *J. Mol. Neurosci.* 7:229–234, 1996.

16. Liu, B., and Gick, G. Characterization of the 5′ flanking region of the rat Na^+/K^+-ATPase β1 subunit gene. *Biochim. Biophys. Acta.* 1130: 336–338, 1992.

17. Peng, M., Huang, L., Xie, Z., Huang, W. H., and Askari, A. Partial inhibition of Na^+/K^+-ATPase by ouabain induces the Ca^{2+}-dependent expressions of early-response genes in cardiac myocytes. *J. Biol. Chem.* 271:10372–10378, 1996.

18. Yamamoto, K., Ikeda, U., Seino, Y., et al. Regulation of Na,K-adenosine triphosphatase gene expression by sodium ions in cultured neonatal rat cardiocytes. *J. Clin. Invest.* 92:1889–1895, 1993.

19. Carafoli, E. The calcium pumping ATPase of the plasma membrane. *Annu. Rev. Physiol.* 53: 531–547, 1991.

20. Stahl, W. L., Eakin, T. J., Owens, J. W. M., et al. Plasma membrane Ca^{2+}-ATPase isoforms: Distribution of mRNAs in rat brain by *in situ* hybridization. *Brain Res. Mol. Brain Res.* 16:223–231, 1992.

21. Harris, Z. L., and Gitlin, J. D. Genetic and molecular basis for copper toxicity. *Am. J. Clin. Nutr.* 63:836S–841S, 1996.

22. Boyer, P. D. The ATP synthase—a splendid molecular machine. *Annu. Rev. Biochem.* 66:717–749, 1997.

23. Hyde, S. C., Emsley, P., Hartshorn, M. J., et al. Structural model of ATP-binding proteins associated with cystic fibrosis, multidrug resistance and bacterial transport. *Nature* 346:362–365, 1990.

24. Higgins, C. F., and Gottesman, M. M. Is the multidrug transporter a flippase? *Trends Biochem. Sci.* 17:18–21, 1992.

25. van Helvoort, A., Smith, A. J., Sprong, H., et al. MDR1 P-glycoprotein is a lipid translocase of broad specificity, while MDR3 P-glycoprotein specifically translocates phosphatidylcholine. *Cell* 87:507–517, 1996.

26. Beaulieu, E., Demeule, M., Ghitescu, L., and Beliveau, R. P-glycoprotein is strongly expressed in the luminal membranes of the endothelium of blood vessels in the brain. *Biochem. J.* 326(Pt. 2):539–544, 1997.

27. Pardridge, W. M., Golden, P. L., Kang, Y. S., and Bickel, U. J. Brain microvascular and astrocyte localization of P-glycoprotein. *J. Neurochem.* 68:1278–1285, 1997.

28. Senior, A. E., al-Shawi, M. K., and Urbatsch, I. L. The catalytic cycle of P-glycoprotein. *FEBS Lett.* 377:285–289, 1995.

29. Gill, D. R., Hyde, S. C., Higgins, C. F., Valverde, M. A., Mintenig, G. M., and Sepulveda, F. V. Separation of drug transport and chloride channel functions of the human multidrug resistance P-glycoprotein. *Cell* 71:23–32, 1992.

30. Croop, J. M., Tiller, G. E., Fletcher, J. A., et al. Isolation and characterization of a mammalian homolog of the *Drosophila* white gene. *Gene* 185:77–85, 1997.

31. Shani, N., and Valle, D. A. *Saccharomyces cerevisiae* homolog of the human adrenoleukodystrophy transporter is a heterodimer of two half ATP-binding cassette transporters. *Proc. Natl. Acad. Sci. USA* 93:11901–11906, 1996.

32. Becker, K. F., Allmeier, H., and Hollt, V. New mechanisms of hormone secretion: MDR-like gene products as extrusion pumps for hormones? *Horm. Metab. Res.* 24:210–213, 1992.

33. Zerangue, N., Arriza, J. L., Amara, S. G., and Kavanaugh, M. P. Differential modulation of human glutamate transporter subtypes by arachidonic acid. *J. Biol. Chem.* 270:6433–6435, 1995.

34. Tanaka, K., Watase, K., Manabe, T., et al. Epilepsy and exacerbation of brain injury in mice lacking the glutamate transporter GLT-1. *Science* 276:1699–1702, 1997.

35. Rothstein, J. D., Dykes-Hoberg, M., Pardo, C. A.,

et al. Knockout of glutamate transporters reveals a major role for astroglial transport in excitotoxicity and clearance of glutamate. *Neuron* 16:675–686, 1996.

36. Zerangue, N., and Kavanaugh, M. P. Flux coupling in a neuronal glutamate transporter. *Nature* 383:634–637, 1996.

37. Mager, S., Kleinberger-Doron, N., Keshet, G., Davidson, N., Kanner, B., and Lester, H. Ion binding and permeation at the GABA transporter GAT1. *J. Neurosci.* 16:5405–5414, 1996.

38. Sonders, M. S., and Amara, S. G. Channels in transporters. *Curr. Opin. Cell Biol.* 6:294–302, 1996.

39. Erickson, J. D., Schafer, M. K., Bonner, T. I., Eiden, L. E., and Weihe, E. Distinct pharmacological properties and distribution in neurons and endocrine cells of two isoforms of the human vesicular monoamine transporter. *Proc. Natl. Acad. Sci. USA* 93:5166–5171, 1996.

40. Nilius, B., and Reichenbach, A. Efficient K^+ buffering by mammalian retinal glial cells is due to cooperation of specialized ion channels. *Pflugers Arch.* 411:654–660, 1988.

41. Payne, J. A., Stevenson, T. J., and Donaldson, L. F. Molecular characterization of a putative K-Cl cotransporter in rat brain. A neuronal-specific isoform. *J. Biol. Chem.* 271:16245–16252, 1996.

42. Gerencser, G., Purushotham, K., and Meng, H. An electrogenic chloride pump in a zoological membrane. *J. Exp. Zool.* 275:256–261, 1996.

43. Owens, D. F., Boyce, L. H., Davis, M. B., and Kriegstein, A. R. Excitatory GABA responses in embryonic and neonatal cortical slices demonstrated by gramicidin perforated-patch recordings and calcium imaging. *J. Neurosci.* 16:6414–6423, 1996.

44. Siesjö, B. K., von Hanwehr, R., Nergelius, G., Nevander, G., and Ingvar, M. Extra- and intracellular pH in the brain during seizures and in the recovery period following the arrest of seizure activity. *J. Cereb. Blood Flow Metab.* 5:47–57, 1985.

45. Voipio, J., Paalasmaa, P., Taira, T., and Kaila, K. Pharmacological characterization of extracellular pH transients evoked by selective synaptic and exogenous activation of AMPA, NMDA, and GABAA receptors in the rat hippocampal slice. *J. Neurophysiol.* 74:633–642, 1995.

46. Deitmer, J., and Rose, C. pH regulation and proton signalling by glial cells. *Prog. Neurobiol.* 48:73–103, 1996.

47. Hardy, S. P., Goodfellow, H. R., Valverde, M. A., Gill, D. R., Sepulveda, V., and Higgins, C. F. Protein kinase C-mediated phosphorylation of the human multidrug resistance P-glycoprotein regulates cell volume-activated chloride channels [published erratum appears in *EMBO J.* 14:1844, 1995]. *EMBO J.* 14:68–75, 1995.

48. Strange, K. Regulation of solute and water balance and cell volume in the central nervous system [editorial]. *J. Am. Soc. Nephrol.* 3:12–27, 1992.

49. Palmiter, R. D., Cole, T. B., Quaife, C. J., and Findley, S. D. ZnT-3, a putative transporter of zinc into synaptic vesicles. *Proc. Natl. Acad. Sci. USA* 93:14934–14939, 1996.

50. Vannucci, S. J., Maher, F., and Simpson, I. A. Glucose transporter proteins in brain: Delivery of glucose to neurons and glia. *Glia* 21:2–21, 1997.

51. Toyosima, C., Sasabe, H., and Stokes, D. L. Three-dimensional cryo-electron microscopy of the calcium ion pump in the sarcoplasmic reticulum membrane. *Nature* 362:469–471, 1993.

52. Yonekura, K., Stokes, D. L., Sasabe H., et al. The ATP-binding site of Ca^{2+}-ATPase revealed by electron image analysis. *Biophys. J.* 72:997–1005, 1997.

52a. Zhang, P., Toyoshima, C., Yonekura, K., Green, N. M., and Stokes, D. L. Structure of the calcium pump form sarcoplasmic reticulum at 8-Å resolution. *Nature* 392:835–839, 1998.

53. Siegel, G. J., Holm, C., Schreiber, J. H., Dermond, T., and Ernst, S. A. Purification of mouse brain Na,K-ATPase catalytic unit and immunocytochemical localization. *J. Histochem.* 34:189, 1986.

54. Ernst, S. A., Palacios, J. R., and Siegel, G. J. Immunocytochemical localization of Na,K-ATPase in mouse choroid plexus. *J. Histochem.* 66:1742–1751, 1986.

55. Chauhan, N. B., and Siegel, G. J. Differential expression of Na,K-ATPase α subunit mRNAs in the aging rat cerebellum. *J. Neurosci. Res.* 47:287–299, 1997.

56. Chauhan, N. B., and Siegel, G. J. In situ analysis of Na,K-ATPase α1- and α2-isoform mRNAs in aging rat hippocampus. *J. Neurochem* 66:1742–1751, 1996.

57. Chauhan, N. B., Lee, J. M., and Siegel G. J. Na,K-ATPase mRNA levels and plaque load in Alzheimer's disease, *J. Molecular Neuroscience* 9:151–166, 1997.

CHAPTER

6

Electrical Excitability and Ion Channels

Bertil Hille and William A. Catterall

Basic Neurochemistry: Molecular, Cellular and Medical Aspects, 6th Ed., edited by G. J. Siegel et al. Published by Lippincott–Raven Publishers, Philadelphia, 1999. Correspondence to Bertil Hille, Department of Physiology and Biophysics, University of Washington School of Medicine, Box 357290, Seattle, Washington 98195-7290.

The nervous system enables animals to receive and act on internal and external stimuli with speed and in a coordinated manner. Activity of the nervous system is reflected in a variety of electrical and chemical signals that arise in the receptor organs, the nerve cells and the effector organs, including the muscles and secretory glands. Consider, for example, a simple reflex arc mediating reflex withdrawal of the hand from a hot surface. Four cell types are involved in a network shown diagrammatically in Figure 6-1. The message travels from skin receptors through the network as a volley of electrical disturbances, terminating in the contraction of some muscles. This chapter concerns the origin of electrical potentials in such excitable cells. As we shall see, potentials are generated by the passive diffusion of ions such as Na$^+$, K$^+$, Ca^{2+} and Cl$^-$ through highly selective molecular pores in the cell surface membrane called ion channels. Over 100 genes coding for subunits of ion channels have been identified. Ion channels play a role in membrane excitation as central as the role of enzymes in metabolism. The opening and closing of specific channels shape the membrane potential changes and give rise to characteristic electrical messages. The interested reader is referred to Hodgkin [1], Armstrong [2], Nicholls et al. [3] and Hille [4,5] for more detailed treatment of this subject.

ELECTRICAL PHENOMENA IN EXCITABLE CELLS

All excitable cells have a membrane potential

At rest, the entire cytoplasm is electrically more negative than the external bathing fluid by 30 to 100 mV. All of this potential drop appears across the extremely thin external cell membrane, as may be ascertained by recording with an electrolyte-filled glass pipette microelectrode. When such an electrode is used to probe potentials around an excitable cell, a sudden negative drop appears at the moment the narrow tip of the pipette breaks through the cell surface. By convention, the membrane potential is always reported in terms of "inside" minus "outside," so the resting potential is a negative number, for example, -70 mV in a myelinated nerve fiber. Signals that make the cytoplasm more positive are said to depolarize the membrane, and those making it more negative are said to hyperpolarize the membrane.

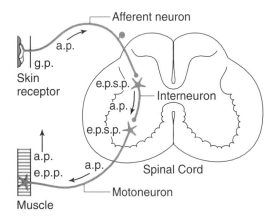

FIGURE 6-1. Path of excitation in a simplified spinal reflex that mediates withdrawal of the arm from a painful stimulus. In each of the three neurons and in the muscle cell, excitation starts with a localized slow potential and is propagated via an action potential *(a.p.)*. Slow potentials are the generator potential *(g.p.)* at the skin, the excitatory postsynaptic potentials *(e.p.s.p.)* at the interneuron and motoneuron and the end-plate potential *(e.p.p.)* at the neuromuscular junction. Each neuron makes additional connections to other pathways, which are not shown.

Electrical signals recorded from cells are basically of two types: stereotyped action potentials characteristic of each cell type and a variety of slow potentials

The action potential of axons is a brief, spike-like depolarization that propagates regeneratively as an electrical wave without decrement and at a high, constant velocity from one end of the axon to the other [3]. It is used for all rapid signaling over a distance. For example, in the reflex arc of Figure 6-1, action potentials in motor axons might carry the message from spinal cord to arm, telling the muscle fibers of the biceps to contract. In large mammalian axons at body temperature, the action potential at any one patch of membrane may last only 0.4 msec as it propagates at a speed of 100 m/sec. The action potential normally is elicited when the cell membrane is depolarized by some type of stimulus to beyond a threshold level; it is said to be produced in an all-or-nothing manner because a subthreshold stimulus gives no propagated response, whereas every suprathreshold stimulus elicits the stereotyped propagating wave. Underlying the propagated action potential is a regenerative wave of opening and closing of voltage-gated ion channels that sweeps along the axon. Action potentials also are frequently referred to as spikes or impulses. Most nerve cell and muscle cell membranes can make action potentials and are said to be electrically excitable, but a few cannot.

By contrast, slow potentials are localized membrane depolarizations and hyperpolarizations, with time courses ranging from several milliseconds to minutes. They are associated with a variety of transduction mechanisms. For example, slow potentials arise at the synaptic site of action of neurotransmitter molecules (see Chap. 10) and of some hormones, as well as in sensory endings of chemosensors, mechanosensors and photoreceptors (see Chaps. 47 and 48). These electrical signals in sensory endings frequently are called generator or receptor potentials, and the signals arising postsynaptically at chemical synapses are called postsynaptic potentials. Slow potentials are graded in relation to their stimulus and sum with each other both spatially and temporally within the cell, while decaying passively over an intracellular distance of no more than a few millimeters from the site of generation. Underlying the slow potential is a graded and local opening or closing of ion channels, reflecting the intensity of the stimulus. These channels are gated by stimuli other than voltage. The natural stimulus for the initiation of propagated action potentials is a depolarizing slow potential exceeding the firing threshold. For example, impulses in a wide variety of presynaptic cells often give rise to a barrage of excitatory, or depolarizing, and inhibitory, or hyperpolarizing, postsynaptic potentials in the dendrites of a postsynaptic neuron. These slow potentials sum within the dendrites and cell body to provide the drive stimulating or suppressing initiation of action potentials at the axon hillock, which then propagate down the axon. In each of the four cell populations involved in the reflex arc in Figure 6-1, depolarizing slow potentials give rise to propagating action potentials as the message moves forward.

THE IONIC HYPOTHESIS AND RULES OF IONIC ELECTRICITY

In the late nineteenth century, physiologists realized that the currents and potentials in excitable cells might be due to the diffusion of ions. Before we can discuss this hypothesis in detail, we must review the physical chemistry of electrodiffusion.

How do membrane potentials arise?

Consider the electrolyte system represented in Figure 6-2 (left), where a porous membrane separates aqueous solutions of unequal concentrations of a fictitious salt, KA. Two electrodes permit the potential difference between the two solutions to be measured. Now, assume that the membrane pores are permeable exclusively to K^+ so that K^+ begins to diffuse across the membrane but A^- does not. For simple statistical reasons, the movement of K^+ from the concentrated side to the dilute side initially will exceed the movement in the reverse direction, and we

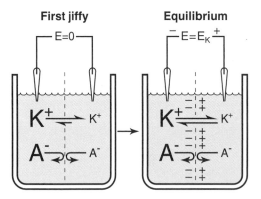

FIGURE 6-2. Origin of the membrane potential in a purely K^+-permeable membrane. The porous membrane separates unequal concentrations of the dissociated salt K^+A^-. In the first "jiffy," the membrane potential, E, recorded by the electrodes above is zero and K^+ diffuses to the right down the concentration gradient. The anion A^- cannot cross the membrane, so a net positive charge builds up on the right and a negative charge on the left. At equilibrium, the membrane potential, caused by the charge separation, has built up to the Nernst potential, E_K, and the fluxes of K^+ become equal in the two directions.

expect a net flux of K^+ down its concentration gradient. However, this process does not continue long since K^+ carries a positive charge from one compartment to the other and leaves a net negative charge behind. The growing separation of charge creates an electrical potential difference, the membrane potential, between the two solutions; and a positive charge appears on the side into which the K^+ ions diffuse, thereby setting up an electrical force that tends to oppose further net movement of K^+.

Equilibrium potential is the membrane potential at which there are no net ion movements

The membrane potential reached in a system with only one permeant ion and no perturbing forces is the equilibrium, or Nernst, potential for that ion; thus, the final membrane potential for the system in Figure 6-2 is the potassium equilibrium potential E_K. At that potential, there is no further net movement of K^+ and, unless otherwise disturbed, the membrane potential and ion gradient will remain stable indefinitely. The value of the Nernst potential is derived from thermodynamics by recognizing that the change

of electrochemical potential, $\Delta \mu_j$, for moving the permeant ion j^{+z} across the membrane must be zero at equilibrium:

$$\Delta\mu_j = 0 = RT\ln\frac{[j]_o}{[j]_i} - zFE \qquad (1)$$

where R is the gas constant (8.31 J/degree/mol), T is absolute temperature in Kelvin (°C + 273.2) and F is Faraday's constant (96,500 C/mol). Using terms appropriate to biology, $[j]_o$ and $[j]_i$ represent activities of ion j^{+z} outside and inside a cell, z is the ionic valence and E is the membrane potential defined as "inside minus outside." Solving for E and calling it E_j to denote the ion at equilibrium gives the Nernst equation for ion j:

$$E_j = \frac{RT}{zF} \ln \frac{[j]_o}{[j]_i} \qquad (2)$$

For practical use at 20°C, the Nernst equation can be rewritten:

$$E_j = \frac{58 \text{ mV}}{z} \log \frac{[j]_o}{[j]_i} \qquad (3)$$

showing that for a 10:1 transmembrane gradient, a monovalent ion can give 58 mV of membrane potential. Table 6-1 gives approximate intracellular and extracellular concentrations of the four electrically most important ions in a mammalian skeletal muscle cell and the Nernst potentials calculated from these numbers at 37°C, neglecting possible activity coefficient corrections. Experimentally, it is found that the resting muscle membrane is primarily permeable to K^+ and Cl^-, and therefore, the resting potential in muscle is −90 mV, close to the equilibrium potentials E_K and E_{Cl}. During a propagated action potential, ion channels permeable to Na^+ open, some Na^+ enters the muscle fiber and the membrane potential swings transiently toward E_{Na}. When these pores close again, the membrane potential returns to near E_K and E_{Cl}. To summarize, membrane potentials arise by diffusion of a small number of ions down their concentration gradient across a permselective membrane.

TABLE 6-1. **APPROXIMATE FREE ION CONCENTRATIONS IN MAMMALIAN SKELETAL MUSCLE**

Ion	Extracellular concentration (mM)	Intracellular concentration (mM)	[Ion]$_o$/[Ion]$_i$	Nernst potential[a] (mV)
Na$^+$	145	12	12	+66
K$^+$	4	155	0.026	−97
Ca^{2+}	1.5	<10^{-3}	>1,500	>97
Cl$^-$	120	4[b]	30[b]	−90[b]

[a]Equilibrium potentials calculated at 37°C from the Nernst equation.
[b]Calculated assuming a −90 mV resting potential for the muscle membrane and that Cl$^-$ ions are at equilibrium.

Real cells are not at equilibrium

Although the concept of equilibrium potentials is essential to understand and predict the membrane potentials generated by ion permeability, real cells are never at equilibrium because different ion channels open and close during excitation and even at rest several types of channel are open simultaneously. Under these circumstances, the ion gradients are dissipated constantly, albeit slowly, and ion pumps are always needed in the long run to maintain a steady state (see Chap. 5). The net passive flux, M_j, of each ion is proportional to the permeability, P_j, for that ion and often is given, at least approximately, by an empirical formula called the Goldman-Hodgkin-Katz flux equation [3–5]:

$$M_j = P_j z_j \frac{EF}{RT} \frac{[j]_o - [j]_i \exp(z_j EF/RT)}{1 - \exp(z_j EF/RT)} \quad (4)$$

Experimentally, these fluxes may be measured as an electrical current or by using radioactive tracers or with sensitive indicator substances responding to the ion in question by fluorescence or other optical changes. In most cases, the fluxes are too small to detect by the less sensitive classical method of chemical analysis for the total amount of an ion.

When the membrane is permeable to several ions, the steady-state potential is given by the sum of contributions of the permeant ions, weighted according to their relative permeabilities:

$$E = \frac{RT}{F} \ln \frac{P_{Na}[Na^+]_o + P_K[K^+]_o + P_{Cl}[Cl^-]_i}{P_{Na}[Na^+]_i + P_K[K^+]_i + P_{Cl}[Cl^-]_o} \quad (5)$$

The Goldman-Hodgkin-Katz voltage equation often is used to determine the relative permeabilities to ions from experiments where the bathing ion concentrations are varied and changes in the membrane potential are recorded. It has the same form as the equation usually used to describe the responses of ion-selective electrodes in analytical work in the laboratory.

During excitation, ion channels open or close, ions move and the membrane potential changes

The extra ion fluxes during activity act as an extra load on the Na$^+$-K$^+$ and the Ca^{2+} pumps, consuming ATP and stimulating an extra burst of cellular oxygen consumption until the original gradients are restored (see Chap. 5). How large are these fluxes? The physical minimum, calculated from the rules of electricity, is a very small number. Only 10^{-12} equivalents of charge need be moved to polarize 1 cm^2 of membrane by 100 mV, meaning that ideally the movement of 1 pmol/cm^2 of monovalent ion would be enough to depolarize the membrane fully. This quantity, related to the electrical capacitance of the membrane, is a constant throughout the animal and plant kingdoms, as would be the case if the effective thickness and dielectric constant of the hydrophobic, insulating part of all cell plasma membranes were similar. In practice, unmyelinated axons gain about 4 to 8 pmol of Na$^+$ and lose about the same amount of K$^+$ per square centimeter for one action potential. The figure is higher than the physical ideal because the oppositely directed fluxes of Na$^+$ and K$^+$

overlap considerably in time, working against each other. With this kind of Na^+ gain, an unmyelinated squid giant axon of 1-mm diameter could be stimulated 10^5 times and a mammalian fiber of 0.2-μm diameter only 10 to 15 times before the internal Na^+ concentration would be doubled, assuming that the Na^+-K^+ pump had been blocked. In myelinated nerve, the Na^+ gain in one impulse is very small, amounting to only 2×10^{-7} mol/kg of nerve because of the special low-capacitance properties of myelin.

Transport systems also may produce membrane potentials

The equations just discussed are those for passive electrodiffusion in ion channels, where the only motive forces on ions are thermal and electrical, and they do indeed explain almost all of the potentials of excitable cells. However, there is another type of electrical current source in cells that can generate potentials: the ion pumps and other membrane devices that couple ion movements to the movements of other molecules. In excitable cells, the most prominent is the Na^+-K^+ pump (see Chap. 5), which gives a net export of positive charge and, hence, tends to hyperpolarize the cell surface membrane in proportion to the rate of pumping [3]; but hyperpolarization from this electrogenic pumping is typically only a modest few millivolts. By contrast, mitochondria, as well as plant, algal and fungal cells, have powerful current sources in their proton-transport system. Their membrane potentials often are dominated by this electrogenic system and, thus, are not describable in terms of diffusion in simple passive channels.

ELECTRICALLY EXCITABLE CELLS

Permeability changes of the action potential

Given the rules of ionic electricity, the major biological problem in understanding action potentials is to describe and explain the ion permeability mechanisms in the membrane. The opening and closing of ion channels involves conformational changes driven by electrical field changes or ligand binding but not by direct consumption of metabolic energy. The independence of immediate metabolic input can be demonstrated in studies with internally perfused cells and with channels reconstituted into lipid bilayers. For example, the great majority of the axoplasm can be squeezed from one cut end of a squid giant axon and the axon reinflated with a continuously flowing salt solution that enters at one end and leaves at the other, and the axon can continue to fire $>100,000$ impulses. Analogous experiments using dialysis techniques or excised patches of membrane have been done with many other excitable cells. These experiments prove that ATP and other intracellular, small molecules of metabolism are not required either for many cycles of opening and closing of Na^+, K^+ or Ca^{2+} channels or for the resulting depolarizing and repolarizing ionic current flows. They also show that intracellular ATP, cGMP and Ca^{2+}, as well as phosphorylation by a variety of protein kinases, can be powerful modulators of channel activities. In the long term, ATP and other molecules also are needed to fuel the Na^+-K^+ and Ca^{2+} pumps and for synthesis and trafficking of membrane components. We must emphasize that channels differ from pumps (see Chap. 5) in their structure, mechanism of ion flux, function and regulation.

Gating mechanisms for Na^+ and K^+ channels in the axolemma are voltage dependent

In a classic series of experiments, Hodgkin, Huxley, and Katz [1,3–6] measured the kinetics of ion permeability changes in squid giant-axon membranes by a direct electrical method called the voltage clamp. The method controls the membrane voltage electrically, usually with step changes of potential, while ion movements are recorded directly as electrical current flowing across the membrane. The recorded current may be resolved into individual ionic components by changing the ions in the solutions that bathe the membrane. The voltage clamp is a rapid and sensitive assay for studying the opening and closing of ion channels. A widely used miniature version of the voltage clamp is the patch clamp, a technique with sufficient sensitivity to study the current flow in a single ion channel [7]. A glass micropipette with a tip diameter <1 μm is fire-polished at the tip and then pressed against the membrane of a cell. Because the tip is smooth, it seals to the membrane in the annular contact zone, rather than piercing the membrane, and defines a tiny patch of the cell surface whose few ion channels can be detected easily by the currents flowing through them. The patch clamp can readily measure a flux of as little as 10^{-20} mol of ion in less than 1 msec.

With the voltage clamp, Hodgkin and Huxley [6] discovered that the processes underlying gating, that is, the opening and closing conformational changes, of axonal Na^+ and K^+ channels are controlled by the membrane potential and, therefore, derive their energy from the work done by the electrical field on charges associated with the channel macromolecule. Hodgkin and Huxley [6] identified currents from two types of ion-selective channel, Na^+ and K^+ channels, which account for almost all of the current in axon membranes; and they made a kinetic model of the opening and closing steps, which may be simplified as shown in Figure 6-3. Depolarization of the membrane is sensed by the voltage sensor of each channel and causes the conformational reactions to proceed to the right. Repolarization or hyperpolarization causes them to proceed to the left. We can understand the action potential in these terms. The action potential, caused by a depolarizing stimulus, begins with a transient, voltage-gated opening of Na^+ channels that al-lows Na^+ to enter the fiber and depolarize the membrane fully, followed by a transient, voltage-gated opening of K^+ channels that allows K^+ to leave and repolarize the membrane. Figure 6-4 shows a calculation of the temporal relation between channel-opening and membrane-potential changes in an axon at 18.5°C, using the model of Hodgkin and Huxley [6].

The action potential is propagated by local spread of depolarization

If there are no chemical or mechanical signals for voltage-gated channels to open, how does the action potential propagate smoothly down an axon, bringing new channels into play ahead of it? Any electrical depolarization or hyperpolarization of a cell membrane spreads a small distance in either

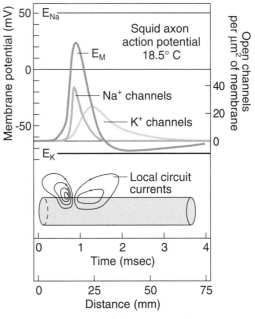

FIGURE 6-4. Events of the propagated action potential calculated from the Hodgkin-Huxley [7] kinetic model. Because the action potential is a nondecrementing wave, the diagram shows equivalently the time course of events at one point in the axon, or the spatial distribution of events at one time as the excitation propagates to the left. **Upper:** Action potential (E_M) and the opening and closing of Na^+ and K^+ channels. The Nernst potentials for Na^+ and K^+ are indicated by E_{Na} and E_K. **Lower:** Local circuit currents. The intense loop on the left spreads the depolarization to the left into the unexcited membrane.

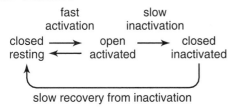

Na⁺ Channels

$$\text{closed} \xrightarrow[\text{resting}]{\text{fast activation}} \text{open activated} \xrightarrow{\text{slow inactivation}} \text{closed inactivated}$$

slow recovery from inactivation

K⁺ Channels

$$\text{closed} \underset{}{\overset{\text{slow}}{\rightleftharpoons}} \text{open}$$

FIGURE 6-3. Simplified kinetic model for opening and closing steps of Na^+ and K^+ channels. (Adapted from Hodgkin and Huxley [7].)

direction inside an axon from its source by a purely passive process often called cable, or electrotonic, spread. The spread occurs because the intracellular and extracellular media are much better conductors than the membrane, so any charges injected at one point across the membrane repel each other and disperse along the membrane surface. The lower part of Figure 6-4 shows diagrammatically the so-called local circuit currents that spread the depolarization forward. In this way, an excited depolarized membrane area smoothly depolarizes the next unexcited region ahead of the action potential, bringing it above firing threshold, opening Na^+ channels there and advancing the wave of excitation. The action potential in the upper part of Figure 6-4 is calculated by combining the known geometry of the squid giant axon with the rules of ionic electricity and the kinetic Hodgkin-Huxley equations for the voltage-dependent gating of Na^+ and K^+ channels. The success of the calculations means that the factors described are sufficient to account for action-potential propagation.

Membranes at nodes of Ranvier are characterized by high concentrations of Na⁺ channels

A wide variety of cells have been studied by voltage clamp methods, and quantitative descriptions of their permeability changes are available. All axons, whether vertebrate or invertebrate, operate on the same principles: they have a small background permeability, primarily to K^+, which sets the resting potential and display brief, dramatic openings of Na^+ and K^+ channels in sequence to shape the action potentials. Chapter 4 describes myelin, a special adaptation of large (1- to 20-μm diameter) vertebrate nerve fibers for higher conduction speed. In myelinated nerves, like unmyelinated ones, the depolarization spreads from one excitable membrane patch to another by local circuit currents; but because of the insulating properties of the coating myelin, the excitable patches of axon membrane, the nodes of Ranvier, may be more than 1 mm apart, so the rate of progression of the impulse is faster. Nodes of Ranvier have Na^+ channels similar to those of other axon membranes, but nodal membranes have at least ten times as many

channels per unit area to depolarize the long, passive, internodal myelin. The Na^+-K^+ pump may be distributed similarly (see Chap. 5). The internodal axon membrane has K^+ channels but far fewer Na^+ channels. After experimental demyelination by diphtheria toxin, which takes several days, and probably in the course of several demyelinating diseases (see Chap. 39), Na^+ channels and excitability can develop in a formerly unexcitable internodal section of axon.

A wide repertoire of voltage-sensitive channels is found among cell types

A diversity of channel types is found in the different cell types in any one organism, where the repertoire of functioning channels is adapted to the special role each cell plays in the body. We know of more than 50 genes for the pore-forming subunits of channels in the voltage-gated family. In many cell types, it is not uncommon to find several Ca^{2+} channels that open with depolarization, supplementing the depolarizing effect of Na^+ channels by adding a slower depolarizing Ca^{2+} influx or sometimes even acting alone to depolarize the membrane without Na^+ channels [8]. Ca^{2+} channels have a special importance because the entering Ca^{2+} often plays the role of a chemical messenger to activate exocytosis, or secretion; contraction; gating of other channels; ciliary reorientation; metabolic pathways; gene expression; and other processes. Indeed, whenever an electrical message activates any nonelectrical event, a change of the intracellular free Ca^{2+} concentration acts as an intermediary. Ca^{2+} channels are particularly concentrated in nerve terminals, where a Ca^{2+} influx is required for release of chemical neurotransmitters.

FUNCTIONAL PROPERTIES OF VOLTAGE-GATED ION CHANNELS

Ion channels are macromolecular complexes that form aqueous pores in the lipid membrane

We have learned much about ion channel function from voltage clamp and patch clamp studies on channels still embedded in the cell membrane

[1–5]. Figure 6-5A summarizes the major functional properties of a voltage-gated macromolecular channel in terms of a fanciful cartoon. The pore is narrow enough in one place, the ionic selectivity filter, to "feel" each ion and to distinguish among Na^+, K^+, Ca^{2+} and Cl^-. The channel also contains charged components that sense the electrical field in the membrane and drive conformational changes that, in effect, open and close gates controlling the permeability of the pore. In Na^+, K^+ and Ca^{2+} channels, the gates seem to close the axoplasmic mouth of the pore and the selectivity filter seems to be near the outer end of the pore.

How do we know that a channel is a pore? By far the most convincing evidence is the large ion flux a single channel can handle. It is not unusual in patch clamp work to measure ionic currents of 2 to 10 pA flowing each time one channel in the patch is open. This would correspond to 12 to 60 × 10^6 monovalent ions moving per second. Such a turnover is several orders of magnitude faster than known carrier mechanisms and agrees well with the theoretical properties of a pore of atomic dimensions. Similar fluxes have been observed with pore-forming antibiotic peptides in model systems, including gramicidin A, alamethicin and monazomycin.

Water molecules break and make hydrogen bonds with other waters 10^{11} to 10^{12} times per second, and alkali ions exchange water molecules or other oxygen ligands at least 10^9 times per second. In these terms, the progress of an ion across the membrane is not the movement of a fixed hydrated complex; rather, it is a continual exchange of oxygen ligands as the ion dances through the sea of relatively free water molecules and polar groups that form the wall of the pore. It is generally assumed that polar and charged groups are in the pore to provide stabilization energy to the permeating ion, compensating for those water molecules that must be left behind as the ion enters into the pore. Evidence for important negative charges in the selectivity filter of Na^+, K^+ and Ca^{2+} channels comes from a block of their permeability as the pH of the external medium is lowered below 5.5 [5] and from site-directed mutagenesis of aspartate and glutamate residues in cloned channels (see below).

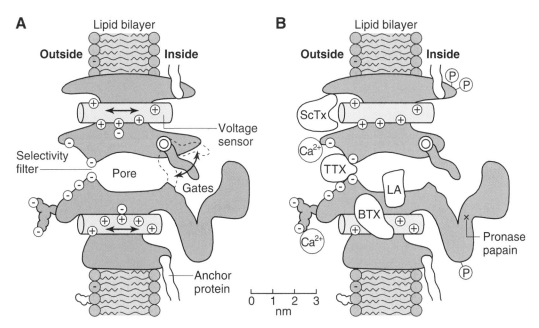

FIGURE 6-5. **A:** Diagram of the functional units of an ion channel and **B:** the hypothesized binding sites for several drugs and toxins affecting Na^+ channels. The drawing is fanciful, and the dimension and shapes of the parts are not known. Drug receptors: *TTX*, tetrodotoxin and saxitonin; *ScTx*, scorpion toxins and anemone toxins; *BTX*, batrachotoxin, aconitine, veratridine and grayanotoxin; *LA*, local anesthetics; *Ca²⁺*, divalent ions screening and associating with surface negative charge.

The minimum size of ion channels has been determined from the van der Waals dimensions of ions that will go through them [5]. Voltage-gated channels with considerable ion selectivity seem to be so narrow that ions need to shed several, though not all, water molecules to pass through. The ion fluxes often are described by models with temporary binding to attractive sites and jumps over energy barriers. Formally, the kinetics of flux through channels are construed similarly to enzyme kinetics. It is assumed that the channel passes through a sequence of "channel–ion complexes" as it catalyzes the progression of an ion across the membrane. Such theories also can describe other properties of ion channels, such as selectivity, saturation, competition and block by permeant ions [5].

Voltage-dependent gating requires voltage-dependent conformational changes in the protein component(s) of ion channels

On theoretical grounds, a membrane protein that responds to a change in membrane potential must have charged or dipolar amino acid residues, located within the membrane electrical field and acting as voltage sensors, as illustrated in Figure 6-5A. Changes in the membrane potential then exert a force on these protein-bound charges. If the energy of the field–charge interactions is great enough, the protein may be induced to undergo a change to a new stable conformational state in which the net charge or the location of charge within the membrane electrical field has been altered. For such a voltage-driven change of state, the steepness of the state function versus membrane potential curve defines the equivalent number of charges that move according to a Boltzmann distribution. On this basis, activation of Na^+ channels would require the movement of six to 12 positive charges from the intracellular to the extracellular side of the membrane. The movement of a larger number of charges through a proportionately smaller fraction of the membrane electrical field would be equivalent. Good candidates for such gating charges have been identified in the amino acid sequences of voltage-gated channels.

Such movements of membrane-bound charge give rise to tiny "gating" currents, which can be detected electrophysiologically [9]. Their voltage and time dependence are consistent with the multistep changes of channel state from resting to active. In contrast to activation, fast inactivation from the open state of Na^+ channels and certain K^+ channels does not seem to be a strongly voltage-sensitive process. This inactivation can be blocked irreversibly by proteolytic enzymes acting from the intracellular side of the channel. Regions of ion channels that are exposed at the intracellular surface of the membrane are important in mediating the process of inactivation.

Pharmacological agents acting on ion channels help define their functions

The Na^+ channel is so essential to successful body function that it has become the target in the evolution of several potent poisons. The pharmacology of such agents has provided important insights to the further definition of functional regions of the channel [2,4,5]. Figure 6-5B shows the supposed sites of action of four prominent classes of Na^+ channel agents. At the outer end of the channel is a site where the pufferfish poison, tetrodotoxin (TTX), a small lipid-insoluble charged molecule, binds with a K_i of 1 to 10 nM and blocks Na^+ permeability. A second important class of Na^+ channel blockers includes such clinically useful local anesthetics as lidocaine and procaine and related antiarrhythmic agents. They are lipid-soluble amines with a hydrophobic end and a polar end, and they bind to a hydrophobic site on the channel protein, where they also interact with the inactivation-gating machinery. The relevant clinical actions of local anesthetics are explained fully by their mode of blocking Na^+ channels. Two other classes of toxins either open Na^+ channels spontaneously or prevent them from closing normally once they have opened. These are lipid-soluble steroids, such as the frog-skin poison, batrachotoxin (BTX); the plant alkaloids, aconitine and veratridine, both acting at a site within the membrane; and peptide toxins from scorpion and anemone venoms, which act at two sites on the outer surface of the membrane. Most scorpion and anemone toxins specifically block the inactivation-gating step. It is interesting to note that the affinity of the channel for each of these classes of toxins depends on the gating conformational state of the channel.

Similarly specific agents affect K^+ and Ca^{2+} channels. Most K^+ channels can be blocked by tetraethylammonium ions, by Cs^{2+} and Ba^{2+} and by 4-aminopyridine. Except for 4-aminopyridine, there is good evidence that these ions become lodged within the channel at a narrow place, from which they may be dislodged by K^+ coming from the other side [2]. In addition, certain K^+ channels can be distinguished by their ability to be blocked by polypeptide toxins, such as charybdotoxin from scorpion, apamin from bee or dendrotoxin from snake. Ca^{2+} channels can be blocked by externally applied divalent ions, including Mn^{2+}, Co^{2+}, Cd^{2+} and Ni^{2+}. Different Ca^{2+} channel subtypes can be distinguished by their block by the dihydropyridines, nifedipine, ω-conotoxins from the cone snail and agatoxins from spider [8].

MOLECULAR COMPONENTS OF VOLTAGE-GATED ION CHANNELS

Why should we study the structural properties of the channel macromolecules themselves? Although biophysical techniques clearly define the functional properties of voltage-sensitive ion channels, it is important to relate those functional properties to the structure of the channel proteins. Understanding the structural basis for function should help to establish the basic physical and chemical principles underlying electrical excitation and signal transmission in excitable cells. Although much is now known about the structure and function of Na^+, Ca^{2+} and K^+ channels, we focus on the Na^+ channel here to illustrate how the molecular structure of an ion channel was first analyzed.

Radiolabeled neurotoxins that act on Na^+ channels are used as molecular probes to tag the channel proteins, allowing their identification

Neurotoxins act at several different sites on Na^+ channels to modify their properties (Fig. 6-5B) [10]. Photoreactive derivatives of the polypeptide toxins of scorpion venom have been at-

tached covalently to Na^+ channels in intact cell membranes, allowing direct identification of channel components without purification. Reversible binding of saxitoxin and TTX to their common receptor has been used as a biochemical assay for the channel protein. Solubilization of excitable membranes with nonionic detergents releases the Na^+ channel, and the solubilized channel can be purified by chromatographic techniques that separate glycoproteins by size, charge and composition of covalently attached carbohydrate. Using this general strategy, Na^+ channels have been purified from the electric organ of the electric eel and from mammalian brain and skeletal muscle [11–13].

Covalent labeling of Na^+ channels in intact excitable cells or membranes and purification of channels solubilized by nonionic detergents result in identification of a large glycoprotein with a molecular weight of 260,000 as the principal component. In eel electroplax, it appears to be the only protein component, but in mammalian brain this large α subunit is associated with two additional polypeptides: β_1, with a molecular weight of 36,000 and β_2, with a molecular weight of 33,000. In skeletal muscle, the α subunit is associated with only the β_1 subunit.

Figure 6-6A illustrates the most probable arrangement of the subunits of the Na^+ channel from brain. The α subunit is a transmembrane polypeptide since it has sites for attachment of several carbohydrate chains and for binding of neurotoxins on the external surface of the channel and sites for phosphorylation by protein kinases on the intracellular surface. Since this single polypeptide suffices to form a channel by itself (see below), a transmembrane orientation is essential to its function. The β_1 and β_2 subunits also are glycosylated heavily. The β_1 subunit is attached noncovalently to the α subunit, while the β_2 subunit is attached covalently via a disulfide bond. The β subunits are integral membrane glycoproteins that interact with the phospholipid bilayer. Much of the carbohydrate on the channel subunits is sialic acid, which contributes to their strong net negative charge. Glycosylation is required for normal biosynthesis and assembly of the functional channel in neurons. If glycosylation is inhibited, newly synthesized α subunits are degraded rapidly and are not inserted into the cell surface membrane.

A

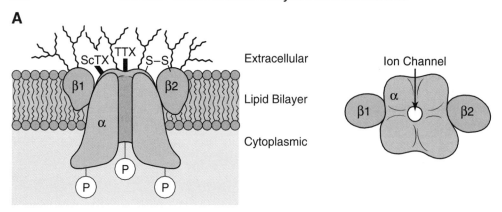

Extracellular

Lipid Bilayer

Cytoplasmic

Ion Channel

B

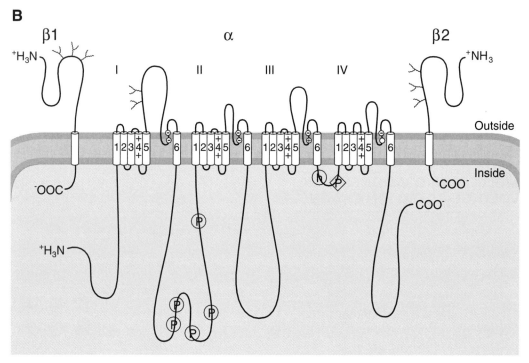

Outside

Inside

C

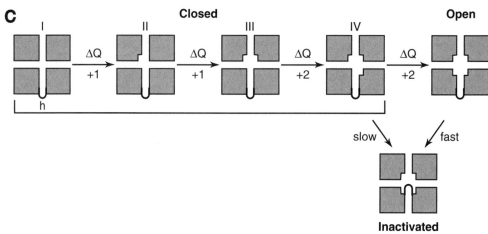

Purified Na^+ channels are functional after reconstitution

An important step in the study of a purified membrane protein is to reconstitute its function in the pure state. This has been accomplished in two ways for the Na^+ channel. In the first approach, purified channels were incorporated into vesicles of pure phospholipid. Activation of the reconstituted channels by treatment with the neurotoxin veratridine markedly increased the permeability of the vesicles to Na^+. The purified channels retain the ion selectivity and pharmacological properties of native channels. In the second approach, ion conductance mediated by single purified channels was measured electrically. Channels reconstituted in phospholipid vesicles were studied directly with patch-clamp methods or incorporated into planar phospholipid bilayer membranes by fusion. The individual purified channels retained the single-channel conductance, ion selectivity and voltage dependence of activation and inactivation that are characteristic of native channels. Hence, purified Na^+ channels seem to contain all of the functional components necessary for electrical excitability.

Primary structures of Na^+- channel subunits have been determined using cDNA cloning

The amino acid sequences of the Na^+ channel α, β_1 and β_2 subunits have been determined by cloning DNA complementary to the mRNA encoding them using antibodies and oligonucleotides developed from work on purified Na^+ channels. The amino acid sequence of the subunits is then deduced from the nucleotide sequence of the mRNA encoding them [14,15]. The primary structures of these subunits are illustrated as topological models in Figure 6-6B. The large α subunits are composed of 1,800 to 2,000 amino acids and contain four repeated domains having greater than 50% internal sequence identity. This sequence similarity implies similar secondary and tertiary structures for the four domains. Each domain contains six segments that are predicted to form transmembrane α helices and additional hydrophobic sequences that are thought to be membrane-associated and to contribute to formation of the outer mouth of the transmembrane pore (see below). In contrast, the smaller β_1 and β_2 subunits of Na^+ channels consist of a large extracellular N-terminal segment, a single transmembrane segment and a short intracellular segment (Fig. 6-6B).

Ca^{2+} channels have a similar structure to Na^+ channels

The general experimental strategy used in studies of the Na^+ channel also has been applied to voltage-gated Ca^{2+} channels. Drugs and neurotoxins that act on Ca^{2+} channels have been used to identify and purify their protein components [16], and experiments to restore their function in purified form and to determine their primary structures have been completed (Fig. 6-7A)

FIGURE 6-6. Structural model of the sodium channel. **A, Left:** A topological model of the rat brain Na^+ channel illustrating the probable transmembrane orientation of the three subunits, the binding sites for tetrodotoxin *(TTX)* and scorpion toxin *(ScTX)*, oligosaccharide chains *(wavy lines)* and cAMP-dependent phosphorylation sites *(P)*. **Right:** An *enface* view of the protein from the extracellular side illustrating the formation of a transmembrane ion pore in the midst of a square array of four transmembrane domains of the α subunit. **B:** A transmembrane folding model of the α and β subunits of the Na^+ channel. The amino acid sequence is illustrated as a *narrow line,* with each segment approximately proportional to its length in the molecule. Transmembrane α-helices are illustrated as cylinders. The positions of amino acids required for specific functions of Na^+ channels are indicated: ++, positively charged voltage sensors in the S4 transmembrane segments; ◯, residues required for high-affinity binding of TTX with their charge characteristics indicated by −, + or open field; ⓗ, residues required for fast inactivation; Ⓟ, sites for phosphorylation by cAMP-dependent protein kinase; and ⬦Ⓟ, sites for phosphorylation by protein kinase C. **C:** Sequential gating of the Na^+ channel. A reaction pathway from closed to open Na^+ channels is depicted. Each square represents one homologous domain of the α subunit. Each domain undergoes a conformational change initiated by a voltage-driven movement of its S4 segment, leading eventually to an open channel. Inactivation of the channel occurs from the final closed state and the open state by folding of the intracellular loop connecting domains III and IV into the intracellular mouth of the transmembrane pore.

[17,18]. Ca^{2+} channels have a principal subunit, α_1, which is structurally analogous to Na^+ channel α subunits. Ca^{2+} channels in neurons have associated α_2 and δ subunits, which form a disulfide-linked transmembrane glycoprotein complex, and β subunits, which are intracellular (Fig. 6-7A). In addition, Ca^{2+} channels in skeletal muscle have a transmembrane γ subunit. The auxiliary subunits of Ca^{2+} channels are not related in primary structure to the Na^+ channel β subunits. Co-expression with the auxiliary α_2, β, γ and δ subunits modulates the properties of the expressed Ca^{2+} channel and can greatly increase its expression. Since voltage-gated ion channels are likely to have evolved from common ancestor proteins, comparison of the conserved structural and functional features among the principal subunits of many different channels will sharpen our view of the molecular basis of their function, as illustrated by the comparison of the mechanisms of ion permeation and gating outlined below.

K^+ channels have been identified by genetic means

Genes that harbor mutations causing an easily detectable altered phenotype in the fruit fly *Drosophila* can be cloned directly from genomic DNA without information about the protein they encode. The *Shaker* mutation in *Drosophila* causes flies to shake under ether anesthesia and is accompanied by loss of a specific K^+ current in the nerve and muscle of mutant flies. By cloning successive pieces of genomic DNA from the region of the chromosome that specifies this mutation, DNA clones that encoded a protein related in amino acid sequence to the α subunit of Na^+ channels were isolated [19]. The K^+ channel protein is analogous to one of the homologous domains of Na^+ or Ca^{2+} channels [19] and is thought to function as a tetramer of four separate subunits in analogy to the structure of Na^+ and Ca^{2+} channels (Fig. 6-7B). K^+ channels may be the ancestral voltage-gated ion channels from which the larger Na^+ and Ca^{2+} channels evolved by two cycles of gene duplication [5]. Like the Na^+ and Ca^{2+} channels, K^+ channels have an auxiliary β subunit, which is an

intracellular protein distantly related to Ca^{2+} channel β subunits [20].

How do the primary structures of the ion channel subunits carry out their functions?

Cloning of the cDNA encoding the Na^+ channel subunits permits detailed tests of the functional properties of the polypeptides. cDNA clones can be used to synthesize mRNA encoding the subunits or to isolate the natural mRNA by specific hybridization. When injected into appropriate recipient cells, such as frog oocytes, isolated mRNAs can be translated to yield functional proteins. In such experiments, mRNA encoding only the α subunit of the channel is capable of directing the synthesis of functional channels in oocytes [21,22]. The α subunits, therefore, seem sufficient to carry out the basic functions of the channel. However, coexpression of the β_1 and β_2 subunits accelerates inactivation and shifts voltage dependence toward more negative membrane potentials, conferring more physiologically correct functional properties on the expressed channel [15]. Similar experiments with Ca^{2+} and K^+ channels also show that only the principal subunits are required for channel function but that the auxiliary subunits modulate channel function [16–20]. These results indicate that the principal subunits of the voltage-gated ion channels are functionally autonomous but that the auxiliary subunits improve expression and modulate physiological properties.

How does the structure of the α subunit of the Na^+ channel allow it to mediate selective ion transport and voltage-dependent gating? The answer remains unknown, but working hypotheses have been developed from extensive structure–function studies that help to guide current research on this problem. Both the gap junction channel and the nicotinic acetylcholine receptor (see Chap. 10) are high-conductance ion channels that form a transmembrane pore at the center of a pseudosymmetrical array of subunits. By analogy, it is believed that the transmembrane pore of the Na^+ channel may be formed at the center of a square array of its four homologous domains (Fig. 6-6A). Formation of a transmembrane pore in the center of a symmetrical or

A

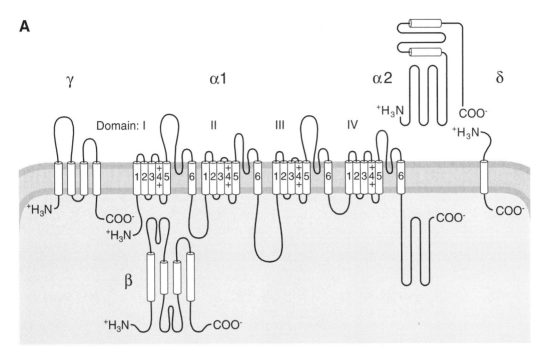

B

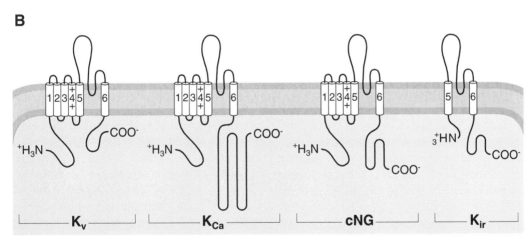

FIGURE 6-7.   Transmembrane organization of voltage-gated Ca^{2+} channels, K^+ channels and relatives. **A:** The primary structures of subunits of the voltage-gated Ca^{2+} channel are illustrated. *Cylinders* represent probable α-helical transmembrane segments. *Bold lines* represent the polypeptide chains of each subunit, with length approximately proportional to the number of amino acid residues. **B:** The primary structures of the plasma membrane cation channels related to K^+ channels are illustrated as transmembrane folding diagrams based on analysis of the hydrophobicity of the amino acid sequence. Predicted transmembrane α helices are illustrated as *cylinders*. The remainder of the polypeptide chain is illustrated as a *bold line*, with the length of each segment approximately proportional to the length of its amino acid sequence. K_v, voltage-gated K^+ channel; K_{Ca}, Ca^{2+}-activated K^+ channel; *cNG*, cyclic nucleotide-gated channel; K_{ir}, inward rectifying K^+ channel.

pseudosymmetrical array of homologous structural units may be a common theme in the structure of high-conductance ion channels.

Which amino acid sequences are involved in forming the pore? For Na^+ channels, insight into this question has come from studies of the amino acid residues required for binding of TTX, which is thought to block the outer mouth of the transmembrane pore (Fig. 6-5B). Site-directed mutagenesis experiments show that pairs of amino acid residues required for high-affinity TTX binding are located in analogous positions in all four domains near the carboxyl ends of the short hydrophobic segments between transmembrane α helices S5 and S6 [23] (Fig. 6-6B). Six of these eight residues are negatively charged and may interact with permeant ions as they approach and move through the channel. In agreement with this idea, mutation of the only two of these residues that are not negatively charged (see domains III and IV, Fig. 6-6B) to glutamic acid residues, as present in the analogous positions in the Ca^{2+} channel, confers Ca^{2+} selectivity on the Na^+ channel [24]. Parallel results also implicated these same regions of the K^+ channel in determining ion selectivity and conductance [25]. Evidently, these membrane-associated segments form the outer mouth and at least part of the walls of the transmembrane pore of the voltage-gated ion channels.

Structural models for voltage-dependent gating of ion channels must identify the voltage sensors, or gating charges (Fig. 6-4A), within the channel structure and suggest a plausible mechanism for transmembrane movement of gating charge and its coupling to the opening of a transmembrane pore. The S4 segments of the homologous domains have been proposed as voltage sensors [13,14,26]. These segments, which are conserved among Na^+, Ca^{2+} and K^+ channels, consist of repeated triplets of two hydrophobic amino acids followed by a positively charged residue. In the α-helical configuration, these segments would form a spiral staircase of positive charge across the membrane, a structure that is well suited for transmembrane movement of gating charge (Fig. 6-5). Each positive charge is proposed to be neutralized by a negative charge in one of the surrounding transmembrane segments to form a spiral array of ion pairs

(Fig. 6-5). Direct evidence in favor of designating the S4 segments as voltage sensors comes from mutagenesis studies of Na^+ and K^+ channels [19,27]. Neutralization of positive charges results in progressive reduction of the steepness of voltage-dependent gating and of the apparent gating charge, as expected if the S4 segments are indeed the voltage sensors. At the resting membrane potential, the force of the electrical field would pull the positive charges inward. Depolarization would abolish this force and allow an outward movement of the S4 helix. A simple spiral movement, as suggested in a sliding helix model of gating [13], would have the net effect of transferring these gating charges across the membrane. Direct evidence for an outward movement of the gating charges in the S4 segments has come from experiments in which cysteine residues substituted at these positions by site-directed mutagenesis were shown to become available for chemical reaction outside the cell upon depolarization [28]. This movement of the S4 helix is proposed to initiate a more general conformational change in each domain. After conformational changes have occurred in all four domains, the transmembrane pore can open and conduct ions (Fig. 6-6C).

Shortly after opening, many voltage-gated ion channels inactivate. The inactivation process of Na^+ channels can be prevented by treatment of the intracellular surface of the channel with proteolytic enzymes [2] or antibodies against the intracellular segment connecting domains III and IV (h in Fig. 6-6B) [29], and expression of the Na^+ channel as two pieces with a cut between domains III and IV greatly slows inactivation [27]. A single cluster of three hydrophobic residues in this intracellular loop is required for fast inactivation [30], and inactivation is eliminated if these three hydrophobic residues are mutated to hydrophilic ones. The phenylalanine at position 1,489 is the critical residue; mutation of this single amino acid to a hydrophilic residue nearly completely blocks fast inactivation of the channel. The segment of the Na^+ channel between domains III and IV is therefore proposed to serve as the inactivation gate by forming a hinged lid, which folds over the intracellular mouth of the pore after activation (Fig. 6-8A). The cluster of hydrophobic residues including

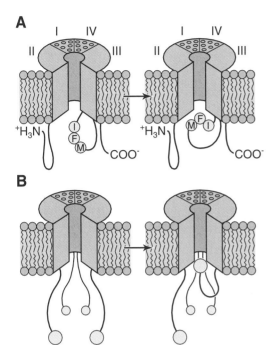

A

B

FIGURE 6-8. Mechanisms of inactivation of Na$^+$ and K$^+$ channels. **A:** A hinged-lid model for Na$^+$ channel inactivation illustrating the inactivation gate formed by the intracellular segment connecting domains III and IV and the critical cluster of hydrophobic residues that forms a latch holding the inactivation gate closed. *IFM,* isoleucine-phenylalanine-methionine. **B:** A ball-and-chain model of K$^+$ channel inactivation. Each of the four subunits of a K$^+$ channel has a ball-and-chain structure at its N-terminus. Any one of the four can bind to the intracellular mouth of the open channel and inactivate it.

phenylalanine 1,489 is thought to enter the intracellular mouth of the pore and to bind there as a latch to keep the channel inactivated.

A detailed model of K$^+$ channel inactivation has been derived from mutagenesis experiments [31,32]. The N-terminus of the K$^+$ channel serves as an inactivation particle, and both charged and hydrophobic residues are involved. A ball-and-chain mechanism [9,31,32] has been proposed in which the N-terminal segment serves as a loosely tethered ball and inactivates the channel by diffusion and binding to the intracellular mouth of the pore (Fig. 6-8B). Consistent with this mechanism, synthetic peptides with amino acid sequences corresponding to that of the inactivation particle region can restore inactivation to channel mutants in which

the N-terminus has been removed. The mechanisms of inactivation of Na$^+$ and K$^+$ channels are similar in that hydrophobic amino acid residues seem to mediate binding of an inactivation particle to the intracellular mouth of the transmembrane pore of the activated channel in each. They differ in that charged amino acid residues are important in the inactivation particle of K$^+$ channels but not Na$^+$ channels and also in that the inactivation particle is located over 200 residues from the membrane at the N-terminus of the K$^+$ channel compared to only 12 residues from the membrane between domains III and IV of the Na$^+$ channel. It is likely that the hinged-lid mechanism of Na$^+$-channel inactivation evolved from the ball-and-chain mechanism of K$^+$ channels.

These models for formation of a voltage-gated transmembrane pore by the voltage-gated ion channel proteins remain speculative at this time. However, they illustrate a general scientific method: new data, such as the amino acid sequences of the ion channel subunits, inevitably lead to the formulation of specific hypotheses, which then spawn a new generation of experiments designed to test their merit. The next phase of research on the molecular properties of ion channels should give us clearer insight into the molecular basis for two of the critical functions of ion channels: selective ion conductance and voltage-dependent gating. However, our understanding will be incomplete until we know the three-dimensional structure of an ion channel at high resolution from x-ray crystallography. We can expect to see the fruits of ion-channel crystallography in the immediate future.

OTHER CHANNELS

K$^+$ channels have many relatives

K$^+$ channels have many different roles in cells. For example, in neurons they terminate the action potential by repolarizing cells, set the resting membrane potential by dominating the resting membrane conductance, determine the length and frequency of bursts of action potentials and respond to neurotransmitters by opening or closing and causing prolonged changes in membrane potential [5]. These channels are regulated by a combination of voltage, G proteins and intracellular second messengers. Remarkably, evolution has created a diverse array of ion channels based on variations of the structure of voltage-gated K^+ channels (K_v) to serve this broad range of functions (Fig. 6-7B) [33,34]. All contain the pore structure of the voltage-gated K^+ channel attached to different regulatory domains: a G protein-binding domain in the inward rectifying K^+ channels (K_{ir}), a Ca^{2+}-binding domain in the Ca^{2+}-activated K^+ channels (K_{Ca}), a cyclic nucleotide-binding domain in the cyclic nucleotide-gated channels or a specialized gating domain in the ether-a-go-go-related K^+ channels (K_{erg}). Moreover, channels of presently unknown function which have the structure of fused K_{ir} and K_v channels have been detected in yeast [35]. Evidently, the K^+ channel structure presents a flexible building block of many ion channels which are specialized for specific functions in cells as different as yeast and vertebrate myocytes and neurons.

There are many other kinds of ion channels

The channels used in the action potential contrast with those generating slow potentials at synapses and sensory receptors by having strongly voltage-dependent gating. The other channels have gates controlled by chemical transmitters, intracellular messengers or by energy sources, such as mechanical deformations in touch and hearing (Box 47-1). In general, less is known about these channels than about Na^+, Ca^{2+} and K^+ channels of action potentials, with the exception of the nicotinic acetylcholine receptor channel of the neuromuscular junction (see Chap. 11). The ionic selectivity of these channels includes a very broad, monovalent anion permeability at inhibitory synapses; a cation permeability that is about equal for Na^+ and K^+ at excitatory synapses, at the neuromuscular junction and at many sensory transducers; and other more selective Ca^{2+} and Na^+ permeabilities in other synapses. The acetylcholine recep-

tors of the neuromuscular junction and brain, the excitatory glutamate receptors and the inhibitory GABA and glycine receptors have been solubilized and chemically purified and the amino acid sequences of their subunits determined by methods of molecular genetics (see Chap. 10). The structural features responsible for the function of these ligand-gated channels are being elucidated rapidly.

As this research shows, there is a great diversity of ion channels playing many roles in cells throughout the body. We can speculate that hundreds of genes code for structural components of channels. Beyond their functions in the nervous system, channel activity in endocrine cells regulates the episodes of secretion of insulin from the pancreas and epinephrine from the adrenal gland. Channels initiate and regulate muscle contraction and cell motility. Channels form part of the regulated pathway for the ion movements underlying absorption and secretion of electrolytes by epithelia. Channels also participate in cellular signaling pathways in many other electrically inexcitable cells. Thus, while they are especially prominent in the function of the nervous system, ion channels are actually a basic component of all animal cells, indeed of all eukaryotic cells [5].

ACKNOWLEDGMENTS

The preparation of this chapter was supported by Grants NS-08174 and NS-15751 from the National Institutes of Health.

REFERENCES

1. Hodgkin A. L. *The Conduction of the Nervous Impulse.* Springfield, IL: Charles C. Thomas, 1964.
2. Armstrong, C. M. Ionic pores, gates, and gating currents. *Q. Rev. Biophys.* 7:179–210, 1975.
3. Nicholls, J. G., Martin, A. R., and Wallace, B. G. *From Neuron to Brain,* 3rd ed. Sunderland, MA: Sinauer Associates, 1992.
4. Hille, B. Ionic basis of resting and action potentials. In J. M. Brookhart, and V. B. Mountcastle, eds. *Handbook of Physiology.* Washington, D.C.:

American Physiological Society, 1977, Vol. 1, pp. 99–136.

5. Hille, B. *Ionic Channels of Excitable Membranes*, 2nd ed. Sunderland, MA: Sinauer Associates, 1992.

6. Hodgkin, A. L., and Huxley, A. F. A quantitative description of membrane current and its application to conduction and excitation in nerve. *J. Physiol. (Lond.)* 117:500–544, 1952.

7. Hamill, O. P., Marty, A., Neher, E., Sakmann, B., and Sigworth, F. J. Improved patch-clamp techniques for high-resolution current recording from cells and cell-free membrane patches. *Pflugers Arch.* 391:85–100, 1981.

8. Tsien R. W. Reflections on Ca^{2+} channel diversity, 1988–1994. *Trends Neurosci.* 18:52–54, 1995.

9. Armstrong, C. M. Sodium channels and gating currents. *Physiol. Rev.* 61:644–683, 1981.

10. Catterall, W. A. Neurotoxins acting on sodium channels. *Annu. Rev. Pharmacol. Toxicol.* 20:15–43, 1980.

11. Agnew, W. S. Voltage-regulated sodium channel molecules. *Annu. Rev. Biochem.* 46:517–530, 1984.

12. Barchi, R. L. Voltage-sensitive sodium ion channels. Molecular properties and functional reconstitution. *Trends Biochem. Sci.* 9:358–361, 1984.

13. Catterall, W. A. Molecular properties of voltage-sensitive sodium channels. *Annu. Rev. Biochem.* 55:953–985, 1986.

14. Noda, M., Ikeda, T., Kayano, T., et al. Existence of distinct sodium channel messenger RNAs in rat brain. *Nature* 320:188–192, 1986.

15. Isom, L., De Jongh, K., Patton, D. E., et al. Primary structure and functional expression of the β_1-subunit of the rat brain sodium channel. *Science* 256:839–842, 1992.

16. Catterall, W. A. Functional subunit structure of voltage-gated calcium channels. *Science* 253:1499–1500, 1991.

17. Hofmann, F., Biel, M., and Flockerzi, V. Molecular basis for Ca^{2+} channel diversity. *Annu. Rev. Neurosci.* 17:399–418, 1994.

18. Catterall, W. A. Structure and function of voltage-gated ion channels. *Annu. Rev. Biochem.* 65:493–531, 1995.

19. Jan, L. Y., and Jan, Y. N. Structural elements involved in specific K^+ channel functions. *Annu. Rev. Physiol.* 54:537–555, 1992.

20. Rettig, J., Heinemann, S. H., Wunder, F., et al. Inactivation properties of voltage-gated K^+ channels altered by presence of β-subunit. *Nature* 369:289–294, 1994.

21. Noda, M., Ikeda, T., Suzuki, H., et al. Expression of functional sodium channels from cloned cDNA. *Nature* 322:826–828, 1986.

22. Goldin, A. L., Snutch, T., Lubbert, H., et al. Messenger RNA coding for only the α-subunit of the rat brain Na channel is sufficient for expression of functional channels in *Xenopus* oocytes. *Proc. Natl. Acad. Sci. USA* 83:7503–7507, 1986.

23. Terlau, H., Heinemann, S. H., Stühmer, W., et al. Mapping the site of block by tetrodotoxin and saxitoxin of sodium channel II. *FEBS Lett.* 293:93–96, 1991.

24. Heinemann, S. H., Terlau, H., Stühmer, W., Imoto, K., and Numa, S. Calcium channel characteristics conferred on the sodium channel by single mutations. *Nature* 356:441–443, 1992.

25. Miller, C. Annus mirabilis for potassium channels. *Science* 252:1092–1096, 1990.

26. Guy, H. R., and Conti, F. Pursuing the structure and function of voltage-gated channels. *Trends Neurosci.* 13:201–206, 1990.

27. Stühmer, W., Conti, F., Suzuki, H., et al. Structural parts involved in activation and inactivation of the sodium channel. *Nature* 339:597–603, 1989.

28. Yang, N. B., George, A. L., Jr., and Horn, R. Molecular basis of charge movement in voltage-gated sodium channels. *Neuron* 16:113–122, 1996.

29. Vassilev, P., Scheuer, T., and Catterall, W. A. Inhibition of inactivation of single sodium channels by a site-directed antibody. *Proc. Natl. Acad. Sci. USA* 86:8147–8151, 1989.

30. West, J. W., Patton, D. E., Scheuer, T., Wang, Y.-L., Goldin, A. L., and Catterall, W. A. A cluster of hydrophobic amino acid residues required for fast sodium channel inactivation. *Proc. Natl. Acad. USA* 89:10910–10914, 1992.

31. Hoshi, T., Zagotta, W., and Aldrich, R. W. Biophysical and molecular mechanisms of Shaker potassium channel inactivation. *Science* 250:533–538, 1990.

32. Zagotta, W., Hoshi, T., and Aldrich, R. W. Restoration of inactivation in mutants of *Shaker* potassium channels by a peptide derived from Sh B. *Science* 250:568–571, 1990.

33. Deal, K. K., England, S. K., and Tamkun, M. M. Molecular physiology of cardiac potassium channels. *Physiol. Rev.* 76:49–67, 1996.

34. Doupnik, C. A., Davidson, N., and Lester, H. A. The inward rectifier potassium channel family. *Curr. Opin. Neurobiol.* 5:268–277, 1995.

35. Ketchum, K. A., Joiner, W. J., Sellers, A. J., Kaczmarek, L. K., and Goldstein, S. A. A new family of outwardly rectifying potassium channel proteins with two pore domains in tandem. *Nature* 376:690–695, 1995.

Cell Adhesion Molecules

David R. Colman and Marie T. Filbin

OVERVIEW

Cell adhesion molecules (CAMs) play critical roles in all facets of nervous system development and maintenance. Important phenomena in which CAMs are involved include initial formation of the neural tube and the neural crest, migration of all neurons and glial cells, axonal out-

Basic Neurochemistry: Molecular, Cellular and Medical Aspects, 6th Ed., edited by G. J. Siegel et al. Published by Lippincott–Raven Publishers, Philadelphia, 1999. Correspondence to David R. Colman, Brookdale Center for Molecular Biology, Box 1126, Mount Sinai School of Medicine, One Gustave L. Levy Place, New York, New York 10029.

growth and guidance, target selection, synaptic stabilization and plasticity, myelination and nerve regeneration after injury (see Chaps. 4, 28, 29 and 50). Adhesion molecules interact with each other and with nonadhesive cell-surface and/or cytoplasmic molecules, and in the two most extreme situations, may produce diametrically opposite results. For example, under certain circumstances, adhesion can vigorously encourage movement or growth along a preferred pathway, or in contrast, it can completely immobilize a cell or membrane and prevent further movement or growth. How can membrane adhesion molecules mediate these very different effects? The answer to this question is not straightforward, but to reduce the answer to simple terms, a number of factors sum to yield the net effect of all adhesive forces acting on cell surfaces. There are always many adhesion molecules expressed at the same time on a given cell surface but in different concentrations. Furthermore, each adhesion molecule subtype is unique in terms of adhesive preference and adhesive strength. An additional complication is that, in some cases, an individual adhesion molecule may display more than one binding site, with each site specific for a different peptide ligand protruding from an opposing cell surface or membrane. Also, the post-translational addition of certain charged carbohydrate moieties, for example, sialic acid, to adhesion proteins may interfere with the adhesive properties of the polypeptide. The post-translationally modified protein is rendered nonadhesive through charge repulsion and may actually repel abutting membrane surfaces. The reality in many systems is that the net result of all adhesion molecule interactions on the cell surface at a given time yields an averaged effect.

Cell adhesion molecules comprise several "families"

These families are defined by individual members which are related to each other by common primary sequences, structural motifs and binding properties. In spite of differences in the biochemistry and function of each CAM, we can make certain generalizations about how they function in nervous tissue. First, CAMs act at the cell surface, where they interact with either identical molecules, termed *homophilic interaction,* or different molecules, termed *heterophilic interaction,* expressed on an opposing cell surface or in the extracellular matrix (ECM). Second, adhesion has consequences for the cells involved, usually by virtue of adhesion molecule interactions with the underlying cytoskeleton [1]. Third, adhesive events between cells vary in strength, "strong" vs. "weak" adhesion, and the strength of adhesion is influenced by a wide range of factors. For example, the sum of all adhesive forces acting on a growing neurite is likely to be weaker than that of all the forces causing permanent adherence of pre- and postsynaptic membranes. Fourth, intercellular adhesion may be modulated, depending on the situation. Last, because the nervous system is not a homogeneous organ, it is important to consider when and where each CAM is expressed. In other words, the temporal and spatial expression patterns of CAMs sharply focus and limit their interactions.

The three major groups of CAMs found in the nervous system are the members of the immunoglobulin (Ig) gene superfamily (IgCAMs), the integrins and the cadherins. Another family of carbohydrate-binding CAMs, the selectins, is important in other tissues, particularly in the immune system [2]. However, the selectins seem not to be expressed by neurons or glia. To date, these proteins have been detected only in the nervous system when expressed by invading immune cells in pathological states. The cadherins and IgCAMs engage exclusively in cell–cell or membrane–membrane interactions, while integrins, for the most part, interact with components of the ECM. Within each of these adhesion molecule families, membership has been defined largely by amino acid sequence similarity, which is reflected in common structural features. Consequently, distinct binding requirements also characterize each family. For example, cadherins interact in a Ca^{2+}-dependent, usually homophilic manner. Binding of the members of the Ig family is Ca^{2+}-independent and, although frequently homophilic, can be heterophilic. Integrin binding is also divalent cation-dependent (Ca^{2+}, Mg^{2+}) but always heterophilic.

Another, but less well defined, class of adhesion molecules is the four-transmembrane domain family, whose members share similar hydropathy plots and may have similar dispositions with respect to the phospholipid bilayer, for example, the myelin proteolipid proteins, the connexins of gap junctions, the ryanodine receptor and others.

THE IMMUNOGLOBULIN GENE SUPERFAMILY

The best studied group of recognition/adhesion molecules expressed in the nervous system is that of the IgCAMs (Fig. 7-1), which are defined by regions that have sequence similarity with Igs, termed the Ig domains [3,4]. Ig domains contain alternating hydrophobic and hydrophilic stretches of residues, which form a series of antiparallel β strands. The β strands come together to form two β sheets. The folding of the β sheets is, in most cases, stabilized by the formation of a disulfide bond between the sheets. There are three subclasses of Ig-like domains, which are defined by their similarity to variable (V) or constant (C) regions of Igs. For V-like domains, there are 70 to 110 amino acids spanning the two cysteines that form the disulfide bond, allowing formation of seven to nine β strands. C-like domains have about 50 amino acids spanning the

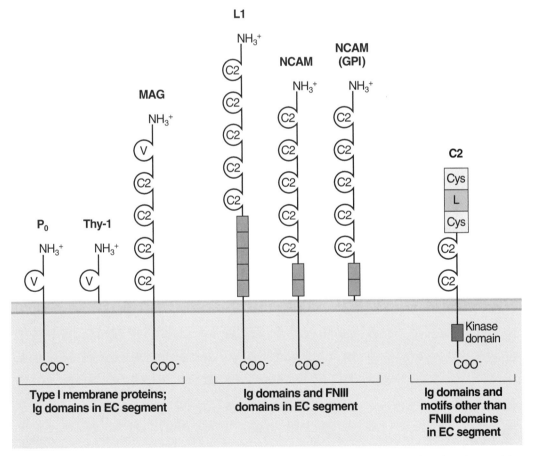

FIGURE 7-1. The immunoglobulin (Ig) gene family of molecules. Several varieties of Ig domain-containing molecules are contained within the Ig gene superfamily. Most are type I membrane proteins; some have only Ig domains or other moieties which may convey function (see text). *V*, variable Ig domain; *C*, constant Ig domain; *MAG*, myelin associated glycoprotein; *NCAM*, neural cell adhesion molecule; *GPI*, glycosylphosphatidyl-inositol; *EC*, extracellular domain; *FN*, fibronectin.

stabilizing cysteines and, consequently, carry seven β sheets. The third class of Ig-like domains is termed a C2 domain. This class of IgCAM has the β strand distribution of a C-like domain but bears more sequence similarity to V-like domains.

The formation of immunoglobulin-like domains may confer characteristics important for extracellular presentation and interaction with other molecules

First, because of the folding pattern, Ig domains are stabilized by both inward-pointing hydrophobic amino acids and the intersheet disulfide bond, making them relatively resistant to proteolysis and, hence, ideal molecules to present to the external cellular environment. Second, the folding of the β strands provides a good platform for the presentation of amino acids, carried in the loops between the strands, for interaction with an opposing molecule. The loops between β strands, in antibodies, carry the antigen-recognition sites and, in Ig-like domains, contain the regions of greatest variability, allowing for distinct and specific interactions.

Members of this family of molecules may have only one Ig-like domain, as is the case for the myelin protein P_0, or, as for most of the family, have many Ig domains. In addition to the subclassification of Ig domains into V-, C- and C2-like domains, Ig family members can be broadly divided into three general classes [5]: (i) those that have only Ig-like domains; (ii) those that have Ig domains and additional domains that resemble regions of the ECM component fibronectin, termed FN-like domains; and (iii) those that have Ig domains and motifs other than FN-like domains. Moreover, any one Ig family member may have many isoforms, which may differ in the length of the cytoplasmic domain, in their post-translational modifications and whether they are membrane-spanning or glycophosphatidylinositol (GPI)-anchored proteins (see Box 3-1). Also, additional amino acid sequences inserted in the extracellular domain may distinguish isoforms of a particular IgCAM. While it is not known how the majority of different isoforms of a particular IgCAM affect its functioning, differ-

ences in effect have been described for molecules that carry some of the isoform-distinguishing amino acid sequences in the extracellular domain of the neural cell adhesion molecule (NCAM). For example, a sequence of ten amino acids, termed the variable alternative spliced exon (VASE) sequence, in the fourth Ig domain of some isoforms of NCAM alters the response of axonal growth to this adhesion molecule; NCAM proteins with the VASE sequence are much less effective at promoting axonal growth than are NCAM proteins without this sequence. However, a puzzling question is: How do IgCAMs that have identical extracellular domains, but are either GPI-linked or membrane-spanning, differ in function? Similarly, how differences in the cytoplasmic domain affect function is still not known. Presumably, the cytoplasmic domains interact with signal-transduction cascades and cytoskeletal proteins and in this way transduce adhesion into an intracellular response.

The siglecs constitute a novel subfamily of immunoglobulin-like molecules that bind to sialosides

These molecules, previously termed sialoadhesins, share considerable sequence similarity among the first four amino-terminal Ig domains [6]. More importantly, all members of this subfamily bind to sialoglycoconjugates. To date, only two siglecs have been identified in the nervous system: the myelin-associated glycoprotein (MAG) and the Schwann cell myelin protein (SMP) (see Chap. 4). All other family members are specific to the immune system. An additional common feature of this IgCAM subfamily is that they bind sialic acid with relatively low affinity. Because of this, it is suggested that siglecs must be clustered within the membrane and that the molecule(s) with which siglecs interact must either be clustered or carry multimeric sialic acid residues to be effective. It should be noted, however, that although both MAG and SMP have been shown to be sialic acid-binding proteins, the identity of a possible sialoglycoconjugate(s) with which they interact and the functional relevance of such an interaction have yet to be described.

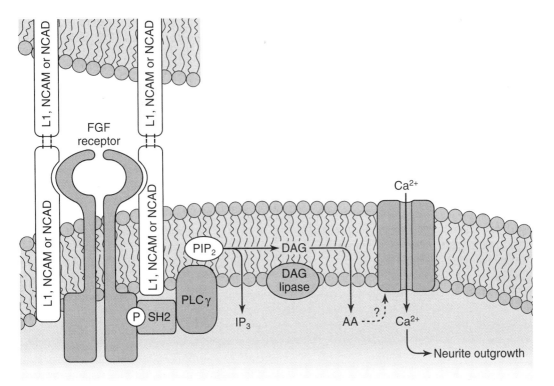

FIGURE 7-2. Signaling events in cell adhesion molecule *(CAM)*-stimulated neurite outgrowth. It has been postulated that a signaling cascade is stimulated by homophilic interactions of neural cell adhesion molecule *(NCAM)*, N-cadherin *(NCAD)* or L1, which dimerizes the fibroblast growth factor *(FGF)* receptor and activates phospholipase C-γ *(PLCγ)* to generate diacylglycerol *(DAG)*, conversion of DAG to arachidonic acid *(AA)* by a DAG lipase and an AA-induced increase in Ca^{2+} influx into the neurons via Ca^{2+} channels. SH2, src homology 2 domain; PIP_2, phosphatidylinositol 4,5-bisphosphate; IP_3, inositol (1,4,5)-trisphosphate.

Immunoglobulin-like cell adhesion molecules signal to the cytoplasm

In some instances, adhesion may act primarily to bind membranes to surfaces, but it now seems clear that some IgCAMs act via the cytoplasmic domain after engaging with a cognate partner molecule to initiate a signal-transduction cascade as a direct consequence of an adhesive interaction. A good example of this is the Trk receptors, which have two Ig domains in their extracellular sequences, or the fibroblast growth factor (FGF) receptor with four Ig-like domains, which first bind a neurotrophin, such as nerve growth factor (NGF), brain-derived growth factor (BDNF), neurotrophin 3 (NT3) or FGF (Chap. 19), after which signal transduction is triggered by dimerization and autophosphorylation of the cytoplasmic domains by endogenous

tyrosine kinases (see Chap. 24). In contrast, in molecules such as NCAM and L1, which have multiple Ig domains, and P_0, which has a single Ig domain, all of which are known to interact homophilically, there is no obvious mechanism whereby a signaling cascade could be initiated after interaction. None of these proteins carries endogenous tyrosine kinase activity or any motifs that might indicate an interaction with G proteins. A novel mechanism for signaling [7,8] has been suggested for NCAM, L1 and N-cadherin (see below) in that these molecules are believed, in certain circumstances, to cluster with the FGF receptor and induce autophosphorylation of that receptor in the absence of its usual ligand, FGF (Fig. 7-2). In contrast, the myelin P_0 protein, although it has been suggested [9] to cluster within its membrane and interact, initially, with the cytoskeleton, is unlikely to initiate a signal-transduction cascade. The primary, if not the only, role of P_0 is to hold the myelin membranes in a tightly compacted state (Chap. 4).

THE INTEGRIN FAMILY

Integrin receptors (Fig. 7-3) on cell surfaces mediate cell–ECM and cell–cell adhesion, and they function in virtually every tissue [10]. Integrins exist as heterodimers composed of noncovalently bound α and β subunits. The α subunits have three or four divalent cation-binding regions in the extracellular domain, and in some, two disulfide-linked heavy and light chains constitute a single subunit. The extracellular domain is followed by a single transmembrane segment and an intracellular carboxyl-terminal, cytoplasmic domain that may contain potential phosphorylation sites. The cytoplasmic domains of integrins are involved in interactions with the cytoskeleton [11].

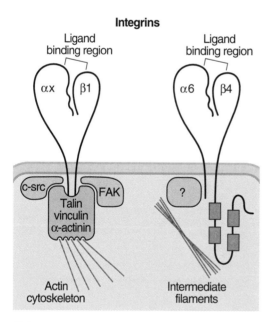

Integrins

Ligand binding region

Ligand binding region

αx $\beta 1$

$\alpha 6$ $\beta 4$

c-src   FAK

Talin
vinculin
α-actinin

?

Actin cytoskeleton

Intermediate filaments

FIGURE 7-3. Integrins are heterodimers. Integrins consist of α and β subunits noncovalently linked, which interact via their cytoplasmic domains with a number of cytoplasmic proteins. The $\alpha x \beta 1$ integrin complex on the left binds to a complex which includes focal adhesion kinase *(FAK)*. The $\alpha 6 \beta 4$ integrin complex contains fibronectin *(FN)* III repeats, which mediate binding to intermediate filaments.

Heterogeneity of integrin subunits increases the complexity of this family

There are at least eight β-integrin subunits that are homologous to each other and more than a dozen α-integrin subunits. This suggests that the interactions within the integrin family must be very complex indeed because of the number of possibilities of linking a given α with any β to make a functional cell-surface integrin. Furthermore, to add to the complexity, different integrins may bind to the same ligand, for example, an ECM protein, using different recognition sequences within the ligand. As an example, the $\alpha 5 \beta 1$ integrin recognizes a sequence in FN, arginine-glycine-aspartic acid (RGD), while an $\alpha 4 \beta 1$ integrin also binds to FN but to a region that does not contain the RGD sequence. Clearly, the integrins are a large and versatile family of CAMs geared for the recognition of an even wider variety of extracellular signals. All integrin receptors mediate links between the extracellular environment and the cytoskeleton, and they are geared for rapid response to changes in the ECM.

THE CADHERIN FAMILY

The cadherins (Fig. 7-4) are a superfamily of adhesion molecules which function in cell recognition [12,13], tissue morphogenesis and tumor suppression [14]. As a group, the cadherins are Ca^{2+}-dependent adhesion molecules, and within the group, the classic cadherins are the best studied. These include neural cadherin (N-cadherin), epithelial cadherin (E-cadherin), placental cadherin (P-cadherin) and retinal cadherin (R-cadherin). Although the classic cadherins were originally named for the tissue in which they were first found, their distributions are in no way limited to these tissues. Brain tissue expresses at least 20 [15,16], and possibly many more, individual cadherins which are used in differential neurite outgrowth, cell–cell interactions and "locking in" pre- and postsynaptic membranes at the synaptic junctional complex.

In general, the cadherins have a common primary structure in that they all contain an

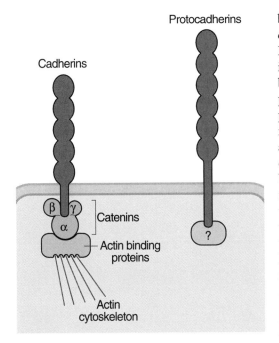

FIGURE 7-4. Basic cadherin structure. Two types of cadherins are present in the nervous system: the classic cadherins with five extracellular domains and the protocadherins with six extracellular domains. For the classic cadherins, the binding partners on the cytoplasmic side include the α, β and γ catenins. The binding partners for the protocadherins have not yet been identified.

amino-terminal extracellular domain, a single transmembrane domain and a conserved carboxyl-terminal cytoplasmic region, which is responsible for interactions with signaling pathways and with cytoplasmic and cytoskeletal proteins. The extracellular domain can be divided into five homologous regions, referred to as extracellular domains 1 through 5 (EC1–EC5). All of the extracellular domains are highly homologous to one another, and between the extracellular domains, Ca^{2+} articulates with binding sites and serves to rigidify the extracellular domain into a rod-like conformation.

The classic cadherins are homophilic adhesion molecules

That is, E-cadherin expressed on one cell surface binds to E-cadherin expressed on an apposed cell surface, N-cadherin binds to N, P to P and so forth. This is particularly true of E-cadherins. It was originally thought that all cadherins would

behave completely homophilically, but it is now clear that, for example, N-cadherin can bind to R-cadherin, although perhaps more weakly than it would to N-cadherin. A crystal structure-based model [17] for a cadherin "adhesion zipper" has been presented (Fig. 7-5). The model postulates that in addition to the broad adhesive interface in EC1, which interacts with a partner adhesive interface protruding from the opposite cell bilayer, there is also a strand dimer formed by two identical cadherin molecules protruding from the same surface. This strand dimer orients the adhesive interfaces in the two strands such that they can interact with identical dimers on the opposite membrane surface, thus creating a linear zipper of tightly adherent cadherin molecules. The strand dimer itself is mediated by a tryptophan in position 2 in the mature classic cadherin molecule. Interestingly, this tryptophan, which is proposed to fit into a hydrophobic pocket on the partner strand, is found in the classic cadherins in the same position. The implications of the existence of the strand dimer are several. First, the cadherin strand dimer, whose formation produces cadherin clustering and concentration in a particular region of plasma membrane, is probably likely to be in a very stable conformational state, which allows for the maintenance of adherens junctions in epithelial cells and, perhaps, the synaptic junctions in the CNS [18,19]. Secondly, it is possible that on a given cell surface which expresses one or more classic cadherins, a monomer (nonadhesive)/dimer (very adhesive) dynamic equilibrium exists, which can be altered as the cell needs more or less adhesion.

The first cadherin to be expressed in the nervous system is N-cadherin

This molecule appears around the time the neural tube closes [20]. As the neural tube expands and develops, a variety of cadherins can be detected in cell bodies, outgrowing neurites and synaptic endings. Many adhesion/recognition molecules have been implicated in guiding axons to their appropriate targets. Once the target axon has arrived in the vicinity of its ultimate destination, it has been suggested [21,22] that expression of identical cadherin molecules on both pre-

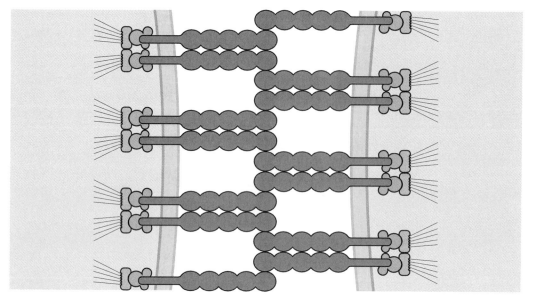

FIGURE 7-5.   Cadherins may form "adhesion zippers" to mediate cell adhesion. A globular model of the adhesion zipper is presented, illustrating the strand dimer postulated to exist between two cadherin molecules emanating from the same cell surface.

and postsynaptic membranes ultimately links up and locks in these membranes to the synaptic junctional complex. According to this proposed mechanism, neurons in the brain would utilize the same mechanisms to produce pre- and post-synaptic membrane adhesion as do other cells in forming junctions, such as the cadherin-based mechanisms of the epithelial adherens junction. In the brain, neural transmitter release mechanisms, neurotransmitter receptors, second-messenger systems and other uniquely synaptic elements are superimposed on this adhesive scaffold. These complex elements expand the function of this "neural adherens junction."

CELL ADHESION MOLECULES AND AXONAL OUTGROWTH

Cell adhesion molecules influence axonal outgrowth

During development, axons extend from the neuronal cell body and grow, frequently over long distances, in order to make very precise connections with a target. Despite the complexity of the nervous system, where over 10^{12} axons

must find their targets, the pattern of axonal outgrowth for any one axon is highly reproducible from one individual to another. The flattened tip of a growing axon is called the growth cone, which resembles the palm of the hand, with processes extending from it like fingers (see Chaps. 8 and 27). It is the growth cone that responds to the environment and determines what direction the growing axon will take. Environmental cues that the growth cone encounters can be either fixed or diffusible, and it is the integration of these signals that determines the final direction. The majority of fixed signals are CAMs, expressed by glia, other cells or older axons that have already traversed that particular pathway. In addition, growth cones use integrins to select a pathway of ECM molecules on which to extend processes.

This has been demonstrated from both tissue culture studies and studies *in vivo* [23–25]. In culture, members of all three families of adhesion molecules found in the nervous system have been shown to promote axonal growth. This was carried out by transfecting the cDNA for the molecule to be tested in a cell line that does not normally express it, usually a fibroblast cell line. Isolated neurons are then grown on a monolayer of the CAM-expressing cells, and neurite length is compared to that obtained by contact with cells not expressing the adhesion molecule. Experiments like these have shown that CAMs, including the cadherins, the integrins and members of the Ig family, in particular NCAM and L1, are very potent promoters of axonal growth from a variety of primary neurons. The same neuron has been shown to respond to different CAMs, indicating that there is not any one unique "CAM cue" for a particular neuron. Instead, it is likely that a variety of CAMs contribute to the effect on axonal growth. As well as being able to promote axonal growth when fixed in the ECM, some CAMs, such as L1, have been shown to promote axonal growth when added in a soluble form to neurons in culture. This strengthens the suggestion that CAMs are not just "sticky" molecules but can exert their effects by activation of a signal-transduction pathway. Indeed, a number of soluble forms of various CAMs, including L1, NCAM, MAG and cadherins, have been found in the extracellular milieu of living cells. It remains to be determined whether these soluble CAMs in fact influence axonal growth *in vivo*.

In addition to CAM-expressing fibroblasts, another more physiological cell substrate has been used to demonstrate the effects of CAMs on axonal growth in culture. When dorsal root ganglion neurons are grown on a monolayer of non-myelinating Schwann cells, which are very permissive for growth *in vivo* when not synthesizing myelin proteins, there is robust axonal outgrowth. Only when a combination of antibodies against NCAM, L1, cadherins and integrins was added to the cultures was outgrowth significantly reduced. Together, these experiments indicate that axonal outgrowth at any one time can be influenced by several CAMs.

This concept is supported by observations *in vivo*. Knockout mice lacking NCAM expression are viable and display subtle abnormalities in the nervous system. These abnormalities include a reduction in the size of the olfactory bulb, which is attributed to a decrease in migration of the neuronal cells that form this structure. Possibly, the inability to migrate normally reflects an increase in cellular adhesivity, due to the absence of the highly sialylated form of

NCAM, which in the wild-type or normal animal tends to repel apposed membranes on which it is expressed. Also, a reduction in the density of mossy fibers in the hippocampus has been noted in the NCAM knockout mouse, revealing a defect in axonal growth. The subtle phenotype in these mice, relative to the dramatic effect of NCAM on axonal growth in culture, suggests that there may be a certain amount of redundancy in nervous tissue, whereby another CAM or combination of CAMs can in part compensate for the absence of NCAM.

Cell adhesion molecules are responsible for axonal fasciculation

Usually, when growing toward their target, axons fasciculate (Fig. 7-6) and grow in bundles. However, there are points along the pathway where axons must defasciculate and different ax-

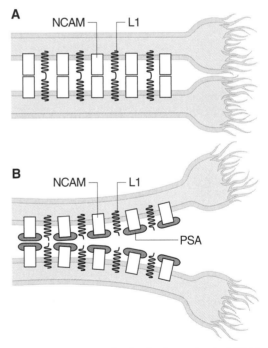

FIGURE 7-6. Neural cell adhesion molecule *(NCAM)* carries different levels of polysialic acid. **A:** NCAM is depicted on a growing axon, without polysialic acid. Under these conditions, NCAM and L1 molecules interact homophilically and axons fasciculate. **B:** NCAM carries polysialic acid (PSA), and NCAM and L1 molecules are far apart and cannot, therefore, interact. Growing axons do not fasciculate under these circumstances.

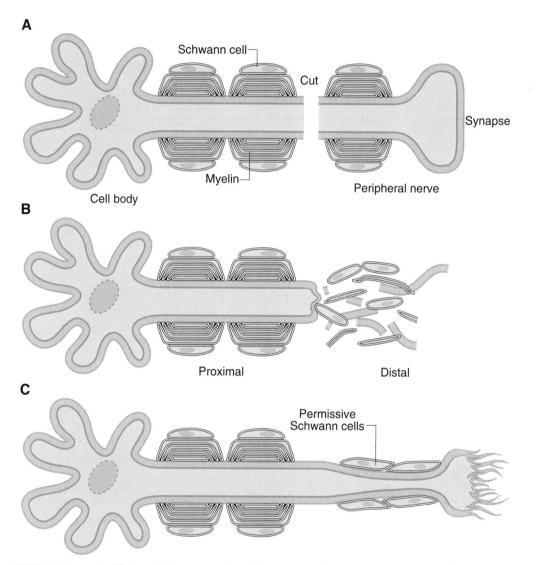

FIGURE 7-7. A simplified model for regeneration. **A:** Transection of a peripheral nerve causes degeneration. **B:** Schwann cells divide and dedifferentiate. Myelin debris is cleared by the Schwann cells and macrophages. **C:** The axon regenerates by growing over the growth-permissive Schwann cells.

ons must take different paths. Hence, in addition to promoting axonal outgrowth, CAMs can affect the direction an axon takes at key decision points along the way. One model that has been proposed for explaining how an axon is selected to remain fasciculated with respect to other axons or to separate from the bundle and grow alone is based on the relative adhesiveness of the substrate vs. the adhesiveness of other axons. This model was proposed based on observations

of adhesion and axonal growth with two forms of NCAM: one form that carries the highly charged sialic acid and polysialic acid (PSA) and another form with very little or no PSA. It has been suggested that the high negative charge on PSA–NCAM renders it less adhesive than its unsialylated counterpart [26]. Because the negatively charged sialic acid moieties tend to sequester water, occupy a large volume in the extracellular space and strongly repel one another across the bilayer, they probably keep plasma membranes sufficiently far apart so as to prevent other adhesion molecules, such as L1 and the cadherins, from getting close enough to interact. Following from this, fasciculated axons, which adhere tightly to each other, express the adhesive form of NCAM that does not carry PSA. In contrast, the PSA form of NCAM is more effective than the unsialylated form at promoting axonal growth.

As stated above, the complexity and precision of connections within the nervous system would appear to require a very rigid set of rules or cues. The ubiquitous expression of individual CAMs throughout the nervous system and during development implies that they could not provide the specificity required for such a precise signal for individual neurons. However, the full repertoire of CAMs used *in vivo* for any single axon to reach its target has yet to be characterized. It is likely, as suggested from both *in vivo* and *in vitro* results, that many CAMs affect the growth of any one axon. In addition, as demonstrated by studies with different isoforms of NCAM, that is, with and without the VASE sequence or with and without PSA, it is highly likely that subtle differences in isoform expression of any single CAM can have dramatic effects on axonal response. What has been determined regarding the role of adhesion molecules in axonal guidance during development to date is most likely an underestimate of their full involvement.

Cell adhesion molecules may also function in regeneration

As well as growing during development, axons grow and regenerate under certain conditions after injury [27]. Axonal regeneration is often successful in the PNS, where it may be accompanied by full restoration of function. In contrast, in the mammalian CNS, there is usually little or no regrowth and function is often lost. The main difference between axonal growth during development and during regeneration is in whether the damaged axon is allowed by the existing conditions to regrow, not if it is able (Chap. 29). In the PNS, after injury, damaged tissue, consisting mostly of myelin debris, is cleared away by

macrophages. Coincident with this event, Schwann cells downregulate the expression of the myelin-specific proteins and upregulate a number of growth-promoting adhesion molecules, including L1 and NCAM. These Schwann cells now resemble Schwann cells in the developing nervous system and are very permissive for axonal growth (Fig. 7-7). In contrast, myelin is not cleared from the CNS after injury and the myelin-forming cells in the CNS, oligodendrocytes, continue to express myelin proteins and do not upregulate any growth-promoting adhesion molecules. There is now substantial evidence to support the idea that the presence of myelin and the absence of growth-promoting molecules are two factors largely responsible for the lack of regeneration in the mammalian CNS [28]. Myelin membranes have been shown to be inhibitory for regeneration both *in vitro* and *in vivo*, and a number of myelin-specific molecules have been shown to be potent inhibitors of axonal growth. One of these is MAG, which is a member of the siglec subfamily. MAG can promote as well as inhibit axonal growth depending on the age and type of neuron. The ability of MAG to inhibit or promote regeneration when presented to the neuron either as a substrate or in a soluble form strongly suggests that MAG binds to a neuronal receptor and activates a signal-transduction mechanism in the neuron that effects changes in axonal growth [29,30].

CELL ADHESION MOLECULES IN MYELINATION

Myelin is formed by the compaction of oligodendrocyte plasma membranes in the CNS or Schwann cell plasma membranes in the PNS as the plasma membrane spirals around the axon. For myelin to function efficiently, a tight apposition of these membranes must be maintained, which, when viewed by electron microscopy, displays a uniform and reproducible spacing between the layers (see Chap. 4). Given the close association of myelin membranes, it is not surprising that CAMs play major roles in the formation and maintenance of this plasma membrane organelle. There is strong evidence

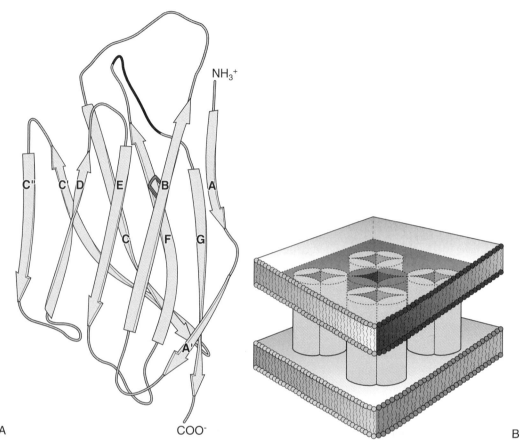

FIGURE 7-8. Structure of the P_0 protomer. **A:** In this ribbon diagram of the extracellular domain of P_0, each β strand is labeled with a letter and two antiparallel β sheets are formed. The disulfide bridge is indicated in dark orange and a hypothetical path for disordered amino acids 103–106 is shown in black in the FG loop. **B:** Lattice formation by P_0. A view of the intraperiod line, or extracellular apposition, of myelin in the PNS. The *orange* tetramer sets emanate from one bilayer and the *black* tetramer interacts with all four of them. This is a view perpendicular to the plane of the myelin membrane.

supporting a role for CAMs in the initiation of myelination, in the compaction of myelin membranes and in the stability of the noncompacted as well as the compact layers of myelin, the axon-myelin interface and the nodes of Ranvier.

The myelinating cell, when brought into contact with a large axon, begins to synthesize vast amounts of plasma membrane. The molecular trigger that starts this process is not yet known, but the interaction of MAG with some axonal component has been suggested to play an important role. The next steps in myelin formation are membrane synthesis, axonal wrapping and compaction. While MAG in both the CNS and PNS is located at the axon-myelin interface

and is therefore likely to play a role in membrane spiraling, different molecules are responsible for membrane compaction in the two systems. In PNS myelin, the most abundant protein is P_0, a small protein containing a single extracellular Ig domain [31] (see Chap. 4). The P_0 protein is responsible for adhesion at the apposition of extracellular surfaces, or intraperiod line, via homophilic interactions of its Ig domain, and at the major dense line, where cytoplasmic surfaces come together via interactions of the highly negatively charged cytoplasmic domain of P_0 with the acidic lipids, mostly phosphatidylserine, of the opposing membrane. Therefore, P_0 protein can be regarded as a "bifunctional" adhesion molecule. It is interesting that P_0 is an "obligatory" adhesion molecule in that it induces strong cell–cell adhesion between any cells in which it is expressed [32–34].

In the CNS of mammals, two proteins are needed to accomplish the dual role of adhesion at both myelin bilayer surfaces that P_0 effects in the PNS. The four-transmembrane-domain proteolipid protein (PLP) is likely to be responsible for adhesion of the extracellular surfaces, while the very basic cytoplasmic myelin basic protein (MBP) holds membranes together at the inner cytoplasmic surfaces in the CNS. Although MBP is also present in the PNS, it is much less abundant than in the CNS and its absence does not have a dramatic effect on PNS myelin compaction.

The importance of P_0 in PNS myelin has been clearly demonstrated. In P_0 gene knockout experiments in mice [35], severe hypomyelination and a virtual absence of compact myelin in the PNS is observed. In humans, there are two disease states associated with mutations in the P_0 gene: *Charcot-Marie-Tooth type I* disease (see Chaps. 39 and 40) and Dejerine-Sottas disease, both dysmyelinating diseases that exhibit a spectrum of severity depending on the particular mutation.

The crystal structure of the extracellular domain of P_0 has also been determined [36]. The arrangement of molecules in the crystal indicates that P_0 may exist on the membrane surface as a tetramer (Fig. 7-8) that can link to other tetramers from the opposing membrane to form an adhesive lattice, like a "molecular Velcro." The structure also suggests that P_0 mediates adhesion through the direct interaction of apically directed tryptophan side chains with the opposing membrane [37], in addition to homophilic protein–protein interaction.

Functional myelin not only depends on compact myelin in the internodes but also requires maintenance of a stable structure in the membranes adjacent to the nodes of Ranvier, termed the paranodes, which are sinuous, open cytoplasmic channels that are continuous with each other throughout the myelin sheath. In the plasma membrane subdomains that surround these channels, a number of adhesion molecules have been localized, namely, MAG, certain inte-

grins [38] and cadherins. The paranodal loops interact across their extracellular surfaces, and it is clear that certain cadherins at least participate in holding them firmly in place against each other [39]. In particular, E-cadherin is expressed by Schwann cells and is localized to these cytoplasmic compartments. This cadherin is not present in the underlying axon. Thus, in peripheral nerve, E-cadherin is unusual in that it does not mediate adhesion between two cells but, instead, mediates adhesion between two regions of a single plasma membrane elaborated by a single Schwann cell.

SUMMARY

Adhesion molecules are indispensible components of nervous tissue. They adhere cell membranes to each other with varying degrees of strength and "translate" adhesion into cellular responses via signal-transduction pathways (see, for example, [40]). The major classes of adhesion molecules, the integrins, IgCAMs and cadherins, act cooperatively [41] and in concert to coordinate brain development and maturation and, in adulthood, to maintain the normal tissue architecture.

REFERENCES

1. Gumbiner, B. M. Proteins associated with the cytoplasmic surface of adhesion molecules. *Neuron* 11:551–564, 1993.
2. Springer, T. A. Adhesion receptors of the immune system. *Nature* 346:425–434, 1990.
3. Williams, A. F., and Barclay, A. N. The immunoglobulin superfamily—Domains for cell surface recognition. *Annu. Rev. Immunol.* 6:381–405, 1988.
4. Edelman, G. M. CAMs and Igs: Cell adhesion and the evolutionary origins of immunity. *Immunol. Rev.* 100:11–45, 1987.
5. Kelm, S., Pelz, A., Schauer, R., et al. Sialoadhesin, myelin-associated glycoprotein and CD22 define a new family of sialic acid-dependent adhesion molecules of the immunoglobulin superfamily. *Curr. Biol.* 4:965–972, 1994.
6. Brummendorf, T., and Rathjen, F. G. Axonal glycoproteins with immunoglobulin and fibronectin

type II-related domains in vertebrates: Structural features, binding activities and signal transduction. *J. Neurochem.* 61:1207–1219, 1993.

7. Walsh, F. S., and Doherty, P. Neural cell adhesion molecules of the immunoglobulin superfamily: Role in axon growth and guidance. *Annu. Rev. Cell. Dev. Biol.* 13:425–456, 1997.

8. Doherty, P., and Walsh, F. CAM–FGF interactions: A model for axonal growth. *Mol. Cell. Neurosci.* 8:99–111, 1996.

9. Filbin, M. T., D'Urso, D., Zhang, K., Wong, M., Doyle, J. P., and Colman, D. R. Protein zero of peripheral nerve myelin: Adhesion properties and functional models. *Adv. Mol. Cell. Biol.* 16: 159–192, 1996.

10. Hynes, R. O. Integrins: Versatility, modulation and signaling in cell adhesion. *Cell* 69:11–25, 1992.

11. Ylänne, J., Chen, Y. L., O'Toole, T. E., Loftus, J. C., Takada, Y., and Ginsburg, M. H. Distinct functions of integrin α and β subunit cytoplasmic domains in cell spreading and formation of focal adhesions. *J. Cell Biol.* 122:223–234, 1993.

12. Takeichi, M. Cadherin cell adhesion receptors as a morphogenetic regulator. *Science* 25: 1451–1455, 1993.

13. Geiger, B., and Ayalon, O. Cadherins. *Annu. Rev. Cell Biol.* 8:307–322, 1993.

14. Takeichi, M. Cadherins in cancer: Implications for invasion and metastasis. *Curr. Opin. Cell Biol.* 5:806–811, 1993.

15. Suzuki, S., Sano, K., and Tanihara, H. Diversity of the cadherin family: Evidence for eight new cadherins in nervous tissue. *Cell. Regul.* 2:261–270, 1991.

16. Sano K., Tanihara, H., Heimark, R. L., et al. Protocadherins: A large family of cadherin-related molecules in central nervous system. *EMBO J.* 12:2249–2256, 1993.

17. Shapiro, L., Fannon, A. M., Kwong, P. D., et al. Structural basis of cell–cell adhesion by cadherins. *Nature* 374:327–337, 1995.

18. Serafini, T. An old friend in a new home: Cadherins at the synapse. *Trends Neurosci.* 20:322–323, 1997.

19. Colman, D. R. Neurites, synapses and cadherins reconciled. *Mol. Cell. Neurosci.* 10:1–6, 1997.

20. Kintner, C. Regulation of embryonic cell adhesion by the cadherin cytoplasmic domain. *Cell* 69:225–236, 1997.

21. Fannon, A. M., and Colman, D. R. A model for central synaptic junctional complex formation based on the differential adhesive specificities of the cadherins. *Neuron* 17:423–434, 1996.

22. Uchida, N., Honjo, Y., Johnson, K. R., Wheelock, M. J., and Takeichi, M. The catenin/cadherin adhesion system is localized in synaptic junctions bordering transmitter release zones. *J. Cell. Biol.* 135:767–779, 1996.

23. Tomaselli, K. J., Neugebauer, K. N., Bixby, J. L., Lilien, J., and Reichardt, L. F. N-Cadherin and integrins: Two receptor systems that mediate neurite outgrowth on astrocyte surfaces. *Neuron* 1:33–43, 1988.

24. Matasunaga, M., Hatta, K., Nagafuchi, A., and Takeichi, M. Guidance of optic nerve fibers by N-cadherin adhesion molecules. *Nature* 334:62–64, 1988.

25. Inouye, A., and Sanes, J. R. Lamina-specific connectivity in the brain: Regulation by N-cadherin, neurotrophins, and glycoconjugates. *Science* 276:1428–1431, 1997.

26. Rutishauser, J. NCAM and its polysialic acid moiety: A mechanism for pull/push regulation of cell interactions during development? *Dev. Suppl.* 99–104, 1992.

27. Fawcett, J. W., and Keynes, R. J. Peripheral nerve regeneration. *Annu. Rev. Neurosci.* 13:43–60, 1990.

28. Keynes, R. J., and Cook, G. M. W. Repulsive and inhibitory signals. *Curr. Opin. Neurobiol.* 5: 75–82, 1995.

29. Filbin, M. T. Myelin-associated glycoprotein: A role in myelination and in the inhibition of axonal regeneration? *Curr. Opin. Neurobiol.* 5:588–595, 1995.

30. Filbin, M. T. The muddle with MAG. *Mol. Cell. Neurosci.* 8:84–92, 1996.

31. Lemke, G., Lamar, E., and Patterson, J. Isolation and analysis of the gene encoding peripheral myelin-protein zero. *Neuron* 1:73–83, 1988.

32. Filbin, M., Walsh, F. S., Trapp, B. D., Pizzy, J. A., and Tennekoon, G. I. Role of myelin P_0 protein as a homophilic adhesion molecule. *Nature* 344:871–872, 1990.

33. D'Urso, D., Brophy, P. J., Staugaitis, S. M., et al. Protein zero of peripheral myelin: Biosynthesis, membrane insertion, and evidence for homotypic interactions. *Neuron* 4:449–460, 1990.

34. Filbin, M. T., and Tennekoon, G. I. Myelin P_0-protein, more than just a structural protein? *Bioessays* 14:541–546, 1992.

35. Giese, K. P., Martini, R., Lemke, G., Soriano, P., and Schachner, M. Mouse P_0 gene disruption leads to hypomyelination, abnormal expression of recognition molecules, and degeneration of myelin and axons. *Cell* 71:565–576, 1992.

36. Shapiro, L., Doyle, J. P., Hensley, P., Colman, D.

R., and Hendrickson, W. A. Crystal structure of the extracellular domain from P_0, the major structural protein of peripheral nerve myelin. *Neuron* 17:435–449, 1996.

37. Wells, C. A., Saavedra, R. A., Inouye, H., and Kirschner, D. A. Myelin P_0-glycoprotein: Predicted structure and interactions of extracellular domain. *J. Neurochem.* 61:1987–1995, 1993.

38. Einheber, S., Milner, T., Giancotti, F., and Salzer, J. Axonal regulation of Schwann cell integrin expression suggests a role for $\alpha 6\ \beta 4$ in myelination. *J. Cell. Biol.* 123:1223–1235, 1993.

39. Fannon, A. M., Sherman, D. L., Ilyina-Gragerova, G., Brophy, P. J., Friedrich, V. L., Jr., and Colman, D. R. Novel E-cadherin mediated adhesion in peripheral nerve: Schwann cell architecture is stabilized by intracellular signals elicited by autotypic adherens junctions. *J. Cell. Biol.* 129:189–202, 1995.

40. Brady-Kalnay, S., Rimm, D., and Tonks, N. Receptor protein tyrosine phosphatase PTPm associates with cadherins and catenins *in vivo*. *J. Cell Biol.* 130:977–986, 1995.

41. Monier-Gavell, F., and Duban, J.-L. Cross talk between adhesion molecules: Control of N-cadherin activity by intracellular signals elicited by $\beta 1$ and $\beta 3$ integrins in migrating neural crest cells. *J. Cell. Biol.* 137:1663–1681, 1997.

8

Cytoskeleton of Neurons and Glia

Laura L. Kirkpatrick and Scott T. Brady

Basic Neurochemistry: Molecular, Cellular and Medical Aspects, 6th Ed., edited by G. J. Siegel et al. Published by Lippincott–Raven Publishers, Philadelphia, 1999. Correspondence to Scott T. Brady, Department of Cell Biology and Neuroscience, University of Texas Southwestern Medical Center, 5323 Harry Hines Boulevard, Dallas, Texas 75235-9111.

Neurons and glia exhibit a remarkable diversity of shapes. These different morphologies are so characteristic and distinctive that they have been used since the time of Ramón y Cajal to define neural functions. For example, Purkinje cells in the cerebellum have such distinctive morphologies that they are readily identifiable in any vertebrate. Neurons do not divide, so their distinctive morphologies are maintained throughout life. Biochemical and immunological markers are now used to delineate neuronal populations. Their distributions correlate well with populations previously defined on morphological grounds. The evidence indicates that the shape of cells in the nervous system is closely connected to their functions. Understanding the proteins and cellular structures that underlie cell morphology is essential for understanding the neural functions.

Proteins of the cytoskeleton play a central role in the creation and maintenance of cell shapes in all tissues. They serve multiple roles in eukaryotic cells. First, they provide structural organization for the cell interior, helping to establish metabolic compartments. Second, cytoskeletal structures serve as tracks for intracellular transport, which creates and maintains differentiated cellular functions. Finally, the cytoskeleton comprises the core framework of cellular morphologies.

Methods for visualizing individual neurons and glia *in vivo* have depended for more than 100 years on histochemical reactions with cytoskeletal elements, and even now these methods have not been surpassed. Because cytoskeletal structures play a particularly prominent role in the nervous system, cytoskeletal proteins represent a large fraction of total brain protein, comprising perhaps a third or more of the total. In fact, much of our knowledge about cytoskeletal biochemistry is based on studies of proteins purified from the brain. The aims of this chapter are twofold: first, to provide an introduction to the cytoskeletal elements themselves and, second, to examine their role in neuronal function. Throughout, the emphasis will be on the cytoskeleton as a vital, dynamic component of the nervous system.

MOLECULAR COMPONENTS OF THE NEURONAL CYTOSKELETON

The cytoskeleton is one of several biological elements that define eukaryotic cells

Other defining elements include the nucleus and mitochondria. The term "cytoskeleton" is often used as if it described a single, unified structure, but the cytoskeleton of neurons and other eukaryotic cells comprises three distinct, interacting structural complexes that have very different properties: microtubules (MTs), neurofilaments (NFs) and microfilaments (MFs). Each has a characteristic composition, structure and organization that may be further specialized in a particular cell type or subcellular domain. The defining structural elements have long been identifiable in electron micrographs (Fig. 8-1), and a considerable amount is known about the detailed organization of these components in neurons and glia. Each set of cytoskeletal structures is considered in turn.

Microtubules act as both dynamic structural elements and tracks for organelle traffic

Neuronal MTs are structurally similar to those found in other eukaryotic cells [1]. The core structure is a polymer of 50-kDa tubulin subunits. Heterodimers of α- and β-tubulin align end to end to form protofilaments, 13 of which join laterally to form a hollow tube with an outer diameter of 25 nm (Fig. 8-2). Examples also exist of MTs with 12 and 14 protofilaments. The α- and β-tubulins are the best known members of a unique protein family, the members of which have significant sequence similarity [2]. There is approximately 40% sequence identity between α- and β-tubulins and even greater identity within the α and β gene subfamilies. Conservation of the primary sequence for tubulins is also high across species so that tubulins from yeast can readily co-assemble with tubulins from human brain. Tubulin dimers bind two molecules of GTP and exhibit GTPase activity that is closely linked to assembly and disassembly of MTs [1,3]. While many questions remain about tubulin and its interactions, the structure of the αβ-tubulin dimer has recently been derived from electron diffraction studies [3], providing a basis for dissection of the functional architecture of MTs.

Heterodimers in a MT are oriented in the same direction, so the resulting MT has asymmetrical ends that differ in assembly properties [4]. The β-tubulin subunit is exposed at the "plus" end, which is the preferred end for addition of tubulin dimers. The opposite, "minus," end grows more slowly at physiological concentrations of tubulin. In the case of free MTs, the balance between assembly and disassembly at each end defines a critical concentration for net growth. MT assembly under *in vitro* conditions

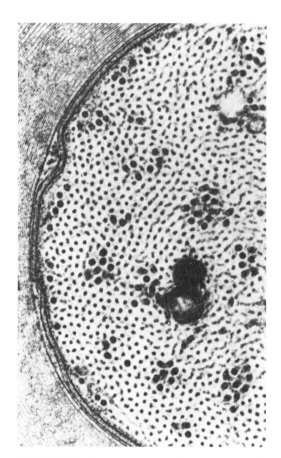
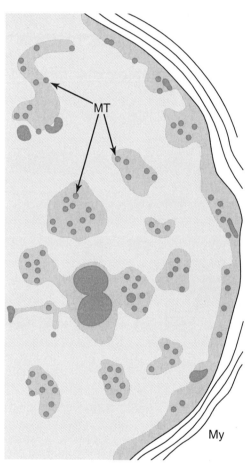

FIGURE 8-1.   The cytoskeleton and organization of the axon in cross-section. **Left:** Electron micrograph of a myelinated toad axon in cross-section taken near a Schmidt-Lanterman cleft; axon diameter is slightly reduced and the different domains within the axoplasm are emphasized. **Right:** Diagram highlighting key features of the axoplasm. Portions of the myelin sheath surrounding the axon can be seen *(My)*. Most of the axonal diameter is taken up by the neurofilaments *(clear area)*. There is a minimum distance between neurofilaments and other cytoskeletal structures that is determined by the side arms of the neurofilaments. (These side arms are visible between some of the neurofilaments in the electron micrograph, **left.**) The microtubules *(MT)* tend to be found in bundles and are more irregularly spaced. They are surrounded by a fuzzy material that is also visible in the region just below the plasma membrane *(stippled areas,* **right**). These areas are thought to be enriched in actin microfilaments and presumably contain other slow component b (SCb) proteins as well. The *stippled regions* with embedded microtubules are also the location of membranous organelles in fast axonal transport *(larger, filled, irregular shapes,* **right**). Both microtubule and microfilament networks need to be intact for the efficient movement of organelles in fast transport. (Electron micrograph provided by Dr. Alan Hodge. From [34], with permission.)

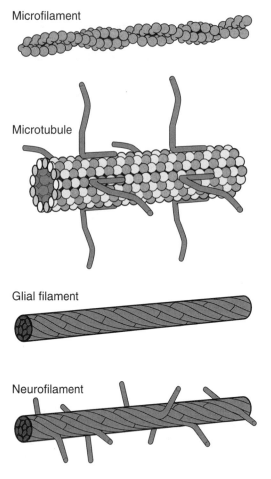

Microfilament

Microtubule

Glial filament

Neurofilament

FIGURE 8-2.   Microfilaments, microtubules and intermediate filaments in the nervous system. Each cytoskeletal structure has a distinctive ultrastructure. This schematic illustrates the major features of the core fibrils. The microfilament consists of two strands of actin subunits twisted around each other like strings of pearls. The individual subunits are asymmetrical, globular proteins that give the microfilament its polarity. The microtubule is also made from globular subunits, but in this case the basic building block is a heterodimer of α- and β-tubulins. These αβ dimers are organized into linear strands, or protofilaments, with β-tubulin subunits oriented toward the plus end of the microtubule. Protofilaments form sheets *in vitro* that roll up into a cylinder with 13 protofilaments forming the wall of the microtubule. Assembly of both microfilaments and microtubules is coupled to slow nucleotide hydrolysis, ATP for microfilaments and GTP for microtubules. The subunits of both glial filaments and neurofilaments are rod-shaped molecules that will self-assemble without nucleotides. The core filament structure is thought to be a ropelike arrangement of individual subunits. Glial filaments are typical type III intermediate filaments in that they form homopolymers without side arms. In contrast, neurofilaments are heteropolymers formed from three subunits, NFH, NFM and NFL for the high-, medium- and low-molecular-weight subunits. The NFH and NFM subunits have extended carboxy-terminal tails that project from the sides of the core filament and may be heavily phosphorylated.

involves a slow nucleation step followed by a more rapid, net growth phase interspersed with occasional, rapid shrinkage, a kinetic pattern described as dynamic instability. In glia and most other non-neuronal cells, however, the minus ends of MTs are usually bound at the site of nucleation, which is associated with the pericentriolar complex of the cell, a site often called the microtubule-organizing center (MTOC) [5]. Anchoring of MT minus ends helps to establish and maintain the polarity of cellular MTs. Anchoring and nucleation of MTs appear to require a third class of tubulin, γ-tubulin, which is detectable only as part of the pericentriolar complex [5].

The organization of MTs in neurons differs in several ways from that seen in non-neuronal cells (Fig. 8-3) [6]. Axonal and dendritic MTs are not continuous back to the cell body nor are they associated with any visible MTOC. Axonal MTs can be more than 100 μm long, but they have uniform polarity, with all plus ends distal to the cell body. Dendritic MTs are typically shorter and often exhibit mixed polarity, with only about 50% of the MTs oriented with the plus end distal. Recent work suggests that MTs in both axons and dendrites are nucleated normally at the MTOC but are then released from the MTOC and delivered to neurites [7].

While MTs in neurons are composed of the same basic constituents as those in non-neuronal cells, they are strikingly more diverse (Table 8-1). Brain MTs contain tubulins of many different isotypes, with many different post-translational modifications and a variety of microtubule-associated proteins (MAPs). MT

Axonal and Dendritic Cytoskeletons

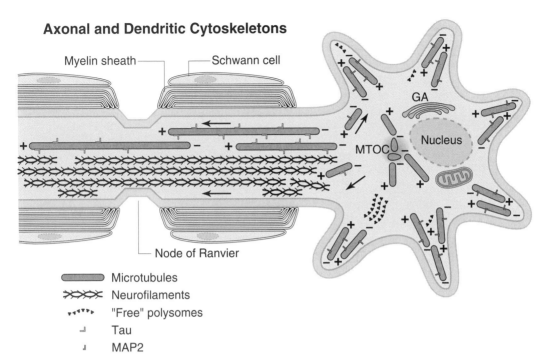

FIGURE 8-3. The axonal and dendritic cytoskeletons differ in both composition and organization. The major differences are illustrated diagramatically in this diagram. With one exception, all cytoskeletal proteins are synthesized on free polysomes in the cell body, then transported to their different cellular compartments. The exception is MAP2, which is the major microtubule-associated protein of dendrites. While some MAP2 is synthesized in the cell body, MAP2 mRNA is specifically enriched in the dendritic compartment and a significant fraction is thought to be synthesized there. The microtubules of cell bodies, dendrites and axons are thought to be nucleated at the microtubule-organizing center *(MTOC)*, then released and delivered to either the dendrites or axon. In the dendrite, microtubules often have mixed polarities with both plus and minus ends distal to the cell body. The functional consequence of this organization is uncertain but may help explain why dendrites taper with distance from the cell body. In contrast, all axonal microtubules are oriented with the plus end distal to the cell body and exhibit uniform distribution across the axon. Although some tau protein can be detected in cell bodies and dendrites, axonal microtubules are enriched in tau and axonal tau is differentially phosphorylated. MAP2 appears to be absent from the axon. Neurofilaments are largely excluded from the dendritic compartments but are abundant in large axons. The spacing of neurofilaments is sensitive to the level of phosphorylation. Microtubules and neurofilaments both stop and start in the axon rather than being continuous back to the cell body. The microfilaments are more dispersed in their organization and may be difficult to visualize in the mature neuron. They are most abundant near the plasma membrane but are also enriched in presynaptic terminals and dendritic spines. *GA*, golgi apparatus.

composition varies according to location, such as in axons or dendrites, suggesting that brain MTs exist in specialized forms to perform designated tasks in the unique environments of the neuron. For example, axonal MTs contain stable segments that are unusually resistant to treatments that depolymerize MTs in other cells. Such stable domains are preserved as short MT segments and may serve to nucleate or organize MTs in axons, particularly during regeneration [8]. This and other specializations of axonal MTs

(see below) may reflect the unusual requirements of the neuronal cytoskeleton, where remarkably long MTs are maintained at considerable distances from sites of new protein synthesis in the cell body.

Multiple genes exist for both α- and β-tubulin. Tubulin isotypes differ primarily at the carboxy terminus, the region where most posttranslational modifications and MAP interactions occur. While most α- and β-tubulin isotypes are expressed in all tissues, some are

TABLE 8-1.   **MAJOR MICROTUBULE CYTOSKELETAL PROTEINS OF THE NERVOUS SYSTEM**

Protein	Expression pattern and distribution	Modifications
α-Tubulin (multigene family)	In all cells but some isoforms preferentially expressed in brain	Acetylation, tyrosination
β-Tubulin (multigene family)	In all cells but some isoforms preferentially expressed in brain	Phosphorylation, polyglutamylation
γ-Tubulin	In all cells, pericentriolar region/MTOC	?
MAP1a (multigene family)	Appears late, wide distribution	Phosphorylation
1b	Appears early, then declines, enriched in axons	Phosphorylation
MAP2a (single gene)	High MW, dendritic in mature neurons	Phosphorylation
2b	High MW, dendritic expressed throughout lifetime	Phosphorylation
2c	Low MW, dendritic in developing neurons	Phosphorylation
Tau (single gene)		Phosphorylation
High MW	Peripheral axons with distinctive phosphorylation pattern	
Low MW	Enriched in CNS axons with distinctive phosphorylation pattern	Phosphorylation
MAP4	Primarily non-neuronal, multiple forms, widespread distribution	Phosphorylation at mitosis

MAP, microtubule-associated protein; MTOC, microtubule-organizing center; MW, molecular weight.

expressed preferentially in different tissues. For example, class III and IVa β-tubulins are neuron-specific [9]. It is not known if such examples of tissue-specific expression imply that different isotypes are structurally suited to function in different tissues or merely that different tubulin genes are part of different tissue-specific developmental programs. Where they can be evaluated, all isotypes available in a given cell appear capable of coassembly and typically can be detected in all cellular MTs [9].

Brain MTs also contain a variety of post-translational modifications. When purified, mammalian tubulin is analyzed by isoelectric focusing and over 20 different isoforms can be seen [9]. These are explained by a combination of multiple genes and various post-translational modifications. The two best studied post-translational modifications of tubulin are α-tubulin detyrosination and acetylation [9]. Most α-tubulins are expressed with a carboxy-terminal tyrosine residue. This tyrosine can be removed by tubulin carboxypeptidase and then replaced by tubulin tyrosine ligase, in a rapid cycle that occurs on the majority of available tubulin. Since the carboxypeptidase acts only on assembled tubulin and the ligase acts on unassembled tubulin, this tyrosination/detyrosination cycle is linked to MT dynamics. Typically, newly assem-

bled MTs will contain Tyr-tubulin. The longer an MT remains polymerized, the higher its content of de-Tyr-tubulin, or Glu-tubulin. A second prominent post-translational modification of neuronal α-tubulin is lysine ε–acetylation. The enzyme responsible for acetylation, tubulin acetyltransferase, like tubulin carboxypeptidase, acts only on assembled tubulin. Neuronal β-tubulin isotypes appear to be subject to fewer post-translational modifications [9]. The β$_{III}$ isotype of brain is phosphorylated, and while the function of this modification is not clear, correlations with neurite outgrowth in neuroblastoma cells have been made. Another modification of β-tubulin is polyglutamylation, the addition of one to five glutamyl units to the γ-carboxyl group of a glutamate residue near the C terminus. Despite the plethora of neuronal tubulin post-translational modifications, to date, none is known to have a direct effect on MT properties.

MTs *in vivo* invariably include members of a heterogeneous set of proteins known as MAPs [10]. MAPs interact with MTs rather than with free tubulin and maintain constant stoichiometry with the tubulin in MTs through cycles of assembly and disassembly. Several categories of brain MAPs can be distinguished: the high-molecular-weight MAPs, which include MAPs

1A, 1B, 2A and 2B (>270 kDa); the tau proteins; MAPs of intermediate molecular weight, such as MAP3 and MAP4; and the molecular motors kinesin and dynein, which drive the intracellular transport of membrane-bound organelles along MT tracts (see Chap. 28). The other groups of MAPs are collectively known as "fibrous" or "structural" because they have been observed to form lateral extensions between adjacent MTs and between MTs and other cytoskeletal elements [10]. Such extensions do not generally represent stable cross-links but, rather, reflect transient interactions which facilitate MT function. One exception is the formation of stably cross-linked axonemal MTs of cilia and flagella, such as occur on ependymal cells in the CNS.

The high molar ratio of MAPs to tubulin in brain suggests that MAPs may play an important role in determining MT properties. Some MAPs are differentially distributed in neurons [10]. For example, MAP2 is found primarily in cell bodies and dendrites, and tau is enriched in axons. Additionally, changes in MAP expression and MAP phosphorylation during development suggest that they may play a role in modulating MT function in the developing brain [10]. For example, MAPs 1A and 1B occur in both axons and somatodendritic domains, but MAP1B is preferentially phosphorylated in axons and especially in developing axons. As many as six different tau proteins are derived by alternative splicing from a single tau gene [11]. Both the expression and the phosphorylation of the different tau isoforms are regulated throughout development. While MAPs affect nucleation and stability of MTs *in vitro*, these may not be their primary functions *in vivo*. Other likely functions include roles in MT spacing and organization, compartmentation and interaction with other cellular structures.

MTs serve multiple roles in neurons [6,8]. Besides acting as the substrate for the transport of membrane-bound organelles, MTs are necessary for the extension of neurites during development; they provide the scaffolding for maintaining neurites after extension, and they help maintain the definition and integrity of intracellular compartments. The diversity of these functions is reflected in differences in the biochemistry and metabolic stability of different MTs.

Neuronal and glial intermediate filaments provide support for neuronal and glial morphology

As a class of cytoskeletal structures, intermediate filaments (IFs) display an unusual degree of cell specificity and are often used as markers of cellular differentiation. They comprise a family of related genes that have been classified in five types. All five share homology in a core rod domain, which contains multiple α-helical domains that can form coiled coils. The sequence homology in this conserved domain is sufficient that some antibodies recognize all known IFs from mammals through a wide range of invertebrates. IFs are also ultrastructurally similar regardless of type, forming 8- to 10-nm rope-like filaments that may be several micrometers long. However, NFs differ from the other IFs because they have sidearms that project from the surface (Fig. 8-2). The result is that IFs in non-neuronal cells are often seen in densely packed bundles, while NFs are widely spaced (Fig. 8-4).

IF types I and II are the keratins which are found in various combinations in epithelial cells throughout the body. Keratin IFs must include representative subunits of both type I and type II, with each tissue having a characteristic combination. In contrast, type III IF subunits typically form homopolymers. They include IFs that are characteristic of less differentiated cells like glial or neuronal precursors, as well as those seen in more specialized cell types like smooth muscle cells and mature astrocytes. These three types of IF not only share sequence homology within their rod domains, but their genes exhibit similar exon and intron structure. All type IV IFs are neuron-specific and have a common pattern of exons and introns that differs from that seen in types I–III. Finally, type V polypeptides are the nuclear lamins which form the walls of the nuclear envelope structure, rather than typical IF structures. While all eukaryotes express type V lamins, the other IF types are not found in plants, many unicellular organisms and the arthropods. Cytoplasmic IFs are, however, nearly ubiquitous in vertebrate cells, and some cells contain more than one type of IF in the cytoplasm. Curiously, oligodendrocyte precursors contain vimentin IFs, but these are lost during

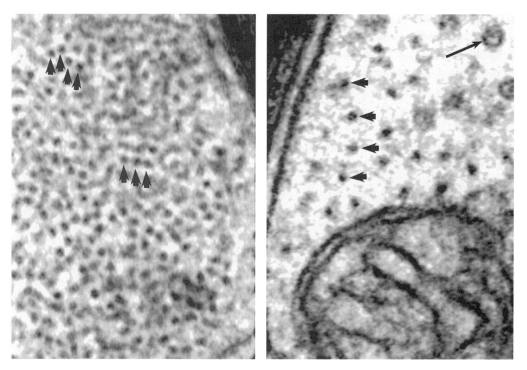

FIGURE 8-4.   Glial filaments and neurofilaments are easily recognized in electron micrographs. The glial filaments lack side arms and often appear to be densely packed, with neighboring subunits almost touching (*large arrows* in **left** panel). In contrast, the spacing between neurofilaments is typically much greater (*large arrows* in **right** panel). This spacing is due to the side arms of neurofilaments formed by the tails of the high- and medium-molecular-weight neurofilaments (NFH and NFM, respectively). These tails are heavily phosphorylated in large axons such that NFH tails may have 50 or more phosphates added to the multiple repeats of a consensus phosphorylation site. NFM tails have fewer sites and typically only ten to twelve phosphates. Charges on the surface of phosphorylated neurofilaments are thought to repel neighboring filaments, creating the large spacing. For comparison, a 25-nm microtubule is indicated in the **right** panel *(thin arrow)*. (Micrograph provided by H. Ross Payne and Scott Brady.)

differentiation, making mature oligodendrocytes one of the few vertebrate cell types that lack cytoplasmic IFs.

The nervous system contains an unusually diverse set of IFs (Table 8-2) with distinctive cellular distributions and developmental expression [12,13]. Despite their molecular heterogeneity, all IFs appear as solid ropelike fibers, 8 to 12 nm in diameter. NFs can be hundreds of micrometers long and have characteristic sidearm projections, while filaments in glia or other non-neuronal cells are shorter and lack sidearms (Fig. 8-4). The existence of NFs was established long before much was known about their biochemistry or properties. As stable cytoskeletal structures, NFs were noted in early electron micrographs, and many traditional histological procedures that visualize neurons are

based on a specific interaction of metal stains with NFs.

The primary type of IF in large myelinated axons is formed from three subunit proteins known as the NF triplet: NF high-molecular-weight subunit (NFH, 180 to 200 kDa), NF middle-molecular-weight subunit (NFM, 130 to 170 kDa) and NF low-molecular-weight subunit (NFL, 60 to 70 kDa) [12,13]. Each of the subunit proteins is coded for by a separate gene. The NF triplet proteins are type IV IF proteins which are expressed only in neurons and have a characteristic domain structure. The amino-terminal regions of all three subunits interact via α-helical coiled coils to form the core of the filament. NFM and NFH also have long carboxy-terminal regions, which project from the core filaments as sidearms. NFH and, to a lesser extent, NFM have

TABLE 8-2.   INTERMEDIATE FILAMENT (IF) PROTEINS OF THE NERVOUS SYSTEM

IF type	Subunit	Cell type
Type III	Vimentin	Neural and glial precursors
	GFAP	Astrocytes, some Schwann cells
	Peripherin	Subset of neurons, particularly in PNS, may coassemble with NFH/NFM/NFL
	Desmin	Smooth muscle cells in vasculature
Type IV	NFH	Most neurons, most abundant in large neurons
	NFM	
	NFL	
	α-Internexin	Subset of neurons, particularly parallel fibers in cerebellum, may also coassemble with NFH/NFM/NFL
Type IV?	Nestin	Neuroectodermal precursors in developing brain

GFAP, glial fibrillary acidic protein; NFH, NFM and NFL, neurofilaments of high, medium and low molecular weight, respectively.

a large number of consensus phosphorylation sites for proline-directed kinases in this carboxy-terminal extension (>50 on NFH and >10 on NFM in many species). In large myelinated axons, most, if not all, of these sites are phosphorylated [12,13]. This phosphorylation of NFH and NFM sidearms alters the charge density on the NF surface, repelling adjacent NFs with similar charge. Such mutual repulsion by the sidearms of NFs is thought to be a major determinant of axonal caliber [8].

Other IFs are also found in the nervous system [12,13]. Vimentin is the most widely expressed type III IF and is found in a variety of cell types, like fibroblasts, microglia and smooth muscle cells, as well as in embryonic cell types, including neuronal and glial precursors. Astrocytes and some Schwann cells contain the type III IF glial fibrillary acidic protein (GFAP). This distribution has led to the widespread use of GFAP immunoreactivity to identify astrocytes in culture and in tissue. In contrast to NFs, type III IFs like GFAP lack sidearms and often appear to be tightly bundled.

At least three other IFs occur in selected neurons or neuronal precursors: α-internexin, peripherin and nestin. All of these are most prominently expressed during development, then downregulated. Based on sequence and gene structure, peripherin is a type III IF, while α-internexin is a type IV IF. While the NF triplet proteins and α-internexin may be components of both CNS and PNS neurons, peripherin ap-

pears to be expressed preferentially in PNS neurons. Both can co-assemble with the NF triplet proteins *in vitro* and may do so *in vivo* but can also form homopolymeric filaments. Both are expressed at higher levels in a variety of developing neurons, and expression becomes more restricted as neurons mature. Many neurons cease to express α-internexin during maturation. However, a few neurons retain the expression of IFs containing α-internexin. Notably, IFs of parallel fibers in the cerebellar cortex contain only α-internexin subunits. Peripherin continues to be expressed in some peripheral neurons in maturity. Nestin is the most divergent of the IFs that form filaments and is sometimes considered to be a distinct IF type. Although nestin is specific to the nervous system, it is expressed in multipotent neuroectodermal precursors and suppressed during subsequent development. For this reason, it can be used as an early marker for differentiation of precursor cells.

Not all neurons have NFs. Indeed, one entire phylum in the animal kingdom, arthropods, expresses only type V nuclear lamins, so arthropod cells have no IF cytoskeletal structures at all. In addition, mature oligodendrocytes lack IFs, although their embryonic precursors contain vimentin. Clearly, the IFs are not essential for cell survival; yet in large myelinated fibers, NFs make up the bulk of axonal volume and represent a substantial fraction of total protein synthesis in the brain. In most organisms, IFs in both glia and neurons contribute to the distinctive morphologies of these cells. They are thought to provide mechanical strength and a stable cytoskeletal framework. In neurons, NFs play an important role in regulating cellular and axonal volumes and are a primary determinant of axonal caliber in large fibers. Finally, NFs exhibit an unusual degree of metabolic stability, which makes them well suited for a role in stabilizing and maintaining neuronal morphology [14].

Actin microfilaments and the membrane cytoskeleton play critical roles in neuronal growth and secretion

This major class of cytoskeletal elements is perhaps the oldest. Certainly, the actin cytoskeleton has the most diverse composition and organization. MFs are formed from 43-kDa actin monomers that are arranged like two strings of pearls intertwined into fibrils 4 to 6 nm in diameter (Fig. 8-2) [15]. A remarkable variety of proteins have been found to interact with actin MFs, ranging from myosin motors to cross-linkers, bundling proteins to anchoring proteins and sequestration proteins to small GTPase regulatory proteins [16,17].

Actin MFs are found throughout neurons and glia [18], but they are enriched in cortical regions near the plasmalemma and are particularly concentrated in presynaptic terminals, dendritic spines and growth cones. Under most circumstances in the nervous system, MFs are short oligomers organized into a meshwork most apparent near the plasma membrane and in the vicinity of axonal MTs. MFs are the main components of the membrane cytoskeleton [19,20], and this may be their primary role in mature neurons. The prominent actin bundles, termed stress fibers, seen in fibroblasts and many other non-neuronal cells in culture are not characteristic of neurons *in vivo* or *in vitro*. Most neuronal MFs are less than 1 μm in length. However, growth cones contain many longer MFs, with bundles of MFs in the filopodia and lamellipodia in addition to the typically more dispersed actin network (Fig. 8-5) [21]. The role of actin MFs in the growth cone will be considered in greater detail below.

Many MF-associated proteins [16] have been described in the nervous system (Table 8-3). In general, a good deal is known about their distribution and function in primary cultures of neurons and glia, but less is known about their role in the mature nervous system. Two that have been characterized more extensively are the major nonactin structural elements of the membrane cytoskeleton: spectrin and ankyrin. Spectrin is a flexible, rod-shaped molecule composed of homologous α and β subunits and was originally characterized as a component

---

TABLE 8-3.   SOME MICROFILAMENT-ASSOCIATED PROTEINS IN THE NERVOUS SYSTEM

Protein	Activity	Cellular location
Actin	Core subunit of MFs	Throughout neurons and glia, enriched in growth cones and in membrane cytoskeleton
Tropomyosin	Stabilize MFs	Codistributed with most MFs
Spectrin/fodrin	Cross-link MFs in membrane cytoskeleton	Enriched in membrane cytoskeleton
Ankyrin	Links MF/spectrin to membrane proteins	Membrane cytoskeleton, distinct forms in axon, dendrite and nodes of Ranvier
Fimbrin	MF bundling and cross-linking	Growing neurites
Gelsolin	Fragments MFs and nucleates assembly, regulated by Ca^{2+}	Growing neurites, glia, mature neurons
β-Thymosins	Binds actin monomers and regulates MF assembly	Growing neurites
Profilin	Binds actin monomers, inhibits MF formation, regulated by selected signal-transduction pathways	Growing neurites, glia, mature neurons

MF, microfilament.

of the erythrocyte membrane cytoskeleton. Neurons were the first cell type, other than erythrocytes, that were shown to contain spectrins, and the brain form was initially called fodrin. Spectrin heterodimers align end to end to form tetramers, which are cross-linked by short actin MFs. This spectrin–actin meshwork is tightly coupled to the plasma membrane through direct binding to membrane proteins. Some of these interactions occur via the protein ankyrin, which has separate binding sites for specific membrane proteins and β-spectrin (see Fig. 2-5). In neurons, specific isoforms of spectrin and ankyrin are localized to axons, dendrites and paranodal regions. The spectrin and ankyrin isoforms in perikarya and dendrites tend to be highly homologous to the erythrocyte forms and distinct from the spectrin and ankyrin isoforms that occur in axons.

A variety of additional MF bundling or linking proteins have been described in the nervous system. For example, fimbrin may play a role in the formation of MF bundles in growth cone filopodia. Still other actin-binding proteins may regulate MF assembly [22,23]. Gelsolin fragments MFs in a Ca^{2+}-sensitive manner but also caps and nucleates MFs. In contrast, profilin and β-thymosins bind to actin monomers and may act in part by sequestering actin subunits, although this oversimplifies the effects of these proteins. The list of MF-associated proteins has become quite long, and this diversity reflects the many forms of MF-based cytoskeletal structures.

MFs in the nervous system appear to have a variety of functions. The neuronal membrane cytoskeleton plays a role in maintaining the distribution of plasma membrane proteins, establishing cell morphologies and segregating axonal and dendritic proteins into their respective compartments [20]. MFs and the membrane cytoskeleton also mediate the interactions between neurons and the external world, including extracellular matrix components and neighboring cells (see Chap. 7). In neurons and glia, cell adhesion sites, such as tight junctions and focal adhesion plaques, interact with the MF cytoskeleton either directly or indirectly. The cortical MF meshwork also restricts access of organelles to the plasma membrane and is involved in both regulated and constitutive secretion (see Chap. 9). Finally, MFs are the basis of filopodia and lamellipodia that are essential for cell migration, growth cone motility and myelination.

ULTRASTRUCTURE AND MOLECULAR ORGANIZATION OF NEURONS AND GLIA

A dynamic neuronal cytoskeleton provides specialized functions in different regions of the neuron

The cytoskeleton in different regions of a neuron differs with regard to both composition and function. While both neurons and glia exhibit distinctive specializations in their cytoskeletal elements, distinct domains are most easily visualized within the neuron. In order to maintain the polarized morphology of a neuron, cytoskeletal, cytoplasmic and membranous elements must be assembled and targeted in a characteristic and consistent manner. The biochemical diversity of each of these elements is striking as the composition of proteins in the axon differs significantly from that in cell bodies and dendrites. There is diversity even along the length of a single axon. In this section, several examples are given which illustrate how characteristic features of the somatodendritic and axonal cytoskeletons are generated and maintained. A common theme underlying each example is the dynamic nature of the cytoskeleton.

Both the composition and organization of cytoskeletal elements in axons and dendrites become specialized early in differentiation

A brief description of how the cytoskeletal elements within axons and dendrites are established illustrates the dynamic nature of the cytoskeleton. The sequence of events has been described for neurons in primary culture [6,24]. Postmitotic neurons initially extend and retract multiple neuritic processes. These early, short neurites are comparable in length and growth rate. All contain MTs oriented with plus ends distal to the cell body and all have both MAP2 and tau MAPs. Eventually, in neurons that elaborate an axon, one neurite outgrows the others. This first long neurite continues to grow without tapering and becomes the single axon. Under culture conditions that lack directional information, the selection of the neurite that becomes the axon appears to be stochastic. Cues in the local environment are likely to specify a particular direction for neurite outgrowth *in vivo*. As the axon grows, it loses MAP2, while tau is enriched and becomes differentially phosphorylated. Subsequent to axonal outgrowth, some of the other neurites are stabilized and begin to extend. The number of dendrites varies with the type of neuron, ranging from the single dendritic process that partially fuses with the axon, producing the single branched process of the dorsal root ganglion pseudo-unipolar neuron, to the elaborate branching dendrite of the Purkinje cell, to the multipolar motor neurons that have both apical and basal dendritic arbors. Most neurites that develop into dendrites become tapered as they grow. When dendrites reach this stage, they begin to contain MTs in both orientations. More or less concurrently, MAP2 becomes enriched in the dendritic processes. Initially, the smallest form of MAP2 is abundant, but a shift to predominantly high-molecular-weight isoforms occurs with maturation.

As axons and dendrites mature, their differences become more apparent [6]. In axons, MTs have a uniform orientation, with plus ends distal to the cell body, but dendrites contain MTs in both orientations. Dendrites and, to a lesser extent, perikarya contain MAP2, which is excluded from axons at an early stage. Curiously, MAP2 mRNA is one of several mRNAs that are specifically transported into the dendrite and translated locally. No other cytoskeletal protein has been found to display a similar expression pattern. Protein synthetic machinery is excluded from the axon. Expression of dendritic mRNAs is affected by synaptic activity, but its physiological function is uncertain. In contrast, tau is enriched in axons and NFs similarly occur primarily in axons. Phosphorylation of MAP1B, tau and NFs is maintained at a high level in axons [10,12,13]. Neuron-specific isoforms of spectrin and ankyrin exist only in axons [20].

While tau is not restricted to the growing axonal process, tau expression appears to be crit-

ical for the initial elongation event which defines an axon-to-be. If tau expression is blocked through use of antisense oligonucleotides before the commitment to axonal outgrowth, no axon is formed [6,10]. If tau expression is blocked after commitment, the axon is retracted, suggesting that tau–MT interactions are necessary for axonal differentiation. Similarly, reduction in MAP2 expression inhibits dendritic differentiation. That MAP2 and tau seem to bestow upon MTs the ability to form "dendrite-like" or "axon-like" processes, respectively, has also been suggested by experiments in which these MAPs have been expressed in non-neuronal cells. MAP2 and tau differentially affect the packing density of MTs, so while these MAPs may not trigger the initial polarization of neurons, they no doubt contribute to maintenance of the polarized phenotype [24,25]. For both axons and dendrites, cytoskeletal composition and organization are carefully orchestrated during differentiation and maturation.

Although axonal and dendritic MTs differ in their associated proteins and organization, both are thought to originate in the cell body. MTs are likely to continue to grow after entry into the axon or dendrite, but there is little evidence for *de novo* formation of MTs in either region. The evidence suggests that both are nucleated at the MTOC, as in other cell types (Fig. 8-3). Instead of remaining associated with the MTOC, neuritic MTs are released from the MTOC and transported into the neurite. The sites where most elongation occurs and where specific MAPs are added remain a matter of dispute. Similarly, the molecular mechanisms by which different cytoskeletal compositions are maintained in different neuronal compartments are unknown.

As the size and shape of neurons change during development, the composition of the IF cytoskeleton varies coordinately. Different types of neurons and neurons in different stages of development vary in the number and composition of their IFs [12,13]. For example, in many neurons, peripherin and α-internexin are expressed very early in neuronal differentiation, then downregulated [26]. NFL and NFM are detectable during initial neurite outgrowth, while NFH is not expressed significantly until much later. Phosphorylation of NFH and NFM occurs even later in development and reaches its full extent only in large myelinated axons. Additionally, NFs in different neuronal populations may not contain the same subunit stoichiometry for NFL, NFM and NFH.

CYTOSKELETAL STRUCTURES IN THE NEURON HAVE COMPLEMENTARY DISTRIBUTIONS AND FUNCTIONS

While each set of cytoskeletal elements has a distinctive spectrum of composition, stability and distribution, all three interact with each other. They have complementary functions and may be coordinately regulated. Such interactions can be seen during development of the nervous system, in mature neuron–glia interactions and in neuropathology.

Microfilament and microtubule dynamics underlie growth cone motility and function

The mechanisms by which neurons make appropriate synaptic connections is a subject of great interest. The first stages of this process are neurite elongation and pathfinding. As the growing tip of a growth cone advances across a substrate, the growth cone must interpret extracellular cues to steer the growing neurite in the right direction [21,27]. Growth cones receive both attractive and repulsive cues and respond by selectively stabilizing, destabilizing or rearranging actin and MT cytoskeletons to allow for directed growth. This section briefly describes how extracellular signals mediate rearrangements of the cytoskeleton.

Growth cones can be roughly divided into three domains [21]: filopodia are long, thin, spike-like projections that grow and retreat rapidly from the growth cone surface; lamellipodia are web-like veils of cytoplasm that also spread and retract, often between filopodia; and the body of the growth cone itself is the area of cytoplasm beyond the cylindrical neurite which adheres to the substratum. Filopodia and lamellipodia sample the environment for favorable conditions, then the body of the growth cone

will move forward as the axon elongates. The distribution of the three cytoskeletal elements in the growth cone is well established (Fig. 8-5) [21,28]. In neurites, MTs occur as bundles, which then splay out into single filaments in the body of the growth cone, but MTs do not extend into the filopodia. NFs are limited to the shaft of the neurite and do not extend beyond the proximal edge of the growth cone body. Actin MFs make up the majority of the growth cone cytoskeleton. They form a complex meshwork that includes a number of actin-associated proteins beneath the entire plasma membrane of lamellipodia and the growth cone body. Bundles of actin MFs form the cores of filopodia. Forces generated by rearrangement of the actin MFs help to realign the MTs and eventually the NFs to the preferred direction for growth.

The diameter of a growth cone is often much greater than that of the neurite, allowing it to sample a large volume of the environment. Typically, the shape of a growth cone is constantly changing, with filopodia and lamellipodia extending and retracting, receiving signals from the surface of other cells, the extracellular matrix or the surrounding media. A number of factors may elicit a growth response, including soluble neurotrophins and membrane- or matrix-bound ligands. In addition, repulsive signals have been identified that lead to collapse of filopodia or lamellipodia and to retraction of growth cones. The extension of filopodia and lamellipodia seems to be regulated in part by members of the Rho family of low-molecular-weight GTPases (Chap. 20) but the exact pathways by which this occurs remain unknown [17].

Although it is not entirely clear how extracellular signals cause growth cones to steer, the following model accounts for the majority of observations [6,21,27]. When one or a few filopodia receive an attractive cue, the growth cone will turn in that direction. At least two things occur in the region of the growth cone chosen for further growth. First, extracellular signals activate cell-surface receptors to recruit a multiprotein complex that links the receptor to the actin meshwork beneath the surface. This is likely to involve local Ca^{2+} current transients and phosphorylation of cytoskeletal proteins in the vicin-

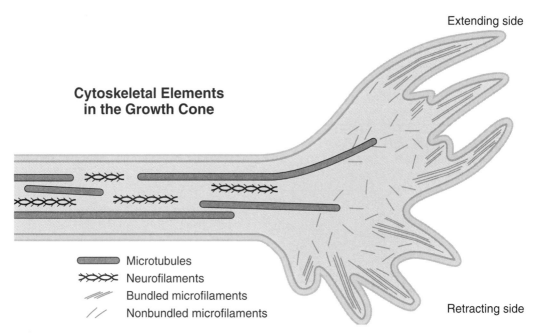

Extending side

Cytoskeletal Elements
in the Growth Cone

Retracting side

Microtubules
Neurofilaments
Bundled microfilaments
Nonbundled microfilaments

FIGURE 8-5.   The cytoskeletal elements of a growth cone are organized for motility. In this diagram of a growth cone, a typical distribution of major cytoskeletal structures is shown. The microfilaments are longer and more prominent in the growth cone than in other regions of a neuron. They are bundled in the lamellipodia and particularly in the filopodia. A combination of actin assembly, microfilament cross-linking and myosin motors (see Chap. 28) is thought to mediate this movement. In the central core of the growth cone, the microfilaments may interact with axonal microtubules which do not extend to the periphery. These microtubules may be pulled toward the preferred direction of growth and appear to be necessary for net advance. In the absence of microtubules, filopodia extend and retract but the growth cone does not advance. Microtubule movements are thought to be a combination of assembly and contractility. Finally, the neurofilaments appear to stabilize the neurite and consolidate advances but appear to be excluded from the growth cone proper.

ity. There is continued polymerization of actin MFs and a protrusion of the membrane at the site of future growth. This burst of actin polymerization is probably due to the concerted actions of a number of different actin-binding proteins, and the membrane protrusion may involve actin-based motors like myosins (see Chap. 28). More or less concurrent with MF rearrangements, the splayed MTs in the growth cone body begin to invade the selected site. This invasion may involve both MT elongation and MT movements. Once MTs form an ordered bundle oriented in the new direction, the membrane of the growth cone collapses around the MT bundle to create an extension of the neurite cylinder and the NFs are advanced to consolidate new growth. Then the growth cone begins looking for the next signal. While this description is an oversimplification of growth cone-

steering events, it nevertheless illustrates that growth cones are highly motile and very dynamic entities.

The axonal cytoskeleton may be influenced by glia

In cross-sections of large myelinated axons, most of the volume is occupied by NFs separated from each other by side-arm spacers. Spaces between fields of NFs are occupied by one of two specialized regions: MTs with membrane-bound organelles or electron-dense regions adjacent to MTs and to the plasma membrane cortex (Fig. 8-1). These electron-dense areas are enriched in short actin MFs. Such images suggest a static, cross-linked cytoskeleton and do not reveal the underlying dynamics of the axonal cytoskeleton. In fact, fully mature neurons also have a dynamic cytoskeleton that is both engaged in axonal transport (see Chap. 28) and responsive to the local environment.

The relationships between an axon and its myelinating glia are both intimate and extensive. Originally, these relationships were thought to be specified by signals from the axon that elicited specific responses in glial cells after contact, including proliferation and myelination [8]. Little thought was given to the possibility of glia influencing neurons. However, more recent studies indicate that the axonal cytoskeleton is also altered locally by glial contacts. Axonal cytoskeletal elements are subject to constant modulation via signals from the axonal environment, including both target cells and cells forming the myelin sheath. Such signals appear to influence axonal branching, synapse formation and axonal caliber.

The response of the axon to loss of myelin is instructive. In the *trembler* mutant mouse, the axon undergoes a continuing cycle of partial myelination followed by demyelination (see Chap. 39). The result is a thin or absent peripheral myelin sheath and a reduction in axonal caliber (Fig. 8-6). Remarkably, this reduction in axonal caliber is highly localized to segments of the axon with disrupted myelin. The local nature of these changes was proven by studies in which regions of sciatic nerve from *trembler* mutants were grafted into normal nerves. Only those axon segments surrounded by Schwann cells from *trembler* mutants have reduced diameters. More importantly, the reduction in axon caliber is due to a twofold increase in NF density in nerves of *trembler* mutants, even though the actual amount of NF protein is not changed. The increased NF packing density means that the same number of NFs now occupy a smaller volume, producing a smaller axon. This change in density appears to be due to a reduction in the phosphorylation of NFH and NFM tail domains, which allows the individual NFs to be packed more tightly [8]. Such changes are restricted to axons in contact with mutant Schwann cells. Thus, it is the direct interaction between the axons and the Schwann cells that modulates the axonal cytoskeleton. The influence of myelinating Schwann cells is not restricted to NFs because the stability, organization and composition of

the MT cytoskeleton are also altered in nerves of *trembler* mutants.

The effects of myelin can be observed in intact normal nerve as well. A similar change in cytoskeletal organization occurs in normal myelinated nerves at the nodes of Ranvier of peripheral nerves [29]. Beginning in the paranodal regions, where compact myelin is lost, the diameter of the axon is reduced, the packing density of NFs is increased and NF phosphorylation is reduced. Thus, the axonal cytoskeleton is constantly being influenced by the myelinating glial environment, providing a dramatic example of the dynamic nature of the neuronal cytoskeleton.

Levels of cytoskeletal protein expression change after injury and during regeneration

As described above, there are substantial changes in the composition and organization of neuronal and glial cytoskeletal elements during development. Changes are equally dramatic following injury to the nervous system. Some of these changes reflect the switch from maintaining cellular structures to growth or repair modes. The response of PNS neurons during regeneration may fall into this category (Chap. 36). In other cases, the response is incomplete or may be reactive to the injury. For example, after CNS injury, astrocytes become reactive, rapidly proliferate and frequently form a glial scar. The hallmark of this glial scar is a dramatic increase in GFAP IF bundles, which allows the astrocytes to fill the injured zone and provide mechanical support for surrounding uninjured tissues. Unfortunately, the glial scar often represents a physical barrier to neuronal elongation and repair (Chap. 29).

The neuronal response to injury has been studied in some detail to gain a better understanding of why mammalian CNS neurons regenerate poorly or not at all, while PNS neurons regenerate effectively. Although regeneration is often described as paralleling developmental growth of neurons, the distinctive pattern of changes in the neuronal cytoskeleton during regeneration differs in some important ways from that during development. First, there is a coordinate downregulation in NF subunit expression following injury. NFH, NFM and NFL protein

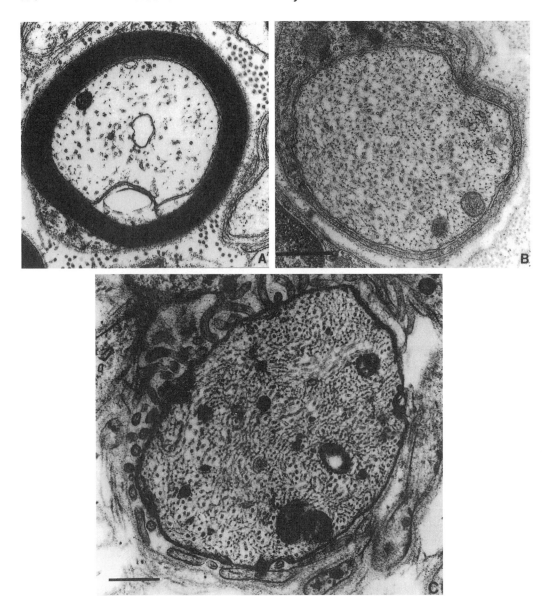

FIGURE 8-6.   The local environment can alter the organization of the axonal cytoskeleton. **A:** In a normal myelinated axon of the sciatic nerve, neurofilaments and microtubules are widely spaced, so they occupy considerable volume. **B:** In contrast, a comparably sized axon from the sciatic nerve of the demyelinating *trembler* mutant mouse has a denser cytoplasm, with neurofilaments densely packed. This has been shown to result from a shift in the net dephosphorylation of neurofilaments produced by demyelination. This effect on the axonal cytoskeleton is highly localized. **C:** Similar changes in the organization and phosphorylation of the axonal cytoskeleton occur even over the short gap in the myelin sheath which occurs at the node of Ranvier. Such changes illustrate the dynamic nature of the axonal cytoskeleton. Bars represent 0.5 μm with **A** and **B** at the same magnification. (Micrographs supplied by Sylvie de Waegh and Scott Brady.)

and mRNA levels in the perikarya decline rapidly after injury and do not recover until after reconnection with an appropriate target cell has occurred. Unlike during development, where NFH expression lags behind the other two, all three NF subunits decline and recover coordinately during regeneration. Concurrent with the reduction in NF protein following injury, both tubulin and actin increase significantly. While NF proteins are low throughout the elongation phase of regeneration, tubulin and actin expression remains high during neurite growth and synaptogenesis. As might be expected, there are associated changes in the expression of MAPs and MF-associated proteins during regeneration as well.

The observation that selected tubulin genes are preferentially upregulated during regeneration has led to proposals that some tubulin isoforms are better suited for neurite growth. While this idea is attractive, there is little evidence for a significant functional difference among the various tubulin genes [9]. Nonetheless, the idea that changes in cytoskeletal protein are required for effective regeneration is consistent with observations that changes in cytoskeletal protein expression after injury are limited or altered in CNS neurons that fail to regenerate after injury. The precise regulation of cytoskeletal gene expression during both development and regeneration suggests the importance of these structures for neuronal growth.

Alterations in the cytoskeleton are frequent hallmarks in neuropathology

A definitive diagnosis for many neurological disorders depends on a histological examination. The identifying characteristic for a number of neuropathological conditions is a disrupted or aberrant cytoskeleton. This is a feature of many toxic neuropathies and a number of neurodegenerative conditions, including motor neuron disease and Alzheimer's disease (see Chap. 46). Although other neuronal functions may also be affected and the initial cause of the disease may not directly involve the cytoskeleton, the associated pathogenic disruption of cytoskeletal function may be a key element in the loss of neurons or neuronal function [30].

In some cases, the primary pathogenic mechanism is an effect on one or more cytoskeletal structures. For example, some chemotherapeutic agents widely used for the treatment of tumors act by disrupting MT function in the spindles of rapidly dividing cancer cells. Such drugs can affect MTs in both neural and non-neuronal cells. Perhaps the two best known examples are vincristine and paclitaxel (Taxol). While these two compounds have opposite actions on MTs, long-term or high-dosage treatment with either leads to a high frequency of associated neuropathies. Vincristine is a classic anti-MT drug that destabilizes existing MTs and blocks assembly of new MTs. In contrast, paclitaxel stabilizes MTs and leads to formation of numerous short MTs in inappropriate sites. Despite these differences, peripheral neuropathies are a troublesome side effect of both drugs. Neuronal viability is compromised because MT function is compromised. Other environmental toxins or chemicals may interfere with NFs. For example, in rabbits, exposure to some aluminum salts leads to accumulation of NFs in the initial segments of the axon.

In fact, a number of diseases with diverse pathogenic mechanisms have associated disruptions in axonal NFs. NFs accumulate in the cell bodies of motor neurons in patients with amyotrophic lateral sclerosis and related motor neuron diseases. The latter example is particularly interesting because the symptoms of motor neuron disease can be produced in animal models in several very different ways. Some of these animal models have little obvious relevance to the cytoskeleton, such as those resulting from point mutations in a superoxide dismutase gene. Others directly involve NFs, such as transgenic mice that express defective NF subunits or overexpress normal NF subunits. Regardless of how these animal models are produced, a characteristic feature of motor neuron pathology is the accumulation of poorly phosphorylated NFs in cell bodies and initial segments [13,31].

Other diseases with disruptions in NF organization include diabetic neuropathy and Charcot-Marie-Tooth disease (see Chaps. 36 and 40). For these diseases, the disruption of NFs is a secondary effect. In most cases, neuronal degeneration is an eventual consequence, but neuronal function may be impaired prior to substantial loss of neurons. Generally, disruption of NFs has the most severe consequences in large motor neurons, which is consistent with the fact that the largest neurons have the highest NF expression.

Phosphorylation of cytoskeletal proteins is involved in both normal function and neuropathology

An entire book could be devoted to research just on the phosphorylation of cytoskeletal proteins. Phosphorylation of cytoskeletal components may affect their assembly and organization as well as their associated function. As described above, the level of phosphorylation on NFs is a major determinant in the regulation of axonal caliber, and a specific set of phosphorylations is a hallmark of tau protein in axons. The phosphorylation of other MAPs is carefully regulated during development and maturation of the nervous system. Similarly, many MF-associated proteins are regulated by phosphorylation, so the local action of kinases and phosphatases may underlie many changes in the membrane cytoskeleton and growth cone motility.

Phosphorylation of cytoskeletal proteins has also been linked to various neuropathological conditions. For example, the NF accumulations seen in many diseases have aberrant phosphorylation patterns. A more significant change may be the hyperphosphorylation of a MAP such as tau, which appears to be a key step in the formation of neurofibrillary tangles in Alzheimer's disease [11]. These tangles contain distinctive paired helical filaments that are extremely resistant to solubilization and analysis. They were initially thought to be aberrant NFs based on their dimensions, but a careful immunochemical and biochemical dissection showed that the primary polypeptide present in the tangles was tau, the axonally enriched MAP [32]. The tau in neurofibrillary tangles is differentially phosphorylated, and this misphosphorylation is thought to play a role in the formation of tangles. While the precise etiology of neurofibrillary tangles and their relationship to the deposition of amyloid are not yet certain, the appearance of these tangles is closely correlated with loss of neurons and their number is a good indication of how far the disease has advanced. Clearly, disruption of the cytoskeleton is an important component of the Alzheimer's disease neuropathology [33] (see Chap. 46).

CONCLUSIONS

The different architecture of neurons and glia is generated by the diverse specializations of MTs, NFs and MFs [14]. Each of these components forms a set of structures that are constantly changing and subject to the influence of extracellular signals. While the importance of the cytoskeleton for development, maintenance and regeneration of nerve fibers is now well documented, many details about its activities remain to be delineated [8]. Continued exploration of these phenomena will provide the basis for a deeper understanding of neuronal development, regeneration and neuropathology.

REFERENCES

1. Hyams, J. S., and Lloyd, C. W. (eds). *Microtubules, Modern Cell Biology*, vol. 13. New York: Wiley-Liss, 1994.
2. Burns, R. G., and Surridge, C. D. Tubulin: Conservation and structure. In J. S. Hyams and C. W. Lloyd (eds.), *Microtubules, Modern Cell Biology*, vol. 13. New York: Wiley-Liss, 1994, pp. 3–31.
3. Nogales, E., Wolf, S. G., and Downing, K. H. Structure of the $\alpha\beta$ tubulin dimer by electron crystallography. *Nature* 391:199–203, 1998.
4. Bayley, P. M., Sharma, K. K., and Martin, S. R. Microtubule dynamics *in vitro*. In J. S. Hyams and C. W. Lloyd (eds.), *Microtubules, Modern Cell Biology*, vol. 13. New York: Wiley-Liss, 1994, pp. 111–137.
5. Joshi, H. C. Microtubule organizing centers and gamma-tubulin. *Curr. Opin. Cell Biol.* 6:54–62, 1994.
6. Heidemann, S. R. Cytoplasmic mechanisms of axonal and dendritic growth in neurons. *Int. Rev. Cytol.* 165:235–296, 1996.
7. Yu, W., Centonze, V. E., Ahmad, F. J., et al. Microtubule nucleation and release from the neuronal centrosome. *J. Cell Biol.* 122:349–359, 1993.
8. Brady, S. T. Axonal dynamics and regeneration. In A. Gorio (ed.), *Neuroregeneration.* New York: Raven Press, 1993, pp. 7–36.

9. Luduena, R. F. Are tubulin isotypes functionally significant? *Mol. Biol. Cell* 4:445–447, 1993.

10. Schoenfeld, T. A., and Obar, R. A. Diverse distribution and function of fibrous microtubule-associated proteins in the nervous system. *Int. Rev. Cytol.* 151:67–137, 1994.

11. Mandelkow, E.-M., Schweers, O., Drewes, G., et al. Structure, microtubule interactions, and phosphorylation of tau protein. *Ann. N.Y. Acad. Sci.* 777:96–106, 1996.

12. Fliegner, K. H., and Liem, R. K. H. Cellular and molecular biology of neuronal intermediate filaments. *Int. Rev. Cytol.* 131:109–167, 1991.

13. Lee, M. K., and Cleveland, D. W. Neuronal intermediate filaments. *Annu. Rev. Neurosci.* 19: 187–217, 1996.

14. Lasek, R. J. Studying the intrinsic determinants of neuronal form and function. In R. J. Lasek and M. M. Black (eds.), *Intrinsic Determinants of Neuronal Form and Function.* New York: Alan R. Liss, 1988, pp. 1–60.

15. Theriot, J. A. Regulation of the actin cytoskeleton in living cells. *Semin. Cell Biol.* 5:193–199, 1994.

16. Vandekerchhove, J., and Vancompernolle, K. Structural relationships of actin-binding proteins. *Curr. Opin. Cell Biol.* 4:36–42, 1992.

17. Mackay, D. J. G., Nobes, C. D., and Hall, A. The rho's progress: A potential role during neuritogenesis for the rho family of GTPases. *Trends Neurosci.* 18:496–501, 1995.

18. Kuczmarski, E. R., and Rosenbaum, J. L. Studies on the organization and localization of actin and myosin in neurons. *J. Cell Biol.* 80:356–371, 1979.

19. Hitt, A. L., and Luna, E. J. Membrane interactions with the actin cytoskeleton. *Curr. Opin. Cell Biol.* 6:120–130, 1994.

20. Beck, K. A., and Nelson, J. The spectrin-based membrane skeleton as a membrane protein-sorting machine. *Am. J. Physiol.* 270:C1263–C1270, 1996.

21. Sobue, K. Actin-based cytoskeleton in growth cone activity. *Neurosci. Res.* 18:91–102, 1993.

22. Schafer, D. A., and Cooper, J. A. Control of actin assembly at filament ends. *Annu. Rev. Cell Dev. Biol.* 11:497–518, 1995.

23. Sun, H. Q., Kwiatkowska, K., and Yin, H. L. Actin monomer binding proteins. *Curr. Opin. Cell Biol.* 7:102–110, 1995.

24. Mandell, J. W., and Banker, G. A. The microtubule cytoskeleton and the development of neuronal polarity. *Neurobiol. Aging* 16:229–238, 1995.

25. Tucker, R. P. The roles of microtubule associated proteins in brain morphogenesis: A review. *Brain Res. Rev.* 15:101–120, 1990.

26. Nixon, R. A., and Shea, T. B. Dynamics of neuronal intermediate filaments: A developmental perspective. *Cell Motil. Cytoskeleton* 22:81–91, 1992.

27. Tanaka, E., and Sabry, J. Making the connection: Cytoskeletal rearrangements during growth cone guidance. *Cell* 83:171–176, 1995.

28. Shaw, G., Osborne, M., and Weber, K. Neurofilaments, microtubules, and microfilament-associated proteins in cultured dorsal root ganglion cells. *Eur. J. Cell Biol.* 24:20–27, 1981.

29. Zimmerman, H. Accumulations of synaptic vesicle proteins and cytoskeletal specializations at the peripheral node of Ranvier. *Microsc. Res. Tech.* 34:462–473, 1996.

30. Griffin, J. W., George, E. B., Hsieh, S., et al. Axonal degeneration and disorders of the axonal cytoskeleton. In S. G. Waxman, J. D. Kocsis, and P. K. Stys (eds.), *The Axon: Structure, Function and Pathophysiology.* New York: Oxford University Press, 1995, pp. 375–390.

31. Brady, S. T. Motor neurons and neurofilaments in sickness and in health. *Cell* 73:1–3, 1993.

32. Kosik, K. S., Orecchio, L. D., Binder, L., et al. Epitopes that span the tau molecule are shared with paired helical filaments. *Neuron* 1:817–825, 1988.

33. Lee, V. M.-Y. Disruption of the cytoskeleton in Alzheimer's disease. *Curr. Opin. Neurobiol.* 5: 663–668, 1995.

34. Hodge, A., and Adelman, W. In *Structure and Function in Excitable Cells.* New York: Plenum, 1983, pp. 75–111.

9

Intracellular Trafficking

Thomas C. Südhof

Basic Neurochemistry: Molecular, Cellular and Medical Aspects, 6th Ed., edited by G. J. Siegel et al. Published by
Lippincott–Raven Publishers, Philadelphia, 1999. Correspondence to Thomas C. Südhof, Center for Basic Neuroscience,
Howard Hughes Medical Institute and Department of Molecular Genetics, The University of Texas Southwestern Medical
School, 5323 Harry Hines Blvd., Dallas, Texas 75235.

INTRACELLULAR MEMBRANE TRAFFIC

Intracellular membrane traffic is a universal process in all eukaryotic cells. At any given time, every cell performs many different membrane-trafficking reactions simultaneously. Based on these considerations, it is not surprising that membrane traffic is very important for nervous system function.

Two types of intracellular membrane traffic can be distinguished in the nervous system

First, maintenance or constitutive membrane traffic closely resembles membrane traffic in other cells and is required for the general viability and functionality of all cells (see Chap. 2), including neurons, glia and supporting cells. Second, specialized or regulated membrane traffic functions in intercellular signaling and, although present in most cells, is most highly developed in neurons. The most abundant and important membrane-trafficking event of the second type in neurons consists of the intracellular trafficking of synaptic vesicles that forms the basis for synaptic vesicle exocytosis and neurotransmitter release [1].

All intracellular membrane traffic is based on the same fundamental operations

First, transport vesicles bud from the membrane of origin, either empty or filled with cargo. Second, the transport vesicles move to their destination point, their target organelle. Finally, the transport vesicles dock at the membrane of their target organelle, that is, attach to it, and fuse with the membrane. Because of the fundamental similarities between all membrane-trafficking processes, most of them are likely to be mechanistically similar. However, there are many different kinds of membrane traffic in all cells at any given time, such as traffic from the endoplasmic reticulum to the Golgi apparatus or from endosomes to lysosomes. Cells normally manage to keep the different types of membrane traffic well separated and controlled. Errors in trafficking, for example, loss of membrane components, are avoided, and there are no membrane traffic jams under physiological conditions. Each membrane-trafficking event is well regulated and has identifying features that distinguish it from others. Although all forms of intracellular membrane traffic are essential for brain function, this chapter focuses on synaptic membrane traffic.

Synaptic membrane traffic leading to neurotransmitter release is of central importance for brain function

Synaptic transmission can be divided into presynaptic and postsynaptic components (see Chap. 10). The presynaptic neuron emits a signal by the regulated release of neurotransmitters, and the postsynaptic cell receives that signal by receptors that are localized precisely opposite to the point of neurotransmitter release. Membrane traffic is important for both the pre- and postsynaptic components. In the presynaptic nerve terminal, neurotransmitter release is mediated by the exocytosis of synaptic vesicles, small secretory organelles that contain high concentrations of neurotransmitters. Thus, membrane traffic is involved directly in signal transmission on the presynaptic side. It forms the basis for the release of neurotransmitters, and the nerve terminal can be considered a specialized secretory organ of neurons. In the postsynaptic cell, membrane traffic is essential for delivery of the receptors to their appropriate place and for regulation of receptor numbers. Consequently, membrane traffic is important for setting up and regulating postsynaptic function without being involved directly in signal transmission.

Because membrane traffic forms the basis for neurotransmitter release, any understanding of synaptic transmission and neuronal information processing depends in part on an understanding of presynaptic membrane traffic. This chapter discusses presynaptic mechanisms as a model system for membrane traffic and as a process fundamental for neuronal signaling.

THE SYNAPTIC VESICLE CYCLE IN THE NERVE TERMINAL

The synaptic vesicle cycle forms the basis for neurotransmitter release by the terminal

When an action potential arrives at a nerve terminal, Ca^{2+} flows into the terminal via voltage-gated Ca^{2+} channels and triggers neurotransmitter release by synaptic vesicle exocytosis [2]. Synaptic vesicles undergo a membrane-trafficking cycle in the presynaptic nerve terminal that prepares them for neurotransmitter release. This cycle is depicted schematically in Figure 9-1.

Central synapses in vertebrates have three morphological hallmarks as viewed in the electron microscope [3]: (i) the presynaptic nerve terminal contains abundant accumulations of synaptic vesicles, small electron-lucent vesicles of approximately 40 nm; (ii) at the point of synaptic contact, the presynaptic plasma membrane is thickened into an active zone, to which several synaptic vesicles are attached; and (iii) facing the presynaptic active zone, the postsynaptic cell also forms a thickening in the plasma membrane, which is referred to as postsynaptic density. Morphological analysis of central synapses of the hippocampus or cerebellum has shown that nerve terminals typically have a volume of 0.1 to 0.3 μm^3 and contain approximately 200 to 500 synaptic vesicles per terminal. Since a mammalian brain has on the order of 10^{14} to 10^{15} synapses, synaptic vesicles are extremely abundant. The presynaptic active zones and postsynaptic densities of a synapse always correspond in size, are precisely aligned and occupy an area of approximately 5 to 20 μm^2. They are separated by a synaptic cleft of 13 to 16 nm, which is slightly wider than the usual intercellular space and morphologically is filled with an unidentified material. Although the number of synaptic vesicles attached to the active zone in a nerve terminal varies, there are usually no more than ten to 30 synaptic vesicles bound to the active zone at a synapse, and most synaptic vesicles are free in the cytosol of the nerve terminal.

Active transport of neurotransmitters into synaptic vesicles is an energy-driven process that requires ATP

Neurotransmitter uptake is mediated by specialized transporter proteins in the synaptic vesicle membrane (step *1* in Fig. 9-1). A vacuolar proton pump (see Chap. 5) in the synaptic vesicle membrane builds up an electrochemical gradient across the synaptic vesicle membrane. This gradient provides the energy for neurotransmitter uptake. After filling with transmitters, synaptic vesicles are moved to the active zone of the presynaptic plasma membrane by a translocation process that may be either diffusion-limited or dependent on molecular motors (step *2* in Fig. 9-1). Synaptic vesicles then attach to the active zone in a process requiring a recognition event since they do not attach to other parts of the presynaptic plasma membrane (step *3* in Fig. 9-1, docking). Docked synaptic vesicles are primed for Ca^{2+}-dependent release by an ATP-dependent process that could involve a partial fusion reaction (step *4* in Fig. 9-1). Ca^{2+} then triggers the completion of the fusion process in a rapid reaction that occurs in as little as 100 μsec and that involves the binding of multiple Ca^{2+} at a cooperative Ca^{2+}-binding site (step *5* in Fig. 9-1). After completion of exocytosis, synaptic vesicles are endocytosed rapidly by coated pits (step 6 in Fig. 9-1) and recycled to the backfield of the synaptic nerve terminal (step *7* in Fig. 9-1). Synaptic vesicles then restart the cycle either via passing through an endosomal intermediate

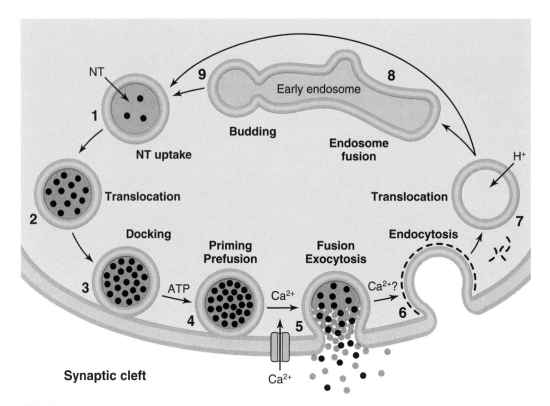

FIGURE 9-1. The synaptic vesicle cycle. The pathway of synaptic vesicles in the nerve terminal is divided into 9 stages. *1:* Empty synaptic vesicles take up neurotransmitters by active transport into their lumen using an electrochemical gradient that is established by a proton pump activity. *2:* Filled synaptic vesicles are translocated to the active zone. *3:* Synaptic vesicles attach to the active zone of the presynaptic plasma membrane but, to no other component of the presynaptic plasma membrane, in a targeted reaction (docking). *4:* Synaptic vesicles are primed for fusion in order to be able to respond rapidly to a Ca^{2+} signal later. Priming probably is a complicated, multicomponent reaction that can be subdivided further into multiple steps. *5:* Ca^{2+} influx through voltage-gated channels triggers neurotransmitter release in less than 1 msec. Ca^{2+} stimulates completion of a partial fusion reaction initiated during priming. *6:* Empty synaptic vesicles are coated by clathrin and associated proteins in preparation for endocytosis. Ca^{2+} may be involved in this process. *7:* Empty synaptic vesicles shed their clathrin coat, acidify via proton pump activity and retranslocate into the backfield of the nerve terminal. *8:* Synaptic vesicles fuse with early endosomes as an intermediate sorting compartment to eliminate aged or mis-sorted proteins. *9:* Synaptic vesicles are freshly generated by budding from endosomes. Although some synaptic vesicles may recycle via endosomes (steps *8* and *9*), it is likely that the endosomal intermediate is not obligatory for recycling and that synaptic vesicles can go directly from step *7* to step *1*. (Adapted from [2], with permission.)

(steps *8* and *9* in Fig. 9-1) or directly, without this trafficking intermediate.

Synaptic vesicles need approximately 60 sec to go through the whole cycle [2]. Of these 60 sec, Ca^{2+}-triggered fusion (step *5* in Fig. 9-1) occurs in less than 1 msec. Docking and priming (steps *3* and *4* in Fig. 9-1) have been estimated to require approximately 10 to 20 msec and endocytosis (step *6* in Fig. 9-1) a few seconds. Thus, the major part of the time a given synaptic vesicle needs to traverse the cycle is spent on neurotransmitter uptake and recycling back to the active zone. This correlates

with the morphological finding that most synaptic vesicles in nerve terminals are free in the cytosol rather than docked or endocytosing [3].

The synaptic vesicle cycle includes basic processes characteristic of all intracellular trafficking

Budding of transport vesicles occurs from the plasma membrane and endosomes (steps *6* and *9* in Fig. 9-1), vesicles move from originating to target organelles (steps *2* and *7* in Fig. 9-1) and transport vesicles dock and fuse with target membranes (steps *3* and *8* in Fig. 9-1). Although the synaptic vesicle cycle involves many independent molecular reactions, it is relatively simple compared to other intracellular trafficking pathways, for example, the trafficking of newly synthesized proteins through the endoplasmic reticulum and Golgi complex. If the endosomal intermediate is bypassed during recycling (Fig. 9-1), the whole synaptic vesicle cycle consists only of single translocation, docking/fusion and budding reactions. The local recycling of synaptic vesicles allows the synaptic vesicle cycle in nerve terminals to be independent of the cell nucleus. This functional autonomy is essential because a nerve terminal can be separated from the nucleus by more than 100 cm, such as in the neuromuscular junctions in the foot belonging to spinal cord neurons. Thus, neurotransmitter release is based on an autonomous intracellular trafficking pathway that is simple relative to the constitutive pathways (see Chap. 2).

The synaptic vesicle cycle as the basis for neurotransmitter release is much more complicated than, for example, the gating of a single ion channel. Why is neurotransmitter release performed by an intracellular trafficking cycle instead of a gated neurotransmitter channel? The great advantage of synaptic vesicle exocytosis over a neurotransmitter channel as a mechanism of release is that synaptic vesicle exocytosis allows the explosive simultaneous release of a packet of neurotransmitters within less than 1 msec [4]. This results in a rapid onset and decline of the signal, a characteristic that would be impossible to achieve with a channel mechanism. Although a channel would have been a mechanistically simpler solution, exocytosis allows a faster release of more signals and a faster signal termination. These characteristics are essential for the information content of synaptic transmission.

COMPOSITION OF SYNAPTIC VESICLES

Synaptic vesicles are abundant organelles of uniform size. Their diameter is ~40 nm as judged by electron microscopy, but they are probably slightly larger under native conditions [3]. As relatively small organelles, synaptic vesicles can accommodate only a limited number of proteins and phospholipids. This restricts the number of molecules present on synaptic vesicles to the number that can be fit into a sphere of 40 nm and the complexity of synaptic vesicles. Although direct measurements are lacking, calculations indicate that synaptic vesicles contain approximately 10,000 molecules of phospholipids per vesicle with a combined molecular weight of proteins approximately 5,000,000 to 10,000,000 [5]. This would mean that with an average molecular weight of 50,000 for a protein, a maximum of 200 protein molecules are present in one synaptic vesicle.

The only known function of synaptic vesicles is neurotransmitter release

Their simplicity allows us, in principle, to obtain a complete description of synaptic vesicles as an organelle and to correlate structure with function for all of its components. The abundance of synaptic vesicles and their relatively uniform small size has made it possible to make exhaustive biochemical studies of them. As a consequence, synaptic vesicles may be the best described organelle in biology. The structures of most, but not all, of their proteins are now known, and an as yet incomplete list of synaptic vesicle proteins is presented in Table 9-1. In spite of this detailed structural information and the relative simplicity of synaptic vesicles, the functions of many of the synaptic vesicle proteins are still obscure.

The proteins of synaptic vesicles are divided into two classes based on function

The first class includes transport proteins, which execute the uptake of neurotransmitters and other components into synaptic vesicles; the second class includes trafficking proteins, which mediate the intracellular traffic of synaptic vesicles. The transport class of synaptic vesicle proteins includes the proton pump, which acidifies the synaptic vesicle interior and thereby establishes an electrochemical transmembrane gradient (see Chap. 5). The proton pump of synaptic vesicles is of the vacuolar type and composed of at least 12 subunits. Probably only a single copy of the proton pump is present in each synaptic vesicle. The proton pump

TABLE 9-1.	GLOSSARY OF SYNAPTIC PROTEINS

1. Synaptic vesicle proteins (see Fig. 9-2)

Cysteine string protein (CSP)	Peripheral membrane protein that is palmitoylated on more than ten cysteines and contains a DNA-J homology domain. Function unknown.
Cytochrome b561	Electron-transport protein required for intravesicular monooxygenases in subsets of secretory vesicles. Required for dopamine-β-hydroxylase and peptide amidase activity.
Neurotransmitter transporters	There are probably at least five types of transport protein specific for glutamate, acetylcholine, catecholamines, glycine/GABA and ATP. The type of transporter contributes to determining the transmitter specificity of a synapse. Only acetylcholine and catecholamine transporters were cloned before 1997.
Rab and ra1 proteins	Rab3A, rab3C, rab5, rab7 and ra1. Since rab proteins cycle between cytosolic and membrane-bound forms, not all synaptic vesicles contain all rab proteins at the same time. Rab proteins regulate docking and fusion processes.
Rabphilin-3A	Peripheral membrane protein that binds to rab3A and rab3C as a function of GTP, is substrate for multiple protein kinases and contains two C-terminal C_2 domains which may bind Ca^{2+}.
Secretory carrier membrane proteins (SCAMPs)	Ubiquitous integral membrane proteins of secretory and transport vesicles of unknown function.
SV2s	Highly glycosylated proteins with at least three isoforms (SV2A, B and C) containing 12 transmembrane regions and homology to bacterial and eukaryotic transporters. Function unknown.
Synapsins Ia, Ib, IIa and IIb	Monotopic membrane proteins that have common N-terminal domains, including phosphorylation sites for CaMKI and protein kinase A, but diverge C-terminally. Synapsins Ia/b contain C-terminal phosphorylation sites for CaMKII and CDK 5. They interact with actin microfilaments, neurofilaments, microtubules, SH3 domains, calmodulin and annexin VI *in vitro*.
Synaptobrevins (VAMPs)	Small-membrane proteins that are cleaved by tetanus toxin and by botulinum toxins B, D, F and G.
Synaptogyrin	Polytopic membrane protein that is tyrosine-phosphorylated. Function unknown.
Synaptophysins	Polytopic membrane proteins, including synaptoporin, that are tyrosine-phosphorylated and bind to synaptobrevins. Function unknown.
Synaptotagmins	Membrane proteins with at least 12 isoforms that contain C_2 domains; bind Ca^{2+} and phospholipids; and interact with neurexins, AP2 and syntaxins. Synaptotagmins I and II probably function as Ca^{2+} sensors in fast Ca^{2+}-dependent neurotransmitter release; functions of other synaptotagmins are unknown.
Transport proteins (channels) for chloride and zinc	Components of synaptic vesicles to mediate the chloride flux for glutamate uptake and zinc uptake in most synaptic vesicles. Zinc transporter is homologous to endosomal and plasma membrane zinc transporters; chloride transporters remain to be identified.
Vacuolar proton pump	Protein complex of more than 12 subunits. Constitutes the largest component of synaptic vesicles and establishes electrochemical gradient for neurotransmitter uptake.

2. Proteins that associate with synaptic vesicles

Amphiphysin	Nerve-terminal protein that associates with synaptic vesicles probably via AP2 bound to synaptotagmin. May function in endocytosis.
AP2 and clathrin	AP2 is a protein complex that binds to a specific receptor on synaptic vesicles and plasma membranes to trigger assembly of clathrin for endocytosis.
Ca^{2+}, calmodulin-dependent protein kinases I and II (CaMKI and CaMKII)	May transiently associate with synaptic vesicles to phosphorylate synapsins and rabphilin-3A. Function unknown.

TABLE 9-1.	**GLOSSARY OF SYNAPTIC PROTEINS** *(continued)*
Dynamin-1	GTPase required for endocytosis that is phosphorylated by protein kinase C and dephosphorylated by calcineurin upon membrane depolarization and binds to AP2. Important for budding but function unknown.
Dynein	Motor protein mediating microtubule-based synaptic vesicle transport. May be involved in retrograde axonal transport to the cell body.
GDP-dissociation inhibitors (GDIs)	Bind isoprenylated rab proteins in the GDP-bound form, resulting in a cytoplasmic complex.
Kinesins	Motor proteins for microtubule-based synaptic vesicle transport. In *Caenorhabditis elegans,* a kinesin encoded by *unc-104* is essential for transport of synaptic vesicles to nerve terminals.
MSS4	Ubiquitous protein that tightly binds to a subgroup of rab proteins, including rab1, rab3 and rab8. Function unknown.
pp60^{src}	Tyrosine kinase that phosphorylates synaptophysin and synaptogyrin.

3. Synaptic plasma membrane proteins

Munc13s	Mammalian homologs (13–1, 13–2 and 13–3) of the *C. elegans unc-13* gene that is essential for exocytosis. Binds phorbol esters but is not a protein kinase. Function unknown.
Neurexins	Cell surface proteins with more than 1,000 isoforms generated by alternative splicing from three genes. Neurexins include one of the receptors for α-latrotoxin and may function in cell–cell recognition between neurons.
SNAP-25	Palmitoylated peripheral membrane protein that is cleaved by botulinum toxins A and E and binds to syntaxins.
Syntaxins (originally named HPC-1)	Ubiquitous membrane proteins that are cleaved by botulinum toxin C1 and bind to synaptotagmins, SNAP-25, synaptobrevins, complexins, munc13s, SNAPs, Ca^{2+} channels and munc18s.
Voltage-gated Ca^{2+} channels	Mediate Ca^{2+} influx for neurotransmitter release at the active zone.
RIM	Binds to rab3 in a GTP-dependent manner and may mediate rab3 action in regulating fusion.

4. Proteins that reversibly associate with plasma membrane proteins

Munc18s	Mammalian homologs of the *C. elegans unc-18* gene and the sec1, sly 1 and slp1 products of yeast. Bind tightly to syntaxins.
N-ethylmaleimide-sensitive factor (NSF)	Trimeric ATPase required for *in vitro* membrane fusion during vesicular transport. Probably function as chaperones in synaptic vesicle recycling.
$\alpha/\beta/\gamma$-SNAPs	Soluble NSF-attachment proteins required to recruit NSF to membranes in an ATP-dependent manner.

has a total size of approximately 600 to 700 kDa, suggesting that a single copy on the synaptic vesicle would account for approximately 10% of the total synaptic vesicle protein. The electrochemical gradient that is established by the proton pump fuels uptake of neurotransmitters via neurotransmitter transporters, which significantly contribute to establishing the transmitter type of a synapse. In addition, synaptic vesicles contain ancillary transport proteins required for Zn^{2+} transport, Cl^{-} flux and possibly other activities.

Most of the trafficking proteins of synaptic vesicles are depicted schematically in Figure 9-2.

There are nine families of proteins that are bound directly to synaptic vesicles and that have putative functions in membrane traffic. It is possible that one or two additional protein families remain to be identified, but it is unlikely that many more protein families are yet undiscovered. Figure 9-2 illustrates that the proteins of synaptic vesicles share no common structural theme. Similar to other organelles, synaptic vesicles contain monotopic and polytopic proteins (see Chap. 2) as well as associated membrane proteins, including synapsins, cysteine string protein (CSP) and rab proteins. The number of

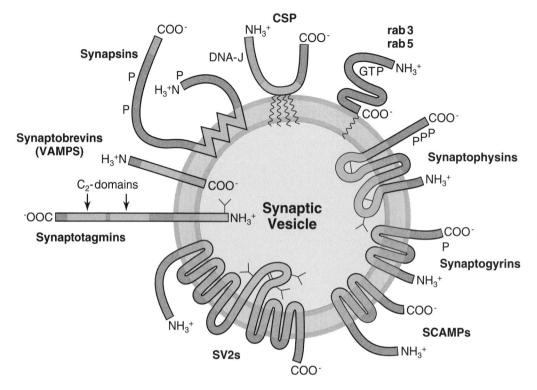

FIGURE 9-2. Trafficking proteins of synaptic vesicles (see Table 9-1). The structures of the major trafficking proteins of synaptic vesicles are shown schematically. Trafficking proteins are defined as those proteins with a likely function in the synaptic vesicle cycle and not in neurotransmitter uptake. Only proteins tightly associated with synaptic vesicles are pictured; although the type of membrane attachment is well established for most proteins, it is completely unclear for synapsins, which may bind to synaptic vesicles via their N- or C-terminal regions instead of the middle region shown here. Only cysteine string protein (*CSP*) and synaptogyrin have each a single isoform present on synaptic vesicles. In contrast, synapsins, synaptobrevins, synaptophysins and rab3s are encoded by at least two genes whose products are located on synaptic vesicles; SV2 proteins are encoded by three genes; secretory membrane carrier proteins (SCAMPs) are encoded by an unknown number of genes; and synaptotagmins are encoded by at least 11 genes, although it is unclear if their products are localized to synaptic vesicles. Only one isoform of the multigene families is shown in each case. (Adapted from [2], with permission.)

proteins containing four transmembrane regions in synaptic vesicles is striking. This topology is the only one that is repeated independently in multiple families of synaptic vesicle proteins; all other transmembrane topologies occur in only a single protein family. There are three distinct protein families with the same topology of four transmembrane regions: synaptophysins, synaptogyrins and secretory carrier membrane proteins (SCAMPs) (Table 9-1). The functions of these proteins, however, are unclear. Taken together, synaptic vesicles are composed of a limited number of membrane proteins, which exhibit a great variety of topologies and structures (Fig. 9-2).

Most trafficking proteins are members of gene families containing multiple isoforms

Typically, these gene families include both proteins that are expressed primarily in neurons on synaptic vesicles and proteins that are found ubiquitously in many different tissues. The transcripts of different trafficking genes of a family often are expressed differentially in the brain in a pattern that does not correlate with neurotransmitter type or functional brain regions. To complicate matters, no two families exhibit the same differential distribution. For example, the four synapsin isoforms generated by alternative splicing from the transcripts of two genes are co-expressed in all brain areas, with rare exceptions [6], whereas synaptotagmins I and II are expressed almost always in different neurons [7]. Rab3A and rab3C, however, are expressed in such a manner that rab3A is the dominant isoform present almost everywhere, whereas rab3C is expressed selectively at high levels in subgroups of neurons, such as the synapses of the perforant pathway of the hippocampus [8].

The specific functions of most synaptic vesicle proteins are unknown. Some synaptic vesicle proteins exhibit interesting homologies. For example, SV2s are homologous to bacterial transporter proteins but perform no known transport activity, and CSP contains a DNA-J domain and interacts with HSP70. However, most synaptic vesicle proteins do not have similarities to other known proteins. The relative simplicity of the synaptic vesicle protein composition has important functional implications. Synaptic vesicles are subject to a life cycle that is simple with respect to its biological function but complicated in that it contains many discrete steps (Fig. 9-1). All of these steps consist of sequential interactions of one synaptic vesicle protein with another. Since synaptic vesicles contain only nine to eleven different families of trafficking proteins, many proteins must have multiple functions. Furthermore, the limited number of synaptic vesicle proteins means that all of them can be manipulated genetically. Thus, it will be possible to perform a genetic saturation analysis of the complete organelle in mice and invertebrates, an opportunity that could have major implications for our understanding of intracellular trafficking.

CHARACTERISTICS OF SYNAPTIC VESICLE EXOCYTOSIS

The most important step in the synaptic vesicle cycle is the Ca^{2+} triggered synaptic vesicle fusion reaction

This exocytotic release of neurotransmitter (step 5 in Fig. 9-1) is followed by rapid endocytosis to allow reuse of synaptic vesicles. Synapses need to transmit signals in a highly localized and rapid manner. These two requirements are met by exclusive targeting of the exocytosis to the active zone and by the speed of Ca^{2+}-triggered synaptic vesicle exocytosis.

Figure 9-3 gives a more detailed representation of synaptic vesicle exo- and endocytosis and provides a tentative assignment of the steps at which selected proteins function. Synaptic vesicles interact with the active zone of the presynaptic plasma membrane. Neurotransmitter release involves at least three steps: docking attaches synaptic vesicles to the active zone of the presynaptic plasma membrane, priming makes the synaptic vesicles competent to react to a Ca^{2+} signal and a pulse of Ca^{2+} triggers completion of the fusion reaction. Since docking occurs only at the active zone and nowhere else, it must involve a recognition reaction between the synaptic vesicles and the active zone. The nature of this signal is, at present, unclear.

The Ca^{2+} triggered step that leads to neurotransmitter release occurs in less than one millisecond

In fact, this process may be as fast as 100 μsec. The speed of neurotransmitter release compares favorably with the time constant of ion channel gating. In contrast to channels that mediate ion flux in single file, the fusion reaction releases thousands of transmitter molecules at once. Ca^{2+} triggers release at high local concentrations, which have been estimated to exceed 100 μM at the point of action. For activation, at least three or four Ca^{2+} are required, suggesting that Ca^{2+} acts cooperatively at binding sites close to the release site.

Whenever an action potential reaches a nerve terminal, voltage-gated Ca^{2+} channels open and Ca^{2+} flows into the nerve terminal. Although every action potential seems to lead to the opening of Ca^{2+} channels and Ca^{2+} influx into nerve terminals, not every Ca^{2+} signal leads to synaptic vesicle exocytosis.

Central nervous system synapses differ in the probability that neurotransmitter will be released by an action potential. This probability is considerably lower than 0.5 in most synapses, suggesting that the response to Ca^{2+} is stochastic and unreliable [9,10]. A second important characteristic of synapses is that although many

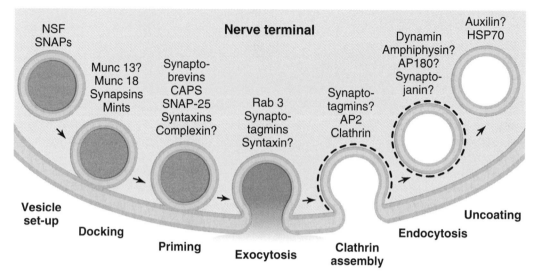

FIGURE 9-3. Tentative assignment of functions to selected proteins in synaptic vesicle exo- and endocytosis. The figure represents schematically the interaction of synaptic vesicles with the active zone of the synapse in seven stages. Tentative assignments of the points of action of identified proteins are listed above each stage. *N*-Ethylmaleimide-sensitive factor (*NSF*) and soluble NSF-attachment proteins (SNAPs) are thought to act as chaperones prior to docking and fusion (or after fusion) to transform fusion proteins such as syntaxin into an active state. Docking requires a targeting mechanism that assures that synaptic vesicles dock only at the active zone; only the requirement for munc18 in this step has been established, whereas the other assignments are more tentative. After docking, synaptic vesicles during priming require the activity of syntaxin, synaptobrevin and SNAP-25, as shown by the ability of botulinum toxins, which selectively cleave these proteins, to disrupt this step. The other assignments of proteins to this step are putative. Ca^{2+}-triggered fusion (exocytosis) is dependent on synaptotagmin I and II, which are required for fast synchronous Ca^{2+}-stimulated exocytosis, possibly via an interaction with syntaxin. In addition, rab3 is required to regulate the number of synaptic vesicles that fuse. After exocytosis, synaptic vesicles are coated with clathrin by the action of the adaptor protein complex AP2, which may be recruited by synaptotagmin to the empty synaptic vesicles. Synaptic vesicles then endocytose in a reaction that requires dynamin and may involve AP180, amphiphysin and synaptojanin. Finally, synaptic vesicles are uncoated by the concerted action of auxilin and HSP70. This is a tentative initial assignment to illustrate the function of protein networks in membrane traffic as the underlying principle.

synaptic vesicles appear to be docked at the active zone at any given time, ready to fuse, Ca^{2+} usually triggers exocytosis of only one. This suggests an unusual degree of regulation, which limits the responsiveness of docked synaptic vesicles to Ca^{2+}.

Fusion is a complex process involving both the inner and outer leaflets of both the plasmalemma and the vesicle membrane

The high speed of Ca^{2+}-triggered exocytosis suggests that Ca^{2+} acts in a shorter time period than it would take to execute a complete fusion process [11]. This indicates that Ca^{2+} triggers only the final stage of a fusion reaction which has been largely executed before Ca^{2+} acts. Thus, before Ca^{2+} acts, synaptic vesicles are thought to undergo a priming reaction, during which synaptic vesicles become competent to respond to Ca^{2+} and undergo a partial fusion reaction. Studies in endocrine cells suggest that priming consists of a series of several steps whose rate also may be Ca^{2+}-regulated [12]. Definition of the molecular nature of these steps will depend greatly on further insight into the biophysics of membrane fusion. It is possible that priming involves hemifusion, fusion of only one of the two lipid bilayers. At the synapse, this would involve the cytoplasmic layers of the synaptic vesicle and plasma membranes without the outer layers, but this idea has not been tested.

PROTEINS THAT FUNCTION IN SYNAPTIC VESICLE EXOCYTOSIS

Although the details of how membrane fusion occurs are unknown, a number of proteins with essential functions in synaptic vesicle exocytosis have been discovered. These proteins are included in Table 9-1, and the hypothetical points of action for some of them are shown in Figure 9-3.

Synapsins may function in the docking of synaptic vesicles

This conclusion is based on results from synapsin-gene knockout studies in mice: their phenotype suggests that synaptic vesicles may be destabilized in the absence of synapsins and that the upregulation of release during synaptic plasticity may be defective [13]. Synapsins interact *in vitro* with microtubules, microfilaments, neurofilaments and spectrin. Attractive speculative models have been proposed based on one or another of these interactions. However, it seems unlikely that all of these interactions are physiological, and the *in vivo* mechanism of action of synapsins remains to be discovered. In addition to synapsins, indirect evidence indicates a role in docking for the plasma membrane proteins munc18, munc13 and mints.

After docking, synaptic vesicles undergo a priming reaction that prepares them for Ca^{2+}-triggered release

Clostridial bacteria synthesize a series of toxins called botulinum toxins and tetanus toxins, which are taken up by nerve terminals and inhibit synaptic vesicle exocytosis [2]. These toxins act intracellularly as proteases, and only a single molecule of a toxin is required to poison a whole nerve terminal. They produce neuropathy in humans (Chaps. 36 and 43). These toxins do not inhibit docking of synaptic vesicles but severely impair Ca^{2+}-triggered release, suggesting that they act during priming. They appear to act before the actual Ca^{2+}-triggered step because they also inhibit the release of neurotransmitters that can be triggered by hypertonic solutions, a nonphysiological manipulation that bypasses the Ca^{2+} step since hypertonicity also works in the absence of Ca^{2+}.

Botulinum and tetanus toxins are very specific proteases. Most have only a single known substrate. Botulinum toxins B, D, F, G and H and tetanus toxin cleave only a single protein, the synaptic vesicle protein synaptobrevin (VAMP). By contrast, botulinum toxins A and E cleave only the protein SNAP-25, found both on the plasma membrane and on synaptic vesicles. Only one toxin, botulinum toxin C1, cleaves two substrates, SNAP-25 and syntaxin, which are codistributed with SNAP-25. The identification of these three synaptic proteins as substrates for these toxins revealed that these proteins must act during the priming reaction (Fig. 9-3). Since the priming reaction involves a partial fusion reaction, it seems likely that these three proteins are involved directly in the fusion of synaptic vesicles. In support of this notion, the three proteins interact with each other to form a stable trimeric complex.

After fusion, this trimeric complex has to be dissolved and its component proteins must be returned to an active conformation for the next fusion reaction. An ATPase called *N*-ethylmaleimide-sensitive factor (NSF) performs this function by acting as a chaperone in conjunction with attachment proteins called soluble-NSF attachment proteins (SNAPs) [14]. NSF originally was thought to participate directly in the fusion reaction, but it is now clear that this enzyme probably is required to recycle the components of the membrane fusion apparatus into an active conformation [15].

Ca^{2+}-triggered release may result from binding of multiple calcium ions to synaptotagmin, a relatively low-affinity sensor

Synaptotagmin is an intrinsic synaptic vesicle membrane protein that fulfills these postulates [7]. It contains two cytoplasmic Ca^{2+}-binding domains of the C_2-domain family, each of which binds at least two Ca^{2+}. Studies of mice with a knockout of synaptotagmin I showed that without this protein fast Ca^{2+}-triggered synaptic vesicle exocytosis is severely impaired, whereas exocytosis triggered by hypertonic sucrose is normal, suggesting that synaptotagmin I is essential for the Ca^{2+}-triggered step after priming

[16]. Although the mechanism of action of synaptotagmin is unclear, Ca^{2+} binding to synaptotagmin triggers the interaction of its first C_2 domain with phospholipids and with syntaxin, both of which are involved in the fusion reaction. Ca^{2+} binding to the second C_2 domain causes self-association of synaptotagmin into larger structures, possibly pore-like structures. Thus, synaptotagmin is an excellent candidate for mediating the Ca^{2+} triggering of the release process.

All synaptic vesicles contain synaptotagmins, and many synaptic vesicles are docked at the active zone at any given time. Why do not all docked synaptic vesicles fuse when Ca^{2+} influx into the nerve terminal occurs? Synaptic vesicle exocytosis appears to be limited to few synaptic vesicles by the action of rab3, a low-molecular-weight G protein of synaptic vesicles [17] (see Chap. 20). In the absence of rab3, more synaptic vesicles fuse as a function of Ca^{2+}, suggesting that rab3 regulates the number of synaptic vesicles that are able to respond to Ca^{2+}. The mechanism of action is unclear, but at least two proteins interact with rab3 only when rab3 is bound to GTP but not when it is bound to GDP. One of these putative effectors, rabphilin, is recruited to synaptic vesicles by rab3, to become a peripheral synaptic vesicle protein. The second putative effector, called RIM, is a plasma membrane protein that can interact with rab3 on synaptic vesicles only when synaptic vesicles are close to the active zone before or after docking. It seems likely that one or both of these effectors mediate the regulation of synaptic vesicle fusion by rab3 [18].

CHARACTERISTICS AND PROTEINS OF SYNAPTIC VESICLE ENDOCYTOSIS

After exocytosis, synaptic vesicles undergo rapid endocytosis, which likely is mediated by clathrin-coated pits and coated vesicles

Clathrin is highly enriched in nerve terminals. A large percentage of the coated vesicles isolated from brain are, in fact, coated synaptic vesicles [19].

Synaptic vesicle endocytosis is probably very similar mechanistically to the receptor-mediated endocytosis in fibroblasts that has been described elegantly for the low-density lipoprotein receptor. Similar proteins are involved, and it seems likely that the mechanism of coated pit assembly is comparable. Nevertheless, synaptic vesicle endocytosis has characteristics that are different from those of fibroblasts. The most striking difference is that endocytosis is much faster at synapses than in fibroblasts, suggesting that it is triggered. The protein composition of synaptic vesicles is different from that of the active zone and other parts of the presynaptic plasma membrane. Therefore, after exocytosis, synaptic vesicle proteins and plasma membrane proteins apparently do not mix with each other by diffusion but remain separated. One property that prevents intermixing of these proteins is that endocytosis is fast and occurs immediately after exocytosis. Another advantage of fast endocytosis is that it allows the synapse to reuse its synaptic vesicles as quickly as possible in order to sustain high rates of repeated exocytosis during repetitive firing.

An efficient mechanism to couple exo- to endocytosis might be to employ the same proteins for two consecutive steps and to utilize Ca^{2+} as a regulatory trigger for both processes. Both coupling mechanisms appear to be used at the synapse. The first step in endocytosis is the recruitment of clathrin to form a coated pit. Adaptor protein 2 (AP2) is a soluble protein complex that is central to forming coated pits by assembling clathrin on the membrane (see also Fig. 2-9). First, AP2 is bound to the membrane at the position of the future coated pit, then clathrin is bound (see Chap. 2). The protein with the highest affinity and binding capacity for AP2 at the synapse is synaptotagmin, which also is required for Ca^{2+} triggering of exocytosis [16,20]. This suggests that the same protein may trigger consecutively exocytosis and then endocytosis. Synaptotagmin binding to AP2 must be regulated. Normally, synaptotagmin must not bind AP2 because otherwise all membranes containing synaptotagmin would be coated. Thus, AP2 binding to synaptotagmin must be activated in conjunction with exocytosis. The mechanism for this is unknown.

Dynamin may be responsible for the rapid endocytosis of synaptic vesicles

This protein is a GTPase that binds to components of the endocytic machinery and to phospholipids [21,22]. Endocytosis is inhibited in a temperature-sensitive mutant of *Drosophila* called *shibire,* which blocks budding of coated vesicles without interfering with the assembly of coated pits. The *shibire* gene encodes dynamin. The *shibire* mutation demonstrates that dynamin is essential for endocytosis downstream of the assembly of coated pits. Interestingly, dynamin is phosphorylated stoichiometrically in the nerve terminal by protein kinase C and rapidly dephosphorylated by calcineurin upon Ca^{2+} influx [23]. It is the single most prominent phosphoprotein in nerve terminals, and it undergoes a stimulation-dependent change, indicating that its function is regulated by phosphorylation. In view of the role of dynamin in endocytosis, its rapid dephosphorylation as a function of an action potential raises the possibility that the rapid nature of synaptic vesicle endocytosis is facilitated by triggering endocytosis via dynamin dephosphorylation.

The mechanism of action of dynamin and, in particular, the significance of its GTPase activity are unknown. Phosphorylation regulates the GTPase activity of dynamin, and GTP-binding mutations influence endocytosis. Thus, dynamin GTPase is likely to be involved directly in endocytosis. One possibility is that dynamin severs the neck of the coated pit after it has been contracted; a second possibility is that it is involved mechanically in the contraction of the pit to a vesicle. After coated vesicles have been formed, they are uncoated rapidly by the action of auxilin, a DNA-J domain protein, in conjunction with HSP70 [24].

Synaptojanin is another protein that has been implicated in synaptic vesicle endocytosis

Although its link to endocytosis is very indirect [25], synaptojanin is a fascinating protein because it hydrolyzes phosphatidylinositol phosphates (see Chap. 21). Accumulating evidence suggests a role for phosphatidylinositol phosphates in membrane traffic, including the synaptic vesicle cycle. The function of phosphatidylinositols in membrane traffic is obscure. However, the action of a phosphatase in endocytosis would be ideally suited to terminate the phosphatidylinositol phosphate signal. This would provide an attractive mechanism for inactivating a fusion machinery and activating an endocytic process. In support of this hypothesis, synaptojanin, similar to dynamin, is dephosphorylated during nerve terminal stimulation, suggesting that dynamin and synaptojanin are regulated coordinately.

IMPLICATIONS FOR INTRACELLULAR TRAFFICKING

Neurotransmitter release is based on a specialized pathway of intracellular trafficking, the synaptic vesicle cycle. As the process that initiates synaptic transmission, neurotransmitter release is of central importance for brain function. To serve the special needs of synaptic secretion, the synaptic vesicle cycle differs from many other intracellular trafficking pathways. The major difference is in the high degree of regulation of intracellular trafficking in the nerve terminal: the exclusive targeting of synaptic vesicle exocytosis to active zones, the high speed with which Ca^{2+} can trigger release, the tight coordinate regulation of all steps of the cycle and the restriction of synaptic vesicle exocytosis in any given nerve terminal to one synaptic vesicle at a time. In spite of these differences, however, the synaptic vesicle cycle has all of the basic characteristics of other intracellular trafficking pathways and shares the same fundamental mechanisms.

REFERENCES

1. Katz, B. *The Release of Neural Transmitter Substances.* Liverpool: Liverpool University Press, 1969.
2. Südhof, T. C. The synaptic vesicle cycle: A cascade of protein–protein interactions. *Nature* 375:645–653, 1995.
3. Peters, A., Palay, S. L., and Webster, H. de F. *The Fine Structure of the Nervous System.* Oxford: Oxford University Press, 1991.

4. Palade, G. E. Intracellular aspects of the process of protein secretion. *Science* 89:347–358, 1975.

5. Jahn, R., and Südhof, T. C. Synaptic vesicle traffic: Rush hour in the nerve terminal. *J. Neurochem.* 61:12–21, 1993.

6. Südhof, T. C., Czernik, A. J., Kao, H. T., et al. Synapsins: Mosaics of shared and individual domains in a family of synaptic vesicle phosphoproteins. *Science* 245:1474–1480, 1989.

7. Südhof, T. C., and Rizo, J. Synaptotagmins: C_2-domain proteins that regulate membrane traffic. *Neuron* 17:379–388, 1996.

8. Castillo, P. E., Janz, R., Südhof, T. C., Malenka, R. C., and Nicoll, R. A. The synaptic vesicle protein rab3A is essential for mossy fiber long term potentiation in the hippocampus. *Nature* 388:590–593, 1997.

9. Hessler, N. A., Shirke, A. M., and Malinow, R. The probability of transmitter release at a mammalian central synapse. *Nature* 366:569–572, 1993.

10. Rosenmund, C., Clements, J. D., and Westbrook, G. L. Nonuniform probability of glutamate release at a hippocampal synapse. *Science* 262:754–757, 1993.

11. White, J. M. Membrane fusion. *Science* 258:917–924, 1992.

12. Heinemann, C., Chow, R. H., Neher, E., and Zucker, R. S. Kinetics of the secretory response in bovine chromaffin cells following flash photolysis of caged Ca^{2+}. *Biophys. J.* 67:2546–2557, 1994.

13. Rosahl, T. W., Spillane, D., Missler, M., et al. Essential functions of synapsins I and II in synaptic vesicle fusion. *Nature* 375:488–493, 1995.

14. Rothman, J. D. Mechanisms of intracellular protein transport. *Nature* 372:55–63, 1994.

15. Mayer, A., Wickner, W., and Haas, A. Sec18p (NSF)-driven release of Sec17p (alpha-SNAP) can precede docking and fusion of yeast vacuoles. *Cell* 85:83–94, 1996.

16. Geppert, M., Goda, Y., Hammer, R. E., et al. Synaptotagmin I: A major Ca^{2+} sensor for transmitter release at a central synapse. *Cell* 79:717–727, 1994.

17. Geppert, M., Goda, Y., Stevens, C. F., and Südhof, T. C. Rab3A regulates a late step in synaptic vesicle fusion. *Nature* 387:810–814, 1997.

18. Wang, Y., Okamoto, M., Schmitz, R., Hofmann, K., and Südhof, T. C. RIM: A putative rab3 effector in regulating synaptic vesicle fusion. *Nature* 388:593–598, 1997.

19. Pfeffer, S. R., and Kelly, R. B. The subpopulation of brain coated vesicles that carries synaptic vesicle proteins contains two unique polypeptides. *Cell* 40:949–957, 1985.

20. Li, C., Ullrich, B., Zhang, J. Z., Anderson, R. G. W., Brose, N., and Südhof, T. C. Ca^{2+}-dependent and Ca^{2+}-independent activities of neural and nonneural synaptotagmins. *Nature* 375:594–599, 1995.

21. van der Bliek, A. M., and Meyerowitz, E. M. Dynamin-like protein encoded by the *Drosophila* shibire gene associated with vesicular traffic. *Nature* 351:411–414, 1991.

22. Chen, M. S., Obar, C. C., Schroeder, C. C., et al. Multiple forms of dynamin are encoded by shibire, a *Drosophila* gene involved in endocytosis. *Nature* 351:583–586, 1991.

23. Robinson, P. J., Sontag, J. M., Liu J. P., et al. Dynamin GTPase regulated by protein kinase C phosphorylation in nerve terminals. *Nature* 365:163–166, 1993.

24. Ungewickell, E., Ungewickell, H., Holstein, S. E. H., et al. Role of auxilin in uncoating clathrin-coated vesicles. *Nature* 378:632–635, 1995.

25. McPherson, P. S., Garcia, E. P., Slepnev, V. I., et al. A presynaptic inositol-5-phosphatase. *Nature* 379:353–357, 1996.

Intercellular Signaling

10

Synaptic Transmission and Cellular Signaling: An Overview

Ronald W. Holz and Stephen K. Fisher

Basic Neurochemistry: Molecular, Cellular and Medical Aspects, 6th Ed., edited by G. J. Siegel et al. Published by Lippincott–Raven Publishers, 1999. Correspondence to Ronald W. Holz, Department of Pharmacology, University of Michigan Medical School, MSRB III, Room 2301, Ann Arbor, Michigan 48109-0632.

SYNAPTIC TRANSMISSION

Chemical transmission between nerve cells involves multiple steps

Until the late nineteenth century, many physiologists believed that there were direct physical connections between nerves and that an impulse from one nerve was communicated to another through a direct physical connection. However, studies by Golgi, Ramon y Cajal and others convinced many histologists that most connections, which we now know as synapses, were close but not continuous. The pioneering work of Oliver and Shäfer, of Langley and of Elliot beginning in the 1890s provided data that raised the possibility of chemical transmission between nerves. Chemical transmission was convincingly demonstrated in the historic experiments of Otto Loewi. He electrically stimulated the vagus nerve of an isolated frog heart to decrease the strength and rate of contractions. The bathing solution caused a decrease in the strength and rate of contractions when subsequently applied to a second heart. We now know that the inhibition was caused by the neurotransmitter acetylcholine (ACh) that had been released by the nerve terminals of the vagus nerve. (See Davenport [1] for an entertaining and excellent review of the early history of chemical transmission.)

Chemical transmission is the major means by which nerves communicate with one another in the nervous system. The pre- and postsynaptic events are highly regulated and subject to use-dependent changes that are the basis for plasticity and learning in the CNS. Although direct electrical connections also occur, these account for transmission of information between nerves only in specialized cases.

Chemical transmission requires the following steps:

1. Synthesis of the neurotransmitter in the presynaptic nerve terminal.
2. Storage of the neurotransmitter in secretory vesicles.
3. Regulated release of neurotransmitter in the synaptic space between the pre- and postsynaptic neurons.

4. The presence of specific receptors for the neurotransmitter on the postsynaptic membrane, such that application of the neurotransmitter to the synapse mimics the effects of nerve stimulation.
5. A means for termination of the action of the released neurotransmitter.

An overview of some of the processes involved in synaptic transmission is shown in Figure 10-1. Many of the processes are discussed below or in other chapters of this book. Many different types of substances are neurotransmitters. "Classical" neurotransmitters, such as ACh (Chap. 11) and norepinephrine (NE) (Chap. 12), are low-molecular-weight substances that have no other function but to serve as neurotransmitters. The predominant excitatory neurotransmitter in the brain, glutamate, and the inhibitory neurotransmitter in the spinal cord, glycine, are common and essential amino acids (Chaps. 15 and 16). They can function as neurotransmitters because the membranes of secretory vesicles in glutamatergic and glycinergic nerve terminals have specific transport systems that concentrate and store these amino acids so that they can be released by exocytosis in a highly regulated manner. Aminergic neurotransmitters, ACh and GABA, the predominant inhibitory amino acid in brain, also enter synaptic vesicles through specific transport proteins. Synaptic vesicles have an acidic interior, pH ~5.5, which is maintained by a vacuolar-type, proton-translocating ATPase (see Chap. 5). The uptake of low-molecular-weight neurotransmitters is coupled via the transporters to the electrochemical H^+ gradient (for reviews, see [2,3]).

Neurotransmitter release is a highly specialized form of the secretory process that occurs in virtually all eukaryotic cells

The fundamental similarity between the events in the nerve terminal that control neurotransmitter release and the ubiquitous vesicular trafficking reactions in all eukaryotic cells is described in Chapter 9. This similarity has important implications for the biochemistry of synaptic transmission. Many of the proteins es-

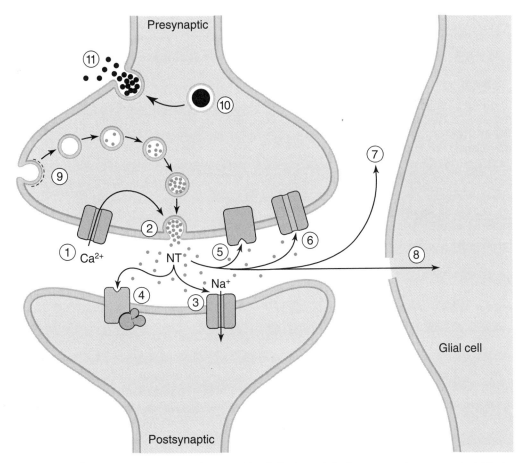

FIGURE 10-1. ① Depolarization opens voltage-sensitive Ca^{2+} channels in the presynaptic nerve terminal. The influx of Ca^{2+} and the resulting high Ca^{2+} concentrations at active zones on the plasma membrane trigger ② the exocytosis of small synaptic vesicles that store neurotransmitter *(NT)* involved in fast neurotransmission. Released neurotransmitter interacts with ③ receptors in the postsynaptic membrane, which couple directly with ion channels and with receptors that act through second messengers, such as ④ G-protein coupled receptors. ⑤ Neurotransmitter receptors, also in the presynaptic nerve terminal membrane, either inhibit or enhance exocytosis upon subsequent depolarization. Released neurotransmitter is inactivated by reuptake into the nerve terminal by ⑥ a transport protein coupled to the Na^+ gradient, for example, dopamine, norepinephrine, glutamate and GABA; by ⑦ degradation (acetylcholine, peptides); or by ⑧ uptake and metabolism by glial cells (glutamate). The synaptic vesicle membrane is recycled by ⑨ clathrin-mediated endocysosis. Neuropeptides and proteins are stored in ⑩ larger, dense core granules within the nerve terminal that are released from ⑪ sites distinct from active zones after repetitive stimulation.

sential for constitutive secretion and endocytosis in yeast and mammalian cells are similar to those involved in the presynaptic events of synaptic transmission (Chap. 9).

Peptides and proteins can also be released from nerve terminals. Their biosynthetic and storage processes are similar to those in other protein secretory cells [4]. They utilize the endoplasmic reticulum, Golgi and trans-Golgi network, which are present in the cell body but not in the nerve terminal. The peptide- and protein-containing vesicles must be transported into the nerve terminal by axonal transport (Chap. 28). Examples of peptide neurotransmitters include substance P, thyrotropin-releasing hormone (TRH), vasopressin, oxytocin, enkephalins and endorphins (endogenous opiate-like agonists), vasoactive intestinal peptide (VIP) and luteinizing hormone–releasing hormone (LHRH) (Chap. 18). The interior of mature secretory granules in neuroendocrine cells in the regulated pathway has a pH of 5.3 to 5.5, similar to the pH in synaptic vesicles. The low pH influences intravesicular protein processing and the conformation of the stored proteins, as well as the transport of other substances into the granules.

A variety of methods have been developed to study exocytosis

Neurotransmitter and hormone release can be measured by electrical effects of released neurotransmitter or hormone on postsynaptic membrane receptors, such as the neuromuscular junction (NMJ) (see below), and directly by biochemical assay. Another direct measure of exocytosis is the increase in membrane area due to the incorporation of the secretory granule or vesicle membrane into the plasma membrane. This can be measured by increases in membrane capacitance (C_m). C_m is directly proportional to membrane area and is defined as: $C_m = QA_m/V$, where C_m is the membrane capacitance in farads (F), Q is the charge across the membrane (coulombs), V is voltage (volts) and A_m is the area of the plasma membrane (cm^2). The specific capacitance, Q/V, is the amount of charge that must be deposited across 1 cm^2 of membrane to change the potential by 1 volt. The specific capacitance is mainly determined by the thickness and dielectric constant of the phospholipid bilayer membrane and is similar for intracellular organelles and the plasma membrane. It is approximately 1 $\mu F/cm^2$. Therefore, the increase in plasma membrane area due to exocytosis is proportional to the increase in C_m.

The electrophysiological technique used to measure changes in membrane capacitance is the patch clamp [5,6] in the whole-cell recording mode, where the plasma membrane patch in the pipet is ruptured. In another configuration of the patch clamp, the plasma membrane patch is maintained intact. In this case, small currents due to the opening of individual channels can be measured in the membrane patch. The whole-cell patch clamp technique establishes a high resistance seal between the glass rim of the micropipet and the plasma membrane that allows low noise, high sensitivity, electrical measurements across the entire plasma membrane. An example of the use of membrane capacitance to measure exocytosis in chromaffin cells is shown in Figure 10-2 [7].

Sensitive electrochemical techniques have also been developed to directly measure the release of oxidizable neurotransmitters such as catecholamines (CAs) and serotonin (5-hydroxytryptamine; 5-HT). Current flows in the circuit when the potential of the electrode is positive enough to withdraw electrons from, that is, oxidize, the released neurotransmitter. The technique is very sensitive and readily detects the release of individual quanta of neurotransmitter resulting from the fusion of single secretory granules (Fig. 10-2).

A variety of different types of tissue preparations are used to study neurosecretion and synaptic transmission. A classical preparation is the frog NMJ (discussed below). The brain slice has been used for many years for biochemical studies of CNS metabolism and is a useful preparation for electrophysiological studies of synaptic transmission in the CNS. Slices can be oriented to maintain the local neuronal circuitry and can be thin, ~0.3 mm, to minimize anoxia. The transverse hippocampal slice is widely used as an electrophysiological preparation to study synaptic plasticity (see Chap. 50). Primary cultures of neurons from selected CNS areas and sympathetic ganglia are also frequently used. They permit excellent visual identification of individual neurons and control of the extracellular milieu, but the normal neuronal connections are disrupted.

Gentle homogenization of brain tissue results in suspensions of intracellular organelles and pinched-off nerve terminals, *synaptosomes*. Homogenization shears off nerve terminals from axons, especially in brain regions with clearly defined anatomical layers, such as the cerebral cortex and hippocampus. Synaptosomes can be partially separated from other organelles by centrifugation techniques. Each of these remarkable structures is 0.5 to 1.0 μm in diameter, contains hundreds of synaptic vesicles and one or more mitochondria and is often associated with postsynaptic membrane fragments. Synaptosomes remain functional for several hours and can be used to study biochemical events, including energy and Ca^{2+} metabolism,

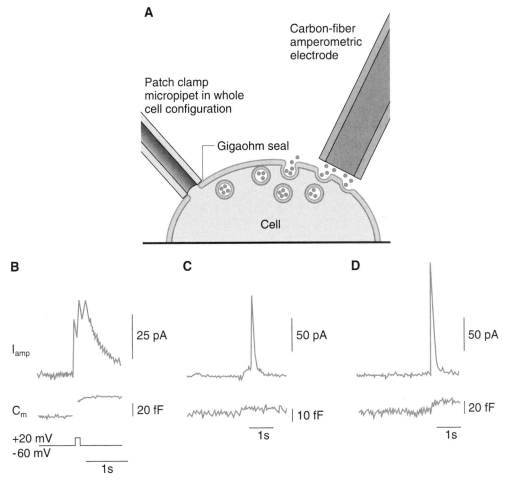

FIGURE 10-2.   Secretory events monitored by simultaneous amperometric *(I_{amp})* and capacitance *(C_m)* measurements demonstrate typical patterns of release. **A:** Configuration of the recording setup. **B:** shows a wide amperometric response composed of multiple spikes due to the fusion of several secretory vesicles triggered by a 50-ms depolarization to +20 mV from a holding potential of −60 mV. From the magnitude of the capacitance response (24 fF), it is estimated that 2 to 24 vesicles fused with the plasma membrane. The exact number of vesicles that fused is not known since there is a distribution in their size. The amperometric response shows at least three to five discernible peaks that lag the capacitance step. However, the broad amperometric response **(B)** is likely to be composed of many more spikes. Two particularly large, isolated fusion events are shown in **C** and **D**. A clear lag between the fusion of a vesicle and the main spike of release can sometimes be observed **(C)**; however, it is not always present **(D)**. This foot contributes to make multiple fusion events, like those of **B,** seem wider than those resulting from single vesicle fusion (compare **B** with **C** and **D**).

neurotransmitter synthesis, transport and secretion. A related preparation is the neurosecretosome, from the posterior pituitary. These nerve terminals originate in the hypothalamus and contain vasopressin and oxytocin in large dense core granules. They are obtained in high purity from the neurohypophysis, which does not contain cell bodies. Neurosecretosomes are some-

what larger than synaptosomes and can be used for biochemical and patch clamp studies.

Several types of cells related to sympathetic neurons can be maintained and studied in tissue culture. Adrenal medullary chromaffin cells have the same precursor cells as postganglionic sympathetic neurons. These excitable neuroendocrine cells store, in large dense core granules called chromaffin granules, epinephrine or NE, together with ATP, and a variety of proteins (chromogranins, opiate peptides and precursors and dopamine β-hydroxylase). Relatively pure primary cultures can be prepared by collagenase digestion of bovine adrenal glands followed by cell-purification techniques. Various aspects of neurotransmitter metabolism and secretion have been extensively studied with these cells. They are amenable to both biochemical and electrophysiological experiments. A clonal cell line, PC12, is derived from a rat pheochromocytoma, a tumor of the adrenal medulla. Upon incubation with nerve growth factor (NGF), PC12 cells differentiate within days into neurons with axons and terminals (Chap. 19). Thus, they are used not only for biochemical and secretion studies but also for investigation of neuronal differentiation.

The neuromuscular junction is a well-defined structure that mediates the release and postsynaptic effects of acetylcholine

The first detailed studies of synaptic transmission were performed at the NMJ. The NMJ is a beautiful example of how structure and function are intimately entwined. The myelinated axon originating from the motor neuron in the spinal cord forms unmyelinated terminals that run longitudinally along the muscle fiber. Specialized transverse release sites, or active zones, occur periodically along the terminals and are oriented opposite invaginations of the postsynaptic membrane (Fig. 10-3). There are approximately 300 active zones per NMJ. The active zones in the nerve terminal display a cloud of clear vesicles, 50 to 60 nm in diameter, that contain ACh (Fig. 10-3). There are approximately 500,000 vesicles in all of the active zones at one NMJ. It is estimated that on the average a vesicle contains 20,000 ACh molecules. A small subset of the vesicles is attached in rows to the presynaptic membrane (Fig. 10-3A, B). These are thought to be docked vesicles that are able to undergo exocytosis upon Ca^{2+} influx. In freeze fracture, these rows coincide with rows of intramembrane particles that may be Ca^{2+} channels (Fig. 10-3C). Ca^{2+} entry that occurs upon stimulation of

the nerve causes exocytosis that is seen as pits in freeze-fracture micrographs (Fig. 10-3D) or as "omega" figures in thin-section electron microscopy (Fig. 10-4). The vesicle membranes in the nerve terminal are recycled by endocytosis (see below).

The postsynaptic membrane opposite release sites is also highly specialized, consisting of folds of plasma membrane containing a high density of nicotinic ACh receptors (nAChRs). Basal lamina matrix proteins are important for the formation and maintenance of the NMJ and are concentrated in the cleft. Acetylcholinesterase (AChE), an enzyme which hydrolyzes ACh to acetate and choline to inactivate the neurotransmitter, is associated with the basal lamina (see Chap. 11).

Quantal analysis defines the mechanism of release as exocytosis

Stimulation of the motor neuron causes a large depolarization of the motor end plate. In 1952, Fatt and Katz [8] observed that spontaneous potentials of approximately 1 mV occur at the motor end plate. Each individual potential change has a time course similar to the much larger evoked response of the muscle membrane that results from electrical stimulation of the motor nerve. These small spontaneous potentials were therefore called miniature end-plate potentials (MEPPs). Because the MEPPs are reduced by the nicotinic antagonist D-tubocurarine and increased in amplitude and duration by the AChE inhibitor prostigmine, it was concluded that they are initiated by the release of ACh. Because the potential changes are too large to be accounted for by the interaction of individual molecules of ACh with the end plate, Fatt and Katz [8] postulated that they reflect the release of packets, or *quanta*, of ACh molecules from the nerve terminal.

A "curious effect" was observed by Fatt and Katz [8]: when the Ca^{2+} concentration is reduced and the Mg^{2+} increased, the evoked end-plate potential (EPP) is diminished without altering the size of the spontaneous MEPPs. With sufficiently low Ca^{2+}, the evoked EPP is similar in size to MEPPs and varies in a stepwise manner. A single nerve impulse results in either no

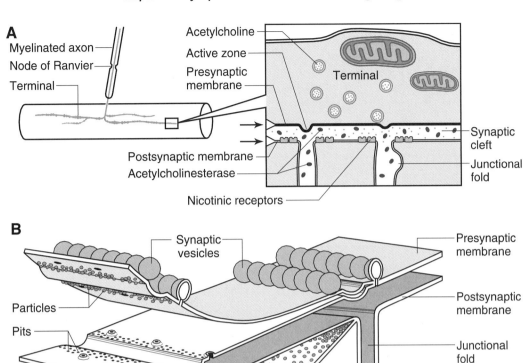

FIGURE 10-3.   Synaptic membrane structure. **A:** Entire frog neuromuscular junction (NMJ, **left**) and longitudinal section through a portion of the nerve terminal **(right)**. *Arrows* indicate planes of cleavage during freeze-fracture. **B:** Three-dimensional view of presynaptic and postsynaptic membranes with active zones and immediately adjacent rows of synaptic vesicles. Plasma membranes are split along planes indicated by the *arrows* in **A** to illustrate structures observed by freeze-fracture. The cytoplasmic half of the presynaptic membrane at the active zone shows on its fracture face protruding particles whose counterparts are seen as pits on the fracture face of the outer membrane leaflet. Vesicles that fuse with the presynaptic membrane give rise to characteristic protrusions and pores in the fracture faces. The fractured postsynaptic membrane in the region of the folds shows a high concentration of particles on the fracture face of the cytoplasmic leaflet; these are probably acetylcholine receptors (AChRs). (Courtesy of U. J. McMahan; from [9], with permission). (*Figure continues on next page.*)

C

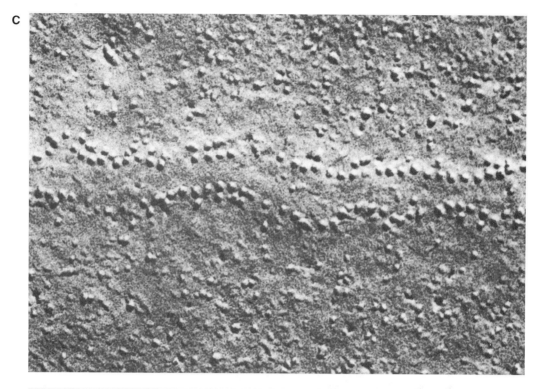

D

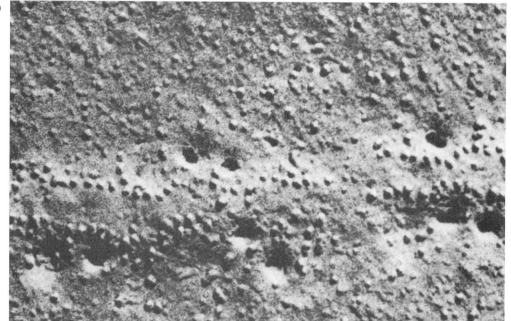

FIGURE 10-3. *(Continued)* Freeze-fractured active zones from frog resting and stimulated NMJ. **C:** The active zone is the region of presynaptic membrane surrounding double rows of intramembrane particles, which may be channels for Ca^{2+} entry that initiates transmitter release. **D:** Holes that appear in active zones during transmitter release are openings of synaptic vesicles engaged in exocytosis. This muscle was prepared by quick-freezing, and transmitter release was augmented with 4-aminopyridine so that the morphological events, such as the opening of synaptic vesicles, could be examined at the exact moment of transmitter release evoked by a single nerve shock ($\times$120,000). (From [10], with permission.)

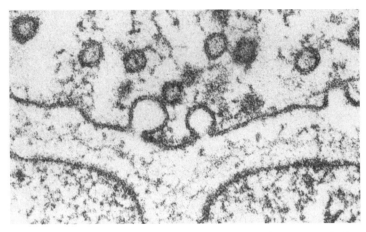

FIGURE 10-4. High-magnification ($\times$145,000) view of freeze-substituted neuromuscular junctions in a muscle frozen during the abnormally large burst of acetylcholine release that is provoked by a single nerve stimulus of 2 mM 4-aminopyridine, in this case delivered 5.1 msec before the muscle was frozen. The section was cut unusually thin (~200 Å) to show the fine structure of the presynaptic membrane, which displayed examples of synaptic vesicles apparently caught in the act of exocytosis. In all cases, these open vesicles were found just above the mouths of the postsynaptic folds, hence, at the site of the presynaptic active zones. (From [11], with permission.)

EPP or EPPs the approximate size of one, two, three or more MEPPs in an apparently random manner. The results of this type of experiment are shown in Figure 10-5. The frequency histogram shows that the amplitudes of evoked potentials are clustered in multiples of the mean spontaneous MEPP value. Statistical analysis [12] demonstrates that the release is a random process described by a Poisson distribution. Each event is unaffected by the preceding events. The model assumes n release sites capable of responding to a nerve impulse, each with a probability, p, of releasing a quantum of ACh. The mean number of quanta (m), or quantal content, released per nerve impulse is $m = np$. For a Poisson distribution, p must be small, <0.05, and n large, >100. The probability of evoked release of x quanta is $P_x = (m^x/x!)e^{-m}$. (See Martin [13] for a review of the Poisson distribution in the analysis of synaptic transmission.)

One critical test for the validity of the Poisson distribution as a description of release in the presence of reduced Ca^{2+} was the excellent agreement of two measures of m. One was derived empirically:

$$m = \text{mean amplitude of EPP/mean amplitude of MEPPS}$$

The other was derived from the Poisson equation and the observed probability of no response, or failures, upon nerve stimulation:

$$P_0 = e^{-m} \text{ and } m = -\ln(P_0)$$

A more stringent test of the model is its ability to predict the histogram in Figure 10-5.

The quantal size m differs for different types of synapses. For a single impulse at the NMJ, 100 to 300 quanta are released. The large number of quanta that are released during a single impulse reflects the need for a large safety factor in the all-or-none response of muscle contraction. Where integration of inputs is important, quantal size is much less. At single terminals in sympathetic ganglia, at inhibitory and excitatory inputs on spinal motor neurons and at individual boutons of cultured hippocampal neurons, m is 1 to 3.

Ca^{2+} is necessary for transmission at the neuromuscular junction and other synapses and plays a special role in exocytosis

In most cases in the CNS and PNS, chemical transmission does not occur unless Ca^{2+} is present in the extracellular fluid. Katz and Miledi

[14] elegantly demonstrated the critical role of Ca^{2+} in neurotransmitter release. The frog NMJ was perfused with salt solution containing Mg^{2+} but deficient in Ca^{2+}. A twin-barrel micropipet, with each barrel filled with either 1.0 M $CaCl_2$ or NaCl, was placed immediately adjacent to the terminal. The sodium barrel was used to depolarize the nerve terminal electrically and the calcium barrel to apply Ca^{2+} ionotophoretically. Depolarization without Ca^{2+} failed to elicit an

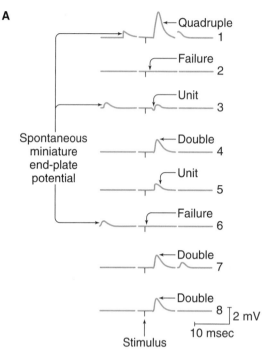

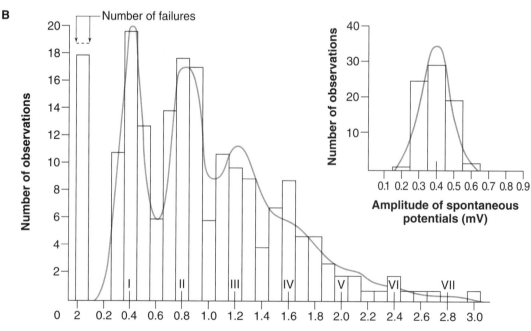

EPP (Fig. 10-6A). If Ca^{2+} was applied just before the depolarization, EPPs were evoked (Fig. 10-6B). In contrast, EPPs could not be elicited if the Ca^{2+} pulse immediately followed the depolarization (Fig. 10-6C). EPPs occurred when a Ca^{2+} pulse as short as 1 msec preceded the start of the depolarizing pulse by as little as 50 to 100 μsec. The experiments demonstrated that Ca^{2+} must be present when a nerve terminal is depolarized in order for neurotransmitter to be released.

The normal extracellular Ca^{2+} concentration is approximately 2 mM. The basal cytosolic Ca^{2+} concentration is 0.1 μM or less. In nerve terminals, the rise of intracellular Ca^{2+} caused by depolarization of the plasma membrane opens voltage-sensitive Ca^{2+} channels. Ca^{2+} influx and the resultant rise in the cytosolic Ca^{2+} concentration adjacent to release sites along the plasma membrane trigger exocytosis. The sites of exocytosis are closely associated with Ca^{2+} channels (Fig. 10-3C). Ca^{2+} channels may, in fact, be components of multimeric protein complexes involved in exocytosis. Intracellular $[Ca^{2+}]$ immediately adjacent to Ca^{2+} channels is probably in the range 50 to 100 μM [17–19]. It is this high Ca^{2+} concentration that triggers exocytosis. Neuroendocrine cells, such as chromaffin cells from the adrenal medulla, also release hormones, such as epinephrine and opioid peptides, upon Ca^{2+} influx through membrane channels.

It is thought that in this type of cell, release sites are usually not closely associated with Ca^{2+} channels and that $[Ca^{2+}]$ in the 0.5 to 10 μM range can trigger exocytosis. It should be noted that other types of cells, such as exocrine cells (for example, pancreatic acinar cells), also release stored protein by exocytosis upon a rise in cytosolic Ca^{2+}. In many cases, Ca^{2+} is released from intracellular stores by inositol trisphosphate (IP_3), which is generated by the hormonal activation of G protein–linked receptors that activate phosphoinositide-specific phospholipase C (PI-PLC) (Chap. 21). In this case, extracellular Ca^{2+} sustains secretion by refilling the intracellular, IP_3-sensitive Ca^{2+} stores rather than by directly triggering secretion.

Presynaptic events during synaptic transmission are rapid, dynamic and interconnected

The time between Ca^{2+} influx and exocytosis in the nerve terminal is very short. At the frog NMJ at room temperature, 0.5 to 1 msec elapses between the depolarization of the nerve terminal and the beginning of the postsynaptic response. In the squid giant synapse, recordings can be made simultaneously in the presynaptic nerve terminal and in the postsynaptic cell. Voltage-sensitive Ca^{2+} channels open toward the end of

FIGURE 10-5. Comparison of the amplitudes of the spontaneous miniature end-plate potentials and the evoked end-plate potentials indicates that transmitter is released in quantal packages that are fixed in amplitude but variable in number. **A:** Intracellular recording from a rat nerve-muscle synapse shows a few spontaneous miniature end-plate potentials and the synaptic responses, or end-plate potentials, evoked by eight consecutive stimuli to the nerve. The stimulus artifact evident in the records is produced by current flowing between the stimulating and recording electrodes in the bathing solution. In a Ca^{2+}-deficient and Mg^{2+}-rich solution designed to reduce transmitter output, the end-plate potentials are small and show considerable fluctuations: two impulses produce complete failures (*2* and *6*), two produce a unit potential (*3* and *5*) and still others produce responses that are two to four times the amplitude of the unit potential. Comparison of the unit potential and the spontaneously occurring miniature end-plate potential illustrates that they are the same size. (Adapted from [15], with permission.) **B:** Distribution of amplitudes of the spontaneous miniature end-plate potentials and the evoked end-plate potentials. Synaptic transmission has again been reduced, this time with only a high-Mg^{2+} solution. The histograms of the evoked end-plate potential illustrate peaks that occur at 1, 2, 3 and 4 times the mean amplitude of the spontaneous potentials (0.4 mV). The distribution of the spontaneous miniature end-plate potentials shown in the **inset** is fitted with a Gaussian curve. The Gaussian distribution for the spontaneous miniature potentials is used to calculate a theoretical distribution of the evoked end-plate potential amplitudes, based on the Poisson equation, that predicts the number of failures, unit potentials, twin and triplet responses and so on. The fit of the data to the theoretical distribution is remarkably good *(solid line)*. Thus, the actual number of failures *(dashed line at 0 mV)* was only slightly lower than the theoretically expected number of failures *(arrows above dashed line)*. (Adapted from [16], with permission.)

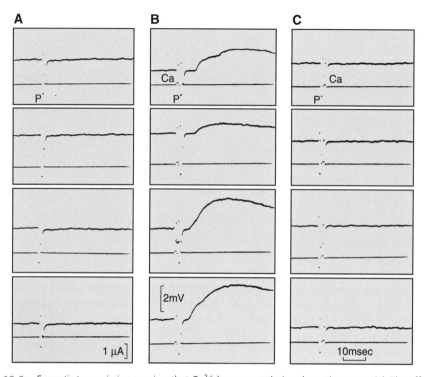

FIGURE 10-6. Synaptic transmission requires that Ca^{2+} be present during the action potential. The effects of iontophoretic pulses of Ca^{2+} on end-plate response are shown. Depolarizing pulses *(P)* and Ca^{2+} were applied from a double-barrel micropipet to a small part of a frog sartorius neuromuscular junction. Intracellular recording was from the end-plate region of the muscle fiber. **Top traces** show the postsynaptic membrane potential responses. **Bottom traces** show current pulses through the pipet. **A:** Depolarizing pulses alone. **B:** Short-duration, approximately 1 msec, Ca^{2+} pulses applied less than 1 msec before the depolarizing pulse. **C:** Short Ca^{2+} pulses immediately following depolarizing pulses. The acetylcholinesterase inhibitor prostigmine was present to enhance the response. Temperature 3°C. Depolarization elicited end-plate potentials only if the Ca^{2+} pulse preceded the depolarizing pulse **(B).** (From [14], with permission.)

the action potential. The time between Ca^{2+} influx and the postsynaptic response is 200 μsec (Fig. 10-7). Recent studies of synaptic transmission between CNS neurons using optical methods to record presynaptic events indicate a delay of only 60 μsec between Ca^{2+} influx and the postsynaptic response at 38°C [20].

The short delays between Ca^{2+} influx and exocytosis have important implications for the mechanism of fusion of synaptic vesicles (Chap. 9). In this short time, a synaptic vesicle cannot move significantly and must be already at the release site. From the diffusion constant of Ca^{2+} in squid axoplasm, one calculates that Ca^{2+} could diffuse only 850 Å, somewhat greater than the diameter of a synaptic vesicle. Therefore, in fast synapses, release sites must be close to the Ca^{2+}

channels that trigger exocytosis. Vesicles are exposed to $[Ca^{2+}]$ of a few hundred micromolar near the mouth of the channels.

The supply of synaptic vesicles in the nerve terminal is limited. With continuous stimulation of the NMJ, the number of quanta released can exceed by many fold the number available in the nerve terminal. Possible transport of secretory vesicles from the cell body would be much too slow to maintain fast synaptic transmission in the terminal. Instead, the synaptic vesicle membrane which fuses with the plasma membrane is rapidly recycled via clathrin-mediated endocytosis (reviewed in [21]) (see Chap. 9). Hence, the vesicle membrane is a reusable container for neurotransmitter storage and exocytosis. The process of membrane recycling at the nerve terminal is

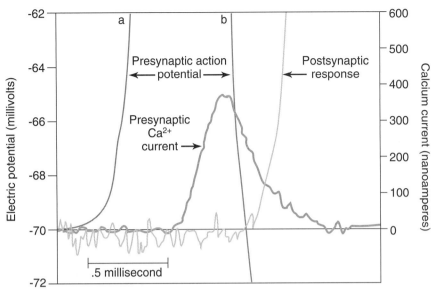

FIGURE 10-7.   The delay between Ca^{2+} influx into the nerve terminal and the postsynaptic response is brief. The temporal relationships between the Ca^{2+} current and the action potential in the nerve terminal and the postsynaptic response in the squid giant synapse are shown. The rapid depolarization *(a)* and repolarization *(b)* phases of the action potential are drawn. A major fraction of the synaptic delay results from the slow-opening, voltage-sensitive Ca^{2+} channels. There is a further delay of approximately 200 μsec between Ca^{2+} influx and the postsynaptic response. (From [22], with permission.)

closely related to the general process of endocytosis that occurs in non-neuronal cells. Strong evidence for this process came from electron micrographs of horseradish peroxidase uptake from the extracellular medium into the nerve terminal of the frog NMJ following nerve stimulation [23,24]. Endocytosis is dispersed along the membrane away from active zones. It was originally proposed that clathrin-coated vesicles bud from the plasma membrane, lose their triskelion clathrin coat and fuse to an intermediary endosomal compartment, from which new synaptic vesicles bud. Synaptic vesicles then take up neurotransmitter and recycle to release sites. However, recent studies suggest an alternative pathway that bypasses the intermediate endosomal compartment. It would allow more rapid endocytic recycling of the synaptic vesicle membrane. Clathrin-coated vesicles bud from the plasma membrane, become uncoated, take up neurotransmitter and recycle to the plasma membrane. Strong stimulation of the nerve terminal may cause invaginations of the plasma membrane, from which clathrin-coated vesicles can also bud (see Chap. 2).

The development of amphipathic fluorescent dyes that label endocytic vesicles has permitted the study of endocytosis in nerve terminals in real time [25]. The probe FM1-43 equilibrates between the aqueous phase and the membrane but is not membrane-permeant. The plasma membrane becomes fluorescent (Fig. 10-8). Upon endocytosis, the labeled membrane is internalized. When removed from the extracellular medium, the dye is retained by the endocytic vesicles but lost from the plasma membrane. Endocytic vesicles are transformed into synaptic vesicles containing FM1-43. Importantly, recycled synaptic vesicles lose the probe upon exocytosis.

This technique has permitted the dynamics of the exocytic/endocytic cycle to be investigated. At the NMJ, a complete cycle of exocytosis and endocytosis requires approximately 1 min. The recycled vesicles mix homogeneously with, and have the same probability of again undergoing exocytosis as, unlabeled vesicles. A single nerve impulse releases 0.1% of the recycling pool. The dynamics of recycling are similar in cultured hippocampal neurons [26]. Endocyto-

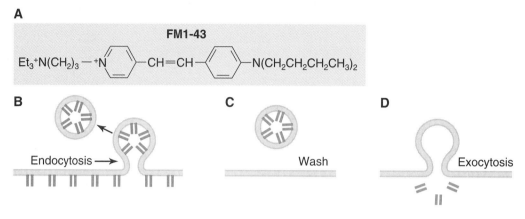

A

FM1-43

$Et_3{}^+N(CH_2)_3 - {}^+N$ ⬡ $-CH=CH-$ ⬡ $-N(CH_2CH_2CH_2CH_3)_2$

B

Endocytosis ⟶

C

Wash

D

Exocytosis

E

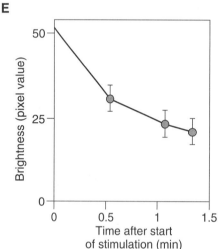

Brightness (pixel value)

Time after start of stimulation (min)

FIGURE 10-8. The probe FM1-43 was used to visualize endocytosis and exocytosis at the neuromuscular junction (NMI). **A:** Structure of the amphipathic membrane probe FM1-43. **B:** Labeling of the plasma membrane by FM1-43 in the extracellular medium. The amphipathic probe is present during electrical stimulation of the NMJ. Note that membrane originating from synaptic vesicles that have undergone exocytosis is labeled. **C:** A brief wash of the NMJ after electrical stimulation removes FM1-43 from the plasma membrane but not from intracellular endocytic vesicles that had formed following exocytosis in the presence of FM1-43. **D** and **E:** A second round of exocytosis stimulated by exocytosis in the absence of extracellular FM1-43 results in loss of the fluorescent probe from newly formed synaptic vesicles that have undergone exocytosis. In **E,** the fluorescence intensity of vesicle populations at the NMJ was followed over time during a 10 Hz stimulation. Note the decline of fluorescence as FM1-43-labeled vesicles undergo exocytosis and release the probe into the extracellular medium (25).

sis follows approximately 20 sec after exocytosis. The transformation of the endocytic vesicle into a functioning synaptic vesicle requires about 15 sec. About 0.5% of the recycling pool is released by a nerve impulse. This corresponds to approximately one vesicle per synaptic bouton.

The importance of endocytosis for the normal function of the nerve terminal is demonstrated by the *shibire* mutant of *Drosophila*. When these mutant flies, bearing a temperature-sensitive allele, are exposed to high temperature, they become paralyzed within 1 min but rapidly recover when returned to the permissive temperature. Electron microscopy demonstrates that the paralysis results from a block of synaptic vesicle endocytosis at the NMJ. The *shibire* allele encodes dynamin, a GTPase that is essential for the fission of the endocytic bud from the plasma membrane.

There are important differences between fast synaptic transmission at nerve terminals and the release of proteins and peptides from nerve terminals and neuroendocrine cells

Because fast synaptic transmission involves recycling vesicles, the neurotransmitter must be replenished locally. Thus, fast synaptic transmission uses neurotransmitters such as ACh, glutamate, GABA, glycine, dopamine (DA) and NE, all of which can be synthesized within the nerve terminal or transported rapidly across the nerve terminal plasma membrane. In contrast, proteins are inserted into secretory granules in the cell body. The secretory granules must then be transported by fast axonal transport into the nerve terminal, a process that can take many hours or days depending on the distance of the nerve terminal from the soma (see Chap. 28). Nerve terminals that are specialized for fast synaptic transmission may have peptidergic granules as well as the recycling vesicles of fast synaptic transmission. For example, nerve terminals can contain VIP as well as ACh, enkephalin as well as NE and substance P as well as 5-HT. The peptidergic granules are usually far less numerous than the smaller vesicles involved in fast exocytosis and are not localized at active zones (Fig. 10-1). The exocytosis of protein-containing granules in nerve terminals may be closely related to exocytosis of protein-containing granules in endocrine and exocrine cells. While a single nerve impulse will release vesicles at active zones, exocytosis of peptidergic granules in nerve terminals can require multiple or high-frequency stimulation. This may reflect the need for sustained elevations of Ca^{2+} that extend into the interior of the nerve terminal. Peptides and proteins released from nerves may have slower and longer-lasting effects on postsynaptic cells than fast neurotransmitters and can modulate the response to fast neurotransmitters.

Discrete steps in the regulated secretory pathway can be defined in neuroendocrine cells

The rapid presynaptic events of synaptic transmission produce closely coordinated exocytosis and endocytosis. Insights into the steps involved in the exocytotic limb of the pathway have come from the studies of kinetics of secretion of protein-containing granules from adrenal chromaffin cells and PC12 cells. Adrenal chromaffin cells are excitable and contain a large number of secretory or chromaffin granules. In bovine chromaffin cells, a neuronal-type nAChR and voltage-sensitive Ca^{2+} channels permit Ca^{2+} entry, which stimulates secretion. The intracellular milieu of chromaffin cells can be directly controlled by extracellular solutions in cells with plasma membranes rendered leaky by the detergent digitonin, by streptolysin-O [27] or by mechanically disrupting the plasma membrane by passage of the cells through a steel cylinder partially blocked by a precision steel bearing [28]. PC12 cells contain far fewer granules than adrenal chromaffin cells, and many are closely associated with the plasma membrane. An analysis of the effects of Ca^{2+}, ATP and temperature suggests that ATP hydrolysis occurs before Ca^{2+} is able to cause secretory granules to secrete. Two distinct Ca^{2+}-dependent steps have been identified. One triggers exocytosis with maximal effects at 100 to 300 μM Ca^{2+}, whereas the other enhances the ability of ATP to prime secretion, with maximal effects at approximately 1 μM Ca^{2+}. Electrophysiological studies have identified additional steps associated with the triggering of exocytosis that may reflect the dynamics of inter-related pools of granules [29].

What is the function of ATP in secretion? While protein phosphorylation can modulate the secretory response, there is compelling evidence that the effect of ATP in priming involves other processes. ATP is necessary for the function of *N*-ethylmaleimide-sensitive factor (NSF). This protein is an ATPase that acts as a molecular chaperone to dissociate complexes of the SNARE proteins VAMP (synaptobrevin), syntaxin and SNAP-25 (see Chap. 9). This may permit their subsequent reassociation as part of the exocytotic response. Another function of ATP in priming exocytosis is the maintenance of the polyphosphoinositides, phosphatidylinositol 4,5-bisphosphate (PIP_2) and phosphatidylinositol 4-phosphate (PIP), by phosphorylation of lipid precursors via phosphatidylinositol 4-kinase and PIP kinase [30–32]. Interestingly, phosphatidylinositol 4-kinase is an integral membrane protein of chromaffin granules. The polyphosphoinositides appear to function in the priming step not as precursors for the formation of IP_3 and diacylglycerol (DAG) but, rather, in some other capacity (see Chap. 21). PIP_2 binds specifically to the vesicle or granule proteins synaptotagmin and rabphilin 3a. PIP_2 also regulates numerous proteins that control the cytoskeleton, such as profilin, gelsolin, scinderin and myosin I. Therefore, the polyphosphoinositides on the secretory granule membrane may coordinate the function in secretion of several secretory granule proteins or may modulate dynamic changes in the cytoskeletal network that are important for exocytosis.

CELLULAR SIGNALING MECHANISMS

Largely as a result of the studies of Langley, the possibility that biological tissues possess receptor molecules that are specific for each neurotransmitter was first entertained in the early 1900s. Langley noted the high degree of specificity and potency with which some agents elicit a biological response and postulated the existence of "receptor" or "acceptor" molecules. This concept has subsequently been fully validated. Many receptors have been isolated and purified biochemically, and many have also been cloned and sequenced. In several cases, the activity of purified receptors has been reconstituted in artificial systems.

Three phases of receptor-mediated signaling can be identified

The first is the binding component in which an extracellular ligand, usually a polar molecule, forms a complex with a cell-surface receptor, which can be localized on either a pre- or a postsynaptic membrane. The second phase is that in which the activated receptor–ligand complex elicits an increase in either the formation of second messengers, the opening or closing of ion channels or the recruitment of cytoplasmic proteins. The third phase typically involves the activation of enzymes, typically protein kinases or phosphatases, which mediate the biological response. Thus, the initial interaction of a ligand with a receptor results in amplification of the signal by means of a cascade of responses.

Four distinct molecular mechanisms that link agonist occupancy of cell-surface receptors to functional responses have been identified

Traditionally, receptors have been classified according to the mediator to which they respond. The first example, proposed by Sir Henry Dale in 1914, was that the neurotransmitter ACh can interact with two types of AChRs, termed either nicotinic or muscarinic AChRs based on the similarity of action of ACh to the plant alkaloids nicotine and muscarine. Similarly, Ahlquist pro-

posed the division of adrenergic receptors into α and β subtypes, based on the potency of a series of natural and synthetic agonists to elicit a biological response. Although the pharmacological characterization of receptors provided a useful starting point, it rapidly became apparent that extensive subclassification of receptors would be required. For example, it is now recognized that there are both neural and non-neural forms of the nAChR, which can be distinguished pharmacologically and biochemically. In addition, multiple adrenergic receptor subtypes, including α_1, α_2, β_1, β_2 and β_3, can be distinguished based on the ability of selective agonists and antagonists to bind to them. Although the pharmacological division of receptors remains that most commonly employed, an alternative classification is based on the effector mechanism to which receptors are linked.

This classification leads to four distinct groups based on the types of primary effector to which they couple [33] (Fig. 10-9). The first group is comprised of receptors which possess intrinsic ion channels that are composed of multiple subunits. Upon the binding of an agonist to these ligand-gated ion channels, the receptors undergo a conformational change which facilitates opening of the intrinsic ion channel. The permeability to specific ions is a characteristic of the receptor; for example, both the neuronal nAChR and NMDA receptors are selectively permeable to Na^+ and Ca^{2+} ions, whereas $GABA_A$ and glycine receptors are primarily permeable to Cl^- ions. As a result of the changes in ion conductance, the membrane potential may become either depolarized, as in nAChR or NMDA receptors, or hyperpolarized, as in $GABA_A$ or glycine receptors. Receptors in this category include those that are activated by synaptically released neurotransmitter and occur on the cell surface. The responses to these cell-surface receptors are extremely rapid, occurring in milliseconds, and do not require either the subsequent generation of second-messenger molecules or protein phosphorylation events. Thus, ligand-gated ion channels mediate "fast synaptic" transmission events in the CNS. The intracellular ligand-gated receptor for IP_3 also opens within milliseconds upon binding of IP_3 (see Chap. 21).

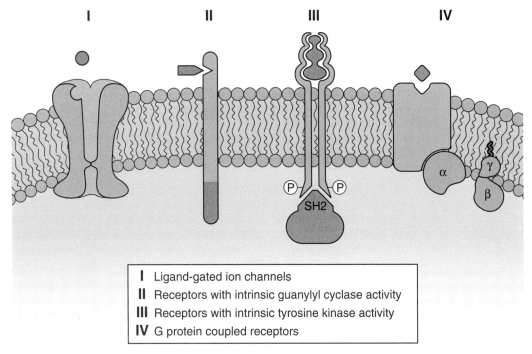

FIGURE 10-9. Cell-surface receptors utilize four distinct molecular mechanisms for transmembrane signaling. *I:* Ligand-gated ion channels. *II:* Receptors which possess intrinsic guanylyl cyclase activity. *III:* Receptors with intrinsic tyrosine kinase activity. *IV:* G protein–coupled receptors, which are linked to the opening/closing of ion channels, modulation of adenylyl cyclase and phosphoinositide-specific phospholipase C activities. *SH2,* src homology 2 domain.

Receptors in the second group possess intrinsic guanylyl cyclase activity and generate cGMP upon receptor activation, for example, brain natriuretic peptide receptor. These receptors consist of an extracellular binding domain, a single transmembrane-spanning domain (TMD), a protein kinase-like domain and a guanylyl cyclase catalytic domain. Ligand binding results in a conformational change in the receptor and activation of the guanylyl cyclase catalytic region. Membrane-bound guanylyl cyclase activity does not require Ca^{2+} and can be modulated by ligand addition to cell-free preparations. A different, cytoplasmic form of guanylyl cyclase is activated by micromolar concentrations of Ca^{2+}. Receptors with intrinsic guanylyl cyclase activity are often very highly phosphorylated in the absence of agonist and rapidly undergo dephosphorylation upon activation (see Chap. 24).

Receptors in the third group possess intrinsic receptor tyrosine kinase (RTK) activity. RTKs, such as epidermal growth factor receptor (EGFR) and platelet-derived growth factor receptor (PDGFR), are found in all multicellular eukaryotic organisms and are involved in the regulation of cellular growth and differentiation (see Chaps. 19 and 25). Structurally, RTKs possess an extracellular ligand-binding domain, a single TMD and an intracellular catalytic kinase domain. Three distinct events underlie signal transduction at RTKs. Initially, upon ligand binding to an RTK, the receptor undergoes a dimerization which results in the juxtaposition of the two cytoplasmic domains. Contact between these domains is thought to result in a stimulation of catalytic activity, which in turn results in an intermolecular autophosphorylation of tyrosine residues both within and outside of the kinase domain. The significance of the phosphorylation of tyrosine residues lies in the subsequent ability of the RTK to recruit cytoplasmic proteins which possess src homology 2 (SH2) domains. These regions of the molecule are 60 to 100 amino acids in length, are globular in structure, protrude from the surface of the protein and permit high-affinity protein–protein interactions to occur. In the case of the SH2 domain, a key arginine residue buried deep in a specific binding pocket interacts with the phosphate group of the tyrosine residue. The presence of an SH2 domain can increase the affinity of a peptide for a phosphorylated tyrosine residue by 1,000-fold. Once autophosphorylated, RTKs can recruit a number of cytoplasmic proteins and initiate a series of reactions involving protein–protein interactions. The best studied pathway of this type is the mitogen-activated protein kinase (MAPK) pathway. RTKs, via the recruitment of an adaptor protein complex such as growth factor receptor–binding protein 2 (Grb2)/son of sevenless (SOS) or SHC (see Chap. 25) can activate Ras, a low-molecular-weight, monomeric G protein. The role of Ras is to recruit and activate Raf (MAPKKK), a serine/threonine kinase, which in turn activates MEK (MAPKK), a dual-specificity tyrosine/ threonine kinase. MEK subsequently activates MAPK, also known as ERK or extracellular signal–regulated kinase, which is a serine/threonine kinase with multiple substrates. ERK can enter the nucleus and regulate gene transcription by phosphorylating nuclear proteins (see Chap. 24).

The fourth group of receptors involves G proteins. Numerically, more diverse types of receptors have been demonstrated to operate via an intervening G protein than by any other mechanism. These G protein–coupled receptors (GPCRs), which have a characteristic seven TMD structure, can be further divided into three categories. Some GPCRs, such as $GABA_B$, α_2-adrenergic, D2-dopaminergic or muscarinic M2, regulate the changes in K^+ conductance independently of second-messenger production (see Chap. 20). A second group of GPCRs is linked to the modulation of adenylyl cyclase activity. This regulation may be either positive, as in the case of activation of the β_2-adrenergic receptor, or negative, as occurs following activation of the α_2-adrenergic receptor. Changes in the concentrations of cAMP regulate the activity of protein kinase A (PKA) (Chap. 22). A third group of GPCRs is linked to the activation of PI-PLC with the attendant breakdown of PIP_2 and formation of IP_3 and DAG (see Chap. 21). These receptors are linked to changes in Ca^{2+} homeostasis and protein phosphorylation via the action of protein kinase C (PKC). Other effector enzymes that may be regulated by IP_3-linked GPCRs include phospholipases A_2 and D.

Cross-talk can occur between intracellular signaling pathways

Most cells possess receptors that operate through each of these four distinct effector mechanisms. Receptors within each class may be subject to further regulation during persistent agonist occupancy. One way that this can occur is via phosphorylation of the receptor, which results in its uncoupling from the effector enzyme, as has been demonstrated for the β-adrenergic receptor (see Chap. 12). This has been called *homologous regulation*. In addition, signaling pathways do not operate in isolation but may regulate and be regulated by one another, which has been termed *heterologous regulation*. In this way, the output of the cell is fine-tuned via subtle modulation of the relevant intracellular signaling mechanisms. There are numerous examples in which the activity of one receptor can regulate, either positively or negatively, the activity of a second; for example, increases in cAMP mediated by PKA can depress or potentiate PI-PLC activity (reviewed in [34]). Conversely, activation of PI-PLC can result in modulation of the activity of other pathways via the activation of PKC. An additional complexity is that the same ligand may activate multiple pathways in a given tissue. For example, NE can activate β_2-adrenergic receptors, which increase adenylyl cyclase; α_2-adrenergic receptors, which are coupled to inhibition of adenylyl cyclase; and α_1-adrenergic receptors, which are linked to the activation of PI-PLC. Similarly, ACh can activate muscarinic cholinergic receptors, which either inhibit adenylyl cyclase, activate PI-PLC or activate K^+ channels. In addition, ACh can directly activate nAChRs, which are linked to changes in Na^+ and Ca^{2+} permeability. Thus, although individual signaling mechanisms are most frequently studied in isolation, their activity *in vivo* is likely to be highly regulated by other signal-transduction events.

A further consideration is that receptors which primarily activate one pathway may, on occasion, activate a second pathway (Fig. 10-10). An example is the ability of GPCRs, such as α_2-adrenergic receptors or mAChRs, to activate the MAPK cascade. Activation of adenylyl cyclase-linked receptors results in the release of G protein $\beta\gamma$ subunits, which, probably via an intermediary protein tyrosine kinase (PTK-X), stimulates phosphorylation of the adaptor protein SHC [35]. This in turn recruits the Grb2–SOS complex and activates the MAPK pathway.

Activation of PI-PLC-linked receptors, such as the mAChR, results in increased PKC activity. Since the addition of phorbol esters, which are PKC agonists (Chap. 21), results in phosphorylation of Raf, this mechanism may provide an explanation for the ability of PI-PLC-coupled receptors to activate MAPK. A recently discovered protein tyrosine kinase PYK2, which is enriched in the CNS, is also activated by PKC. Like PTK-X, PYK2 phosphorylates SHC and recruits the Grb2–SOS complex, which results in activation of the MAPK cascade. PYK2 is also activated by Ca^{2+}, raising the possibility that the activity of ligand-gated ion channels can also modulate the MAPK pathway. However, to date, there is no evidence to suggest that this regulation is reciprocal, that is, that activation of the MAPK pathway can modulate the activity of either GPCRs or ligand-gated ion channels.

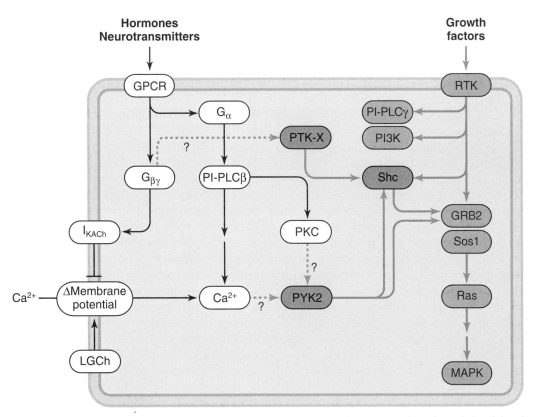

FIGURE 10-10. Cross-talk between G protein–coupled receptors *(GPCRs)*, ligand-gated ion channels *(LGChs)* and receptor protein tyrosine kinases *(RTKs)*. GPCRs, via activation of PTK-X or PYK2, can activate the mitogen-activated protein kinase *(MAPK)* pathway. LGChs, via an increase in $[Ca^{2+}]_i$, may also activate PYK2. Note that the key "go-between" molecule is the adaptor protein Shc, which in turn can interact with growth factor receptor–binding protein 2 *(GRB2)*/son of sevenless *(Sos1)* to activate the MAPK pathway. Question marks indicate that the pathways of activation still need to be firmly established. I_{KACh}, inwardly rectifying, acetylcholine-regulated channel; *PI3K,* phosphatidylinositol 3-kinase; *PKC,* protein kinase C; *PI-PLC,* phosphoinositide-specific phospholipase C. (Adapted from [35], with permission.)

Signaling molecules can activate gene transcription

In addition to their ability to elicit acute effects within cells, second-messenger molecules, such as cAMP, Ca^{2+} and DAG, can regulate gene transcription. The transcription factors cAMP response element–binding (CREB) protein, fos and jun, which respond to these signaling molecules, are members of the amphipathic helix family of proteins, and each contains a characteristic "leucine zipper," which mediates dimerization (Chap. 26). The best studied of these transcription factors is CREB, which becomes phosphorylated on Ser^{133} in response to increases in the intracellular concentration of cAMP and subsequent activation of PKA. CREB can also be phosphorylated by Ca^{2+}/calmodulin-dependent protein kinase IV. In its phosphorylated form, CREB binds to an eight-base *cis*-regulatory sequence called cAMP response element (CRE) and stimulates transcription. CREB has been implicated in long-term potentiation and memory (see Chap. 50). Increased concentrations of cytoplasmic Ca^{2+} and DAG activate PKC, which can also activate gene transcription via fos and jun. Activation of the MAPK pathway also leads to increased expression of jun and fos. Because increases in mRNA for fos and jun are observed very rapidly following a variety of stimuli, they have been termed *immediate early genes*. The fos–jun heterodimers, termed AP-1, bind to a seven-base pair *cis*-regulatory element called tetradecanoyl-phorbol acetate (TPA) response element (TRE). The latter has been demonstrated to control the transcription of several genes coding for neuropeptide modulators. Thus, despite major differences in the initial molecular mechanisms that underlie activation of RTKs or receptors coupled to either adenylyl cyclase or PI-PLC, these diverse groups of receptors share at least one common end point, that of gene regulation.

Nitric oxide acts as an intercellular signaling molecule in the central nervous system

Because cells rarely act in isolation, a signaling event in one cell may have a significant impact on the activity of neighboring cells. Initial evidence for intercellular, nonsynaptic signaling was obtained from experiments with blood vessels, in which it was observed that the addition of ACh increased cGMP concentrations and resulted in vasodilation and relaxation of the vascular smooth muscle. The increases in cGMP concentrations were dependent on the presence of Ca^{2+} and could not be demonstrated in tissue homogenates. A key observation was that removal of the endothelium abolished the relaxing effect of ACh, indicating the existence of an *endothelium-derived relaxing factor* (EDRF). Subsequently, it was discovered that EDRF was a short-lived gaseous molecule, nitric oxide (NO). NO is synthesized from arginine via the Ca^{2+} activation of nitric oxide synthase (NOS), an enzyme that requires NADPH as coenzyme and tetrahydrobiopterin as cofactor. Three distinct forms of NOS have been identified. An inducible form (iNOS), which is present in glia; a neuronal form (nNOS), which is widespread in distribution throughout the CNS; and an endothelial enzyme (eNOS) [36]. The activity of both nNOS and eNOS is Ca^{2+}/calmodulin-dependent, whereas that of iNOS is Ca^{2+}-insensitive. More recent evidence suggests that the activity of nNOS can be increased by brain lesions or ischemia (see Chap. 34). As a signaling molecule, NO differs from conventional neurotransmitters in that (i) it is not present in synaptic vesicles, (ii) it is not released by exocytosis and (iii) no specific extracellular synaptic receptors for NO exist. Rather, NO is released upon stimulation and diffuses from its site of production, which can be either neuronal or glial cells, to affect neurons up to 100 μm away. At these locations, NO activates a soluble form of guanylyl cyclase through electron transfer to the heme group on the enzyme. The increase in cGMP concentration subsequently activates cGMP-dependent protein kinases. In the CNS, NO has been speculated to play a role in both long-term potentiation (LTP) and long-term depression, although the precise mechanism remains to be defined. One counterargument for a role of NO in LTP is the observation that the latter persists in transgenic mice lacking nNOS. Recent evidence suggests that NO can also post-translationally modify sulfhydryl groups on synaptic vesicle proteins, thereby facilitating synaptic vesicle exocytosis [37].

It is conceivable that other gaseous molecules may also act as intercellular messengers. One putative candidate is carbon monoxide, which is generated from the conversion of heme to biliverdin, a reaction catalyzed by an oxygenase. One form of the enzyme, heme oxygenase-2, is constitutive and is found in high concentrations in various brain regions. Like NO, CO increases the production of cGMP.

Intercellular signaling may also occur via other mechanisms. For example, cell–cell propagation of Ca^{2+} signals can result from the gap junctional transfer of IP_3 [38]. Alternatively, the release of humoral factors such as 5-HT, glutamate and nucleotides can initiate intercellular signaling. Thus, ATP and ADP released from human neuroepithelioma cells in response to a rise in the concentration of intracellular Ca^{2+} serves to further the propagation of intercellular Ca^{2+} signals [39]. Within the CNS, glutamate released from glia can activate receptors on neurons [40]. An additional consideration is that the secreted factor may act in an autocrine fashion. Thus, prostaglandins released from myenteric neurons in response to the addition of bradykinin can modulate the subsequent Ca^{2+} influx mediated by bradykinin receptors [40].

ACKNOWLEDGMENTS

This work was supported by NS 23831 and MH46252 (SKF) and DK 27959 (RWH).

REFERENCES

1. Davenport, H. W. Early history of the concept of chemical transmission of the nerve impulse. *Physiologist* 34:129–190, 1991.
2. Njus, D., Kelley, P., and Harnadek, G. J. Bioenergetics of secretory vesicles. *Biochim. Biophys. Acta* 853:237–265, 1987.
3. Schuldiner, S., Shirvan, A., and Michal, L. Vesicular neurotransmitter transporters: From bacteria to humans. *Physiol. Rev.* 75:369–391, 1995.
4. Palade, G. Intracellular aspects of the process of protein synthesis. *Science* 189:347–358, 1975.
5. Neher, E., and Marty, A. Discrete changes of cell membrane capacitance observed under conditions of enhanced secretion in bovine adrenal chromaffin cells. *Proc. Natl. Acad. Sci. USA* 79:6712–6716, 1982.
6. Cahalan, M., and Neher, E. Patch clamp techniques: An overview. *Methods Enzymol.* 207:3–14, 1992.
7. Robinson, I. M., Finnegan, J. M., Monck, J. R., Wightman, R. M., and Fernandez, J. M. Colocalization of calcium entry and exocytotic release sites in adrenal chromaffin cells. *Proc. Natl. Acad. Sci. USA* 92:2474–2478, 1995.
8 Fatt, P., and Katz, B. Spontaneous subthreshold activity at motor nerve endings. *J. Physiol. (Lond.)* 117:109–128, 1952.
9. Nichols, J. G., Martin, A. R., and Wallace, B. G. *From Neuron to Brain.* Sunderland, MA: Sinauer Associates, 1992.
10. Heuser, J. E., and Reese, T. S. Structure of the synapse. In E. R. Kandel (ed.), *Handbook of Physiology. The Nervous System. Cellular Biology of Neurons.* Bethesda: American Physiological Society, 1977, Sect. 1, Vol. I, pp. 261–294.
11. Heuser, J. E. Synaptic vesicle exocytosis revealed in quick-frozen frog NMJ treated with 4-aminopyridine and given a single electric shock. In W. M. Cowan and J. Ferrendelli (eds.), *Approaches to the Cell Biology of Neurons.* Bethesda: Society for Neuroscience, 1976, pp. 215–239.
12. Del Castillo, J., and Katz, B. Quantal components of the end-plate potential. *J. Physiol. (Lond.)* 124:560–573, 1954.
13. Martin, A. R. Junctional transmission II. Presynaptic mechanisms. In E. R. Kandel (ed.), *Handbook of Physiology. The Nervous System. Cellular Biology of Neurons.* Bethesda: American Physiological Society, 1977, Sect. 1, Vol. I, pp. 329–355.
14. Katz, B., and Miledi, R. The timing of calcium action during neuromuscular transmission. *J. Physiol. (Lond.)* 189:535–544, 1967.
15. Liley, A. W. The quantal components of the mammalian end-plate potential. *J. Physiol. (Lond.)* 133:571–587, 1956.
16. Boyd, I. A., and Martin, A. R. The end-plate potential in mammalian muscle. *J. Physiol. (Lond.)* 132:74–91, 1956.
17. Simon, S. M., and Llinás, R. R. Compartmentalization of the submembrane calcium activity during calcium influx and its significance in transmitter release. *Biophys. J.* 48:485–498, 1985.
18. Augustine, G. J., Adler, E. M., and Charlton, M. P. The calcium signal for transmitter secretion from presynaptic nerve terminals. *Ann. N. Y. Acad. Sci.* 635:365–381, 1991.
19. Zucker, R. S. Exocytosis: A molecular and physiological perspective. *Neuron* 17:1049–1055, 1996.

20. Sabatini, B. L., and Regehr, W. G. Timing of neurotransmission at fast synapses in mammalian brain. *Nature* 384:170–172, 1996.

21. De Camilli, P., and Takei, K. Molecular mechanisms in synaptic vesicle endocytosis and recycling. *Neuron* 16:481–486, 1996.

22. Llinás, R. R. Calcium in synaptic transmission. *Sci. Amer.* 247(4):56–65, 1982.

23. Heuser, J. E., and Reese, T. S. Evidence for recycling of synaptic vesicle membrane during transmitter release at the frog NMJ. *J. Cell Biol.* 57:315–344, 1973.

24. Ceccarelli, B., Hurlbut, P., and Mauro, A. Turnover of transmitter and synaptic vesicles at the frog NMJ. *J. Cell Biol.* 57:499–524, 1973.

25. Betz, W. J., and Bewick, G. S. Optical analysis of synaptic vesicle recycling at the frog NMJ. *Science* 255:200–203, 1992.

26. Ryan, T. A., and Smith, S. J. Vesicle pool mobilization during action potential firing at hippocampal synapses. *Neuron* 14:983–989, 1995.

27. Holz, R. W., Bittner, M. A., and Senter, R. A. Regulated exocytotic fusion I: Chromaffin cells and PC12 cells. *Methods Enzymol.* 219:165–178, 1992.

28. Martin, T. F. J., and Walent, J. H. A new method for cell permeabilization reveals a cytosolic protein requirement for Ca^{2+}-activated secretion in GH_3 pituitary cells. *J. Biol. Chem.* 264:10299–10308, 1989.

29. Neher, E., and Zucker, R. S. Multiple calcium-dependent processes related to secretion in bovine chromaffin cells. *Neuron* 10:21–30, 1993.

30. Eberhard, D. A., Cooper, C. L., Low, M. G., and Holz, R. W. Evidence that the inositol phospholipids are necessary for exocytosis: Loss of inositol phospholipids and inhibition of secretion in permeabilized cells caused by a bacterial phospholipase C and removal of ATP. *Biochem. J.* 268:15–25, 1990.

31. Hay, J. C., and Martin, T. F. J. Phosphatidylinositol transfer protein required for ATP-dependent priming of Ca^{2+}-activated secretion. *Nature* 366:572–575, 1993.

32. Hay, J. C., Fisette, P. L., Jenkins, G. H., et al. ATP-dependent inositide phosphorylation required for Ca^{2+}-activated secretion. *Nature* 374:173–177, 1995.

33. Neubig, R. R., and Thomsen, W. J. How does a key fit a flexible lock? Structure and dynamics in receptor function. *Bioessays* 11:136–141, 1989.

34. Fisher, S. K. Homologous and heterologous regulation of receptor-stimulated phosphoinositide hydrolysis. *Eur. J. Pharmacol.* 288:231–250, 1995.

35. Bourne, H. R. Team blue sees red. *Nature* 376:727–729, 1995.

36. Bredt, D. S., and Snyder, S. H. Nitric oxide: A physiological messenger molecule. *Annu. Rev. Biochem.* 63:175–195, 1994.

37. Meffert, M. K., Calakos, N. C., Scheller, R. H., and Schulman, H. Nitric oxide modulates synaptic vesicle docking/fusion reactions. *Neuron* 16:1229–1236, 1996.

38. Boitano, S., Dirksen, E. R., and Sanderson, M. J. Intercellular propagation of calcium waves mediated by inositol trisphosphate. *Science* 258:292–295, 1992.

39. Palmer, R. K., Yule, D. I., Shewach, D. S., Williams, J. A., and Fisher, S. K. Paracrine mediation of calcium signaling in human SK-N-MCIXC neuroepithelioma cells. *Am. J. Physiol.* 271 *(Cell Physiol.* 40):C43–C53, 1996.

40. Parpura, V., Basarsky, T. A., Liu, F., Jeftinija, K., Jeftinija, S., and Haydon, P. G. Glutamate-mediated astrocyte–neuron signalling. *Nature* 369:744–747, 1994.

41. Gelperin, D., Mann, D., Del Valle, J., and Wiley, J. Bradykinin (BK) increases cytosolic calcium in cultured rat myenteric neurons via BK-2 type receptors coupled to mobilization of extracellular and intracellular sources of calcium: Evidence that calcium influx is prostaglandin dependent. *J. Pharmacol. Exp. Ther.* 271:507–514, 1994.

11

Acetylcholine

Palmer Taylor and Joan Heller Brown

Basic Neurochemistry: Molecular, Cellular and Medical Aspects, 6th Ed., edited by G. J. Siegel et al. Published by Lippincott–Raven Publishers, Philadelphia, 1999. Correspondence to Palmer Taylor and Joan Heller Brown, Department of Pharmacology, 0636, University of California, San Diego, La Jolla, California 92093.

There is considerable evidence that acetylcholine (ACh) arrived within the evolutionary scheme long before the design of the nervous system and functional synapses. Bacteria, fungi, protozoa and plants store ACh and possess biosynthetic and degradative capacities for turnover of the molecule. Even in higher organisms, ACh distribution is far wider than the nervous system. For example, ACh is found in the cornea, certain ciliated epithelia, the spleen of ungulates and the human placenta [1]. Although definitive evidence is lacking, ACh has been proposed to play a role in development and tissue differentiation.

ACh was first proposed as a mediator of cellular function by Hunt in 1907, and in 1914 Dale [2] pointed out that its action closely mimicked the response of parasympathetic nerve stimulation (see Chap. 10). Loewi, in 1921, provided clear evidence for ACh release by nerve stimulation. Separate receptors that explained the variety of actions of ACh became apparent in Dale's early experiments [2]. The nicotinic ACh receptor was the first transmitter receptor to be purified and to have its primary structure determined [3,4]. The primary structures of several subtypes of both nicotinic and muscarinic receptors have been ascertained, as have the structures of cholinesterases, choline and ACh transporters and choline acetyltransferase (ChAT).

CHEMISTRY OF ACETYLCHOLINE

Torsional rotation in the ACh molecule can occur around bonds τ_1, τ_2 and τ_3 (Fig. 11-1). Since the methyl groups are disposed symmetrically around τ_3 and constraints may be placed on τ_1 by the planar acetoxy group, the most important torsion angle determining ACh conformation in solution is τ_2. A view from the β-methylene carbon of the molecule (Fig. 11-1) shows the lowest energy configurations around τ_2. Nuclear magnetic resonance (NMR) studies indicate that the *gauche* conformation is predominant in solution [5,6]. Studies of the activities of rigid analogs of ACh suggest that the *trans* conformation may be the active conformation at muscarinic receptors [7], while results of NMR studies show that the

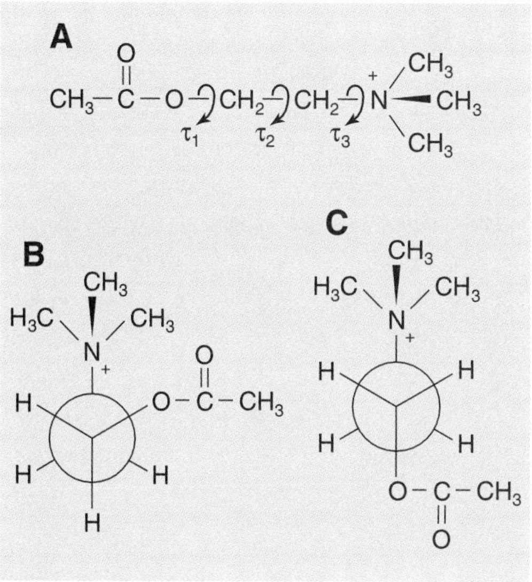

FIGURE 11-1. Structure of acetylcholine. **A:** The three torsion angles τ_1, τ_2 and τ_3. **B:** Newman projection of the *gauche* conformation. **C:** Newman projection of the *trans* conformation. The molecule is viewed in the plane of the paper from the left side, and the bond angles around τ_2 are compared.

naturally occurring agonists were determined (Fig. 11-3). The greatly different activities of the antagonists atropine on muscarinic receptors and *d*-tubocurarine on nicotinic receptors further supported the argument that multiple classes of receptors exist for ACh. Subsequently, it was found that all nicotinic receptors are not identical. Nicotinic receptors in the neuromuscular junction, sometimes denoted as N_1 receptors, show selectivity for phenyltrimethylammonium as an agonist; elicit membrane depolarization in the presence of bisquaternary agents, with decamethonium being the most potent; are preferentially blocked by the competitive antagonist *d*-tubocurarine; and are blocked irreversibly by the snake α-toxins. Nicotinic receptors in ganglia, N_2 receptors, are stimulated preferentially by 1,1-dimethyl-4-phenylpiperazinium; blocked competitively by trimethaphan; blocked noncompetitively by bisquaternary agents, with hexamethonium being the most potent; and resistant to the snake α-toxins [9]. A large number of distinct neuronal nicotinic receptors are found in the central nervous system (CNS); they are closer relatives of the nicotinic receptors in ganglia than of those in muscle.

Muscarinic receptors also exhibit distinct subtypes. The antagonist pirenzepine (PZ) has the highest affinity for one subtype, M_1, which is found mainly in neuronal tissues. Another antagonist, methoctramine, has a higher affinity for M_2 receptors, which are the predominant muscarinic receptor subtype in mammalian heart. Hexahydrosiladifenidol is relatively selective for the M_3 receptors present in smooth muscle and glands, whereas himbacine exhibits high affinity for M_4 receptors. With this level of multiplicity of receptor subtypes, limitations on specificity preclude a single antagonist defining a distinct subtype.

acetoxy and quaternary nitrogens in the bound state of ACh are too close together for this conformation to exist when ACh is bound to the nicotinic receptor [6]. Hence, the bound conformations of this flexible molecule appear to differ substantially with receptor subtype. This finding should not emerge as a great surprise since it has been known for years that the structural modifications that enhance or diminish activity on muscarinic receptors are very different from those modifications that influence activity on nicotinic receptors [8].

ORGANIZATION OF THE CHOLINERGIC NERVOUS SYSTEM

Acetylcholine receptors have been classified into subtypes based on the pharmacology of the receptors

Initially, subtyping of the receptors in the cholinergic nervous system was based on the pharmacological activity of two alkaloids: nicotine and muscarine (Fig. 11-2). This classification occurred long before the structures of these

The intrinsic complexity and the multiplicity of cholinergic receptors became evident upon elucidation of their primary structures

In the CNS, at least eight different sequences of α subunits and three different sequences of β subunits of the nicotinic receptor have been

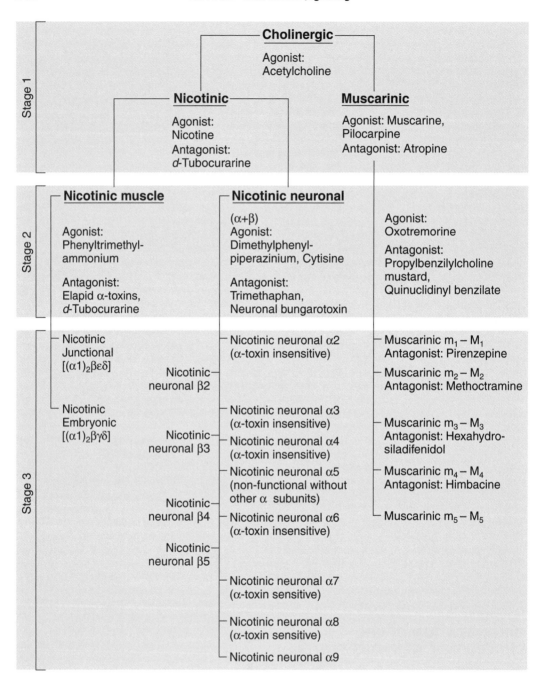

FIGURE 11-2. Classification of cholinergic receptors. The diagram shows a historical classification of receptors analyzed on the basis of distinct responses with crude alkaloids **(stage 1),** the partial resolution of receptor subtypes with chemically synthesized agonists and antagonists **(stage 2)** and the distinction of primary structures of the receptors principally through cloning by recombinant DNA techniques **(stage 3).**

FIGURE 11-3. Structure of compounds important to the classification of receptor subtypes at cholinergic synapses. Compounds are subdivided as nicotinic *(N)* and muscarinic *(M).* The compounds interacting with nicotinic receptors are subdivided further according to whether they are neuromuscular *(N$_1$)* or ganglionic *(N$_2$)*. Those compounds with greatest muscarinic subtype selectivity *(M$_1$, M$_2$, M$_3$, M$_4$)* are also noted.

Nicotinic and muscarinic agonists

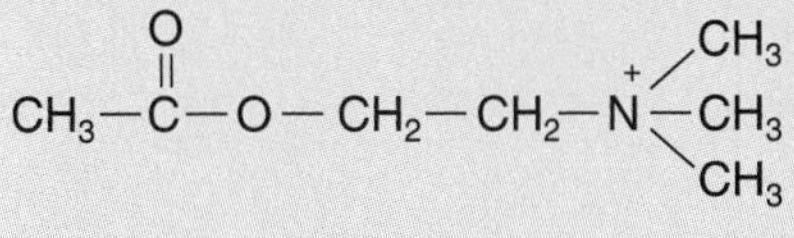

Acetylcholine (N + M)

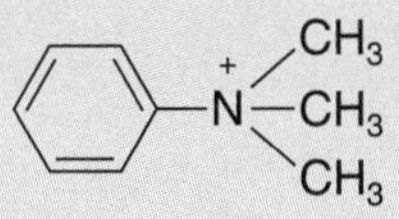

Phenyltrimethylammonium (N₁)

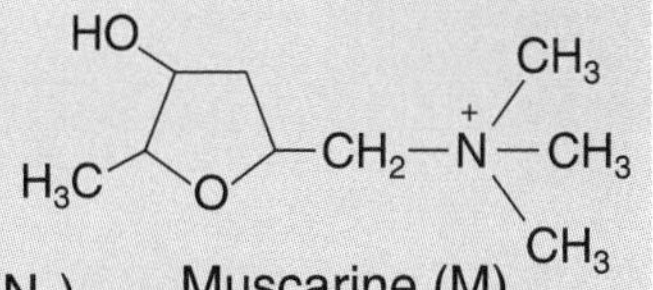

Muscarine (M)

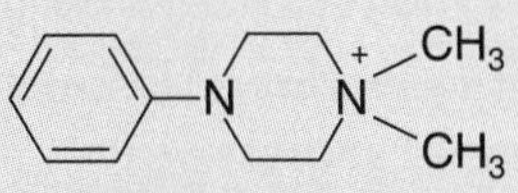

1,1-Dimethyl-4-phenylpiperazinium (N₂)

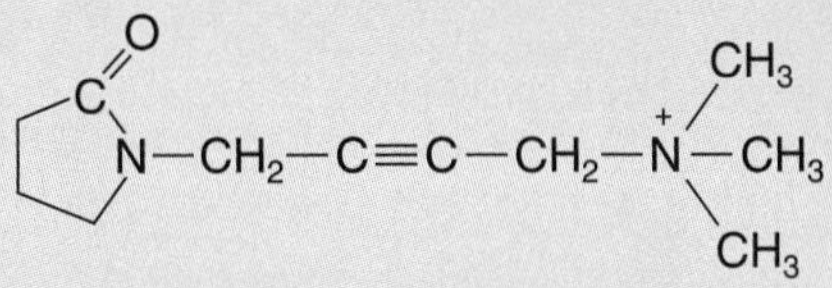

Oxotremorine-M (M)

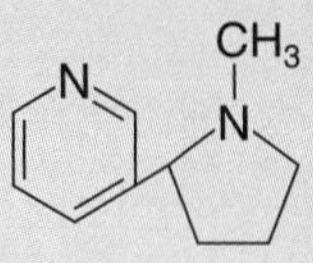

Nicotine (N₁ + N₂)

Nicotinic antagonists

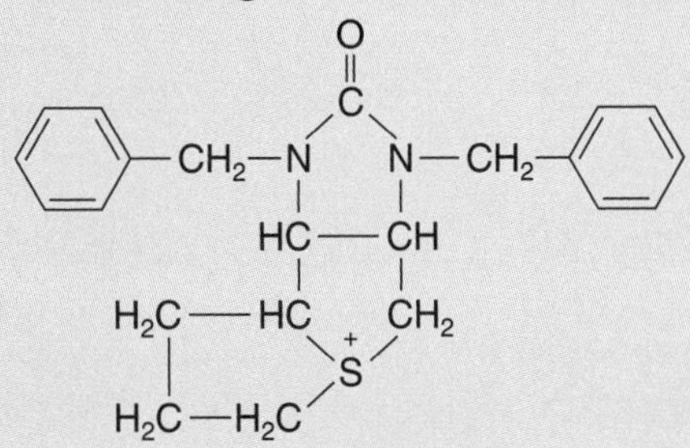

Trimethaphan (N₂)

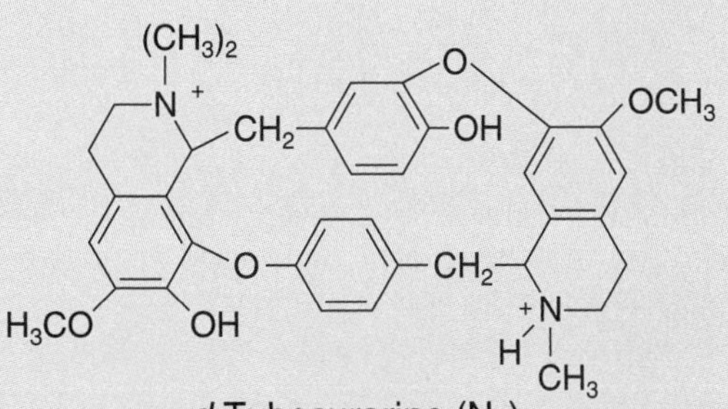

d-Tubocurarine (N₁)

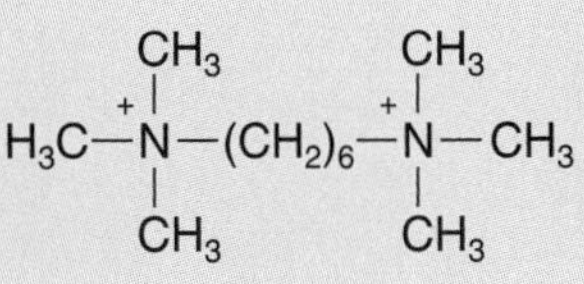

Hexamethonium (N₂)

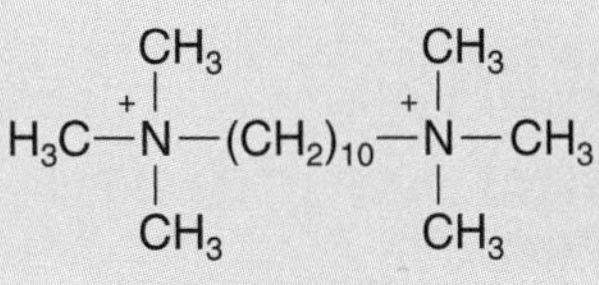

Decamethonium (N₁)

Muscarinic antagonists

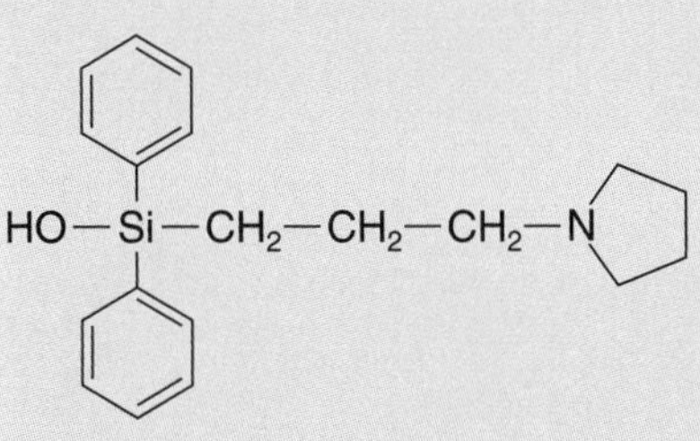

Hexahydrosiladifenidol (M₃)

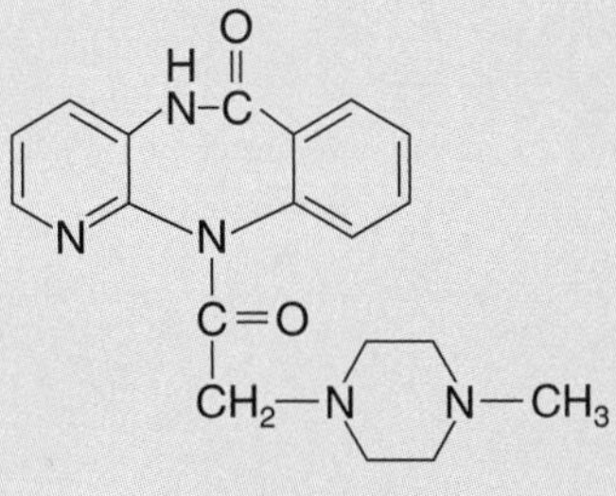

Pirenzepine (M₁)

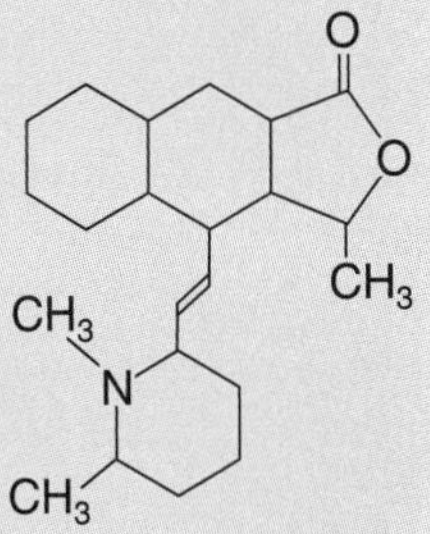

Himbacine (M₄)

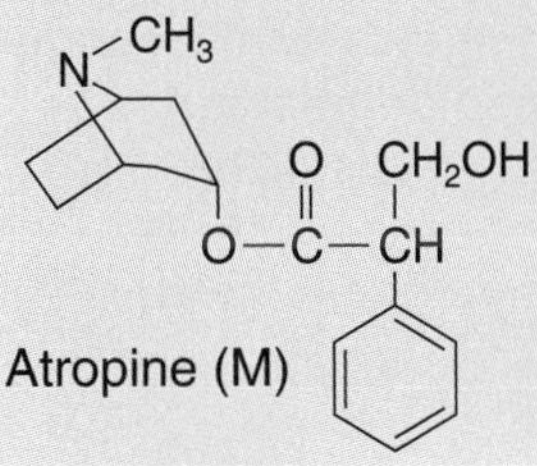

Atropine (M)

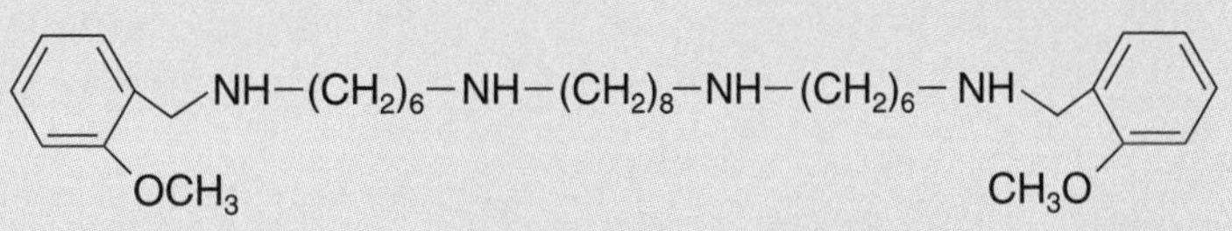

Methoctramine (M₂)

identified [10,11]. Expression of the cloned genes encoding certain subunit combinations yields functional receptors with different sensitivities toward various toxins and agonists.

At least five distinct muscarinic receptor genes have been cloned and sequenced. The genes are called m_1 to m_5. The m_1 to m_4 clones correlate with the M_1 to M_4 receptors identified pharmacologically. The subtypes differ in their ability to couple to different G proteins and, hence, to elicit cellular signaling events. The muscarinic and nicotinic receptor subtypes exhibit distinct regional locations of their mRNAs, based on *in situ* hybridization.

Thus, cholinergic receptor classification can be considered in terms of three stages of development. Initially, Dale [2] distinguished nicotinic and muscarinic receptor subtypes with crude alkaloids. Then, chemical synthesis and structure–activity relationships clearly revealed that nicotinic and muscarinic receptors were heterogeneous but could not come close to uncovering the true diversity of receptor subtypes. Lastly, analysis of subtypes comes from molecular cloning, which makes possible the classification of receptors on the basis of primary structure (Fig. 11-2).

FUNCTIONAL ASPECTS OF CHOLINERGIC NEUROTRANSMISSION

The individual subtypes of receptors often show discrete anatomical locations in the peripheral nervous system, and this has facilitated their classification. Nicotinic receptors are found in peripheral ganglia and skeletal muscle. Upon innervation of skeletal muscle, receptors congregate in the junctional or postsynaptic endplate area. Upon denervation or in noninnervated embryonic muscle, the receptors are distributed across the surface of the muscle, and these extrajunctional receptors are synthesized and degraded rapidly. Junctional receptors exhibit far slower rates of turnover and are distinguished by an ∈ subunit replacing a γ subunit in the assembled pentameric receptor.

Ganglionic nicotinic receptors are found on postsynaptic neurons in both parasympathetic and sympathetic ganglia and in the adrenal gland. Ganglionic nicotinic receptors

appear in tissues of neural crest embryonic origin and exhibit identical properties in sympathetic and parasympathetic ganglia.

Muscarinic receptors are responsible for postganglionic parasympathetic neurotransmission. Some responses originating in the sympathetic nervous system, such as sweating and piloerection, also are mediated through muscarinic receptors.

Both muscarinic and nicotinic responses are found in brain and spinal cord

A few specific central cholinergic pathways have been characterized. For example, Renshaw cells in the spinal cord play a role in modulating motoneuron activity by a feedback mechanism. Stimulation of Renshaw cells occurs through branches of the motoneuron, and the transmitter is ACh acting on nicotinic receptors. Both nicotinic and muscarinic receptors are widespread in the CNS. Muscarinic receptors with a high affinity for PZ, M_1 receptors, predominate in the hippocampus and cerebral cortex, whereas M_2 receptors predominate in the cerebellum and brainstem and M_4 receptors are most abundant in the striatum. Nicotinic receptors may be largely prejunctional. The mapping of cholinergic pathways in the brain continues to be pursued actively and relies on several techniques [12]. Histochemical studies utilizing antibodies selective for ChAT and presynaptic transport proteins, along with receptor autoradiography with labeled ligands, have produced detailed maps of the CNS. In addition, the nerve cell bodies containing the mRNA encoding these proteins have been defined through *in situ* hybridization with a cDNA or antisense mRNA. Studies involving iontophoretic application of transmitter, local stimulation and intracellular or cell-surface measurements of responses establish appropriate functional correlates.

Neurotransmission in autonomic ganglia is more complex than depolarization mediated by a single transmitter

In autonomic ganglia, the primary electrophysiological event following preganglionic nerve stimulation is the rapid depolarization of postsynaptic sites by released ACh acting on nicotinic receptors. This activation gives rise to an initial excitatory postsynaptic potential (EPSP), which is due to an inward current through a cation channel (see Chaps. 6 and 10). This mechanism is virtually identical to that in the neuromuscular junction, with an immediate onset of the depolarization and decay within a few milliseconds. Nicotinic antagonists such as trimethaphan competitively block ganglionic transmission, whereas agents such as hexamethonium produce blockade by occluding the channel. An action potential is generated in the postganglionic nerve when the initial EPSP attains a critical amplitude.

Several secondary events amplify or suppress this signal. These include the slow EPSP; the late, slow EPSP; and an inhibitory postsynaptic potential (IPSP). The slow EPSP is generated by ACh acting on muscarinic receptors and is blocked by atropine. It has a latency of approximately 1 sec and a duration of 30 to 60 sec. The late, slow EPSP can last for several minutes and is mediated by peptides found in ganglia, including substance P, angiotensin, leutinizing hormone-releasing hormone (LHRH) and the enkephalins. The slow EPSP and late, slow EPSP result from decreased K^+ conductance and are believed to regulate the sensitivity of the postsynaptic neuron to repetitive depolarization [13]. The IPSP seems to be mediated by the catecholamines, dopamine and/or norepinephrine and is blocked by α-adrenergic antagonists and atropine. ACh released from presynaptic terminals may act on a catecholamine-containing interneuron to stimulate the release of norepinephrine or dopamine. As in the case of the slow EPSP, the IPSP has a longer latency and duration of action than the fast EPSP. These secondary events vary with the individual ganglia and are believed to modulate the sensitivity to the primary event. Hence, drugs that selectively block the slow EPSP, such as atropine, will diminish the efficiency of ganglionic transmission rather than eliminate it. Similarly, drugs such as muscarine and the ganglion-selective muscarinic agonist McN-A-343 are not thought of as primary ganglionic stimulants. Rather, they enhance the initial EPSP under conditions of repetitive stimulation.

Since parasympathetic and sympathetic ganglia exhibit comparable sensitivities to nicotine and ACh in producing the initial EPSP, the pharmacological action of ganglionic stimulants depends on the profile of innervation to particular organs or tissues (Table 11-1). For example, blood vessels are innervated only by the sympathetic nervous system; thus, ganglionic stimulation should produce only vasoconstriction. Similarly, the pharmacological effects of ganglionic blockade will depend on which component of the autonomic nervous system is exerting the predominant tone at the effector organ.

Muscarinic receptors are widely distributed at postsynaptic parasympathetic effector sites

The response of systemically administered ACh is characteristic of stimulation of postganglionic ef-

---

TABLE 11-1.   **PREDOMINANCE OF SYMPATHETIC OR PARASYMPATHETIC TONE AT EFFECTOR SITES: EFFECTS OF AUTONOMIC GANGLIONIC BLOCKADE**

Site	Predominant tone	Primary effects of ganglionic blockade
Arterioles	Sympathetic (adrenergic)	Vasodilation, increased peripheral blood flow, hypotension
Veins	Sympathetic (adrenergic)	Dilation, pooling of blood, decreased venous return, decreased cardiac output
Heart	Parasympathetic (cholinergic)	Tachycardia
Iris	Parasympathetic (cholinergic)	Mydriasis
Ciliary muscle	Parasympathetic (cholinergic)	Cycloplegia (focus to far vision)
Gastrointestinal tract	Parasympathetic (cholinergic)	Reduced tone and motility of smooth muscle, constipation, decreased gastric and pancreatic secretions
Urinary bladder	Parasympathetic (cholinergic)	Urinary retention
Salivary glands	Parasympathetic (cholinergic)	Xerostomia
Sweat glands	Sympathetic (cholinergic)	Anhidrosis

fector sites rather than of ganglia. This is a consequence of the greater abundance of muscarinic receptors at effector sites in innervated tissues and the relatively poor blood flow to ganglia. Muscarinic receptors are found in visceral smooth muscle, in cardiac muscle, in secretory glands and in the endothelial cells of the vasculature. Except for endothelial cells, each of these sites receives cholinergic innervation. Responses can be excitatory or inhibitory, depending on the tissue. Even within a single tissue the responses may vary. For example, muscarinic stimulation causes gastrointestinal smooth muscle to depolarize and contract, except at sphincters, where hyperpolarization and relaxation are seen (Table 11-2). Smooth muscle in many tissues innervated by the cholinergic nervous system exhibits intrinsic electrical and/or mechanical activity. This activity is modulated rather than initiated by cholinergic nerve stimulation. Cardiac muscle and smooth muscle exhibit spikes of electrical activity that are propagated between cells. These spikes are initiated by rhythmic fluctuations in resting membrane potential. In intestinal smooth muscle, cholinergic stimulation will cause a partial depolarization and increase the frequency by spike production. In contrast, cholinergic stimulation of atria will decrease the generation of spikes through hyperpolarization of the membrane.

Membrane depolarization typically results from an increase in Na^+ conductance. In addi-

tion, mobilization of intracellular Ca^{2+} from the endoplasmic or sarcoplasmic reticulum and the influx of extracellular Ca^{2+} appear to be elicited by ACh acting on muscarinic receptors (see Chap. 23). The resulting increase in intracellular free Ca^{2+} is involved in activation of contractile, metabolic and secretory events. Stimulation of muscarinic receptors has been linked to changes in cyclic nucleotide concentrations. Reductions in cAMP concentrations and increases in cGMP concentrations are typical responses (see Chap. 22). These cyclic nucleotides may facilitate contraction or relaxation, depending on the particular tissue. Inhibitory responses also are associated with membrane hyperpolarization, and this is a consequence of an increased K^+ conductance. Increases in K^+ conductance may be mediated by a direct receptor linkage to a K^+ channel or by increases in intracellular Ca^{2+}, which in turn activate K^+ channels. The mechanisms through which muscarinic receptors couple to multiple cellular responses are considered later.

Stimulation of the motoneuron for skeletal muscle results in the release of acetylcholine and contraction of the skeletal muscle fibers

Contraction and associated electrical events can be produced by intra-arterial injection of ACh close to the muscle. Since skeletal muscle does

---

TABLE 11-2. **EFFECTS OF ACETYLCHOLINE (ACh) STIMULATION ON PERIPHERAL TISSUES**

Tissue	Effects of ACh
Vasculature (endothelial cells)	Release of endothelium-derived relaxing factor (nitric oxide) and vasodilation
Eye iris (pupillae sphincter muscle)	Contraction and miosis
Ciliary muscle	Contraction and accommodation of lens to near vision
Salivary glands and lacrimal glands	Secretion—thin and watery
Bronchi	Constriction, increased secretions
Heart	Bradycardia, decreased conduction (atrioventricular block at high doses), small negative inotropic action
Gastrointestinal tract	Increased tone, increased gastrointestinal secretions, relaxation at sphincters
Urinary bladder	Contraction of detrusor muscle, relaxation of the sphincter
Sweat glands	Diaphoresis
Reproductive tract, male	Erection
Uterus	Variable, dependent on hormone influence

not possess inherent myogenic tone, the tone of apparently resting muscle is maintained by spontaneous and intermittent release of ACh. The consequences of spontaneous release at the motor endplate of skeletal muscle are small depolarizations from the quantized release of ACh, termed *miniature endplate potentials* (MEPPs) [14] (see Chap. 10). Decay times for the MEPPs range between 1 and 2 msec, a value of about the same duration as the mean channel open time seen with ACh stimulation of individual receptor molecules. Stimulation of the motoneuron results in the release of several hundred quanta of ACh. The summation of MEPPs gives rise to a postsynaptic excitatory potential (PSEP), also termed *motor endplate potential*. A sufficiently large and abrupt potential change at the endplate will elicit an action potential by activating voltage-sensitive Na^+ channels. The action potential propagates in two-dimensional space across the surface of the muscle to release Ca^{2+} and elicit contraction. Therefore, the PSEP may be thought of as a generator potential. It is found only in junctional regions and arises from the opening of the receptor channel. Normal resting potentials in endplates are about -70 mV. The PSEP causes the endplate to depolarize partially to about -55 mV. It is the rapid and transient changes from -70 to -55 mV in localized areas of the endplate that triggers action potential generation [9,14].

Competitive blocking agents cause muscle paralysis by preventing access of acetylcholine to its binding site on the receptor

Competitive blockade with agents such as *d*-tubocurarine result in maintenance of the endplate potential at -70 mV. Without frequent PSEPs, action potentials are not triggered and there is flaccid paralysis of the muscle. The actions of competitive blocking agents can be surmounted by excess ACh. Depolarizing neuromuscular blocking agents, such as decamethonium and succinylcholine, produce depolarization of the endplate such that the endplate potential is -55 mV. The high concentrations of depolarizing agent that are maintained in this synapse do not allow regions of the end-plate to repolarize, as would occur with a labile transmitter such as ACh. Since it is the transition between -70 and -55 mV that triggers the action potential, flaccid paralysis also will occur with a depolarizing block [9]. Excess ACh will not reverse the paralysis by depolarizing blocking agents. As might be expected if depolarization occurs in a nonuniform manner in microscopic areas within individual endplates and in individual motor units, the onset of depolarization blockade is characterized by muscle twitching and fasciculations that are not evident in competitive block. Once paralysis occurs, the overall pharmacological actions of competitive and depolarizing blocking agents are similar, yet intracellular measurements of endplate potential can distinguish these two classes of agent.

SYNTHESIS, STORAGE AND RELEASE OF ACETYLCHOLINE

Acetylcholine is synthesized from its two immediate precursors, choline and acetyl coenzyme A

The synthesis reaction is a single step catalyzed by the enzyme ChAT (EC 2.3.1.6):

$$\text{Choline} + \text{Acetyl coenzyme A}$$
$$\rightleftharpoons \text{Acetylcholine} + \text{Coenzyme A}$$

ChAT, first assayed in a cell-free preparation in 1943, subsequently has been purified and cloned from several sources [15]. The purification of ChAT has allowed production of specific antibodies. Whereas acetylcholinesterase (AChE), the enzyme responsible for degradation of ACh, is produced by cells containing cholinoreceptive sites as well as in cholinergic neurons, ChAT is found in the nervous system specifically at sites where ACh synthesis takes place. Within cholinergic neurons, ChAT is concentrated in nerve terminals, although it is also present in axons, where it is transported from its site of synthesis in the soma. When subcellular fractionation studies are carried out, ChAT is recovered in the synaptosomal fraction, and within synaptosomes it is primarily cytoplasmic. It has been suggested that ChAT also binds to the outside of the storage vesicle under physiological conditions and that ACh synthesized in that location may be situated favorably to enter the vesicle.

Brain ChAT has a K_D for choline of approximately 1 mM and for acetyl coenzyme A (CoA) of approximately 10 μM. The activity of the isolated enzyme, assayed in the presence of optimal concentrations of cofactors and substrates, appears far greater than the rate at which choline is converted to ACh *in vivo*. This suggests that the activity of ChAT is repressed *in vivo*. Inhibitors of ChAT do not decrease ACh synthesis when used *in vivo;* this may reflect a failure to achieve a sufficient local concentration of inhibitor but also suggests that this step is not rate-limiting in the synthesis of ACh.

The acetyl CoA used for ACh synthesis in mammalian brain comes from pyruvate formed from glucose. It is uncertain how the acetyl CoA, generally thought to be formed at the inner membrane of the mitochondria, accesses the cytoplasmic ChAT, and it is possible that this is a rate-limiting step.

Acetylcholine formation is limited by the intracellular concentration of choline, which is determined by uptake of choline into the nerve ending

Choline is present in the plasma at a concentration of about 10 μM. A "low-affinity" choline uptake system with a K_m of 10 to 100 μM is present in all tissues, but cholinergic neurons also have an Na^+-dependent "high-affinity" choline uptake system, with a K_m for choline of 1 to 5 μM [16]. The high-affinity uptake mechanisms should be saturated at 10 μM choline, so the plasma choline concentration is probably adequate for sustained ACh synthesis even under conditions of high demand, as observed in ganglia. Since the plasma concentration of choline is above the K_m of the high-affinity choline-transport system, it is not expected that choline concentrations in the nerve ending would be increased by increasing the plasma concentration of choline or by changing the K_m of the uptake system. However, neuronal choline content might be changed by altering the capacity of the high-affinity choline-uptake mechanism, such

as changing the maximum velocity (V_{max}) for transport, and this has been reported to occur in some brain regions in response to increased or decreased neuronal activity. There is some dispute about whether the capacity of the uptake system is increased or whether choline influx is regulated by changes in the intraterminal concentration of choline; it is agreed, however, that some event associated with neuronal activity enhances choline entry into neurons [16]. If the K_m of ChAT for choline *in vivo* is as high as that seen with the purified enzyme, one would expect ACh synthesis to increase in proportion to the greater availability of choline. Conversely, ACh synthesis should be diminished when high-affinity choline uptake is blocked. Hemicholinium-3 is a potent inhibitor of the high-affinity choline-uptake system, with a K_i in the submicromolar range (Fig. 11-4). Treatment with this drug decreases ACh synthesis and leads to a reduction in ACh release during prolonged stimulation; these findings lend support to the notion that choline uptake is the rate-limiting factor in the biosynthesis of ACh. To date, the high-affinity choline-uptake system has not been cloned successfully.

A second transport system concentrates acetylcholine in the synaptic vesicle

ACh is transported into storage vesicles following its synthesis by ChAT in the nerve ending [16]. The vesicular ACh transporter (VAChT) has been cloned and expressed. Its sequence places it in the 12-membrane-spanning family characteristic of other biogenic amine transporters found in adrenergic nerve endings [17,18]. Interestingly, the gene encoding the transporter is located within an intron of the ChAT gene, suggesting a mechanism for coregulation of gene expression for ChAT and VAChT. ACh uptake in the vesicle is driven by a proton-pumping ATPase. Coupled countertransport of H^+ and ACh allows the vesicle to remain iso-osmotic and electroneutral [16].

A selective inhibitor of ACh transport, vesamicol (Fig. 11-4), inhibits vesicular ACh uptake with an IC_{50} of 40 nM [16–18]. Inhibition appears noncompetitive, suggesting that it acts on some site other than the ACh-binding site on the transporter. Vesamicol blocks the evoked release

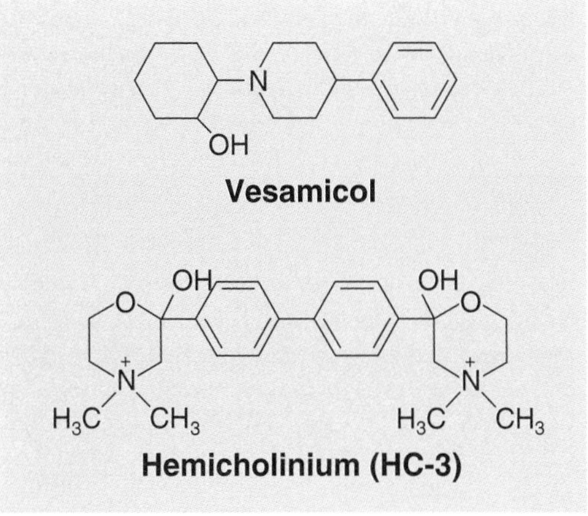

FIGURE 11-4. Structures of hemicholinium (HC-3) and vesamicol.

of newly synthesized ACh without significantly affecting high-affinity choline uptake, ACh synthesis or Ca^{2+} influx. The fact that ACh release is lost secondary to the blockade of uptake by the vesicle strongly suggests that the vesicle is the site of ACh release. The expressed transporter from the cloned cDNA also is inhibited by vesamicol [17,18].

Choline is supplied to the neuron either from plasma or by metabolism of choline-containing compounds

At least half of the choline used in ACh synthesis is thought to come directly from recycling of released ACh, hydrolyzed to choline by cholinesterase. Presumably, uptake of this metabolically derived choline occurs rapidly, before the choline diffuses away from the synaptic cleft. Another source of choline is the breakdown of phosphatidylcholine, which may be stimulated by locally released ACh. Choline derived from these two sources becomes available in the extracellular space and is then subject to high-affinity uptake into the nerve ending. In the CNS, these metabolic sources of choline appear to be particularly important because choline in the plasma cannot pass the blood–brain barrier. Thus, in the CNS, the high-affinity uptake of choline into cholinergic neurons might not be saturated and ACh synthesis could be limited by the supply of choline, at least during sustained activity. This would be consistent with the find-

ing that ACh stores in the brain are subject to variation, whereas ACh stores in ganglia and muscles remain relatively constant.

A slow release of acetylcholine from neurons at rest probably occurs at all cholinergic synapses

This was described first by Fatt and Katz, who recorded small, spontaneous depolarizations at frog neuromuscular junctions that were subthreshold for triggering action potentials. These MEPPs were shown to be due to the release of ACh. When the nerve was stimulated and endplate potentials recorded and analyzed, the magnitude of these potentials always was found to be some multiple of the magnitude of the MEPPs. It was suggested that each MEPP resulted from a finite quantity or quantum of released ACh and that the endplate potentials resulted from release of greater numbers of quanta during nerve stimulation (see Chap. 10).

A possible structural basis for these discrete units of transmitter was discovered shortly thereafter when independent electron microscopic and subcellular fractionation studies by de Robertis and Whittaker revealed the presence of vesicles in cholinergic nerve endings. Subcellular fractionation of mammalian brain and *Torpedo* electric organs yields resealed nerve endings, or synaptosomes, that can be lysed to release a fraction enriched in vesicles. More than half of the ACh in the synaptosome is associated with particles that look like the vesicles seen under an electron microscope. Therefore, it is clear that ACh is associated with a vesicle fraction, and it is likely that it is contained within the vesicle. The origin of the free ACh within the synaptosome is less clear. It may be ACh that is normally in the cytosol of the nerve ending, or it may be an artifact of release from the vesicles during their preparation (see Chap. 10).

The relationship between the amount of acetylcholine in a vesicle and the quanta of acetylcholine released can only be estimated

Estimates of the amount of ACh contained within cholinergic vesicles vary, and there is obviously some subjectivity in correcting the values obtained, such as the percent of vesicles that are cholinergic or how much ACh may be lost during their preparation [19]. Whittaker estimated that there are about 2,000 molecules of ACh in a cholinergic vesicle from the CNS. A similar estimate of about 1,600 molecules of ACh per vesicle was made using sympathetic ganglia. The most abundant source of cholinergic synaptic vesicles is the electric organ of *Torpedo*. Vesicles from *Torpedo* are far larger than those from mammalian species and are estimated to contain up to 100 times more ACh, that is, 200,000 molecules per vesicle. The *Torpedo* vesicle also contains ATP and, in its core, a proteoglycan of the heparin sulfate type. Both of these constituents may serve as counter-ions for ACh, which otherwise would be at a hyperosmotic concentration.

The amount of ACh in a quantum has been estimated by comparing the potential changes associated with MEPPs to those obtained by iontophoresis of known quantities of ACh. Based on such analysis, the amount of ACh per quantum at the snake neuromuscular junction was estimated to be something less than 10,000 molecules [19]. Given the possible error in these calculations, this would be within the range of that estimated to be contained in a vesicle. Therefore, it is likely that quanta are defined by the amount of releasable ACh in the vesicle. An alternative favored by some investigators is that ACh is released directly from the cytoplasm. In this model, definable quanta are evident because channels in the membrane are open for finite periods of time when Ca^{2+} is elevated. A presynaptic membrane protein suggested to mediate Ca^{2+}-dependent translocation of ACh has been isolated [18]. Although there are some compelling arguments in support of this model, most investigators favor the notion that the vesicle serves not only as a unit of storage but also as a unit of release. The vesicle hypothesis and release of neurotransmitters are discussed also in Chapter 10.

Depolarization of the nerve terminal by an action potential increases the number of quanta released per unit time

Release of ACh requires the presence of extracellular Ca^{2+}, which enters the neuron when it is depolarized. Most investigators are of the opinion that a voltage-dependent Ca^{2+} current is the initial event responsible for transmitter release, which occurs about 200 μsec later. The mechanism through which elevated Ca^{2+} increases the probability of ACh release is not yet known; phosphorylation or activation of proteins that causes the vesicle to fuse with the neuronal membrane, are among the possibilities. Dependence on Ca^{2+} is a common feature of all exocytotic release mechanisms, and it is likely that exocytosis is a conserved mechanism for transmitter release. There is good evidence that adrenergic vesicles empty their contents into the synaptic cleft because norepinephrine and epinephrine are released along with other contents of the storage vesicle. Although less rigorous data are available for cholinergic systems, cholinergic vesicles contain ATP, and release of ATP has been shown to accompany ACh secretion from these vesicles. Furthermore, Heuser and Reese demonstrated, in electron microscopic studies at frog nerve terminals, that vesicles fuse with the nerve membrane and that vesicular contents appear to be released by exocytosis; it has been difficult to ascertain, however, whether the fusions are sufficiently frequent to account for release on stimulation. The nerve ending also appears to endocytose the outer vesicle membrane to form vesicles that subsequently are refilled with ACh [19].

All of the acetylcholine contained within the cholinergic neuron does not behave as if in a single compartment

Results of a variety of neurophysiological and biochemical experiments suggest that there are at least two distinguishable pools of ACh, only one of which is readily available for release. These have been referred to as the "readily available," or "depot," pool and the "reserve," or "stationary," pool. The reserve pool refills the readily available pool as it is utilized. Unless the rate of mobilization of ACh into the readily available pool is adequate, the amount of ACh that can be released may be limited. It is also likely that newly synthesized ACh is used to fill the readily available pool of ACh because it is the newly synthesized ACh that is released preferentially during nerve stimulation. The precise relationship between these functionally defined pools and ACh storage vesicles is not known. It is possible that the readily available pool resides in vesicles poised for release near the nerve ending membrane, whereas the reserve pool is in more distant vesicles. Although cholinergic vesicles appear to be homogeneous, there may be subpopulations of vesicles that differ in size and density.

ACETYLCHOLINESTERASE AND THE TERMINATION OF ACETYLCHOLINE ACTION

Cholinesterases are widely distributed throughout the body in both neuronal and non-neuronal tissues

Based largely on substrate specificity, the cholinesterases are subdivided into the acetylcholinesterases (AChEs) (EC 3.1.1.7) and the butyryl or pseudocholinesterases (BuChE) (EC 3.1.1.8) [20,21]. Acetylcholines with an acyl group the size of butyric acid or larger are hydrolyzed very slowly by the former enzyme; selective inhibitors for each enzyme have been identified. BuChE is made primarily in the liver and appears in plasma; however, it is highly unlikely that appreciable concentrations of ACh diffuse from the locality of the synapse and elicit a systemic response. The distribution of BuChE mutations showing resistance to naturally occurring inhibitors suggests that this enzyme hydrolyzes dietary esters of potential toxicity. Although BuChE is localized in the nervous system during development, the existence of nonexpressing mutations in the BuChE gene within the human population demonstrates that this enzyme is not essential for nervous system function. In general, AChE distribution correlates with innervation and development in the nervous system. The AChEs also exhibit synaptic localization upon synapse formation. Acetyl- and butyrylcholinesterases are encoded by single, but distinct, genes.

Acetylcholinesterases exist in several molecular forms

These forms differ in solubility and mode of membrane attachment rather than in catalytic activity. One class of molecular forms exists as a homomeric assembly of catalytic subunits that appear as monomers, dimers or tetramers (Fig. 11-5). These forms also differ in their degree of hydrophobicity, and their amphiphilic character arises from a post-translational addition of a glycophospholipid on the carboxyl-terminal amino acid. The glycophospholipid allows the enzyme to be tethered on the external surface of the cell membrane. Soluble globular forms of the enzyme have been identified in brain.

The second class of AChEs exists as heteromeric assemblies of catalytic and structural subunits. One form consists of up to 12 catalytic subunits linked by a disulfide bond to filamentous, collagen-containing structural subunits. These forms are often termed *asymmetric,* since the tail unit imparts substantial dimensional asymmetry to the molecule. The asymmetric species are localized to synaptic areas. The collagenous tail unit is responsible for this molecular form being associated with the basal lamina of the synapse rather than the plasma membrane. Asymmetric forms are particularly abundant in the neuromuscular junction. A second type of structural subunit, to which a tetramer of catalytic subunits is linked by disulfide bonds, has been characterized in brain. This subunit contains covalently attached lipid, enabling this form of the enzyme to associate with the plasma membrane. The different subunit assemblies and post-translational modifications lead to distinct localization of AChE on the cell surface but appear not to affect the intrinsic catalytic activities of the individual forms.

The primary and tertiary structures of the cholinesterases are known

The primary structures of the cholinesterases define a large and functionally eclectic family of extracellular proteins that function not only catalytically as hydrolases and dehalogenases but also in forming heterologous cell contacts, as seen in the structurally related proteins neurotactin, glutactin, gliotactin and neuroligin. A sequence homologous to the cholinesterases and a presumed common structural matrix are found in thyroglobulin, in which tyrosine residues become iodinated and conjugated to form thyroid

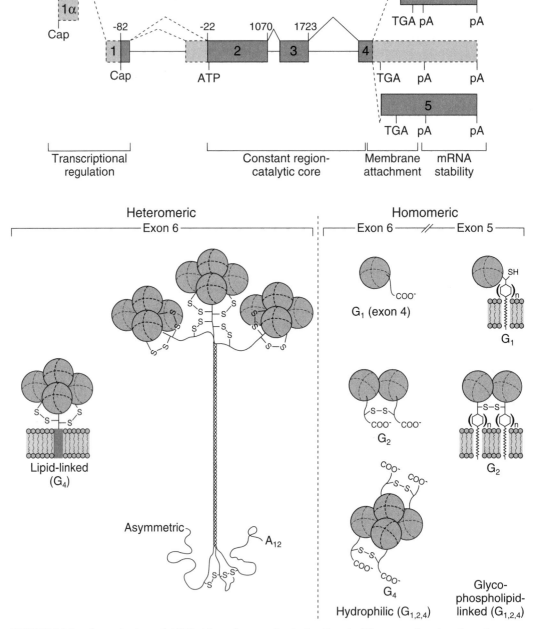

FIGURE 11-5.   Gene structure of AChE. Alternative cap sites in the 5' end of the gene allow for alternative promoter usage in different tissues. Exons 2, 3 and 4 encode an invariant core of the molecule that contains the essential catalytic residues. Just prior to the stop codon, three splicing alternatives are evident: *1*, a continuation of exon 4; *2*, the 4–5 splice; and *3*, the 4–6 splice. The catalytic subunits produced differ only in their carboxy-termini and are shown in the lower panel. (Modified from [20] with permission.)

hormone [20]. The heterologous contacts formed by the tactin and neuroligin members of the family suggest that the cholinesterases also may have nonhydrolase functions.

The initial solution of the crystal structure of the *Torpedo* enzyme [22], followed by the mammalian enzyme [23], revealed that the active center serine lies at the base of a rather narrow gorge that is lined heavily with aromatic residues (Fig. 11-6). The enzyme carries a net negative charge, and an electrostatic dipole is oriented on the enzyme to facilitate diffusional entry of cationic ligands. Crystal structures of several inhibitors in a complex with AChE also have been elucidated.

The open reading frame in mammalian AChE genes is encoded by three invariant exons (exons 2, 3 and 4) followed by three splicing al-

ternatives. Continuation through exon 4 gives rise to a monomeric species. Splicing to exon 5 gives rise to the carboxyl-terminal sequence signal for addition of glycophospholipid, while splicing to exon 6 encodes a sequence containing a cysteine that links to other catalytic or structural subunits. These species of AChE differ only in the last 40 residues in their carboxy-termini.

The catalytic mechanism for acetylcholine hydrolysis involves formation of an acyl enzyme, followed by deacylation

The acylation step proceeds through the formation of a tetrahedral transition state. Alkylphosphate inhibitors, such as diisopropyl-fluorophosphate, are tetrahedral in configura-

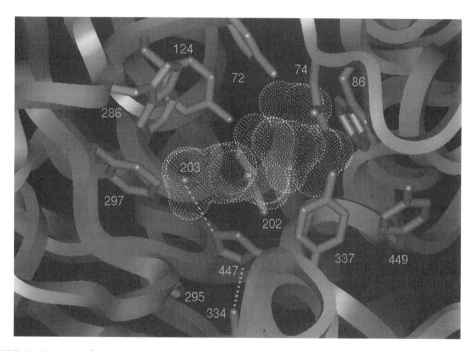

FIGURE 11-6.   View of the active center gorge of mammalian acetylcholinesterase looking into the gorge cavity. The gorge is 18 to 20 Å in depth in a molecule of 40 Å diameter and is heavily lined with aromatic amino acid side chains. Side chains from several sets of critical residues are shown emanating from the α carbon of the α carbon-amide backbone: (i) A catalytic triad between Glu 334, His 447 and Ser 203 is shown by dotted lines to denote the hydrogen-bonding pattern. This renders Ser 203 more nucleophilic to attack the carbon of acetylcholine (shown in white with the van der Waals surface). This leads to formation of an acetyl enzyme, which is deacetylated rapidly, (ii) The acyl pocket outline by Phe 295 and 297 is of restricted size in acetylcholinesterase. In butyrylcholinesterase, these side chains are aliphatic, increasing the size and flexibility in the acyl pocket, (iii) The choline subsite lined by the aromatic residues Trp 86, Tyr 337 and Tyr 449 and the anionic residue Glu 202. (iv) A peripheral site which resides at the rim of the gorge encompasses Trp 286, Tyr 72, Tyr 124 and Asp 74. This site modulates catalysis by binding inhibitors or, at high concentrations, a second substrate molecule.

tion, and this geometric resemblance to the transition state in part accounts for their effectiveness as inhibitors of AChE. Acylation occurs on the active-site serine, which is rendered nucleophilic by proton withdrawal by Glu 334 through His 447. The acetyl enzyme that is formed is short-lived, lasting approximately 10 μsec; this accounts for the high catalytic efficiency of the enzyme (Fig. 11-6). The availability of a crystal structure of AChE has enabled investigators to assign residues and domains in the cholinesterase responsible for catalysis and inhibitor specificity [22,23].

Inhibition of acetylcholinesterase occurs by several distinct mechanisms

Some AChE inhibitors are useful therapeutically, whereas others have proven useful as insecticides. Still others have been manufactured for a more insidious use in chemical warfare. Inhibitors such as edrophonium bind reversibly to the active site of the enzyme and prevent access of the substrate. Other reversible inhibitors, such as gallamine, propidium and the three-fingered peptide from snake venom, fasciculin, bind to a peripheral site on the enzyme. The carbamoylating agents, such as neostigmine and physostigmine, form a carbamoyl enzyme by reacting with the active-site serine. The carbamoyl enzymes are more stable than the acetyl enzyme; their deacylation occurs over several minutes. Since the carbamoyl enzyme will not hydrolyze ACh, the carbamoylating agents are alternative substrates that are effective inhibitors of ACh hydrolysis. The alkylphosphates, such as diisopropylfluorophosphate or echothiophate, act in a similar manner; however, the alkylphosphorates and alkylphosphonates form extremely stable bonds with the active-site serine on the enzyme. The time required for their hydrolysis often exceeds that for biosynthesis and turnover of the enzyme. Accordingly, inhibition with the alkylphosphates is typically irreversible.

Consequences of acetylcholinesterase inhibition differ between synapses

At postganglionic parasympathetic effector sites, AChE inhibition enhances or potentiates the action of administered ACh or ACh released by nerve stimulation. In part, this is a consequence of stimulation of receptors extending over a larger area from the point of transmitter release. Similarly, ganglionic transmission is enhanced by cholinesterase inhibitors. Since atropine and other muscarinic antagonists are effective antidotes of the toxicity of inhibitors of AChE, at least some CNS manifestations result largely from excessive muscarinic stimulation.

By prolonging the residence time of ACh in the synapse, AChE inhibition in the neuromuscular junction promotes a persistent depolarization of the motor endplate. The decay of endplate currents or potentials resulting from spontaneous release of ACh is prolonged from 1 to 2 msec to 5 to 30 msec. This indicates that the transmitter activates multiple receptors before diffusing from the synapse. Excessive depolarization of the endplate, resulting from slowly decaying endplate potentials, leads to a diminished capacity to initiate coordinated action potentials. In a fashion similar to depolarizing blocking agents, fasciculations and muscle twitching are observed initially with AChE inhibition, followed by flaccid paralysis.

NICOTINIC RECEPTORS

The nicotinic acetylcholine receptor is the best characterized neurotransmitter receptor

The nicotinic receptor was purified about a decade before purification of other neurotransmitter receptors. The electric organ of *Torpedo*, consisting of stacks of electrocytes that have differentiated from tissue of embryonic origin common to that of skeletal muscle, is a rich source of nicotinic receptors. Upon differentiation, the electrogenic bud in the electrocyte proliferates, but the contractile elements atrophy. The excitable membrane encompasses the entire ventral surface of the electrocyte rather than being localized to small, focal junctional areas, as found in skeletal muscle. The electrical discharge in *Torpedo* relies solely on a PSEP resulting from depolarization of the postsynaptic membrane, rather than propagation from an action potential. The density of receptors in the *Torpedo* electric organ approaches 100 pmol/mg protein, which may be compared with 0.1 pmol/mg protein in skeletal muscle.

In the early 1960s, it was established that snake α-toxins, such as α-bungarotoxin, irreversibly inactivate receptor function in intact skeletal muscle, and this finding led directly to the identification and subsequent isolation of the nicotinic ACh receptor from *Torpedo* [3]. By virtue of their high affinity and very slow rates of dissociation, labeled α-toxins serve as markers of the receptor during solubilization and purification.

Purification of the nicotinic acetylcholine receptor facilitated examination of its overall structure

Antibodies were raised to the purified protein, and sufficient amino acid sequence of the receptor itself became available to permit the cloning and sequencing of the genes encoding the individual subunits of the receptor [4]. As a consequence of the high density of nicotinic ACh receptors in the postsynaptic membranes of *Torpedo,* sufficient order of the receptor molecules is achieved in isolated membrane fragments such that image reconstructions from electron microscopy have allowed a more detailed analysis of structure [24]. Finally, labeling of functional sites, determination of subunit composition and structure modification through mutagenesis contributed to our understanding of the structure of nicotinic receptors [25].

The nicotinic acetylcholine receptor consists of five subunits arranged around a pseudoaxis of symmetry

The subunits display homologous amino acid sequences with 30 to 40% identity of amino acid residues [4]. In muscle, one subunit, designated α, is expressed in two copies; the other three, β, γ and δ, are present as single copies (Fig. 11-7). Thus, the receptor is a pentamer of molecular mass of approximately 280 kDa. Structural studies show the subunits to be arranged around a central cavity, with the largest portion of the protein exposed toward the ex-

tracellular surface. The central cavity is believed to lead to the ion channel, which in the resting state is impermeable to ions; upon activation, however, it opens to a diameter of 6.5 Å. The open channel is selective for cations. The two α subunits and the opposing face of the γ and δ subunits form the two sites for binding of agonists and competitive antagonists and provide the primary surface with which the larger snake α-toxins associate. The sites for ligand binding are localized toward the external perimeter of each of the α subunits; occupation of both sites is necessary for receptor activation. Electrophysiological and ligand-binding measurements together with analysis of the functional states of the receptor indicate positive cooperativity in the association of agonists; Hill coefficients greater than unity have been described for agonist-elicited channel opening, agonist binding and agonist-induced desensitization of the receptor [3,25]. Noncompetitive inhibitor sites within various depths of the internal channel also have been defined and are the sites of local anesthetic inhibition of receptor function.

Sequence identity among the subunits appears to be greatest in the hydrophobic regions. Various models for the disposition of the peptide chains have been proposed on the basis of hydropathy and reactivity of certain residues to modifying agents and antibodies (Fig. 11-8). Four candidate membrane-spanning regions are predicted, although only one clear α-helical segment is evident in the electron microscopic reconstruction of the channel [24]. All of these potential membrane-spanning domains appear after residue 210, with the amino-terminal portion of the molecule on the extracellular surface. The homology among the four subunits strongly suggests that the same folding pattern is found in all subunits.

Site-directed labeling, chemical cross-linking, homology modeling, antibody association, fluorescence energy transfer and site-specific mutagenesis represent techniques that have made incremental contributions to the understanding of nicotinic receptor structure [25]. Analysis with techniques achieving atomic level resolution has not been possible for an integral membrane protein of this size.

A

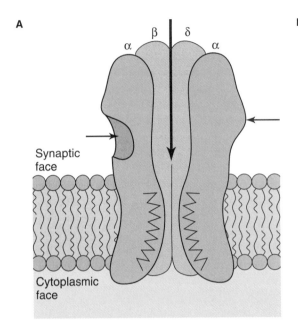

Synaptic face

Cytoplasmic face

B

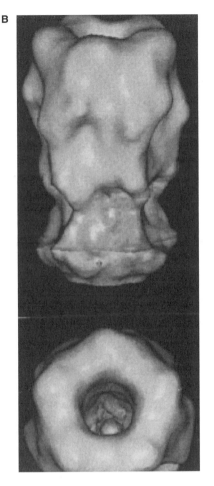

C

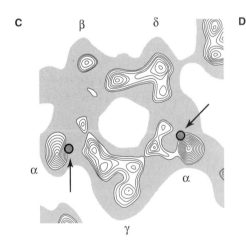

D

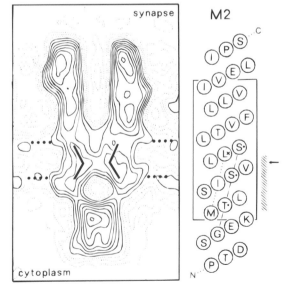

synapse

cytoplasm

M2

A disulfide loop between Cys 128 and 142 in the α subunit is conserved in the entire receptor channel family (Fig. 11-8A). A second disulfide is found in the α subunits between vicinal Cys 192 and 193, and this structural feature has been used to identify α subunits. Early studies showed that reduction of the Cys 192–193 bond allowed for labeling by the site-directed sulfhydryl-reactive agonist and antagonist, respectively, bromoacetylcholine and *m*-maleimidobenzyl trimethylammonium (Fig. 11-8B) [25]. Subsequent studies involving photolytic labeling, labeling by the natural coral toxin lophotoxin and site-specific mutagenesis identified the region between residues 185 and 200 in the α subunit as being important for forming part of the agonist- and antagonist-binding surface. Two other segments of sequence in the α subunit and four discrete segments on the opposing face of the γ and δ subunits also have been identified as forming loops that contribute to the binding surfaces at the αγ and αδ interfaces [26].

Four candidate membrane-spanning regions are found after residue 210 with a large cytoplasmic loop between membrane spans 3 and 4 (Fig. 11-8A). Based on labeling experiments and site-specific mutagenesis, membrane span 2 was found to be proximal to the ion channel. This span, when constructed as an α helix, is amphipathic, with an abundance of serine and threonine residues pointed toward the channel lumen. Positions corresponding to α-Thr 244, α-Leu 251, α-Val 255 and α-Glu 262 in this transmembrane span have been labeled with the noncompetitive, channel-blocking inhibitors chlorpromazine and tetraphenyl phosphonium [3,25]. Mutation of several of the hydroxyl groups on residues at these positions affects channel kinetics. The channel gate, or constriction, is thought to lie deep within the channel either at the boxed leucine in Figure 11-8C or even farther to the cytoplasmic side. The ion selectivity of the channels appears to be controlled in part by rings of charges formed by all five subunits at the extracellular surface of the channel corresponding to α-Glu 262 and at the cytoplasmic exit corresponding to α-Glu241. Exposed amide backbone hydrogens and carbonyl groups and a ring of hydroxylated amino acids corresponding to α-Thr 244 also contribute to ion selectivity and permeation [25].

Analysis of the opening and closing events of individual channels has provided information about ligand binding and activation of the receptor

Electrophysiological studies utilize high-resistance patch electrodes of 1 to 2 μM diameter, which form tight seals on the membrane surface [27]. They have the capacity to record conductance changes of individual channels within the lumen of the electrode (see Chap. 10). The patch of membrane affixed to the electrode may be excised, inverted or studied on the intact cell. The individual opening events for ACh achieve a conductance of 25 pS across the membrane and

---

FIGURE 11-7.   A: Longitudinal view of the muscle nicotinic acetylcholine receptor with the γ subunit removed. The remaining subunits, two copies of α, one of β and one of δ, surround an internal channel with outer vestibule and its constriction or gating locus deep within the membrane bilayer region. Spans of α helices with bowed structures from the M_2 region of the sequence form the perimeter of the channel (see D). Acetylcholine-binding sites, denoted by *arrows*, are found at the αγ- and αδ (not visible)-subunit interfaces. C and D show the data on which this structure is based. (Adapted from [24] with permission.) **B:** Image reconstruction of electron micrographs yielding a structure at 9 Å resolution. Shown are side and synaptic views. (Adapted from [24] with permission.) **C:** Electron-density image of a section of the receptor molecule on the synaptic side taken 30 Å above the plane of the membrane and normal to the pseudo fivefold axis of symmetry. *Arrows* show route of entry of the neurotransmitter. Red circles indicate the respective positions of the bungarotoxin-binding sites and the two α subunits. The pentameric structure of the receptor is evident with a presumed clockwise orientation of subunits α, γ, α, β and δ. (Adapted from [24] with permission.) **D:** Longitudinal view of the electron density of the receptor. The transmembrane area is shown between the *dots*. The visible transmembrane-spanning helixes are shown by the *V-shaped solid lines*. This helix is believed to be the M_2 region, the sequence of which is shown. The area inside the rectangle is the transmembrane-spanning region. The "X" denotes the conserved leucine (see C). The additional density in the cytoplasmic region arises from an associated 43-kDa protein, rapsyn. The *shaded area* to the right indicates the zone of narrowest constriction.

A

Receptor

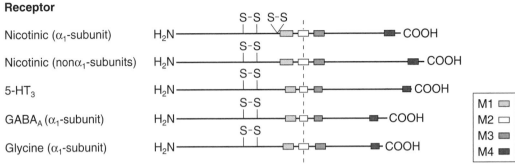

B

Sequence in the α subunit of various nicotinic acetylcholine receptors of muscle (α1) and neuronal origin (α2-α9)[a] between residues 179 and 207

```
                  179                                                        207
Torpedo c.  α1    K D Y R G W K H W V Y Y T C C P D T P Y L D I T Y H F I M
Xenopus l.  α1α   K D Y R G W K H W V Y Y D C C P E T P Y L D I T Y H F L L
Xenopus l.  α1β   K D Y R G W K H W V Y Y T C C P D K P Y L D I T Y H F V L
Chicken     α1    K D Y R G W K H W V Y Y A C C P D T P Y L D I T Y H F L M
Calf        α1    K E S R G W K H W V F Y A C C P S T P Y L D I T Y H F V M
Mouse       α1    K E A R G W K H W V F Y S C C P T T P Y L D I T Y H F V M
Human       α1    K E S R G W K H S V T Y S C C P D T P Y L D I T Y H F V M
Cobra       α     K D Y R G F W H S V N Y S C C L D T P Y L D I T Y H F I L
Natrix t.   α     K D Y R G F W H S V N Y S C C L D T P Y L D I T Y H F I L
Drosophila  α     M R V P A V R N E K F Y S C C - E E P Y L D I T Y N L T L
Chicken     α2    I N A I G R Y N S K K Y D C C - T E I Y P D I V F Y F V I
Chicken     α3    I K A P G Y K H D I K Y N C C - E E I Y T D I T F S L Y I
Chicken     α4    I N S V G N Y N S K K Y E C C - T E I Y P D I T Y S F I I
Rat         α2    I N A T G T Y N S K K Y D C C - E E I Y Q D I T Y S L Y I
Rat         α3    I K A P G Y K H E I K Y N C C - E E I Y Q D I T Y S L Y I
Rat         α4    V D A V G T Y M T R K Y E C C - A E I Y P D I T Y A F I I
Rat         α5    M S A M G S K G N R T D S C C W - - - Y P Y I T Y S F V I
Rat         α6    V D A S G Y K H D I K Y N C C - E E I Y I D I T Y S F Y I
Rat         α7    M G I P G K R N E K E Y E C C - E E P Y P D V T Y T V T M
Rat         α8    V G V P G K R N E L Y Y E C C - E E P Y P D V T Y T I T M
Rat         α9    H G M F A V K N V I S Y G C C - S E P Y P D V T F T L L L
```

To date, no activity has been observed with rat α5 when expressed with other subunits of muscle or neuronal origin.

C

Charged amino acids (circled) and conserved leucine (boxed) on M2 are shown in relation to estimated position of bilayer

```
Torpedo AChR  α    G Ⓔ Ⓚ M T L S I S V L [L] S L T V F L L V I V Ⓔ L
Torpedo AChR  β    G Ⓔ Ⓚ M S L S I S A L [L] A T V V F L L L L A Ⓓ Ⓚ
Torpedo AChR  γ    G Q Ⓚ C T L S I S V L [L] A Q T I F L F L I A Q Ⓚ
Torpedo AChR  δ    G Ⓔ Ⓚ M S T A I S V L [L] A Q A V F L L L T S Q Ⓡ
Rat AChR      α1   G Ⓔ Ⓚ I T L S I S V L [L] S L T V F L L V I V Ⓔ L
Rat AChR      α2   G Ⓔ Ⓚ I T L C I S V L [L] S L T V F L L L I T Ⓔ I
Rat AChR      β2   G Ⓔ Ⓚ M T L C I S V L [L] A L T V F L L L I S Ⓚ I
GABAA         α1   P A Ⓡ T V F G V T T V [L] T M T T L S I S A Ⓡ N S
GABAA         β1   A A Ⓡ V A L G I T T V [L] T M T T I S T H L Ⓡ Ⓔ T
Glycine       α1   P A Ⓡ V G L G I T T V [L] T M T T Q S S G S Ⓡ A S
Glycine       β1   A A Ⓡ V P L G I F S V L [L] S L A S Ⓔ C T T L A A Ⓔ
5-HT3         G Ⓔ Ⓡ V S F Ⓚ I T L L L [L] G Y S V F L I V S Ⓓ T L
```

Bilayer

have an opening duration that is distributed exponentially around a value of about 1 msec. The duration of channel opening is dependent on the particular agonist, whereas the conductance of the open-channel state is usually agonist-independent. Analyses of the frequencies of opening events have permitted an estimation of the kinetic constants for channel opening and ligand binding, and these numbers are in reasonable agreement with estimates of ligand binding and activation from rapid kinetic, or stopped-flow, studies. Overall, activation events can be described by Scheme 1 [3,27].

$$2L + R \underset{k_{-1}}{\overset{2k_{+1}}{\rightleftharpoons}} LR \underset{2k_{-1}}{\overset{k_{+1}}{\rightleftharpoons}} L_2R \underset{k_{-2}}{\overset{k_{+2}}{\rightleftharpoons}} L_2R^*$$

(Closed) (Closed) (Closed) (Open)

Scheme 1

Two ligands (L) associate with the receptor (R) prior to the isomerization step to form the open-channel state L_2R^*. For ACh, the forward rate constant for binding, k_{+1}, is 1 to 2×10^8 M^{-1} sec^{-1}; k_{+2} and k_{-2}, forward and reverse rate constants for isomerization, yield rates of isomerization consistent with opening events in the millisecond time frame. Since k_{+2} and k_{-2} are greater than k_{-1}, the rate constant for ligand dissociation, several opening and closing events with the fully liganded receptor occur prior to dissociation of the first ligand. Binding of the first and second ligands appears not to be identical, even allowing for the statistical differences arising from the two sites. Such a conclusion is consistent with receptor structure since different subunits, such as the γ and δ subunits in muscle, are adjacent to the same face of the α subunits in the pentamer.

Continued exposure of nicotinic receptors to agonist leads to desensitization of the receptors

This diminution of the response occurs even though the concentration of agonist available to the receptor has not changed. Katz and Thesleff examined the kinetics of desensitization with microelectrodes and found that a cyclic scheme in which the receptor existed in two states, R and R′, prior to exposure to the ligand best described the process.

To achieve receptor desensitization and activation by a single ligand, multiple conformational states of the receptor are required. The binding steps represented in horizontal equilibria are rapid; vertical steps reflect the slow, unimolecular isomerizations involved in desensitization (Scheme 2). Rapid isomerization to the open channel state (Scheme 1) should be added. To accommodate the additional complexities of the observed fast and slow steps of desensitization, additional states have to be included.

FIGURE 11-8.   Features of the sequence of the acetylcholine receptor. **A:** Schematic drawing of the sequence showing candidate regions for spanning the membrane. The region M_2 is believed to be an α helical segment and lines the internal pore of the receptor. M_1, M_3 and M_4 contain hydrophobic sequences, but it is not known whether they traverse the membrane as α helices. The nicotinic β, γ and δ subunits contain homologous M_1 through M_4 hydrophobic domains at similar positions in the linear sequence. Two disulfide loops, 128–142 and 192–193, in the α subunits are shown. While the other subunits contain the larger disulfide loop, they lack cysteines 192 and 193 and tyrosine 190. Sequences of other homologous subunits in ligand-gated channel (5-hydroxytryptamine [5-HT-3], GABA and glycine) receptors are shown. The amino-terminal portion is found on the extracellular (synaptic) surface. (Modified from [24] with permission.) **B:** Amino acid sequence between residues 179 and 207 in the α subunit of various nicotinic receptors. Cysteines 192 and 193 and tyrosines 190 and 198 have been shown by chemical labeling and site-specific mutagenesis to be in the vicinity of the ligand-binding site. **C:** Amino acid sequence of the M_2-spanning domain for the homologous series of ligand-gated ion channels. The conformation is believed to be α-helical, with the amino-terminal portion (left-hand side) entering from the cytoplasmic side. The membrane-spanning region is largely hydrophobic but with hydroxylated residues positioned at strategic positions in the α-helical wheel. Charged residues are found bordering the hydrophobic membrane-spanning region. The helices from each of the five subunits form the internal perimeter outlining the channel (see Fig. 11-7) and are believed to assume a bowed, hourglass shape, with the boxed leucine being near the constriction point (cf. [24,25]).

A simplified scheme, in which only one desensitized and one open-channel state of the receptor exist, is represented in Scheme 2, where R is the resting (activatable) state, R* the active (open channel) state and R′ the desensitized state of the receptor; M is an allosteric constant defined by R′/R, and K and $K′$ are equilibrium dissociation constants for the ligand.

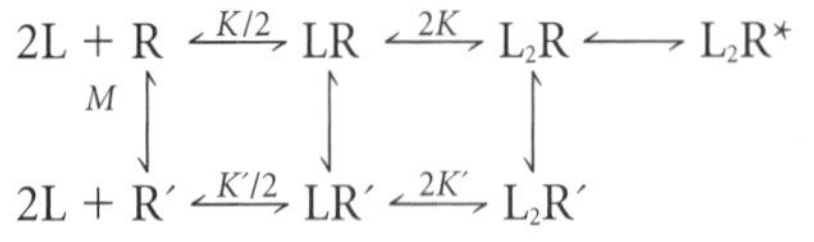

$$2L + R \xrightarrow{K/2} LR \xrightarrow{2K} L_2R \longleftrightarrow L_2R^*$$
$$M \updownarrow \qquad \updownarrow \qquad \updownarrow$$
$$2L + R' \xrightarrow{K'/2} LR' \xrightarrow{2K'} L_2R'$$

Scheme 2

In this scheme, $M < 1$ and $K′ < K$. Addition of ligand eventually will result in an increased fraction of R′ species due to the values dictated by the equilibrium constants. Direct binding experiments have confirmed the generality of this scheme for nicotinic receptors. Thus, distinct conformational states govern the different temporal responses that ensue on addition of a ligand to the nicotinic receptor. No direct energy input or covalent modification of the receptor channel is required.

Nicotinic receptor subunits are part of a large superfamily of ligand-gated channels

Nicotinic receptors on neurons, such as those originating in the CNS or neural crest, show ligand specificities distinct from the nicotinic receptor in the neuromuscular junction. One of the most remarkable differences is the resistance of most nicotinic neuronal receptors containing α2 through α6 subunits to α-bungarotoxin and related snake α-toxins. This fact and the lack of an abundant source of neuronal CNS receptors limited initial progress in their isolation and characterization. However, low-stringency hybridization with cDNAs encoding the subunits of electric organ and muscle receptors provided a means to clone neuronal nicotinic receptor genes. Isolation of the candidate cDNA clones, their expression in cell systems to yield functional receptors and the discrete regional localizations of the endogenous mRNAs encoding

these receptor subunits revealed that the nicotinic receptor subunits are part of a large and widely distributed gene family. They are related in structure and sequence to receptors for inhibitory amino acids (GABA and glycine), to 5-hydroxytryptamine type 3 ($5HT_3$) receptors and, somewhat more distantly, to glutamate receptors.

At least 11 distinct genes encoding neuronal nicotinic receptor subunits α2 through α9 and β2 through β4 have been identified in the central and peripheral nervous systems (Fig. 11-2). The α subunits are similar in sequence to the muscle α1 subunit and contribute to the ligand-binding interface. The β subunits fulfill the role of β1, γ and δ subunits in the muscle receptor. When certain pairs or triplets of cDNAs encoding neuronal α and β subunits are cotransfected into cells or their corresponding mRNAs are injected into oocytes, characteristic ACh-gated channel function can be achieved. The α5 subunit appears unique in that it will not contribute to function in the absence of other α subunits; its global sequence features are more similar to those of the β subunits. The α7 and α8 subunits display function as homologous pentamers. Receptors containing α7 subunits have a high Ca^{2+} permeability, and Ca^{2+} entry may be integral to their function *in vivo*. While not all combinations of α and β mRNAs lead to the expression of functional receptors on the cell surface, the number of permutations is large [10,11,25]. A future challenge is the assignment of pharmacological and biophysical signatures to all of the subunit combinations found *in vivo*.

The α3 subunit is prevalent in peripheral ganglia, usually with β2, β4, and α5 subunits, while the α4β2 subunit combination predominates in the CNS. The α6 subunit appears to localize with biogenic amine-containing neurons, while α9 is found in vestibular sensory and cochlear hair cells. Receptors containing the α9 subunit may have some muscarinic receptor characteristics.

Substantial evidence points to nicotinic receptors in the CNS functioning at presynaptic locations to regulate release of several CNS transmitters [10]. Electrophysiological and microdialysis studies provide evidence that glutamatergic, dopaminergic, serotonergic, peptidergic and cholinergic pathways are under the control of presynaptic nicotinic receptors. Hence, nicotinic receptors appear to play an important amplification and modulatory role in the CNS.

Both nicotinic receptors and acetylcholinesterase are regulated tightly during differentiation and synapse formation

At present, we understand more about tissue-specific gene expression in muscle than in nerve [28,29]. Both of the above proteins show enhanced expression during myogenesis upon differentiating from a mononucleated myoblast to a multinucleated myotube. Curiously, enhanced receptor expression occurs largely by transcriptional activation, while the increase in cholinesterase expression arises from stabilization of the mRNA [30]. The receptor appears to cluster spontaneously, which involves a protein on the cytoplasmic side of the membrane, termed 43K or rapsyn [28,29]. This protein links the receptor to cytoskeletal elements and restricts its diffusional mobility. Following innervation and synaptic activity, expression of the receptor and AChE persists in endplate, or junctional, regions and disappears in extrajunctional regions. The collagen-tail-containing species of AChE is localized to the basal lamina in the neuromuscular synapse.

With innervation and the development of electrically excitable synapses, the γ subunit of the receptor is replaced by an ϵ subunit; small changes in the biophysical properties of the receptor occur concomitantly. Upon denervation, many of the developmental changes associated with innervation are reversed and there is again an increase in expression of extrajunctional receptors containing the γ subunit. In multinucleated muscle cells, particular subsynaptic nuclei drive the expression of these synapse-specific proteins. The factors controlling these regulatory events are incompletely understood, but calcitonin gene-related peptide (CGRP) and the protein ACh receptor-inducing activity (ARIA) may be extracellular mediators of expression. In addition, intracellular Ca^{2+}, membrane depolarization and protein kinase C play distinct roles in maintaining junctional expression of synapse-localized proteins.

A neurally derived signaling protein, agrin, acts through a receptor tyrosine kinase, MuSK, in the formation of the specialized postsynaptic endplate by interaction with rapsyn. Thus, MuSK–rapsyn interactions are critical in forming the local scaffold for postsynaptic components in the motor endplate [29,31].

MUSCARINIC RECEPTORS

Muscarinic and nicotinic receptors are related more closely to other receptors in their respective families than to one another, both structurally and functionally. The nicotinic receptor is far more similar to other ligand-gated ion channels, such as the GABA receptor, than to the muscarinic receptor. The muscarinic receptor in turn belongs to a group of seven transmembrane-spanning receptors that includes the adrenergic receptors [32], which transduce their signals across membranes by interacting with GTP-binding proteins (see Chap. 20). Several macromolecular interactions are involved in the responses triggered by activation of the muscarinic receptor. These associations contribute to the 100 to 250 msec latency characteristic of muscarinic responses, which are slow compared with those mediated by nicotinic receptors.

Muscarinic receptor stimulation causes inhibition of adenylyl cyclase, stimulation of phospholipase C and regulation of ion channels

Many types of neurons and effector cells respond to muscarinic receptor stimulation. Despite the diversity of responses that ensue, the initial event that follows ligand binding to the muscarinic receptor may be, in all cases, the interaction of the receptor with a G protein. Depending on the nature of the G protein, the receptor–G protein interaction can initiate any of several early biochemical events seen with muscarinic receptor occupation, including inhibition of adenylyl cyclase, stimulation of phosphoinositide hydrolysis or regulation of potassium channels (Fig. 11-9) [33].

Primary biochemical responses
mediated by muscarinic acetylcholine receptors

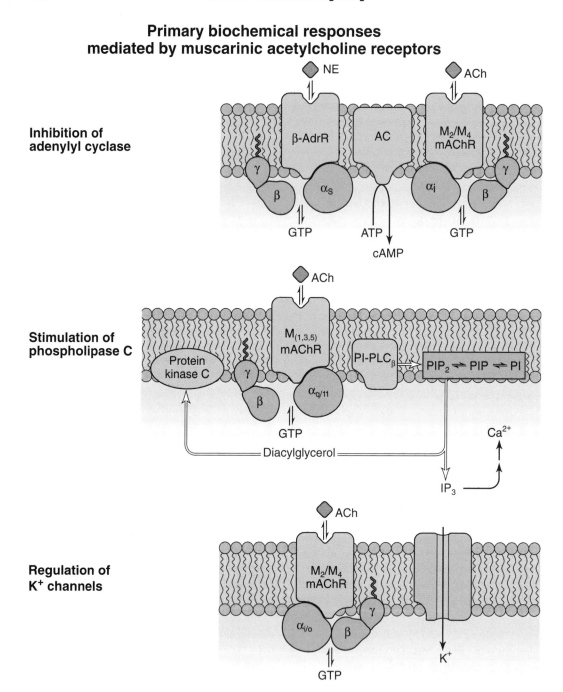

FIGURE 11-9.   Acetylcholine (ACh) interacts with a muscarinic receptor of the subtypes indicated to induce various responses. The M_2 and M_4 muscarinic acetylcholine receptors (mAChRs) interact with the α subunit of GTP-binding protein, G_i. When ACh binds, $G\alpha_i$ dissociates from $\beta\gamma$ and inhibits adenylyl cyclase *(AC)*. The M_1, M_3 and M_5 mAChRs interact with GTP-binding proteins in the G_q and G_{11} family. The $G\alpha_q$ and α_{11} subunits activate phosphoinositide-specific phospholipase C *(PI-PLC)*. The M_2 and M_4 mAChRs regulate inwardly rectifying K^+ channels through the $\beta\gamma$ subunit of G_i or G_o. Diffusible second messengers formed within the cell include cAMP, inositol trisphosphate *(IP₃)* and diacylglycerol (DAG). IP_3 is generated from phosphatidylinositol bisphosphate (PIP₂). *NE*, norepinephrine; *β-AdrR*, β-adrenergic receptor; *PI*, phosphatidylinositol; *PIP*, phosphatidylinositol-4-phosphate; *PIP₂*, phosphatidylinositol-4,5-bisphosphate.

Decreased cAMP formation is caused by muscarinic receptor stimulation. This effect is most apparent when adenylyl cyclase is stimulated, for example, by activation of adrenergic receptors with catecholamines or forskolin. Simultaneous addition of cholinergic agonists decreases the amount of cAMP formed in response to the catecholamine, in some tissues almost completely. The result is diminished activation of cAMP-dependent protein kinase (PKA) and decreased substrate phosphorylation catalyzed by this kinase. The mechanism by which the muscarinic receptor inhibits adenylyl cyclase is through activation of an inhibitory GTP-binding protein, G_i. The α subunit of G_i competes with the α subunit of the G protein activated by stimulatory agonists (G_S) for regulation of adenylyl cyclase (see Chaps. 20 and 22). Although muscarinic receptors do not interact with G_s, increases in cAMP formation are seen under some circumstances. These may result from stimulatory effects of $\beta\gamma$ subunits released from G_i or effects of elevated intracellular Ca^{2+} on specific isoforms of adenylyl cyclase.

Activation of phosphoinositide-specific phospholipase C by muscarinic agonists stimulates phosphoinositide hydrolysis. Activation of the β_1 isoform of phosphoinositide-specific phospholipase C (PI-PLC) is mediated through the α subunit of a GTP-binding protein, $G_{q/11}$ [34]. This is the primary mechanism by which muscarinic receptors regulate this enzyme. However, some PLC isoforms, most clearly β_2, also are activated by $\beta\gamma$ subunits. This probably accounts for the pertussis toxin-sensitive, G_i/G_o-mediated activation of PI-PLC seen when high levels of cloned M_2 receptors are expressed stably in some cell lines. The hydrolysis of phosphatidylinositol 4,5-bisphosphate yields two potential second messengers, inositol 1,4,5-trisphosphate (IP_3) and diacylglycerol (DAG) (see Chap. 21). DAG increases the activity of the Ca^{2+} and phospholipid-dependent protein kinase (PKC). IP_3 mobilizes Ca^{2+} from intracellular stores in the endoplasmic reticulum and thereby elevates cytosolic free Ca^{2+}. Subsequent responses are triggered by direct effects of Ca^{2+} on Ca^{2+}-regulated proteins and by phosphorylation mediated through Ca^{2+}/calmodulin-dependent kinases and PKC. Stimulation of a phospholipase D, which hydrolyzes phosphatidylcholine, also occurs in response to muscarinic receptor activation. This appears to be secondary to activation of PKC and contributes to a secondary rise in DAG.

Regulation of K^+ channels. Muscarinic agonists cause rapid activation of G protein-coupled, inwardly rectifying potassium channels (GIRKs). This muscarinic effect can be mimicked by GTP analogs in whole-cell clamp experiments, and the response is sensitive to pertussis toxin, which ribosylates and inactivates G_i and a related protein, G_o (see Chap. 20). It is now generally agreed that GIRK1 and GIRK2 are activated directly by binding $\beta\gamma$ subunits released from G_i or G_o. This is a primary mechanism by which muscarinic agonists cause hyperpolarization of cardiac atrial cells, as well as of neurons [35]. This pathway contrasts with muscarinic inhibition of the M-current in sympathetic ganglia; suppression of this K^+ channel is mediated indirectly through muscarinic formation of a diffusible second messenger.

Intracellular mediators of muscarinic receptor action. The three events described above, inhibition of adenylyl cyclase, stimulation of PLC and regulation of K^+ channels, occur within the plasma membrane. They can be triggered directly by muscarinic receptor occupation independent of changes in cytosolic mediators. However, these primary events in turn affect the generation of diffusible second messengers such as cAMP, DAG, IP_3 and Ca^{2+}, which generate other metabolic sequelae. For example, an increase in cytosolic free Ca^{2+} probably contributes to activation of phospholipase A_2, generating arachidonic acid, prostaglandins and related eicosanoids (see Chap. 35). These products in turn can stimulate cGMP formation and can regulate ion channel activity. Increased Ca^{2+} also can activate Ca^{2+}-dependent ion channels (K^+, Cl^-), regulate cAMP phosphodiesterase and activate Ca^{2+}/calmodulin kinase-dependent protein phosphorylation. PKC is activated by DAG, generally in concert with Ca^{2+}, and has effects on ion-channel activity, as well as on cholinergic secretory and contractile responses.

Given the obviously complex set of possible interactions between the intracellular mediators, it is easy to explain how diverse cellular responses can be mediated through a single receptor activating relatively few primary responses (see Chap. 10).

Radioligand-binding studies have been used to characterize muscarinic receptors

In membranes or homogenates from heart, brain and other tissues, muscarinic agonists compete for antagonist-binding sites with Hill slopes of less than unity, suggesting that these agonists interact with more than a single population of muscarinic receptors [32]. Direct binding experiments with radiolabeled agonists also show multiple binding sites for agonists. Competition curves are best fit by a model in which there are sites with low, high and in some cases, superhigh affinity for agonists. Addition of GTP to the binding assay can have a dramatic effect on the agonist competition curve or on direct agonist binding. The effect of GTP is to decrease the apparent affinity of the receptor for agonists. This results from a change in the interaction of the receptor with the GTP-binding protein that transduces its effects.

Agonists vary in their binding properties. Some, like ACh, carbamylcholine and methacholine, bind with high affinity to a large percentage of the total sites. Others, like oxotremorine and pilocarpine, appear to bind to a single class of sites and may show relatively little high-affinity binding. The capacity of an agonist to induce high-affinity binding correlates with the efficacy of that agonist for eliciting responses such as contraction or phosphoinositide breakdown. It therefore appears that interaction of the receptor and G protein is critical to production of the cellular response.

Unlike agonists, most muscarinic antagonists, such as quinuclidinylbenzilate, *N*-methylscopolamine and atropine, bind to the receptor with Hill slopes of unity, as expected for a mass-action interaction with a single receptor type. There is little difference in affinity for these ligands in various tissues. Similar findings with other antagonists initially suggested that all muscarinic receptors were the same. However, a number of functional studies have suggested that muscarinic receptors are heterogeneous, and several putative subtype-selective antagonists have been described throughout the years.

The binding properties of the antagonist pirenzepine led to the initial classification of muscarinic receptors

Pirenzepine (PZ) binds to muscarinic receptors in cortex, hippocampus and ganglia with relatively high affinity; these sites have been termed M_1, as mentioned earlier. Heart, gland and smooth muscle muscarinic receptors, as well as those in brainstem, cerebellum and thalamus, show 30- to 50-fold lower affinity for PZ [32,33]. The affinity for classic antagonists like *N*-methylscopolamine is the same in all of these regions, emphasizing the unique selectivity of PZ. Direct binding studies using [^{3}H]PZ confirm that only certain tissues and brain regions have receptors with high affinity for this antagonist. Results of pharmacological studies also indicate that PZ blocks muscarinic responses in ganglia better than responses in heart. Brain and heart subsequently were used to purify M_1 and M_2 muscarinic receptors, and cDNA clones corresponding to these receptors were isolated from rat brain and heart libraries.

The cDNAs for the muscarinic receptors encode apparent glycoproteins of 55 to 70 kDa, which contain seven predicted transmembrane-spanning regions, similar to what is seen for the β-adrenergic receptor and other receptors that couple to G proteins (Fig. 11-10). There is only 38% amino acid identity between the proteins cloned from porcine brain and heart. The cDNA encoding the receptor initially cloned from the brain has been termed m_1, whereas that cloned from the heart has been termed m_2.

The human and rat homologs of these receptor genes, as well as three additional subtypes termed m_3, m_4 and m_5, subsequently have been cloned and expressed. Comparison of the amino acid sequences of the five muscarinic receptor subtypes suggests that they are members of a highly conserved gene family. The greatest sequence identity is in the transmembrane-span-

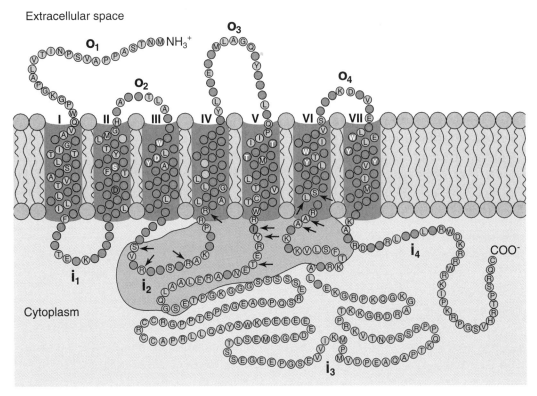

FIGURE 11-10.   Predicted amino acid sequence and transmembrane domain structure of the human M_1 muscarinic receptor. Amino acids that are identical among the m_1, m_2, m_3 and m_4 receptors are dark orange. The *shaded cloud* represents the approximate region that determines receptor–G protein coupling. *Arrows* denote amino acids important for specifying G protein coupling. Amino acids predicted to be involved in agonist or antagonist binding are denoted by white letters [36].

ning regions, whereas the long cytoplasmic loop (i_3) between transmembrane domains V and VI varies among the receptor subtypes [32,36]. The cloned receptors, expressed in mammalian cells, show differences in antagonist affinity similar to those of the pharmacologically defined receptors. Thus, the expressed m_1 receptor is blocked selectively by PZ, the m_2 receptor is blocked by AFDX-116 and methoctramine and the m_3 receptor is blocked by hexahydrosiladifenidol [33]. The regions in the receptor responsible for differences in antagonist affinity have not yet been identified clearly. Ligands are believed to bind to the receptor at sites facing the extracellular space but located in a central cavity deep within the bundle formed by transmembrane domains III through VII. The binding site for the covalent antagonist propylbenzilylcholine mustard has been mapped to a particular aspartic acid residue in the third transmembrane region.

This amino acid is conserved in all biogenic amine G-protein-coupled receptors. Mutagenesis of this amino acid profoundly affects both agonist and antagonist binding to muscarinic receptors. It is hypothesized that this residue participates in ionic bonding with the ammonium headgroup of the cholinergic ligand [32].

Expression of the cloned receptors in Chinese hamster ovary cells, other mammalian cells and *Xenopus* oocytes has demonstrated differential coupling of these receptors to cellular responses. In general the m_1, m_3 and m_5 receptors regulate phosphoinositide hydrolysis by stimulating PLC. This occurs through selective coupling of the receptor to a pertussis toxin-insensitive G protein, probably $G_{q/11}$, which can activate the β isoform of PLC [34]. Calcium-dependent K^+ and Cl^- channels are activated secondarily to the PLC-mediated increase in intracellular Ca^{2+}. In contrast, the m_2 and m_4

receptors couple through a pertussis toxin-sensitive G protein (G_i) to inhibition of adenylyl cyclase. Regulation of K^+ channels also is mediated through m_2 or m_4 receptor interaction with specific pertussis toxin-sensitive G proteins.

Chimeric receptors have been used to determine the regions critical for specifying coupling to particular responses. These studies demonstrate that it is the third intracellular (i_3) loop that defines functional specificity [33,36]. A series of amino acids proximal to the transmembrane domain, that is, at the amino- and the carboxy-terminal ends of the i_3 loop, carry most of this information. These particular regions are similar in the m_1, m_3 and m_5 receptors and in the m_2 and m_4 receptors but distinguish these two groups from one another. Both site-directed and random mutagenesis studies have identified specific amino acids at the amino-terminus of the i_3 loop which are required for G protein recognition and activation [36,37]. These critical noncharged amino acids are predicted to reside on the hydrophobic face of an α-helical extension of transmembrane domain V. Conserved amino acids in the carboxy-terminus of the i_3 loop and adjacent transmembrane domain VI also have been demonstrated to specify coupling to G_i- versus G_q-mediated responses. The hydrophobic regions at the two ends of the i_3 loop thus are suggested to form a surface that binds to and discriminates between different classes of G protein [36]. Other regions, including a portion of the second intracellular loop, also contribute to specifying correct G protein coupling.

The selectivity in muscarinic receptor coupling is not absolute. Overexpression of receptors or of particular G proteins supports interactions that may differ from those described above. For example, m_2 receptors expressed in Chinese hamster ovary cells not only inhibit adenylyl cyclase but also can stimulate phosphoinositide hydrolysis through a pertussis toxin-sensitive G protein [38]; this is not seen, however, when m_2 receptors are expressed in Y1 cells. These findings indicate that caution must be exercised in interpreting data obtained when receptors are expressed, often at high levels, in cells in which they normally do not function.

Muscarinic receptors of the m_1, m_3 and m_5 subclasses induce transformation or cell proliferation, a feature not shared by m_2 and m_4 receptors [39]. This property has been exploited to develop a high-throughput assay for screening effects of receptor mutations [37]. Mitogen-activated protein kinases (MAP kinases) also are activated by muscarinic receptors, but unlike transformation, this response occurs with receptors of the m_2/m_4 subtype as well as of the m_1/m_3 subtype. Notably, induction of cell growth by muscarinic receptor stimulation is cell type-specific and is seen only at high levels of receptor expression [39]. Thus, it is questionable whether there is a physiological role for ACh in growth regulation.

Transgenic mice are being generated to assess the functions of receptor subtypes *in vivo*

Knowledge of the anatomical distribution and coupling properties of receptor subtypes can indicate which physiological responses they mediate *in vivo*. However, the lack of good subtype-selective antagonists limits the use of pharmacological approaches to address this question. Generation of transgenic mice in which muscarinic receptors are overexpressed or receptor genes are disrupted by homologous recombination provides a new approach for evaluation of muscarinic receptor function. The m_1 gene has been targeted selectively, and m_1 receptor expression in the forebrain was eliminated [40]. Homozygous m_1 receptor-deficient mice are completely resistant to seizures produced by pilocarpine, implicating the m_1 receptor in this model of epilepsy. Furthermore, inhibition of the M-current in sympathetic ganglia, suggested by previous pharmacological experiments to be m_1 receptor-coupled, is ablated in knockout mice. Future development of this approach should provide considerable insight into the distinct roles of the m_1, m_2 and other muscarinic receptor subtypes in peripheral and central nervous system function.

REFERENCES

1. Rama-Sastry, B. V., and Sadavongvivad, C. Non-neuronal acetylcholine. *Pharmacol. Rev.* 30:65–132, 1979.

2. Dale, H. H. The action of certain esters and ethers of choline and their relation to muscarine. *J. Pharmacol.* 6:147–190, 1914.

3. Changeux, J. P. Chemical signaling in the brain. *Sci. Am.* 269:58–62, 1993.

4. Numa, S., Noda, M., Takahashi, H., et al. Molecular structure of the acetylcholine receptor. *Cold Spring Harb. Symp. Quant. Biol.* 48:57–69, 1983.

5. Partington, P., Feeney, J., and Burgen, A. S. V. The conformation of acetylcholine and related compounds in aqueous solutions as studied by nuclear magnetic resonance spectroscopy. *Mol. Pharmacol.* 8:269–277, 1972.

6. Behling, R. W., Yamane, T., Navon, G., and Jelinski, L. W. Conformation of acetylcholine bound to the nicotinic acetylcholine receptor. *Proc. Natl. Acad. Sci. USA* 85:6721–6724, 1988.

7. Portoghese, P. S. Relationships between stereostructure and pharmacological activity. *Annu. Rev. Pharmacol.* 10:51–76, 1970.

8. Baker, R. W., Pauling, P., and Petcher, T. J. Structure and activity of muscarinic stimulants. *Nature* 230:439–445, 1971.

9. Lefkowitz, R. J., Hoffman, B. B., and Taylor, P. Neurohumoral transmission: The autonomic and somatic motor nervous systems. In J. G. Hardman and L. E. Limbird (eds.), *Goodman & Gilman's Pharmacological Basics of Therapeutics.* New York: Macmillan, 1996, pp. 105–140.

10. Role, L. W., and Berg, D. K. Nicotinic receptors in the development and modulation of CNS synapses. *Neuron* 16:1077–1085, 1996.

11. Lindstrom, J. Neuronal nicotinic receptors. In T. Narahashi (ed.), *Ion Channels,* Vol. 4. New York: Plenum Press, 1996, pp. 377–450.

12. Kasa, P. The cholinergic systems in brain and spinal cord. *Prog. Neurobiol.* 26:211–272, 1986.

13. Adams, P. R., Brown, D. A., and Constitini, A. Pharmacological inhibition of the M-current. *J. Physiol. (Lond.)* 332:223–262, 1982.

14. Van der kloot, W., and Molgo, J. Quantal acetylcholine release at the vertebrate neuromuscular junction. *Physiol. Rev.* 74:898–991, 1994.

15. Wu, D., and Hersh, L. B. Choline acetyltransferase: Celebrating its fiftieth year. *J. Neurochem.* 62:1653–1663, 1994.

16. Parsons, S. M., Bahr, B. A., Gracz, M., et al. Acetylcholine transport: Fundamental properties and effects of pharmacologic agents. *Ann. N. Y. Acad. Sci.* 493:220–233, 1987.

17. Erickson, J. D., Weihe, E., Schafer, M. K. M., et al. The VAChT/ChAT "cholinergic gene locus": New aspects of genetic and vesicular regulation of cholinergic function. *Prog. Brain Res.* 109:69–82, 1996.

18. Varoqui, H., Mennier, F.-M., Mennier, F. A., et al. Expression of the vesicular acetylcholine transporter in mammalian cells. *Prog. Brain Res.* 109:83–95, 1996.

19. Kuffler, S. W., Nicholls, J., and Martin, R. A. *From Neuron to Brain: A Cellular Approach to the Function of the Nervous System.* Sunderland, MA: Sinauer Associates, 1984.

20. Taylor, P., and Radic, Z. The cholinesterases: From genes to proteins. *Annu. Rev. Pharmacol. Toxicol.* 34:281–320, 1994.

21. Massoulié, J., Pezzementi, L., Bon, S., Krejci, E., and Vallette, F.-M. Molecular and cellular biology of cholinesterases. *Prog. Neurobiol.* 41:31–91, 1993.

22. Sussman, J. L., Harel, M., Frolow, F., et al. Atomic structure of acetylcholinesterase from *Torpedo californica.* A prototypic acetylcholine-binding protein. *Science* 253:872–878, 1992.

23. Bourne, Y., Taylor, P., and Marchot, P. Acetylcholinesterase inhibition by fasciculin. Crystal structure of the complex. *Cell* 83:503–512, 1995.

24. Unwin, N. Nicotinic acetylcholine receptor at 9 Å resolution. *J. Mol. Biol.* 229:1101–1124, 1993.

25. Karlin, A., and Akabas, M. H. Towards a structural basis for the function of nicotinic acetylcholine receptors and their cousins. *Neuron* 15:1231–1244, 1995.

26. Tsigelny, I., Sugiyama, N., Sine, S. M., and Taylor, P. A model of the nicotinic receptor extracellular domain based on sequence identity and residue location. *Biophys. J.* 73:52–56, 1997.

27. Sakmann, B. Elementary steps in synaptic transmission revealed by currents through single ion channels. *Science* 256:503–512, 1992.

28. Changeux, J. P. Compartmentalized transcription of acetylcholine receptor genes during motor end-plate epigenesis. *New Biol.* 3:413–429, 1991.

29. Sanes, J. R. Genetic analysis of postsynaptic differentiation at the vertebrate neuromuscular junction. *Curr. Opin. Neurobiol.* 7:93–100, 1997.

30. Fuentes, M. E., and Taylor, P. Control of acetylcholinesterase gene expression during myogenesis. *Neuron* 10:679–687, 1993.

31. Fischbach, G. D., and Rosen, K. M. ARIA: A neuromuscular junction neuregulin. *Annu. Rev. Neurosci.* 20:420–458, 1997.

32. Hulme, E., Birdsall, N., and Buckley, N. Muscarinic receptor subtypes. *Annu. Rev. Pharmacol. Toxicol.* 30:633–673, 1990.

33. Caulfield, M. D. Muscarinic receptors—characterization, coupling and function. *Pharmacol. Ther.* 58:319–379, 1993.

34. Berstein, G., Blank, J. L., Smrcka, A. V., et al. Reconstitution of agonist stimulated phosphatidylinositol 4-5 bisphosphate hydrolysis using purified m_1 muscarinic receptor, $G_{q/11}$, and phospholipase C-β1. *J. Biol. Chem.* 267: 8081–8088, 1992.

35. Kofuji, P., Davidson, N., and Lester, H. Evidence that neuronal G-protein gated inwardly rectifying K^+ channels are activated by G protein $\beta\gamma$ subunits and function as heteromultimers. *Proc. Natl. Acad. Sci. USA* 92:6542–6546, 1995.

36. Wess, J. Molecular biology of muscarinic acetylcholine receptors. *Crit. Rev. Neurobiol.* 10:69–99, 1996.

37. Hill Eubank, D., Burstein, E., Spalding, T., Brauner-Osborne, H., and Brann, M. Structure of a G-protein coupling domain of a muscarinic receptor predicted by random saturation mutagenesis. *J. Biol. Chem.* 271:3058–3065, 1996.

38. Ashkenazi, A., Winslow, J. W., Peralta, E. G., et al. An M_2 muscarinic receptor subtype coupled to both adenylyl cyclase and phosphoinositide turnover. *Science* 238:672–675, 1987.

39. Gutkind, J. S., Novotny, E. A., Brann, M. R., and Robbins, K. C. Muscarinic acetylcholine receptor subtypes as agonist-dependent oncogenes. *Proc. Natl. Acad. Sci. USA* 88:4703–4707, 1991.

40. Hamilton, S. E., Loose, M. D., Qi, M., et al. Disruption of the m1 receptor gene ablates muscarinic receptor-dependent M current regulation and seizure activity in mice. *Proc. Natl. Acad. Sci. USA*, 94:13311–13316, 1997.

12

Catecholamines

Michael J. Kuhar, Pastor R. Couceyro and Philip D. Lambert

Basic Neurochemistry: Molecular, Cellular and Medical Aspects, 6th Ed., edited by G. J. Siegel et al. Published by
Lippincott–Raven Publishers, Philadelphia, 1999. Correspondence to Michael J. Kuhar, Division of Neuroscience, Yerkes
Regional Primate Research Center of Emory University, Atlanta, Georgia 30322.

The catecholamines dopamine (DA), norepinephrine (NE) and epinephrine are neurotransmitters and/or hormones in the periphery and in the central nervous system (CNS) (for reviews, see [1,2]). NE is a neurotransmitter in the brain as well as in postganglionic, sympathetic neurons. DA, the precursor of NE, has biological activity in the periphery, most particularly in the kidney, and serves as a neurotransmitter in several important pathways in the CNS. Epinephrine, formed by the N-methylation of NE, is a hormone released from the adrenal gland, and it stimulates catecholamine receptors in a variety of organs. Small amounts of epinephrine are also found in the CNS, particularly in the brainstem.

BIOSYNTHESIS OF CATECHOLAMINES

The enzymatic processes involved in the formation of catecholamines have been characterized. The component enzymes in the pathway have been purified to homogeneity, which has allowed for detailed analysis of their kinetics, substrate specificity and cofactor requirements and for the development of inhibitors (Fig. 12-1). Studies with knockout mice clearly indicate the importance of these enzymes since absence of at least some of them results in loss of viability (Table 12-1).

Tyrosine hydroxylase is the rate-limiting enzyme for the biosynthesis of catecholamines

Tyrosine hydroxylase (TH) is found in all cells that synthesize catecholamines and is a mixed-function oxidase that uses molecular oxygen and tyrosine as its substrates and biopterin as its co-factor [3]. TH is a homotetramer, each subunit of which has a molecular weight of approximately 60,000. It catalyzes the addition of a hydroxyl group to the *meta* position of tyrosine, thus forming 3,4-dihydroxy-L-phenylalanine (L-DOPA). TH can also hydroxylate phenylalanine to form tyrosine, which is then converted to L-DOPA; this alternative synthetic route may be of significance in patients affected with phenylketonuria, a condition in which phenylalanine hydroxylase activity is depressed (see Chap. 44). TH has a K_m for tyrosine in the micromolar range. As a result, it is virtually saturated by the high tissue concentrations of endogenous tyrosine. The cofactor, biopterin, may be at subsaturating concentrations within catecholamine-containing neurons and, thus, may play an important role in regulating NE biosynthesis. TH is primarily a soluble enzyme; however, interactions with membrane constituents, such as phosphatidylserine, or with polyanions, such as heparin sulfate, have been shown to alter its kinetic characteristics. Analogs of tyrosine, such as α-methyl-*p*-tyrosine (AMPT), are competitive inhibitors of TH. Sequence analysis [4] reveals consensus sequences for phosphorylation primarily in the N-terminal portion of the molecule. The gene reveals considerable sequence homology with phenylalanine hydroxylase and tryptophan hydroxylase.

DOPA decarboxylase catalyzes the removal of the carboxyl group from DOPA to form dopamine

DOPA decarboxylase (DDC) is a pyridoxine-dependent enzyme that has a low K_m and a high V_{max} with respect to L-DOPA; thus, endogenous L-DOPA is efficiently converted to DA [5]. DDC

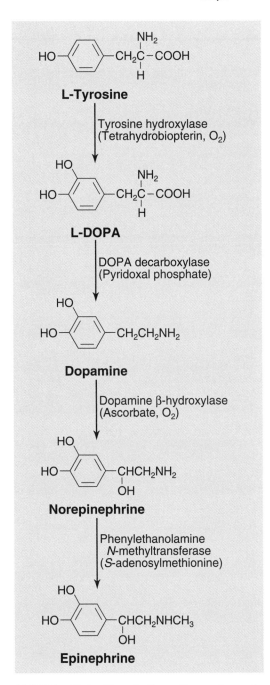

FIGURE 12-1. Biosynthetic pathway for catecholamines.

the body, where it is found both in catecholamine- and serotonin-containing neurons and in non-neuronal tissues, such as kidney and blood vessels. In DA-containing neurons, this enzyme is the final step in the pathway. α-Methyldopa inhibits DDC *in vitro* and leads to a reduction in blood pressure after being converted to the false transmitter α-methylnorepinephrine *in vivo*.

For neurons that synthesize epinephrine or norepinephrine, dopamine β-hydroxylase is the next step in the biosynthetic pathway

Like TH, dopamine β-hydroxylase (DBH) is a mixed-function oxidase that uses molecular oxygen to form the hydroxyl group added to the β carbon on the side chain of DA [6]. Ascorbate, reduced to dihydroascorbate during the reaction, provides a source of electrons. DBH contains Cu^{2+}, which is involved in electron transfer in the reaction; accordingly, copper chelators, such as diethyldithiocarbamate, are potent inhibitors of the enzyme. DBH is a tetrameric glycoprotein containing subunits of 77 and 73 kDa, as determined by sodium dodecyl sulfate (SDS) gel electrophoresis. A full-length clone encodes a polypeptide chain of 578 amino acids [7]. The enzyme is concentrated within the vesicles that store catecholamines; most of the DBH is bound to the inner vesicular membrane, but some is free within the vesicles. DBH is released along with catecholamines from nerves and from the adrenal gland and is found in plasma.

In cells that synthesize epinephrine, the final step in the pathway is catalyzed by the enzyme phenylethanolamine *N*-methyltransferase

This enzyme is found in a small group of neurons in the brainstem that utilize epinephrine as their neurotransmitter and in the adrenal medullary cells, for which epinephrine is the primary neurohormone. Phenylethanolamine *N*-methyltransferase (PNMT) transfers a methyl group from *S*-adenosylmethionine to the nitrogen of NE, forming a secondary amine [8]. The

can also decarboxylate 5-hydroxytryptophan, the precursor of serotonin, as well as other aromatic amino acids; accordingly, it has also been called aromatic amino acid decarboxylase (AADC). DDC is widely distributed throughout

TABLE 12-1.	STUDIES WITH KNOCKOUT MICE	
Tyrosine hydroxylase	Not viable	[32]
Dopamine hydroxylase	Not viable	[33]
Dopamine transporter	Hyperlocomotion, no effect of MPTP or psychostimulants	[34]
Vesicular transporter	Not viable	[35]
α_{2B}-Adrenergic receptor	Apparently normal	[36]
β_1-Adrenergic receptor	Most die prenatally, survivors have altered cardiovascular responses	[37]
β_3-Adrenergic receptor	Altered leptin and insulin concentrations after agonist treatment	[38]
		[39]
Dopamine 1 (D1) receptor	Lack responses to agonists, hyperlocomotion, altered striatal peptides	[40]
		[41]
Dopamine 2 (D2) receptor	Impaired movements	[42]
Dopamine 3 (D3) receptor	Hyperlocomotion	[43]

See Chap. 40 for a discussion of knockout mice. MPTP, *N*-methyl-4-phenyl-1,2,3,6-tetrahydropyridine.

coding sequence of bovine PNMT is contained in a single open reading frame encoding a protein of 284 amino acids [9]. PNMT activity is regulated by corticosteroids.

STORAGE AND RELEASE OF CATECHOLAMINES

Catecholamines are concentrated in storage vesicles that are present at high density within nerve terminals

Ordinarily, low concentrations of catecholamines are free in the cytosol, where they may be metabolized by enzymes including monoamine oxidase (MAO). Thus, conversion of tyrosine to L-DOPA and L-DOPA to DA occurs in the cytosol; DA then is taken up into the storage vesicles. In NE-containing neurons, the final β hydroxylation occurs within the vesicles. In the adrenal gland, NE is *N*-methylated by PNMT in the cytoplasm. Epinephrine is then transported back into chromaffin granules for storage.

cDNA clones encoding vesicular amine transporters have been obtained. The sequence suggests that the proteins have 12 transmembrane domains and are homologous to a family of bacterial drug-resistance transporters. The expressed protein, referred to as vesicular membrane transporter 2 (VMAT2), has a high affinity for reserpine, which blocks vesicular uptake *in vivo* [10]. The mechanism that concentrates catecholamines within the vesicles is an ATP-depen-

dent process linked to a proton pump. The intravesicular concentration of catecholamines is approximately 0.5 M, and they exist in a complex with ATP and acidic proteins known as chromogranins. The vesicular uptake process has broad substrate specificity and can transport a variety of biogenic amines, including tryptamine, tyramine and amphetamines; these amines may compete with endogenous catecholamines for vesicular storage sites. Reserpine is a specific, irreversible inhibitor of the vesicular amine pump that blocks the ability of the vesicles to concentrate the amines. Treatment with reserpine causes a profound depletion of endogenous catecholamines in neurons. The effect of reserpine is to inhibit the uptake of DA and other catecholamines into vesicles. Knockout mice lacking VMAT2 are not viable (Table 12-1).

The vesicles play a dual role: they maintain a ready supply of catecholamines at the terminal available for release, and they mediate the process of release. When an action potential reaches the nerve terminal, Ca^{2+} channels open, allowing an influx of the cation into the terminal; increased intracellular Ca^{2+} promotes the fusion of vesicles with the neuronal membrane (see Chap. 9). The vesicles then discharge their soluble contents, including NE, ATP and DBH, into the extraneuronal space [11]. The demonstration that DBH is released concurrently and proportionately with NE established that release occurs by the process of exocytosis since proteins would not be expected to diffuse across cell membranes. Exocytotic release from sympathetic neurons may be the source of some of the DBH found in the plasma and cerebrospinal fluid (CSF) of animals and humans. Indirectly acting sympathomimetics, like tyramine and amphetamine, release catecholamines by a mechanism that is neither dependent on Ca^{2+} nor associated with release of DBH. These drugs displace catecholamines from storage vesicles, resulting in leakage of neurotransmitter from the nerve terminals.

The concentration of catecholamines within nerve terminals remains relatively constant

Despite the marked fluctuations in the activity of catecholamine-containing neurons, efficient regulatory mechanisms modulate the rate of synthesis of catecholamines [12]. A long-term process affecting catecholamine synthesis involves alterations in the amounts of TH and DBH present in nerve terminals [1]. When sympathetic neuronal activity is increased for a prolonged period of time, the amounts of mRNA coding for TH and DBH are increased in the neuronal perikarya. DDC does not appear to be modulated by this process. The newly synthesized enzyme molecules are then transported down the axon to the nerve terminals.

Alteration in the rate of synthesis of TH and DBH provides a mechanism to modulate synthesis of catecholamines in response to persistent changes in neuronal activity. In addition, two mechanisms operative at the level of the nerve terminal play important roles in the short-term modulation of catecholamine synthesis and are responsive to momentary changes in neuronal activity [13]. TH, the rate-limiting enzyme in the synthesis pathway, is modulated by end-product inhibition [12]. Thus, free intraneuronal catecholamines inhibit the further activity of TH by competing at the site that binds the pterin cofactor; conversely, neuronal activity results in the release of catecholamines, a decrease in cytoplasmic concentrations and disinhibition of the enzyme. An additional and probably more important effect of depolarization of catecholaminergic terminals is activation of TH. The kinetic characteristics of the enzyme change so that it has a higher affinity for the pterin co-

factor and is less sensitive to end-product inhibition. Activation of the enzyme is associated with reversible phosphorylation of the enzyme (Fig. 12-2) [14]. Protein kinase C (PKC), cAMP-dependent protein kinase (PKA) and Ca^{2+}/calmodulin-dependent protein kinases (CaMKs) are all capable of inducing phosphorylation of the enzyme, leading to an increase in activity (see Chaps. 21 and 22).

Monoamine oxidase and catechol-*O*-methyltransferase are primarily responsible for the inactivation of catecholamines

MAO and catechol-*O*-methyltransferase (COMT) are widely distributed throughout the body (Fig. 12-3). MAO is a flavin-containing enzyme located on the outer membrane of the mitochondria [15]. This enzyme oxidatively deaminates catecholamines to their corresponding aldehydes; these can be converted, in turn, by aldehyde dehydrogenase to acids or by aldehyde reductase to form glycols. Because of its intracellular localization, MAO plays a strategic role in inactivating catecholamines that are free within the nerve terminal and not protected by storage vesicles. Accordingly, drugs that interfere with vesicular storage, such as reserpine, or indirectly acting sympathomimetics, such as amphetamines, which displace catecholamines from vesicles, cause a marked increase in deaminated metabolites. Isozymes of MAO with differential substrate specificities have been identified: MAO-A preferentially deaminates NE and serotonin and is selectively inhibited by clorgyline, whereas MAO-B acts on a broad spectrum of phenylethylamines, including β-phenylethylamine. MAO-B is selectively inhibited by deprenyl. MAO in the gastrointestinal tract and liver plays an important protective role by preventing access to the general circulation of ingested, indirectly acting amines, such as tyramine and phenylethylamine, that are contained in food; however, patients being treated for depression or hypertension with MAO inhibitors are not afforded this protection and can suffer severe hypertensive crises after ingesting foods that contain large amounts of tyramine. Such foods include port wine, Stilton cheese and herring. A methyl substituent on the α carbon of the phenylethyl-

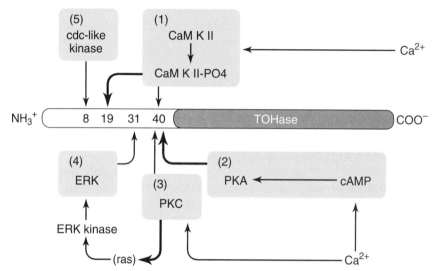

FIGURE 12-2. Schematic diagram of the phosphorylation sites on each of the four 60-kDa subunits of tyrosine hydroxylase (TOHase). Serine residues at the N-terminus of each of four subunits of TOHase can be phosphorylated by at least five protein kinases. *(1)*, Calcium/calmodulin-dependent protein kinase II *(CaM K II)* phosphorylates serine residue 19 and to a lesser extent serine 40. *(2)*, cAMP-dependent protein kinase *(PKA)* phosphorylates serine residue 40. *(3)*, Calcium/phosphatidylserine-activated protein kinase *(PKC)* phosphorylates serine 40. *(4)*, Extracellular receptor-activated protein kinase *(ERK)* phosphorylates serine 31. *(5)*, A cdc-like protein kinase phosphorylates serine 8. Phosphorylation on either serine 19 or 40 increases the activity of TOHase. Serine 19 phosphorylation requires the presence of an "activator protein," also known as 14-3-3 protein, for the expression of increased activity. Phosphorylation of serines 8 and 31 has little effect on catalytic activity. The model shown includes the activation of ERK by an ERK kinase. The ERK kinase is activated by phosphorylation by PKC. (From [44], with permission.)

amine side chain protects against deamination by MAO; the prolonged action of amphetamine and related indirectly acting stimulants is in part a consequence of the presence of an α-methyl group, which prevents their inactivation by MAO.

COMT is found in nearly all cells, including erythrocytes [16]; thus, the enzyme can act on extraneuronal catecholamines. Most studies of COMT are carried out with enzyme purified from homogenates of liver. The enzyme, which requires Mg^{2+}, transfers a methyl group from the cosubstrate *S*-adenosylmethionine to the 3-hydroxy group on the catecholamine ring. This enzyme has broad substrate specificity, methylating virtually any catechol regardless of the side-chain constituents; for this reason, competitive inhibitors of the enzyme that are of pharmacological significance have not been developed.

Measurement of catecholamine metabolites can provide insight into the rate of release or turnover of catecholamines in the brain. In clinical studies, metabolites of catecholamines are generally assayed in the CSF because the large quantities derived from the peripheral sympathomedullary system obscure the small contribution from the brain to urinary concentrations. However, acid metabolites are actively excreted from the CSF; more reliable estimates of turnover in the brain are obtained when this transport process is blocked by pretreatment with the drug probenecid.

4-Hydroxy-3-methoxy-phenylacetic acid, more commonly known as homovanillic acid (HVA), is a major metabolite of DA. Spinal fluid concentrations of HVA provide insight into the turnover of DA in the striatum. Concentrations of HVA are decreased, for example, in CSF of patients with Parkinson's disease (see Chap. 45). A metabolite of NE formed relatively selectively in the brain is 3-methoxy-4-hydroxyphenylglycol (MHPG). Because this is a minor metabolite of the much larger amounts of NE metabolized in the periphery, it is estimated that between 30 and 50% of the MHPG excreted in urine is derived from the brain. MHPG has been measured in

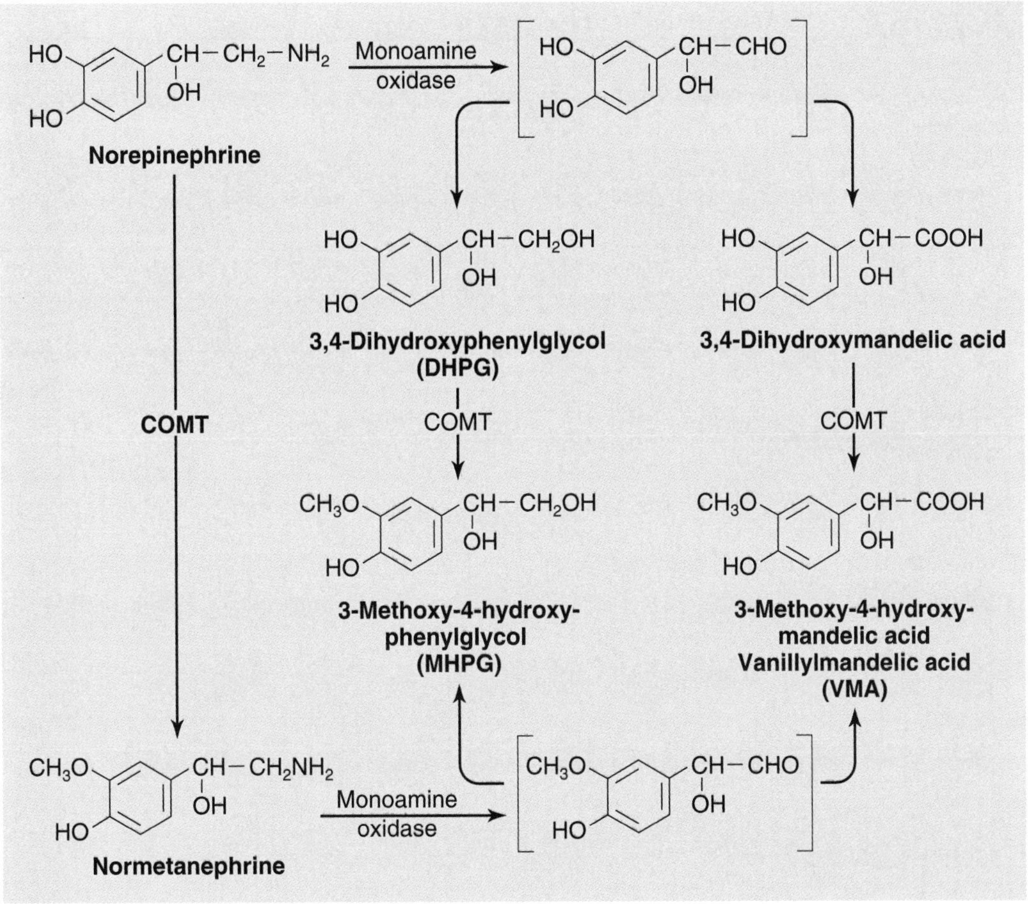

FIGURE 12-3. Pathways of norepinephrine degradation. Unstable glycol aldehydes are shown in brackets. COMT, catechol-O-methyltransferase.

CSF and in urine to provide an index of NE turnover in the brain and concentrations of MHPG have been shown to be decreased in certain forms of depression (see Chap. 52).

The action of catecholamines released at the synapse is terminated by diffusion and reuptake into presynaptic nerve terminals

Catecholamines diffuse from the synaptic cleft and are taken up or transported back into the nerve terminal. Some of the catecholamine molecules may be catabolized by MAO and COMT. The catecholamine-reuptake process was originally described by Axelrod [17]. He observed that when radioactive NE was injected intravenously, it accumulated in tissues in direct proportion to the density of the sympathetic innervation in the tissue. The amine taken up into the tissues was protected from catabolic degradation, and studies of the subcellular distribution of catecholamines showed that they are localized in synaptic vesicles. Ablation of the sympathetic input to organs abolished the ability of vesicles to accumulate and store radioactive NE. Subsequent studies demonstrated that this Na^+ and Cl^--dependent uptake process is a characteristic feature of catecholamine-containing neurons in both the periphery and the brain; the transport process has been extensively studied in sheared-off nerve terminals or synaptosomes isolated from the brain (Table 12-2).

The uptake process is mediated by a carrier or transporter located on the outer membrane of the catecholaminergic neurons. It is saturable

TABLE 12-2.   PROPERTIES OF AMINE TRANSPORTERS

	NET	DAT	VMAT-2
Mechanism	NaCl-dependent	NaCl-dependent	H^+-dependent
Transmembrane segments	12	12	12
Amino acids	617	620	742
Chromosome	16	5	10
Blockers	Nisoxetine, desipramine	GBR12909, RTI-121	Reserpine, tetrabenazine

The neuronal membrane norepinephrine transporter (NET), the dopamine transporter (DAT) and the vesicular membrane transporter (VMAT-2), which is the same in all catecholamine-containing neurons, have similar numbers of predicted transmembrane segments. They have different numbers of amino acids, pharmacological properties and chromosomal localizations.

and obeys Michaelis-Menten kinetics. A transport process selective for NE is found only in noradrenergic neurons, whereas a transporter with different specificity is found in DA-containing neurons. Cloning of genes for transporters responsible for uptake of NE and DA has been accomplished, revealing proteins with conserved structural features [18]. The presence of 11 to 13 transmembrane domains is a recurrent theme (Fig. 12-4, Table 12-2). Transmembrane domains 1, 2 and 4–8 show the highest degree of sequence identity. The transporters are part of a larger family of neurotransporters (Chap. 5) [18]. They have consensus sites for phosphorylation, although the importance of phosphorylation has not been elucidated. The uptake process is energy-dependent since it can be inhibited by incubation at a low temperature or by metabolic inhibitors. The energy requirements reflect a coupling of the uptake process with the Na^+ gradient across the neuronal membrane. The process is also Cl^--dependent. Drugs such as ouabain, which inhibits Na,K-ATPase, or veratridine, which opens Na^+ channels, inhibit the uptake process. The linkage of uptake to the Na^+ gradient may be of physiological significance since transport temporarily ceases at the time of depolarization-induced release of catecholamines. The transport of catecholamines can be inhibited selectively by such drugs as tricyclic antidepressants and cocaine. In addition, a variety of phenylethylamines, such as am-

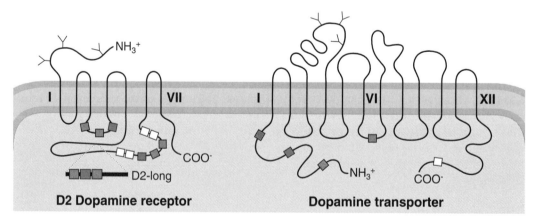

FIGURE 12-4.   Schematic of the D2 receptor and dopamine transporter. The amino acid chain is depicted as a line crossing the membrane. The D2 receptor has the typical seven transmembrane domains, while the dopamine transporter has approximately 12. The D2 dopamine receptor has two alternatively spliced mRNA variants that result in a short and a long form of the receptor. The longer variant has the insertion in the second intracellular loop. Putative glycosylation sites are indicated with *Y-shaped symbols* on extracellular sequences. Possible phosphorylation sites are indicated with *boxes* for various protein kinases: *gray boxes,* protein kinase A; *orange boxes,* protein kinase C; *white boxes,* calcium-calmodulin protein kinase. The dopamine transporter has a large glycosylated extracellular loop between transmembrane regions III and IV.

phetamine, are substrates for carrier; thus, they can be concentrated within catecholamine-containing neurons and can compete with the catecholamines for transport. Neurotoxins such as mercaptopyrazide pyrimidine (MPP$^+$) and 6-hydroxydopamine are also taken up by transporters, and this is required for the neurotoxic effect. Mice have been prepared with their transporter genes "knocked out" (see Chap. 40). Extensive studies with these mice confirm the important role of transporters (see Table 12-1).

Once an amine has been taken up across the neuronal membrane, it can be taken up by adrenergic storage vesicles. Neuronal uptake is Na$^+$-dependent and is not affected by drugs like reserpine; uptake across the vesicle membrane requires H$^+$ and is inhibited by reserpine (Table 12-2). Once a compound is taken up into the vesicles, it can be released in place of NE. Such substances are called false transmitters.

ANATOMY OF CATECHOLAMINERGIC SYSTEMS

Our understanding of the function of catecholamine-containing neurons has been aided by neuroanatomical methods of visualizing these neurons

Nearly two decades ago, Falck and Hillarp took advantage of the fact that in the presence of formaldehyde catecholamines cyclize to form intensely fluorescent products [19]. With a fluorescence microscope, neurons containing catecholamines could be visualized in thin sections obtained from tissue previously exposed to formaldehyde vapor. A modification of the method uses glyoxylic acid and has resulted in enhanced sensitivity and a more stable fluorophor for even better visualization of the fine axons and terminals.

Once the enzymes that synthesize catecholamines were purified, it was possible to elicit antisera against each enzyme and to localize the enzyme by immunocytochemistry. Thin sections of tissue can be incubated with antibody against a particular enzyme, for example, rabbit anti-DBH, and then incubated with a second antibody linked to a marker, such as fluorescein or horseradish peroxidase. These markers can be readily visualized and examined with a microscope. By using this technique, the PNMT-containing neurons that synthesize epinephrine can be distinguished from the noradrenergic neurons that are devoid of PNMT; similarly, noradrenergic neurons that contain DBH can be separated from the DA-containing neurons that do not possess this enzyme. Cloning the genes that encode for catecholaminergic biosynthetic enzymes makes it possible to use *in situ* hybridization to localize mRNAs within particular neurons.

Finally, experimental advantage has been taken of the highly selective uptake process for catecholamines. Thus, after incubation with radioactive NE, noradrenergic axons can be demonstrated at the ultrastructural level by autoradiographic techniques. Alternatively, after administration of the congener 5-hydroxydopamine, which is taken up actively and stored within the vesicles, catecholamine-containing terminals can be distinguished by the presence of dense precipitates of 5-hydroxydopamine within their vesicles. Also, antibodies against transporters have been used in immunocytochemistry and their mRNAs mapped by *in situ* hybridization. These studies generally confirm the findings of earlier ones.

Cell bodies of noradrenergic neurons are clustered in the medulla oblongata, pons and midbrain and are considered to be anatomically part of the reticular formation

On the basis of their major axonal projections, noradrenergic fibers can be divided into two major pathways: the dorsal and ventral bundles (Fig. 12-5). The cell bodies of origin for the dorsal bundle are contained in a dense nucleus known as the locus ceruleus, located on the lateral aspect of the fourth ventricle. Axons of neurons in the locus ceruleus have endings in the spinal cord and cerebellum and course anteriorly through the medial forebrain bundle to innervate the entire cerebral cortex and hippocampus. The ventrally located cell bodies send fibers that innervate the brainstem and hypothalamus. As demonstrated by immunocytochemical tech-

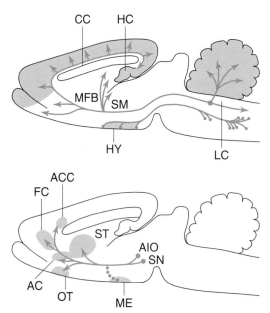

FIGURE 12-5. Some catecholaminergic neuronal pathways in the rat brain. **Upper**: Noradrenergic neuronal pathways. **Lower**: Dopaminergic neuronal pathways. *AC*, nucleus accumbens; *ACC*, anterior cingulate cortex; *CC*, corpus callosum; *FC*, frontal cortex; *HC*, hippocampus; *HY*, hypothalamus; *LC*, locus ceruleus; *ME*, median eminence; *MFB*, median forebrain bundle; *OT*, olfactory tubercle; *SM*, stria medullaris; *SN*, substantia nigra; *ST*, striatum. (Courtesy of J. T. Coyle and S. H. Snyder.)

niques, in the ventral portion of the pons and medulla there are a small number of neurons that contain PNMT; the axons of these epinephrine-containing neurons terminate primarily in the brainstem and hypothalamus.

Large numbers of cell bodies of dopamine-containing neurons are located in the midbrain

Some of the DA-containing neurons can be divided into three groups: nigrostriatal, mesocortical and tuberohypophysial. A major dopaminergic tract in brain originates in the zona compacta of the substantia nigra and sends axons that provide a dense innervation to the caudate nucleus and putamen of the corpus striatum; nearly 80% of all DA in the brain is found in the corpus striatum. In Parkinson's disease, the nigrostriatal tract degenerates (see Chap. 45). This accounts for a profound depletion of DA from the striatum and for the symptoms of this disorder.

DA-containing cell bodies that lie medial to the substantia nigra in the ventral tegmental area provide a diffuse, but modest, innervation to the forebrain, including the frontal and cingulate cortex, septum, nucleus accumbens and olfactory tubercle. It has been hypothesized that these neurons are critical for the action of antipsychotic drugs, antihyperactivity drugs and psychostimulant drugs.

DA-containing cell bodies in the arcuate and periventricular nuclei of the hypothalamus send axons that innervate the intermediate lobe of the pituitary and the median eminence. These neurons play an important role in regulating the release of pituitary hormones, especially prolactin (see Chap. 18). In addition to these major pathways, DA-containing interneurons have been found in the olfactory bulb and in the neural retina.

TABLE 12-3.	PROPERTIES OF CLONED DOPAMINE RECEPTOR SUBTYPES				
	D1	D5	D2S/D2L	D3	D4
Amino acids (human)	446	477	415/444	400	387
Chromosome	5	4	11	3	11
Effector pathways	↑cAMP	↑cAMP	↓cAMP ↑K$^+$ channel ↓Ca^{2+} channel	↓cAMP	↓cAMP ↑K$^+$ channel
mRNA distribution	Caudate putamen, nucleus accumbens, olfactory tubercle	Hippocampus, hypothalamus	Caudate putamen, nucleus accumbens, olfactory tubercle	olfactory tubercle, hypothalamus, nucleus accumbens	Frontal cortex, medulla, midbrain

TABLE 12-4. SUBTYPES OF α_1-ADRENERGIC RECEPTOR

	α_{1D}	α_{1B}	α_{1A}
Pharmacology			
Antagonists	BMY7378, SKF105854		SNAP-5089, indoramin
Distribution	Aorta	Liver, spleen, DDT$_1$ cells, MF-2 cells	Kidney
Effector mechanism	Ca^{2+} channel	IP$_3$	?
Structure (cloning, human)			
Number of amino acids	560	515	466
Human gene chromosome number	C2B	C5	C8

Modified from [26,27] with permission.

CATECHOLAMINE RECEPTORS

The brain contains multiple classes of receptors for catecholamines

Effects of DA are mediated through interaction with D1-like (D1 and D5) and D2-like (D2, D3 and D4) receptors (Table 12-3), while effects of NE and epinephrine are mediated through α_1- and α_2-adrenergic receptors (Tables 12-4, 12-5) and through β-adrenergic receptors (Table 12-6). As of the present time, three subtypes of α_1-, three subtypes of α_2- and three subtypes of β-adrenergic receptors have been identified (Tables 12-4–12-6). Mice lacking these receptors can have significant physiological deficits (Table 12-1). The postsynaptic receptors on any given neu-ron receive information from transmitters re-leased by another neuron. Typically, postsynaptic receptors are located on dendrites or cell bodies of neurons, but they may also occur on axons or nerve terminals; in the latter case, an axoaxonic synaptic relationship may cause presynaptic inhi-bition or excitation. In contrast, autoreceptors are situated on a given neuron and respond to transmitter molecules released from the same neuron. Autoreceptors may be widely distributed on the surface of the neuron. At the nerve termi-nal, they respond to transmitter molecules re-leased into the synaptic cleft; on the cell body, they may respond to transmitter molecules re-leased by dendrites. Functionally, most autore-ceptors appear to regulate transmitter release in such a way that the released transmitter, acting

TABLE 12-5. SUBTYPES OF α_2-ADRENERGIC RECEPTOR

	α_{2A}	α_{2B}	α_{2C}
Pharmacology			
Selective antagonists	Oxymetazoline, BAM 1303	ARC 239, prazosin, spiroxatrine	BAM 1303, WB-4101
Prototypic tissues and cell lines	Human platelet, HT29 cells	Neonatal rat lung, NG108 cells	Opossum kidney, OK cells
Effector mechanism	All three subtypes have been shown to inhibit adenylyl cyclase		
Structure (cloning, human)			
Number of amino acids	450	450	461
Human gene chromosome number	10	2	4

Modified from [26] with permission.

TABLE 12-6.   SUBTYPES OF β-ADRENERGIC RECEPTOR

Type	Potency (antagonist)	Characteristics	No. of amino acids	Second messenger	Introns
β_1	ISO > EPI = NE (Practolol, ICI 89,406)	Fatty acid mobilization from adipose tissue, cardiac stimulation	477-C10 (human)	↑cAMP	No
β_2	ISO > EPI > NE (Butoxamine, ICI 118,551)	Bronchodilation, vasodepression, inhibition of uterine contraction, glycogenolysis	410-C5 (human)	↑cAMP	No
β_3	ISO > EPI (BRL-37344, Pindolol)	Lipolysis	402 (human)	↑cAMP	Yes

on autoreceptors, regulates additional release. Autoreceptors have been identified for NE-, DA-, serotonin- and GABA-containing neurons. A major type of inhibitory autoreceptor described in both the sympathetic PNS and the brain has pharmacological properties resembling those of the α_2-adrenergic receptor [20].

In the sympathetic PNS, autoreceptors of the β-adrenergic type have also been described. These differ from most other known autoreceptors in that NE acting on these receptors facilitates transmitter release and thus amplifies the effects of neuronal firing. This effect contrasts with the inhibitory action of α-adrenergic and DA autoreceptors, which exert negative feedback control on transmitter release. The DA autoreceptors in the nigrostriatal pathway appear to be of the D2 subtype.

DOPAMINE RECEPTORS

Multiple dopamine receptor subtypes exist

Two subtypes of DA receptor were initially identified on the basis of pharmacological and biochemical criteria. D1 receptors were shown to couple to stimulation of adenylyl cyclase activity, while D2 receptors inhibited enzyme activity (Fig. 12-6). More recently, multiple D1-like and D2-like receptors have been identified (Table 12-3) [21,22] and amino acid sequences determined. The known subtypes of DA receptor are members of the G protein-linked receptor family with seven hydrophobic domains, an extracellular N terminus and an intracellular C termi-

nus (Fig. 12-4). Consensus sequences for phosphorylation are found in the second (i_2) and third intracellular (i_3) loops and the C-terminal tail. The D1-like receptors have relatively small i_3 loops and long C-terminal tails, while the D2-like receptors have large i_3 loops and short C-terminal tails.

The D1-like receptors include the D1 and D5 receptors [21,22]. The D1-like receptors have a high affinity for benzazepines like SCH-23390 and a low affinity for benzamides and are coupled to stimulation of adenylyl cyclase activity. The most striking pharmacological difference among them is the high affinity of D5 receptors for DA.

Molecular genetic studies have demonstrated the presence of two forms of mRNA coding for D2 receptors, designated D2L and D2S. These two forms differ by 87 bases, corresponding to a 29-amino-acid insert in the i_3 loop of the receptor (Fig. 12-4). The two species of D2 receptor mRNA appear to arise through alternative splicing. Both D2L and D2S receptors are coupled to inhibition of adenylyl cyclase activity, although D2S stimulation causes a greater inhibition. The D3 receptor, a second member of the D2-like receptor family, has been cloned and expressed in COS-7 cells. D3 receptor mRNA is found in limbic areas of the brain, including the nucleus accumbens. Comparison of the properties of D2 and D3 receptors shows that the D3 receptor has a relatively high affinity for atypical neuroleptics and for DA autoreceptor inhibitors, including (+)-UH232 and (+)-AJ76. Cloning of the D4 receptor has introduced an additional level of complexity to the study of DA receptors. Of particular interest is the high affinity of D4 re-

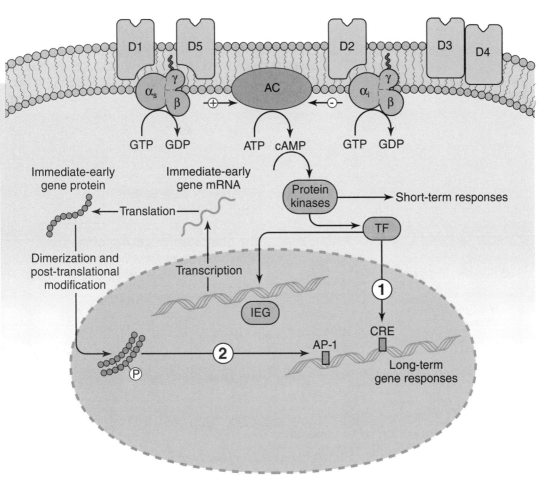

FIGURE 12-6. Effect of dopamine on intracellular signaling pathways. Stimulation of receptors by agonists can change enzyme activities as well as gene expression. Five subtypes of dopamine receptor have been identified. The D1 and D5 receptors are coupled to adenylyl cyclase *(AC)* via a stimulatory G protein (G_S). The D2 receptor inhibits cyclase activity via coupling to an inhibitory G protein (G_i). Activation of D3 and D4 receptors also inhibits cAMP production. Adenylyl cyclase catalyzes the conversion of ATP into cAMP, which in turn causes dissociation of the regulatory and catalytic subunits of protein kinase A. The activated catalytic subunit catalyzes conversion of protein substrates into phosphoproteins. This is turn can lead to a short-term response within the cell or activate transcription factors (TF) which enter the nucleus and alter gene expression. Long-term gene responses can be initiated by the action of constitutively expressed TFs either directly on DNA ① or via a mechanism involving transcription of an immediate-early gene (IEG) and cytoplasmic production of its protein. This protein can then act on DNA via an adaptor protein 1 *(AP-1)*-binding site ②. *TF,* constitutively expressed transcription factors, such as a cAMP-response element (CRE), *IEG,* immediate-early genes, such as c-*fos,* c-*jun* and *knox.*

ceptors for the atypical neuroleptic clozapine. D4 receptor mRNA has been detected in the frontal cortex, midbrain, amygdala and medulla, with lower concentrations detected in the basal ganglia. The use of molecular approaches in the study of the D4 receptor has been hampered by the high G/C content of its coding sequences. D3 and D4 receptors inhibit adenylyl cyclase, and D4 receptors are positively coupled to K^+ channels.

The number of D1 and D2 receptors can be modulated by antagonists or neurotoxins

The density of D2 receptors in rat striatum is increased following lesions with the neurotoxin 6-hydroxydopamine or by administration of antagonists. Similar results for D1 receptors were obtained following chronic administration of the D1-selective antagonist SCH-23390. Subtypes of DA receptor may be coregulated since the D2 antagonist sulpiride attenuated the ability of SCH-23390 to increase the density of D1 receptors. The increase in the density of D2 receptors following chronic administration of antagonists may be responsible for the development of a movement disorder called tardive dyskinesia (see Chap. 45).

Available behavioral data suggest that either acute or repeated administration of agonists acting at DA receptors results in augmentation of the behavioral effects of the drugs. This phenomenon, known as reverse tolerance or sensitization, is characterized by a selective increase in the intensity or duration or a shift to an earlier time of onset of stereotypical behaviors such as locomotion, sniffing, rearing, licking and gnawing. Sensitization to indirect DA agonists like amphetamine or cocaine also occurs. The mechanisms underlying behavioral sensitization are likely to be complex. It is known, for example, that stereotypical behavior and locomotor hyperactivity are critically dependent on activation of both D1 and D2 receptors.

Direct and indirect agonists at dopamine receptors, including amphetamine, bromocriptine and lisuride, have been shown to induce psychotic episodes

A strong correlation exists between the clinical doses of neuroleptics and their affinity for brain D2 receptors. This has led to the hypothesis that psychotic disorders result from overstimulation of D2 receptors. Long-term administration of neuroleptics to humans or experimental animals can result in an increase in the density of striatal D2 receptors and in the appearance of extrapyramidal side effects, including parkinsonian movement disorders and tardive dyskinesia. A panel of antipsychotic drugs referred to as atypical neuroleptics, including clozapine, melperone and fluperlapine, have been reported to produce fewer extrapyramidal side effects and have been useful in the treatment of patients with schizophrenia who respond poorly to typical antipsychotics such as haloperidol. The relative affinities of D2, D3 and D4 receptors for typical and atypical neuroleptics together with the selec-

tive expression of D3 receptor mRNA in limbic areas of the brain have led to the hypothesis that the clinical utility of neuroleptics in the treatment of psychiatric illness may be due, at least in part, to their ability to antagonize stimulation of D3 or D4 receptors, while the motor dysfunction observed following chronic treatment with typical neuroleptics could be due to alterations in the density of D2 receptors in the striatum.

α- AND β-ADRENERGIC RECEPTORS

The pharmacological responses to catecholamines were ascribed to effects of α- and β-adrenergic receptors in the late 1940s

NE and epinephrine act at both α and β receptors, but isoproterenol, a synthetic agonist, acts only at β receptors (Tables 12-4–12-6). Numerous antagonists also differentiate between α and β receptors. The prototypic β-adrenergic receptor antagonist propranolol is essentially inactive at α receptors; the α-adrenergic receptor antagonist phentolamine is very weak at β receptors.

Distinct subtypes of β-adrenergic receptor exist and have important pharmacological consequences. β_1-Adrenergic receptors predominate in the heart and in the cerebral cortex, whereas β_2-adrenergic receptors predominate in the lung and cerebellum. However, in many cases, β_1- and β_2-adrenergic receptors coexist in the same tissue, sometimes mediating the same physiological effect. A major side effect of β_2-selective agonists like metaproterenol, used to treat bronchial asthma, is cardiac acceleration. This is due to the coexistence of β_1- and β_2-adrenergic receptors in the heart. Both classes of receptor are coupled to the electrophysiological effects of catecholamines in the heart.

The brain contains both β_1 and β_2 receptors, which cannot be differentiated in terms of their physiological functions. Moreover, radioactive drugs that bind exclusively to one or the other type of β receptor are not yet available. However, one can label all of the β-adrenergic receptors in a given tissue with a nonselective radioligand and then selectively inhibit binding to one of the β-receptor subtypes with increasing concentrations of β_1- or β_2-selective agents [21]. ICI 89,406 and ICI 118,551 are highly selective antagonists at β_1- and β_2-adrenergic receptors, respectively. A similar approach can be used to define the anatomical localization of β_1- and β_2-adrenergic receptors using the technique of quantitative autoradiography. The density of β_1 receptors varies in different brain areas to a greater extent than does that of β_2 receptors. It has been suggested that this is due to the presence of β_2-adrenergic receptors on glia or blood vessels.

A third subtype of β-adrenergic receptor has been identified. This receptor has pharmacological properties distinct from those of β_1- and β_2-adrenergic receptors. Agonists that are selective for β_3 receptors exist and cause nonshivering thermogenesis in rodents. The β_3 receptor in humans has been linked to hereditary obesity, control of lipid metabolism and the development of diabetes. mRNA for β_3-adrenergic receptors is selectively expressed in brown adipose tissue present in rodents and in newborn humans. Message can be detected in white adipose tissue, but expression is very low.

The amino acid sequences of β-adrenergic receptors in brain and various tissues have been determined

A striking structural feature of the β-adrenergic receptors that have been cloned and sequenced, from turkey erythrocytes, hamster lung and human placenta and brain, and of the other members of the G protein-linked receptor family is their topographical orientation with respect to the membrane [23,24] (see Fig. 12-4). Hydropathicity analysis suggests that there are seven hydrophobic regions, each of 20 to 25 amino acids. These are potentially membrane-spanning. Other structural features of β-adrenergic receptors include a long C-terminal hydrophilic sequence thought to be intracellular, a somewhat shorter N-terminal hydrophilic sequence thought to be extracellular and a long cytoplasmic loop between presumptive transmembrane segments V and VI. Sites for *N*-linked glycosylation are found in the N-terminal extracellular portion of the molecule, while numerous sites that may be phosphorylated are found in the C-

terminal portion of the molecule and on the i_2 and i_3 loops (see Chap. 22). Evidence from studies involving limited proteolysis and site-directed mutagenesis has led to the conclusion that the hydrophobic transmembrane helices are involved in the formation of the binding site for catecholamines, and the i_3 loop together with the C terminus may play a role in the interaction of the receptor with GTP-binding proteins (see Chap. 20). A conserved aspartate residue in transmembrane 3 and a pair of serines in transmembrane 5 are thought to provide counterions for the amino and catechol hydroxyl groups, respectively [24].

Multiple serine and threonine residues on the i_3 loop and C terminus and consensus sequences for cAMP-dependent phosphorylation may be important in explaining processes including agonist-induced receptor sequestration and desensitization (see also below). cAMP- and non-cAMP-dependent phosphorylations of β-adrenergic receptors have been observed. β-adrenergic receptor-stimulated synthesis of cAMP results in activation of PKA. The phosphorylated receptor is functionally uncoupled. Other receptors coupled to activation of adenylyl cyclase can also cause what is known as heterologous desensitization. In addition, occupancy of β-adrenergic receptors by agonists results in the activation of β-adrenergic receptor kinase (βARK), which leads to phosphorylation of the receptor. The uncoupling of the receptor from G_s also appears to involve a protein called β-arrestin, which is similar to a 48-kDa protein in the retina (see Chap. 47).

The proposed structure of the β-adrenergic receptor is strikingly similar in sequence and topography to that of bacterial rhodopsin (see Chap. 47) and the other members of the G protein-linked receptor family whose cDNAs have recently been cloned (see Chap. 20). Although these proteins mediate widely disparate biological effects, they show a high degree of homology. This is almost certainly related to the fact that, in each case, the immediate consequence of receptor activation is to promote an interaction between the receptor and a GTP-binding protein. The homologies between the members of the extended family of proteins are most evident within the presumed membrane-spanning helices.

Two families of α-adrenergic receptors exist

Radiolabeled agonists and antagonists have been used to label α receptors in both the brain and the peripheral tissues. As with β receptors, the binding properties of α receptors are essentially the same in the brain and the periphery. Some tissues possess only postsynaptic α_1 receptors, others postsynaptic α_2 receptors, and some organs have a mixture of both. Results of pharmacological and physiological studies have led to the suggestion that there are multiple types of α_1 and α_2 receptors. Of particular clinical importance are differences in the properties of junctional and extrajunctional α receptors. The proportions of α_1 and α_2 receptors also vary in different brain regions [25,26]. The physiological consequences of the two types of α receptor in the brain are unclear at the present time. It is striking that the drug specificity of postsynaptic α_2 receptors closely resembles that of adrenergic autoreceptors, which are therefore also referred to as α_2 receptors.

Studies involving the binding of radioligands are also consistent with the suggestion that there are subtypes of both α_1- and α_2-adrenergic receptors (Tables 12-4 and 12-5). The suggestion that there are subtypes of α_1-adrenergic receptor was initially based on a comparison of the properties of [3H]prazosin and [3H]WB4-101 binding to α_1-adrenergic receptors in rat brain and uterus. Heterogeneity of α_2-adrenergic receptors was initially based on a comparison between the binding of [3H]clonidine and [3H]yohimbine in a variety of tissues and species. The observation that prazosin is more potent in neonatal rat lung [25,26] and cerebral cortex than in the human platelet, the prototypic tissue for the study of α_2 receptors, was interpreted as indicating a heterogeneity in the pharmacological characteristics of α_2-adrenergic receptors. Cloning and sequence analysis suggest that there are three subtypes of α_1-adrenergic receptor and three subtypes of α_2-adrenergic receptor [26,27]. In some instances, the α_{1D} receptor has been linked to activation of Ca^{2+} channels, while the α_{1B} receptor has been shown to activate phosphoinositide-specific phospholipase C (PI-PLC), resulting in liberation of di-acylglycerol (DAG) and inositol trisphosphate (IP_3) (see Chap. 20). Prototypic tissues expressing each of the subtypes of α_2 receptor have been identified. All three of the known subtypes of α_2-adrenergic receptor are linked to inhibition of adenylyl cyclase activity. As seen with other receptors linked to inhibition of adenylyl cyclase activity, the α_2-adrenergic receptors have long i_3 loops and relatively short C-terminal tails.

Not surprisingly, the known subtypes of α-adrenergic receptor share structural features with DA receptors (Fig. 12-4) and the other members of the G protein-linked receptor family. The degree of sequence identity is greater when the subtypes of α_1 or α_2 receptors are compared with each other than when α_1 and α_2 receptors are compared. The sequences of α_1 and α_2 receptors are not more closely related to each other than either is to the three known members of the β-adrenergic receptor family. Nomenclature notwithstanding, it is appropriate to think of three families of adrenergic receptor called α_1, α_2 and β. Sequence similarities both within and between families of adrenergic receptors are greater when the sequences of the putative transmembrane helices are compared than when one looks at overall sequence identity. It is sometimes difficult to distinguish between receptor subtypes and species homologs of the same receptor. Small differences in amino acid sequence can sometimes lead to large changes in the pharmacological specificity of an expressed receptor. The possibility that additional catecholamine receptors remain to be identified clearly exists.

DYNAMICS OF CATECHOLAMINE RECEPTORS

Changes in the number of receptors appear to be associated with altered synaptic activity

Neurotransmitter receptors are not static entities; in both the sympathetic PNS and the brain, destruction of catecholamine-containing nerves is associated with functional supersensitivity of postsynaptic sites. Conversely, administration of tricyclic antidepressants or inhibitors of MAO leads to functional subsensitivity. These changes appear to be a compensatory response involving changes in the density of β-adrenergic receptors (see below). Destruction of the DA-containing nigrostriatal pathway also has well-described behavioral consequences. Unilateral nigrostriatal lesion causes asymmetry in DA innervation between the two cerebral hemispheres. Behavioral studies demonstrate that the DA receptors in the denervated corpus striatum are supersensitive. Apomorphine, a DA agonist that stimulates DA receptors selectively, causes rotational behavior in rats with unilateral lesions in a direction contralateral to the lesion. In contrast, indirect agonists such as cocaine cause rotation in the opposite direction.

The extent of receptor supersensitivity can be quantified by measuring the amount of rotational behavior. After selective nigrostriatal lesions have been produced in rats by injections of 6-hydroxydopamine in the substantia nigra, the number of DA receptors in the ipsilateral corpus striatum increases markedly, and the increase in the number of receptors may correlate with the extent of behavioral supersensitivity as monitored by rotational behavior [28]. Thus, the increase in receptor density appears to play a role in the behavioral supersensitivity of these animals.

Changes in the number of dopamine receptors may also be involved in pharmacological actions of neuroleptic drugs

One of the most serious side effects of the neuroleptic drugs is tardive dyskinesia, a disfiguring, excessive motor activity of the tongue, face, arms and legs in patients treated chronically with large doses of the drugs (see Chap. 45). Paradoxically, reduction of the dosage worsens the symptoms, whereas increasing the dosage alleviates the symptoms. It has been suggested that tardive dyskinesia reflects a supersensitivity of DA receptors that have been chronically blocked. This hypothesis gains support from the direct demonstration that chronic treatment with neuroleptics leads to an increase in the number of DA receptors in the corpus striatum. Moreover, the ability of neuroleptics to elicit this increase correlates with their ability to block DA receptors.

The number of α_1 and α_2 receptors increases after the noradrenergic neurons in the brain have been destroyed by injections of 6-hydroxydopamine. It is interesting that after this induced destruction of NE-containing neurons the number of β_1 receptors increases markedly but no changes occur in the number of β_2 receptors [23]. This may be a consequence of the fact that β_2 receptors have a low affinity for NE and that the concentration of epinephrine in the brain is relatively low. Similarly, chronic administration of tricyclic antidepressants, which block the reuptake of NE, leads to a selective decrease in the density of β_1-adrenergic receptors in the cerebral cortex. This suggests that the β_1-adrenergic receptors in the cortex are functionally innervated.

Exposure of cells to agonists results in diminished responsiveness, referred to as desensitization

The phenomenon of desensitization has been most extensively explored for β_2-adrenergic receptors. Within minutes of exposure to an agonist, β receptors are phosphorylated by βARK. This promotes the binding of another protein, β-arrestin, to the receptor, which uncouples the β receptors from the G protein. The uncoupling stops signaling and is followed by a sequestration of cell-surface β receptors into intracellular compartments. There is some evidence that β receptors are then recycled back to the surface of the cell. It is not clear if this regulatory process involving βARKs and β-arrestins [29–31] applies to all catecholamine receptors, but it is a reasonable hypothesis.

Other mechanisms of receptor regulation have been most thoroughly investigated on transformed and transfected cell lines expressing subtypes of β-adrenergic receptor. Transcriptional, post-transcriptional and post-translational regulatory phenomena have been described. Exposure of such cells to an agonist like isoproterenol results in an unexpected increase in mRNA levels. This is thought to be a consequence of the presence of a cAMP-response element (CRE) located approximately 50 bases upstream from the initiation codon. Exposure of cells to isoproterenol results in increases in cAMP and activation of PKA. A CRE-binding protein is then phosphorylated, resulting in activation of the CRE. The resulting increase in mRNA levels is transient and does not have an obvious effect on the synthesis of receptor protein. Over a somewhat longer time scale, post-transcriptional regulatory mechanisms are activated. In particular, mRNA concentrations decline, apparently as a consequence of a decrease in mRNA stability. The mechanism underlying this change in message stability has not been elucidated. Transcriptional and post-transcriptional types of regulation of β-adrenergic receptor synthesis are superimposed on the post-translational phenomena described above (see also Chap. 22).

ACKNOWLEDGMENTS

Support was provided by NIH grant RR00165. This chapter is a modification of the earlier one in the fifth edition, and the extensive contributions of Drs. P. Molinoff and N. Weiner are acknowledged.

REFERENCES

1. Molinoff, P. B., and Axelrod, J. Biochemistry of catecholamines. *Annu. Rev. Biochem.* 40:465–500, 1971.
2. Goldstein, D. S., Eisenhofer, G., and McCarty, R. (eds.) *Catecholamines: Bridging Basic Science with Clinical Medicine.* New York: Academic Press, 1998.
3. Shiman, R., Akino, M., and Kaufman, S. Solubilization and partial purification of tyrosine hydroxylase from bovine adrenal medulla. *J. Biol. Chem.* 246:1330–1340, 1971.
4. Grima, B., Lamouroux, A., Blanot, F., Biguet, N. F., and Mallet, J. Complete coding sequence of rat tyrosine hydroxylase mRNA. *Proc. Natl. Acad. Sci. USA* 82:617–621, 1985.
5. Christenson, J. G., Dairman, W., and Udenfriend, S. Preparation and properties of homogeneous aromatic L-amino acid decarboxylase from hog kidney. *Arch. Biochem. Biophys.* 141:356–367, 1970.
6. Craine, J. E., Daniels, G., and Kaufman, S. Dopamine β-hydroxylase: The subunit structure and anion activation of the bovine adrenal enzyme. *J. Biol. Chem.* 248:7838–7844, 1973.
7. Lamouroux, A., Vigny, A., Biguet, N. F., et al. The primary structure of human dopamine β-hydroxylase: Insights into the relationship between the soluble and the membrane-bound forms of the enzyme. *EMBO J.* 6:3931–3937, 1987.
8. Connett, R. J., and Kirshner, N. Purification and properties of bovine phenylethanolamine-N-methyltransferase. *J. Biol. Chem.* 245:329–334, 1970.
9. Baetge, E. E., Suh, Y. H., and Joh, T. H. Complete nucleotide and deduced amino acid sequence of bovine phenylethanolamine N-methyltransferase: Partial amino acid homology with rat tyrosine hydroxylase. *Proc. Natl. Acad. Sci. USA* 83:5454–5458, 1986.
10. Liu, Y., Peter, D., Roghani, A., et al. A cDNA that suppresses MPP⁺ toxicity encodes a vesicular amine transporter. *Cell* 70:539–551, 1992.
11. Weinshilboum, R. M., Thoa, N. B., Johnson, D. G., Kopin, I. J., and Axelrod, J. Proportional release of norepinephrine and dopamine β-hydroxylase from sympathetic nerves. *Science* 174:1349–1351, 1971.
12. Alousi, A., and Weiner, N. The regulation of norepinephrine synthesis in sympathetic nerves: Effect of nerve stimulation, cocaine and catecholamine-releasing agents. *Proc. Natl. Acad. Sci. USA* 56:1491–1496, 1966.
13. Goldstein, M. Long- and short-term regulation of tyrosine hydroxylase. In F. E. Bloom and D. J. Kupfer (eds.), *Psychopharmacology: The Fourth Generation of Progress.* New York: Raven Press, 1995, pp. 189–196.
14. Zigmond, R. E., Schwarzschild, M. A., and Rittenhouse, A. R. Acute regulation of tyrosine hydroxylase by nerve activity and by neurotransmitters via phosphorylation. *Annu. Rev. Neurosci.* 12:415–461, 1989.
15. Costa, E., and Sandler, M. *Monoamine Oxidase: New Vistas.* New York: Raven, 1972.
16. Nikodejevic, B., Sinoh, S., Daly, J. W., and Creveling, C. R. Catechol-O-methyltransferase II: A new class of inhibitors of catechol-O-methyltransferase; 3,5-dihydroxy-4-methoxybenzoic acid and related compounds. *J. Pharmacol. Exp. Ther.* 174:83–93, 1970.
17. Axelrod, J. Noradrenaline: Fate and control of its biosynthesis. *Science* 173:598–606, 1971.
18. Amara, S. G., and Kuhar, M. J. Neurotransmitter transporters: Recent progress. *Annu. Rev. Neurosci.* 16:73–93, 1993.
19. Bjorklund, A., and Hokfelt, T. (eds.) *Handbook of Chemical Neuroanatomy.* New York: Elsevier, 1984.

20. Langer, S. Z. Presynaptic regulation of catecholamine release. *Biochem. Pharmacol.* 23:1793–1800, 1974.

21. Gingrich, J. A., and Caron, M. G. Recent advances in the molecular biology of dopamine receptors. *Annu. Rev. Neurosci.* 16:299–321, 1993.

22. Sibley, D. R., and Monsma, F. J., Jr. Molecular biology of dopamine receptors. *Trends Pharmacol. Sci.* 13:61–68, 1992.

23. Minneman, K. P., Dibner, M. D., Wolfe, B. B., and Molinoff, P. B. β_1- and β_2-adrenergic receptors in rat cerebral cortex are independently regulated. *Science* 204:866–868, 1979.

24. Kobilka, B. Adrenergic receptors as models for G protein-coupled receptors. *Annu. Rev. Neurosci.* 15:87–114, 1992.

25. U'Prichard, D. C., and Snyder, S. H. Distinct α-noradrenergic receptors differentiated by binding and physiological relationships. *Life Sci.* 24:79–88, 1979.

26. Bylund, D. B. Subtypes of α_1- and α_2-adrenergic receptors. *FASEB J.* 6:832–839, 1992.

27. Hieble, J. P., Bylund, D. B., Clarke, D. E., et al. International Union of Pharmacology recommendation for nomenclature of α_1-adrenoceptors: Consensus update 1995. *Pharmacol. Rev.* 47:267–270, 1995.

28. Creese, I., Burt, D. R., and Snyder, S. H. Biochemical actions of neuroleptic drugs: Focus on the dopamine receptor. In L. L. Iversen, S. D. Iversen, and S. H. Snyder (eds.), *Handbook of Psychopharmacology.* New York: Plenum, 1978, Vol. 10, pp. 37–90.

29. Lefkowitz, R. J. G protein-coupled receptor kinases. *Cell* 74:409–412, 1993.

30. Ferguson, S., Barak, S. G., Zhang, L. S., and Caron, M. G. G protein-coupled receptor regulation: Role of G protein-coupled receptor kinases and arrestins. *Can. J. Physiol. Pharmacol.* 74:1095–1110, 1996.

31. Sterne-Marr, R., and Benovic, J. L. Regulation of G protein-coupled receptors by receptor kinases and arrestins. *Vitam. Horm.* 51:193–234, 1995.

32. Zhou, Q.-Y., Quaife, C. J., and Palmiter, R. D. Targeted disruption of the tyrosine hydroxylase gene reveals that catecholamines are required for mouse fetal development. *Nature* 374:640–643, 1995.

33. Thomas, S. A., and Palmiter, R. D. Disruption of the dopamine beta-hydroxylase gene in mice suggests roles for norepinephrine in motor function, learning, and memory. *Behav. Neurosci.* 111:579–589, 1997.

34. Giros, B., Jaber, M., Jones, S. R., Wightman, R. M., and Caron, M. G. Hyperlocomotion and indifference to cocaine and amphetamine in mice lacking the dopamine transporter. *Nature* 379:606–612, 1996.

35. Takahashi, N., Miner, L. L., Sora, I., et al. VMAT2 knockout mice: Heterozygotes display reduced amphetamine-conditioned reward, enhanced amphetamine locomotion, and enhanced MPTP toxicity. *Proc. Natl. Acad. Sci. USA* 94:9938–9943, 1997.

36. Link, R. E., Stevens, M. S., Kulatunga, M., Scheinin, M., Barsh, G. S., and Kobilka, B. K. Targeted inactivation of the gene encoding the mouse $\alpha(2C)$-adrenoceptor homol. *Mol. Pharmacol.* 48:48–55, 1995.

37. Rohrer, D. K., Desai, K. H., Jasper, J. R., et al. Targeted disruption of the mouse β-1-adrenergic receptor gene: Developmental and cardiovascular effects. *Proc. Natl. Acad. Sci. USA* 93:7375–7380, 1996.

38. Mantzoros, C. S., Qu, D., Frederich, R. C., et al. Activation of $\beta(3)$ adrenergic receptors suppresses leptin expression and mediates a leptin-independent inhibition of food intake in mice. *Diabetes* 45:909–914, 1996.

39. Grujic, D., Susulic, V. S., Harper, M. E., et al. $\beta3$-Adrenergic receptors on white and brown adipocytes mediate $\beta3$-selective agonist-induced effects on energy expenditure, insulin secretion, and food intake. A study using transgenic and gene knockout mice. *J. Biol. Chem.* 272:17686–17693, 1997.

40. Xu, M., Hu, X. T., Cooper, D. C., et al. Elimination of cocaine-induced hyperactivity and dopamine-mediated neurophysiological effects in dopamine D1 receptor mutant mice. *Cell* 79:945–955, 1994.

41. Drago, J., Gerfen, C. R., Westphal, H., and Steiner, H. D1 dopamine receptor-deficient mouse: Cocaine-induced regulation of immediate-early gene and substance P expression in the striatum. *Neuroscience* 74:813–823, 1996.

42. Baik, J. H., Picetti, R., Saiardi, A., et al. Parkinsonian-like locomotor impairment in mice lacking dopamine D2 receptors. *Nature* 377:424–428, 1995.

43. Accili, D., Fishburn, C. S., Drago, J., et al. A targeted mutation of the D3 dopamine receptor gene is associated with hyperactivity in mice. *Proc. Natl. Acad. Sci. USA* 93:1945–1949, 1996.

44. Waymire, J. C., and Craviso, G. L. Multiple site phosphorylation and activation of tyrosine hydroxylase. *Adv. Prot. Phosphatases* 7:501–513, 1993.

13

Serotonin

Alan Frazer and Julie G. Hensler

Basic Neurochemistry: Molecular, Cellular and Medical Aspects, 6th Ed., edited by G. J. Siegel et al. Published by Lippincott–Raven Publishers, Philadelphia, 1999. Correspondence to Alan Frazer, Department of Pharmacology, University of Texas Health Science Center at San Antonio, 703 Floyd Curl Drive, San Antonio, Texas 78284-7764.

SEROTONIN

The indolealkylamine 5-hydroxytryptamine, serotonin, was identified initially because of interest in its cardiovascular effects

It has been known since the mid-nineteenth century that after blood clots the resulting serum possesses a substance that constricts vascular smooth muscle so as to increase vascular tone. Around the turn of this century, platelets were identified as the source of this substance. In the late 1940s, Rapport and collaborators [1] isolated, purified and identified this "tonic" substance in "serum" (hence, serotonin) as the substituted indole 5-hydroxytryptamine (5-HT).

The structures of serotonin and related compounds are shown in Figure 13-1. The combination of the hydroxyl group in the 5 position of the indole nucleus and a primary amine nitrogen serving as a proton acceptor at physiological pH makes 5-HT a hydrophilic substance. As such, it does not pass the lipophilic blood–brain barrier readily. Thus, its discovery in brain indicated that 5-HT is synthesized in brain, where it might play an important role in brain function. The observation, at about the same time, that the psychedelic drug ($+$)lysergic acid diethylamide (LSD) antagonized a response produced by 5-HT further substantiated the idea that 5-HT might have important behavioral effects, even though the response was contraction of gastrointestinal smooth muscle. Subsequently, various theories arose linking abnormalities of 5-HT function to the development of a number of psychiatric disorders, particularly schizophrenia and depression. Psychotherapeutic drugs are now available that are effective in depression (see Chap. 52), anxiety disorders and schizophrenia; some of these drugs have potent, and in some cases selective, effects on serotonin neurons in brain.

Understanding the neuroanatomical organization of serotonergic cells in brain provides insight into the functions of this neurotransmitter

Serotonin-containing neuronal cell bodies are restricted to discrete clusters or groups of cells located along the midline of the brainstem. Their axons, however, innervate nearly every area of the CNS (Fig. 13-2). In 1964, Dahlstrom and Fuxe (discussed in [2]), using the Falck-Hillarp technique of histofluorescence, observed that the majority of serotonergic soma are found in cell body groups, which previously had been designated as the raphe nuclei. This earlier description of the raphe nuclei was based on cell body structural characteristics and organization. Dahlstrom and Fuxe described nine groups of serotonin-containing cell bodies, which they designated B_1 through B_9, and which correspond for the most part with the raphe nuclei (discussed in [2]) (Table 13-1). Some serotonergic neuronal cell bodies, however, are found outside the raphe nuclei, and not all of the cell bodies in the raphe nuclei are serotonergic. In most of the raphe nuclei, the majority of neurons are non-

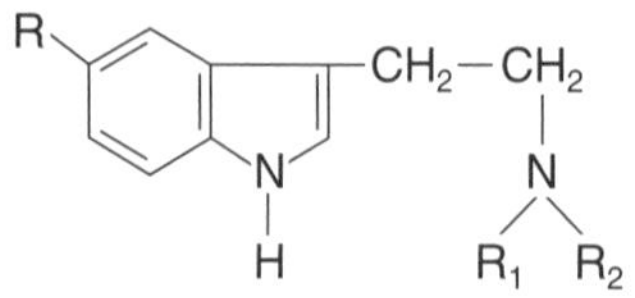

Compound	Position		
	R	R_1	R_2
Tryptamine	H	H	H
Serotonin	OH	H	H
Melatonin	OCH_3	$COCH_3$	H
Diethyltryptamine (DET)*	H	CH_3CH_2	CH_3CH_2
Dimethyltryptamine (DMT)*	H	CH_3	CH_3
Bufotenine*	OH	CH_3	CH_3

*Psychotropic (modifies mental activity)

FIGURE 13-1.   Chemical structures of 5-hydroxytryptamine and related indolealkylamines. The indole ring structure consists of the benzene ring and the attached five-member ring structure containing nitrogen.

TABLE 13-1.	**CLASSIFICATION OF SEROTONERGIC CELL BODY GROUPS ACCORDING TO DAHLSTROM AND FUXE AND CORRESPONDING ANATOMICAL STRUCTURE**
Groups of serotonin-containing cell bodies	**Anatomical structure**
B_1	Raphe pallidus nucleus, caudal ventrolateral medulla
B_2	Raphe obscurus nucleus
B_3	Raphe magnus nucleus, rostral ventrolateral medulla, lateral paragigantocellular reticular nucleus
B_4	Raphe obscurus nucleus, dorsolateral part
B_5	Median raphe nucleus, caudal part
B_6	Dorsal raphe nucleus, caudal part
B_7	Dorsal raphe nucleus principal, rostral part
B_8	Median raphe nucleus, rostral main part; caudal linear nucleus; nucleus pontis oralis
B_9	Nucleus pontis oralis, supralemniscal region

Modified from [3] with permission.

serotonergic. For example, the dorsal raphe contains the largest number of serotonergic neurons; however, only 40 to 50% of the cell bodies in the dorsal raphe are serotonergic (Fig. 13-3).

Since the late 1960s, a variety of techniques have been used to characterize the neuronal circuitry of serotonin cells in the CNS. The density of serotonergic innervation in the forebrain was underestimated initially because the original histofluorescence method was limited in sensitivity and did not permit the detection of many fine axons and terminals. Subsequent anatomical techniques, such as immunohistochemical localization of either 5-HT or tryptophan hy-

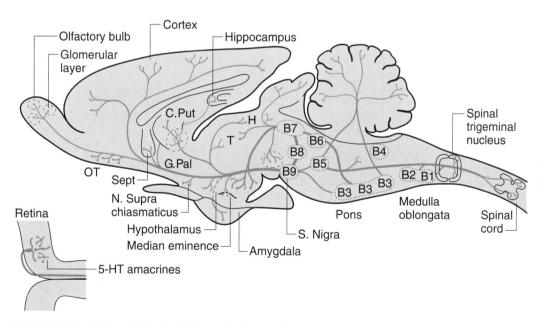

FIGURE 13-2.   Schematic drawing depicting the location of the serotonergic cell body groups in a sagittal section of the rat central nervous system and their major projections. *OT,* olfactory tuberculum; *Sept,* septum; *C. Put,* nucleus caudate-putamen; *G. Pal,* globus pallidus; *T,* thalamus; *H,* habenula; *S. Nigra,* substantia nigra. Modified from [40].

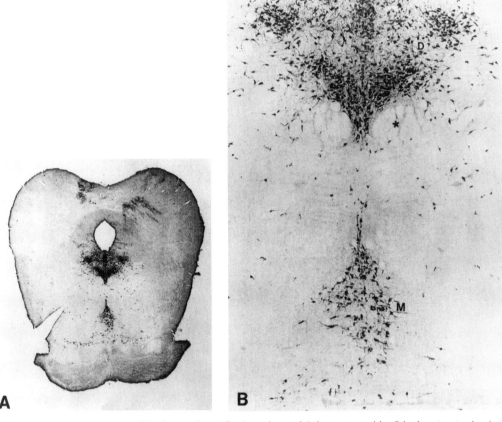

FIGURE 13-3. Serotonergic cell bodies in the midbrain raphe nuclei demonstrated by 5-hydroxytryptamine immunocytochemistry. **A:** Low magnification of transverse section through rat midbrain. The serotonergic cell body groups shown give rise to widespread serotonergic projections to cerebral cortex and forebrain structures. **B:** Higher magnification micrograph showing serotonergic cell bodies in dorsal and median raphe nuclei. The dorsal raphe nucleus lies in the central gray matter just beneath the cerebral aqueduct. In the transverse plane, the dorsal raphe can be subdivided further into a ventromedial cell cluster between and just above the medial longitudinal fasciculus (MLF)*, a smaller dorsomedial group just below the aqueduct and large bilateral cell groups. The median raphe nucleus lies in the central core of the midbrain, below the MLF. *D,* dorsal raphe; *M,* median raphe; *A,* aqueduct. (From [2], with permission.)

droxylase, an enzyme unique to the synthesis of 5-HT, in addition to retrograde and anterograde axonal transport studies, have allowed a more complete and accurate characterization of the serotonergic innervation of forebrain areas.

The largest group of serotonergic cells is B_7 (Fig. 13-2), which is continuous with a smaller group of serotonergic cells, B_6. Groups B_6 and B_7 often are considered together as the dorsal raphe nucleus, with B_6 being its caudal extension. Another prominent serotonergic cell body group is B_8, which corresponds to the median raphe nu-

cleus, also termed the nucleus central superior. Group B_9, part of the ventrolateral tegmentum of the pons and midbrain, forms a lateral extension of the median raphe (Fig. 13-2) and, therefore, is not considered one of the midline raphe nuclei. Ascending serotonergic projections innervating the cerebral cortex and other regions of the forebrain arise primarily from the dorsal raphe, median raphe and B_9 cell group.

Two distinct ascending projections arise from the rostral serotonergic system. The two main ascending serotonergic pathways emerging from the midbrain raphe nuclei to the forebrain are the dorsal periventricular path and the ventral tegmental radiations. Both pathways converge in the caudal hypothalamus, where they join the medial forebrain bundle. Axons of both dopaminergic and noradrenergic neurons course anteriorly through the medial forebrain bundle as well (see Chap. 12).

Ascending projections from the raphe nuclei to forebrain structures are organized in a topographical manner. The dorsal and median raphe nuclei give rise to distinct projections to forebrain regions (Fig. 13-4). The median raphe projects heavily to hippocampus, septum and hypothalamus, whereas the striatum is innervated predominantly by the dorsal raphe. The dorsal and median raphe nuclei send overlapping neuronal projections to the neocortex. Within the dorsal and median raphe, cells are organized in particular zones or groups that send axons to specific areas of brain. For example, the frontal cortex receives heavy innervation from the rostral and lateral subregions of the dorsal raphe nucleus. Raphe neurons send collateral axons to areas of brain that are related in function, such as the amygdala and hippocampus or the substantia nigra and caudate putamen. The specific and highly organized innervation of forebrain structures by raphe neurons implies independent functions of sets of serotonergic neurons dependent on their origin and terminal projections, as opposed to a nonselective or general role for serotonin in the CNS.

Serotonergic axon terminals, labeled by uptake of [³H]5-HT or studied with immunohistochemical techniques, appear to exhibit morphological differences related to the raphe nucleus of origin (Fig. 13-4). Serotonergic axons from the median raphe nucleus, type M, look relatively coarse with large spherical varicosities. By contrast, axons from the dorsal raphe, type D, are very fine and typically have small, pleomorphic varicosities. Dorsal raphe axons appear to be more vulnerable to certain neurotoxic amphetamine derivatives, such as d-fenfluramine, 3,4-methylenedioxymethamphetamine (MDMA, commonly termed Ecstasy) or parachloroamphetamine (PCA). Median raphe axons appear to be more resistant to the neurotoxic effects of these drugs. Blockade of the sero-

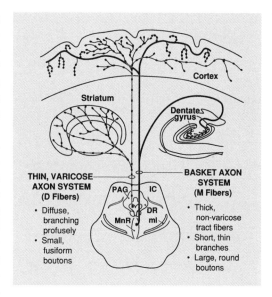

FIGURE 13-4. Simplified diagram of the main features of the dual serotonergic system innervating the forebrain. The thin varicose axon system (D fibers) arises from the dorsal raphe (DR) nucleus with fibers that branch profusely in their target areas. It is difficult to demonstrate the synaptic connections of these fibers, and therefore, the incidence of synapses on these fibers is still being debated. The basket axon system (M fibers) arises from the median raphe nucleus (MnR) with thick, nonvaricose axons, giving rise to branches with characteristic axons that appear beaded, with round or oval varicosities. These large terminals make well-defined synapses with target cells. (From [2], with permission.) *PAG*, periaqueductal gray matter; *IC*, inferior colliculus; *ml*, medial lemniscus.

tonin transporter prevents the neurotoxic effects of these amphetamine derivatives, indicating that activity of this transporter is critical for the neurotoxic effects of these drugs.

As expected, serotonergic terminals make the usual specialized synaptic contacts with target neurons and release serotonin following nerve stimulation. In some areas of the mammalian CNS, there are sites where 5-HT is released and no evidence for synaptic specialization has been found. For example, it is difficult to demonstrate the synaptic contacts of the fine varicose fibers, whereas large terminals make well defined synapses with target cells. The percentage of 5-HT terminals associated with synaptic specializations appears to vary in particular brain regions. This may have important implications for the type of information processing in which 5-HT is involved in these brain areas. The appearance of specialized synaptic contacts suggests relatively stable and strong associations between a presynaptic neuron and its target. Conversely, the lack of synaptic specialization implies a dynamic, and perhaps less specific, interaction with target neurons. For example, neurotransmitter is released and then diffuses over distances as great as several hundred microns. In this case, 5-HT may act as a neuromodulator to adjust or tune ongoing synaptic activity.

The other raphe nuclei, B_1 to B_4, are situated more caudally in the midpons to caudal medulla and contain a smaller number of serotonergic cells. These cell body groups give rise to serotonergic axons that project within the brainstem and to the spinal cord (Fig. 13-2). The spinal cord receives a strong serotonergic innervation. Three principal descending pathways have been described: (i) from the raphe magnus nucleus (B_3) to laminae I and II of the dorsal horn, (ii) from the raphe obscurus nucleus (B_2, B) to lamina IX of the ventral horn and (iii) from the rostral ventrolateral medulla and the lateral paragigantocellular reticular nucleus (B_3) to the interomediolateral cell column. Projections from the caudal ventrolateral medulla (B_1) are not known at present [3].

Afferent connections to the raphe nuclei include those between the dorsal and median raphe nuclei, B_9, B_1 and B_3. Connections between the raphe nuclei have been described by retrograde tracing techniques using horseradish peroxidase and wheat germ agglutinin. Such innervation may have considerable physiological and/or pharmacological importance as serotonin released in the vicinity of serotonergic cell bodies regulates the firing of serotonergic neurons through the activation of somatodendritic autoreceptors. The raphe nuclei also receive input from other cell body groups in the brainstem, such as the substantia nigra and ventral tegmental area (dopamine), superior vestibular nucleus (acetylcholine), locus ceruleus (norepinephrine) and nucleus prepositus hypoglossi and nucleus of the solitary tract (epinephrine). Other afferents include neurons from the hypothalamus, thalamus and limbic forebrain structures (see [2–4] for a comprehensive review of serotonergic neuroanatomy).

The amino acid L-tryptophan serves as the precursor for the synthesis of 5-hydroxytryptamine

Not all cells that contain 5-HT synthesize it. For example, platelets do not synthesize 5-HT; rather, they accumulate 5-HT from plasma by an active-transport mechanism found on the platelet membrane. Certain brain cells do synthesize 5-HT. The synthesis and primary metabolic pathways of 5-HT are shown in Figure 13-5. The initial step in the synthesis of serotonin is the facilitated transport of the amino acid L-tryptophan from blood into brain. The primary source of tryptophan is dietary protein. Certain other neutral amino acids, such as phenylalanine, leucine and methionine, are transported into brain by the same carrier. The entry of tryptophan into brain is related not only to its concentration in blood but is also a function of its concentration in relation to the concentrations of other neutral amino acids. Consequently, lowering the dietary intake of tryptophan while raising intake of the amino acids that tryptophan competes with for transport into brain lowers the content of 5-HT in brain and changes certain behaviors associated with 5-HT function. This strategy for lowering the brain content of 5-HT has been used clinically to evaluate the importance of brain 5-HT in the mechanism of action of psychotherapeutic drugs [5].

Serotonergic neurons contain the enzyme L-tryptophan-5-monooxygenase (EC 1.14.16.4), more commonly termed tryptophan hydroxylase, which converts tryptophan to 5-hydroxytryptophan (5-HTP) (Fig. 13-5). This enzyme is synthesized in serotonergic cell bodies of the raphe nuclei and is found only in cells that synthesize 5-HT; its distribution in brain is similar to that of 5-HT itself. The enzyme requires both molecular oxygen and a reduced pteridine cofactor, such as L-erythro-tetrahydrobiopterin (BH_4), for activity. In the enzymatic reaction, one atom of oxygen is used to form 5-HTP and the other is reduced to water. The pteridine cofactor donates electrons, and the unstable quinonoid dihydrobiopterin that results is regenerated immediately to the tetrahydrobiopterin form by a NADPH-linked enzymatic reaction:

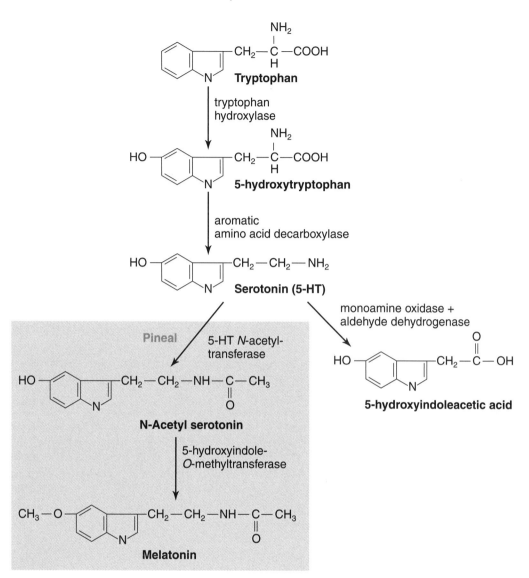

FIGURE 13-5. The biosynthesis and catabolism of serotonin. Note that in the pineal gland, serotonin is converted enzymatically to melatonin.

$$\text{L-Tryptophan} + BH_4 + O_2 \rightarrow$$
$$\text{L-5-HTP} + \text{quinonoid } BH_4 + H_2O$$

The K_m of partially purified tryptophan hydroxylase for tryptophan is approximately 30 to 60 μM, a concentration comparable to that of tryptophan in brain. If the concentration of tryptophan in serotonergic neurons is assumed to be comparable to that in whole brain, the enzyme would not be saturated with substrate and the

formation of 5-HT in brain would be expected to rise as the brain concentration of tryptophan increases. This occurs specifically in response to raising the dietary intake of tryptophan. However, the relationship among tryptophan availability, total tissue 5-HT concentration and 5-HT release is not fully understood.

cDNAs encoding tryptophan hydroxylase from both brain and pineal gland have been cloned and sequenced. Some biochemical differences between the enzyme(s) obtained from brain and from pineal gland, such as molecular weight, substrate specificity and isoelectric point, have been reported previously. However, cDNAs isolated from both tissue sources appear to have identical nucleotide sequences, making it likely that tissue-specific differences in the properties of tryptophan hydroxylase result from differential post-translational processing. Tryptophan hydroxylase contains 444 amino acids, corresponding to a molecular weight of about 51,000, and is 50% homologous with tyrosine hydroxylase, the rate-limiting enzyme in catecholamine (CA) biosynthesis (see Chap. 12). The greatest homology resides in the central and C-terminus regions of these enzymes, making it likely that these areas contain the catalytic site. Substrate specificity may reside in those amino acids nearer the N-terminus.

The other enzyme involved in the synthesis of serotonin, aromatic L-amino acid decarboxylase (AADC) (EC 4.1.1.28), is a soluble pyridoxal-5′-phosphate-dependent enzyme which converts 5-HTP to 5-HT (Fig. 13-5). It has been demonstrated that administration of pyridoxine increases the rate of synthesis of 5-HT in monkey brain, as revealed using position emission tomography. This presumably reflects a regulatory effect of pyridoxine on AADC activity and raises the interesting issue of the use of pyridoxine supplementation in situations associated with 5-HT deficiency.

AADC is present not only in serotonergic neurons but also in catecholaminergic neurons, where it converts 3,4-dihydroxyphenylalanine (DOPA) to dopamine (see Chap. 12). However, different pH optima or concentrations of substrate or cofactor are required for optimal activity of the enzyme in brain homogenates when using either 5-HTP or DOPA as the substrate. cDNAs encoding AADC have been cloned from various species. The encoded protein contains 480 amino acids and has a molecular weight of 54,000 but it appears to exist as a dimer. Characterization of the protein expressed in cells transfected with the cDNA shows that it decarboxylates either DOPA or 5-HTP. Also, *in situ* hybridization of the mRNA for the enzyme revealed its presence both in serotonergic cells in the dorsal raphe nucleus and in catecholaminergic cells in brain regions containing catecholaminergic soma [6]. Taken together, these results support the idea that the enzymatic decarboxylation of both DOPA and 5-HTP is catalyzed by the same enzyme.

Because the decarboxylase enzyme is not saturated with 5-HTP under physiological conditions, that is, the concentration of 5-HTP is much less than the K_m of 10 μM, it is possible to raise the content of 5-HT in brain not only by increasing the dietary intake of tryptophan but also by raising the intake of 5-HTP. This procedure, though, results in the formation of 5-HT in cells that would not normally contain it, such as catecholaminergic neurons, because of the nonselective nature of AADC.

The initial hydroxylation of tryptophan, rather than the decarboxylation of 5-HTP, appears to be the rate-limiting step in serotonin synthesis. Evidence in support of this view includes the fact that 5-HTP is found only in trace amounts in brain, presumably because it is decarboxylated about as rapidly as it is formed. As might be expected if the hydroxylation reaction is rate-limiting, inhibition of this reaction results in a marked depletion of the content of 5-HT in brain. The enzyme inhibitor most widely used in experiments is parachlorophenylalanine (PCPA). *In vivo*, PCPA irreversibly inhibits tryptophan hydroxylase, presumably by incorporating itself into the enzyme to produce an inactive protein. This results in a long-lasting reduction of 5-HT levels. Recovery of enzyme activity and 5-HT biosynthesis requires the synthesis of new enzyme. Marked increases in levels of mRNA for tryptophan hydroxylase are found in the raphe nuclei 1 to 3 days after administration of PCPA [7].

The synthesis of 5-hydroxytryptamine can increase markedly under conditions requiring a continuous supply of the neurotransmitter

Plasticity is an important concept in neurobiology. In general, this refers to the ability of neuronal systems to conform to either short- or long-term demands placed upon their activity or function. One of the processes contributing to neuronal plasticity is the ability to increase the rate of neurotransmitter synthesis and release in response to increased neuronal activity. Serotonergic neurons have this capability; the synthesis of 5-HT from tryptophan is increased in a frequency-dependent manner in response to electrical stimulation of serotonergic soma [8]. The increase in synthesis results from the enhanced conversion of tryptophan to 5-HTP and has an absolute dependence on extracellular Ca^{2+}. It is likely that the increased synthesis results in part from alterations in the kinetic properties of tryptophan hydroxylase, perhaps due to calcium-dependent phosphorylation of the enzyme. The enzyme can be phosphorylated directly by the action of calmodulin-dependent protein kinase II; an activator protein appears to be required for this interaction. In the presence of the activator, tryptophan hydroxylase also may be a substrate for cAMP-dependent protein kinase (PKA). The increased activity of tryptophan hydroxylase does not result from the removal of enzyme inhibition caused by either 5-HT or 5-HTP.

Short-term requirements for increases in the synthesis of 5-HT can be met by processes that change the kinetic properties of tryptophan hydroxylase, such as phosphorylation, without necessitating the synthesis of more molecules of tryptophan hydroxylase. By contrast, situations requiring long-term increases in the synthesis and release of 5-HT result in the synthesis of tryptophan hydroxylase protein. For example, partial but substantial destruction of >60% of central serotonergic neurons results in an increase in the synthesis of 5-HT in residual terminals. The increase in synthesis initially results from activation of existing tryptophan hydroxylase molecules, but the increased synthesis of 5-HT seen weeks after the lesion results from more tryptophan hydroxylase being present in the residual terminals. An increase in tryptophan hydroxylase mRNA has been reported in residual raphe serotonergic neurons after partial lesioning, consistent with the idea of an increase in the synthesis of tryptophan hydroxylase molecules in residual neurons.

As with other biogenic amine transmitters, 5-hydroxytryptamine is stored primarily in vesicles and released by an exocytotic mechanism

Peripheral sources of monoamine-containing cells have been utilized to study the properties of storage vesicles, such as chromaffin cells of the adrenal medulla for CAs and parafollicular cells of the thyroid gland for 5-HT. In some respects, the vesicles that store 5-HT resemble those that store CAs. For example, drugs such as reserpine and tetrabenazine, which inhibit the activity of the transporter localized to the vesicular membrane, deplete the brain content of 5-HT as well as of CAs. Storage of 5-HT in vesicles requires its active transport from the cytoplasm. The vesicular transporter uses the electrochemical gradient generated by a vesicular H^+-ATPase to drive transport, such that a cytoplasmic amine is exchanged for a luminal proton; that is, uptake of 5-HT is coupled to efflux of H^+ (Fig. 13-6).

Two synaptic vesicle transporters have been cloned, with the predicted amino acid sequence containing 12 transmembrane domains. The first transporter, cloned from chromaffin granules, has been termed vesicular membrane transporter$_1$ (VMAT$_1$). It contains 521 amino acids and a large loop between transmembrane domains 1 and 2, which faces the lumen of the vesicle, contains sites for glycosylation. Both the NH$_2$ and COOH termini face the cytoplasm. A second vesicular transporter (VMAT$_2$), cloned from rat brain, is 62% identical to VMAT$_1$. Human chromosome 8 contains the gene for VMAT$_1$ and chromosome 10 contains the gene for VMAT$_2$. These transporters show homology to a family of drug-resistant transporters in bacteria and yeast. All members of this family function as antiporters to remove toxic compounds from the cytoplasm. It has been suggested that this family, including VMAT$_1$ and VMAT$_2$, be termed *Toxin-Extruding Antiporters* (TEXANs) [9].

Although there are clear structural differences between the vesicular transporter and the Na^+-dependent plasma membrane transporter for 5-HT (described below), there are also striking structural similarities. Nevertheless, drugs that inhibit the vesicular transporter generally do not block the plasma membrane transporter and *vice versa*. However, two drugs that have effects at both the vesicular transporter and the plasma membrane transporter are the anorectic agent fenfluramine and MDMA. Fenfluramine inhibits the vesicular transporter directly by competing for its substrate-binding site. It also dissipates the transmembrane pH gradient to inhibit further 5-HT uptake into the vesicle

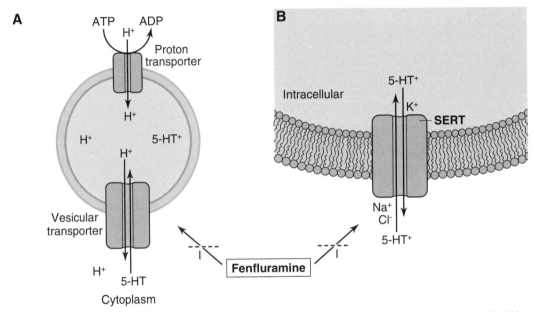

FIGURE 13-6.   The substituted amphetamine fenfluramine inhibits the transport of 5-hydroxytryptamine *(5-HT)* by both **(A)** the vesicular transporter and **(B)** the serotonin transporter *(SERT)*. Substituted amphetamines, such as fenfluramine and 3,4-methylenedioxymethamphetamine (MDMA), stimulate the release of 5-HT from serotonergic terminals. These drugs block the vesicular transporter and disrupt the proton gradient across the vesicle membrane. The increase in intracellular 5-HT favors the release of 5-HT by the reverse action of the SERT. These drugs also act as substrates for the SERT so as to inhibit the transport of 5-HT into cells.

(Fig. 13-6). MDMA has these pharmacological effects as well. The effects of these drugs on the plasma membrane transporter are described below. The consequence of such pharmacological actions is stimulation of 5-HT release by a nonexocytotic mechanism.

Vesicles storing 5-HT exhibit some differences from those storing CAs. In contrast to CA-containing vesicles, there is virtually no ATP in serotonin vesicles. Also, serotonergic synaptic vesicles, but not chromaffin granules, contain a specific protein that binds 5-HT with high affinity. This serotonin-binding protein is present in serotonergic cells derived ontogenetically from the neuroectoderm [10]. It binds 5-HT with high affinity in the presence of Fe^{2+}. There are three isoforms of serotonin-binding protein. The 45-kDa isoform appears to be packaged in secretory vesicles along with 5-HT, which probably accounts for the observation that newly taken up [^{3}H]5-HT is rapidly complexed with this isoform in brain *in situ*. This isoform is secreted along with 5-HT by a calcium-dependent process.

There is considerable evidence that the release of 5-HT occurs by exocytosis, that is, by the discharge from the cell of the entire contents of individual storage vesicles. First, 5-HT is ionized sufficiently at physiological pH so that it does not cross plasma membranes by simple diffusion. Second, most intraneuronal 5-HT is contained in storage vesicles and other contents of the vesicle, including serotonin-binding protein (SPB), are released together with serotonin. By contrast, cytosolic proteins do not accompany electrical stimulation-elicited release of 5-HT. Third, the depolarization-induced release of 5-HT occurs by a calcium-dependent process; indeed, it appears that the influx of Ca^{2+} with or without membrane depolarization can increase the release of 5-HT. Ca^{2+} has been reported to stimulate the fusion of vesicular membranes with the plasma membrane.

The rate of serotonin release is dependent on the firing rate of serotonergic soma in the raphe nuclei. Numerous studies have revealed that an increase in raphe cell firing enhances the release of 5-HT in terminal fields. The opposite effect is observed when raphe cell firing decreases. This means that drugs that change the firing rate of serotonergic soma modify the release of serotonin as well. An important target for such drugs is the somatodendritic autoreceptor, which, as discussed later, is the 5-HT_{1A} receptor subtype (see Fig. 13-8). Administration of 5-HT_{1A} agonists, such as 8-hydroxy-2-(di-*n*-propylamino)-tetralin (8-OH-DPAT), into the dorsal raphe nucleus slows the rate of firing of serotonergic soma. Using the technique of *in vivo* microdialysis, application of 8-OH-DPAT in the dorsal raphe nucleus decreases the release of 5-HT in the striatum. Depending on the species, serotonergic autoreceptors in terminal fields appear to be either the 5-HT_{1B} or the 5-HT_{1D} subtype. Administration of agonists of these receptors into areas receiving serotonergic innervation decreases the synthesis and release of 5-HT measured *in vitro* or *in situ*, using the technique of microdialysis. However, in contrast to the activation of somatodendritic autoreceptors, such effects are not due to decreases in the firing rate of serotonergic soma.

The activity of 5-hydroxytryptamine in the synapse is terminated primarily by its re-uptake into serotonergic terminals

Synaptic effects of many amino acid and monoaminergic neurotransmitters, including 5-HT, are terminated by binding of these molecules to specific transporter proteins. The serotonin transporter (SERT) is located on serotonergic neurons. Evidence for this comes from studies showing that the selective lesioning of serotonergic neurons in brain markedly reduces both the high-affinity uptake of [^{3}H]5-HT in areas of brain receiving serotonergic innervation and the specific binding of radioligands to the serotonin transporter. Activity of the SERT regulates the concentration of 5-HT in the synapse, thereby influencing synaptic transmission.

The uptake system for 5-HT is saturable and of high affinity, with a K_m value for 5-HT of approximately 0.2 to 0.5 μM. Uptake of 5-HT is an active process that is temperature-dependent and has an absolute requirement for external Na^+ and Cl^-; it is inhibited by metabolic inhibitors as well as by inhibitors of Na/K ATPase

activity. From these and other data, it has been inferred that the energy requirement for 5-HT uptake is not used directly to transport 5-HT but rather is necessary to maintain the gradient of Na^+ across the plasma membrane, upon which 5-HT uptake is dependent. The current model of transport has one Na^+, one Cl^- and one protonated 5-HT binding to the transporter extracellularly prior to translocation to form a quaternary complex that subsequently undergoes a conformational change to release the neurotransmitter and the ions into the cytoplasm. The conformational change may involve the "opening" of a pore formed by some portion of the transmembrane domains of the SERT (see below). In the cytoplasm, K^+ associates with the SERT to promote reorientation of the unloaded carrier for another transport cycle (Fig. 13-6).

The cloning, sequencing and expression of several transporter proteins, including that for 5-HT, has aided considerably in understanding structure/function relationships of transporter proteins [11,12]. The cDNA for the SERT isolated from rat brain predicts a protein containing 630 amino acids with a molecular weight of about 68,000. The SERT is encoded by a single gene on the long arm of chromosome 17. The mRNA for the SERT has been localized in brain exclusively to the serotonergic cells in the raphe nuclei. Of interest is the fact that mRNA for the SERT has not yet been detected in glia, even though primary cultures of astrocytes *in vitro* can take up 5-HT. The inability to detect message for the SERT in glia raises questions about the physiological relevance of the uptake of 5-HT by glia *in vitro*.

The putative structure of the SERT has 12 transmembrane domains (TMDs) with both the amino- and carboxy-termini being intracellular, and a large extracellular loop containing canonical glycosylation sites connecting TMDs 3 and 4 (Fig. 13-7). Glycosylation seems necessary for optimal stability of the transporter in the membrane but not for 5-HT transport or ligand binding. There are also six potential sites of phosphorylation by PKA and protein kinase C (PKC) on the human SERT. The predicted structure of the serotonin transporter is similar to that of other cloned neurotransmitter transporters and quite distinct, for example, from the seven-transmem-

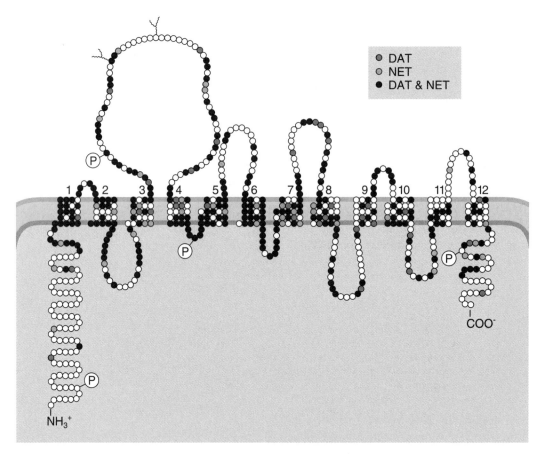

FIGURE 13-7. Putative structure of the rat serotonin transporter showing homologous amino acids with the rat dopamine transporter *(DAT)*, human norepinephrine transporter *(NET)* or both. Possible phosphorylation ⓟ sites are shown, as are possible glycosylation sites on the large second extracellular loop. Note the considerable degree of homology in the 12 transmembrane-spanning regions. (Diagram courtesy of Dr. Beth J. Hoffman, Laboratory of Cell Biology, NIMH, Bethesda, MD.)

brane domain structure of G protein-linked receptors. These transporters are considered members of the Na^+ and Cl^--dependent neurotransporter family, distinct from the vesicular transporter family described earlier. All members of this family are fragmented by multiple introns, raising the possibility of multiple transcripts by alternative RNA processing.

SERT exhibits about 50% absolute homology with the transporters for norepinephrine (NET) and dopamine (DAT), with the greatest homology being found in TMDs 1 and 2 and TMDs 4-8. The least conserved regions are the intracellular amino- and carboxy-terminal tails (Fig. 13-7). It has been proposed that the conserved regions may be involved in general transport functions and the least conserved regions in the unique attributes of each carrier, such as pharmacological specificity. However, studies in which the terminal regions were exchanged between the SERT and the NET revealed no alternation in substrate or antagonist selectivity. Thus, the NH_2 and COOH termini may not be important for ligand recognition.

Of considerable interest is whether the SERT is subject to physiological regulation. Such regulation could occur at the level of transcription or translation or by post-translational modifications, such as glycosylation or phosphorylation. The focus of much of this research, carried out *in vitro* using cells that naturally express the SERT or cells stably transfected with the SERT, has been on the role of second-messenger systems, particularly those activating protein kinases. It has been established that SERT gene expression is (i) influenced by cAMP-dependent pathways and (ii) rapidly regulated by changes in intracellular Ca^{2+}, treatment with calmodulin inhibitors or activation of PKC as well as nitric oxide synthase (NOS)/cGMP pathways. Most of the kinetic alterations reflect changes in maximal transport capacity (V_{max}) rather than in apparent affinity (K_m). Activation of PKC causes a loss of SERT protein on the cell surface. It remains to be established, however, whether such processes contribute to modulation of SERT activity *in vivo*.

Although there is structural homology among the transporters for 5-HT, NE and DA, some drugs exhibit great selectivity at inhibiting the activity of just one of these proteins. For example, secondary amine tricyclic antidepressants, such as desipramine, are 25- to 150-fold more potent at inhibiting transport of NE than 5-HT. By contrast, some of the newer antidepressants, appropriately termed *selective serotonin reuptake inhibitors* (SSRIs), such as fluoxetine, sertraline and paroxetine, are 15 to 75 times more potent at inhibiting the uptake of 5-HT than the uptake of NE. However, there are also drugs, such as cocaine, that are nonselective inhibitors of all three transporters.

In addition to facilitating the removal of transmitters from the synapse, plasma membrane transporters function under certain circumstances to release transmitter by a non-Ca^{2+}-dependent, that is, nonexocytotic, process. In contrast to exocytotic release, this release process is not modulated by presynaptic receptors. However, such transporter-mediated release is Na^+-dependent and sensitive to transport inhibitors. The role of such transporter-mediated release in physiological circumstances is speculative. However, certain drugs elicit the release of 5-HT, at least in part, through such a mechanism. For example, both fenfluramine and MDMA act as substrates for the SERT and not only inhibit the transport of 5-HT into the cell but also facilitate its outward transport. The action of these drugs on 5-HT-storing vesicles raises cytoplasmic 5-HT and facilitates SERT-mediated efflux of 5-HT (Fig. 13-6). The release of 5-HT caused by drugs such as fenfluramine is prevented by inhibitors of the SERT.

The primary catabolic pathway for 5-hydroxytryptamine is oxidative deamination by the enzyme monoamine oxidase

Monoamine oxidase (MAO) (E.C.1.4.3.4.) converts serotonin to 5-hydroxyindoleacetaldehyde, and this product is oxidized by an NAD^+-dependent aldehyde dehydrogenase to form 5-hydroxyindoleacetic acid (5-HIAA) (Fig. 13-5). The intermediate acetaldehyde also can be reduced by an NADH-dependent aldehyde reductase to form the alcohol 5-hydroxytryptophol. Whether oxidation or reduction takes place depends on the ratio of NAD^+ to NADH in the tissue. In brain, 5-HIAA is the primary metabolite of serotonin.

There are at least two isoenzymes of MAO, referred to as MAO-A and MAO-B. These isoenzymes are integral flavoproteins of outer mitochondrial membranes in neurons, glia and other cells. Evidence for the existence of isoenzymes was based initially on differing substrate specificities and sensitivities to inhibitors of MAO. For example, both 5-HT and NE are metabolized preferentially by MAO-A. Selective inhibitors of each form of MAO exist: clorgyline or moclobemide for type A and deprenyl for type B. Definitive proof of the existence of these two forms of MAO comes from the cloning of cDNAs encoding subunits of MAO-A and MAO-B from human liver [13]. The deduced amino acid sequences of MAO-A and MAO-B show about 70% homology and have masses of 59.7 and 58.8 kDa, respectively. When each cDNA was cloned into an expression vector and transfected independently into a cell line, the activity of the proteins expressed resembled that of the endogenous enzymes from human brain, such that the expressed MAO-A preferred 5-HT as a substrate and was inhibited preferentially by clorgyline. From such data it was inferred that the functional differences between these two enzymes exist in their primary structures.

Several different techniques have been used to study the neuroanatomical localization of the two forms of MAO in brain. Originally, both histochemical and immunohistochemical techniques were used. More recently, *in situ* hybridization histochemistry has been used to demonstrate the location of the mRNAs for the two isoenzymes. The development of radioligands selective for each form has enabled their distribution to be revealed by quantitative autoradiography. In general, the results from the use of these different techniques are similar. It is of interest that there is more MAO-A than MAO-B throughout rat brain, whereas human brain contains more MAO-B than MAO-A. Serotonergic cell bodies contain predominantly MAO-B, for which 5-HT is not a preferred substrate. This has led to the hypothesis that MAO-B in serotonergic neurons prevents the cell from accumulating various other natural substrates, such as DA, that could interfere with the storage, release and uptake of 5-HT. Furthermore, treatment of rats with clorgyline, a selective inhibitor of MAO-A, raises the brain content of 5-HT and reduces the conversion of 5-HT to 5-HIAA in brain. Thus, 5-HT may well be oxidized preferentially by MAO-A *in vivo*, as it is *in vitro*, even though serotonergic neurons do not contain much of this form of the enzyme.

The use of transgenic mice permits the selective elimination, or "knockout," of either MAO type [14]. In the brains of mice deficient in MAO-A, the content of 5-HT is elevated markedly for about 12 days after birth and then slowly declines, reaching values comparable to those in normal mice after about 7 months. In MAO-A-deficient mice, the selective inhibitor of MAO-B, deprenyl, had a greater effect on serotonin metabolism than it did in normal mice. Such observations indicate that, in the absence of MAO-A, MAO-B can metabolize 5-HT *in vivo*. However, mice lacking the MAO-B isoenzyme do not have elevated levels of 5-HT in brain. Of interest are the aggressive behaviors exhibited by mice deficient in MAO-A, consistent with a postulated role of serotonergic neurons in human aggressive behaviors.

SEROTONIN RECEPTORS

Pharmacological and physiological studies have contributed to the definition of the many receptor subtypes for serotonin

The initial suggestion that there might be more than one type of receptor for serotonin came from experiments on the isolated guinea pig ileum, which demonstrated that only a portion of the contractile response to serotonin could be blocked by high concentrations of morphine, whereas the remainder of the response could be blocked by low concentrations of dibenzyline (phenoxybenzamine). Similarly, when maximally effective concentrations of dibenzyline were present, the remaining contractile response elicited by serotonin was blocked by low concentrations of morphine. It was speculated that there were two different receptors for 5-HT in the ileum: D receptors, which are blocked by dibenzyline, and M receptors, which are blocked by morphine. The D receptor was thought to be on the smooth muscle of the ileum, whereas the M receptor was considered to be on ganglia or nerves within the muscle.

In the 1970s, the development of radioligand-binding assays furthered our understanding of subtypes of receptors for serotonin. Initially, a number of radioligands, such as [^{3}H]5-HT, [^{3}H]LSD and [^{3}H]spiperone, were used to label sites related to serotonin receptors. These radioligands originally were proposed to label two classes of serotonin receptor in brain. Binding sites that were labeled with high affinity by [^{3}H]5-HT were designated 5-HT$_1$ receptors; binding sites labeled with high affinity by [^{3}H]spiperone were termed 5-HT$_2$ receptors. Many subsequent experiments have shown that the D receptor and the 5-HT$_2$ receptor are pharmacologically indistinguishable.

The binding of [^{3}H]5-HT to 5-HT$_1$ receptors was shown to be displaced by spiperone in a biphasic manner, suggesting that what was termed the 5-HT$_1$ receptor might be a heterogeneous population of receptors. The [^{3}H]5-HT-binding site that showed high affinity for spiperone was termed the 5-HT$_{1A}$ subtype, whereas the component of [^{3}H]5-HT binding that showed low affinity for spiperone was called the 5-HT$_{1B}$ subtype. A high density of binding sites for [^{3}H]5-HT was found in the choroid plexus. These [^{3}H]5-HT-binding sites were termed the 5-HT$_{1C}$ subtype as they did not show the pharmacological characteristics used to classify the 5-HT$_{1A}$, 5-HT$_{1B}$ or 5-HT$_2$ binding sites. Subsequently, a fourth binding site for [^{3}H]5-HT was identified in bovine brain and called the 5-HT$_{1D}$ receptor. The 5-HT$_{1D}$ receptor was identified by pharmacological criteria only in brains of species devoid of the $5\text{-}HT_{1B}$ receptor, such as pig, cow, guinea pig and human.

Bradley and associates in 1986 proposed a classification scheme with three major types of receptors for serotonin, using pharmacological criteria and functional responses primarily in peripheral tissues [15]. The receptors were called "$5\text{-}HT_1$-like," $5\text{-}HT_2$ and $5\text{-}HT_3$. The development of potent and selective antagonists of the $5\text{-}HT_2$ receptor, such as ketanserin, facilitated the assignment of certain effects mediated by 5-HT to the $5\text{-}HT_2$ receptor. The M receptor, originally described in guinea pig ileum, is pharmacologically distinct from all of the binding sites associated with the serotonin receptors just described. Bradley and associates renamed this the $5\text{-}HT_3$ receptor. The development of potent selective antagonists and an agonist, 2-methyl-5-HT, provided useful tools for the pharmacological characterization of $5\text{-}HT_3$ receptors.

Molecular biological techniques have led to the rapid discovery of additional serotonin-receptor subtypes and their properties

The first 5-HT receptor to be cloned was the $5\text{-}HT_{1C}$ receptor. Over the course of the next 5 years, the $5\text{-}HT_{1A}$, $5\text{-}HT_{1B}$, $5\text{-}HT_{1D}$, $5\text{-}HT_2$ and $5\text{-}HT_3$ receptors also were cloned. The $5\text{-}HT_{1A}$, $5\text{-}HT_{1B}$, $5\text{-}HT_{1C}$, $5\text{-}HT_{1D}$ and $5\text{-}HT_2$ receptors are single-subunit proteins that are members of the G protein receptor superfamily. This receptor family is characterized by the presence of seven transmembrane domains, an intracellular carboxy-terminus and an extracellular amino-terminus. It is the interaction of the receptor with the G protein that allows the receptor to modulate the activity of different effector systems, such as ion channels, phospholipase C and adenylyl cyclase. The transmembrane domains of G protein-coupled receptors are the most highly conserved regions of these proteins. The $5\text{-}HT_3$ receptor differs from all other known subtypes of serotonin receptor in that it is a member of the ligand-gated ion channel superfamily. Members of this receptor superfamily consist of five subunits, each of which possesses four transmembrane segments and a large, extracellular N-terminal region.

The rapid discovery of additional subtypes of receptor for serotonin made it necessary to establish an unambiguous system of nomenclature. The current classification scheme takes into account not only operational criteria, such as drug-related characteristics, but also information about intracellular signal-transduction mechanisms and amino acid sequence of the receptor protein. For example, the $5\text{-}HT_{1C}$ receptor was reclassified as a $5\text{-}HT_2$ receptor based on the sequence homology, similar pharmacological characteristics and effector coupling of the $5\text{-}HT_2$ and $5\text{-}HT_{1C}$ receptors. The $5\text{-}HT_2$ receptor was renamed $5\text{-}HT_{2A}$ and the $5\text{-}HT_{1C}$ receptor was renamed the $5\text{-}HT_{2C}$ [16]. The amino acid sequence of several new serotonin receptors has been reported. However, the classification of these receptors remains tentative due to limited knowledge of their operational and tranductional characteristics, which have only been described in transfected cell systems for these recombinant receptors. Because the functions mediated by these serotonin receptors in intact tissue are unknown, lowercase appellations are presently used [16].

The three serotonin receptor subfamilies, the $5\text{-}HT_1$ family; the $5\text{-}HT_2$ family; and the family that includes the $5\text{-}HT_4$, $5\text{-}ht_6$ and $5\text{-}HT_7$ receptors, represent the three major classes of serotonin receptor that are members of the G protein-coupled receptor superfamily. As mentioned above, the $5\text{-}HT_3$ receptor is a ligand-gated ion channel and is a separate subfamily. Although each serotonin receptor can be activated potently by serotonin, differences in signal-transduction mechanisms, neuroanatomical distribution and affinities for synthetic chemicals create opportunities for drug discovery and make each serotonin receptor subtype a potential therapeutic target.

The $5\text{-}HT_1$ receptor family contains receptors that are negatively coupled to adenylyl cyclase and includes the $5\text{-}HT_{1A}$, $5\text{-}HT_{1B}$, $5\text{-}HT_{1D}$, $5\text{-}ht_{1E}$ and $5\text{-}ht_{1F}$ receptors. The $5\text{-}HT_{1A}$ receptor is coupled via G proteins to two distinct effector systems: (i) inhibition of adenylyl cyclase activity and (ii) the opening of K^+ channels, which results in neuronal hyperpolarization. In terminal field areas of serotonergic innervation, such as the hippocampus, $5\text{-}HT_{1A}$ receptors are

TABLE 13-2. **SEROTONIN RECEPTORS PRESENT IN THE CENTRAL NERVOUS SYSTEM**

Receptor[a]	Human locus	Distribution	Effector mechanism
5-HT_{1A}	5q11.2–13	Hippocampus, amygdala, septum, entorhinal cortex, hypothalamus, raphe nuclei	Inhibition of adenylyl cyclase, opening of K^+ channels
$5\text{-HT}_{1D\alpha}$	1p34.3–36.3	Not distinguishable from $5\text{-HT}_{1D\beta}$	Inhibition of adenylyl cyclase
$5\text{-HT}_{1D\beta}$	6q13	Substantia nigra, basal ganglia, superior colliculus	Inhibition of adenylyl cyclase
5-ht_{1E}	?	?	Inhibition of adenylyl cyclase
5-ht_{1F}	3p11	Cerebral cortex, striatum, hippocampus, olfactory bulb	Inhibition of adenylyl cyclase
5-HT_{2A}	13q14–21	Claustrum, cerebral cortex, olfactory tubercle, striatum, nucleus accumbens	Stimulation of phosphoinositide-specific phospholipase C, closing of K^+ channels
5-HT_{2B}	2q36.3–37.1	?	Stimulation of phosphoinositide-specific phospholipase C
5-HT_{2C}	Xq24	Choroid plexus, globus pallidus, cerebral cortex, hypothalamus, septum, substantia nigra, spinal cord	Stimulation of phosphoinositide-specific phospholipase C
5-HT_3	?	Hippocampus, entorhinal cortex, amygdala, nucleus accumbens, solitary tract nerve, trigeminal nerve, motor nucleus of the dorsal vagal nerve, area postrema, spinal cord	Ligand-gated cation channel
5-HT_4	?	Hippocampus, striatum, olfactory tubercle, substantia nigra	Stimulation of adenylyl cyclase
5-ht_{5A}	7q36	?	Inhibition of adenylyl cyclase
5-HT_{5B}	2q11–13	?	?
5-ht_6	?	?	Stimulation of adenylyl cyclase
5-HT_7	10q23.3–24.3	Cerebral cortex, septum, thalamus, hypothalamus, amygdala, superior colliculus	Stimulation of adenylyl cyclase

[a]Lower-case appellations are used in some cases because the functions mediated by these receptors in intact tissue are presently unknown.

coupled to both effector systems (Table 13-2). However, in the dorsal raphe nucleus, 5-HT_{1A} receptors are coupled only to the opening of potassium channels.

The 5-HT_{1B} and 5-HT_{1D} receptor subtypes are also linked to inhibition of adenylyl cyclase activity (Table 13-2). Binding sites that have been defined pharmacologically as 5-HT_{1B} receptors have been characterized in the rat, mouse and hamster, whereas the 5-HT_{1D} receptor has been characterized using pharmacological criteria in species such as guinea pig, pig, cow and human. In the substantia nigra, where a high density of 5-HT_{1B} or 5-HT_{1D} receptors has been demonstrated by radioligand-binding studies, these serotonin receptors are linked to the inhibition of adenylyl cyclase through a G protein.

An issue raised by the use of molecular biological techniques for the study of neurotransmitter receptors is whether a receptor is a subtype or a species homolog, that is, an equivalent receptor in different species. For example, the 5-HT_{1B} and 5-HT_{1D} receptors originally were considered to be species variants of the same receptor because the pharmacological profiles of these two receptors are similar, although not identical; the distribution of these two receptors in brain is very similar; and both receptors are coupled to the inhibition of adenylyl cyclase. Although biochemical, pharmacological and functional data suggest that the 5-HT_{1B} receptor found in rats and mice and the 5-HT_{1D} receptor found in other species, including humans, are functionally equivalent species homologs, the story has been complicated somewhat by the discovery of two genes encoding the human 5-HT_{1D} receptor, 5-$HT_{1D\alpha}$ and 5-$HT_{1D\beta}$ [16].

Radioligand-binding studies currently do not allow the differentiation of 5-$HT_{1D\alpha}$ and 5-$HT_{1D\beta}$ receptors, and the binding profiles of these receptor subtypes match the previously described 5-HT_{1D}-binding site. Furthermore, a rat homolog of the human 5-$HT_{1D\alpha}$ receptor has been isolated and shown to encode a receptor with a 5-HT_{1D}-binding site profile, suggesting that the 5-HT_{1B} and 5-HT_{1D} receptors may not be species homologs but distinct 5-HT receptor subtypes. There is still some debate as to whether a common appellation should be used to refer to the protein products of two distinct genes, the 5-$HT_{1D\alpha}$ and the 5-$HT_{1D\beta}$ receptor, and whether the human 5-$HT_{1D\beta}$ receptor should be called the human 5-HT_{1B} receptor, even though it has a distinct pharmacological profile from that of the rat 5-HT_{1B} receptor. Because there are no compounds currently available to differentiate between the 5-$HT_{1D\alpha}$ and the 5-$HT_{1D\beta}$ receptors, we will refer to them in this chapter as 5-HT_{1D}. Furthermore, because of distinct pharmacological profiles of the 5-HT_{1B} receptor found in rat and the 5-HT_{1D} receptor found in other species, we will not refer to the 5-$HT_{1D\beta}$ as the human 5-HT_{1B} receptor.

The 5-ht_{1E} receptor originally was identified in homogenates of human frontal cortex by radioligand-binding studies with [^{3}H]5-HT in the presence of 5-carboxamidotryptamine (5-CT) to block 5-HT_{1A} and 5-HT_{1D} receptor sites. Because of the lack of specific radioligands for the 5-ht_{1E} receptor, the overall distribution in brain is unknown. With the cloning of the various subtypes of receptors for serotonin, knowledge of receptor sequences can be used to generate radioactive probes for mRNAs encoding individual serotonin receptor subtypes. Using *in situ* hybridization histochemistry, the localization of these mRNAs and, thus, the distribution of cells expressing the mRNAs for serotonin receptors can be established in brain. 5-ht_{1E} receptor mRNA has been found in the caudate putamen, parietal cortex and olfactory tubercle [17]. The function of the 5-ht_{1E} receptor in intact tissue is not known due to the lack of selective agonists or antagonists. In trans-

fected cells, the 5-ht_{1E} receptor is coupled to the inhibition of adenylyl cyclase activity. The 5-ht_{1E} receptor displays a higher degree of homology with the 5-HT_{1D} receptor (64%) than any other 5-HT_1 receptors [16].

The 5-HT_{1F} receptor was cloned and sequenced in 1993 and shares the greatest sequence homology with the 5-ht_{1E} receptor (61%). 5-ht_{1F} receptor mRNA is found in cortex, hippocampus, dentate gyrus, nucleus of the solitary tract, spinal cord, trigeminal ganglion neurons, uterus and mesentery. In transfected cells, the 5-ht_{1F} receptor is coupled to the inhibition of adenylyl cyclase [16]. Because selective agonists or antagonists for the 5-ht_{1F} receptor have not been available until very recently, little is known about the distribution or function of the 5-ht_{1F} receptor in brain. The selective agonist radioligand [^{3}H]LY334370 has been used to demonstrate the presence of 5-ht_{1F} receptor sites in cortex, striatum, hippocampus and olfactory bulb [18]. Activation of 5-ht_{1F} receptors *in vivo* inhibits neurogenic dural inflammation and dural protein extravasation.

The 5-HT_2 receptor family stimulates phosphoinositide-specific phospholipase C (PI-PLC) and includes the 5-HT_{2A}, 5-HT_{2B} and 5-HT_{2C} (formerly the 5-HT_{1C}) receptors. 5-HT_{2A} receptor-mediated stimulation of phosphoinositide hydrolysis has been well characterized in cerebral cortex. 5-HT_{2C} receptor-mediated stimulation of inositol lipid hydrolysis has been studied in the choroid plexus (Table 13-2). Stimulation of phosphoinositide turnover by 5-HT in these tissues is not dependent on the activity of lipoxygenase or cyclooxygenase pathways, nor is it blocked by agents that inhibit neuronal firing, suggesting that coupling of the 5-HT_{2A} or 5-HT_{2C} receptor to the enzyme PI-PLC mediates the enhanced response (see Chap. 21). Activation of 5-HT_{2A} receptors also mediates neuronal depolarization, a result of the closing of potassium channels. The 5-HT_{2A} receptor was first cloned in the rat by homology with the rat 5-HT_{2C} receptor. The rat 5-HT_{2A} receptor is 49% homologous to the rat 5-HT_{2C} receptor.

Cloning of the 5-HT_{2A} receptor has been used to gain insight into a controversy over the nature of agonist binding to the 5-HT_{2A} receptor. The hallucinogenic amphetamine derivative [³H]2,5-Dimethoxy-4-bromoamphetamine (DOB), an agonist, binds to a small number of sites with properties very similar to those of the receptor labeled with the antagonist [³H]ketanserin. Agonists, though, have higher affinities for the receptor labeled with [³H]DOB than for that labeled with [³H]ketanserin. Some investigators have interpreted these and other data as evidence for the existence of a new subtype of 5-HT$_{2A}$ receptor, whereas others have interpreted these data as indicative of agonist high-affinity and agonist low-affinity preferring states of the 5-HT$_{2A}$ receptor. In experiments in which the cDNA encoding the 5-HT$_{2A}$ receptor was transfected into clonal cells, binding sites for both the 5-HT$_{2A}$ receptor antagonist [³H]ketanserin and the 5-HT$_2$ receptor agonist [³H]DOB were found. Furthermore, agonists had higher affinities for [³H]DOB binding than for [³H]ketanserin binding. Thus, a single gene produces a protein with both binding sites, substantiating the view that agonist and antagonist binding are to different states, rather than to two different subtypes, of the 5-HT$_{2A}$ receptor.

Although the 5-HT$_{2B}$ receptor is the most recently cloned of the 5-HT$_2$ receptor class, it was among the first of the serotonin receptors to be characterized using pharmacological criteria. The first report of the sensitivity of rat stomach fundus to serotonin was published by Vane in 1959. This receptor, whose activation results in the contraction of fundus smooth muscle, originally was placed in the 5-HT$_1$ receptor class by Bradley and associates [15] because of its sensitivity to serotonin and because responses mediated by it were not blocked by 5-HT$_2$ or 5-HT$_3$ receptor antagonists. It has been reclassified as a 5-HT$_2$ receptor because of its similar pharmacological profile to the 5-HT$_{2C}$ receptor (Table 13-2). The recombinant receptor expressed in clonal cells is coupled to the stimulation of inositol lipid hydrolysis. However, in rat stomach fundus, the 5-HT$_{2B}$ appears not to be coupled to phosphoinositide hydrolysis. 5-HT$_{2B}$ receptor-mediated contraction of rat stomach fundus is dependent on the influx of calcium through voltage-sensitive channels, intracellular calcium release and activation of PKC [19]. The effector system to which this receptor is coupled in the CNS remains to be established. Using quantitative polymerase chain reaction (PCR), 5-HT$_{2B}$ mRNA has been detected in the rat stomach fundus, intestine, kidney, heart, lung and dura mater but not in rat brain. In humans, 5-HT$_{2B}$ receptor mRNA has been found peripherally and in cerebellum, cerebral cortex, amygdala, substantia nigra, caudate, thalamus, hypothalamus and retina [16].

The 5-HT$_3$ receptor is homomeric and belongs to the ligand-gated ion channel superfamily. As mentioned above, the 5-HT$_3$ receptor is a serotonin-gated cation channel that causes the rapid depolarization of neurons (Table 13-2). The depolarization mediated by 5-HT$_3$ receptors is caused by a transient inward current, specifically the opening of a channel for cations. A single subunit of the 5-HT$_3$ receptor, the 5-HT$_3$-A receptor subunit, has been cloned. An alternatively spiced variant, the 5-HT$_3$-As receptor subunit, has been identified in mouse, rat and human. The cloned receptor subunit exhibits sequence similarity to the α subunit of the nicotinic acetylcholine receptor and to the β$_1$ subunit of the GABA$_A$ receptor. It is not known whether the native 5-HT$_3$ receptor is composed of this single subunit or several different subunits. Although single subunits of members of the ligand-gated ion channel receptor family can form functional homomeric receptors, they generally lack some of the properties of the native, multisubunit receptor. The cloned subunit of the 5-HT$_3$ receptor has been studied in *Xenopus* oocytes injected with mRNA encoding this receptor. Although the expressed 5-HT$_3$-A and 5-HT$_3$-As receptors are functional, they do not display all of the characteristics of native 5-HT$_3$ receptors. The 5-HT$_3$ receptor, like other members of the ligand-gated ion channel superfamily, appears to possess additional pharmacologically distinct recognition sites for alcohols and anesthetic agents, by which the function of this receptor can be allosterically modulated [20].

5-HT$_4$, 5-ht$_6$ and 5-HT$_7$ receptors are included in a family of serotonin receptors coupled to the stimulation of adenylyl cyclase. The 5-HT$_4$ receptor originally was described in cultured murine collicular neurons as a serotonin receptor coupled to the stimulation of adenylyl cyclase activity, possessing pharmacological characteristics distinct from those of the $5-HT_1$, $5-HT_2$ or $5-HT_3$ receptors. The $5-HT_4$ receptor gene has been cloned from rat brain RNA by reverse transcriptase (RT)-PCR [21]. Two different cDNA clones, the long isoform, 5.5-kb $5-HT_{4l}$, and the short isoform, 4.5-kb $5-HT_{4s}$, have been isolated and are most likely the result of alternative splicing of $5-HT_4$ receptor mRNA.

The $5-ht_6$ receptor is approximately 30% homologous to other serotonin receptors. When expressed in transfected cells, it shows high affinity for $[^{125}I]LSD$ and $[^3H]5-HT$. The pharmacology of this recombinant receptor is unique. Interestingly, this receptor has high affinity for various antipsychotic and antidepressant drugs, such as clozapine, amitriptyline, clomipramine, mianserin and ritanserin. The $5-ht_6$ receptor stimulates adenylyl cyclase when expressed in some, but not all, cell systems. The function of the $5-ht_6$ receptor in intact tissue has not been characterized due to the lack of selective agonists or antagonists. Expression of $5-ht_6$ receptor mRNA has been detected in the striatum, nucleus accumbens, olfactory tubercle, hippocampus and cerebral cortex [16].

Two rat $5-HT_7$ receptor clones, which differ only in the C terminus and presumably result from alternative mRNA splicing, have been identified. The $5-HT_7$ receptor shows the highest amino acid sequence homology with the *Drosophila* $5-HT_{1A}$ receptor, 42%, and approximately 35% homology with all other serotonin receptors. To date, no selective agonists or antagonists have been described for the $5-HT_7$ receptor. In transfected cells, the $5-HT_7$ receptor stimulates adenylyl cyclase. $5-HT_7$ receptors have been identified in human vascular smooth muscle cells and frontal cortical astrocytes in primary culture, where they are coupled to the stimulation of adenylyl cyclase.

The $5-ht_{5A}$ and $5-HT_{5B}$ receptors may constitute a new family of serotonin receptors since neither is coupled to adenylyl cyclase or PI-PLC; their effector systems are currently unknown. Both the $5-ht_{5A}$ and $5-HT_{5B}$ receptors were cloned by using degenerate oligonucleotides derived from TMDs III and VI of G protein-coupled serotonin receptors. Both genomic clones possess one intron in the middle of the third cytoplasmic loop. The receptor proteins are 77% identical to each other, whereas the homology to other serotonin receptors is low.

$5-ht_{5A}$ receptor mRNA transcripts have been detected by *in situ* hybridization in the cerebral cortex, hippocampus, granule cells of the cerebellum, medial habenula, amygdala, septum, several thalamic nuclei and olfactory bulb of the rat and mouse. $5-HT_{5B}$ mRNA has been detected by *in situ* hybridization in the hippocampus, habenula and the dorsal raphe nucleus of rat and human [16].

Immunohistochemical studies with antibodies to the $5-ht_{5A}$ receptor have shown this receptor to be expressed predominantly by astrocytes, although some neurons in cortex were labeled as well. In transfected cells expressing the $5-ht_{5A}$ receptor, 5-HT does not stimulate the formation of cAMP as it does in wild-type cells. Furthermore, 5-HT inhibits forskolin-stimulated cAMP formation, an effect not seen in wild-type cells. Thus, the $5-ht_{5A}$ receptor appears to be coupled to the inhibition of adenylyl cyclase activity [22]. At the present time, the functional correlate and transductional properties are unknown for the $5-HT_{5B}$ receptor.

The many serotonin-receptor subtypes are differentiated by their localization in the central nervous system

$5-HT_{1A}$ receptors are present in high density in the hippocampus, septum, amygdala, hypothalamus and neocortex (Table 13-2). Destruction of serotonergic neurons with the neurotoxin 5,7-dihydroxytryptamine (5,7-DHT) does not reduce $5-HT_{1A}$ receptor number in forebrain areas, indicating that $5-HT_{1A}$ receptors are located postsynaptically in these brain regions. Many of these serotonergic terminal field areas are components of the limbic system, the pathway thought to be involved in the modulation of emotion. The presence of $5-HT_{1A}$ receptors in high density in the limbic system indicates that the reported effects of 5-HT or serotonergic drugs on emotional states could be mediated by $5-HT_{1A}$ receptors. The presence of $5-HT_{1A}$ receptors in the neocortex suggests that this receptor also may be involved in cognitive or integrative functions of the cortex. 5-HT_{1A} receptors are also present in high density in serotonergic cell body areas, in particular the dorsal and median raphe nuclei, where they function as somatodendritic autoreceptors, modulating the activity of serotonergic neurons. Activation of these autoreceptors causes a decrease in the rate of firing of serotonergic neurons and a reduction in the release of 5-HT from serotonergic terminals. Neurotoxin-induced destruction of serotonergic cell bodies dramatically reduces the number of 5-HT_{1A} receptors in these areas, consistent with their location on serotonergic soma.

The 5-HT_{1B} receptor in rats and mice and the 5-HT_{1D} receptor in bovine and human brain are located in high density in the basal ganglia, particularly in the globus pallidus and the substantia nigra (Table 13-2). Functional studies indicate that the 5-HT_{1B} and 5-HT_{1D} receptors are located on presynaptic terminals of serotonergic neurons and modulate the release of serotonin. Release of 5-HT from the dorsal raphe nucleus also appears to be under the control of $5\text{-HT}_{1B/1D}$ receptors, although it is unclear whether these receptors are located on serotonergic terminals or cell bodies. The 5-HT_{1B} and 5-HT_{1D} receptors also are located postsynaptically, where they may modulate the release of other neurotransmitters, such as acetylcholine (ACh) in the hippocampus and DA in the prefrontal cortex. The presence of these receptors in high density in the basal ganglia raises the interesting possibility that they may play a role in diseases of the brain which involve the basal ganglia, such as Parkinson's disease.

A high density of 5-HT_{2A} receptors is found in many cortical areas. These receptors are particularly concentrated in the frontal cortex. 5-HT_{2A} receptors also are found in high density in the claustrum, a region which is connected to the visual cortex; in parts of the limbic system; and in the basal ganglia and the olfactory nuclei (Table 13-2). 5-HT_{2A} receptors in the cortex are thought to be located postsynaptically on intrinsic cortical neurons as destruction of projections to the cortex does not reduce 5-HT_{2A} receptors. Because of the lack of selective agonists to differentiate between members of the 5-HT_2 receptor family, many of the functional and clinical correlates of the 5-HT_{2A} receptor may very well involve or be attributed to the 5-HT_{2C} receptor.

5-HT_{2C} receptors are present in high density in the choroid plexus. High-resolution autoradiography has shown that they are enriched on the epithelial cells of the choroid plexus. It has been proposed that 5-HT-induced activation of 5-HT_{2C} receptors could regulate the composition and volume of the cerebrospinal fluid. 5-HT_{2C} receptors also are found throughout the brain, particularly in areas of the limbic system, including the hypothalamus, hippocampus, septum, neocortex and regions associated with motor behavior, including the substantia nigra and globus pallidus. 5-HT_{2C} receptors are present in much lower concentrations in these areas than in the choroid plexus (Table 13-2). The lack of truly selective 5-HT_{2C} receptor agonists and antagonists has limited our knowledge about the functional role of these receptors in brain.

5-HT_3 receptors initially appeared to be confined to peripheral neurons, where they mediate depolarizing actions of 5-HT and modulate neurotransmitter release. 5-HT_3 receptors are found in high density in peripheral ganglia and nerves, including the superior cervical ganglion and vagus nerve, as well as in the substantia gelatinosa of the spinal cord. Their localization in spinal cord and medulla suggests that 5-HT could modulate nociceptive mechanisms via the 5-HT_3 receptor. 5-HT_3 receptors facilitate the release of substance P in the spinal cord [23]. The localization of 5-HT_3 receptor-binding sites in cortical and limbic areas of the brain is consistent with behavioral studies in animals which suggest that 5-HT_3 receptor antagonists may have potential anxiolytic, antidepressant and cognitive effects. 5-HT_3 receptors are located postsynaptically, where they modulate the release of neurotransmitters such as ACh or DA. 5-HT_3 receptors modulate the activity of dopaminergic neurons in the ventral tegmental area. In the cortex and hippocampus, the majority of neurons expressing 5-HT_3 receptor mRNA are GABAergic. The highest density of 5-HT_3 receptor sites in the brain is in the area postrema, the site of the chemoreceptor trigger zone (Table 13-2).

Studies of the 5-HT_4 receptor, originally characterized by measuring cAMP production in cultured mouse collicular neurons, have been hampered by the absence of a high-affinity radioligand. The synthesis and development of specific radioligands, [³H]GR 113808 and [¹²⁵I]SB 207710, have provided the necessary tools for the study and characterization of the 5-HT$_4$ receptor. 5-HT$_4$ receptor binding sites are localized with high densities in the striatum, substantia nigra and olfactory tubercle and have been reported in the hippocampus as well (Table 13-2). The 5-HT$_4$ receptor indirectly mediates the enhancement of striatal DA release by 5-HT, although 5-HT$_4$ receptors do not appear to be located on striatal DA terminals. In the alimentary tract, 5-HT$_4$ receptors are located on neurons, for example, the myenteric plexus of the ileum, smooth muscle cells and secretory cells, where they evoke secretions and the peristaltic reflex.

Although there is no known selective agonist or antagonist available for the 5-HT$_7$ receptor, the distinct pharmacological profile of 5-HT$_7$ receptor sites, that is, the potent agonism by the 5-HT$_1$ receptor agonist 5-CT and antagonism by methiothepin, clozapine and a variety of ergot compounds, has been used to delineate the function and distribution of this receptor *in vivo*. 5-HT$_7$ receptor-binding sites in the rat brain have been described using receptor autoradiography in layers 1–3 of the cortex, septum, thalamus, hypothalamus, amygdala and superior colliculus [24] (Table 13-2). In the periphery, the 5-HT$_7$ receptors mediate relaxation of vascular smooth muscle.

An atypical 5-HT receptor exists on the enteric neurons of the gut. This receptor has high affinity for [³H]5-HT and mediates a slow depolarization of particular myenteric neurons that is not blocked by selective 5-HT$_3$ antagonists. It has been termed the 5-HT$_{1P}$ receptor as it has a high affinity for 5-HT and is found in the periphery. The available functional and radioligand-binding data confirm the orphan status of the 5-HT$_{1P}$ receptor and emphasize the need to establish a rigorous basis for its positive identification [16].

Many serotonin-receptor subtypes do not appear to undergo compensatory regulatory changes

Classically, a decrease in exposure of a tissue to its endogenous transmitter leads to a supersensitive, or exaggerated, response to exogenous agonist, which may be accounted for by an increase in the density or upregulation of postsynaptic receptors for the transmitter. Conversely, increased exposure of a tissue to agonists overtime will result in a decreased responsiveness, or desensitization, to the agonist, which may be due, at least in part, to a decrease, or downregulation, in receptor density. Central β_1-noradrenergic and D2-dopaminergic receptors undergo such regulatory processes.

Chronic or repeated administration of antidepressant drugs, such as MAO inhibitors or inhibitors of serotonin uptake, or 5-HT$_{1A}$ receptor agonists to laboratory rats results in a desensitization of behavioral and electrophysiological responses believed to be mediated by 5-HT$_{1A}$ receptors. Lesioning serotonergic neurons results in increased behavioral and electrophysiological responses. However, these treatments do not result in changes in 5-HT$_{1A}$ receptors as measured with binding assays. Some investigators have reported diminished 5-HT$_{1A}$ receptor-mediated inhibition of adenylyl cylcase following repeated administration of some antidepressant drugs to rats. However, desensitization of second-messenger function has not been observed consistently after chronic antidepressant or agonist treatments.

Lesions of serotonergic neurons do not cause detectable changes in 5-HT$_{1B}$ receptors in forebrain areas and have been reported to cause upregulation, downregulation or not to effect the density of 5-HT$_{1B}$ receptors in substantia nigra. Interpretation of these reports may be complicated by the fact that the 5-HT$_{1B}$ receptor is located both pre- and postsynaptically. Cells maintained in culture represent an alternative to *in vivo* systems. The 5-HT$_{1B}$ receptor is found on an epithelial cell line from opossum kidney (OK cells). Exposure of OK cells to 5-HT results in a time- and dose-dependent decrease in the density of 5-HT$_{1B}$ receptors and a desensitization of the 5-HT$_{1B}$ receptor-mediated inhibition of forskolin-stimulated cAMP accumulation [25]. It seems, then, that the 5-HT$_{1B}$ receptor can downregulate in response to prolonged exposure to an agonist.

5-HT$_{2A}$ receptors do not respond to changes in agonist exposure in the classic manner. Specifically, no change in $5\text{-}HT_{2A}$ receptor density is observed after lesioning serotonergic neurons or after depletion of serotonin stores. $5\text{-}HT_{2A}$ receptor-mediated phosphoinositide hydrolysis is also unchanged after such treatments, suggesting that denervation supersensitivity does not occur. Thus, it appears that neither the $5\text{-}HT_{2A}$ receptor nor its second-messenger pathway is regulated by a decrease in neurotransmitter exposure. After administration of hallucinogenic $5\text{-}HT_2$ receptor agonists or chronic administration of selective inhibitors of serotonin uptake, $5\text{-}HT_{2A}$ receptor-mediated inositol lipid hydrolysis becomes desensitized and $5\text{-}HT_{2A}$ receptors downregulate. Surprisingly, $5\text{-}HT_{2A}$ receptor desensitization and downregulation also occur following administration of drugs that are antagonists at $5\text{-}HT_{2A}$ receptors, such as ketanserin, the atypical antidepressant mianserin and atypical antipsychotic drugs. Given that agonist exposure causes desensitization of $5\text{-}HT_2$ receptors, it has been proposed that the absence of supersensitivity after denervation may reflect low tonic activity at synapses innervating $5\text{-}HT_2$ receptors [26].

Following the lesioning of serotonergic neurons with neurotoxin, $5\text{-}HT_{2C}$ receptor-mediated phosphoinositide hydrolysis in choroid plexus is increased, indicating that these receptors undergo denervation supersensitivity. However, radioligand-binding studies fail to show an increase in $5\text{-}HT_{2C}$ receptor number or in receptor upregulation. Paradoxically, chronic administration of the $5\text{-}HT_2$ receptor antagonist mianserin to rats results in downregulation of the $5\text{-}HT_{2C}$ receptor. In a fibroblast cell line transfected with $5\text{-}HT_{2C}$ receptor cDNA, phosphorylation is increased by agonist treatment and accompanies agonist-mediated desensitization [27].

$5\text{-}HT_3$ receptors, located on neurons in the periphery and in the CNS, mediate fast, excitatory responses, that is, membrane depolarization to serotonin. Like many other receptors that are ligand-gated ion channels, the $5\text{-}HT_3$ receptor exhibits rapid desensitization after sustained agonist exposure. In addition to preparations of peripheral neurons, cultured hippocampal cells and neuroblastoma cells have been used to study this phenomenon.

Studies of $5\text{-}HT_7$ receptor regulation have been performed on rat frontal cortical astrocytes in primary culture. In these cells, $5\text{-}HT_7$ receptors are coupled to the stimulation of adenylyl cyclase. Exposure of astrocytes in culture to the atypical antidepressant mianserin or to the tricyclic antidepressant amitriptyline for 3 days increased the stimulation of cAMP accumulation in response to $5\text{-}HT$ [28]. Whether such effects are relevant for the therapeutic effects of these drugs is a topic for future research.

SEROTONIN INVOLVEMENT IN PHYSIOLOGICAL FUNCTION AND BEHAVIOR

Serotonin may set the tone of brain activity in relationship to the state of behavioral arousal/activity

Serotonin has been implicated in practically every type of behavior, such as appetitive, emotional, motor, cognitive and autonomic. However, from a physiological perspective, it is not clear whether $5\text{-}HT$ affects such behaviors specifically or more generally by coordinating the activity of the nervous system, particularly to set the tone of activity in conjunction with the amount of arousal.

The primary body of data that has contributed to the view that $5\text{-}HT$ has a general effect on behavior by modulating the tone of nervous system activity comes from studies of the firing rate of serotonergic soma in raphe nuclei [29]. Under quiet waking conditions, serotonergic neurons display a slow, clock-like activity of about 1 to 5 spikes/sec, which shows a gradual decline as the animal becomes drowsy and enters slow-wave sleep. A decrease in the regularity of firing accompanies this overall slowing of neuronal activity. During rapid eye movement (REM) sleep, the activity of these neurons becomes silent. In response to certain types of arousing stimuli, the firing rate of these serotonergic neurons increases. Not surprisingly, such data led to the idea that the activity of serotonergic neurons is related to the level of behavioral arousal/activity. Such data also have contributed to the idea that the activity of serotonergic neurons is associated with motor output since atonia of the major skeletal muscle groups occurs during REM sleep. Also oral–buccal motor activity, such as chewing, biting, licking or grooming, causes a marked increase in the firing rate of a subgroup of serotonergic soma that are also activated by somatosensory stimuli applied to the head, neck and face. However, exposing a cat to environmental stressors, such as a loud noise or seeing a dog, although producing strong sympathetic activation and typical behavioral responses, does not alter the firing rate of serotonergic neurons. Thus, the type of motor activity that activates serotonergic soma seems to be repetitive, like that mediated by central pattern generators. Furthermore, activation of serotonergic transmission inhibits information processing in afferent systems. From all such data, it has been suggested that the serotonergic neuronal system functions at the organismic level to integrate functions needed for behavioral output, that is, facilitation of motor output with suppression of activity in sensory systems irrelevant to the ongoing behavior.

Serotonin appears to be involved in a wide variety of physiological functions and behaviors, such as eating, sleep, circadian rhythmicity and neuroendocrine function

Perturbation of the 5-HT system by different types of drugs can elicit alterations in behaviors. Drugs affecting serotonergic neurons and their receptors are used to treat diseases such as depression, anxiety disorders and schizophrenia. In part because of this, 5-HT also has been speculated to be involved specifically in the regulation of all types of behaviors and physiological processes. The possible involvement of 5-HT in three areas, neuroendocrine function, circadian rhythms and feeding behavior, will be highlighted for illustrative purposes.

The hypothalamus secretes several releasing factors and release-inhibiting factors to control the secretion of hormones from the anterior pituitary gland. Serotonin is among the many neurotransmitters that participate in the hypothalamic control of pituitary secretion, particularly in the regulation of adrenocorticotropin (ACTH), prolactin and growth hormone secretion. A direct synaptic connection between serotonergic terminals and corticotropin-releasing hormone (CRH)-containing neurons in the paraventricular nucleus of the hypothalamus has been described. Precursors of 5-HT or drugs that enhance the effect of 5-HT increase CRH in portal blood and ACTH in plasma. In addition to effects at the hypothalamus, 5-HT may have direct effects on the anterior pituitary to stimulate the release of ACTH and at the level of the adrenal cortex to regulate release of corticosterone or cortisol. Actions of serotonin on 5-HT_{1A}, 5-HT_2, 5-HT_3 and 5-HT_4 receptors seem to be involved in these effects on the hypothalamic–pituitary–adrenal axis [30]. However, what role, if any, is played by serotonin in regulating stress-induced elevations of CRH or the circadian periodicity of the hypothalamic–pituitary–adrenal axis is unclear.

Measurement of these endocrine responses after administration of drugs that increase brain serotonin function provides one of the few methods currently available for assessing such function in humans. Precursors of 5-HT, releasing agents, reuptake inhibitors and receptor agonists and antagonists have been used to probe serotonergic function. For example, intravenous administration of the serotonin precursor L-tryptophan consistently increases plasma concentrations of prolactin and growth hormone but not of ACTH or cortisol. Fenfluramine causes a dose-dependent increase in plasma prolactin. When administered to humans, serotonin agonists that stimulate 5-HT_{1A} and 5-HT_2 receptors also increase plasma concentrations of ACTH, cortisol, prolactin and perhaps growth hormone. The neuroendocrine response in humans to such agents has been used clinically to assess the functioning of the central serotonergic system in patients with psychiatric disorders.

Serotonin also appears to be involved in the regulation of circadian rhythms. The suprachiasmatic nuclei (SCN) of the hypothalamus generate electrophysiological and metabolic cycles which repeat approximately every 24 hr. When isolated *in vitro*, the SCN continue to produce 24-hr rhythms in metabolism, vasopressin secretion and spontaneous electrical activity, indicating that circadian time-keeping functions or pacemaker activity are endogenous characteristics of the SCN. Ordinarily, this rhythm is synchronized or entrained to the environmental photoperiod, also about 24 hr. A serotonergic contribution to circadian rhythm regulation has been postulated because the SCN receive very dense serotonergic innervation from the midbrain raphe nuclei. In addition, there is a serotonergic innervation to the intergeniculate leaflet (IGL), an area of brain through which photic information indirectly accesses the SCN.

Serotonin appears to function as an inhibitory transmitter that modulates the effects of light on circadian rhythmicity. Direct application of 5-HT or receptor agonists to the SCN blocks light-induced phase shifts during the subjective night but causes phase advances during the subjective day. Such agents inhibit the excitatory effect of light, measured electrophysiologically, in either the SCN or the lateral geniculate complex. The nonselective 5-HT agonist quipazine resets or shifts the rhythm of spontaneous electrical activity of single cells recorded extracellularly in SCN isolated in brain slices.

Lesions of serotonergic neurons in laboratory animals have been reported by some investigators to disrupt locomotor rhythms or result in loss of the daily rhythm of corticosterone. In the hamster, the median raphe nucleus projects to the SCN, whereas the dorsal raphe nucleus innervates the IGL; furthermore, serotonergic innervation to the SCN, and not the IGL, is necessary for the photic entrainment of locomotor activity [31]. It appears, then, that the SCN circadian pacemaker, or clock, is modulated by stimulation of serotonergic receptors in the SCN and that serotonergic projections to the SCN may modulate the phase of the SCN in intact animals.

The possible involvement of 5-HT in feeding behavior has been an active area of research for many years. Pharmacological studies have contributed primarily to the idea that 5-HT has an inhibitory effect on feeding behavior. Drugs that either directly or indirectly activate postsynaptic 5-HT receptors decrease food consumption, whereas agents that inhibit serotonergic transmission increase food intake. Precisely how this occurs is controversial, with claims that 5-HT governs the selection of macronutrients in the diet, influences responses to the taste qualities of food or modulates gastric activity to reduce feeding. Perhaps the most comprehensive

and enduring view is that enhanced serotonergic activity enhances satiety, particularly by increasing the rate of satiation and prolonging the state of satiety [32].

Fenfluramine, originally the racemate and more recently the *d*-isomer, has been the prototypical drug for studying serotonergic mechanisms in feeding behavior. As mentioned previously, fenfluramine elicits the release of 5-HT and inhibits its reuptake (Fig. 13-7). *d*-Fenfluramine has an active de-ethylated metabolite, *d*-norfenfluramine, that contributes to the appetite-suppressant effects of the parent compound. Fenfluramine decreases meal size, rate of eating and eating between meals. This probably is related to its ability in humans to decrease the sensation of hunger and to increase the feeling of "fullness." Serotonin-reuptake inhibitors, such as fluoxetine and serotonin precursors, mimic these effects. The effects of fenfluramine on feeding behavior are blocked by the nonselective serotonin receptor antagonist metergoline.

Multiple mechanisms in brain appear to be responsible for the effects of serotonergic drugs on satiety; for example, postsynaptic 5-HT_{1B} receptors are involved in regulating the size of meals eaten, but 5-HT_{2C} receptors influence the rate of eating. The sites in brain where these drugs, and presumably 5-HT, cause such effects remain to be identified. The paraventricular nucleus (PVN) of the hypothalamus may be an important site, although there are data indicating that actions on the PVN may be sufficient, but not necessary, to reduce caloric intake. In addition to brain mechanisms, 5-HT may act through peripheral mechanisms to produce satiety.

The pharmacological effects produced by drugs such as fenfluramine on feeding behavior in animals have led to its use in the treatment of obesity in humans. In many double-blind, placebo-controlled trials, chronic administration of fenfluramine causes greater weight loss than placebo. Although not as extensively studied clinically, fluoxetine produces similar effects. Weight gain occurs when fenfluramine is stopped, which indicates that the weight loss was related to its administration [33]. Given all of the medical problems associated with obesity, anorectic agents are valuable tools to be used in association with other modalities, such as diet and exercise, in the treatment of the truly obese individual.

5-Hydroxytryptamine not only has important physiological effects of its own but also is the precursor of the hormone melatonin

The human pineal gland weighs about 150 mg and occupies the depression between the superior colliculi at the posterior border of the corpus callosum. Although there are physical connections between the pineal gland and brain, the pineal gland lies "outside" the blood–brain barrier (see Chap. 32) and is innervated primarily by sympathetic nerves arising from the superior cervical ganglia.

Extracts of the pineal gland were reported as early as 1917 to lighten frog skin *in vitro;* in the late 1950s, the pineal hormone, melatonin, which produces this effect was isolated and its chemical structure, 5-methoxy-*N*-acetyltryptamine, described (Fig. 13-5). Melatonin is synthesized from serotonin, and the pineal gland contains all of the enzymes necessary to synthesize serotonin from tryptophan as well as two additional enzymes required to convert serotonin to melatonin (Fig. 13-5). The rate-limiting enzyme, serotonin *N*-acetyltransferase (EC 2.31.87), or arylalkylamine *N*-acetyltransferase (AANAT), converts serotonin to *N*-acetylserotonin; this product is converted to melatonin by the enzyme 5-hydroxyindole-*O*-methyltransferase (HIOMT), which uses *S*-adenosylmethionine as the methyl donor. The human AANAT gene has been cloned and has considerable sequence identity to the sheep and rat genes. The human gene is localized on chromosome 17. The gene product is a 23.2-kDa protein that contains putative phosphorylation sites. Such sites are likely to be involved in the cAMP-dependent regulation of enzyme activity.

A unique feature of pineal gland physiology is that the synthesis and secretion of melatonin is influenced markedly by the light–dark cycle, acting through a multisynaptic pathway that relays in the superior cervical ganglia of the sympathetic nervous system. During daylight, the synthesis and secretion of melatonin are reduced, as is impulse flow along the sympathetic nerves innervating the pineal gland. At the onset of darkness, there is activation of these nerves, and the increased release of NE from them activates β adrenoceptors on the pineal gland to increase the formation of cAMP, with activation of α_1 adrenoceptors further amplifying the response. This second messenger causes activation of AANAT so as to increase the synthesis of melatonin. The extent of the nighttime increase in AANAT activity is very species-dependent, being, for example, as much as 150-fold in rats but only 1.5-fold in sheep. What type of rhythm is exhibited by humans is not yet known, although mRNA for AANAT is abundant in the pineal gland of humans during the day, as it is in sheep, whereas the transcript is nearly undetectable during the day in the rat pineal gland.

Thus, the pineal gland functions as a neuroendocrine transducer. In mammals, photosensory information impinging on the retina influences the activity of its neuronal projections, which ultimately inhibits or stimulates the secretion of melatonin. A circadian rhythm of melatonin secretion persists in animals housed in continuous darkness. Thus, melatonin synthesis is turned on by an endogenous "clock," probably located within the SCN of the hypothalamus, with the daily rhythm normally being entrained to the day–night, light–dark cycle [34].

The exact physiological and behavioral effects of melatonin in humans are unclear. Such effects primarily result from the actions of melatonin on the SCN to influence the timing of circadian rhythms. The effects of melatonin are mediated by its activation of specific receptors. Two mammalian receptors for melatonin have been cloned [35], both of which belong to the G protein-coupled receptor family. A third subtype has been cloned from chickens but not yet in mammals. The melatonin$_{1A}$ receptor is expressed in the hypophyseal pars tuberalis (PT) and the SCN, presumed sites of the reproductive and circadian effects of melatonin. The human melatonin$_{1B}$ receptor is 60% identical to, and exhibits similarity in, its pharmacological profile and second-messenger coupling to the melatonin$_{1A}$ receptor. It is found most abundantly in retina and to a lesser extent in brain. It has not been detected in the PT or the SCN. It seems likely that the ability of melatonin to act in the retina to affect some light-dependent functions, such as photopigment disc shedding and phagocytosis, may be due to its activation of the melatonin$_{1B}$ receptor.

Perhaps the strongest case can be made for melatonin playing a role in reproduction, particularly in seasonally breeding mammals such as hamsters or sheep, which time their reproductive cycles via changes in the photoperiod. Information on day length may be relayed to the hypothalamic–pituitary–gonadal axis by the pattern of melatonin production. Although the effects of melatonin on reproduction were believed to be solely antigonadotropic, melatonin has been shown to be capable of causing progonadotropic effects. The type of effect caused by melatonin is dependent on the time point in the photoperiod when it is administered, the length of the photoperiod, the species and the dose administered. In general, the effects of melatonin are most robust when given around the time of the light-to-dark transition.

Melatonin has potent sedative and hypnotic activity. This has been demonstrated in double-blind, placebo-controlled studies. The hypnotic effect of melatonin seems to be separable from its effects on circadian rhythms. Although far from being fully understood, the entraining effect of melatonin on biological rhythms has led to its being used by humans for disorders that may be related to disturbances of circadian rhythms. For example, it is used to alleviate symptoms of jet lag as well as alertness-related problems in shift workers. Much more research will be needed to establish its efficacy in such conditions. Unfortunately, claims of its usefulness for these types of problems far exceed any controlled clinical data demonstrating such effects. At a different level, but one receiving comparable attention in the popular press as those mentioned above, is the purported antiaging properties of melatonin due to its antioxidant properties. Based on its demonstrated antioxidant properties, seen both *in vitro* and *in vivo,* melatonin has been speculated to be part of the natural defense system of the body against the toxic effects caused by free radicals.

SEROTONIN NEURONS AND RECEPTORS AS DRUG TARGETS

Serotonin neurons and receptors are targets for a wide variety of therapeutic drugs. The most widely used class of antidepressant drugs is commonly referred to as the tricyclic antidepressants. It has been known for about 25 years that many of these drugs, such as imipramine and amitriptyline, are potent inhibitors of the uptake of both NE and 5-HT. Some tricyclic antidepressants, such as desipramine and protriptyline, inhibit the uptake of NE much more potently than the uptake of 5-HT. Thus, it was unclear whether the inhibition of serotonin uptake played any role in the antidepressant action of those tricyclic drugs that possessed this pharmacological property. However, effective antidepressants, such as fluoxetine, paroxetine and sertraline, have been marketed; these drugs, referred to as selective serotonin reuptake inhibitors (SSRIs), are much more potent inhibitors of the uptake of 5-HT than of NE [36] (Fig. 13-8). Thus, selective inhibition of the uptake of either NE or 5-HT can result in an antidepressant effect.

Another class of antidepressant drug is the MAO inhibitors (MAOIs), including phenelzine and tranylcypromine. These drugs irreversibly inhibit the activity of MAO (Fig. 13-8). Because MAO catabolizes biogenic amines, such as 5-HT, DA and NE, these neurotransmitters have been implicated in the mechanism of action of these drugs. Interestingly, studies have been carried out from which it was inferred that serotonin is needed for SSRIs or MAOIs to produce a beneficial clinical response in depressed patients. Such data are consistent with the idea that drug-induced enhancement of serotonergic transmission can produce amelioration of depressive symptomatology.

Inhibition of serotonin uptake not only can cause an antidepressant effect but also may reduce the symptoms of obsessive-compulsive disorder (OCD) (see Chap. 52). This clinical effect also is produced by SSRIs but is not found with drugs that inhibit the uptake of NE, such as desipramine. A tricyclic antidepressant, clomipramine, which is somewhat selective *in vivo* as an inhibitor of 5-HT uptake, does produce clinically significant amelioration of the symptoms associated with OCD.

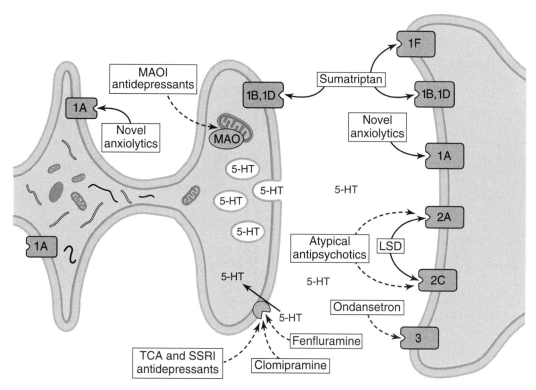

FIGURE 13-8. Effects of psychoactive drugs on serotonergic neurotransmission. Drugs that act as agonists are indicated by *solid-line arrows,* whereas antagonists or inhibitors are shown with *broken-line arrows.* The 5-hydroxy-tryptamine *(5-HT)*$_{1A}$ receptor acts as both the somatodendritic autoreceptor and a postsynaptic receptor. Anxiolytic drugs, such as buspirone, are agonists at this receptor. In terminal fields, the autoreceptor is either the 5-HT$_{1B}$ or 5-HT$_{1D}$ subtype; these receptors also function as postsynaptic receptors. The antimigraine drug sumatriptan is an agonist at these receptors as well as at the 5-HT$_{1F}$ receptor. Hallucinogenic drugs, such as LSD, are agonists at 5-HT$_{2A}$ and 5-HT$_{2C}$ receptors, whereas atypical antipsychotic drugs, such as clozapine and olanzapine, are antagonists. The 5-HT$_3$ receptor, a ligand-gated ion channel, is blocked by drugs effective in the treatment of chemotherapy-induced nausea and emesis, such as ondansetron. Another important target for psychotherapeutic drugs is the serotonin transporter, which is blocked by drugs effective in the treatment of depression or obsessive-compulsive disorder, such as clomipramine. The enzyme responsible for the catabolism of serotonin, monoamine oxidase *(MAO),* is inhibited by another class of antidepressants. *MAOI,* monoamine oxidase inhibitor; *TCA,* tricyclic antidepressant; *SSRI,* selective serotonin reuptake inhibitor.

The drugs most widely used for the treatment of generalized anxiety disorder are the benzodiazepines, such as diazepam and lorazepam. These drugs act by enhancing the activity of the inhibitory amino acid transmitter GABA. Novel anxiolytics that seem to act initially through serotonergic mechanisms have become available. These drugs include substituted azapirones, such as buspirone and gepirone, and are agonists at the 5-HT$_{1A}$ receptor. As mentioned previously, this receptor functions both as the somatodendritic autoreceptor and the postsynaptic receptor, and research is currently

under way to determine which anatomical locus is primarily involved in the anxiolytic activity of these drugs (Fig. 13-8).

Antipsychotic drugs effective in the treatment of schizophrenia are believed to act primarily by inhibiting central dopaminergic transmission by virtue of their being DA receptor antagonists. Atypical antipsychotic drugs, such as clozapine and olanzapine, share this property but are more potent antagonists at 5-HT$_{2A}$ receptors than classic or typical antipsychotic drugs, such as chlorpromazine and haloperidol. Some, but not all, atypical antipsychotic drugs also exhibit high affinity for the structurally similar 5-HT_{2C} receptor. The balance between the effects of antipsychotic drugs on dopaminergic and serotonergic function has been hypothesized to be important in their clinical effects. The relatively greater potency of atypical antipsychotic drugs on 5-HT_{2A}/5-HT_{2C} receptors may play some role in the ability of the atypical drugs to produce fewer extrapyramidal side effects than the more typical compounds or to be more effective for some symptoms of schizophrenia, such as loss of energy or the inability to experience pleasure. The hallucinogenic activity of drugs such as LSD appears to be related to agonist activity at 5-HT_{2A} and/or 5-HT_{2C} receptors [37] (Fig. 13-8).

Drugs acting at other 5-HT receptors also have important therapeutic properties. Serotonin appears to play a role in the pathogenesis of migraine, either directly or indirectly. In particular, neurogenic inflammation of the dura is thought to be an important component of migraine pain, and a reduction in serotonergic tone may contribute to this. The drug sumatriptan is effective in the acute treatment of migraine headaches. Whether the beneficial clinical effect of sumatriptan is related to its ability to cause cerebral vasoconstriction or to block neurogenic extravasation from blood vessels within dura mater or to some other mechanism remains to be determined. This drug originally was thought to cause its beneficial effect by being an agonist at 5-HT_{1D} receptors. Its agonism at the 5-HT_{1F} receptor also may be important for its efficacy [38] (Fig. 13-8).

Finally, antagonists at 5-HT_3 receptors, such as ondansetron and granisetron (Fig. 13-8), are an important class of drugs for the treatment of nausea and vomiting in cancer patients receiving chemotherapy [39]. By an unknown mechanism, chemotherapeutic drugs, such as cisplatin and dacarbazine, induce the release of 5-HT from enterochromaffin cells of the gastrointestinal tract. Large amounts of 5-HT are found in the enterochromaffin cells, and the enteric nerves innervating the smooth muscle of the gastrointestinal tract contain 5-HT_3 receptors. The released 5-HT activates 5-HT_3 receptors, causing depolarization of visceral afferent nerves and increasing

their rate of firing. The enhanced afferent input leads to stimulation of the chemoreceptor trigger zone, which produces nausea and vomiting. Antagonism of 5-HT_3 receptors would prevent or reduce this chain of events. The site of action of these drugs appears to be the 5-HT_3 receptors in the gastrointestinal tract, even though the central area regulating emesis, the chemoreceptor trigger zone, possesses a high density of 5-HT_3 receptors. Unfortunately, there is a more prolonged and often milder form of emesis caused by chemotherapeutic drugs, which is not dependent on the release of 5-HT and is resistant to improvement with 5-HT_3 receptor antagonists.

REFERENCES

1. Rapport, M. M., Green, A. A., and Page, I. H. Serum vasoconstrictor (serotonin). IV. Isolation and characterization. *J. Biol. Chem.* 176:1243–1251, 1948.
2. Molliver, M. E. Serotonergic neuronal systems: What their anatomic organization tells us about function. *J. Clin. Psychopharmacol.* 7 (6 Suppl.): 3s–23s, 1987.
3. Tork, I. Anatomy of the serotonergic system. *Ann. N. Y. Acad. Sci.* 600:9–34, 1990.
4. Jacobs, B. L., and Azmitia, E. C. Structure and function of the brain serotonin system. *Physiol. Rev.* 72:165–229, 1992.
5. Heninger, G. R., Delgado, P. L., and Charney, D. S. The revised monoamine theory of depression: A modulatory role for monoamines, based on new findings from monoamine depletion experiments in humans. *Pharmacopsychiatry* 29:2–11, 1996.
6. Eaton, M. J., Gudehithlu, K. P., Quach, T., Silvia, C. P., Hadjiconstantinou, M., and Neff, N. H. Distribution of aromatic L-amino acid decarboxylase mRNA in mouse brain by *in situ* hybridization histology. *J. Comp. Neurol.* 337:640–654, 1993.
7. Cortes, R., Mengod, G., Celada, P., and Artigas, F. *p*-Chlorophenylalanine increases tryptophan-5-hydroxylase mRNA levels in the rat dorsal raphe: A time course study using *in situ* hybridization. *J. Neurochem.* 60:761–764, 1993.
8. Boadle-Biber, M. C. Regulation of serotonin synthesis. *Prog. Biophys. Mol. Biol.* 60:1–15, 1993.

9. Schuldiner, S. A molecular glimpse of vesicular monamine transporters. *J. Neurochem.* 62:2067–2078, 1994.

10. Tamir, H., Liu, K., Hsiung, S., Adlersberg, M., and Gershon, M. D. Serotonin binding protein: Synthesis, secretion, and recycling. *J. Neurochem.* 63:97–107, 1994.

11. Blakely, R. D., DeFelice, L. J., and Hartzell, H. C. Molecular physiology of norepinephrine and serotonin transporters. *J. Exp. Biol.* 196:263–281, 1994.

12. Borowsky, B., and Hoffman, B. J. Neurotransmitter transporters: Molecular biology, function, and regulation. *Int. Rev. Neurobiol.* 38:139–199, 1995.

13. Shih, J. C. Molecular basis of human MAO A and B. *Neuropsychopharmacology* 4:1–3, 1991.

14. Cases, O., Seif, I., Grimsby, J., et al. Aggressive behavior and altered amounts of brain serotonin and norepinephrine in mice lacking MAO A. *Science* 268:1763–1766, 1995.

15. Bradley, P. B., Engel, G., Feniuk, W., et al. Proposals for the classification and nomenclature of functional receptors for 5-hydroxytryptamine. *Neuropharmacology* 25:563–576, 1986.

16. Hoyer, D., Clarke, D. E., Fozard, J. R., et al. International union of pharmacology classification of receptors for 5-hydroxytryptamine (serotonin). *Pharmacol. Rev.* 46:157–203, 1994.

17. Lucas, J. J., and Hen, R. New players in the 5-HT receptor field: Genes and knockouts. *Trends Pharmacol. Sci.* 16:246, 1995.

18. Wainscott, D. B., Krushinski, J. H., Schaus, J. M., et al. [^{3}H]LY334370, a selective radioligand for labeling the serotonin$_{1F}$ (5-HT$_{1F}$) receptor. *Soc. Neurosci. Abstr.* 22:1331, 1996.

19. Cox, D. A., and Cohen, M. L. 5-HT$_{2B}$ receptor signaling in the rat stomach fundus: Dependence on calcium influx, calcium release and protein kinase C. *Behav. Brain Res.* 73:289–292, 1996.

20. Parker, R. M. C., Bentley, K. R., and Barnes, N. M. Allosteric modulation of 5-HT$_3$ receptors: Focus on alcohols and anaesthetic agents. *Trends Pharmacol. Sci.* 17:95–99, 1996.

21. Gerald, C., Adham, N., Kao, H.-T., et al. The 5-HT$_4$ receptor: Molecular cloning and pharmacological characterization of two splice variants. *EMBO J.* 14:2806, 1995.

22. Carson, M. J., Thomas, E. A., Danielson, P. E., and Sutcliffe, J. G. The 5-HT$_{5A}$ serotonin receptor is expressed predominantly by astrocytes in which it inhibits cAMP accumulation: A mechanism for neuronal suppression of reactive astrocytes. *Glia* 17:317–326, 1996.

23. Inoue, A., Hashimoto, T., Hide, I., Nishio, H., and Nakata, Y. 5-Hydroxytryptamine-facilitated release of substance P from rat spinal cord slices is mediated by nitric oxide and cyclic GMP. *J. Neurochem.* 68:128–133, 1997.

24. Gustafson, E. L., Durkin, M. M., Bard, J. A., Zgombick, J., and Branchek, T. A. A receptor autoradiographic and *in situ* hybridization analysis of the distribution of the 5-HT$_7$ receptor in rat brain. *Br. J. Pharmacol.* 117:657–666, 1996.

25. Unsworth, C. D., and Molinoff, P. B. Regulation of the 5-hydroxytryptamine 1B receptor in opossum kidney cells after exposure to agonists. *Mol. Pharmacol.* 42:464–470, 1992.

26. Sanders-Bush, E. Adaptive regulation of central serotonin receptors linked to phosphoinositide hydrolysis. *Neuropsychopharmacology* 3:411–416, 1990.

27. Westphal, R. S., Backstrom, J. R., and Sanders-Bush, E. Increased basal phosphorylation of the constitutively active serotonin 2C receptor accompanies agonist-mediated desensitization. *Mol. Pharmacol.* 48:200–205, 1995.

28. Shimizu, M., Nishida, A., Zensho, H., and Yamawaki, S. Chronic antidepressant exposure enhances 5-hydroxytryptamine 7 receptor-mediated cyclic adenosine monophosphate accumulation in rat frontocortical astrocytes. *J. Pharmacol. Exp. Ther.* 279:1551–1558, 1996.

29. Jacobs, B. L., and Fornal, C. A. 5-HT and motor control: A hypothesis. *Trends Neurosci.* 16:346–352, 1993.

30. Dinan, T. G. Serotonin and the regulation of hypothalamic-pituitary-adrenal axis function. *Life Sci.* 58:1683–1694, 1996.

31. Meyer-Bernstein, E. L., and Morin, L. P. Differential serotonergic innervation of the suprachiasmatic nucleus and the intergeniculate leaflet and its role in circadian rhythm modulation. *J. Neurosci.* 16:2097–2111, 1996.

32. Simansky, K. J. Serotonergic control of the organization of feeding and satiety. *Behav. Brain Res.* 73:37–42, 1996.

33. Bray, G. A. Use and abuse of appetite-suppressant drugs in the treatment of obesity. *Ann. Intern. Med.* 119:707–713, 1993.

34. Reiter, R. J. Melatonin: The chemical expression of darkness. *Mol. Cell. Endocrinol.* 79:C153–C158, 1991.

35. Reppert, S. M., Weaver, D. R., and Godson, C. Melatonin receptors step into the light: Cloning and classification of subtypes. *Trends Pharmacol. Sci.* 17:100–102, 1996.

36. Frazer, A. Pharmacology of antidepressants. *J. Clin. Psychopharmacol.* 17(Suppl. 1):2S–18S, 1997.

37. Glennon, R. A., and Dukat, M. Serotonin receptor subtypes. In F. E. Bloom and D. J. Kupper (eds.), *Psychopharmacology: The Fourth Generation of Progress.* New York: Raven Press, 1995, pp. 415–429.

38. Johnson, K. W., Schaus, J. M., Cohen, M. L., et al. Inhibition of neurogenic protein extravasation in the dura via 5-HT$_{IF}$ receptor activation—implications to migraine therapy. *Soc. Neurosci. Abstr.* 22:1330, 1996.

39. Cubeddu, L. X. Serotoin mechanisms in chemotherapy-induced emesis in cancer patients. *Oncology* 53:18–25, 1996.

40. Consolazione, A., and Cuello, A. C. CNS serotonin pathways. In *The Biology of Serotonergic Transmission.* New York: John Wiley & Sons, Ltd., 1982, pp. 29–61.

14

Histamine

Lindsay B. Hough

Basic Neurochemistry: Molecular, Cellular and Medical Aspects, 6th Ed., edited by G. J. Siegel et al. Published by Lippincott–Raven Publishers, Philadelphia, 1999. Correspondence to Lindsay B. Hough, Department of Pharmacology and Neuroscience, Albany Medical College, A-136, Albany, New York 12208.

HISTAMINE: A MESSENGER MOLECULE WITHIN AND OUTSIDE OF THE NERVOUS SYSTEM

Although the existence of histamine in the brain was known over 50 years ago, a neuromodulatory role for this substance was not widely appreciated until relatively recently. Paradoxically, the existence of well-established roles for histamine outside of the nervous system is one factor that has hampered the acceptance of this amine as a neuronal messenger. Other limitations, mostly methodological, have been surmounted. It is now clear that histamine is formed within and released from CNS neurons and is an important regulator of several brain functions.

The chemical structure of histamine has similarities to the structure of other biogenic amines, but important differences also exist

Chemically, histamine is 2-(4-imidazolyl)ethylamine (Fig. 14-1). The ethylamine "backbone" is a common feature of many of the amine transmitters, such as dopamine, norepinephrine and serotonin. However, the imidazole nucleus, absent from other known transmitters, endows histamine with several distinct

chemical properties. Among these is prototypic tautomerism, a property which permits histamine to exist in two different chemical forms (Fig. 14-1). The tautomeric properties of histamine are thought to be critical in the ability of this molecule to activate some of its receptors (see sections below). Although histamine has more than one basic center, both tautomers exist predominantly as monocations at physiological pH. This tautomerism has also contributed to confusion in naming histamine congeners (Fig. 14-1).

Outside of the central nervous system, histamine is a mediator of several physiological and pathological processes

As a physiological mediator, histamine is best known as an endogenous stimulant of gastric secretion. Histamine is also released from mast cells and basophils by antigens, certain peptides and small basic drugs. In addition, histamine participates in inflammation and in the regulation of immune responses, but these functions are less well understood. Cardiac stores of histamine probably play no physiological role but may be of pathological significance. Endogenous peripheral histamine may also participate in the modulation of sympathetic and/or afferent nerve activity; the storage of this histamine is probably non-neuronal.

HISTAMINERGIC CELLS OF THE CENTRAL NERVOUS SYSTEM: ANATOMY AND MORPHOLOGY

The brain stores and releases histamine from more than one type of cell

Mast cells are a family of bone marrow-derived secretory cells that store and release high concentrations of histamine. They are known to be present within and surrounding the brain of many species [1,2]. In many, but not all, species they are prevalent in the thalamus and hypothalamus, as well as in the dura mater, leptomeninges and choroid plexus [1]. The quantitative contribution made to brain histamine concentrations by mast cells can be substantial in some cases, such as rat thalamus, although various approaches to this problem have not reached the same conclusion. Earlier biochemical studies suggested that histamine in brain mast cells could be distinguished from neuronal histamine by characteristics such as histamine turnover rates, subcellular fractionation and ontogenic pattern [2]. However, activated mast cells may not show a slow histamine turnover rate. Brain and dural mast cells have been characterized histologically and histochemically in detail. Characterization of neuronal histamine has been facilitated by the study of mast cell-deficient mice and rats.

The functions for brain and dural mast cells are not certain, but several hypotheses are being investigated. The close proximity of many of these cells to blood vessels, along with the potent vascular actions of their contents, has led to the suggestion that they regulate blood flow, permeability and/or immunological access to the brain. Dural mast cells are localized in close proximity to sensory nerve fibers and may modulate the release of inflammatory mediators from these cells (see also H_3 receptor section and Table 14-1). Perhaps most intriguing are recent findings showing that behavioral and hormonal alterations can induce dramatic changes in the morphology or distribution of CNS mast cells. Brain and/or dural mast cells may also participate in neurodegenerative diseases, such as multiple sclerosis, Alzheimer's disease or Wernicke's encephalopathy [3,3a]. In addition to mast cells and neurons, other brain cells, such as cerebrovascular endothelial cells [2,4], may synthesize and/or store histamine.

Histaminergic fibers originate from the tuberomammillary region of the posterior hypothalamus

The inability to visualize histaminergic neurons greatly limited the understanding and acceptance of this neuronal system. In 1984, antibodies raised against histamine [5] or its biosynthetic enzyme [6] provided the first detailed anatomical studies of these cells and their distribution. In all mammals studied, including humans, histaminergic neurons are found in the tuberomammillary nucleus of the posterior basal hypothalamus (Fig. 14-2). In the rat brain, five cell clusters have been distinguished, termed E1–E5 [7], although this subdivision does not easily apply to other species.

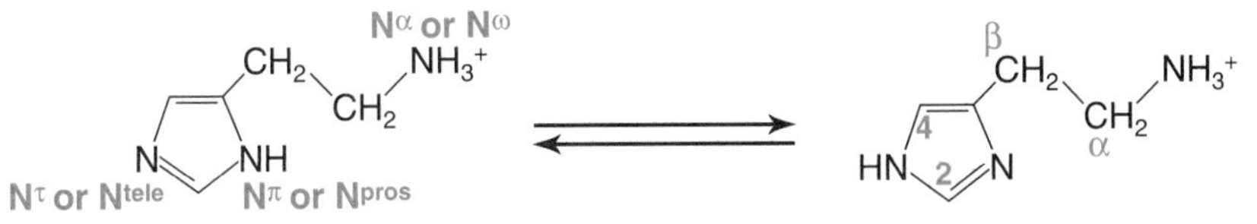

FIGURE 14-1. Chemical structure of histamine, illustrating the two tautomeric forms. The names of the nitrogen atoms are shown on the **left** tautomer, and the numbering scheme for carbon atoms is on the **right**. For example, N^τ-methyl, N^α-methyl and α-methylhistamine are distinct substances and have very different properties (see Fig. 14-3 and Table 14-2). This nomenclature system avoids references to the ring nitrogens as 1- and 3-, a designation that becomes confused by the tautomerism.

TABLE 14-1.   INTERACTIONS BETWEEN HISTAMINE AND OTHER TRANSMITTERS IN THE CNS

| Transmitter | Histaminergic modulation of transmitters | | | Transmitter modulation of histamine | | |
	Transmitter parameter	Receptor	Effect	Histamine parameter	Receptor	Effect
Acetylcholine	Release	H_3	↓[a]	Release	M_1	↓
Acetylcholine	Release[b]	H_2	↑	Release[b]	M_1	↓
Acetylcholine				Turnover	Muscarinic	↓
Acetylcholine				Turnover	Nicotinic	↓
CGRP, substance P	Release[c]	H_3	↓			
Dopamine	Release	H_3	↓	Release[b]	D2	↑
Dopamine	DOPAC levels	H_1	↑[d]	Release[b]	D3	↓
GABA				Release[b]	$GABA_{A,B}$	↓
GABA				Turnover	?	↓
Glutamate				Release[b]	NMDA	↑
Norepinephrine	Release	H_3	↓	Release	α_2	↓
Norepinephrine	Release[b]	H_1	↑			
Norepinephrine	Turnover	H_1	↑			
Opioids				Release	κ	↓
Opioids				Turnover	κ	↓
Opioids				Release[b]	μ	↑
Opioids				Turnover	μ	↑
Serotonin	Release	H_3	↓	Release[b]	$5HT_{2C/2A}$	↑
Serotonin	5-HIAA levels	H_1	↑[e]	Turnover	$5HT_{1A}$	↓

Experiments investigating the interactions between brain histamine and other transmitters are summarized. Unless otherwise specified, "release" experiments were performed *in vitro* with brain slices or synaptosomes.
[a] Inhibition by H_3 receptor may not be direct.
[b] Release measured by *in vivo* techniques.
[c] Release from isolated perfused heart.
[d] Some effects of histamine on dopaminergic parameters are found to depend on noradrenergic activity.
[e] Exogenous, but not endogenous histamine increased 5-hydroxytryptamine (5-HT) metabolite levels.
CGRP, calcitonin gene-related peptide; DOPAC, 3,4-dihydroxyphenylacetic acid; 5-HIAA, 5-hydroxyindoleacetic acid; NMDA, *N*-methyl-D-aspartate. See [37,43,44] for references.

Histaminergic neurons have morphological and membrane properties that are similar to those of neurons storing other biogenic amines

Histaminergic perikarya can be of medium size, but most are large, bipolar or multipolar cells, with diameters of up to 30 μm. Ultrastructural characteristics resemble those of noradrenergic and serotonergic cell bodies [2]. Some of the most ventrally located cells may make direct contact with CSF.

Electrophysiological properties of histaminergic neurons, which have been characterized in both hypothalamic explants and brain slices, show spontaneous activity of about 2 Hz, positive action potentials, a persistent sodium current and both inward and transient outward rectification [8]. Noradrenergic and serotonergic neurons show similar properties.

Histaminergic fibers project widely to most regions of the central nervous system

Two ascending and at least one descending efferent pathways account for the histaminergic innervation of the mammalian brain and spinal cord (Fig. 14-2B). The ascending tracts are predominantly, 70 to 80%, ipsilateral. All cell groups appear to contribute to all pathways. Although nearly all CNS areas contain some histaminergic fibers, the density of innervation is heterogeneous [9,10]. The highest densities are found in several hypothalamic nuclei, the medial septum, the nucleus of the diagonal band and the ventral tegmental area. Moderate densities are found in cerebral cortex, amygdala and basal ganglia. Most areas of the brainstem and spinal cord contain only small numbers of fibers. These densities follow closely the tissue concentrations of histamine and its biosynthetic enzyme found throughout the brain [11]. In the monkey brain, a homogeneous innervation of many areas of the visual system has also been noted. Ultrastructural studies in rat show that histaminergic varicosities form only a few synaptic contacts, implying that most neuronal histamine is released by nonsynaptic mechanisms; this seems to be the case for the other amine transmitter systems as well. However, histaminergic synapses have been characterized in some detail in rat brain, such as in the innervation of the mesencephalic trigeminal nucleus. Histaminergic varicosities also appear to make contact with glia and blood vessels [7].

A number of substances are colocalized with histamine and its biosynthetic enzyme in hypothalamic tuberomammillary neurons [12]. These include glutamate decarboxylase (GAD), GABA, GABA-transaminase (GABA-T), adenosine deaminase, monoamine oxidase-B (MAO-B) and the neuropeptide Met-Enk-Arg[6]-Phe[7]. A subset of cells in rat brain also contain galanin. Thyrotropin-releasing hormone (TRH) is present in some rat histaminergic neurons but is absent from those in mouse and guinea pig. These findings suggest that some of these peptides, as well as GABA and/or adenosine, may function as cotransmitters in this system. Galanin may be a presynaptic inhibitor of neuronal histamine release, similar to its proposed actions on cholinergic and serotonergic fibers. Endogenous GABA appears to regulate neuronal histamine release, but the cellular origin of this GABA is not known (Table 14-1).

Relatively little is known about the afferent connections to the histaminergic tuberomammillary neurons. Double-labeling experiments suggest that these cells receive innervation from the infralimbic prefrontal cortex, several areas within the septum/diagonal band complex and the medial preoptic area of the hypothalamus. These or other afferents seem to contain neuropeptide Y (NPY) or substance P. Other experiments suggest that tuberomammillary cells may also receive monoaminergic input from adrenergic (C1–C3), noradrenergic (A1–A2) and serotonergic (B5–B9) cells. Since some of these

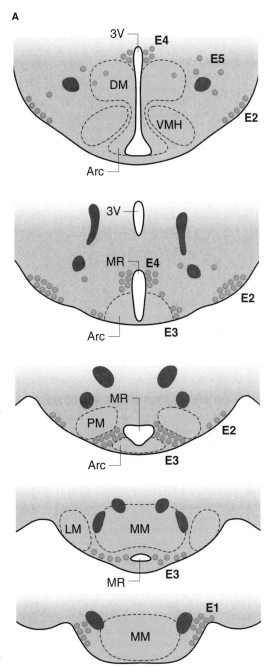

FIGURE 14-2. The histaminergic system of the rat brain. **A:** Frontal sections through the posterior hypothalamus showing the location of histaminergic neurons and the designation of the E1–E5 subgroups. *Arc,* arcuate nucleus; *DM,* dorsomedial hypothalamic nucleus; *LM,* lateral mammillary nucleus; *MM,* medial mammillary nucleus; *MR,* mammillary recess; *PM,* premammillary nucleus; *3V,* third ventricle; *VMH,* ventromedial hypothalamic nucleus. Modified from [45] with permission. *(Figure continues on next page.)*

B

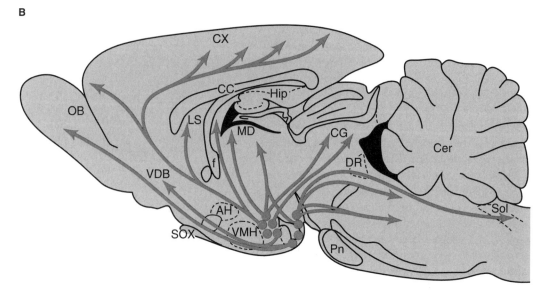

FIGURE 14-2.   *(Continued.)* **B:** A sagittal view illustrating the major ascending and descending fiber projections. *AH*, anterior hypothalamus; *CC*, corpus callosum; *Cer*, cerebellum; *CG*, central grey; *CX*, cerebral cortex; *DR*, dorsal raphe; *f*, fornix; *Hip*, hippocampus; *LS*, lateral septum; *MD*, mediodorsal thalamus; *OB*, olfactory bulb; *Pn*, pontine nuclei; *Sol*, nucleus of solitary tract; *SOX*, supraoptic decussation; *VDB*, vertical limb of the diagonal band; *VMH*, ventromedial hypothalamic nucleus. Modified from [2] with permission.

areas seem to have both input and output connections with histaminergic areas, the possibility of reciprocal control has been considered [2].

Histaminergic neurons are present in many species

Histaminergic neurons have been detected in the hypothalamus or diencephalon in a variety of vertebrate brains, including those of fish, snake, turtle and bird. In invertebrates, histamine also seems to function as a transmitter, for example, in arthropod and insect photoreceptors [13,14,14a]. It is well established that the C2 neuron of *Aplysia* uses histamine as a transmitter [15].

DYNAMICS OF HISTAMINE IN THE BRAIN

Specific enzymes control histamine synthesis and breakdown

Figure 14-3 summarizes the major mechanisms for the synthesis and metabolism of histamine. Biosynthesis is performed in one step by the en-zyme L-histidine decarboxylase (HDC, E.C. 4.1.1.22). Histamine metabolism occurs mainly by two pathways. Oxidation is carried out by diamine oxidase (DAO, E.C. 1.4.3.6), leading to imidazole acetic acid (IAA), whereas methylation is effected by histamine N-methyltransferase (HMT, E.C. 2.1.1.8), producing *tele*-methylhistamine (t-MH). IAA can exist as a riboside or ribotide conjugate. t-MH is further metabolized by MAO-B, producing *tele*-methylimidazole acetic acid (t-MIAA). Note that histamine is a substrate for DAO but not for MAO. Aldehyde intermediates, formed by the oxidation of both histamine and t-MH, are thought to be quickly oxidized to acids under normal circumstances. In the vertebrate CNS, histamine is almost exclusively methylated and only small amounts of DAO are detectable. However, IAA, a GABA agonist, has been detected and can be formed in the rat brain. Although IAA in the brain is probably normally formed by the transamination of histidine, it can also be formed by histamine oxidation under some circumstances. In some invertebrate nervous systems, such as *Aplysia*, histamine is metabolized to γ-glutamylhistamine.

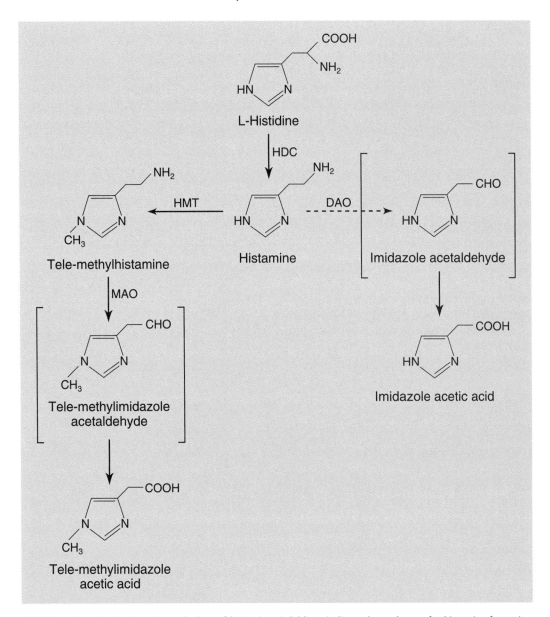

FIGURE 14-3. Synthesis and metabolism of histamine. Solid lines indicate the pathways for histamine formation and catabolism in brain. Dashed lines show additional pathways that can occur outside of the nervous system. *HDC,* histidine decarboxylase; *HMT,* histamine methyltransferase; *DAO,* diamine oxidase; *MAO,* monoamine oxidase. Aldehyde intermediates, shown in brackets, have been hypothesized but not isolated.

Several forms of histidine decarboxylase may derive from a single gene

A single cDNA, cloned from rat [16], mouse and human cells, encodes a 74-kDa protein with functional HDC activity. Two species of HDC mRNA have been found in some cells, but the larger one, which contains an additional insert sequence, does not encode a functional enzyme and is not found in brain. Consistent with the immunohistochemical studies discussed above, HDC mRNA is localized to the caudal hypothalamus in rats. The human HDC gene is large, composed of 12 exons with a size of about 2.4 kb. The enzyme, which requires pyridoxal-5′-phosphate as a coenzyme, shares some homology with DOPA decarboxylase (Chap. 12), another enzyme that requires this cofactor. Protein purification studies have shown HDC to be a dimer composed of two identical 55-kDa subunits. Post-translational modification of the enzyme occurs by an elastase-like enzyme, which converts the 74-kDa form to the smaller protein. Biochemical, biophysical and immunological studies have suggested the existence of HDC isoenzymes [2], now thought to result from either post-translational modification of the protein or, possibly, allelic variants. The rat HDC gene has two potential *N*-glycosylation sites and two recognition sequences for phosphorylation by cAMP-dependent protein kinase (PKA). These potential modulatory sites might contribute to HDC heterogeneity [16].

Histamine synthesis in the brain is controlled by the availability of L-histidine and the activity of histidine decarboxylase

Figure 14-4 depicts the dynamics of histamine in mammalian brain. Although histamine is present in plasma, it does not penetrate the blood–brain barrier. Thus, histamine concentrations in the brain must be maintained by synthesis. With a K_m value of 0.1 mM for *L*-histidine under physiological conditions, HDC is not saturated by histidine concentrations in the brain, an observation which explains the effectiveness of large systemic doses of this amino acid in raising the concentrations of histamine in the brain. The essential amino acid L-histidine is transported into the brain by a saturable, energy-dependent mechanism (see Chap. 32), but there is no evidence for specialized histidine transport into histaminergic neurons [2]. Subcellular fractionation studies show HDC to be localized in cytoplasmic fractions of isolated nerve terminals, that is, synaptosomes.

HDC activity can be regulated by both hormonal and neuronal factors, most of which are poorly understood. Phosphorylation of the enzyme by PKA may be an important regulatory mechanism. Several regulatory sites have recently been found in the promoter region of the gene. Unlike catecholamines and indoleamines, histamine itself is not a direct inhibitor of its

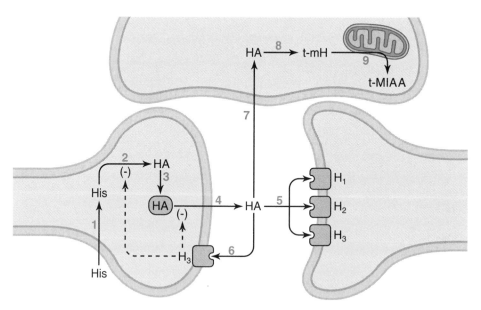

FIGURE 14-4. Dynamics of neuronal histamine. Steps in the synthesis, release and metabolism of histamine are shown: *1*, L-histidine (*His*) transport into nerve terminal; *2*, histamine (*HA*) synthesis by histidine decarboxylase; *3*, formation of histamine containing vesicles; *4*, histamine release by exocytosis; *5*, activation of post-synaptic receptors; *6*, feedback inhibition of histamine synthesis and release by H_3 autoreceptors; *7*, histamine transport by astrocytes (re-uptake by nerve terminals has not been found); *8*, metabolism by histamine-*N*-methyltransferase (*HMT*); *9*, oxidation of t-MH by monoamine oxidase-B. The cellular localization of steps 7–9 remain poorly understood. *t-MH, tele*-methylhistamine; *t-MIAA, tele*-methylimidazoleacetic acid.

biosynthetic enzyme, but it exerts feedback control through the H_3 autoreceptor (discussed below). Perhaps the most powerful tool in the study of the histamine system is S-α-fluoromethylhistidine, a highly selective and potent "suicide" inhibitor of HDC [17]. This compound has been used successfully to study many of the functions of histamine in brain.

Histamine is stored within and released from neurons, but no evidence for active neuronal re-uptake has been discovered

Newly synthesized neuronal histamine is thought to be stored within nerve terminal vesicles. Both *in vivo* and *in vitro* studies show that depolarization of nerve terminals activates the exocytotic release of histamine by a voltage- and calcium-dependent mechanism. Once released, histamine is thought to activate both postsynaptic and presynaptic receptors (discussed below). Unlike the other amine transmitters, however, histaminergic nerve terminals do not exhibit a high-affinity uptake system for histamine [2]. Most of the negative studies were performed with rat brain; studies of the brain in other mammals have shown some evidence for neuronal transport [4]. As depicted (Fig. 14-4), astrocytes may contain a histamine-transport system.

In the vertebrate brain, histamine metabolism occurs predominantly by methylation

HMT, the histamine-methylating enzyme, uses the methyl donor S-adenosyl-L-methionine. The enzyme has a K_m of about 10 μM for both histamine and the methyl cofactor. Antibodies raised against a highly purified kidney enzyme with a molecular weight of 33,000 coprecipitate the brain enzyme, showing strong similarities between the proteins. A 1.3-kb cDNA has been cloned and expressed in *Escherichia coli;* the encoded protein shows the characteristics of the natural enzyme [18]. Several earlier studies suggested that isoforms of HMT exist, but no molecular basis for these findings has yet been discovered. HMT is subject to inhibition by both

its product, t-MH, and, at higher concentrations, its substrate, histamine. Experimental inhibitors of HMT include metoprine and SKF91488. These agents have been used in metabolic studies, as well as to probe functions for CNS histamine. As expected, they increase histamine concentrations in the brain and reduce the concentrations of t-MH and t-MIAA. Many other compounds can also inhibit HMT. For example, tacrine, a cholinesterase inhibitor of possible benefit in treating Alzheimer's disease, also inhibits HMT at therapeutic doses.

Neuronal histamine is probably methylated outside of histaminergic nerve terminals

Several observations support this idea. First, in contrast to the striking regional distribution of histamine and HDC, HMT shows a more even distribution [11]. Second, lesions that destroy histaminergic fibers with large reductions in HDC concentrations have a lesser effect on brain HMT activity. Finally, glial cell lines contain HMT, a finding which also supports an extraneuronal localization for histamine metabolism [2]. Immunocytochemical methods have not yet been successfully applied to brain to confirm this. Given that HMT does not follow the characteristic regional distribution of histamine and HDC, it is surprising that in the brain concentrations of t-MH, the HMT product, show the same regional histaminergic pattern. This finding suggests that the formation of t-MH is limited by the rate of histamine release from neurons. The rate at which histamine is formed and methylated, that is, the histamine turnover rate, also follows the characteristic regional pattern and is thought to reflect the activity of histaminergic neurons. Since histamine is likely to be methylated after its neuronal release and astrocytes may contain both a histamine-transport system and HMT, the idea that histamine methylation occurs following its transport into astrocytes (Fig. 14-4) is a viable hypothesis which requires further study.

In contrast to histamine, t-MH is much less active on known histamine receptors. Thus, a role for t-MH in the brain has not been discovered, although it is active when iontophoretically applied to cerebral cortical neurons. t-MH is a substrate for MAO-B and is ultimately oxidized to t-MIAA, the end product of brain histamine metabolism. Thus, MAO inhibitors increase brain t-MH concentrations and lower t-MIAA concentrations, with little or no effect on histamine concentrations. Both t-MH and t-MIAA are detected in brain and CSF. In the brain, t-MIAA concentrations are unaffected by probenecid, an inhibitor of the brain transport of other transmitter metabolites.

The activity of histaminergic neurons is regulated by H_3 autoreceptors

The observation that histamine can inhibit its own synthesis and release from brain slices and synaptosomes suggested the existence of a histamine autoreceptor, this hypothesis was confirmed by the discovery of unique agonists and antagonists of this receptor (Table 14-2) [19,20]. The prototype H_3 antagonist thioperamide enhances the firing of histaminergic neurons and increases the release of neuronal histamine. The compound also increases the histamine turnover rate and t-MH concentrations in the brain. H_3 agonists, such as R-α-methylhistamine and immepip, produce the opposite effects. In addition to regulating histamine release, the H_3 autoreceptor appears to regulate the activity of HDC. H_3 agonists and antagonists are important tools for understanding the brain histamine system, and several new agents are currently being developed for clinical uses (see below). As discussed

TABLE 14-2. CHARACTERISTICS OF HISTAMINE RECEPTORS[a]

Characteristics	H_1	H_2	H_3
Cloned?	Yes	Yes	No
Gene localization (mouse)	Chromosome 6	Chromosome 13	Unknown
Effectors[a]	PI-PLC: $\uparrow$ IP$_3$ [$\uparrow$Ca^{2+}, $\uparrow$cGMP] PI-PLC: $\uparrow$ DAG [$\uparrow$PKC] PI-PLA$_2$: $\uparrow$ AA, $\uparrow$ TXA$_2$	$\uparrow$ cAMP $\uparrow$ PI-PLC: Ca^{2+}, IP$_3$[e] $\downarrow$ AA[e]	Unknown
Conductances	Excit: $\downarrow$ K$^+$ (mammals) $\uparrow$ Na$^+$ (invertebrates) Inhib: $\uparrow$ I$_{kCa}$2$^+$	Excit: $\downarrow$ I$_{kCa}$2$^+$ Inhib: $\downarrow$ Cl$^-$ (?)	Inhib: $\uparrow$ K$^+$ (?)
Selective agonists	2-Thiazolylethylamine, 2-phenylhistamine	Impromidine amthamine	R-α-Methylhistamine,[b] imetit, immepip[b]
Antagonists	Pyrilamine (mepyramine),[b] terfenadine	Ranitidine Zolantidine[b]	Thioperamide,[b] clobenpropit[b]
Radioligands	^{3}H-Pyrilamine, ^{125}I-Iodobolpyramine	^{125}I-Iodoaminopotentidine	^{3}H-N^α-Methylhistamine, ^{125}I-iodophenpropit, ^{125}I-iodoproxyfan
CNS distribution[d]	Cerebellum, thalamus, hippocampus	Cerebral cortex, striatum, nucleus accumbens	Striatum, nucleus accumbens, cerebral cortex, substantia nigra
Localization[c]	Neurons, astrocytes, blood vessels	Neurons, astrocytes, blood vessels	Presynaptic (auto) and postsynaptic

[a] The characteristics of the three major classes of histamine receptors are summarized. Question marks indicate suggestions from the literature that have not been confirmed. AA, arachidonic acid; TXA$_2$, thromboxane A$_2$; IP$_3$, inositol 1,4,5-trisphosphate; DAG, diacylglycerol; PKC, protein kinase C; PI-PLC, phosphoinositide-specific phospholipase C; I$_{kCa}$2$^+$, calcium-activated potassium current..

[b] Has brain-penetrating characteristics after systemic administration.

[c] All three receptors may exist in non-neuronal brain tissue as well.

[d] Distribution in guinea pig (H_1 and H_2) and rat (H_3) brain. For the H_1 receptor, distribution is very different across species.

[e] Contradictory findings have been reported.

below, H_3 receptors function as heteroreceptors and as autoreceptors.

MOLECULAR SITES OF HISTAMINE ACTION

Histamine acts on at least three receptors in the CNS. Table 14-2 summarizes the characteristics of known histamine receptors. All three receptors are thought to be linked to G proteins, and all have been found inside and outside of the CNS. Within the brain, all have unique regional distributions, but none is localized exclusively to neurons. Selective agonists and antagonists are also available for each of the three receptors [21]. The judicious use of these compounds for receptor classification and discovery has been reviewed extensively [15,15a].

Binding and molecular biological techniques have been used to characterize brain H_1 receptors

The specific binding of radiolabeled pyrilamine, also termed mepyramine, was used to identify the H_1 receptor many years before the molecular properties of the receptor were known [15a,22,23]. Although the original method accurately identifies the receptor in brain, artifactual specific binding was subsequently demonstrated and characterized in other tissues, such as liver. Derivatives of H_1 antagonists have been developed for use in autoradiography and as photoaffinity labels for the receptor [2,21,23]. Other ligands, such as the antidepressant doxepin, have very high affinity for H_1 receptors but bind to more than one class of sites [23]. More recently, H_1 receptors have been visualized and studied in living brain of animals and humans with [^{11}C]-ligands and positron emission tomography. Unlike the regional distributions of other histamine receptors, H_1 receptors show striking differences among animal species in their densities across brain regions (Table 14-2) [22]. Lesion studies suggest that H_1 receptors in different parts of the brain exist on both neurons and non-neuronal cells. The presence of H_1-binding sites on cultured astrocytes and endothelial cells is in agreement with this suggestion [23].

Biochemical analysis of irreversibly labeled H_1 receptor protein from brain suggested a 56-kDa peptide [2]; a larger isoform was detected from guinea pig heart. The protein was successfully cloned from a cDNA library of bovine adrenal medulla [24]. The intronless cDNA encodes a 491-amino-acid protein with an apparent molecular weight of 56,000. Features common to many of the G protein-coupled receptors are present, including seven transmembrane domains, N-terminal glycosylation sites and phosphorylation sites for PKA and protein kinase C (PKC). The third cytoplasmic loop is large, characteristic of other phospholipase C-linked receptors (see below). The H_1 receptor proteins from rat, guinea pig, mouse and human have also been cloned and show some species variations. The mouse H_1 gene has been localized to chromosome 6.

Intracellular messengers. Activated H_1 receptors can generate several intracellular messengers. H_1 receptors are known to activate a pertussis toxin-insensitive G protein, G_q, that stimulates phosphoinositide-specific phospholipase C (PI-PLC), with the subsequent generation of inositol 1,4,5-trisphosphate (IP_3) and diacylglycerol (DAG) (Chap. 21). These two mediators are known to elevate intracellular Ca^{2+} concentrations and to activate PKC, respectively [23,25]. Both internal and external Ca^{2+} sources are required to initiate and maintain responses (Chap. 23). The distribution of H_1-activated IP_3 concentrations in the brain corresponds well to the distribution of H_1-binding sites in the guinea pig [2].

H_1 receptors are also known to stimulate the activity of phospholipase A_2 (PLA_2), with the subsequent release of arachidonate and its metabolites (Chap. 35). In platelets, this response does not require activation of the phosphoinositide cycle and is inhibited by pertussis toxin, suggesting a second, distinct transduction mechanism. In cells transfected with the H_1 receptor, PLA_2 activation is partially inhibited by pertussis toxin, also suggesting at least two transduction systems [21,25]. H_1 receptors in brain slices can also stimulate glycogen metabolism [2] and can positively modulate receptor-linked stimulation of cAMP synthesis (see below).

Activation of brain H_1 receptors also stimulates cGMP synthesis [15,23]. Outside of the brain, histamine is known to relax vascular smooth muscle by activation of endothelial H_1 receptors, thereby increasing endothelial Ca^{2+} concentrations and stimulating the synthesis and release of nitric oxide. The latter, a diffusible agent, then activates the smooth muscle guanylyl cyclase [21]. Although less is known about these mechanisms in the CNS, there is evidence that brain H_1 receptor activation can produce effects that depend on guanylyl cyclase. Lipoxygenase products of arachidonate metabolism may also contribute to the H_1-mediated increase in cGMP concentrations [15].

H_1 receptor activation induces depolarizing responses in many brain areas, notably hypothalamus, thalamus and cerebral cortex. In vertebrate brain, these excitatory effects are mediated by blockade of several K^+ conductances; in invertebrates, activation of inward Na^+ currents has also been implicated [23]. In oocytes, expression of the cloned receptor activates a Ca^{2+}-dependent increase in Cl^- conductance [24]. H_1 receptors are thought to contribute to hyperpolarizing responses by activating a Ca^{2+}-dependent K^+ conductance. This latter mechanism may be most closely related to the synthesis of IP_3.

H_1 receptor domains. Histamine interacts with at least two domains of the H_1 receptor. Site-directed mutagenesis studies have helped to elucidate the mechanisms by which agonists and antagonists act on histamine receptors [21]. As shown in Figure 14-5, both histamine and the catecholamines share positively charged ethylamine side chains, which interact with specific, negatively charged aspartate residues in transmembrane domain 3 (TM3) of the respective receptors. This amino acid residue is required for the actions of agonists and antagonists on H_1 and H_2 receptors. As expected, the imidazole-recognition sites within TM5 of the histamine receptors are different from the catecholamine-binding sites within the β_2-adrenergic receptor (Fig. 14-5). Thus, the two serine residues of the adrenergic receptor have been replaced with threonine and asparagine in the H_1 receptor. For the interaction of histamine with the H_1 receptor, the latter, but not the former, amino acid is

required [21]. However, lysine in TM5 at position 191 in the human receptor (Fig. 14-5) may also be important for activating the H_1 receptor [15a].

H_2 receptors have been studied with biochemical and molecular biological techniques

Although early work showed that radiolabeled H_2 antagonists such as cimetidine could specifically bind to brain components, later studies showed that this binding does not reflect properties of the H_2 receptor [15]. Labeled tiotidine, a more potent antagonist, has been successfully used as an H_2 ligand, although a large amount of nonspecific binding has been observed with this compound [2,15]. Iodopotentidine, a more recently developed radioligand, gives good results for both homogenate and autoradiographic studies of guinea pig brain (Table 14-2) [2]. A photoaffinity derivative of this ligand was used to identify a 59-kDa peptide thought to be the H_2 receptor. Other approaches estimated the molecular weight of the protein to be between 63,000 and 95,000 [21].

The H_2 receptor protein has been cloned from several species [20,21], including dog [26], rat, guinea pig, mouse and human. These intronless genes encode for receptor proteins having 358 to 359 amino acids with a molecular weight of approximately 40,000 and show the typical features of G protein-coupled receptors. Like the H_1 receptor, the H_2 protein has sites for phosphorylation by PKC and for glycosylation. Unlike the former, the latter lacks a consensus site for PKA. Surprisingly, there is only about a 40% homology in the structure of these two histamine receptors. The protein structure of the H_2 receptor, as expected, shows strong resemblance to other receptors known to be positively coupled to adenylyl cyclase. Features include a short third cytoplasmic loop and a long C-terminal cytoplasmic tail [20]. In mice, the H_2 gene has been localized to chromosome 13. When expressed in cells, the cloned H_2 receptor shows binding profiles and biochemical characteristics that closely resemble the natural receptor. Both neurons and non-neuronal cells of brain possess H_2 receptors [2]. H_2 receptors are abundant in

Receptor	TM3													TM5													
α_1	V	W	A	A	V	**D**	V	L	C	C	T	A	S	–	Y	V	L	F	**S**	A	L	G	**S**	F	Y	V	P	–
β_2	F	W	T	S	I	**D**	V	L	C	V	T	A	S	–	Y	A	I	A	S	**S**	I	V	**S**	F	Y	V	P	–
D_2	I	F	V	T	L	**D**	V	M	M	C	T	A	S	–	F	V	V	Y	S	**S**	I	V	**S**	F	Y	V	P	–
H_1	F	W	L	S	M	**D**	Y	V	A	S	T	A	S	–	F	K	V	M	**T**	A	I	I	**N**	F	Y	L	P	–
H_2	I	Y	T	S	L	**D**	V	M	L	C	T	A	S	–	Y	G	L	V	**D**	G	L	V	**T**	F	Y	L	P	–

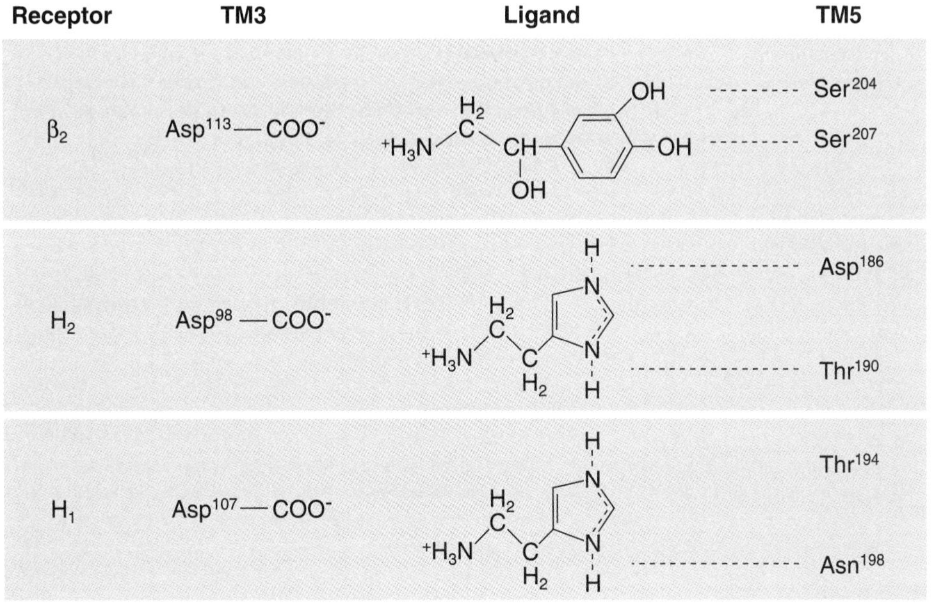

FIGURE 14-5. Recognition of histamine by H_1 and H_2 receptors. Selected components of transmembrane domains 3 and 5 (TM3, TM5) from the H_1 and H_2 receptors are depicted, along with those of several catecholamine receptors. **Top:** Key portions of the amino acid sequences show the similarities and differences between catecholamine and histamine receptor structures. All sequences are from humans except for α_1, which is the bovine α_{1c} receptor. Shaded amino acids are shown in more detail in the bottom diagram. **Bottom:** Essential interactions between selected receptor components and ligands are illustrated. In all three receptors shown, the aspartate residue in TM3 (*D*, **top**, *Asp*, **bottom**) provides an electrostatic interaction with both norepinephrine and histamine at the side chain cationic site. In contrast, serine residues in TM5 of the β_2 receptor, which are necessary for catecholamine binding, have been replaced by other amino acids in the histamine receptors. At TM5 of the H_2 receptor, both Asp^{186} and Thr^{190} are postulated to participate in a proton-transfer reaction initiated by histamine, but this mechanism requires further clarification. The mechanism is different for the binding of histamine to the H_1 receptor, since Asn^{198}, but not Thr^{194} is essential. However, Lys^{191} (*K*) may be important in this case. Asn^{198} is shown interacting with the N^{π} atom of histamine, but this has been questioned.

the cerebral cortex, corpus striatum and nucleus accumbens of the guinea pig brain (Table 14-2). In the rat, characterization of brain H_2 receptors has been hampered by low concentrations of receptor; however, H_2 receptor mRNA has been observed in this species.

H_2 receptors and cAMP. H_2 receptors are linked to increases in cAMP but also to other intracellular signals. It is well established that H_2 receptors lead to increases in cAMP concentrations in many tissues by stimulation of adenylyl cyclase [22,23] (see Chap. 22). Since this effect is blocked by cholera toxin, a G_s-type protein is implicated in its mediation of these effects. Elevated cAMP concentrations then result in the activation of PKA, leading to numerous cellular changes. Outside of the nervous system, cAMP is thought to be responsible for most of the effects of H_2 receptor stimulation. However, this may not be true for brain tissue. For example, H_2 receptors activate adenylyl cyclase in homogenates from several regions of guinea pig brain, but the density of H_2-binding sites does not correlate with the magnitude of cyclase activation across regions. Cells transfected with H_2 receptors demonstrate activation of adenylyl cyclase, confirming that cAMP is an important H_2 messenger. However, these and other experiments suggest that this receptor also uses additional transduction mechanisms, including activation of phospholipase C, increased intracellular Ca^{2+}, increased IP_3 concentrations, increased phospholipid methylation and decreased arachidonate release [20–22]. Both G_s and G_q proteins have been implicated in these responses, suggesting that the same receptor can activate more than one type of G protein. Similar conclusions have been reached in studies of other G protein-linked receptors. It must be emphasized that there are contradictory findings concerning these additional H_2 mechanisms, and further study is needed.

Electrophysiological studies have reported many inhibitory effects of H_2 receptor activation, including hyperpolarization and decreased signal transmission. Some of these inhibitory effects may be due to activation of Cl^- conductances. However, H_2 receptor stimulation of mammalian cortex and hippocampus produces excitation by inhibition of a Ca^{2+}-activated K^+ conductance. This excitation resembles that produced by activation of β-adrenergic receptors in these areas and is probably mediated by increases in cAMP [23].

Agonist recognition sites for histamine receptors differ from each other and from those of other biogenic amines, but specificity is determined by only a few amino acids. Both theoretical and molecular biological studies suggest that histamine interacts with residues in both TM3 and TM5 of the H_2 receptor, similar to the mechanisms postulated for the H_1 receptor and for other biogenic amines (Fig. 14-5). Long before the receptor structure was known, histamine was postulated to activate the H_2 receptor by a three-site mechanism consisting of neutralization of the side chain ethylammonium, with proton donation and proton acceptance from the *tele-* and *pros*-amines, respectively. The mechanism amounts to a proton

transfer between two sites of the receptor [27]. More recent molecular studies suggest an explicit version of this model (Fig. 14-5), in which the three recognition sites are Asp[98] (TM3), Asp[186] (TM5) and Thr[190] (TM5). Although some results from site-directed mutation experiments are consistent with the model, other findings are not easily reconciled, and alternative models are being considered. However, it is clear that receptor specificity is controlled by a small number of amino acids. For example, replacement of Asp[186]-Gly[187] with Ala[186]-Ser[187] yielded a mutant H_2 receptor that was activated by epinephrine and blocked by both H_2 and β-adrenergic antagonists (Fig. 14-5).

Both positive and negative interactions may occur between H_1 and H_2 receptors

The activation of brain cAMP synthesis by histamine is a well-studied phenomenon which reveals a positive interaction between histamine receptors [22,23]. When studied in cell-free preparations, this response shows characteristics of H_2, but not H_1, receptors. When similar experiments are performed in brain slices, however, both receptors appear to participate in the response. Subsequent work showed that H_1 receptors do not directly stimulate adenylyl cyclase but enhance the H_2 stimulation, probably through some type of calcium signaling that requires cellular integrity. Other receptors that act through PI-PLC, such as α_1-adrenergic and serotonergic receptors, are known to enhance adenylyl cyclase-mediated messages, such as histamine H_2 or adenosine A_2, as well, but they do not always do so. The H_1–PI-PLC pathway itself is subject to intracellular modulation as activation of adenylyl cyclase in some tissues decreases this H_1 signal [22]. H_1 and H_2 receptors may also exert opposing influences on other transduction mechanisms, such as arachidonate release (above and Table 14-2). G protein pathways have extensive modulatory interactions with each other, which are being actively explored.

Prolonged exposure of H_1 receptors to high concentrations of histamine decreases concentrations of H_1 second messengers, including inositol phosphates and Ca^{2+}, and reduces H_1-mediated responses in cell lines, smooth muscle preparations and brain slices [21]. Both homologous, that is, H_1 receptor-specific, and heterologous desensitization have been found. Phosphorylation of the H_1 receptor by PKC may be one mechanism for desensitization, but additional mechanisms are also important. H_2 receptors also undergo rapid desensitization and internalization upon exposure to histamine [28]. Site-directed mutagenesis studies have shown that both cAMP-dependent and cAMP-independent mechanisms can contribute to this desensitization [28]. Chronic exposure to H_2 antagonists can induce upregulation of H_2 receptors. The ability of cimetidine, but not all H_2 antagonists, to behave as inverse agonists in systems expressing high receptor numbers has been suggested to account for this upregulation.

There may be more than one type of H_3 receptor

Following the discovery of the H_3 autoreceptor, selective H_3 antagonists, H_3 agonists and H_3 radioligands were developed [20,21] (Table 14-2). The agonist $[^3H]N^\alpha$-methylhistamine has been studied extensively as a radioligand and shows binding properties that are characteristic of H_3 responses. However, both kinetic and equilibrium studies with this ligand under some conditions show complex results that may reflect the existence of more than one receptor subtype. There are considerable pharmacological data that can be interpreted as supportive of the existence of subtypes of the H_3 receptor, but selective compounds that act on the putative subtypes have not been found. Alternatively, some of these complexities may be due to the use of agonist radioligands or certain experimental conditions [21]. Antagonist ligands have also been developed (Table 14-2) but have not yet resolved many of these problems. Autoradiographic studies show high levels of H_3 binding in cerebral cortex, nucleus accumbens and striatum. H_3 binding has also been found in peripheral tissues, including guinea pig lung and human gastric mucosa.

Histamine release, as well as the release of other transmitters, is inhibited by the H_3 receptor. The H_3 receptor, first characterized as an autoreceptor, has been presumed to exist on histaminergic fibers and to regulate histamine synthesis and release in the CNS. There is strong, albeit indirect, evidence for this hypothesis [2,23]. However, attempts to directly demonstrate a presynaptic localization for brain H_3 receptors have not been successful. Lesions that destroy histaminergic fibers fail to reduce H_3 binding. In contrast, chemical lesions of cells that receive histaminergic input in striatum do reduce H_3 binding, suggesting that many H_3 receptors exist as postsynaptic heteroreceptors on histaminergic targets. Many functional studies support this possibility (see transmitter interactions, below). Outside of the CNS, H_3 receptors appear to be present on peripheral afferent fibers, where they may regulate the release of nociceptive/inflammatory neuropeptide transmitters. This hypothesis is consistent with known interactions between afferent fibers, mast cells and histamine.

Transduction mechanisms associated with the H_3 receptor are not well characterized. In comparison to the H_1 and H_2 receptors, much less is known about the H_3 receptor [21]. Binding sites with characteristics of H_3 receptors have been purified from brain homogenates and cell lines. In these and other preparations, binding studies and electrophysiological experiments suggest that the H_3 receptor is coupled to G proteins. However, the identities of these G proteins and their associated transduction mechanisms remain uncertain. H_3 receptors purified from a gastric tumor cell line have an estimated molecular weight of 70,000 and appear to be negatively coupled to PI-PLC, an effect which is inhibited by both cholera and pertussis toxin. Pertussis toxin also alters H_3 binding and guanyl nucleotide interactions with the receptor [28a]. However, in smooth muscle cells, H_3 receptors show an enhancement of voltage-dependent Ca^{2+} channels that is modulated by guanyl nucleotides but resistant to pertussis toxin, suggesting the involvement of a different G protein. Outside of the brain, H_3 receptor stimulation may activate the synthesis and release of nitric oxide.

The best understood function for H_3 receptors, that is, inhibition of transmitter release, depends on extracellular Ca^{2+} concentrations [21].

Thus, it has been inferred that the ultimate consequence of H_3 receptor activation would be to reduce the activity of voltage-dependent Ca^{2+} influx. The ability of H_3 agonists to hyperpolarize isolated tuberomammillary neurons by increases in K^+ conductance seems consistent with this idea, but the relevant channels have not been identified. Molecular cloning of the H_3 receptor, presently being pursued in several labs, will contribute enormously toward solving these problems.

It is likely that histamine acts at sites that are distinct from H_1, H_2 and H_3 receptors, but selective antagonists for these responses are lacking

Histamine has been reported to induce a number of atypical pharmacological responses at several peripheral sites, including liver, platelets, eosinophils and lymphocytes. In the arthropod nervous system, histamine activates a ligand-gated Cl^- channel at photoreceptor synapses [13], but the pharmacology of this response has not been adequately studied. In preparations from mammalian brain, histamine has been shown to enhance excitatory amino acid transmission at NMDA receptors; the effect seems to be independent of known histamine receptors and may be due to an action at the polyamine-binding site on the NMDA receptor. Histamine may act at this site to facilitate the induction of long-term potentiation in hippocampal slices [29]. However, it has not yet been established that endogenous histamine can act at this site. All indications are that many additional histamine receptors remain to be discovered.

HISTAMINE ACTIONS IN THE CENTRAL NERVOUS SYSTEM

Histamine in the brain may act as both a neuromodulator and classical transmitter

Histaminergic neurons appear to provide a variety of signaling mechanisms in the brain. A "neuromodulator" role for histamine has received the most attention. Thus, activation of a small number of tuberomammillary cells is thought to release histamine, which subsequently increases excitability in target cells distributed widely throughout the brain [7]. As mentioned, most of this histamine release is nonsynaptic, implying wide diffusion of the modulator. Such a system is consistent with the characteristics of known histamine receptors, which function through "slow" transmission mechanisms (see Chap. 10) requiring the production of intracellular second messengers (Table 14-2). However, it is becoming clear that neuronal histamine is also capable of providing discrete, fast neurotransmission in the brain. For example, electrical stimulation of the tuberomammillary cells has been shown to evoke fast excitatory postsynaptic potentials in phasically firing supraoptic neurons, effects that are mimicked by application of histamine and blocked by histamine antagonists [30]. These findings imply that, like serotonin (see Chap. 13), histamine may be able to activate both ligand-operated channels and receptors linked to second messengers. The former remain to be identified, however.

Histaminergic neurons can regulate and be regulated by other neurotransmitter systems

A number of other transmitter systems can interact with histaminergic neurons (Table 14-1). As mentioned, the H_3 receptor is thought to function as an inhibitory heteroreceptor. Thus, activation of brain H_3 receptors decreases the release of acetylcholine, dopamine, norepinephrine, serotonin and certain peptides. However, histamine may also increase the activity of some of these systems through H_1 and/or H_2 receptors. Activation of NMDA, μ opioid, dopamine D2 and some serotonin receptors can increase the release of neuronal histamine, whereas other transmitter receptors seem to decrease release. Different patterns of interactions may also be found in discrete brain regions.

Histamine in the central nervous system may participate in a variety of brain functions

Several of the suspected physiological roles for histamine are related to its ability to increase the excitability of CNS neurons. In fact, in the brain, histamine has been suggested to be a regulator of "whole brain" activity [7]. For example, mutant mice lacking the H_1 receptor show defective locomotor and exploratory behaviors [30a]. Closely related may be the role of histamine as a mediator of arousal. All available evidence from several species shows that histaminergic neurons, when activated, increase wakefulness and induce electrographic arousal. The H_1 receptor in the ventrolateral hypothalamus is one important site for this effect [31], but actions on the thalamus and cerebral cortex may also be significant. The onset of sleep has been traced to cells in the ventral preoptic area of the hypothalamus, which, when activated, are thought to turn off the histaminergic tuberomammillary cells. Thus, histamine is an important regulator of sleep–wake cycles and probably contributes to the diurnal changes in other brain functions as well.

Histamine also reduces seizure activity, another H_1 receptor-mediated effect. H_1 antagonists increase seizure onset and/or seizure duration in humans and animals. H_1 receptor numbers are increased in some types of human epileptic foci [12]. Pharmacological studies suggest that centrally administered histamine can also enhance learning and retention of tasks in laboratory animals. However, the role of histaminergic neurons in these tasks is complex, and contradictory findings have been reported [31a].

Histamine is a powerful regulator of many hypothalamic functions. Neuroendocrine responses, especially vasopressin release, are physiologically regulated by histaminergic neurons [30,32]. Hypothalamic histamine may also participate in the physiological regulation of oxytocin, prolactin, adrenocorticotrophic hormone (ACTH) and β-endorphin release. Regulation of the latter two occurs by changes in release of both corticotropin-releasing hormone and vasopressin [33,34]. Both H_1 and H_2 receptors seem to function in the histaminergic control of pituitary function.

Neuronal histamine is also an effective modulator of both food and water intake [12,34a]. Histamine and compounds that increase extracellular histamine concentrations are powerful suppressants of food intake. An action on the H_1 receptor in the ventromedial hypothalamus (VMH) seems to account for these effects [35]. Evidence that histamine contributes to the physiological control of appetite includes findings with genetically obese Zucker rats, which have very low concentrations of hypothalamic histamine. Histamine is also a powerful dipsogen (an agent that induces drinking), whether administered systemically or directly into the hypothalamus. Multiple hormonal and neuronal mechanisms may contribute to these effects [36]. Other suggested roles for histamine in the regulation of vegetative functions include thermoregulation [37], regulation of glucose and lipid metabolism [38] and control of blood pressure.

Histamine also induces antinociceptive, that is, pain-relieving, responses in animals after microinjection into several brain regions [39]. Both neuronal and humoral mechanisms may be involved. Brain H_2 receptors appear to mediate some forms of endogenous analgesic response, especially those elicited by exposure to stressors [40]. Many of the modulatory actions of histamine discussed above appear to be activated as part of stress responses. For reasons that remain unclear, histamine releasers, such as thioperamide, show only mild, biphasic antinociceptive actions, even though histamine is a potent and effective analgesic substance.

Histamine may contribute to brain diseases or disorders

As mentioned above, a role for brain histamine in several neurodegenerative diseases, such as multiple sclerosis, Alzheimer's disease and Wernicke's encephalopathy, is being studied closely [3,12]. Whether from neurons or mast cells, histamine may participate in these processes by contributing to vascular changes, alterations in the blood–brain barrier, changes in immune function or even cell death. The ability of histamine to enhance excitatory transmission at NMDA receptors (discussed above) may explain its neurotoxic actions [3]. However, neuronal histamine does not always enhance brain damage; it seems to exert a protective effect in some models of cerebral ischemia. Histaminergic neurons are also activated by vestibular disturbances, leading to the release of histamine in brainstem emetic centers. Thus, neuronal histamine may be one mediator of motion sickness [41].

SIGNIFICANCE OF BRAIN HISTAMINE FOR DRUG ACTION

The sedative properties of some drugs on the central nervous system are attributable to their H_1-blocking effects

Blockade of brain H_1 receptors induces drowsiness and other signs of CNS depression in humans. For many years, these side effects limited the use of H_1 antagonists in allergic disorders such as hay fever. Newer, non-sedating antihistamines, such as terfenadine or loratadine, relieve peripheral allergic symptoms but have a low brain penetration, eliminating the sedative side effects. However, most over-the-counter sleep aids, such as chlorpheniramine and diphenhydramine, are brain-penetrating H_1 antagonists. These agents are also effective treatments for motion sickness and, in some instances, Meniere's disease. Many other centrally acting drugs have a high affinity for H_1 receptors. Notable are certain tricyclic antidepressants and neuroleptics; some of the former are thought to exert their sedative effects by this mechanism.

Morphine-like analgesics activate histaminergic mechanisms in the brain

Although μ opioid agonists like morphine initiate many neurochemical changes, the release of neuronal histamine and the subsequent activation of brain H_2 receptors are essential features of pain relief by these agents [39]. Other nonanalgesic effects of opiates, such as hormone release, may also be mediated by histaminergic mechanisms. Stress responses also can contribute to opioid analgesia, and histaminergic neurons appear to mediate the stress-induced potentiation of morphine antinociception. Although no new analgesic drugs have yet been developed based on H_2 receptors, a novel analgesic activity was recently discovered in compounds

related to cimetidine, which is an H_2 antagonist, and burimamide, which is a drug with both H_2 and H_3 properties. Although the mechanism for these effects is unknown, existing histamine receptors (H_1, H_2, H_3) and the μ opioid receptor have been excluded [42]. The antinociceptive profile of these compounds suggests that brain-penetrating derivatives of these agents could be useful analgesics.

Brain-penetrating drugs that act on the H_3 receptor are being developed to treat obesity, sleep disturbances, epilepsy, pain and cognitive disorders

Drugs with selective agonist or antagonist activity at the H_3 receptor are being developed for several uses. The ability of histamine to promote arousal, suppress appetite, elevate seizure threshold and stimulate cognitive processes implies that compounds able to enhance the release of neuronal histamine should mimic these effects. Several H_3 antagonists in development demonstrate such activity and show promise as effective and novel therapeutic agents. Because H_3 agonists suppress the release of neuronal histamine, compounds that can activate brain H_3 receptors may become clinically useful sleep-promoting drugs. H_3 agonists also show some anti-inflammatory and antinociceptive properties, consistent with the H_3-mediated inhibition of release of nociceptive/inflammatory peptides from primary afferent nerve fibers (discussed above and in Table 14-1). As noted, pre- and postsynaptic H_3 receptors may contribute to these responses.

ACKNOWLEDGMENTS

The author thanks Prof. Helmut Haas (Dusseldorf, Germany) and Dr. Glen Hatton (Riverside, California) for valuable discussions of electrophysiological experiments. Thanks are also due to members of the author's laboratory for helpful comments on the manuscript. The author apologizes to the many scientists whose research was mentioned in this chapter but not cited due to editorial limitations. Many of these citations appear in the CD-ROM version of this chapter. This work was supported by a grant (DA-03816) from the National Institute on Drug Abuse.

REFERENCES

1. Hough, L. B., Goldschmidt, R. C., Glick, S. D., and Padawer, J. Mast cells in rat brain: Characterization, localization, and histamine content. In C. R. Ganellin and J. C. Schwartz (eds.), *Frontiers in Histamine Research: A Tribute to Heinz Schild. Advances in the Biosciences.* New York: Pergamon Press, 1985, pp. 131–140.

2. Schwartz, J. C., Arrang, J. M., Garbarg, M., Pollard, H., and Ruat, M. Histaminergic transmission in the mammalian brain. *Physiol. Rev.* 71:1–51, 1991.

3. Langlais, P. J., Zhang, S. X., Weilersbacher, G., Hough, L. B., and Barke, K. E. Histamine-mediated neuronal death in a rat model of Wernicke's encephalopathy. *J. Neurosci. Res.* 38:565–574, 1994.

3a. Rouleau, A., Dimitriadou, V., Trung, M. D., et al. Mast cell specific proteases in rat brain: Changes in rats with experimental allergic encephalomyelitis. *J. Neural Transm.* 104(4–5):399–417, 1997.

4. Hough, L. B. Cellular localization and possible functions for brain histamine: Recent progress. In G. A. Kerkut and J. W. Phillis (eds.), *Progress in Neurobiology,* Vol. 30. Oxford: Pergamon Press, 1988, pp. 469–505.

5. Panula, P., Yang, Y. H. T., and Costa, E. Histamine-containing neurons in the rat hypothalamus. *Proc. Natl. Acad. Sci. USA* 81:2572–2576, 1984.

6. Watanabe, T., Taguchi, Y., Shiosaka, S., et al. Distribution of the histaminergic neuron system in the central nervous system of rats: A fluorescent immunohistochemical analysis with histidine decarboxylase as a marker. *Brain Res.* 295:13–25, 1984.

7. Wada, H., Inagaki, N., Yamatodani, A., and Watanabe, T. Is the histaminergic neuron system a regulatory center for whole-brain activity? *Trends Neurosci.* 14:415–418, 1991.

8. Haas, H. L., Reiner, P. B. and Greene, R. W. Histamine and histaminoceptive neurons: Electrophysiological studies in vertebrates. In: T. Watanabe, and H. Wada (eds.) *Histaminergic Neurons: Morphology and Function.* CRC Press, Boca Raton, 1991, pp. 195–208.

9. Inagaki, N., Yamatodani, A., Ando-Yamamoto, M., Tohyama, M., Watanabe, T., and Wada, H. Organization of histaminergic fibers in the rat brain. *J. Comp. Neurol.* 273:283–300, 1988.

10. Panula, P., Pirvola, U., Auvinen, S., and Airaksinen, M. S. Histamine-immunoreactive nerve fibers in the rat brain. *Neuroscience* 28:585–610, 1989.

11. Hough, L. B., and Green, J. P. Histamine and its receptors in the nervous system. In A. Lajtha (ed.), *Handbook of Neurochemistry,* 2nd ed. New York: Plenum Press, 1984, pp. 148–211.

12. Onodera, K., Yamatodani, A., Watanabe, T., and Wada, H. Neuropharmacology of the histaminergic neuron system in the brain and its relationship with behavioral disorders. *Prog. Neurobiol.* 42:685–702, 1994.

13. Hardie, R. C. A histamine-activated chloride channel involved in neurotransmission at a photoreceptor synapse. *Nature* 339:704–706, 1989.

14. Stuart, A. E., and Callaway, J. C. Histamine: The case for a photoreceptor's neurotransmitter. *Neurosci. Res.* (Suppl.) 15:S13–S23, 1991.

14a. Melzig, J., Buchner, S., Wiebel, F., et al. Genetic depletion of histamine from the nervous system of Drosophila eliminates specific visual and mechanosensory behavior. *J. Comp. Physiol. A* 179:763–773, 1996.

15. Prell, G. D., and Green, J. P. Histamine as a neuroregulator. *Annu. Rev. Neurosci.* 9:209–254, 1986.

15a. Hill, S. J., Ganellin, C. R., Timmerman, H., et al. International Union of Pharmacology. XIII. Classification of histamine receptors. *Pharmacol. Rev.* 49:253–278, 1997.

16. Joseph, D. R., Sullivan, P. M., Wang, Y.-M., et al. Characterization and expression of the complementary DNA encoding rat histidine decarboxylase. *Proc. Natl. Acad. Sci. USA* 87:733–737, 1990.

17. Watanabe, T., Yamatodani, A., Maeyama, K., and Wada, H. Pharmacology of α-fluoromethylhistidine, a specific inhibitor of histidine decarboxylase. *Trends Pharmacol. Sci.* 11:363–367, 1990.

18. Takemura, M., Tanaka, T., Taguchi, Y., et al. Histamine N-methyltransferase from rat kidney. *J. Biol. Chem.* 267:15687–15691, 1992.

19. Arrang, J. M., Garbarg, M., Lancelot, J. C., et al. Highly potent and selective ligands for histamine H_3-receptors. *Nature* 327:117–123, 1987.

20. Arrang, J.-M., Drutel, G., Garbarg, M., Ruat, M., Traiffort, E., and Schwartz, J.-C. Molecular and functional diversity of histamine receptor subtypes. *Ann. NY Acad. Sci.* 757:314–323, 1995.

21. Leurs, R., Smit, M. J., and Timmerman, H. Molecular pharmacological aspects of histamine receptors. *Pharmacol. Ther.* 66:413–463, 1995.

22. Hill, S. J. Distribution, properties, and functional characteristics of three classes of histamine receptor. *Pharmacol. Rev.* 42:45–83, 1990.

23. Schwartz, J. C., and Haas, H. L. (eds.), *The Histamine Receptor*. New York: Wiley-Liss, 1992.

24. Yamashita, M., Fukui, H., Sugama, K., et al. Expression cloning of a cDNA encoding the bovine histamine H_1 receptor. *Proc. Natl. Acad. Sci. USA* 88:11515–11519, 1991.

25. Leurs, R., Traiffort, E., Arrang, J. M., Tardivel-Lacombe, J., Ruat, M., and Schwartz, J.-C. Guinea pig histamine H_1 receptor. II. Stable expression in Chinese hamster ovary cells reveals the interaction with three major signal transduction pathways. *J. Neurochem.* 62:519–527, 1994.

26. Gantz, I., Schaffer, M., DelValle, J., et al. Molecular cloning of a gene encoding the histamine H_2 receptor. *Proc. Natl. Acad. Sci. USA* 88:429–433, 1991.

27. Weinstein, H., Mazurek, A. P., Osman, R., and Topiol, S. Theoretical studies on the activation mechanism of the histamine H_2 receptor: The proton transfer between histamine and a receptor model. *Mol. Pharmacol.* 29:28–33, 1989.

28. Smith, M. J. Dynamic regulation of the histamine H_1 and H_2 receptors. Ph.D. Thesis, Vrije Universiteit, Amsterdam, 1995.

28a. Clark, E. A., and Hill, S. J. Sensitivity of histamine H3 receptor agonist–stimulated [35S]GTP-gamma[S] binding to pertussis toxin. *Eur. J. Pharmacol.* 296:223–225, 1996.

29. Brown, R. E., Fedorov, N. B., Haas, H. L., and Reymann, K. G. Histaminergic modulation of synaptic plasticity in area CA1 of rat hippocampal slices. *Neuropharmacology* 34:181–190, 1995.

30. Hatton, G. I., and Yang, Q. Z. Synaptically released histamine increases dye coupling among vasopressinergic neurons of the supraoptic nucleus: Mediation by H_1 receptors and cyclic nucleotides. *J. Neurosci.* 16:123–129, 1996.

30a. Inoue, I., Yanai, K., Kitamura, D., et al. Impaired locomotor activity and exploratory behavior in mice lacking histamine H_1 receptors. *Proc. Natl. Acad. Sci. USA* 93:13316–13320, 1996.

31. Lin, J.-S., Sakai, K., Vanni-Mercier, G., et al. Involvement of histaminergic neurons in arousal mechanisms demonstrated with H_3-receptor ligands in the cat. *Brain Res.* 523:325–330, 1990.

31a. Huston, J. P., Wagner, U., and Hasenöhrl, R. U. The tuberomammillary nucleus projections in the control of learning, memory and reinforcement processes: Evidence for an inhibitory role. *Behav. Brain Res.* 83:97–105, 1997.

32. Kjaer, A., Knigge, U., Rouleau, A., Garbarg, M., and Warberg, J. Dehydration-induced release of vasopressin involves activation of hypothalamic histaminergic neurons. *Endocrinology* 135: 675–681, 1994.

33. Knigge, U., and Warberg, J. The role of histamine in the neuroendocrine regulation of pituitary hormone secretion. *Acta Endocrinol. (Copenh.)* 124:609–619, 1991.

34. Knigge, U., Matzen, S., Bach, F. W., Bang, P., and Warberg, J. Involvement of histaminergic neurons in the stress-induced release of pro-opiomelanocortin-derived peptides in rats. *Acta Endocrinol. (Copenh)* 120:533–539, 1989.

34a. Sakata, T., and Yoshimatsu, H. Homeostatic maintenance regulated by hypothalamic neuronal histamine. *Methods Find. Exp. Clin. Pharmacol.* 17(Suppl. C):51–56, 1995.

35. Ookuma, K., Sakata, T., Fukagawa, K., et al. Neuronal histamine in the hypothalamus suppresses food intake in rats. *Brain Res.* 628:235–242, 1994.

36. Kraly, F. S., Keefe, M. E., Tribuzio, R. A., Kim, Y. M., Finkell, J., and Braun, C. J. H_1, H_2, and H_3 receptors contribute to drinking elicited by exogenous histamine and eating in rats. *Pharmacol. Biochem. Behav.* 53:347–354, 1996.

37. Phillipu, A. Interactions with other neuron systems. In: T. Watanabe and H. Wada (eds) Histaminergic Neurons: Morphology and Function. CRC Press, Boca Raton, 1991, pp 323–344.

38. Sakata, T., Kurokawa, M., Oohara, A., and Yoshimatsu, H. A physiological role of brain histamine during energy deficiency. *Brain Res. Bull.* 35:135–139, 1994.

39. Hough, L. B. Histaminergic mechanisms of antinociception. In G. D. Prell (ed.): *Histamine in Neurobiology*. Clifton, NJ: Humana Press, 1998 (in press).

40. Gogas, K. R., and Hough, L. B. Inhibition of naloxone-resistant antinociception by centrally-administered H_2 antagonists. *J. Pharmacol. Exp. Ther.* 248:262–267, 1989.

41. Takeda, N., Morita, M., Hasegawa, S., Horii, A., Kubo, T., and Matsunaga, T. Neuropharmacology of motion sickness and emesis. A review. *Acta Otolaryngol. (Stockh.)* Suppl. 501:10–15, 1993.

42. Hough, L. B., Nalwalk, J. W., Li, B. Y., et al. Novel qualitative structure–activity relationships for the antinociceptive actions of H_2 antagonists, H_3

antagonists and derivatives. *J. Pharmacol. Exp. Ther.* 283:1534–1543, 1997.

43. Schwartz, J. C., Arrang, J. M., Garbarg, M., Gulat-Marnay, C., and Pollard, H. Modulation of histamine synthesis and release in brain via pre-synaptic autoreceptors and heteroreceptors. *Ann. NY Acad. Sci.* 604:40–54, 1990.

44. Schlicker, E., Malinowska, B., Kathmann, M., and Göthert, M. Modulation of neurotransmitter release via histamine H_3 heteroreceptors. *Fundam. Clin. Pharmacol.* 8:128–137, 1994.

45. Inagaki, N., Toda, K., Taniuchi, I. et al. An analysis of histaminergic efferents of the tuberomaxillary nucleus to the medial preoptic area and inferior colliculus of the rat. *Exp. Brain Res.* 80: 374–380, 1990.

CHAPTER

15

Glutamate and Aspartate

Raymond Dingledine and Chris J. McBain

Basic Neurochemistry: Molecular, Cellular and Medical Aspects, 6th Ed., edited by G. J. Siegel et al. Published by Lippincott–Raven Publishers, Philadelphia, 1999. Correspondence to Raymond Dingledine, Department of Pharmacology, Emory University School of Medicine, 1510 Clifton Road, Atlanta, Georgia 30322-3090.

The amino acids glutamate and aspartate, and perhaps certain of their analogs, mediate most of the excitatory synaptic transmission in the brain. The realization that glutamatergic pathways are involved in such diverse processes as epilepsy, ischemic brain damage and learning and that they play major roles in the development of normal synaptic connections in the brain is of great practical interest. Studies of the functions of excitatory amino acid receptors were dominated by electrophysiological approaches until molecular cloning revealed the sequences of increasingly large and heterogeneous families of receptors. Thus, the neurochemistry and protein chemistry of these receptors, their transmitters and associated transporters have resurfaced as major research thrusts.

In this chapter, we follow the practice of naming this family of receptors after their most prominent neurotransmitter agonist and so use the term "glutamate receptor" to refer to all excitatory amino acid receptors. Reviews covering the pharmacology, physiology, molecular biology and neuropathological involvement of glutamate receptors [1–4] provide a worthwhile supplement to the material presented in this chapter.

THREE CLASSES OF IONOTROPIC GLUTAMATE RECEPTOR

For ionotropic glutamate receptors, the agonist-binding sites and associated ion channels are incorporated into the same macromolecular complex. Agonists increase the probability that the channel will open, and the three classes of ionotropic receptor originally were named after reasonably selective agonists: N-methyl-D-aspartate (NMDA), α-amino-3-hydroxy-5-methyl-4-isoxazole propionic acid (AMPA) and kainate (KA). These functionally defined receptor classes are represented by distinct molecular families of receptor genes.

Five functional families can be defined by structural homologies

The cloning by expression of the first glutamate receptor cDNA, for GluR1 in late 1989 [5] triggered a predictable frenzy of activity that has led to the identification of more than 16 mammalian genes that encode structurally related functional proteins. Currently, six families of ionotropic glutamate receptor subunits have been shown to assemble into functional receptors, as shown in Figure 15-1. Within a given family, members show at least 80% identity at the amino acid level over the ~400-amino-acid stretch of membrane-spanning regions. Between families, however, a lower degree of identity exists, 40 to 55% or less.

Based on analogy with other channel proteins, such as K^+ channels and nicotinic acetylcholine receptors, the ligand-gated ion channel receptors are likely to be multimeric assemblies of individual subunits. A significant feature of the glutamate receptors is that different subunit combinations produce functionally different receptors, as described below. This predicts that a very large family of glutamate receptors may exist in the brain. *In situ* hybridization and immunohistochemistry have highlighted regional differences in expression of subunits encoding glutamate receptors. These differences illustrate the likely heterogeneity of glutamate receptors throughout the CNS. Together with differences in electrophysiological properties of different subunit combinations expressed in cell lines or oocytes, diverse patterns of subunit expression throughout the CNS predict the existence of multiple subtypes of AMPA, KA and NMDA receptors.

AMPA and kainate receptors both are blocked by quinoxalinediones but have different desensitization pharmacology

AMPA receptors are widespread throughout the CNS and appear to serve as synaptic receptors

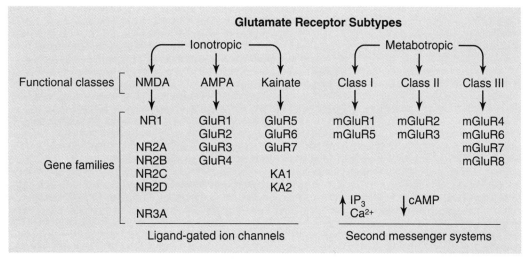

FIGURE 15-1.   Molecular families of glutamate receptors. Each of the two main glutamate receptor divisions comprises three functionally defined groups (classes) of receptor. These are made up of numerous individual subunits, each encoded by a different gene.

for fast excitatory synaptic transmission mediated by glutamate. GluR1 is predicted to be 889 amino acids long, compared to about 480 amino acids for nicotinic-, $GABA_A$- or glycine-receptor subunits. The extra length in GluR1 is due to an unusually large N-terminal extracellular domain. GluR1 through GluR4 subunits, also named GluRA through GluRD or, in mouse, α_1 through α_4, coassemble to form proteins with the pharmacological profile of AMPA receptors (Fig. 15-2). Thus, when *Xenopus* oocytes are injected with mixtures of GluR1 through GluR4 mRNAs, receptors are formed that can be blocked specifically by certain quinoxalinediones, notably 6-nitro-7-sulfamobenzo[f]   quinoxaline-2,3-dione (NBQX). NBQX is a potent and selective competitive antagonist of AMPA receptors but has weak or no effects on other receptors. Drugs in the 2,3-benzodiazepine class are noncompetitive antagonists of AMPA receptors and show some promise as neuroprotective agents for treating stroke. Antibodies to the GluR3 receptor function as antagonists and induce seizure-like activity in rabbits [6]. Of particular interest was the observation that sera obtained from patients with active Rasmussen's encephalitis, a form of pediatric epilepsy, also possessed anti-GluR3 receptor reactivity (see Chap. 37).

Subunits of the GluR5 through GluR7 family appear to coassemble with KA receptor subunits, KA1 or KA2 into functional KA receptors when studied in heterologous expression systems. Results of experiments with radioligands demonstrate that homomeric GluR5, GluR6 and GluR7 receptors expressed in mammalian cell lines bind [^{3}H]KA with an affinity of approximately 80 to 100 nM. Such homomeric receptors may correspond to the "low-affinity" KA-binding sites identified earlier in studies of plasma membranes from brain. Homomeric KA1 receptors bind KA with an affinity of 4 nM and may contribute to the high-affinity KA-binding site in brain. KA1 and KA2 receptors are virtually inactive when expressed alone, and therefore, might be thought of as modulatory subunits. Although none of the homomeric receptors is sensitive to AMPA, heteromeric complexes of GluR6 and KA1 do respond to AMPA with a desensitizing current.

KA receptors desensitize within milliseconds upon exposure to KA, and AMPA receptors likewise desensitize upon exposure to AMPA. Currently, AMPA and KA receptors can be distinguished from one another only by their response to two drugs, the lectin concanavalin A (Con A) and cyclothiazide [4]. Con A relieves desensitization of KA receptors, presumably via interaction with surface sugar chains, but has insignificant effects on AMPA receptors. Con-

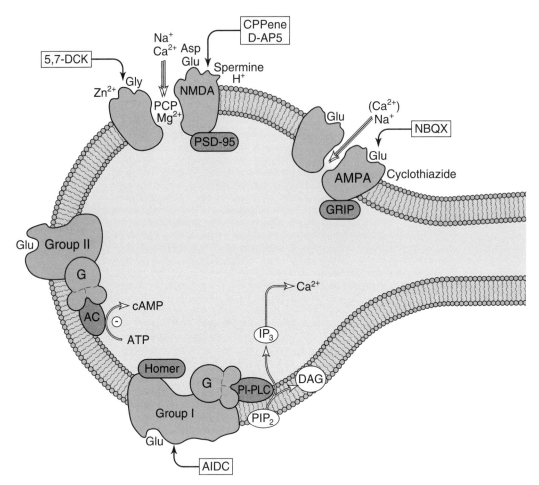

FIGURE 15-2.   Schematic views of four types of glutamate receptor. Two heteromeric ionotropic receptors are shown, the NMDA and AMPA receptors, as well as group I and group II metabotropic receptors. Competitive antagonists of each receptor are boxed. The NMDA receptor channel is additionally blocked by Mg^{2+} and phencyclidine *(PCP)*. Zn^{2+} is both a negative and a positive modulator. Protons suppress NMDA receptor activation, and polyamines, such as spermine, relieve the proton block. Cyclothiazide removes desensitization of AMPA receptors. Both classes of metabotropic receptor are coupled via G proteins *(G)* to intracellular enzymes, phosphoinositide-specific phospholipase C *(PI-PLC)* for group I receptors and adenylyl cyclase *(AC)* for group II receptors. PI-PLC catalyzes the production of inositol-1,4,5-trisphosphate *(IP₃)* and diacylglycerol *(DAG)* from phosphatidylinositol-4,5-bisphosphate *(PIP₂)*. The resulting increase in cytoplasmic IP_3 triggers release of Ca^{2+} from intracellular stores. Activation of group II metabotropic glutamate receptors typically results in inhibition of AC. The cytoplasmic proteins PSD-95, GRIP and Homer anchor the receptors to synaptic membranes [28,29], presumably by forming a bridge between the receptor and cytoskeletal structures. *AIDC,* 1-aminoindan-1,5-dicarboxylate; *5,7-DCK,* 5,7-dichlorokynurenic acid; *D-AP5,* D-2-amino-5-phosphonopentanoic acid; *CPPene,* 3-(2-carboxypiperazin-4-yl)1-propenyl-1-phosphoric acid; *NBQX,* 6-nitro 7-sulfamobenzo[f] quinoxaline-2,3-dione.

versely, cyclothiazide relieves AMPA receptor desensitization, with no effect on KA receptors. Until selective KA receptor antagonists are developed, these two drugs provide the best way to determine if a given synaptic current is mediated by AMPA or KA receptors.

N-Methyl-D-aspartate receptors have multiple regulatory sites

To date, three NMDA receptor subunit families have been identified, one apparently represented by a single gene *(NRI)* and the others by multiple genes *(NR2A–NR2D, NR3A)* (Fig. 15-1) encoding proteins of about 900 and 1,450 amino acids. Homomeric NR1 receptors possess the full complement of pharmacological features of bona fide NMDA receptors. All agonist and regulatory binding sites, thus, are encoded by a single gene. Agonist-induced cation currents are very small in homomeric NR1 receptors but are increased more than 100-fold by coexpression with one of the NR2 subunits. This suggests that most NMDA receptors in the brain are probably heteromeric receptors, as is likely to be the case with AMPA and KA receptors. Inclusion of NR3A reduces the open time and conductance of single NMDA receptor channels, suggesting NR3A plays a regulatory role. The mRNAs encoding most NMDA receptor subunits are distributed differentially, as are those of other glutamate receptors. Expression of *NR1* mRNA is

nearly ubiquitous in the CNS. In contrast, the four *NR2* genes show differential patterns of expression (Fig. 15-3). Like *NR1*, *NR2A* is present throughout the forebrain and cerebellum. However, *NR2B* and *NR2C* have a more limited distribution. Expression of *NR2B* is highest in the forebrain and *NR2C* is expressed most highly in the cerebellum, where *NR2B* mRNA is not detected. Expression of *NR2D* seems virtually complementary to that of *NR2A* in being high in the midbrain and hindbrain but low in the forebrain. NR3A distribution is widespread except in the cerebellum.

NMDA receptors are among the most tightly regulated neurotransmitter receptors. There are no fewer than six distinct binding sites for endogenous ligands that influence the probability of ion-channel opening (Fig. 15-2). These consist of two different agonist-recognition

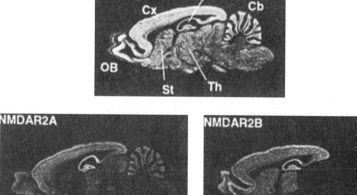

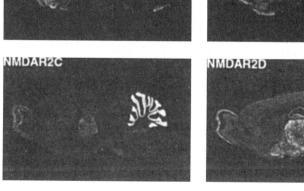

FIGURE 15-3. Regional distribution of mRNAs encoding the five NMDA receptor genes in adult rat brain, by *in situ* hybridization. *OB,* olfactory bulb; *Cx,* cortex; *Hi,* hippocampus; *Cb,* cerebellum; *Th,* thalamus; *St,* striatum. (From [30], with permission.)

sites, one for glutamate and one for glycine, and a polyamine regulatory site, all of which promote receptor activation, and separate recognition sites for Mg^{2+}, Zn^{2+} and H^+ that inhibit ion flux through agonist-bound receptors.

NMDA receptor agonists are typically short-chain dicarboxylic amino acids, such as glutamate, aspartate and NMDA. Acting at the conventional agonist-binding site, glutamate is the most potent agonist endogenous to the mammalian brain. NMDA itself, although a very selective agonist at these receptors, is 30-fold less potent than glutamate in electrophysiological assays. It is important to note that the natural transmitter aspartate appears to recognize only NMDA receptors, being inactive at AMPA and probably at KA receptors.

Competitive antagonists of the glutamate-recognition site are formed from the corresponding agonists by extending the carbon chain, sometimes in a ring structure and often including replacement of the ω-carboxyl group with a phosphonic acid group. Numerous competitive antagonists of this recognition site are available, notably D-2-amino-5-phosphonopentanoic acid (D-AP5) and 3-(2-carboxypiperazin-4-yl)1-propenyl-1-phosphonic acid (2R-CPPene), the latter having a K_d of approximately 40 nM in binding and functional studies. These compounds are polar and penetrate the blood–brain barrier only poorly, although several NMDA receptor blockers have been developed that have better access to the brain from the blood.

The NMDA receptor is unique among all known neurotransmitter receptors in its requirement for the simultaneous binding of two different agonists for activation. In addition to the conventional agonist-binding site typically occupied by glutamate, the binding of glycine appears to be required for receptor activation [7]. Because neither glycine nor glutamate acting alone can open this ion channel, they are referred to as coagonists of the NMDA receptor [7]. The glycine site on the NMDA receptor is pharmacologically distinct from the classical inhibitory glycine receptor (see Chap. 16) in that it is not blocked by strychnine and is not activated by β-alanine. Several small analogs of glycine, including serine and alanine, also act as agonists

at this site. In both cases, the D-isomer is 20- to 30-fold more potent than the L-isomer. Bicyclic compounds and many derivatives of either kynurenic acid or quinoxalinedicarboxylic acid are competitive antagonists of the glycine site. Interestingly, most glycine site antagonists in these two series also competitively block the agonist-recognition site of AMPA receptors, suggesting possible structural similarities in the two ligand-recognition sites. Halogenation of both ring structures typically induces a large increase in potency, with 5,7-dichlorokynurenic acid (5,7-DCK) being a very potent, $K_d = 60$ nM, and highly selective glycine-site antagonist.

Thus, glutamate and glycine act in concert to open NMDA ion channels. In contrast, a very important brake on NMDA receptor activation is provided by extracellular Mg^{2+}, which exerts a voltage-dependent block of the open ion channel [8]. Other voltage-dependent blockers of NMDA receptor channels include MK-801, the anesthetic ketamine and the recreational drug of abuse phencyclidine (PCP). These blockers and Mg^{2+} exhibit varying degrees of voltage dependence and, therefore, probably recognize somewhat different domains in the channel of the NMDA receptor.

Another important endogenous allosteric inhibitor of NMDA receptor activation is pH. The frequency of NMDA receptor channel openings is reduced by protons over the physiological pH range, with a midpoint at pH 7.4, such that at pH 6.0 receptor activation is suppressed nearly completely [9]. This suggests that an ionizable histidine or cysteine may play a key role in receptor activation. One or more modulatory sites that bind polyamines, such as spermine and spermidine, also are found on NMDA receptors. Occupancy of one of the polyamine sites relieves tonic proton block and, thus, potentiates NMDA receptor activation in a pH-dependent manner [9]. At higher concentrations, however, polyamines act on an extracellular site to produce a voltage-dependent block of the ion channel and, thus, inhibit receptor activation.

In addition to the regulatory mechanisms discussed above, an interesting form of Ca^{2+}-dependent inactivation of NMDA receptors is brought about by calmodulin. Activated by Ca^{2+} entry, calmodulin interacts with the C-terminal domain of the NR1 subunit; this interaction causes inactivation of the receptor, manifested by reduced channel opening frequency and reduced channel open time [10]. The Ca^{2+}/calmodulin-dependent phosphatase calcineurin inactivates NMDA receptors [11], suggesting a two-step process for modulation involving dephosphorylation of the NMDA receptor followed by binding of Ca^{2+}/calmodulin.

The transmembrane topology of glutamate receptors differs from that of nicotinic receptors

Knowledge about which segments of a receptor are intracellular, extracellular and transmembrane is necessary for identifying the ligand-recognition sites, for understanding the mechanism by which ligand binding leads to channel opening, for interpreting mutagenesis data and for identifying potential targets for drug development. A variety of experimental approaches indicate that nicotinic-receptor subunits have four transmembrane domains, with both N and C termini facing the extracellular fluid (Chap. 11). However, analysis of the protease sensitivity of the AMPA receptor subunit GluR3 fused at different positions to a large reporter group in-

dicated only three transmembrane domains [12]. Most interestingly, the channel-lining M2 domain, which controls ion permeation was found to be a re-entrant pore loop, with both ends facing the cytoplasm (Fig. 15-4). Homology mapping of the glutamate receptors onto the crystal structure of bacterial amino acid-binding proteins and functional evaluation of GluR3 through GluR6 chimeras suggests that agonist binding requires portions of both the large N terminus and a short region between M3 and M4, as illustrated in Figure 15-4. Subsequent studies of NMDA receptor subunits provided evidence for a similar transmembrane topology [13], suggesting that the glutamate receptor family has a topology different from that of other ligand-gated ion channels, typified by the nicotinic acetylcholine receptors.

Genetic regulation via splice variants and RNA editing further increases receptor heterogeneity

Splice variants that impart functional differences and/or different cellular expression patterns have been found for most of the glutamate receptor subunits. The first splice variants to be described are the so-called flip and flop versions

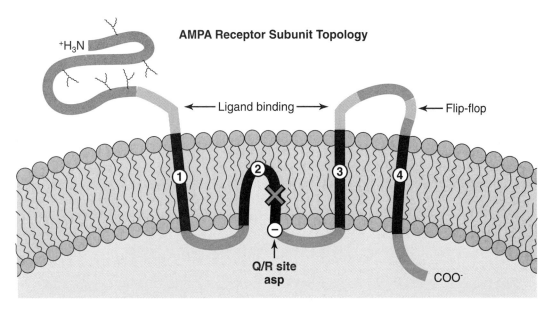

AMPA Receptor Subunit Topology

^+H_3N

← Ligand binding →

← Flip-flop

Q/R site
asp

COO$^-$

FIGURE 15-4. Transmembrane topology and functional domains of AMPA receptors. The *X* represents the location of the Q/R site in the second membrane domain.

of the AMPA receptor subunits GluR1 through GluR4 [14]. The mRNA encoding each of these subunits exists in two versions, differing by a 115-base pair (bp) segment. Within this encoded cassette of 38 amino acids that lie in the M3–M4 extracellular loop (Fig. 15-4), the two alternative versions differ by only nine to eleven amino acids, these being mostly conservative substitutions. The flip and flop splice variants give rise to receptors that differ in desensitization rate and in regional distribution in the brain. Additional C-terminal splice isoforms of GluR4 exist and are differentially expressed in the cerebellum, one predominantly in granule cells and the other in Bergmann glial cells. Alternative splicing of GluR5 near the C terminus also has been demonstrated. Alternative exon selection within the large N-terminal extracellular domain of NR1 influences many modulatory sites, including those sensitive to pH, spermine and Zn^{2+}. Thus, alternative exon selection is used by neurons to fine-tune the properties of all three classes of glutamate receptor.

An important form of regulation appears to be achieved by editing the primary RNA transcripts of the AMPA and KA receptor subunits. For example, AMPA receptors that contain the GluR2 subunit are much less permeable to Ca^{2+} than those assembled without GluR2. This important feature of GluR2 was traced by site-directed mutagenesis techniques to a single amino acid within the second membrane-associated domain [15]. A glutamine (Q) resides in this position in GluR1, GluR3 and GluR4, but an arginine (R) is present in GluR2 (Fig. 15-5); thus, this site has been named the "Q/R site." In addition to Ca^{2+} permeability, the Q/R site influences the single-channel conductance and the sensitivity of the activated receptor to block by polyamine spider toxins and internal polyamines. Voltage-dependent block by internal polyamines gives rise to inward rectification of AMPA receptors with low GluR2 abundance. Interestingly, the genomic DNA sequence has a glutamine codon in the Q/R position, even for subunits such as GluR2, in which the mature mRNA has an arginine codon in this site. A double-stranded RNA adenosine deaminase is employed as an "editor" to control the amino acid encoded by this critical codon [16]. RNA editing and associated changes in ionic permeability also have been demonstrated for some KA receptor subunits. The conditions under which neurons utilize RNA editing to regulate the permeability properties of their glutamate receptors remain to be demonstrated.

Given this combination of internal and C-terminal splice variants and Q/R editing, it appears that four to eight or more mature RNAs can be made from each of the 16 known genes encoding ionotropic receptor subunits. Thus, neurons have a massive degree of flexibility in

AMPA Receptors: Role of Q/R Site in Permeation

	M2
GluR1	Q
GluR2	NEFGIFNSLWFSLGAFMRQGCDISPRSLS
GluR3	Q
GluR4	Q

Receptors	Internal polyamines	Pca	External polyamine spider toxins	γ (pS)
Lacking GluR2	Block	High	Block	7/16/27
+ GluR2 (R)	No block	Low	No effect	4/8
+ GluR2 (Q)	Block	High	Block	7/16/24

FIGURE 15-5. Location and role of Q/R site in ion permeation through AMPA receptors. The amino acid sequences of GluR1-GluR4 are identical within the pore loop (see Fig. 15-4) except for the Q/R site, as shown. The phenotypes of AMPA receptors containing edited or unedited GluR2 or lacking GluR2 are summarized. Pca, calcium permeability; γ(pS), single channel conductance.

constructing a potentially huge number of receptors. The actual degree of glutamate receptor heterogeneity utilized by neurons remains a major unanswered question.

The permeation pathway of all glutamate receptors is similar

Current flow through AMPA receptors containing GluR2 normally is carried largely by the movement of Na^+ from the extracellular face to the intracellular compartment; these receptors have very low Ca^{2+} permeability. However, receptors that lack GluR2 are three to five times more permeable to Ca^{2+} than to the monovalent ions [15], due to the absence of an arginine in the Q/R site, as mentioned above. An asparagine residing in the homologous site of all NMDA receptor subunits confers high Ca^{2+} permeability on these receptors [17]; replacement of this asparagine with an arginine by site-directed mutagenesis produces NMDA receptors with very low Ca^{2+} permeability, similar to that of GluR2-containing AMPA receptors. An arginine or glutamine residing in the Q/R site of all known KA receptor subunits also strongly influences the degree of Ca^{2+} permeability. Thus, it is likely that the critical portion of the pore that forms the cation "selectivity filter" is similar among all glutamate receptors.

The permeation pathway of NMDA receptors has a property that sets them apart from other conventional ligand-gated receptors. At hyperpolarized membrane potentials more negative than about -70 mV, the concentration of Mg^{2+} in the extracellular fluid of the brain is sufficient to virtually abolish ion flux through NMDA receptor channels even in the presence of the coagonists glutamate and glycine [8] (Fig. 15-6C). Thus, although glutamate or aspartate is bound to the receptive site and the channel is "activated," the entry of Mg^{2+} into the channel pore blocks the movement of monovalent ions across the channel (Fig. 15-2). In the presence of Mg^{2+} ions, NMDA receptor channels exhibit a characteristic J-shaped current–voltage relationship (Fig. 15-6C). As the membrane potential is made less negative or even positive, the affinity of Mg^{2+} for its binding site decreases and the

block becomes ineffective. Depolarization-induced relief from voltage-dependent channel block by Mg^{2+} is at the root of several of the most interesting aspects of NMDA receptor function (see below).

METABOTROPIC RECEPTORS MODULATE SYNAPTIC TRANSMISSION

Eight metabotropic glutamate receptors that embody three functional classes have been identified

Metabotropic glutamate receptors (mGluRs) are so named because they are linked by G proteins to cytoplasmic enzymes (see [1] for review). To date, eight mGluRs have been cloned and named mGluR1 through mGluR8. The genes for these receptors appear to encode seven-membrane-spanning proteins, and like the ionotropic receptors, they possess an unusually large extracellular domain preceding the membrane-spanning segments. Metabotropic glutamate receptors have been grouped into three functional classes based on amino acid-sequence homology, agonist pharmacology and the signal-transduction pathways to which they are coupled (Fig. 15-1). Members of each class share ~70% sequence homology, with about 45% homology between classes. Alternatively spliced variants have been described for mGluR1, mGluR4, mGluR5 and mGluR7.

Glutamate itself activates all of the recombinant metabotropic glutamate receptors but with widely varying potencies, ranging from 2 nM, in the case of mGluR8, to 1,000 μM, in the case of mGluR7. Highly selective agonists for each of the three groups have been identified. L-Amino-4-phosphonobutyrate (L-AP4) is a selective agonist of group III; 2R,4R-4-aminopyrrolidine-2-4-dicarboxylate (APDC) is a highly selective and reasonably potent (400 nM) agonist for group II, whereas 3,5-dihydroxyphenylglycine appears to be a selective group I agonist. Some other phenylglycine derivatives are antagonists of metabotropic glutamate receptors, but highly group-selective antagonists have not yet been identified.

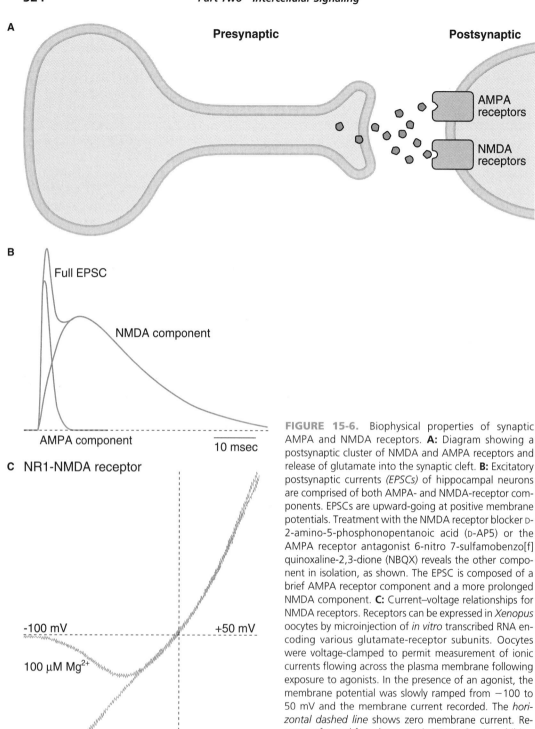

A

Presynaptic   Postsynaptic

AMPA
receptors

NMDA
receptors

B

Full EPSC

NMDA component

AMPA component

10 msec

C NR1-NMDA receptor

-100 mV   +50 mV

100 μM Mg^{2+}

0 Mg^{2+}

FIGURE 15-6. Biophysical properties of synaptic AMPA and NMDA receptors. **A:** Diagram showing a postsynaptic cluster of NMDA and AMPA receptors and release of glutamate into the synaptic cleft. **B:** Excitatory postsynaptic currents *(EPSCs)* of hippocampal neurons are comprised of both AMPA- and NMDA-receptor components. EPSCs are upward-going at positive membrane potentials. Treatment with the NMDA receptor blocker D-2-amino-5-phosphonopentanoic acid (D-AP5) or the AMPA receptor antagonist 6-nitro 7-sulfamobenzo[f] quinoxaline-2,3-dione (NBQX) reveals the other component in isolation, as shown. The EPSC is composed of a brief AMPA receptor component and a more prolonged NMDA component. **C:** Current–voltage relationships for NMDA receptors. Receptors can be expressed in *Xenopus* oocytes by microinjection of *in vitro* transcribed RNA encoding various glutamate-receptor subunits. Oocytes were voltage-clamped to permit measurement of ionic currents flowing across the plasma membrane following exposure to agonists. In the presence of an agonist, the membrane potential was slowly ramped from −100 to 50 mV and the membrane current recorded. The *horizontal dashed line* shows zero membrane current. Receptors formed from homomeric NRIA subunits exhibit a roughly linear current–voltage relationship in the absence of Mg^{2+}, but in the presence of Mg^{2+}, current flux through NMDA receptor channels becomes progressively smaller as the membrane potential is made more negative. At −100 mV, the NMDA-induced current is virtually abolished by Mg^{2+}.

Metabotropic glutamate receptors are linked to diverse effector mechanisms

The classification of metabotropic glutamate receptors into three groups is further supported by a consideration of their signal-transduction mechanisms. Group I receptors stimulate phosphoinositide-specific phospholipase C (PI-PLC) activity and the release of Ca^{2+} from cytoplasmic stores (Figs. 15-1 and 15-2). The ability to increase intracellular Ca^{2+} levels differs between the members of this class and their splice variants, a property probably attributable to the different affinities each receptor has for the G protein. Activation of PI-PLC leads to the formation of not only inositol-1,4,5-trisphosphate (IP_3) but also diacylglycerol (DAG), which in turn activates protein kinase C (PKC) (see Chap. 21). Activation of group II and probably group III receptors results in inhibition of adenylyl cyclase (Figs. 15-1 and 15-2). This response is blocked by pertussis toxin, indicating that a G protein of the G_i family probably is involved (see Chap. 22).

Postsynaptic metabotropic glutamate receptors modulate ion channel activity

Metabotropic glutamate receptors located on the postsynaptic membrane modulate a wide variety of ligand- and voltage-gated ion channels expressed on central neurons, as would be expected if receptor activation is coupled to multiple effector enzymes. Activation of all three classes of mGluRs inhibits L-type voltage-dependent Ca^{2+} channels, and both group I and group II receptors inhibit N-type Ca^{2+} channels (Box 23-1). Metabotropic glutamate receptors also decrease a high-threshold Ca^{2+} current in spiking neurons of *Xenopus* retina. Metabotropic receptor activation closes voltage-dependent, acetylcholine-sensitive and Ca^{2+}-dependent K^+ channels in certain neurons, leading to slow depolarization and consequent neuronal excitation. The exact mechanism of mGluR modulation of K^+ currents is at present unclear. In cerebellar granule cells, stimulation of metabotropic glutamate receptors increases the activity of Ca^{2+} dependent and inwardly rectifying K^+ channels, leading to a reduction in excitability.

A large number of ligand-gated channels also are modulated by metabotropic glutamate receptor activation, including AMPA and NMDA receptors as well as dopamine, $GABA_A$ and norepinephrine receptors. Whether activation of metabotropic glutamate receptors inhibits or potentiates a receptor depends on what component of the signal-transduction mechanism is targeted and often is tissue-specific. For example, in hippocampal pyramidal cells, mGluR activation potentiates currents through NMDA receptors. The effect is reduced by PKC inhibitors and may be caused by a reduction in the affinity of the NMDA channel for its blocking ion, Mg^{2+}. In contrast, in cerebellar granule cells, metabotropic-glutamate receptor activation inhibits NMDA receptor-induced elevations of $[Ca^{2+}]_i$ also by a mechanism thought to involve PKC.

Metabotropic receptors can mediate presynaptic inhibition

Immunohistochemical studies at both the light and electron microscopic level have firmly placed a number of mGluRs at the presynaptic terminals of central neurons. Activation of presynaptic metabotropic glutamate receptors blocks both excitatory glutamatergic and inhibitory GABAergic synaptic transmission in a variety of central structures. For example, mossy fiber-evoked excitatory postsynaptic potentials (EPSPs) onto CA3 hippocampal pyramidal neurons are blocked by activation of mGluR2, which is located on presynaptic granule cell terminals. In contrast, transmission at synapses between Schaffer collaterals and CA1 pyramidal cells is resistant to mGluR2 agonists but is blocked by L-AP4, suggesting activation of mGluR4 or mGluR7. The actual mechanism of how mGluR activation regulates synaptic transmission is unclear. However, because all three mGluR groups inhibit voltage-dependent Ca^{2+} channels, it seems highly probable that presynaptic Ca^{2+} channels are a target for mGluR modulation. This has been demonstrated directly in the presynaptic terminal of the calyx of Held, where mGluR agonists suppress a high voltage-activated P/Q-type Ca^{2+} conductance, thereby inhibiting transmitter release at this glutamatergic synapse [18].

Genetic knockouts provide clues to metabotropic glutamate receptor functions

The ability to ascertain the precise physiological functions of metabotropic glutamate receptors has been hampered, in part, by the lack of sufficiently potent and selective pharmacological agents. The use of alternative strategies for the study of mGluRs, therefore, is clearly warranted. To address this problem, several groups have used gene targeting to produce knockout mice (see Chap. 40) that are devoid of the mGluR subtype of interest. These experiments have strongly suggested a physiological role for a number of receptors. Establishment of specific neuronal connections in the mature nervous system occurs through a process by which redundant connections formed during development are eliminated. In the adult cerebellum, each Purkinje cell is innervated by a single climbing fiber (CF) that originates from the inferior olive of the medulla. This one-to-one relationship is preceded by a developmental stage in which each Purkinje cell is innervated by multiple CFs. Massive elimination of synapses formed by CFs occurs postnatally, and a monosynaptic relationship is established at around postnatal day 20. Mice lacking the mGluR1 gene show symptoms of cerebellar dysfunction, such as ataxic gait, intention tremor and dysmetria, and are impaired in motor coordination and motor learning [19]. These mutant mice are deficient in long-term depression (LTD) at CF–Purkinje cell synapses, a form of synaptic plasticity in the cerebellum thought to be a cellular basis for motor learning (see Chap. 50). In addition, innervation of multiple CFs onto a Purkinje cell persists into adulthood in mGluR1 mutant mice, suggesting that the precise sculpting of these synaptic connections requires activation of mGluR1 during development.

The strong expression of mGluR2 in dentate gyrus granule cells has suggested a role for these receptors in presynaptic regulation of transmission at the mossy fiber–CA3 pyramidal neuron synapses, as described above. In mice lacking the mGluR2 gene, basal synaptic transmission and paired-pulse facilitation at the hippocampal mossy fiber to CA3 pyramidal synapses were indistinguishable from wild-type responses. In contrast, presynaptic inhibition at mossy fiber synapses induced by the mGluR2 agonist DCG-IV was reduced markedly in mutant mice, confirming a role for mGluR2 in the presynaptic regulation of neurotransmission. Interestingly, this mGluR2 deficiency was without effect on the magnitude of long-term potentiation (LTP) induced at these synapses, but LTD was impaired significantly [20]. These data suggest that mGluR2 is not required for mossy fiber LTP but is essential for mossy fiber LTD. In a variety of CNS structures, including the hippocampus, olfactory tract, spinal cord and thalamus, activation of presynaptically located group III mGluRs by L-AP4 inhibits synaptic transmission. One member of this group, mGluR4, is preferentially expressed in the cerebellum and has a role in the presynaptic regulation of synaptic transmission. Targeted elimination of the *mGluR4* gene reveals that mGluR4 is essential in providing a presynaptic mechanism for maintaining synaptic efficacy during repetitive activation and suggests that the presence of *mGluR4* at the parallel fiber–Purkinje cell synapse is required for maintaining normal motor function [21].

GLUTAMATE AND ASPARTATE ARE THE MAJOR EXCITATORY TRANSMITTERS IN THE BRAIN

Historically, the most compelling evidence that glutamate and aspartate function as neurotransmitters came from the observation that at low concentrations they excite virtually every neuron in the CNS. In the adult CNS, L-glutamate and L-aspartate are the most likely candidates for neurotransmitter action at excitatory amino acid receptors, and these amino acids are used by some of the most widely distributed neuronal types. Glutamate and aspartate are present in high concentrations in the CNS and are released in a Ca^{2+}-dependent manner upon electrical stimulation *in vitro*. Both have powerful excitatory effects on neurons when iontophoresed *in vivo*. High-affinity uptake systems have been cloned and are located in nerve terminals and glial cells associated with many neuronal pathways (see below). Selective binding sites can be demonstrated by both autoradiographic immunohistochemical and pharmacological techniques *in vitro*. Although the unequivocal identification of glutamate and aspartate as neurotransmitter candidates has been hampered by their involvement in many other functions, they are accepted universally in this role.

Glutamate and aspartate are nonessential amino acids that do not cross the blood—brain barrier and, therefore, are synthesized from glucose and a variety of other precursors. Synthetic and metabolic enzymes for glutamate and aspartate have been localized to the two main compartments of the brain, neurons and glial cells (Fig. 15-7). Glutamic acid is in a metabolic pool with α-ketoglutaric acid and glutamine. A large

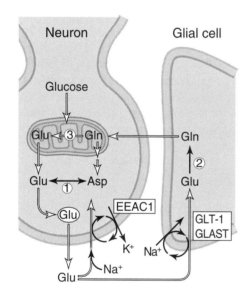

FIGURE 15-7. Metabolism of glutamate in synaptic structures. Glutamate is synthesized and stored within synaptic endings of nerve terminals. Synthesis of transmitter pools of glutamate is likely to involve two major synthetic pathways. The conversion of glutamine to glutamate involves the enzymatic action of glutaminase ③ within the mitochondrial compartment. Glutamate formation also occurs by a process of transamination ①. Newly synthesized glutamate is then packaged and stored in high concentration within synaptic vesicles. After release of glutamate from the nerve terminal into the synaptic cleft, it is taken up into glial cells by glutamate transporter-1 *(GLT-1)* and glutamate–aspartate transporter *(GLAST)* and converted into glutamine ②. Glutamine is then cycled back to the nerve terminal, where it participates in the replenishment of transmitter stores of glutamate. Alternatively, some glutamatergic nerve terminals contain the excitatory amino acid carrier-1 *(EAAC1)*, which recovers glutamate directly.

fraction of the glutamate released from nerve terminals probably is taken up into glial cells, where it is converted into glutamine. Glutamine then cycles back to nerve terminals, where it participates in the replenishment of the transmitter pools of glutamate and GABA. At present, there is little evidence for the extracellular metabolism of glutamate in the CNS.

The transmitter pool of glutamate is stored in synaptic vesicles

Electron-microscopic analysis of glutamate immunoreactive puncta within the cortex has shown that many of these structures are axon terminals. Most glutamate-positive axon terminals form asymmetrical synaptic contacts on small- and medium-caliber dendritic shafts and spines; glutamate-positive axon terminals on cell bodies are extremely rare.

Synaptic vesicles actively accumulate glutamate through a Mg^{2+}/ATP-dependent process. This uptake mechanism is inhibited by substances that destroy the electrochemical gradient. The concentration of glutamate within synaptic vesicles is thought to be very high, in excess of 20 mM. Aspartate is neither an inhibitor nor a substrate for this vesicular uptake mechanism. A vesicular uptake mechanism for aspartate has not yet been demonstrated, somewhat weakening the case for considering aspartate to be a neurotransmitter. In hippocampal slices, however, reduction of the extracellular glucose concentration strongly reduces KCl-evoked glutamate release but enhances aspartate release, suggesting that when glutamate and aspartate metabolism via the tricarboxylic acid cycle is perturbed, aspartate may become preferentially available for release during synaptic transmission.

Glutamate-receptor activation underlies most fast excitatory synaptic transmission in the brain

Both AMPA and NMDA receptors are present on most CNS neurons, although there are a few notable exceptions. Accordingly, activation of AMPA and NMDA receptors appears to underlie the vast majority of "fast" synaptic transmission in the CNS. The concentration of glutamate required to half-maximally activate AMPA receptors is approximately 200 μM, about two orders of magnitude less than the concentration thought to be contained within synaptic vesicles; glutamate is much more potent on NMDA receptors, with an EC_{50} of 10 to 15 μM. Therefore, synaptically released glutamate has a high probability of transiently saturating its receptors on the adjacent cell. Considerable evidence suggests that on many cell types AMPA and NMDA receptors are clustered together within the same postsynaptic densities (Fig. 15-6A). Receptor clustering appears to be mediated by binding of the extreme C-terminal tail of certain glutamate-receptor subunits to a family of proteins that express the PDZ modular protein interaction domain (Fig. 15-2). These PDZ-containing proteins presumably form a scaffold or bridge between receptor and cytoskeletal proteins located near the postsynaptic membrane. This close apposition results in the simultaneous activation of these receptors. The integration of current flow through the two receptor systems endows the cell with a powerful means of regulating neuronal excitation. It should be remembered that aspartate has little or no affinity for AMPA receptors, so synaptically released aspartate will activate only NMDA receptors.

Both NMDA- and AMPA-receptor components of the EPSP are thought to be produced by a brief (1 msec) appearance of free transmitter in the synaptic cleft. Synaptically released glutamate thus results in a two-component excitatory postsynaptic current (EPSC) upon binding to AMPA and NMDA receptors at most central synapses (Fig. 15-6B). Activation of AMPA receptors mediates a component that has a rapid onset and decay, whereas the component mediated by NMDA receptor activation has a slower rise time and a decay lasting up to several hundred milliseconds (Fig. 15-6C). Rapid desensitization of AMPA receptors may control the time course of EPSPs at many synapses. The long time course of NMDA receptor activation, by contrast, provides more opportunities for temporal and spatial summation of multiple inputs. The resulting summed depolarization may allow other synaptic inputs or nonsynaptic membrane channels to initiate action potentials. The decay

time of the NMDA receptor component is approximately 100 times longer than the mean open time of the channel. The more prolonged activation of NMDA receptors is thought to be due to the higher affinity of glutamate for NMDA than AMPA receptors; high affinity often results from a slow dissociation of the agonist from its receptor, which could result in multiple channel activations for each against binding event.

Ca^{2+} influx through *N*-methyl-D-aspartate and AMPA receptors mediates synaptic plasticity

Although activation of NMDA receptors results in appreciable current flow and tends to depolarize the cell membrane toward threshold for an action potential, this is unlikely to be the sole role of this receptor when activated at typical resting membrane potentials because NMDA receptors are highly permeable to Ca^{2+}, as mentioned above. Likewise, AMPA receptors on some interneurons have no GluR2 subunits and are permeable to Ca^{2+} as described above. Thus, an important role of NMDA and some AMPA receptors may be to inject Ca^{2+} into the postsynaptic membrane.

The high permeability of NMDA receptor channels for divalent cations has many implications for cell function. Ca^{2+} concentration within the cell interior is heavily buffered to about 100 nM. The elevation of cytoplasmic Ca^{2+} by Ca^{2+} entry through NMDA-receptor channels may lead to the transient activation of a variety of Ca^{2+}-activiated enzymes, including Ca^{2+}/calmodulin-dependent protein kinase II, calcineurin, PKC, phospholipase A$_2$, PI-PLC, nitric oxide synthase and a number of endonucleases. Activation of each of these enzymes occurs as a result of Ca^{2+} entry following glutamate-receptor activation. Although a variety of forms of synaptic plasticity have been found in the mammalian CNS, LTP and LTD of excitatory synaptic responses in hippocampal CA1 pyramidal cells have been characterized most extensively. LTP and LTD are activity-dependent alterations in synaptic efficacy that can last up to several weeks *in vivo* and are thought to be involved in the acquisition of spatial memories (Chap. 50).

Receptor knockouts reveal clues to ionotropic receptor functions

In most neurons, high expression of the edited GluR2 subunit ensures that synaptic AMPA receptors will permit only insignificant Ca^{2+} influx. However, mice engineered to harbor an editing-incompetent *GluR2* gene expressed AMPA receptors with increased Ca^{2+} permeability [22]. These mice developed seizures and died by 3 weeks of age, demonstrating that GluR2 editing is essential for normal brain development. Deletion of the GluR2 editing enzyme RAD1 by gene targeting produces the same phenotype. Surprisingly, complete deletion of the GluR2 allele, which also increases Ca^{2+} permeability of AMPA receptors in targeted mouse neurons, neither induced seizures nor proved lethal in homozygous mice. Rather, Ca^{2+} entry through GluR2-lacking synaptic AMPA receptors could produce a form of LTP [23]. It is unclear why these two genetic manipulations had such different outcomes, although it is possible that a complete absence of GluR2 impairs AMPA receptor assembly because the density of synaptic AMPA receptors appeared to be low in the latter study.

Conventional gene targeting of the NMDA receptor NR1 subunit interferes with breathing and is lethal within a few hours of birth. However, mouse strains in which the NR1 gene knockout is restricted to the CA1 region of the hippocampus survive and grow normally [24]. This was accomplished by using a clever second-generation cre-loxP strategy for gene targeting. Temporal and spatial restriction of gene knockouts using the cre-loxP system should be applicable to any gene and may circumvent developmental problems associated with conventional strategies. With this approach, 34-bp loxP elements were inserted to flank the NR1 gene, rendering the gene susceptible to the action of the enzyme cre recombinase. Mice with a "floxed" NR1 allele were mated with transgenic mice that harbored a *cre* gene under the control of a calmodulin kinase II promoter, which restricted expression of cre to the CA1 pyramidal neurons, predominantly after postnatal day 21. In these mice, the *NR1* gene was deleted by cre but only in CA1 pyramidal cells. Remarkably, LTP was impaired in the CA1 but not other hippocampal regions, and these mice exhibited impaired spatial memory in a water maze task. These findings demonstrate the essential role of NMDA receptors in LTP in the CA1 region and strongly suggest that LTP in the CA1 region is necessary for the acquisition of spatial memory.

GLUTAMATE TRANSPORTERS

As zwitterionic molecules, glutamate and aspartate are unable to diffuse across membranes. It is now well documented that uptake mechanisms have an important role in regulating the extracellular concentrations of glutamate and aspartate in the brain. At least two families of glutamate transporter have been localized to the plasma membrane of neurons and astrocytes (Fig. 15-7). Only the Na^+-dependent glutamate transporter is coupled to the electrochemical gradient that permits transport of glutamate and aspartate against their concentration gradients. To date, four members of the Na^+-dependent glutamate transporter family have been cloned [25]. Na^+-dependent glutamate transporters transport L-aspartate and L-glutamate with similar apparent affinity and maximum velocity. Unlike many of the other CNS transport systems, this process transports D-aspartate with similar affinity but does not transport D-glutamate.

Three members of this family have been cloned to date: the glutamate–aspartate transporter (GLAST), glutamate transporter-1 (GLT-1) and excitatory amino acid carrier-1 (EAAC1). Human orthologs of these three transporters also have been cloned (EAAT1, EAAT2 and EAAT3). Another member of this family, EAAT4, was cloned from human motor cortex. The glutamate transporters share little or no sequence similarity with other Na^+-dependent transporters, such as those for norepinephrine, dopamine, GABA and serotonin, and therefore, are members of a new gene family. The predicted amino acid sequences of the three proteins share ~50% homology with one another.

In the CNS, GLT-1 and GLAST are expressed preferentially in glial cells. GLT-1 has its highest expression in the thalamus and cerebellum, with lower levels in the hippocampus, cortex and striatum. GLAST immunoreactivity is found predominantly in the cerebellum and less so in the forebrain. In contrast, EAAC1 is expressed predominantly in neurons, most prominently in the hippocampus, and is absent from glial cells. The expression patterns of the three members of this family, therefore, suggest that GLT-1 and GLAST represent the primary transport carrier for glutamate uptake into glia, while EAAC1 is involved predominantly in neuronal glutamate and aspartate uptake (Fig. 15-7). Na^+-dependent glutamate transporters, unlike other amine transporters, are not Cl^--dependent. The net transport of glutamate is increased by high intracellular K^+; upon dissociation of glutamate and Na^+ from the transport machinery, cytoplasmic K^+ binds to be recycled into the extracellular compartment. With each cycle, two Na^+ ions accompany the movement of glutamate or aspartate into the intracellular compartment, with one K^+ ion being transported out, accompanied by either OH^- or HCO_3^-. Therefore, one complete cycle results in a net positive movement of charge into the cell.

A major role for glutamate transporters is to limit the free concentrations of glutamate and aspartate in the extracellular space, thus preventing excessive stimulation of glutamate receptors [26]. It is likely that membrane depolarization during ischemic insult causes reverse transport of glutamate, or aspartate, out of glia and/or neurons. Accumulation of aspartate or glutamate in the extracellular space and the resulting excessive activation of glutamate receptors can result in a number of pathological conditions and, ultimately, cell death.

EXCESSIVE GLUTAMATE RECEPTOR ACTIVATION AND NEUROLOGICAL DISORDERS

Glutamate and aspartate can be excitotoxins, especially when energy metabolism is compromised

Glutamate and other amino acids were first recognized as neurotoxins in the 1970s when these agents were given orally to immature animals. Acute neurodegeneration was observed in those areas not well protected by the blood–brain bar-

rier, notably the arcuate nucleus of the hypothalamus. The mechanisms of neurodegeneration are divergent, and activation of all classes of ionotropic glutamate receptor has been implicated. Neurodegeneration, for example, following an ischemic insult, may involve mechanisms resembling a pathological exaggeration of LTP-like phenomena; that is, the neuronal insult results partially from AMPA receptor activation with concomitant NMDA receptor involvement and Ca^{2+} influx.

Metabolic inhibition that leads to impaired ATP production predisposes neurons to glutamate-mediated neurotoxicity [27]. Numerous mechanisms contribute, including impaired cytoplasmic Ca^{2+} homeostasis and release of oxygen free radicals, which exacerbate damage. Deficits in energy metabolism occur in ischemic tissue and are prominent in some chronic neurodegenerative disorders. Understanding the interplay between mitochondrial function and sensitivity to glutamate overloads may provide new molecular targets for neuroprotective therapy.

Intracerebroventricular injection of kainic acid results in a well-characterized pattern of neuronal cell damage. In the hippocampus, kainic acid causes an axon-sparing selective lesion of the CA3 pyramidal neurons, an area rich in *KA1* and *GluR6* mRNA expression (see above). The consequences of kainic acid lesioning are cell death and epileptiform discharges in cells normally innervated by the damaged pyramidal neurons. Other cell types in the hippocampus are relatively unharmed. This suggests that activation of KA receptors may contribute to this toxic effect of kainic acid.

Glutamate receptors are involved in ischemic cell damage and neuroprotection

Periods of anoxic insult to neuronal tissue that last more than a few seconds, such as during cardiac arrest or thrombotic stroke, often result in neurotoxicity (see Chap. 34). Oxygen deprivation precipitates a depletion of energy stores within neuronal and glial cell compartments with a concomitant acidosis and release of free radicals (Fig. 15-8). Depletion of energy stores affects cellular metabolism, energy-dependent ionic pumps and the ability of cells to maintain resting membrane potential. Consequently, depolarization of cells results in action potentials and the release of glutamate from presynaptic terminals, which activates postsynaptic AMPA and NMDA receptors. Entry of Ca^{2+} through glutamate receptors and voltage-sensitive Ca^{2+} channels increases the intracellular concentration of Ca^{2+}. As described above, an elevation of intracellular Ca^{2+} will trigger a cascade of second-messenger systems, many of which remain activated long after the initial stimulus is removed. The inability of a population of cells to maintain a resting potential thus precipitates a positive feedback loop, leading to neuronal cell injury or death.

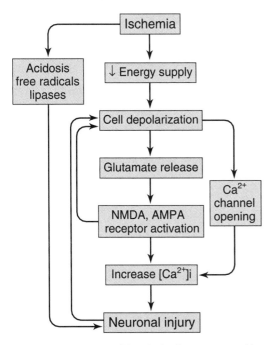

FIGURE 15-8. Potential paths leading to neuronal injury resulting from an episode of ischemic insult. An ischemic episode initiates a complex pathway involving the depletion of cellular energy stores and the release of free radicals. The energy depletion permits sustained activation of glutamate receptors and the consequent entry of Ca^{2+} via NMDA receptors, (GluR2 lacking) AMPA receptors and voltage-gated Ca^{2+} channels. Elevation of intracellular Ca^{2+} causes excessive activation of a variety of Ca^{2+}-dependent enzymes. Excessive neuronal depolarization results in neuronal injury and often cell death.

Animal models of ischemic cell injury have highlighted the potential benefits of suitable neuroprotectants targeted to the glutamate receptor family. In some stroke models, for example, administration of an NMDA receptor blocker even several hours after the initial insult results in substantial protection of the hippocampus and striatum, two of the regions most heavily damaged by interruption in blood supply. Ischemic tissue is acidotic due to release of lactate and other metabolites. The low pH should shut down certain splice variants of NMDA receptors, as described above, perhaps resulting in a natural neuroprotective action. Interestingly, some neuroprotective drugs, such as ifenprodil, appear to inhibit NMDA receptors by shifting the pK for the proton-accepting group in an alkaline direction, such that at physiological pH a larger fraction of the proton sites are occupied by protons, thus rendering a larger fraction of NMDA receptors unavailable for activation.

Epileptiform activity involves glutamate receptor activation

The involvement of excitatory amino acids in epilepsy has been well documented. A large number of animal models of epilepsy have clearly implicated a causal role for the glutamate-receptor family (see Chap. 37). Excessive stimulation of glutamatergic pathways, block of glutamate transporters or pharmacological manipulation resulting in glutamate-receptor activation can precipitate seizures. Epileptiform activity usually begins with excessive AMPA receptor activation; as seizure activity intensifies, an increased involvement of NMDA receptors is observed. Studies with a variety of animal models have shown that NMDA receptor antagonists can reduce the intensity and duration of seizure activity. Antagonism of AMPA-receptor activation usually prevents initiation of the seizure-like event. This suggests that epileptiform activity depends on the interplay between synaptic AMPA and NMDA receptors. Evidence from human tissue supports the role of amino acids in epilepsy. For example, in patients with refractory complex partial seizures with an associated structural focus, surgically removed hippocampal tissue shows an upregulation of AMPA and NMDA receptors.

Some neurodegenerative disorders may involve chronic glutamate receptor activation

Disorders of excitatory amino acid transmission have been implicated in amyotrophic lateral sclerosis (ALS) and the chronic neurodegenerative diseases olivopontocerebellar atrophy and Huntington's chorea. Neurolathyrism is a spastic disorder occurring in East Africa and India. It is associated with the dietary consumption of the legume *Lathyrus sativus*. The glutamate-like excitant β-*N*-oxalylamino-L-alanine has been identified as the toxin in this plant. Its action at AMPA receptors in the spinal cord may be responsible for the observed degeneration of lower and upper motor neurons.

The high incidence of ALS observed in residents of the Pacific island of Guam was determined to be due to the dietary ingestion of the cycad *Cyas circinalis*. This seed contains an amino acid, β-*N*-methylamino-L-alanine, which, in the presence of bicarbonate, becomes excitotoxic through a mechanism involving the activation of AMPA and NMDA receptors. Its action can be blocked by the NMDA receptor antagonist D-AP5. An important topic for future research will be to identify the roles, if any, that overactivation of glutamate receptors plays in such neurological disorders.

FUTURE PROSPECTS

Research directed toward understanding the functions of glutamate receptors has progressed in parallel with the expansion of neuroscience research since the 1980s. Indeed, demonstrations that glutamate receptors are involved in numerous physiological and pathophysiological phenomena continue to fuel a substantial fraction of neuroscience research. With the cloning and mutagenesis of the glutamate receptors, application of the patch voltage clamp and the refinement of neuroanatomical techniques, new opportunities have arisen to address the basic functions of these nearly ubiquitous neurotrans-

mitter receptors. The application of molecular biological approaches has been particularly instructive. For example, the transmembrane topology of subunits is known, the major structural domains responsible for ion permeation and ligand recognition have been identified and we know that different combinations of subunits assemble into receptors with different functional properties. The latter realization is quite important since it suggests that new therapeutic strategies that take advantage of the molecular diversity of these receptors might be devised.

Current and future research will seek to determine which subunit combinations are permissible *in situ*, the genetic regulation of glutamate receptor functions and the precise roles of glutamatergic pathways and receptor subtypes in neurological disorders, development and learning. Realization of these goals will require a coordinated effort from multiple disciplines.

REFERENCES

1. Conn, P. J., and Pin, J.-P. Pharmacology and functions of metabotropic glutamate receptors. *Annu. Rev. Pharmacol. Toxicol.* 37:205–238, 1997.
2. Hollmann, M., and Heinemann, S. Cloned glutamate receptors. *Annu. Rev. Neurosci.* 17:31–108, 1994.
3. Sucher, N. J., Awobuluyi, M., Choi, Y.-B., and Lipton, S. A. NMDA receptors: From genes to channels. *Trends Pharmacol. Sci.* 17:348–355, 1996.
4. Fletcher, E. J., and Lodge, D. New developments in the molecular pharmacology of α-amino-3-hydroxy-5-methyl-4-isoxazole propionate and kainate receptors. *Pharmacol. Ther.* 70:65–89, 1996.
5. Hollmann, M., O'Shea-Greenfield, A., Rogers, S. W., and Heinemann, S. F. Cloning by functional expression of a member of the glutamate receptor family. *Nature* 342:643–648, 1989.
6. Twyman, R. E., Gahring, L.-C., Spiess, J., and Rogers, S.-W. Glutamate receptor antibodies activate a subset of receptors and reveal an agonist binding site. *J. Biol. Chem.* 272:11295–11301, 1997.
7. Kleckner, N. W., and Dingledine, R. Requirement for glycine in activation of NMDA receptors expressed in *Xenopus* oocytes. *Science* 241:835–837, 1988.

8. Nowak, L., Bregestovski, P., Ascher, P., Herbet, A., and Prochiantz, A. Magnesium gates glutamate-activated channels in mouse central neurones. *Nature* 307:462–465, 1984.

9. Traynelis, S. F., Hartley, M., and Heinemann, S. F. Control of proton sensitivity of the NMDA receptor by RNA splicing and polyamines. *Science* 268:873–876, 1995.

10. Ehlers, M. D., Zhang, S., Bernhardt, J. P., and Huganir, R. L. Inactivation of NMDA receptors by direct interaction of calmodulin with the NMDA$_1$ subunit. *Cell* 84:745–755, 1996.

11. Tong, G., Shepard, D., and Jahr, C. E. Synaptic desensitization of NMDA receptors by calcineurin. *Science* 267:1510–1512, 1995.

12. Bennett, J. A., and Dingledine, R. Topology profile for a glutamate receptor: Three transmembrane domains and a channel-lining reentrant membrane loop. *Neuron* 14:373–384, 1995.

13. Kuner, T., Wollmuth, L. P., Karlin, A., Seeburg, P. H., and Sakmann, B. Structure of the NMDA receptor channel M2 segment inferred from the accessibility of substituted cysteines. *Neuron* 17:343–352, 1996.

14. Sommer, B., Keinanen, K., Verdoorn, T. A., et al. Flip and flop: A cell specific functional switch in glutamate-operated channels of the CNS. *Science* 249:1580–1585, 1990.

15. Hume, R. I., Dingledine, R., and Heinemann, S. F. Identification of a site in glutamate receptor subunits that controls calcium permeability. *Science* 253:1028–1032, 1991.

16. Higuchi, M., Single, F. N., Kohler, M., Sommer, B., Sprengel, R., and Seeburg, P. H. RNA editing of AMPA receptor subunit GluRB: A base-paired intron–exon structure determines position and efficiency. *Cell* 75:1361–1370, 1993.

17. Wollmuth, L. P., Kuner, T., Seeburg, P. H., and Sakmann, B. Differential contribution of the NMDA$_1$- and NMDA$_2$ A-subunits to the selectivity filter of recombinant NMDA receptor channels. *J. Physiol. (Lond.)* 491:779–797, 1996.

18. Takahashi, T., Forsythe, I. D., Tsujimoto, T., Barnes-Davies, M., and Onodera, K. Presynaptic calcium current modulation by a metabotropic glutamate receptor. *Science* 274:594–597, 1996.

19. Kano, M., Hashimoto, K., Kurihara, H., et al. Persistent multiple climbing fiber innervation of cerebellar Purkinje cells in mice lacking mGluR1. *Neuron* 18:71–79, 1997.

20. Yokoi, M., Kobayashi, K., Manabe, T., et al. Impairment of hippocampal mossy fiber LTD in mice lacking mGluR2. *Science* 273:645–647, 1996.

21. Pekhletski, R., Gerlai, R., Overstreet, L. S., et al. Impaired cerebellar synaptic plasticity and motor performance in mice lacking the mGluR4 subtype of metabotropic glutamate receptor *J. Neurosci.* 16:6364–6373, 1996.

22. Brusa, R., Zimmerman, F., Koh, D. S., et al. Early-onset epilepsy and postnatal lethality associated with an editing-deficient GluR-B allele in mice. *Science* 270:1677–1680, 1995.

23. Jia, Z., Agopyan, N., Miu, P., et al. Enhanced LTP in mice deficient in the AMPA receptor GluR2. *Neuron* 17:945–956, 1996.

24. Tsien, J. Z., Huerta, P. T., and Tonegawa, S. The essential role of hippocampal CA1 NMDA receptor-dependent synaptic plasticity in spatial memory. *Cell* 87:1327–1338, 1996.

25. Robinson, M. B., and Dowd, L. A. Heterogeneity and functional properties of subtypes of sodium-dependent glutamate transporters in the mammalian nervous system. *Adv. Pharmacol.* 37: 69–115, 1997.

26. Rothstein, J. D., Dykes-Hoberg, M., Pardo, C. A., et al. Knockout of glutamate transporter reveals a major role for astroglial transport in excitotoxicity and clearance of glutamate. *Neuron* 16:675–686, 1996.

27. Greene, J. G., and Greenamyre, T. Bioenergetics and glutamate toxicity. *Prog. Neurobiol.* 48: 613–634, 1996.

28. Dong, H., O'Brien, R. J., Fung, E. T., Lanahan, A. A., Worley, P. F., and Huganir R. L. GRIP: A synaptic PDZ domain-containing protein that interacts with AMPA receptors. *Nature* 386: 279–284, 1997.

29. Brakeman, P. R., Lanahan, A. A., O'Brien, R., et al. Homer: A protein that selectively binds metabotropic glutamate receptors. *Nature* 386: 284–288, 1997.

30. Nakanishi, S. Molecular diversity of glutamate receptors and implications for brain function. *Science* 258:597–603, 1992.

CHAPTER

16

GABA and Glycine

Richard W. Olsen and Timothy M. DeLorey

Basic Neurochemistry: Molecular, Cellular and Medical Aspects, 6th Ed., edited by G. J. Siegel et al. Published by Lippincott–Raven Publishers, Philadelphia, 1999. Correspondence to Richard W. Olsen, Department of Molecular and Medical Pharmacology, UCLA School of Medicine, Center for Health Sciences, 10833 LeConte Avenue, Los Angeles, California 90024-1735.

γ-Aminobutyric acid (GABA) is the major inhibitory neurotransmitter in the mammalian central nervous system (CNS). It was discovered in 1950 by Roberts and Awapara. Electrophysiological studies between 1950 and 1965 suggested a role for GABA as a neurotransmitter in the mammalian CNS. Since then, GABA has met the five classical criteria for assignment as a neurotransmitter: it is present in the nerve terminal, it is released from electrically stimulated neurons, there is a mechanism for terminating the action of the released neurotransmitter, its application to target neurons mimics the action of inhibitory nerve stimulation and specific receptors exist.

In view of the ubiquitous nature of GABA in the CNS, it is perhaps not too surprising that its functional significance should be far-reaching. A growing body of evidence suggests a role for altered GABAergic function in neurological and psychiatric disorders of humans, including Huntington's disease, epilepsy, tardive dyskinesia, alcoholism, schizophrenia, sleep disorders, Parkinson's disease and mental retardation. Pharmacological manipulation of GABAergic transmission is an effective approach for the treatment of anxiety [1]. In addition, it has been demonstrated that the nervous system-depressant actions of barbiturates and other general anesthetics result from an enhancement of inhibitory synaptic transmission mediated by GABA$_A$ receptors [2,3].

GABA SYNTHESIS, UPTAKE AND RELEASE

GABA is formed *in vivo* by a metabolic pathway referred to as the GABA shunt

The GABA shunt is a closed-loop process with the dual purpose of producing and conserving the supply of GABA. GABA is present in high concentrations (millimolar) in many brain regions. These concentrations are about 1,000 times higher than concentrations of the classical monoamine neurotransmitters in the same regions. This is in accord with the powerful and specific actions of GABAergic neurons in these regions. Glucose is the principal precursor for GABA production *in vivo*, although pyruvate and other amino acids also can act as precursors. The first step in the GABA shunt is the transamination of α-ketoglutarate, formed from glucose metabolism in the Krebs cycle by GABA α-oxoglutarate transaminase (GABA-T) into L-glutamic acid [4] (Fig. 16-1). Glutamic acid decarboxylase (GAD) catalyzes the decarboxylation of glutamic acid to form GABA. GAD appears to be expressed only in cells that use GABA as a neurotransmitter. GAD, localized with antibodies or mRNA hybridization probes, serves as an excellent marker for GABAergic neurons in the CNS. Two related but different genes for GAD have been cloned, suggesting independent regulation

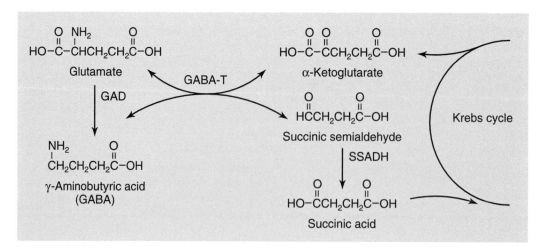

FIGURE 16-1. GABA shunt reactions are responsible for the synthesis, conservation and metabolism of GABA. *GABA-T,* GABA α-oxoglutarate transaminase; *GAD,* glutamic acid decarboxylase; *SSADH,* succinic semialdehyde dehydrogenase.

and properties for the two forms of GAD: GAD_{65} and GAD_{67}. Furthermore, expression of GAD and some GABA receptor subunits has been demonstrated in some non-neural tissues, indicating the likely function of GABA outside of the CNS [5]. GABA is metabolized by GABA-T to form succinic semialdehyde. To conserve the available supply of GABA, this transamination generally occurs when the initial parent compound, α-ketoglutarate, is present to accept the amino group removed from GABA, reforming glutamic acid. Therefore, a molecule of GABA can be metabolized only if a molecule of precursor is formed. Succinic semialdehyde can be oxidized by succinic semialdehyde dehydrogenase (SSADH) into succinic acid and can then re-enter the Krebs cycle, completing the loop.

GABA release into the synaptic cleft is stimulated by depolarization of presynaptic neurons. GABA diffuses across the cleft to the target receptors on the postsynaptic surface. The action of GABA at the synapse is terminated by re-uptake into both presynaptic nerve terminals and surrounding glial cells. The membrane transport systems mediating reuptake of GABA are both temperature- and ion-dependent processes. These transporters are capable of bidirectional neurotransmitter transport. They have an absolute requirement for extracellular Na^+ ions with an additional dependence on Cl^- ions. The ability of the reuptake system to transport GABA against a concentration gradient has been demonstrated using synaptosomes. Under normal physiological conditions, the ratio of internal to external GABA is about 200. The driving force for this reuptake process is supplied by the movement of Na^+ down its concentration gradient [6] (see Chap. 5). GABA taken back up into nerve terminals is available for reutilization, but GABA in glia is metabolized to succinic semialdehyde by GABA-T and cannot be resynthesized in this compartment since glia lack GAD. Ultimately, GABA can be recovered from this source by a circuitous route involving the Krebs cycle [4]; GABA in glia is converted to glutamine, which is transferred back to the neuron, where glutamine is converted by glutaminase to glutamate, which re-enters the GABA shunt (see Chap. 15).

The family of GABA transporters is a set of 80-kDa glycoproteins with multiple transmembrane regions; they have no sequence homology with GABA receptors. Pharmacological and kinetic studies have suggested a variety of subtypes, and at least six separate but related entities have been demonstrated by molecular cloning [6,7]. This has led to rapid developments in understanding the localization, pharmacological specificity, structure–function and mechanism of GABA transport.

GABA RECEPTOR PHYSIOLOGY AND PHARMACOLOGY

GABA receptors have been identified electrophysiologically and pharmacologically in all regions of the brain

Because GABA is widely distributed and utilized throughout the CNS, early GABAergic drugs had very generalized effects on CNS function. The development of more selective agents has led to the identification of at least two distinct classes of GABA receptor, $GABA_A$ and $GABA_B$. They differ in their pharmacological, electrophysiological and biochemical properties. Electrophysiological studies of the $GABA_A$-receptor complex indicate that it mediates an increase in membrane conductance with an equilibrium potential near the resting level of -70 mV. This conductance increase often is accompanied by a membrane hyperpolarization, resulting in an increase in the firing threshold and, consequently, a reduction in the probability of action potential initiation, causing neuronal inhibition. This reduction in membrane resistance is accomplished by the GABA-dependent facilitation of Cl^- ion influx through a receptor-associated channel. On the other hand, increased Cl^- permeability can depolarize the target cell under some conditions of high intracellular Cl^-. This in turn potentially can excite the cell to fire or to activate Ca^{2+} entry via voltage-gated channels and has been proposed as a physiologically relevant event, especially in embryonic neurons.

Electrophysiological data [8] suggest that there are two GABA-recognition sites per $GABA_A$-receptor complex. An increase in the concentration of GABA results in an increase in the mean channel open time due to opening of doubly liganded receptor forms, which exhibit open states of long duration. It has been demonstrated, using a membrane preparation from rat brain, that the increase in the ionic permeability of the GABA$_A$ receptor complex is transient in the continuing presence of agonist [9]. This phenomenon is known as desensitization and is rapidly reversible. The molecular mechanism of desensitization is not understood, and various hypotheses remain under investigation. The existence of GABA-binding sites specific for the initiation of desensitization and distinct from sites mediating opening of the Cl$^-$ channel has been proposed [9].

GABA$_B$ receptors, which are always inhibitory, are coupled to G proteins

Less is known about the GABA$_B$ receptor, primarily due to the limited number of pharmacological agents selective for this site. Originally, GABA$_B$ receptors were identified by their insensitivity to the GABA$_A$ antagonist bicuculline and certain GABA$_A$-specific agonists [1,10]. The GABA analog $(-)$baclofen (β-(4-chlorophenyl)-γ-aminobutyric acid) was found to be a potent and selective GABA$_B$ agonist.

GABA$_B$ receptors are coupled indirectly to K$^+$ channels. When activated, these receptors can decrease Ca^{2+} conductance and inhibit cAMP production via intracellular mechanisms mediated by G proteins. GABA$_B$ receptors can mediate both postsynaptic and presynaptic inhibition. Presynaptic inhibition may occur as a result of GABA$_B$ receptors on nerve terminals causing a decrease in the influx of Ca^{2+}, thereby reducing the release of neurotransmitters. The cloning of the GABA$_B$ receptor [11] and its structural similarity to the metabotropic glutamate receptors should allow rapid progress in the pharmacological characterization of receptor subtypes and the development of new drugs of improved selectivity. Pharmacological responses to GABA that are insensitive to both bicuculline and baclofen have been termed GABA$_C$ receptors. Some, but not all, of these responses can be explained by a structural analog of GABA$_A$ receptors, the ρ subunit [10].

The GABA$_A$ receptor is part of a larger GABA/drug receptor–Cl$^-$ ion channel macromolecular complex

The complex includes five major binding domains (Fig. 16-2). These include binding sites localized in or near the Cl$^-$ channel for GABA, benzodiazepines, barbiturates and picrotoxin as well as binding sites for the anesthetic steroids.

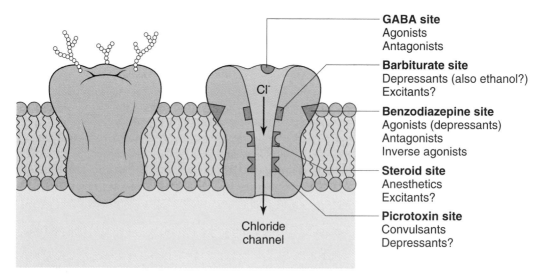

GABA site
Agonists
Antagonists

Barbiturate site
Depressants (also ethanol?)
Excitants?

Benzodiazepine site
Agonists (depressants)
Antagonists
Inverse agonists

Steroid site
Anesthetics
Excitants?

Picrotoxin site
Convulsants
Depressants?

Cl$^-$

Chloride channel

FIGURE 16-2. Structural model of the GABA$_A$ benzodiazepine receptor–chloride (Cl$^-$) ionophore complex. The cut-away view demonstrates targets for a variety of compounds that influence the receptor complex. No specific drug receptor location is implied.

These binding domains modulate receptor response to GABA stimulation. In addition, other drugs, including volatile anesthetics, ethanol and penicillin, have been reported to have an effect on this receptor [3,8]. An integral part of this complex is the Cl^- channel. The GABA-binding site is directly responsible for opening the Cl^- channel. A variety of agonists bind to this site and elicit GABA-like responses. One of the most useful agonists is the compound muscimol, a naturally occurring GABA analog isolated from the psychoactive mushroom *Amanita muscaria*. It is a potent and specific agonist at $GABA_A$ receptors and has been a valuable tool for pharmacological and radioligand-binding studies [10,12]. Other GABA agonists include isoguvacine, 4,5,6,7-tetrahydroisoxazolo-[5,4-*c*]pyridin-3-ol (THIP), 3-aminopropane-sulfonate and imidazoleacetic acid [12]. The classical $GABA_A$-receptor antagonist is the convulsant bicuculline, which reduces current by decreasing the opening frequency and mean open time of the channel [8,10]. It is likely that bicuculline produces its antagonistic effects on $GABA_A$-receptor currents by competing with GABA for binding to one or both sites on the $GABA_A$ receptor.

The $GABA_A$ receptor is the major molecular target for the action of many drugs in the brain

Among these are benzodiazepines, intravenous and volatile anesthetics and possibly ethanol. Benzodiazepine receptor-binding sites copurify with the GABA-binding sites [13]. In addition, benzodiazepine receptors are immunoprecipitated with antibodies that were developed to recognize the protein containing the GABA-binding site [14]. This indicates that the benzodiazepine receptor is an integral part of the $GABA_A$ receptor–Cl^- channel complex.

Benzodiazepine agonists represent the newest group of agents in the general class of depressant drugs, which also includes barbiturates, that show anticonvulsant, anxiolytic and sedative–hypnotic activity. Well-known examples include diazepam and chlordiazepoxide, which often are prescribed for their anti-anxiety effects [1]. The mechanism of action of benzodiazepine

agonists is to enhance GABAergic transmission. From electrophysiological studies, it is known that these benzodiazepines increase the frequency of channel opening in response to GABA, thus accounting for their pharmacological and therapeutic actions [8]. In addition, the benzodiazepine site is coupled allosterically to the barbiturate and picrotoxin sites [2]. Benzodiazepine receptors are heterogeneous with respect to affinity for certain ligands. A wide variety of nonbenzodiazepines, such as the β-carbolines, cyclopyrrolones and imidazopyridines, also bind to the benzodiazepine site.

Barbiturates comprise another class of drugs commonly used therapeutically for anesthesia and control of epilepsy. Phenobarbital and pentobarbital are two of the most commonly used barbiturates. Phenobarbital has been used to treat patients with epilepsy since 1912. Pentobarbital is also an anticonvulsant, but it has sedative side effects. Barbiturates at pharmacological concentrations allosterically increase binding of benzodiazepines and GABA to their respective binding sites [2]. Measurements of mean channel open times show that barbiturates act by increasing the proportion of channels opening to the longest open state (9 msec) while reducing the proportion opening to the shorter open states (1 and 3 msec), resulting in an overall increase in mean channel open time and Cl^- flux [8].

Channel blockers, such as the convulsant compound picrotoxin, cause a decrease in mean channel open time. Picrotoxin works by preferentially shifting opening channels to the briefest open state (1 msec). Thus, both picrotoxin and barbiturates appear to act on the gating process of the $GABA_A$ receptor channel, but their effects on the open states are opposite to each other. Experimental convulsants like pentylenetetrazol and the cage convulsant *t*-butyl bicyclophosphorothionate (TBPS) act in a manner similar to picrotoxin, preventing Cl^- channel permeability. The antibiotic penicillin is a channel blocker with a net negative charge. It blocks the channel by interacting with the positively charged amino acid residues within the channel pore, consequently occluding Cl^- passage through the channel [8].

There have been numerous studies on the role of $GABA_A$ receptors in anesthesia. A considerable amount of evidence has been compiled to suggest that general anesthetics, including barbiturates, volatile gases, steroids and alcohols, enhance GABA-mediated Cl^- conductance. A proper assessment of this phenomenon requires not only a behavioral assay of anesthesia but also *in vitro* models for the study of receptor function. In this regard, not only electrophysiological methods but also neurochemical measurements of Cl^- flux and ligand binding have been useful. For example, a strong positive correlation exists between anesthetic potencies and the stimulation of GABA-mediated Cl^- uptake. This is seen with barbiturates and anesthetics in other chemical classes [3].

Comparison of ligand-gated ion channels that vary in sensitivity to anesthetic modulation, using the chimera and site-directed mutagenesis approach, has identified two amino acids in the membrane-spanning domains that are critical for anesthetic sensitivity [14a]. Direct evidence of ethanol augmentation of $GABA_A$ receptor function, measured either by electrophysiological techniques or agonist-mediated Cl^- flux, has been reported [3,15]. The similarity between the actions of ethanol and sedative drugs such as benzodiazepines and barbiturates that enhance GABA action suggests that ethanol may exert some of its effects by enhancing the function of $GABA_A$ receptors. Ethanol potentiation of $GABA_A$ receptor function appears to be dependent upon the cell type tested and the method of assay. This suggests that the ethanol interaction may be specific for certain receptor subtypes and/or that it may be an indirect action [3].

Neurosteroids, which may be physiological modulators of brain activity, enhance $GABA_A$ receptor function

This enhancement by steroids involves direct action on the membrane receptor protein rather than through the classical genomic mechanism mediated by soluble high-affinity cytoplasmic steroid hormone receptors (see Chap. 49). Chemically reduced analogs of the hormones progesterone and corticosterone derivatives administered to animals and humans exert sedative–hypnotic and anti-anxiety effects. This led

to the development of a synthetic steroid anesthetic, alphaxalone. These neuroactive steroids are potent modulators of $GABA_A$-receptor function *in vitro* [2,3,16]. The neuroactive steroids can be produced in the brain endogenously and may influence CNS function under certain physiological or pathological conditions. Some observations suggesting that neurosteroids physiologically affect the CNS include the rapid behavioral effects of administered steroids; diurnal and estrous cycle effects on behavior; gender-specific pharmacology, especially of GABAergic drugs; and the development of withdrawal symptoms following cessation of chronically administered steroids. Neuroactive steroids have effects similar to those of barbiturates in that they enhance agonist binding to the GABA site and allosterically modulate benzodiazepine and TBPS binding [2,3]. Also, like barbiturates, high concentrations of neurosteroids directly activate the $GABA_A$ receptor Cl^- channel. These observations led to the hypothesis that the neurosteroid-binding site may be similar to the barbiturate site, but the sites of action for the two classes of drugs are clearly not identical [2].

CLONING GABA RECEPTORS

A family of pentameric $GABA_A$-receptor protein subtypes exists

The $GABA_A$ receptor was first cloned using partial protein sequence, and verification of these cDNAs as GABA-receptor subunits was made by expression in *Xenopus* oocytes of GABA-activated channels [17]. Our current understanding of the molecular structure of the $GABA_A$ receptor–ionophore complex is that it is a heteropentameric glycoprotein of about 275 kDa composed of combinations of at least 17 different but closely related polypeptides. The subunits are 50 to 60 kDa and have about 20 to 30% sequence identity between classes α, β, γ, δ, ϵ and ρ [8,14,18–20] (Fig. 16-3A). Variants of most of these subunits have been reported in vertebrate brain, including $\alpha_{1–6}$, $\beta_{1–4}$, $\gamma_{1–4}$, δ, ϵ and $\rho_{1–3}$. β_4 and γ_4 so far have been identified only in birds. About 70% sequence identity is shared between the isoforms of each subunit class (Fig. 16-3A).

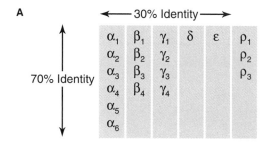

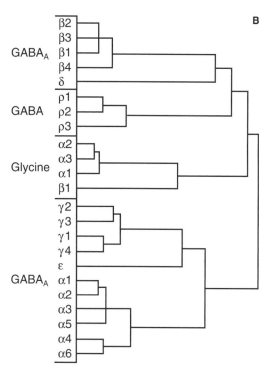

FIGURE 16-3. A: Homology between peptide sequences making up the subunits of the GABA$_A$ receptor. Percentages of sequence identity between polypeptide isoforms of a single subunit class, for example, α_{1-6}, and between different subunit classes, for example, α vs. β, are approximate values. **B:** Dendrogram showing evolutionary relationships between DNA sequences of GABA$_A$ receptor subunits and glycine receptors. The dendrogram is based on data from the literature regarding human cDNAs except for β_4 and γ_4, which are chicken cDNAs, a kind gift from Tim Hales and Ewen Kirkness. (Based on [19].)

This suggests that the genes probably evolved from a common ancestral sequence; the evolutionary relationships are shown in the dendrogram of Figure 16-3B.

Sequencing revealed that the GABA$_A$ receptor is a member of a superfamily of ligand-gated ion channel receptors

This family includes the nicotinic acetylcholine receptor, the strychnine-sensitive glycine receptor and the serotonergic 5-HT$_3$ receptor. About 10 to 20% homology exists among GABA$_A$ subunits and those of other members of the ligand-gated ion channel gene superfamily. In addition, splice variants exist for several of the subunits. In several cases, these variants provide phosphorylation substrates on the intracellular domain [20].

Differential distribution of GABA$_A$-receptor-subunit mRNAs and polypeptides in brain is consistent with data indicating variation in physiological function, pharmacology and biochemistry of different brain regions. It is likely that different combinations with differing pharmacologies and conductances are expressed in different neuronal populations. The subunit composition of native isoforms has been deduced by a combination of determining which polypeptides are present in a given cell, which ones can be isolated together as an oligomer using subunit-specific antibodies and what pharmacological properties can be reconstituted from recombinant subunits of known combinations. Table 16-1 summarizes the most abundant isoforms identified, their localization and their unique pharmacological properties [14,18–20]. The ρ subunits are expressed primarily, if not exclusively, in the retina, where they appear to form Cl$^-$ channels, possibly homomers, with novel pharmacology, notably insensitivity to baclofen, bicuculline and GABA$_A$-positive modulators like benzodiazepines and anesthetics. This has led some to designate these ρ receptors as "GABA$_C$," but structurally they are part of the GABA$_A$ class [10]. The ϵ class produces receptors as heteromers with α and β subunits, resulting in another sort of novel pharmacology including low sensitivity to anesthetics [19].

Each GABA$_A$ subunit contains four putative α-helical membrane-spanning domains (M1–M4) with a predominantly hydrophobic

TABLE 16-1. **DISTRIBUTIONS AND NOVEL PHARMACOLOGICAL AND PHYSIOLOGICAL PROPERTIES OF THE MAJOR GABA$_A$ RECEPTOR SUBTYPES IN THE RAT BRAIN**

Isoform	Relative abundance	Location	Pharmacology/property
α1β2γ2	40%	Most brain areas; hippocampal, cortical interneurons; cerebellar Purkinje cells	Common coassembly BZ-type I Zn-insensitive
α2β3γ2	15%	Spinal cord motoneurons, hippocampal pyramidal cells	BZ-type II Moderately Zn-sensitive
α3βγ2/3	10%	Cholinergic, monaminergic neurons	BZ-type II, abecarnil-sensitive
α2βγ1	10%	Bergmann glia, thalamus, hypothalamus	BZ inverse agonist-enhanced
α5β3γ2/3	3%	Hippocampal pyramidal cells	BZ-type II, zolpidem-insensitive, moderate Zn-sensitivity
α6βγ2	2%	Cerebellar granule cells	BZ agonist-insensitive, moderate Zn-sensitivity
α6βδ	3%	Cerebellar granule cells	Insensitive to all BZ, GABA high affinity, high Zn-sensitivity, steroid-insensitive
α4βγ	2%	Cortical, hippocampal pyramidal cells; striatum	BZ agonist-insensitive, low steroid sensitivity
α4β2δ	4%	Thalamus, dentate granule cells	Insensitive to all BZ, GABA high affinity, high Zn sensitivity, steroid-insensitive
All other	11%	Throughout CNS	

BZ, benzodiazepine.
Modified from McKernan and Whiting [20] with permission.

character. One or more membrane-spanning regions from each subunit, probably M2, form the walls of the channel pore (see also Chap. 11). The sequences of these transmembrane segments are highly conserved between the subunits of the GABA$_A$ receptor as well as between members of the gene superfamily. The region between M3 and M4 contains a long, variable putative intracellular domain. This contributes to the subtype specificity and may participate in intracellular regulatory mechanisms such as phosphorylation and interaction with other cellular constituents [8,17,20].

Photoaffinity-labeling and site-directed mutagenesis of the GABA$_A$ receptors suggest that the binding sites for benzodiazepines are localized at the interface of the α and γ subunits and that those for GABA ligands are located at the interface between the α and β subunits [21,22]. The binding pockets for each class of ligand appear to be formed from three loops of amino acids (Fig. 16-4). These models are consistent with studies on recombinant GABA$_A$ receptors expressed in heterologous cells. Such studies show that the nature of the α and β subunits determines the pharmacological specificity at the GABA and benzodiazepine sites and that the γ subunits are necessary for sensitivity to benzodiazepines and insensitivity to Zn^{2+} inhibition [18]. Combinations including the α$_1$ subunit have a high affinity for certain "type 1-selective" benzodiazepine site ligands, while those with the α$_2$, α$_3$ and α$_5$ subunits have moderate affinity. The α$_5$ subunit has a unique specificity to bind most benzodiazepine ligands but not the sedative drug zolpidem [18]. Some GABA$_A$ receptors apparently lack benzodiazepine-binding sites altogether or have a novel pharmacological profile at this site. Subunit combinations containing the α$_4$ or α$_6$ subunit with a γ subunit bind benzodiazepine inverse agonists but

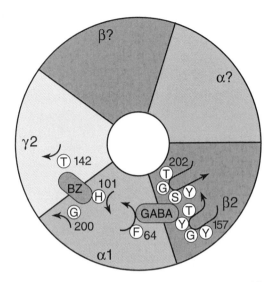

FIGURE 16-4. Model of GABA$_A$ receptor protein with five subunits, indicating amino acid residues implicated in the binding of GABA and benzodiazepines *(BZ)*. The subunit stoichiometry is tentative, as indicated by *question marks*. *Arrows* indicate direction of polypeptide sequence. (Reproduced with permission from [21].) An update of the model for benzodiazepine binding sites recently appeared [27].

not agonists and are moderately sensitive to Zn^{2+} and neurosteroids. Combinations containing α_4 or α_6 with a δ subunit instead of a γ subunit do not bind benzodiazepine-site ligands, are highly sensitive to Zn^{2+} and are relatively insensitive to neurosteroids [8,18,20].

Cloning of the GABA$_A$ receptor subunits and deduction of the corresponding amino acid sequences have led to the finding that phosphorylation sites for one or more kinases are present on virtually all of the subunits. Phosphorylation of the β subunits by cAMP-dependent protein kinase (PKA) and phosphorylation of β and γ subunits by protein kinase C and tyrosine kinase have been reported [8,23]. Current studies are directed toward an understanding of the functional consequences of phosphorylation of GABA$_A$ receptors for both acute and more prolonged time frames.

GLYCINE RECEPTORS

It was first proposed in 1965 that glycine acts as a neurotransmitter in mammalian spinal cord and since then glycine has been demonstrated to meet all of the criteria for that designation. Glycine is widely recognized as a major inhibitory neurotransmitter in the vertebrae CNS, especially the spinal cord [4]. Like GABA, it inhibits neuronal firing by gating Cl$^-$ channels but with a characteristically different pharmacology.

Glycine is synthesized from glucose and other substrates in the brain

The immediate precursor of glycine is serine, which is converted to glycine by the activity of the enzyme serine hydroxymethyltransferase (SHMT). As for GABA, Ca^{2+}-dependent release of glycine and specific postsynaptic receptors have been demonstrated. The action of glycine is terminated by its reuptake by a high-affinity transporter system. Synaptosomal uptake of radioactive glycine has been demonstrated in spinal cord and lower brainstem. In supraspinal regions, glycine can be taken up by transport systems that have lower affinity and specificity for it. It is likely that a family of transporters will be identified for glycine, as for GABA and other neurotransmitters. The metabolic disposal is unclear, but it can be converted to a variety of other substances. However, none of these mechanisms has been associated with glycine neurons.

GLYCINE RECEPTOR PHYSIOLOGY AND PHARMACOLOGY

A number of amino acids can activate, to varying degrees, the inhibitory glycine receptor

The amino acids that can activate the glycine receptor include β-alanine, taurine, L-alanine, L-serine and proline. GABA is inactive at this receptor. There are only few known antagonists of glycine receptors. They include the plant alkaloid strychnine, which is highly selective for the glycine receptor, and the amidine steroid RU 5135, which is less selective. Both compounds bind the glycine receptor with nanomolar affinities. The binding site for glycine is thought to be related closely to the site for antagonist binding, but it may not be identical. Current findings suggest that at least three molecules of glycine are required to activate the glycine receptor. The physiological significance of multiple binding sites for glycine is unclear [24].

Glycine is inhibitory on ligand-gated, strychnine-sensitive Cl⁻ channel receptors but excitatory on N-methyl-D-aspartate receptors

Although acting as a classical neurotransmitter at inhibitory ion channel receptors, glycine is also an activating ligand at a class of excitatory ion channel receptors, the N-methyl-D-aspartate (NMDA) receptors (see Chap. 15). Currently, it is thought that glycine is a necessary cofactor for activation of the NMDA receptor by its neurotransmitter L-glutamate and that glycine is normally present in the extracellular space at suitable concentrations. Regulation of NMDA receptor activity via control of glycine concentrations can be considered more of a neuromodulatory role than a neurotransmitter role. It is curious that common amino acids like glycine and glutamate, which have other roles in metabolism, should be employed as signaling molecules as well and that glycine should be utilized as both an inhibitory and an excitatory signal in the nervous system. It is likely that receptors for signaling molecules evolved from prokaryotic proteins utilized for recognition of nutrients in the environment, including glycine, glutamate and GABA. GABA, a carbon- and nitrogen-storage molecule in plants and algae, appears to act as a colony-stimulating factor for abalone, an invertebrate mollusk.

CLONING GLYCINE RECEPTORS

Glycine receptors belong to the same gene superfamily as the GABA_A receptor

The native receptor is a macromolecular complex of about 250 kDa composed of a combination of two homologous polypeptides identified as α (48 kDa) and β (58 kDa). It has been proposed that the glycine receptor, like the other members of the family, consists of a quasisymmetrical pentameric arrangement forming a central ion pore [24,25] There is approximately 50% amino acid sequence identity between the

α and β subunits; significant homology with GABA_A receptors is also evident (Fig. 16-3B). In addition, a 93-kDa polypeptide, gephyrin, co-purifies with the glycine receptor. Photoaffinity labeling of the glycine receptor shows that the binding sites for glycine and strychnine are found on the 48-kDa polypeptide α subunit [24]. The α and β subunits span the postsynaptic membrane and are believed to be glycosylated. Like the GABA_A receptor and nicotinic acetylcholine receptor subunits, glycine receptor subunits have four hydrophobic segments, M1–M4, which probably span the lipid bilayer as α helices.

Unlike the α and β subunits, the 93-kDa polypeptide gephyrin is a highly hydrophilic protein, cytoplasmically localized at postsynaptic membranes. The 93-kDa polypeptide is a peripheral component anchoring the glycine receptor in the postsynaptic membrane by attaching it to cytoskeletal elements [25] (Fig. 16-5). Such a role appears analogous to that of the ankyrin family of proteins, which restrict lateral mobility of many membrane proteins, including transporters and channels. The 43-kDa protein rapsyn appears to play this cytoskeleton-

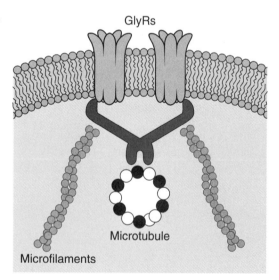

FIGURE 16-5. Model of gephyrin-dependent glycine receptor *(GlyR)* anchoring. Gephyrin *(dark gray)* links the *GlyR* β-subunit *(orange)* to microtubules, which restrict lateral movement. Microfilaments may help disperse receptor clusters after microtubule depolymerization. (Reproduced with permission from [25].)

linking role with acetylcholine receptors (see Chap. 11); gephyrin or related proteins also may be associated with $GABA_A$ receptors.

Site-directed mutagenesis studies of glycine receptor subunits have led to a greater understanding of domains within the ligand-gated ion channel polypeptides that participate in pentamer assembly and interaction with the cytoskeleton, as well as the agonist-binding pocket and ion channel domains [25]. For example, α subunits can produce abnormal homopentamers in recombinant expression systems, while β subunits cannot. The α homomers are abnormal in channel properties and pharmacology in that they are sensitive to the $GABA_A$ antagonist picrotoxin; coexpression of α and β subunits produces a more native receptor that is insensitive to picrotoxin, as are glycine receptors in real cells. Mutagenesis of certain amino acid residues in the extracellular domain of β subunits, making them similar to α subunits, confers the ability to assemble homomeric channels. Mutagenesis of other amino acid residues that differ between α and β subunits has identified domains involved in binding glycine and Zn^{2+} [25].

Currently, four isoforms of the α subunit, but only one form of β, have been cloned. The $α_2$ polypeptide represents a subunit primarily expressed neonatally, whereas $α_3$ is found primarily postnatally. Functional expression of the $α_1$, $α_2$ and $α_3$ transcripts in frog oocytes generates glycine-gated Cl^- channels that are blocked by nanomolar concentrations of strychnine. Mutations of the $α_1$ subunit, namely leucine or glutamine for arginine at position 271, have been associated with hyperekplexia, a rare neurological disease characterized by an exaggerated startle response [26]. A variant of the $α_2$ subunit produces a channel that has a much lower affinity for strychnine and that is thought to correspond with the strychnine-insensitive glycine receptor found neonatally in rat spinal cord. Mutations in both α and β subunits have been implicated in two single-gene mutations in mice that show neurological phenotypes, as well as in one type of human genetic seizure disorder [25].

Immunocytochemical mapping with monoclonal antibodies raised against α-subunit antigen gives results similar to those obtained in autoradiographic studies of [³H]strychnine-binding sites. Although the majority of sites are found in spinal cord and brainstem, a small but significant population is found in more rostral brain regions. Interestingly, β-subunit mRNA is abundant in many brain regions, and even non-neural tissues, where neither [³H]strychnine binding nor known α-subunit mRNAs are found. The implication of this finding is presently unclear.

GABA AND GLYCINE ARE THE MAJOR RAPIDLY ACTING INHIBITORY NEUROTRANSMITTERS IN BRAIN

The roles of these two neurotransmitters are clearly distinct, both chemically and physiologically. The major receptors for both of the two neurotransmitters are inhibitory ligand-gated Cl^- channels with significant structural homology. Diversity of subunit isoforms has been exhibited in both $GABA_A$ and glycine receptors. The data suggest a varied pharmacology and physiology associated with differing isoform combinations. An understanding of the nature of these combinations should assist in the development of a new series of therapeutic agents which interact with GABA or glycine receptors in a more specific manner than currently available drugs. Furthermore, a detailed understanding of the functional domains of the proteins may aid in rational drug design. Gene-targeting studies and analyses of existing mutant mice have revealed important roles for GABA and glycine receptors in nervous system function and development. Finally, plastic changes in subunit composition have been documented as a result of environmental experiences, giving new clues to mechanisms of learning, disease states and drug dependence.

REFERENCES

1. Enna, S. J., and Bowery, N. G. (eds.), *The GABA Receptors*, 2nd ed. Clifton, NJ: Humana Press, 1997.
2. Olsen, R. W., Sapp, D. W., Bureau, M. H., Turner, D. M., and Kokka, N. Allosteric actions of central nervous system depressants including anesthetics on subtypes of the inhibitory γ-aminobutyric

acid$_A$ receptor–chloride channel complex. *Ann. N. Y. Acad. Sci.* 625:145–154, 1991.

3. Harris, R. A., Mihic, S. J., Dildy-Mayfield, J. E., and Machu, T. K. Actions of anesthetics on ligand-gated ion channels: Role of receptor subunit composition. *FASEB J.* 9:1454–1462, 1995.

4. McGeer, P. L., and McGeer, E. G. Amino acid neurotransmitters. In G. Siegel, B. Agranoff, R. W. Albers, and P. Molinoff (eds.), *Basic Neurochemistry*, 4th ed. New York: Raven Press, 1989, pp. 311–332.

5. Kaufman, D. L., Houser, C. R., and Tobin, A. J. Two forms of the GABA synthetic enzyme glutamate decarboxylase have distinct intraneuronal distributions and cofactor interactions. *J. Neurochem.* 56:720–723, 1991.

6. Guastella, J., Nelson, N., Nelson, H., et al. Cloning and expression of a rat brain GABA transporter. *Science* 24:1303–1306, 1990.

7. Smith, K. E., Gustafson, E. L., Borden, L. A., et al. Heterogeneity of brain GABA transporters. In C. Tanaka, and N. Bowery (eds.), *GABA Receptors, Transporters and Metabolism*. Basel: Birkhauser-Verlag, 1996, pp. 63–72.

8. Macdonald, R. L., and Olsen, R. W. GABA$_A$ receptor channels. *Annu. Rev. Neurosci.* 17: 569–602, 1994.

9. Cash, D. J., and Subbarao, K. Desensitization of γ-aminobutyric acid receptor from rat brain: Two distinguishable receptors on the same membrane. *Biochemistry* 26:7556–7562, 1987.

10. Johnston, G. A. R. GABA$_C$ receptors: Relatively simple transmitter-gated ion channels? *Trends Pharmacol. Sci.* 17:319–323, 1996.

11. Kaupmann, K., Huggel, K., Heid, J., et al. Expression cloning of GABA$_B$ receptors uncovers similarity to metabotropic glutamate receptors. *Nature* 386:239–246, 1997.

12. Krogsgaard-Larsen, P., Nielsen, L., and Falch, E. The active site of the GABA receptor. In R. W. Olsen and J. C. Venter (eds.), *Benzodiazepine/ GABA Receptors and Chloride Channels*. New York: Alan R. Liss, 1986, pp. 73–95.

13. Sigel, E., Stephenson, F. A., Mamalaki, C., and Barnard, E. A. A γ-aminobutyric acid/benzodiazepine receptor complex of bovine cerebral cortex: Purification and partial characterization. *J. Biol. Chem.* 258:6965–6971, 1983.

14. Fritschy, J. M., and Möhler, H. GABA$_A$ receptor heterogeneity in the adult rat brain: Differential regional and cellular distribution of seven major subunits. *J. Comp. Neurol.* 359:154–194, 1995.

14a.Mihic, S. J., Ye, Q., Wick, M. J., et al. Sites of alcohol and volatile anesthetic action on GABA$_A$ and glycine receptors. *Nature* 389:385–389, 1997.

15. Suzdak, P. D., Schwartz, R. D., Skolnick, P., and Paul, S. M. Ethanol stimulates gamma-aminobutyric acid receptor-mediated chloride transport in rat brain synaptoneurosomes. *Proc. Natl. Acad. Sci. USA* 83:4071–4075, 1986.

16. Majewska, M. D., Harrison, N. L., Schwartz, R. D., Barker, J. L., and Paul, S. M. Steroid hormone metabolites are barbiturate-like modulators of the GABA receptor. *Science* 232:1004–1007, 1986.

17. Schofield, P. R., Darlison, M. G., Fujita, N., et al. Sequence and functional expression of the GABA$_A$ receptor shows a ligand-gated receptor super-family. *Nature* 328:221–227, 1987.

18. Lüddens, H., Korpi, E., and Seeburg, P. H. GABA$_A$ benzodiazepine receptor heterogeneity: Neurophysiological implications. *Neuropharmacology* 34:245–254, 1995.

19. Davies, P. A., Hanna, M. C., Hales, T. G., and Kirkness, E. F. Insensitivity to anaesthetic agents conferred by a class of GABA$_A$ receptor subunit. *Nature* 385:820–823, 1997.

20. McKernan, R. M., and Whiting, P. J. Which GABA$_A$-receptor subtypes really occur in the brain? *Trends Neurosci.* 19:139–143, 1996.

21. Smith, G. B., and Olsen, R. W. Functional domains of GABA$_A$ receptors. *Trends Pharmacol. Sci.* 16:162–168, 1995.

22. Weiss, D. B., and Amin, J. GABA$_A$ receptor needs two homologous domains of the beta-subunit for activation by GABA but not by pentobarbital. *Nature* 366:565–569, 1993.

23. Moss, S. J., McDonald, B., Gorrie, G. H., Krishek, B. K., and Smart, T. G. Regulation of GABA$_A$ receptors by multiple protein kinases. In C. Tanaka and N. Bowery (eds.), *GABA Receptors, Transporters and Metabolism*. Basel: Birkhauser-Verlag, 1996, pp. 173–184.

24. Grenningloh, G., Rienitz, A., Schmitt, B., et al. The strychnine-binding subunit of the glycine receptor shows homology with nicotinic acetylcholine receptors. *Nature* 328:215–220, 1987.

25. Kuhse, J., Betz, H., and Kirsch, J. The inhibitory glycine receptors: Architecture, synaptic localization and molecular pathology of a postsynaptic ion-channel complex. *Curr. Opin. Neurobiol.* 5:318–323, 1995.

26. Shiang, R., Ryan, S. G., Zhu, Y.-Z., Hahn, A. F., O'Connell, P., and Wasmuth, J. J. Mutations in the α$_1$ subunit of the inhibitory glycine receptor cause the dominant neurologic disorder, hyperekplexia. *Nat. Genet.* 5:351–358, 1993.

27. Sigel, E., and Buhr, A. The benzodiazepine binding site of GABA$_A$ receptors. *Trends Pharmacol. Sci.* 18:425–429, 1997.

Purinergic Systems

Joel M. Linden

Purines such as ATP and adenosine play a central role in the energy metabolism of all life forms. This fact probably delayed recognition of other roles for purines as autocrine and paracrine substances and neurotransmitters. Today it is recognized that purines are released from neurons and other cells and produce widespread effects on multiple organ systems by binding to purinergic receptors on the cell surface. The principal ligands for purinergic receptors are adenosine, ATP, uridine triphosphate (UTP) and diadenosine polyphosphates (two adenosines coupled via ester bonds to three to six phosphates, Ap_nA). Primordial voltage-gated ion channels may have evolved at an early stage to respond to ATP, an early chemical signal. Such a possibility is suggested by the high degree of homology between cloned P2X receptors and epithelial Na^+ channels [1].

Basic Neurochemistry: Molecular, Cellular and Medical Aspects, 6th Ed., edited by G. J. Siegel et al. Published by Lippincott–Raven Publishers, Philadelphia, 1999. Correspondence to Joel M. Linden, Departments of Medicine and Molecular Physiology and Biological Physics, University of Virginia, Box MR4 6012, Health Sciences Center, Charlottesville, Virginia 22902.

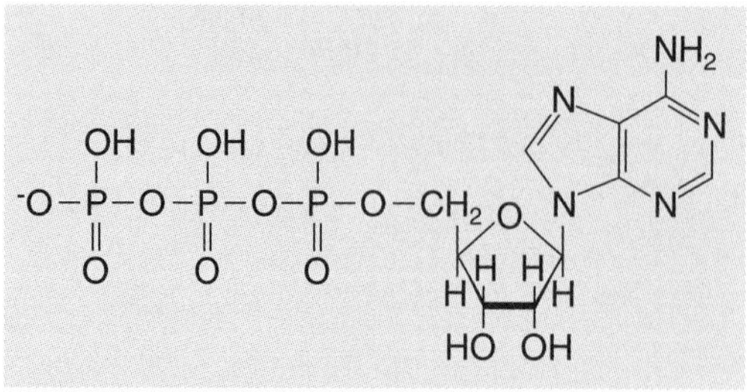

FIGURE 17-1. Adenosine 5′-triphosphate. A purine nucleotide consisting of adenine, ribose and triphosphate.

A nucleoside consists of a purine or pyrimidine base linked to a pentose, either D-ribose to form a ribonucleoside or 2-deoxy-D-ribose to form a deoxyribonucleoside. Three major purine bases and their corresponding ribonucleosides are adenine/adenosine, guanine/guanosine and hypoxanthine/inosine. The three major pyrimidines are cytosine, uracil and thymine. A nucleotide such as ATP (Fig. 17-1) is a phosphate or polyphosphate ester of a nucleoside.

PURINE RELEASE AND METABOLISM

Many cells in the nervous system release adenosine and adenine nucleotides

In addition to having a central role in cellular energy metabolism, ATP and diadenosine polyphosphates are classical neurotransmitters that are packaged into secretory granules of neurons and adrenal chromaffin cells. They are released in quanta in response to action potentials, as illustrated in Figure 17-2A. ATP is released from synaptosomal preparations of cortex, hypothalamus and medulla. In cortical synaptosomes, a portion of the ATP that is released is coreleased with acetylcholine (ACh) or norepinephrine (NE), but the majority is released from neurons that are neither adrenergic nor cholinergic. In affinity-purified cholinergic nerve terminals, ATP and ACh are coreleased in a ratio of 1:10. In addition, it has been proposed that there are membrane proteins that can extrude ATP from non-neuronal cells [2].

Nucleotides can be metabolized in the extracellular space

Ectoenzymes are involved in the rapid metabolism of ATP and other nucleotides [3]. ATP applied to rat brain hippocampal slices is mostly converted to adenosine in less than 1 sec. Some of the enzymes involved in ATP, UTP and nucleoside metabolism are depicted in Figure 17-2B. Inhibitors of these enzymes that are useful as experimental tools are listed in Table 17-1.

EctoATP diphosphohydrolase (ADPase or apyrase) is a plasma membrane-bound enzyme that hydrolyses extracellular ATP and ADP to produce AMP. This enzyme is identical to CD39, an activation marker found on B lymphocytes [4]. A selective inhibitor of ecto-ATPase that has little effect on P2 receptors is ARL67156 (Table 17-1). This compound potentiates the effect of endogenously released as well as exogenously added ATP. Extracellular AMP is converted to adenosine by ecto-5′-nucleotidase, an enzyme that is attached to the cell surface by a glycosyl phosphatidylinositol linker. 5′-Nucleotidases catalyze the conversion of purine and pyrimidine nucleoside monophosphates to the corresponding nucleosides. CD73 is a 5′-nucleotidase that is found on T and B lymphocytes [5]. Ecto-5′-nucleotidase can be blocked by α, β-methylene-adenosine diphosphate (AOPCP) (Table 17-1). In cytochemical studies, ecto-5′-nucleotidase has been associated with plasma membranes of glial cells and astrocytes, particularly synaptic terminals. Soluble cytosolic 5′-nucleotidases also exist. These are involved in the formation of adenosine during increased metabolic activity. Even a small decrease in ATP can lead to a large increase in the substrate for this enzyme, AMP, because under normal conditions the concentration of ATP is about 50 times higher than that of AMP. The differentiation of neural cells is dependent on 5′-nucleotidase activity, suggesting that adenosine formation from continuously released nucleotides is essential for neuronal survival. 5′-Nucleotidase is phosphorylated and activated by protein kinase C (PKC). In rat brain, ischemia results in an upregulation of 5′-nucleotidase on activated astrocytes. This is thought to increase the capac-

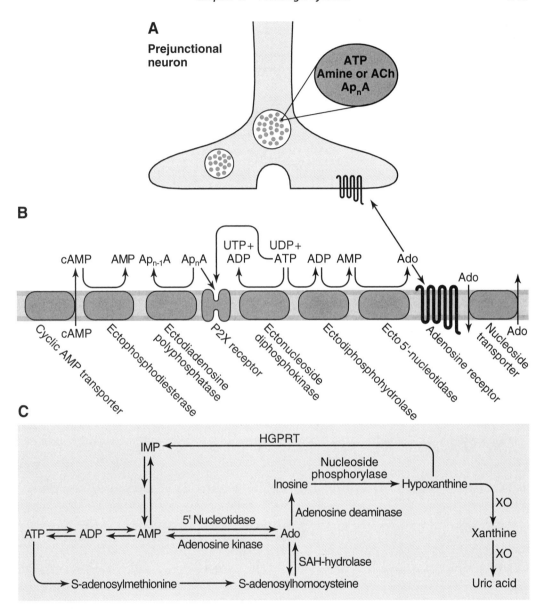

FIGURE 17-2.   Purine release and metabolism. **A, Prejunctional neuron:** Adenine nucleotides are schematically depicted as being stored as cotransmitters in synaptic granules (see *enlargement*). *Amine,* aminergic neurotransmitter; *ACh,* acetylcholine; *Ap$_n$A,* diadenosine polyphosphate. **B, Postjunctional membrane:** Adenine and uridine nucleotides, diadenosine polyphosphates and cAMP are degraded by ectoenzymes. Adenosine *(Ado)* and inosine accumulate in hypoxic, ischemic or metabolically active cells. Cyclic AMP accumulates as a second messenger in response to various neurotransmitters (see Chap. 22). These purines can be transported to the interstitial space by membrane-associated transport proteins. Both **(A)** pre- and **(B)** post-junctional adenosine receptors are depicted as traversing the plasma membrane seven times, as is typical of receptors that interact with GTP-binding proteins, including P1 and P2Y (not shown) receptors. A P2X postjunctional ATP receptor is depicted as a ligand-gated channel. **C, Cytosol:** The major pathways of intracellular adenosine metabolism are shown. *IMP,* inosine monophosphate; *SAH, S*-adenosyl-homocysteine; *XO,* xanthine oxidase; *HGPRT,* hypoxanthine-guanine phosphoribosyl transferase.

TABLE 17-1. **SUBSTRATES AND INHIBITORS OF ENZYMES INVOLVED IN NUCLEOTIDE AND NUCLEOSIDE METABOLISM**

Enzyme	Substrate	Inhibitor
ATP diphosphohydrolase	ATP, ADP	ARL67156
Diadenosine pholyphosphatase	Ap_nA	Suramin[a]
5'-Nucleotidase	AMP	AOPCP
Nucleoside transporter	Adenosine	Dipyridamole, NBTI, mioflazine
Adenosine deaminase	Adenosine	EHNA, 2-deoxycoformycin
Adenosine kinase	Adenosine	5'-Iodotubercidin, 5'-deoxy-5'-amino-adenosine
Xanthine oxidase	Hypoxanthine, xanthine	Allopurinol, CMTA
Nucleoside phosphorylase	Inosine	8-Aminoguanosine

[a] Suramin also is an inhibitor of P2 receptors.
ARL 67156, 6-*N,N*-diethyl-D-β,γ-dibromomethylene ATP; AOPCP, α,β-methylene-adenosine diphosphate; NBTI, nitrobenzylthioinosine; Ap_nA, diadenosine polyphosphate (n = 3–6); EHNA, erythro-9-(2-hydroxy-3-nonyl)adenine; CMTA, 2-(3-cyano-4-isobutoxyphenyl)-4-methyl-5-thiazolecarboxylic acid.

ity of damaged tissue to form neuroprotective adenosine. Extracellular adenosine also can be derived from the metabolism of extracellular cAMP by an ectocAMP phosphodiesterase [6]. Stimulation of receptors that increase cAMP accumulation, such as β-adrenergic or vasoactive intestinal peptide (VIP) receptors, in cultured rat cortical neurons causes the accumulation of extracellular adenosine, which can be blocked by inhibition of cAMP transport, cyclic nucleotide phosphodiesterase or 5'-nucleotidase, indicating that extracellular cAMP is a source of the adenosine.

Diadenosine polyphosphates also are degraded in the extracellular space. In neural tissues, the activity of ectodiadenosine polyphosphatases is lower than that of ectoATP-diphospohydrolase. Hence, the diadenosine polyphosphates have a longer half-life in the extracellular space than does ATP.

UDP and UTP are selective agonists of certain P2Y receptors, suggesting that these pyrimidines may play a physiological role in signaling via P2 receptors. It is not yet clear which factors control the release of uridine nucleotides into the extracellular space. UTP can be formed from UDP in the extracellular space by the action of the enzyme nucleoside diphosphokinase, which catalyzes the transfer of the γ-phosphate of nucleoside triphosphates to nucleoside diphosphates, for example, ATP + UDP → ADP + UTP.

Adenosine is considered to be a neuromodulator

Adenosine is not a classical neurotransmitter because it is not stored in neuronal synaptic granules or released in quanta. It gains access to the extracellular space in part from the breakdown of extracellular adenine nucleotides and in part by translocation from the cytoplasm of cells by nucleoside transport proteins, particularly in stressed or ischemic tissues (Fig. 17-2C). Adenosine thus acts as a metabolic messenger that imparts information about the intracellular metabolic state of a particular cell to extracellular-facing receptors on the same cell and on adjacent cells.

Extracellular adenosine is rapidly removed in part by reuptake into cells and in part by degradation to inosine by adenosine deaminases, enzymes that catalyze the conversion of adenosine and deoxyadenosine to inosine and deoxyinosine, respectively. Adenosine deaminase is mainly cytosolic, but it also occurs as a cell-surface ectoenzyme.

Adenosine and homocysteine are formed from the hydrolysis of *S*-adenosylhomocysteine (SAH) by the enzyme SAH hydrolase (Fig. 17-2C). Attempts to measure intracellular adenosine are complicated by the fact that over 90% of intracellular adenosine may be weakly bound to this enzyme. SAH is formed from *S*-adenosylmethionine (SAM), which is a cofactor in transmethylation reactions. SAH is the precursor of a sizable fraction of adenosine under resting conditions, but most adenosine is derived from the 5′-nucleotidase pathway during conditions of hypoxia, ischemia or metabolic stress. Under these conditions, the accumulation of high concentrations of adenosine and the resultant deamination of adenosine also lead to a large increase in inosine. Intracellular adenosine can be reincorporated into the nucleotide pool upon phosphorylation by the cytosolic enzyme adenosine kinase. In normoxic resting tissues, most adenosine is rephosphorylated since the K_m of adenosine kinase is 10 to 100 times lower than the K_m of adenosine deaminase. Deamination, leading to a large accumulation of inosine, becomes the major pathway of adenosine metabolism when adenosine concentrations are elevated because maximal adenosine kinase activity is much less than maximal adenosine deaminase activity. By elevating adenosine, inhibitors of adenosine kinase or adenosine deaminase produce adenosine-like actions in laboratory animals. Concentrations of adenosine and inosine in the interstitial fluid of brain and other tissues are increased when oxygen supply exceeds oxygen demand. The effect of adenosine is to increase oxygen delivery by dilating most vascular beds and generally to decrease oxygen demand by reducing cellular energy utilization. In the brain, this is usually manifested as a decrease in neuronal firing and in the diminished release of excitatory neurotransmitters.

Adenosine and inosine can be transported across cell membranes in either direction by a membrane-associated, facilitated nucleoside transport protein. Concentrative transporters also have been identified [7]. Messenger RNA for a pyrimidine-selective Na^+-nucleoside cotransporter (rCNT1) and a purine-selective Na^+-nucleoside cotransporter (rCNT2) are found throughout the rat brain. Most degradation of adenosine is intracellular, as evidenced by the fact that inhibitors of adenosine transport, such as dipyridamole, increase interstitial concentrations of adenosine. Dipyridamole is clinically used to elevate adenosine in coronary arteries and to produce coronary vasodilation. In high doses, dipyridamole can accentuate adenosine receptor-mediated actions in the CNS, resulting in sedation and sleep, anticonvulsant effects, decreased locomotor activity and decreased neuronal activity.

Hypoxanthine is derived from inosine by the enzyme nucleoside phosphorylase. Hypoxanthine can be converted to inosine monophosphate (IMP) by hypoxanthine-guanine phosphoribosyl transferase (HGPRT), one of the enzymes of the purine salvage pathway. Lesch-Nyhan syndrome is a severe neurological disorder caused by a deficiency of HGPRT (see Box 17-1). AMP can be formed from IMP by insertion of an amino group at C-6 in place of the carbonyl oxygen. This is a two-step reaction involving the formation of adenylosuccinate as an intermediate. Unsalvaged hypoxanthine is oxidized to xanthine, which is further oxidized to uric acid by xanthine oxidase (Fig. 17-3). Molecular oxygen, the oxidant in both reactions, is reduced to H_2O_2 and other reactive oxygen species. In humans, uric acid is the final product of purine degradation and is excreted in the urine.

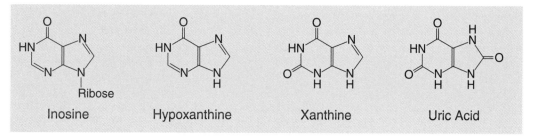

FIGURE 17-3.   Adenosine metabolites. Adenosine is converted to inosine by adenosine deaminase. Removal of the ribose by nucleoside phosphorylase produces hypoxanthine, which is sequentially oxidized to xanthine and uric acid by xanthine oxidase.

Box 17-1

INHERITED DISEASES OF PURINE METABOLISM

Lesch-Nyhan syndrome (LNS) is an X-linked recessive inherited disorder usually evident at six to ten months of age with choreiform movements, compulsive self-mutilation, spasticity, mental retardation, hyperuricemia and gout. LNS is associated with mutations in the gene for the purine salvage enzyme hypoxanthine-guanine phosphoribosyltransferase (HPRT). There is an almost complete deficiency of this enzyme in patients with the full syndrome. However, individuals with a partial deficiency in HPRT generally have hyperuricemia and gout but not the neurologic manifestations. Treatment with allopurinol, which inhibits xanthine oxidase, reduces the levels of uric acid and the attendant symptoms of hyperuricemia but does not ameliorate the neurologic phenomena. Transgenic mouse models made to be genetically deficient in HPRT or doubly deficient in HPRT and in another purine salvage enzyme, adenine phosphoribosyltransferase (APRT), and thus devoid of any purine salvage pathways, do not show

behavioral abnormalities reflective of the LNS phenotype [1]. Mice, in contrast to humans, exhibit uricase activity that might alter the consequences of high uric acid [2]. However, other diseases associated with hyperuricemia, as in gout or phosphoribosylpyrophosphate synthetase deficiency, are not associated with the neurologic phenotype of LNS. Therefore, the neuropsychiatric and behavioral patterns of the phenotype are not explained simply by deficits in a single gene. However, administration of an inhibitor of APRT to HPRT-deficient mice did produce self-injurious behavior [3]. Administration of dopamine agonists to rats with 6-OH-dopamine-induced lesions of catecholamine pathways or to primates with surgical lesions of the nigrostriatal pathway demonstrate stereotypical and self-injurious behaviors. These patterns appear related to supersensitivity of dopamine D1 receptors (see Chap. 12). Positron emission tomography with [18F]-fluorodopa to image dopa decarboxylase activity and dopamine storage in nerve

PURINERGIC RECEPTORS

Receptors for both ATP and adenosine are widely distributed in the nervous system as well as in other tissues. The notion that there are purinergic receptors, that is, proteins on the surface of cells that bind and respond to purines, was slow to evolve. The first evidence was the observation of cardiovascular physiological effects of purines. Drury and Szent-Gyorgyi [8] first noted effects of adenine nucleotides on cardiac and vascular tissues in 1929. Thirty-four years later, Berne [9] identified a physiological role for adenosine as a mediator of coronary vasodilation in response to myocardial hypoxia. In the 1970s, adenosine was found to stimulate cAMP formation in brain slices. Subsequently, physio-

logical effects of adenosine on almost all tissues have been described. Based on the responses of various tissues to purines, Burnstock [10] proposed that there are distinct receptors that bind adenosine or ATP, designated P1 and P2 receptors, respectively. The existence of adenosine receptors was not widely accepted until the 1980s, when saturable binding sites for radioactive adenosine analogs were demonstrated in brain. The existence of adenosine receptors was proved unequivocally when the first adenosine receptors were cloned in 1990 [11]. Originally, the "P" in P1 and P2 was meant to designate purinergic receptors. However, it has been discovered that some of the P2 receptors bind pyrimidines, UTP or UDP, preferentially over the purine, ATP. Hence, the "P" in P2 is now used to designate

Box 17-1 (continued)

terminals (see Chap. 54) has demonstrated abnormally few dopaminergic nerve terminals and cell bodies in the basal ganglia and frontal cortex of LNS patients, suggesting pervasive developmental abnormalities in dopaminergic systems. By the method of single photon emission computed tomography (SPECT), the imaging of dopamine plasmalemma transporters (Chaps. 5 and 12) with a specific ligand also demonstrates diminished numbers of dopamine re-uptake sites in the striatum. Developmental dopaminergic neuronal system abnormalities may be related to the genetic alteration that occurs in the context of a multigene regulation pattern specific for the species.

Another recessive, but autosomal, inherited disorder in purine metabolism, a mutation in the gene for adenylosuccinate lyase (ASL), is associated with severe mental retardation and autistic behavior, but apparently not self-mutilation [4]. This enzyme, as studied in *B. subtilis*, catalyzes *de novo* purine biosynthesis leading to AMP and IMP [5]. Future research into the cellular and regional expression and regulation of enzymes of purine metabolism in the brain during development will contribute to understanding the physiology of these complex behaviors.

—*George J. Siegel*

REFERENCES

1. Engle, S. J., Womer, D. E., Davies, P. M., et al. HPRT-APRT-deficient mice are not a model for Lesch-Nyhan syndrome. *Hum. Mol. Genet.* 5:1607–1610, 1996.
2. Wu, X., Wakamiya, M., Vaishnav, S., et al. Hyperuricemia and urate nephropathy in urate oxidase-deficient mice. *Proc. Natl. Acad. Sci. (USA)* 91:742–746, 1994.
3. Wu, C. L., and Melton, D. W. Production of a model for Lesch-Nyhan syndrome in hypoxanthine phosphoribosyltransferase-deficient mice. *Nat. Genet.* 3:235–240, 1993.
4. Stone, R. L., Aimi, J., Barshop, B. A., et al. A mutation in adenylosuccinate lyase associated with mental retardation and autistic features. *Nat. Genet.* 1:59–63, 1992.
5. Redinbo, M. R., Eide, S. M., Stone, R. L., Dixon, J. E., and Yeates, T. O. Crystallization and preliminary structural analysis of Bacilus subtilis adenylosuccinate lyase, an enzyme implicated in infantile autism. *Protein Sci.* 5:786–788, 1996.

purine or pyrimidine. Despite these exceptions, P1 and P2 receptors collectively are still generally referred to as purinergic receptors.

In addition to adenosine, various synthetic adenosine analogs activate P1, but not P2, receptors and synthetic ATP or UTP analogs activate P2, but not adenosine, receptors. However, not all purines activate P1 or P2 receptors. For example, adenine, guanosine and uric acid do not activate P1 receptors. Inosine, the purine nucleoside product of adenosine deamination, generally has weak activity at P1 receptors but does activate A_3 adenosine receptors in ischemic tissues, particularly in rodent species [12]. This action of inosine may be physiologically significant because inosine accumulates to very high concentrations (>1 mM) in ischemic tissues. The development of synthetic compounds that activate P1 or P2 receptors has been important for elucidating how these receptors function because some of these compounds are more potent and selective than the parent purines and most are more stable than the short-lived endogenous compounds adenosine and ATP.

Adenosine also binds to an intracellular site on adenylyl cyclase

Since P1 and P2 receptors are located on the surface of cells, they bind purines or pyrimidines in the extracellular space. There also is an adenosine-binding site located intracellularly on the enzyme adenylyl cyclase. This is referred to as the "P-site" of adenylyl cyclase; and binding of

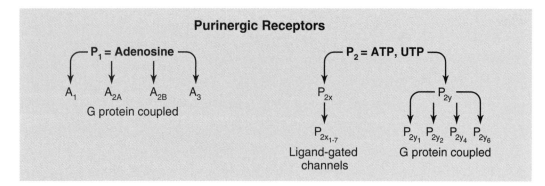

FIGURE 17-4. The purinergic receptor family. The purinergic receptors are divided into two major families: the P1, or adenosine, receptors and P2 receptors, which bind ATP and/or UTP. P1 and P2Y receptors are coupled to GTP-binding proteins. The P2X family of receptors are ligand-gated channels. Additional P2Y receptor subtypes have been claimed, but their identity as purinergic receptors is controversial.

adenosine and other purines, notably 3'-AMP, 2'-deoxy-3'-ATP and 2',5'-dideoxyadenosine, inhibits adenylyl cyclase activity [13]. The P-site of adenylyl cyclase and other intracellular purine-binding sites are not classified as purinergic receptors.

There are four subtypes of adenosine receptor that have been cloned

The four P1 receptors that have been cloned are referred to as A_1, A_{2A}, A_{2B} and A_3 (Fig. 17-4). All four of these belong to the superfamily of recep-

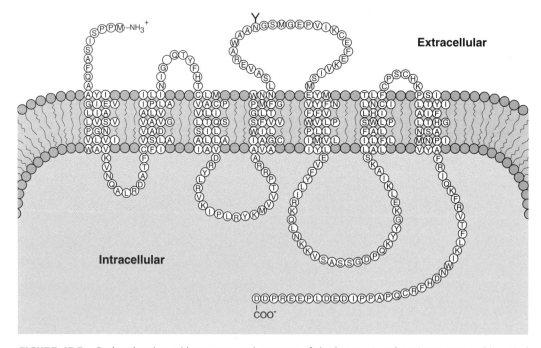

FIGURE 17-5. Deduced amino acid sequence and structure of the human A_1 adenosine receptor. This typical adenosine receptor is a member of the large family of guanine nucleotide-binding, protein-coupled receptors that span the plasma membrane seven times. An unusual feature of adenosine receptors is the short amino termini lacking *N*-linked glycosylation sites. These are found instead on extracellular loop 2 (as pictured). The ligand-binding pocket is thought to be formed by amino acids in transmembrane segments 2, 3 and 7. GTP-binding proteins are thought to interact with juxtamembranous regions of intracellular loops 2 and 3 and the carboxyl terminus.

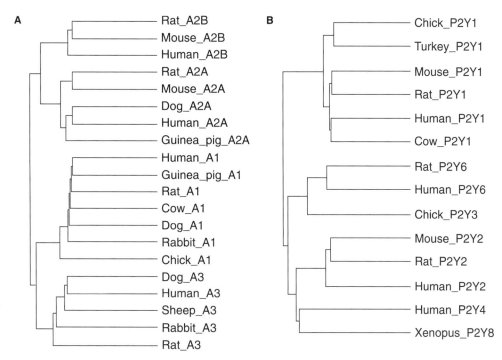

FIGURE 17-6. Dendograms illustrating structural similarities among G protein-coupled purinergic receptor subtypes. Distance along the horizontal axis is proportional to differences between species. **A:** Adenosine receptor subtypes; the rat and rabbit A_3 receptors are 73.2% similar. **B:** P2Y$_2$ receptor subtypes; the *Xenopus* P2Y$_8$ and human P2Y$_4$ receptors are 71.1% similar.

tors that signal via G proteins and contain seven hydrophobic transmembrane-spanning segments, as illustrated in the case of the A_1 adenosine receptor in Figure 17-5. The receptors consist of single subunits that have a molecular weight of 35,000 to 46,000 and one or two consensus sequences for *N*-linked glycosylation (NXS/T) in the second extracellular loop. The human A_3 adenosine receptor also has two sites for *N*-linked glycosylation near the amino terminus. These glycosylation sites may be involved in targeting receptors for expression on the cell surface. Adenosine receptors also contain multiple serine and threonine residues on the third intracellular loop or near the carboxyl terminus. In some cases, these may become phosphorylated and lead to receptor desensitization during prolonged exposure to adenosine. The greatest similarities in the structure of the adenosine receptor subtypes are found in the transmembrane segments, particularly in segments 2, 3 and 7. This suggests that these segments may be aligned next to each other in the plane of the membrane

bilayer to form a ligand-binding pocket. Three of the adenosine receptors, A_1, A_{2B} and A_3, have a cysteine residue, thought to be palmitoylated, located within 25 amino acids of the carboxyl terminus. The addition of this fatty acid is thought to anchor the carboxyl-terminal region of the receptor to the plasma membrane. As illustrated in Figure 17-6, the structure of the G protein-coupled purinergic receptors varies little between species, and there is somewhat greater variability between subtypes, even within a single species. The adenosine receptor subtypes, their effectors and the identity of some selective agonists and antagonists are listed in Table 17-2.

Xanthines block P1, but not P2, receptors

One of the criteria initially used to distinguish between adenosine and ATP receptors was selective blockade of the former by xanthines (Fig. 17-7) such as caffeine (1,3,7-trimethylxanthine) and theophylline (1,3-dimethylxanthine). These

TABLE 17-2. SUBTYPES OF ADENOSINE RECEPTOR, THEIR EFFECTORS AND SELECTIVE AGONISTS AND ANTAGONISTS

Receptor/ (accession #)[a]	Effector[b]	Agonist	Antagonist
A_1 (S45235)	Adenylyl cyclase (−) K$^+$ channels (+) Ca^{2+} channels (−) PI-PLC (+ via βγ)	CPA	WRC-0571, CPX, CVT-124
A_{2A} (S46950)	Adenylyl cyclase (+)	CGS21680	ZM241385, SCH58261, CSC
A_{2B} (M97759)	Adenylyl cyclase (+) PI-PLC (+ via $α_q$)	None	Enprofylline
A_3 (L22607)	Adenylyl cyclase (−) PI-PLC (+ via βγ)	IB-MECA	L-249313
Nonselective ligands		NECA	SPT

[a] Genebank accession numbers are for human clones.
[b] PI-PLC, phosphoinositide-specific phospholipase C; βγ and $α_q$, subunits of GTP-binding proteins activated by these receptors.
CPA, N^6-cyclopenthyadenosine; WRC-0571, C^8-(N-methylisopropyl)-amino-N^6-(5'-endohydroxy)-endonorbornan-2-yl-9-methyladenine; CPX, 1,3-dipropyl-8-cyclopentylxanthine; CVT 124, S-1,3-dipropyl-8[2-(5,6-eoxynorbornyl)]xanthine; CGS21680, 2-[4-(2-carboxyethyl)phenethylamino]-5'-N-ethylcarboxamidoadenosine; ZM241385, 4-(2-[7-amino-2-[2-furyl][1,2,4]triazolo[2,3-α][1,3,5] triazin-5-yl-aminoethyl)phenol; SCH58261, 5-amino-7-(2-phenylethyl) -2-(2-furyl)-pyrazolo [4,3-epsilon]-1,2,4-triazolo[1,5-c]pyrimidine; CSC, 8-(3-chlorostyryl)-caffeine IB-MECA, N^6-(2-iodo)benzyl-5'-N-methylcarboxamidodo adenosine; L-249313, 6-carboxymethyl-5,9-dihydro-9-methyl-2-phenyl-[1,2,4]-triazolo[5,1-α][2,7]naphthyridine; NECA, 5'-N-ethylcarboxamidoadenosine; SPT, p-sulfophenyltheophylline. Xanthines block P1 but not P2 receptors.

xanthines occur naturally in coffee, tea and chocolate, and their well-known stimulant action has been attributed to blockade of adenosine receptors in the CNS. 8-Phenylxanthines, 8-cycloalkylxanthines and nonxanthine synthetic antagonists have been synthesized and characterized as adenosine-receptor antagonists that are thousands of times more potent and, in some cases, more selective for individual adenosine-receptor subtypes than are caffeine and theophylline.

Subtypes of P2 receptors can be classified pharmacologically

Four G protein-coupled P2Y receptors (P2Y$_1$, P2Y$_2$, P2Y$_4$ and P2Y$_6$) have been cloned from mammalian species [14]. The subset of receptors that respond to UTP formerly were referred to as P2U receptors. The P2Y$_1$ receptor is an ADP receptor antagonized by ATP and expressed in platelets and megakaryocytes formerly referred to as P2T [15]. The P2Y$_2$ receptor is activated by UTP and ATP with similar potency and is not activated by nucleoside diphosphates. Diadenosine tetraphosphate is a potent agonist at this receptor. The P2Y$_4$ receptor is highly selective for UTP over ATP and is not activated by nucleoside diphosphates. The P2Y$_6$ receptor is activated most potently by UDP and weakly or not at all by UTP, ADP and ATP.

The P2X receptors are structurally unrelated to the P2Y receptors. They have two transmembrane domains with intracellular N and C termini separated by a large extracellular loop. The P2X receptors generally are activated by ATP and 2-methylthio-ATP. [^{35}S]ATPγS has been used as a radioligand for the direct labeling of cloned P2X receptors. α,β-Methylene-ATP is an agonist of P2X$_1$ and P2X$_3$ receptors but does not activate the other P2X subtypes. ADP is a selective agonist of P2X$_5$ and P2X$_6$ receptors, and benzoyl-ATP is an agonist of the P2X$_7$ receptor, an unusual receptor, previously called P2Z, that can cause cell lysis by promoting the formation of large pores.

FIGURE 17-7. Structures of selective agonists and antagonists of adenosine receptors.

P₁ Receptor Agonists and Antagonists

Parent structures

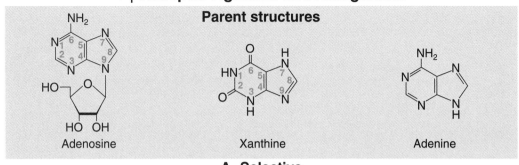

Adenosine   Xanthine   Adenine

A₁ Selective

Agonists	Xanthine Antagonists	Nonxanthine Antagonists

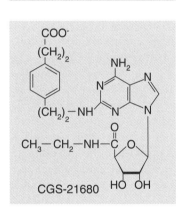

CPA

CVT-124

WRC-0571

A₂ₐ Selective

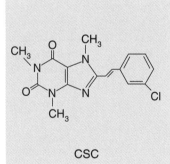

CGS-21680

CSC

ZM 241385

A₃ Selective

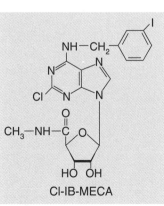

CI-IB-MECA

L-249313

TABLE 17-3.	DISTRIBUTION OF P2 mRNAs IN THE CNS[a]	
Receptor	Accession #[b]	Transcript location
P2X$_1$	X83688	Large motor neurons of the spinal cord
P2X$_2$	—	Sensory and autonomic ganglia, adrenal medulla, dorsal and ventral horns of the spinal cord, thalamus, hypothalamus, preoptic area, red nucleus, oculomotor nucleus, locus ceruleus and dorsal motor nucleus of vagus
P2X$_3$	Y07683	A subset of small cells of sensory neurons
P2X$_4$	Y07684	Widespread in brain and spinal cord
P2X$_5$	U49395	Proprioceptive neurons of mesencephalic trigeminal nucleus, sensory ganglia
P2X$_6$	—	Widespread in brain, spinal cord and sensory ganglia
P2X$_7$	Y09561	Macrophages
P2Y$_1$	Z49205	Telencephalon, diencephalon, mesencephalon and cerebellum
P2Y$_2$	U07225	Found in pituitary but not in human brain
P2Y$_4$	X91852	Not detected in human brain
P2Y$_6$	X97058	Not detected in human brain

[a] From [1] with permission.
[b] Genebank accession numbers of human clones.

A problem that continues to hamper the study of P2 receptors is the absence of receptor subtype-selective antagonists. The compounds that are used as P2 receptor antagonists are non-selective, low-affinity compounds. These include reactive blue 2 (P2Y receptors), suramin (P2Y$_1$ > P2Y$_2$ > P2Y$_4$), NF023 (P2X receptors) and pyridoxalphosphate-6-azophenyl-2',4'-disulfonic acid (PPADS) (P2X > P2Y). ATP and ARL-66,096 are antagonists of P2Y$_1$ receptors. The distribution of mRNA for P2 receptor subtypes in the nervous system of the adult rat is summarized in Table 17-3.

Receptors exist for diadenosine polyphosphates, distinct from P1 or P2 receptors

Radioligand-binding experiments carried out with [^{3}H]Ap4A on synaptosomal preparations give K_D values of about 100 pM for high-affinity binding sites [16]. ApnA induces Ca^{2+} entry into midbrain synaptic terminals. By autoradiography, [^{3}H]Ap4A binds most to gray matter in the seventh cranial nerve, medial superior olive, pontine nuclei, glomerular and external plexiform layers of the olfactory bulb and the granule cell layer of the cerebellar cortex.

EFFECTS OF PURINES IN THE NERVOUS SYSTEM

Adenosine receptors

The adenosine that activates receptors in the nervous system is derived in part from adenine nucleotides packaged in the synaptic granules of nerves and in part from ATP and adenosine derived from sources other than synaptic granules. Adenosine release evoked by electrical stimulation is completely dependent on propagated electrical activity, blocked by tetrodotoxin (TTX) and largely Ca^{2+}-dependent. Adenosine release evoked by anoxia is Ca^{2+}-independent and largely insensitive to TTX. Many of the central actions of adenosine can be attributed to inhibition of Ca^{2+}-dependent excitatory neurotransmitter release. Most of these effects appear to be presynaptic and are mediated by G proteins coupled to inhibition of N-type Ca^{2+} channels or to stimulation of K$^+$ channels. However, in some instances, adenosine produces excitatory effects in the CNS. For example, in the nucleus tractus solitarius, adenosine increases glutamate release and elicits excitatory cardiovascular effects [17]. Both excitatory and inhibitory effects of adenosine have been noted in hippocampal slices. In spinal cord, adenosine can be derived from capsaicin-sensitive, small-diameter, primary afferent neurons and potentiates the antinociceptive action of norepinephrine [18]. Opiates have been shown to induce release of adenosine from brain slices, synaptosomes and the spinal cord; some of the effects of opiates are blocked by adenosine receptor antagonists. It has also been suggested that some of the behavioral effects of alcoholic beverages may be mediated by adenosine because intoxicating concentrations of ethanol can block adenosine transport.

A_1-adenosine receptors were originally characterized on the basis of their ability to inhibit adenylyl cyclase in adipose tissue. A number of other G protein-mediated effectors of A_1 receptors have subsequently been discovered; these include activation of K^+ channels, extensively characterized in striatal neurons [19], and inhibition of Ca^{2+} channels, extensively characterized in dorsal root ganglion cells [20]. Activation of A_1 receptors has been shown to produce a species-dependent stimulation or inhibition of the phosphatidylinositol pathway in cerebral cortex. In other tissues, activation of A_1 receptors results in synergistic activation of the phosphatidylinositol pathway in concert with Ca^{2+}-mobilizing hormones or neurotransmitters [20]. The effectors of A_1 adenosine receptors and other purinergic receptor subtypes are summarized in Table 17-2.

A_1 adenosine receptors are widely distributed in the CNS (Fig. 17-8). These receptors have been extensively characterized in brain because they are expressed at a high density, 0.5 to 1.0 pmol/mg membrane protein, and because of the development of several high-affinity radioligands, including [3H]1,3-dipropyl-8-cyclopentylxanthine (CPX). In the periphery, A_1-

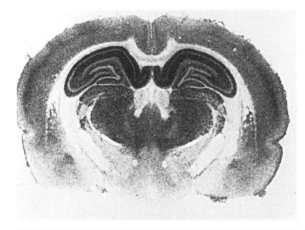

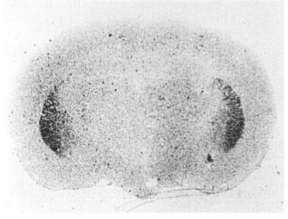

FIGURE 17-8. Distribution of A_1 and A_{2A} receptors in rat brain. **Top:** Autoradiograph of the binding of the A_1-selective radioligand [3H]cyclohexyladenosine to a slice of rat brain. Note the widespread distribution of A_1 receptors and the particularly high density of receptors in the hippocampus. **Bottom:** Autoradiograph of the binding of the A_{2A}-selective radioligand [125I]APE. Note the restricted striatal distribution. (Photograph courtesy of Dr. Kevin Lee of the University of Virginia.)

adenosine receptors are found in the heart, where they produce negative inotropic, chronotropic and dromotropic responses [22]; in adipose tissue, where they inhibit lipolysis and enhance insulin-stimulated glucose transport; and in kidney, where they reduce glomerular filtration pressure and produce an antidiuresis. At the neuromuscular junction, adenosine inhibits ACh release by a prejunctional effect on A_1 adenosine receptors.

Effects of adenosine that have been attributed to activation of A_1 receptors in the CNS include sedation, anticonvulsant activity, analgesia and neuroprotection. Adenosine modulates synaptic plasticity associated with distinct stimulation frequency patterns. Presynaptic A_1-adenosine receptors inhibit neurotransmitter release, especially at high stimulation frequency. Activation of A_1 receptors reduces long-term changes in synaptic efficiency, such as long-term potentiation, in various brain regions; for example, activation of A_1 receptors reduces long-term potentiation of the population spikes evoked in the hippocampal CA1 area by stimulation of the Schaffer fibers. Release of glutamate and aspartate from nerve terminals in the CA1 region of the hippocampus is highly sensitive to inhibition by adenosine. These excitatory amino acids enhance the release of adenosine.

A_2-adenosine receptors were originally classified on the basis of their ability to stimulate cAMP accumulation in neuronal tissues. Based on substantial differences in binding affinity for adenosine, A_2 receptors were subdivided into A_{2A} and A_{2B} subtypes, a division that has subsequently been confirmed by molecular cloning. Adenosine analogs substituted on the 2 position, such as CG2S1680, are agonists that bind with higher affinity to A_{2A} than to A_{2B} receptors. Caffeine, the most widely used psychoactive drug, has some selectivity as an antagonist of A_{2A} receptors. In transgenic mice lacking A_{2A} receptors, caffeine reduces exploratory activity, opposite to its usual effect of stimulating exploratory activity [23]. Potent and selective antagonists of A_{2A} receptors have been developed, including the caffeine derivative, 8-(3-chlorostyryl)-caffeine (CSC), and nonxanthine antagonists ZM241385 and SCH58261.

In the CNS, the high-density expression of A_{2A} receptors is restricted to the striatum, nucleus accumbens and olfactory tubercle (Fig. 17-8). The distribution of A_{2A} receptors closely matches that of dopamine D2 receptors, which are expressed in striatopallidal GABAergic neurons. Antagonistic interactions exist between the A_{2A} and D2 dopamine receptors. Blockade of A_{2A} receptors mimics the action of dopamine D2 receptor agonists. Activation of A_{2A} adenosine receptors enhances cAMP formation, whereas activation of D2 dopamine receptors inhibits cAMP formation. Administration of drugs that stimulate dopamine receptors, such as apomorphine and L-DOPA, to rodents with a unilateral lesion of the nigrostriatal pathway induces a turning behavior contralateral to the lesioned side. This effect is due to the development of supersensitivity of dopamine receptors in the denervated striatum. Compounds that block adenosine receptors also produce such turning behavior and potentiate the effects of dopamine agonists. Moreover, adenosine A_{2A} agonists inhibit D2 mediated behaviors. These findings suggest that modulation of striatal dopaminergic systems by adenosine contributes to the psychomotor depressant effects of adenosine agonists and to the psychomotor stimulatory effects of methylxanthines. A_{2A}-selective adenosine receptor antagonists may have potential as antiparkinsonian drugs [24].

A_2 receptors present on sensory nerves in the carotid body, aortic body, pulmonary circulation and elsewhere produce excitatory sensory input. These receptors have been implicated in the production of dyspnea and pain of angina pectoris, ulcer and the human blister base preparation.

A_3-adenosine receptors. Prior to their cloning, the existence of A_1 and A_2 receptors had been postulated based on results of binding assays with radioligands and the study of physiological and biochemical responses to various ligands. After these receptors were cloned, a search for related genes revealed an unexpected receptor in the adenosine family, designated A_3. The term A_3 was also used to designate a putative A_1-like receptor in heart and autonomic neurons; however, such a receptor has not been proven to exist, and this old, pharmacologically postulated A$_3$ receptor is distinct from the A$_3$ receptor that has been cloned. In current usage, A$_3$ refers to the cloned receptor. In the rat, abundant A$_3$ transcript is found almost exclusively in testes. However, the transcript for homologous sheep and human receptors is modestly expressed throughout the brain and heavily in pineal, lung and spleen tissues. A$_3$ receptor activation may play a role in the generation of neuronal injury. Chronic activation of A$_3$ receptors protects against ischemic damage, possibly due to receptor desensitization.

ATP receptors

P2-ATP receptors have a very wide tissue distribution. Excitatory effects of ATP on neurons in the CNS have been noted in cuneate nucleus, in cerebellar Purkinje cells, in cells in the sensory vestibular and trigeminal nuclei and in cortex. In many instances, ATP has been noted to have biphasic or inhibitory effects, attributed in part to its breakdown to adenosine.

P2X receptors are widespread in the brain (Table 17-3) and have excitatory effects. P2X receptor-mediated responses in central and peripheral neurons indicate that ATP is a fast neurotransmitter that acts by opening ligand-gated channels [25]. These receptors also are found in the gastrointestinal tract, veins and arteries, genitourinary tract, urinary bladder, vas deferens, nictitating membrane, cardiac muscle and pheochromocytoma (PC-12) cells. Effects of P2X antagonists on excitatory postsynaptic currents in CA1 and CA3 pyramidal neurons suggest that they have a role in the facilitation of glutamate release.

P2Y receptors have been extensively characterized in turkey erythrocytes as well as in liver and endothelial cells. They couple via a G protein, G$_q$, to activate phosphoinositide-specific phospholipase C and produce an inositol-1,4,5-trisphosphate-dependent mobilization of intracellular Ca^{2+}. UTP is being examined as a P2Y$_2$ receptor agonist for the treatment of cystic fibrosis.

P2Y receptors found on endothelial cells elicit a Ca^{2+}-dependent release of endothelium-dependent relaxing factor (EDRF) and vasodilation. Secondary activation of a Ca^{2+}-sensitive phospholipase A$_2$ increases the synthesis of endothelial prostacyclin, which limits the extent of intravascular platelet aggregation following vascular damage and platelet stimulation. The P2Y-mediated vasodilation opposes a vasoconstriction elicited by P2X receptors, found on vascular smooth muscle cells, that elicits an endothelium-independent excitation, that is, constriction. P2Y receptors are also found on adrenal chromaffin cells and platelets, where they modulate catecholamine release and aggregation, respectively.

In the brain, P2Y receptors may mediate the ability of ATP to enhance the postsynaptic actions of glutamate. Cotransmitter synergistic actions of ATP on the functional effects of glutamate may play an important role in learning and memory [26].

P2Y$_1$ receptors are found exclusively on platelets, their precursor megakaryocyte cells and certain cultured hematopoietic cells, such as K562 leukemia cells. They can be distinguished from other P2 receptors in that ADP is the most potent natural agonist and ATP is a competitive antagonist. ADP acts via a G protein to inhibit cAMP accumulation, mobilize intracellular Ca^{2+} and stimulate granule secretion. The responses of platelets to ADP are prevented by activators of PKC, such as phorbol 12-myristate 13-acetate. ARL67085 is a selective antagonist of P2Y$_1$ receptors and has antithrombotic activity.

REFERENCES

1. Humphrey, P. P., Buell, G., Kennedy, I., et al. New insights on P2X purinoceptors. *Nauyn Schmiedebergs Arch. Pharmacol.* 352:585–596, 1995.
2. Abraham, E. H., Prat, A. G., Gerweck, L., et al. The multidrug resistance (mdr1) gene product functions as an ATP channel. *Proc. Natl. Acad. Sci. USA* 90:312–316, 1993.
3. Zimmermann, H. Extracellular purine metabolism. *Drug Dev. Res.* 39:337–352, 1996.
4. Kaczmarek, E., Koziak, K., Sevigny, J., et al. Identification and characterization of CD39/vascular ATP diphosphohydrolase. *J. Biol. Chem.* 271: 33116–33122, 1996.

5. Resta, R., and Thompson, L. F. T cell signalling through cd73. *Cell. Signal.* 9:131–139, 1997.

6. Rosenberg, P. A., and Li, Y. Vasoactive intestinal peptide regulates extracellular adenosine levels in rat cortical cultures. *Neurosci. Lett.* 200:93–96, 1995.

7. Anderson, C. M., Xiong, W., Young, J. D., Cass, C. E., and Parkinson, F. E. Demonstration of the existence of mRNAs encoding N1/cif and N2/cit sodium/nucleoside cotransporters in rat brain. *Mol. Brain Res.* 42:358–361, 1996.

8. Drury, A. N., and Szent-Gyorgyi, A. The physiological activity of adenine compounds with special reference to their action upon the mammalian heart. *J. Physiol. (Lond.)* 68:213–237, 1929.

9. Berne, R. M. Cardiac nucleotides in hypoxia: Possible role in regulation of coronary blood flow. *Am. J. Physiol.* 204:317–322, 1963.

10. Burnstock, G. A basis for distinguishing two types of purinergic receptor. In L. Bolis and R. W. Straub (eds.), *Cell Membrane Receptors for Drugs and Hormones: A Multidisciplinary Approach.* New York: Raven Press, 1978, pp. 107–118.

11. Maenhaut, C., Van Sande, J., Liebert, F., et al. RDC8 codes for an adenosine A2 receptor with physiological constitutive activity. *Biochem. Biophys. Res. Commun.* 173:1169–1178, 1990.

12. Jin, X., Shepherd, R. K., Puling, B. R. and Linden, J. Inosine binds to A3 adenosine receptors and stimulates mast cell degranulation. *J. Clin. Invest.* 100:2849–2857, 1997.

13. Johnson, R. A., Desaubry, L., Bianchi, G., et al. Isozyme-dependent sensitivity of adenylyl cyclases to p-site-mediated inhibition by adenine nucleosides and nucleoside 3′-polyphosphates. *J. Biol. Chem.* 272:8962–8966, 1997.

14. Nicholas, R. A., Lazarowski, E. R., Watt, W. C., Li, Q., Boyer, J., and Harden, T. K. Pharmacological and second messenger signalling selectivities of cloned P2Y receptors. *J. Auton. Pharmacol.* 16:319–323, 1996.

15. Leon, C., Hechler, B., Vial, C. et al. The P2Y1 receptor is an ADP receptor antagonized by ATP and expressed in platelets and megakaryoblastic cells. *FEBS Letters* 403:26–30, 1997.

16. Miras-Portugal, M. T., Castro, E., Mateo, J., and Pintor, J. The diadenosine polyphosphate receptors: P_{2D} purinoceptors. *Ciba Found. Symp.* 198:35–52, 1996.

17. Mosqueda-Garcia, R., Tseng, C.-J., Appalsamy, M., Beck, C., and Robertson, D. Cardiovascular excitatory effects of adenosine in the nucleus of the solitary tract. *Hypertension* 18:494–502, 1991.

18. Sawynok, J., Reid, A., and Isbrucker, R. Adenosine mediates calcium-induced antinociception and potentiation of noradrenergic antinociception in the spinal cord. *Brain Res.* 524:187–195, 1990.

19. Trussel, L. O., and Jackson, M. B. Adenosine-activated potassium conductance in cultured striatal neurons. *Proc. Natl. Acad. Sci. USA* 82:4857–4861, 1985.

20. Dolphin, A. C., Forda, S. R., and Scott, R. H. Calcium-dependent currents in cultured rat dorsal root ganglion neurons are inhibited by an adenosine analogue. *J. Physiol. (Lond.)* 373:47–61, 1986.

21. Linden, J. Structure and function of the A_1 adenosine receptor. *FASEB J.* 5:2668–2676, 1991.

22. Bellardinelli, L., Linden, J., and Berne, R. M. The cardiac effects of adenosine. *Prog. Cardiovasc. Dis.* 32:73–97, 1989.

23. Ledent, C., Vaugeois, J. M., Schiffmann, S. N., et al. Aggressiveness, hypoalgesia and high blood pressure in mice lacking the adenosine A(2a) receptor. *Nature* 388:674–678, 1997.

24. Ferre, S., Von Euler, G., Johansson, B., Fredholm, B. B., and Fuxe, K. Stimulation of high-affinity adenosine A_2 receptors decreases the affinity of dopamine D_2 receptors in rat striatal membranes. *Proc. Natl. Acad. Sci. USA* 88:7238–7241, 1991.

25. Edwards, F. A., and Gibb, A. J. ATP—A fast neurotransmitter. *FEBS Lett.* 325:86–89, 1993.

26. Wieraszko, A., and Ehrlich, Y. H. On the role of extracellular ATP in the induction of long-term potentiation in the hippocampus. *J. Neurochem.* 63:1731–1738, 1994.

CHAPTER

18

Peptides

Richard E. Mains and Betty A. Eipper

Basic Neurochemistry: Molecular, Cellular and Medical Aspects, 6th Ed., edited by G. J. Siegel et al. Published by Lippincott–Raven Publishers, Philadelphia, 1999. Correspondence to Richard E. Mains, Departments of Neuroscience and Physiology, Johns Hopkins University School of Medicine, 725 North Wolfe Street, Baltimore, Maryland 21205-2185.

THE NEUROPEPTIDES

Many neuropeptides were originally identified as pituitary or gastrointestinal hormones

Probably the first neuropeptide to be identified was vasopressin, a nine-amino-acid peptide secreted by the nerve endings in the neural lobe of the pituitary. The source of the vasopressin is the magnocellular neurons of the hypothalamus, which send axons to the neurohypophysis, which is the site of release into the blood, in classic neurosecretory fashion. Like vasopressin, a number of gastrointestinal peptides, such as cholecystokinin (CCK), are also found at high concentrations in the nervous system. In the gastrointestinal (GI) system, CCK is secreted by the duodenum and governs the delivery of digestive enzymes and bile acids into the intestine. In contrast to vasopressin and CCK, the hypothalamic releasing factors are peptides released into a special portal blood system that bathes the anterior pituitary, controlling the secretion of pituitary hormones. In this system, "portal" means two successive capillary beds, one in the hypothalamus and one in the anterior pituitary. Substance P was first purified as a "sialogogic peptide," causing salivation in a bioassay. Now substance P is recognized as a major bioactive peptide in many neuronal pathways, including pain signaling. Since there are so many peptides, this chapter focuses on the principles of how neuropeptides are synthesized, stored and released and how they act on the cells they regulate. Comparisons among peptides and smaller, "conventional" neurotransmitters will be emphasized. It is significant to note that the number of known neuropeptides far exceeds the number of classical neurotransmitters.

Peptides can be grouped by structural and functional similarity

Like GABA and glutamate, which differ by only a single carboxyl group yet have very different functions, many neuropeptides with similar structures have very different functions. Vasopressin and oxytocin are the two major neurohypophyseal peptides, and each consists of nine amino acids. These two peptides are identical at seven of those residues and are thought to be the result of gene duplication early in evolution. The actions of the two peptides are distinct: oxytocin causes milk letdown and uterine contraction, while vasopressin causes water retention in the kidney and blood vessel contraction. Likewise, the opiate peptides share a common Tyr-Gly-Gly-Phe-Met/Leu sequence at the NH_2 terminus, and all are potent endogenous opiates but with distinct patterns of selectivity at the various classes of opiate receptor. The three glycoprotein hormones from the anterior pituitary, thyroid stimulating hormone (TSH), luteinizing hormone (LH) and follicle-stimulating hormone (FSH), share a common α subunit but have distinct β subunits, and only the $\alpha\beta$ dimer is biologically active. The tachykinin group includes substance P and various frog skin peptides, all with similar core sequences and -Phe-X-Gly-Leu-Met-NH_2 at the COOH terminus. The GI peptides CCK and gastrin share a common COOH-terminal sequence (Trp-Met-Asp-Phe-NH_2) and are among the few peptides which undergo tyrosine sulfation. The sites of action of CCK and gastrin are distinct: gastrin stimulates gastric acid secretion, while CCK stimulates enzyme and bile acid delivery to the small intestine. Interestingly, the common COOH-terminal tetrapeptide, while inactive in the GI tract, is abundant in the cerebral cortex and has important behavioral actions.

The function of peptides as first messengers is evolutionarily very old

In phylogenetic terms, neuropeptides were established very early as molecules effecting intercellular communication. In coelenterates, such as *Hydra*, there are many peptides used in neurotransmission, but many of the "conventional" neurotransmitter systems, such as acetylcholine (ACh), catecholamines and serotonin, covered in previous chapters, are not found [1,2]. The nerve net is strongly peptidergic in the lowest animal group with a nervous system, the cnidarians, which includes sea anemones, corals, jellyfishes and *Hydra*. Yeast use bioactive peptides such as a- and α-mating factors to communicate.

Various techniques are used to identify additional neuropeptides

Although the list of neuropeptides is already quite long, as seen in the partial listing in Figure 18-1, additional neuropeptides are still being identified. A number of experimental approaches are in use.

Bioassays are the oldest and surest way to identify biologically active peptides: a skin-darkening assay led to the discovery of α-melanotropin, increased salivation was used to identify substance P and CCK was identified as the factor causing bile acid secretion. More recently, with the advent of radioreceptor assays, peptides have been identified by their ability to bind to a

Selected Bioactive Peptides

Hypothalamic releasing factors

CRH: corticotropin releasing hormone
GHRH: growth hormone releasing hormone
GnRH: gonadotropin releasing hormone
Somatostatin
TRH: thyrotropin releasing hormone

Pituitary hormones

ACTH: adrenocorticotropic hormone
αMSH: α-melanocyte stimulating hormone
β-endorphin
GH: growth hormone
PRL: prolactin
FSH: follicle stimulating hormone
LH: luteinizing hormone
TSH: thyrotropin [thyroid stimulating hormone]

GI and brain peptides

CCK: cholecystokinin
Gastrin
GRP: gastrin releasing peptide
Motilin
Neurotensin
Substance K; substance P (tachykinins)

Circulating

Angiotensin
Bradykinin

Frog skin

Bombesin
Caerulein
Ranatensin

Opiate peptides

β-endorphin
Dynorphin
Leu-enkephalin
Met-enkephalin

Neurohypophyseal peptides

Oxytocin
Vasopressin

Neuronal and endocrine

ANF: atrial natriuretic peptide
CGRP: calcitonin gene-related peptide
VIP: vasoactive intestinal peptide

GI and pancreas

Glucagon
PP: pancreatic polypeptide

Neurons only?

Galanin
Neuromedin K
NPY: neuropeptide Y
PYY: peptide YY

Endocrine only?

Calcitonin
Insulin
Secretin
Parathyroid hormone

FIGURE 18-1.   Selected bioactive peptides are grouped by structural similarity or by tissue source.

known receptor and thus to displace a ligand or to produce a biological response. This was one of the methods used to search for opiate peptides, assaying for peptides that could displace [^{3}H]-etorphine or other opiate ligands. Similarly, several of the peptides in Figure 18-1 are routinely assayed by their ability to increase adenylyl cyclase activity in membrane preparations due to their stimulatory interaction with peptide receptors. Use of a relatively homogeneous tissue source, such as adrenal chromaffin granules, enabled identification of peptides derived from chromogranin A. Mass spectrometry is being used to characterize peptides in certain large neurons of invertebrates. As noted above, peptides important in the nervous system were often identified first in some peripheral source, such as CCK in the gut, or even in unusual places, such as frog skin. Since α-amidation of the COOH-terminus of peptides has proven to be a signature of bioactive peptides, assays specific for COOH-terminal α-amides were developed and used to discover neuropeptide Y and several other peptides.

Molecular biological approaches have been used to discover many new peptides. Neuropeptide genes have been cloned from a single identified neuron, such as the R3-14 and L5-67 propeptides of *Aplysia*. Subtractive hybridization and differential display have been used to screen for unique transcripts, allowing identification of both the *c*ocaine and *a*mphetamine-*r*egulated *t*ranscript (CART), and RESP18, a dopamine-regulated transcript [3,4]. Finally, screens using orphan receptors, which have no known ligand, were used to find natural ligands, such as orphanin FQ or prepronociceptin [5].

The neuropeptides exhibit a few key differences from the classical neurotransmitters

First, neuropeptides are present in tissues at much lower concentrations than classical neurotransmitters but are also active at receptors at correspondingly lower concentrations. For example, the concentration of ACh in synaptic vesicles is in the 100 mM range (see Chap. 11), while the concentration of neuropeptide in a large dense core vesicle is 3 to 10 mM at most.

Correspondingly, the affinity of ACh for its receptors is in the 100 μM to 1 mM range, while peptides typically bind to their receptors with nanomolar to micromolar affinities.

Probably the most striking difference between neuropeptides and conventional neurotransmitters is in their biosynthesis (Fig. 18-2). Neuropeptides are derived from larger, inactive precursors that are generally at least 90 amino acid residues in length [6–8]. The simplest example is prolactin, a pituitary product. The signal sequence for prolactin must be removed and disulfide linkages must form, but no further cleavages are necessary. The next simplest case is somatostatin, in which a single cleavage after signal peptide removal produces the bioactive peptide. Neuropeptide Y (NPY) comes from proneuropeptide Y after signal peptide removal, cleavage between NPY and the C-terminal flanking peptide of NPY (CPON) and additional modifications which are discussed below. The pro-opiomelanocortin (POMC) precursor includes several different bioactive peptides, as does the egg-laying hormone (ELH) precursor [8]. One interesting attribute common to peptide precursors in evolutionarily older species is the existence of multiple copies of the same bioactive peptide in one precursor; this is exemplified by the FMRF-NH$_2$ (Phe-Met-Arg-Phe-amide) precursor, with 29 copies of the active peptide [1]. Even in yeast, a similar process is used, so that four copies of α-mating factor are produced from the α-mating factor precursor. Precursors with multiple copies of bioactive peptide are much less common in evolutionarily more advanced species, although the rat TRH precursor contains five copies of the TRH tripeptide.

The supply of conventional neurotransmitters in small synaptic vesicles is replenished in nerve terminals by local synthesis, and many conventional neurotransmitters are recaptured after secretion. In striking contrast, neuropeptides are initially synthesized in the cell soma, sequestered within the lumen of the secretory pathway and transported down the axon while undergoing cleavages and other processing events, after which the peptide-containing, large dense core vesicle (LDCV) is used once. After exocytosis, the membrane components of the

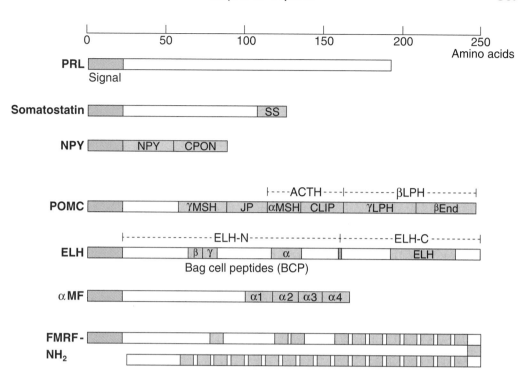

FIGURE 18-2. Structures of selected bioactive peptide precursors are diagrammed. The structures of prolactin *(PRL)*, somatostatin, neuropeptide Y *(NPY)*, pro-opiomelanocortin *(POMC)*, egg-laying hormone *(ELH)*, yeast α-mating factor *(αMF)* and FMRF-amide precursors *(FMRF-NH₂)* are indicated. Signal sequences are shaded and on the left of each precursor. *CPON*, C-terminal flanking peptide of NPY; *ACTH*, adrenocorticotropic hormone; *LPH*, lipotropin; *MSH*, melanocyte-stimulating hormone; *JP*, joining peptide; *SS*, somatostatin; βEnd, β-endorphin; *CLIP*, corticotropin-like intermediate lobe peptide.

LDCV must be reinternalized and either destroyed or reutilized after transport to the cell body. Thus, no synaptic re-use occurs of either the neuropeptides or their immediate precursors.

Release is another area of difference: conventional neurotransmitters are secreted from small secretory vesicles (SSVs) after cytosolic [Ca²⁺] transiently reaches concentrations of 50 to 100 μM, while peptides are released from LDCVs at lower concentrations of cytosolic [Ca²⁺]. Conventional neurotransmitter release is thought to occur very close to the site of Ca²⁺ entry (see Chaps. 9 and 10), while neuropeptides are typically released at a distance from the site of Ca²⁺ entry. Furthermore the Ca²⁺ that stimulates exocytosis from LDCVs may come from either internal stores or the transmembrane current (Fig. 18-3). Thus, the location of LDCVs relative to the site of Ca²⁺ influx can determine the amount of Ca²⁺ necessary for secretion to occur.

Neuropeptides are often found in neurons with conventional neurotransmitters

As diagrammed in Figure 18-3, both conventional neurotransmitters and neuropeptides are found at a majority of the synapses in the nervous system. Neuropeptide expression is extremely plastic, even in the adult. For example, the hypothalamic neurons which express vasopressin and those which synthesize corticotropin-releasing hormone (CRH) are situated close to each other but constitute separate and virtually nonoverlapping populations of neurons in the normal animal. However, after glucocorticoid concentrations are lowered by blockade of adrenal cortical function or removal of the adrenal glands, vasopressin neurons begin to express CRH and CRH neurons begin to synthesize vasopressin. This adaptive response can be understood from a teleological point of view

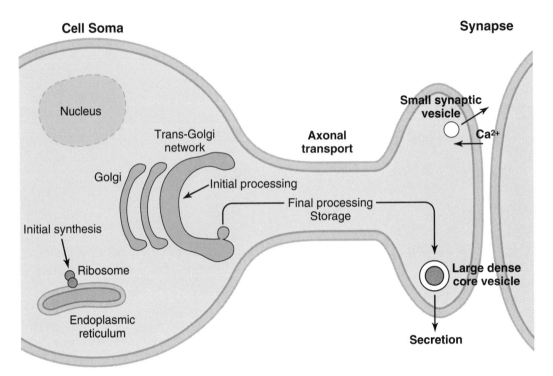

FIGURE 18-3.   Intracellular pathway of bioactive peptide biosynthesis, processing and storage. Neuropeptide precursors are synthesized on ribosomes at the endoplasmic reticulum and processed through the Golgi. Axonal transport of the large dense core vesicle to the synaptic site of release precedes the actual secretion.

by knowing that CRH normally stimulates the adrenocorticotropic hormone (ACTH)-producing cells of the anterior pituitary to secrete ACTH and that ACTH stimulates glucocorticoid production in the adrenal cortex. Vasopressin acts synergistically to increase ACTH secretion in times of need, such as adrenalectomy. In addition to neuropeptides, many LDCVs contain ATP, just as many conventional neurotransmitter vesicles do, so that ATP is released along with neuropeptides. ATP and adenosine can have potent synaptic actions in their own right (see Chap. 17).

The biosynthesis of neuropeptides is fundamentally different from that of conventional neurotransmitters

To add to the complexity discussed above, the processing of neuropeptide precursors is tissue-specific, with a general rule that most precursors are expressed in more than one tissue and that the processing is not identical in different tissues (Fig.

18-4) [6–10]. For example, anterior pituitary corticotropes cleave POMC to ACTH(1–39), a molecule that stimulates adrenal glucocorticoid production. Neurons in the arcuate nucleus cleave ACTH and α-amidate the smaller peptide to create ACTH(1–13)NH_2, which cannot stimulate the adrenal cortex but does have potent behavioral effects in the CNS. Intermediate pituitary melanotropes go one step further and α-*N*-acetylate this molecule to produce α-melanocyte-stimulating hormone (MSH), which has skin-darkening activity, especially in lower vertebrates for which background color adaptation is protective. Similarly, corticotropes produce β-lipotropin (βLPH), which has no activity as an opiate peptide, while melanotropes and CNS neurons cleave βLPH to produce the potent opiate peptide β-endorphin(1–31). In some tissues, the β-endorphin may be shortened at the COOH-terminus, which decreases its opiate activity, or α-*N*-acetylated at the NH_2-terminus, which abolishes opiate activity. The cellular control of these different patterns of processing is beginning to be

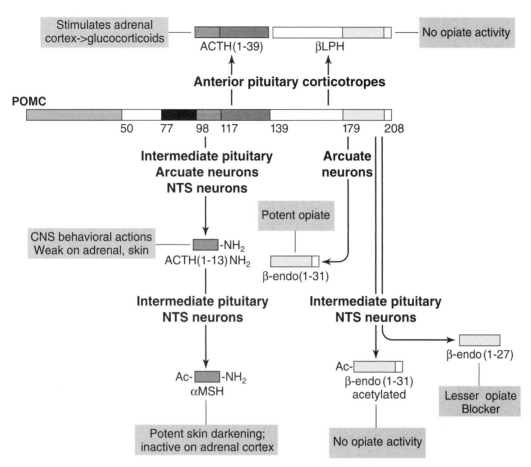

FIGURE 18-4. Tissue-specific processing of the pro-opiomelanocortin *(POMC)* precursor yields a wide array of bioactive peptide products. Processing of the POMC precursor varies in various tissues. In anterior pituitary, adreno-corticotropic hormone [*ACTH (1–39)*] and β-lipotropin *(β-LPH)* are the primary products of post-translational processing. Arcuate neurons produce the potent opiate β-endorphin [*β-endo (1–31)*] as well as *ACTH(1–13)NH₂*. Intermediate pituitary produces α-melanocyte-stimulating hormone *(αMSH)*, acetylated β-endo (1–31) and β-endo (1-27). *NTS*, nucleus tractus solitarii.

understood, with the identification of some of the enzymes that mediate these steps (see below).

Other examples of tissue-specific processing include proenkephalin, proglucagon, procholecystokinin and prosomatostatin. Somatostatin neurons in the hypothalamus primarily produce a 14-residue form of the peptide, while somatostatin endocrine cells of the pancreas and intestine produce a 28-residue form derived from the same precursor [11]. Proenkephalin is processed in the adrenal medulla to a set of opiate peptides of 15 to 35 residues, while proenkephalin in the brain is cleaved primarily to the pentapeptides met-enkephalin and leuenkephalin. Procholecystokinin in the gut is processed to peptides of

approximately 30 residues, which act on the pancreas and gallbladder, while smaller CCK-related peptides with behavioral effects are found in the brain. These smaller CCK-related peptides have no effects when applied to the pancreas or gallbladder [9].

Many of the enzymes involved in peptide biogenesis have been identified

The most common steps in precursor processing and the enzymes involved are shown in Figure 18-5. The endoproteases involved are prohormone convertases 1 and 2 (PC1 and PC2), the exopeptidase is carboxypeptidase E (CPE, also called CPH

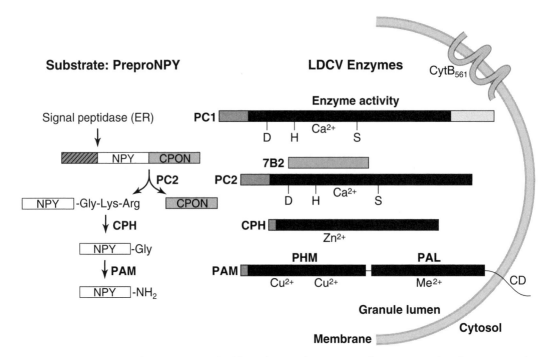

FIGURE 18-5.   Sequential enzymatic steps lead from the peptide precursor to bioactive peptides. The neuropeptide Y *(NPY)* precursor shown at the **left** is processed sequentially by the enzymes of the large dense-core vesicles *(LDCV)* shown at right. *ER*, endoplasmic reticulum; *PC*, prohormone convertase; *CPON*, C-terminal flanking peptide of NPY; *CPH*, carboxypeptidase E; *PAM*, peptidylglycine α-amidating mono-oxygenase; *PHM*, peptidylglycine α-hydroxylating mono-oxygenase; *PAL*, peptidyl-α-hydroxyglycine α-amidating lyase; *CD*, cytoplasmic domain.

and enkephalin convertase) and the α-amidating enzyme is peptidylglycine α-amidating mono-oxygenase (PAM). Many steps in their biosynthesis are not unique to neuropeptides, such as signal peptide cleavage, disulfide bond formation, the addition and subsequent modification of N-linked and O-linked oligosaccharides, phosphorylation and sulfation. As diagrammed in Figure 18-3, many of the post-translational steps occur as the maturing neuropeptides travel down the axon toward the synapse in LDCVs. The later steps in neuropeptide biosynthesis (Fig. 18-5) are unique to neurons and endocrine cells.

Key enzymes in neuropeptide biosynthesis include endoproteases, exoproteases and enzymes modifying the ends of the peptides. The discovery and characterization of Kex2p, the endoprotease that cleaves yeast pro-α-mating factor to produce four copies of the pheromone α-mating factor (Fig. 18-2), were key to the discovery of the mammalian prohormone convertases, including furin, PC1/3, PC2, PC4,

PC5/6, PC7/8/LPC, and PACE4 [6,7]. The prohormone convertases share homology with bacterial subtilisins and have an Asp-His-Ser catalytic triad, which consists of three key amino acids involved in catalysis (denoted *D*, *H*, and *S* in Fig. 18-5). The proregion of each (Fig. 18-5) must be present during biosynthesis for the protease to fold correctly but must be removed to yield an activated protease. For PC1 and furin, removal of the proregion occurs within a few minutes of biosynthesis while the enzyme is in the endoplasmic reticulum and is most likely an autocatalytic event. For the other prohormone convertases removal of the proregion is much slower. Expression of active PC2 requires coexpression of the peptide 7B2 (Fig. 18-5), which appears to perform a chaperone function and may also prevent expression of PC2 endoproteolytic activity until PC2 has been deposited into secretory granules. No corresponding chaperone/inhibitor peptide has been identified for the other prohormone convertases.

The mammalian endoproteases most clearly involved in neuropeptide processing are PC1 and PC2, Ca^{2+}-dependent proteases found in secretory granules whose expression is limited to neurons and endocrine cells (Fig. 18-5). Several other members of this endoprotease family are more widely expressed, while still others are expressed in restricted locations distinct from neurons and endocrine cells. For example, furin is found in virtually all cells and is localized primarily to the *trans*-Golgi network; furin catalyzes cleavages important in peptide function, such as the initial cleavage of the ELH, nerve growth factor and parathyroid hormone precursors, as well as cleavage within the insulin receptor precursor to produce the active $\alpha\beta$ dimer form of the receptor. Furin may also be instrumental in the activation of some of the other processing enzymes, such as PC2 and CPE.

PC1 and PC2 cleave at selected pairs of basic amino acids in peptide precursors: Lys-Arg, Arg-Arg, Lys-Lys and Arg-Lys. PC1 may also catalyze cleavages at the selected single Arg sites present in some precursors, such as prosomatostatin and procholecystokinin. Cleavages in LDCVs by PCs are tightly controlled, often occurring in a very orderly fashion (Fig. 18-6). The initial cleavages of POMC occur in less than 1 hr (Fig. 18-6, steps 1 and 2), while other cleavages occur only after several hours (Fig. 18-6, steps 6 and 7). The endoproteolytic cleavage of propeptides is often the rate-limiting reaction in peptide biosynthetic processing.

The pattern of cleavages catalyzed by PC1, PC2 and furin when expressed in neurons and endocrine cells is much more selective than the pattern of cleavages seen in test tube assays with purified enzymes. For example, although prohormone convertases usually cleave at the COOH-terminus of a pair of basic residues in model peptide substrates, in cells the cleavages can be in the middle of the pairs of basic residues, as in the case of POMC cleavage (Fig. 18-6), where the basic residues are separated and remain with the two resulting mature peptides [8]. It is likely that the Ca^{2+} concentration and internal pH of LDCVs are two variables used by neurons and endocrine cells to regulate endoproteolytic activity in LDCVs.

Additional endoproteases may be shown to play a role in neuropeptide biosynthesis. Leading candidates are the mammalian homolog of the yeast aspartyl protease-3 (YAP-3) and the *N*-arginine dibasic (NRD) convertase [12,13]. An

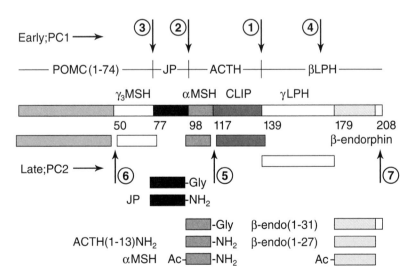

FIGURE 18-6. Processing of the pro-opiomelanocortin *(POMC)* precursor proceeds in an ordered, stepwise fashion. Cleavage of the POMC precursor occurs at seven sites, with some of the reactions being tissue-specific. The circled numbers indicate the temporal order of cleavage in tissues where these proteolytic events occur. *JP,* joining peptide; *ACTH,* adrenocorticotropic hormone; *LPH,* lipotropin; *MSH,* melanocyte-stimulating hormone; *CLIP,* corticotropin-like intermediate lobe peptide; *PC,* prohormone convertase.

additional twist in peptide biosynthesis is seen in the heart, where proatrial natriuretic factor (proANF) is stored in LDCVs and yet mature ANF is released from atrial cells into the circulation. The processing of proANF, which involves cleavage after a single Arg residue in proANF, cannot involve PC1 or PC2 since there are negligible amounts of those PCs in the heart.

CPE is a soluble protein found in virtually all LDCVs in neurons and endocrine cells (Fig. 18-5) [14]. It removes basic residues, Lys or Arg, from the COOH termini of peptide intermediates produced by the prohormone convertases. It was originally identified by its tissue distribution and substrate specificity, along with its specific inhibition by guanidinoethylmercaptosuccinic acid (GEMSA). CPE is a Co^{2+}- and Zn^{2+}-activated enzyme with a short proregion that is normally removed during maturation of the enzyme; unlike the prohormone convertases, CPE is active with the proregion attached. The carboxypeptidase function of peptide processing is not normally rate-limiting since peptide intermediates with COOH-terminal basic residues are detected only at extremely low concentrations in tissue or LDCV extracts. Recently, additional carboxypeptidases have been identified, notably CPD, an integral membrane form of the enzyme with 3 carboxypeptidase domains. The relative importance of CPE and these additional carboxypeptidases to neuropeptide processing *in vivo* is unclear. Given that cleavage at a pair of basic residues can be in the middle of the pair, there is good reason to think that an aminopeptidase will be found in LDCVs.

PAM is a bifunctional enzyme found in nearly all LDCVs (Fig. 18-5) [15]. PAM acts on peptide substrates after endoproteolytic cleavage and exopeptidase action, when a COOH-terminal Gly residue is exposed, and converts the peptidyl-Gly into the corresponding peptide-NH_2. About half of the known bioactive peptides are α-amidated, and α-amidation is generally crucial to biological potency. The peptidyl-Gly and peptide-COOH forms are usually inactive at physiological concentrations. The first step of the α-amidation reaction is performed by peptidylglycine α-hydroxylating mono-oxygenase (PHM), which is the NH_2-terminal portion of the bifunctional PAM protein. PHM binds two Cu^{2+} atoms that participate in catalysis by undergoing cycles of reduction and oxidation. PHM uses ascorbic acid as the reductant, with one atom of oxygen from O_2 incorporated into the peptide during the hydroxylation step. Thus, PHM is enzymatically very similar to dopamine β-mono-oxygenase (DBM), which converts dopamine to norepinephrine (see Chap. 12). The second step of the α-amidation reaction is performed by a second enzymatic domain of PAM, peptidyl-α-hydroxyglycine α-amidating lyase (PAL). The PAL domain constitutes a novel, divalent metal ion-dependent enzyme. Neurons primarily express an integral membrane form of the bifunctional PAM protein (Fig. 18-5), while an additional mRNA-splicing event enables some endocrine cells to express soluble versions of the protein, lacking the transmembrane domain. In the integral membrane forms of PAM, the short COOH-terminal domain extends into the cytoplasm and participates in the routing of PAM between LDCVs and the cell surface. The supply of reduced ascorbate in LDCVs is maintained by cytochrome B_{561}, a protein that has five transmembrane domains and shuttles electrons from cytosolic ascorbate to ascorbate in the lumen of the LDCVs [16]. Cytochrome B_{561} is also found in catecholamine-containing vesicles, where it performs a similar function for DBM (see Chap. 12). Nervous and endocrine tissues maintain concentrations of reduced ascorbate about 100-fold above the blood concentration of ascorbate, while most other tissues do not concentrate ascorbate.

Several peptides have NH_2-terminal pyroglutamic acid residues, also termed cyclic glutamic acid (<Glu), which are essential to bioactivity, for example, thyrotropin-releasing hormone (TRH) and gonadotropin-releasing hormone (GnRH). The enzyme responsible for this step is glutaminyl cyclase, which converts the original NH_2-terminal Gln into <Glu. The regulation and function of glutaminyl cyclase has not yet been extensively studied. Another important but infrequent modification of peptides is α-*N*-acetylation (Figs. 18-6 and 18-7). During POMC processing, α-*N*-acetylation greatly increases the skin-darkening potency of ACTH(1–13)NH_2 while abolishing both the adrenal steroidogenic potency of ACTH and the opiate activity of β-endorphin [8]. The enzyme(s) responsible for this modification has not yet been purified or cloned.

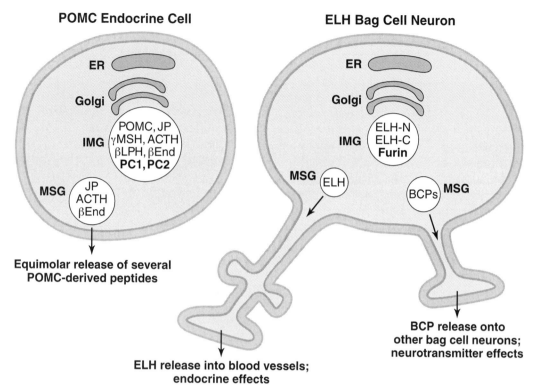

FIGURE 18-7.   Cell-specific packaging of peptides into large dense core vesicles can lead to very different patterns of peptide secretion. Sorting of neuropeptides into distinct mature secretory granules *(MSG)* is shown for bag cell neurons but does not occur for endocrine cells. *ELH,* egg-laying hormone, *POMC,* pro-opiomelanocortin; *ER,* endoplasmic reticulum; *JP,* joining peptide; *MSH,* melanocyte-stimulating hormone; *ACTH,* adrenocorticotropic hormone; *LPH,* lipotropin; *PC,* prohormone convertase; *BCP,* bag cell peptide; *IMG,* immature granules; βEnd, β-endorphin.

As an example, Figure 18-6 shows the pattern of processing steps in the POMC system [8]. The initial endoproteolytic steps (Fig. 18-6, steps 1–4) are mediated by PC1 and occur in all POMC-producing neurons and endocrine cells, usually in the numerical order shown. It is clear that steps 1 and 2 are initiated in the *trans*-Golgi network and continue in LDCVs, while step 4 occurs only in LDCVs. Steps 5–7 occur only in LDCVs and seem to require PC2. In the adult anterior pituitary, corticotropes contain PC1 but not PC2 and perform only cleavages 1–4. However, during early postnatal development, corticotropes also express PC2 and cleavages 5–7 are transiently seen in corticotropes. In the rat, expression of PC2 and cleavage within ACTH (cleavage 5) decline simultaneously a few weeks after birth, at about the time that the adult pattern of ACTH control over adrenal steroidogenesis appears.

Melanotropes and CNS neurons making POMC express both PC1 and PC2 and, thus, the smaller peptide products are seen in these cells. PAM is expressed in all POMC-producing cells, so the α-amidation of joining peptide (JP), a small peptide with no clear biological function, occurs rapidly in all POMC cells (Fig. 18-6). In the melanotropes of the intermediate pituitary and the POMC neurons of the nucleus of the solitary tract, α-*N*-acetylation of ACTH(1–13)NH$_2$ and β-endorphin occurs. In melanotropes, α-*N*-acetylation of ACTH can occur before cleavage 5. As indicated in Figure 18-4, the particular cleavages made and the modifications made to the NH$_2$- and COOH-termini of the peptide products determine the mixture of bioactive peptides released.

Neuropeptides are packaged into large dense core vesicles

In many cases, the peptide products from the processing of a propeptide are packaged together in an equimolar fashion in LDCVs and the peptides and the soluble processing enzymes (PC1, PHM, CPE) are all released together in response to stimuli (Fig. 18-7) [6–8]. By comparison, there are also examples where the products of propeptide processing are sorted into different LDCVs or are subject to degradation. In *Aplysia* bag cell neurons, ELH is formed from the COOH terminus of the pro-ELH precursor (Fig. 18-2), while α, β and γ bag cell peptides (BCPs) are formed from the NH$_2$-terminal portion (Fig. 18-7). The initial cleavage of the pro-ELH precursor occurs in the trans-Golgi network and the peptides are then separated into two distinct types of LDCV, which are sent to different parts of the cell (Fig. 18-7). These two sets of peptides

mediate a coordinated set of behaviors involved in egg laying. Similarly, in TRH neurons, the NH$_2$ and COOH-terminal domains of the pro-TRH precursor are separated from each other and stored in distinct LDCVs.

Diversity is generated by families of propeptides, alternative splicing, proteolytic processing and post-translational modifications

The huge number of biologically active peptides is the result of many factors. First, there are several families of genes which clearly evolved from a common ancestor (Fig. 18-1): examples include the three precursors to β-endorphin, dynorphin and the enkephalins; the precursors to gastrin and CCK; and the precursors to oxytocin and vasopressin. Second, there are several peptide precursors which yield multiple copies of bioactive peptide: examples in-

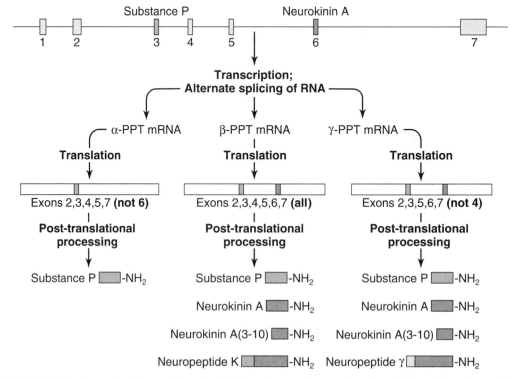

FIGURE 18-8. Several mechanisms through which the substance P gene gives rise to different bioactive peptides in different neurons (adapted from [17]). Alternative splicing of mRNA leads to translation of distinct precursors, and subsequent processing leads to unique mature peptides. *PPT*, pre-protachykinin.

clude the pro-ELH precursor, the α-mating factor precursor, the FMRF-NH$_2$ precursor and the enkephalin precursor. Likewise, several distinct biological activities are found within the POMC and ELH precursors. Third, there is alternative splicing of mRNAs encoding prepro-hormones, first discovered in the calcitonin and calcitonin gene-related peptide precursors but also seen in the case of the prepro-tachykinin precursor, which yields substance P, substance K and several other peptides, depending on the splicing pattern (Fig. 18-8) [17]. Finally, RNA editing can be involved, as in the case of the amphibian bombesin-like peptides, where nucleotides in the mRNA are changed and the final protein is not a direct reflection of the sequence encoded in the gene. RNA editing is also seen in the glutamate and serotonin receptors (Chaps. 13 and 15) and probably will be found elsewhere as detection methods become more sophisticated.

NEUROPEPTIDE RECEPTORS

Most neuropeptide receptors are seven-transmembrane-domain, G protein-coupled receptors

The first neuropeptide receptors characterized were those for substance P and neurotensin, and most have the general architecture shown in Figure 18-9. The basic rules for the function of these seven-transmembrane-domain receptors are the same as the rules established for similar serpentine receptors for conventional small molecule neurotransmitters, such as muscarinic, adrenergic and metabotropic glutamatergic receptors (Chaps. 11–16) [10,11,18,19]. For large glycoprotein ligands, such as TSH and chorionic gonadotropin, the extracellular domain plays a major role in ligand binding (Fig. 18-9). By contrast, the key components of the binding sites for smaller peptides

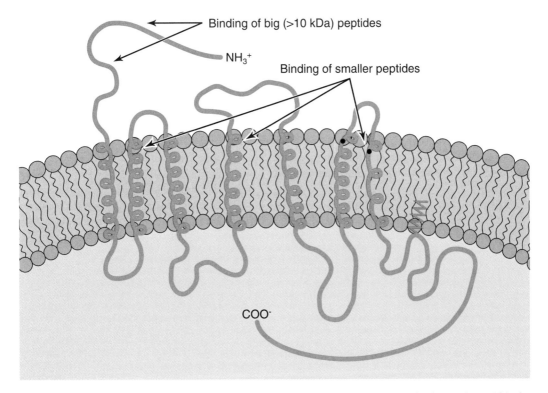

FIGURE 18-9. Serpentine (seven-transmembrane-domain) receptors for peptides have binding regions within the membrane and in the NH$_2$-terminal loop.

are the analogous residues important for binding small nonpeptide ligands to their receptors.

The binding specificity of neuropeptide receptors for a given neuropeptide may vary considerably. Five somatostatin receptors have been identified; they bind somatostatin similarly, and all inhibit adenylyl cyclase. However, these receptors differ substantially with regard to their interaction with various somatostatin analogs used for therapeutic purposes. For example, the receptor called SSTR2 binds a small agonist, the peptide analog octreotide, much more tightly than the other somatostatin receptors. Changing a few amino acids in transmembrane domains VI and VII of SSTR1 to the residues found in SSTR2 (Fig. 18-9) allows the mutant SSTR1 to bind the peptide analog as well as SSTR2. Similar changes in specificity are seen with several other peptide receptor families [11,17–19].

Neuropeptide receptors are not confined to synaptic regions

Peptidergic neurotransmission often operates on a slower time scale than conventional neurotransmitters, so it is not surprising that placement of peptide receptors is often not localized to the synapse. For example, although some substance P terminals contact membranes with substance P receptor, only a small fraction of the substance P receptor-laden membrane is apposed to synaptic terminals. Substance P may diffuse a considerable distance from its release site and still find a receptor with which it can interact.

Expression of peptide receptors and the corresponding peptides is not well matched

Neuropeptides can act at many sites. They may act directly on a postsynaptic target at the synapse; presynaptically on the terminal that released the peptide (autocrine effects); on an immediately adjacent cell (juxtacrine effects); or on a cell a few cell diameters away from the site of release (paracrine effects). In addition, peptides can exert their actions via travel through the circulation to reach their target, termed endocrine effects, as in the case of hypothalamic releasing factors and neurohypophyseal hormones.

There is some correspondence of the peptide families and the families of peptide receptors, but it is certainly not simple. For example, there are three opiate peptide precursors, POMC, proenkephalin and prodynorphin, and three major types of opiate receptor, μ, κ and δ. The best endogenous ligand for the μ receptor is β-endorphin, enkephalins are best for δ receptors and dynorphins are best for κ receptors. However, the sites at which opiate peptides and opiate receptors are expressed in the brain do not show a simple 1:1 correspondence. In addition, the δ receptor is usually in presynaptic locations, while the μ and κ receptors tend to be postsynaptic [20]. Recently, an orphan receptor resembling the opiate receptors was expressed and used to identify its endogenous ligand, called orphanin FQ or nociceptin. This new preprohormone is most similar to the dynorphin precursor and defines a fourth type of opiate-like peptide containing the sequence Phe-Gly-Gly-Phe instead of the Tyr-Gly-Gly-Phe sequence that defined the existing members of the opiate peptide family [5]. The orphanin FQ peptide is hyperalgesic in that it increases pain sensitivity, which is the opposite action to the opiate peptides. Reduction of the level of the orphanin FQ receptor in brain using antisense oligonucleotides leads to analgesia.

Similarly, five closely related melanocortin receptors that respond to various peptides derived from the POMC precursor have been identified, including ACTH, γMSH and αMSH (Fig. 18-6). As expected, the receptor on adrenal cortical cells responds best to ACTH, which normally stimulates adrenal steroidogenesis, and the receptor on melanocytes responds best to αMSH, which causes skin darkening. However, the pattern of melanocortin receptor expression in the brain is not simply explained by the known patterns of the peptide expression in the brain or by the known effects of POMC-derived peptides when applied to various brain regions. With this number of peptide receptors, it is obvious that production of final peptide products must be precisely controlled and that different biosynthetic processing pathways can dramatically affect the biological activity observed (Figs. 18-6 and 18-7).

The amiloride-sensitive FMRF-amide-gated sodium channel was the first peptide-gated ion channel identified

FMRF-amide induces a fast excitatory depolarizing response due to *direct activation* of an amiloride-sensitive sodium channel. Using cDNA from the snail *Helix aspersa* and a *Xenopus* oocyte expression system, an amiloride-sensitive, FMRF-amide-activated sodium channel was identified. The channel has only two transmembrane domains and as such is similar in structure to the directly gated ion channels activated by some purinergic ligands (Chap. 17) and by hydrogen ions.

NEUROPEPTIDE FUNCTIONS AND REGULATION

The study of peptidergic neurons requires a number of special tools

These tools include methods to detect the neuropeptides, the enzymes specific to their biosynthesis and their cognate receptors.

Antibody-based detection includes immunocytochemistry, which gives only qualitative data but has very good spatial resolution. Radioimmunoassay is a second method for neuropeptide detection which provides a quantitative measure of release or content. Sometimes passive immunization has been used successfully to establish the importance of a particular peptide in a physiological interaction between cells. One of the major limitations of all antibody-based methods is the potential for cross-reactivity among the many peptides that are distinct but closely related structurally. For example, some of the most sensitive "gastrin" antisera also detect CCK since the peptides share a common COOH-terminal tetrapeptide sequence.

RNA-based methods for detection of mRNA-encoding neuropeptides include Northern blots and RNase protection assays, which provide quantitative data but lack fine anatomical resolution. Alternatively, *in situ* hybridization preserves anatomical relationships but is not usually considered quantitative.

Direct methods for detection of neuropeptides include metabolic labeling with an appropriate radioactive amino acid and chemical isolation of peptides. Isolation often involves using high-pressure liquid chromatography and sensitive spectroscopic methods of detection along with mass spectroscopy. These approaches make possible measurements of tissue concentrations of peptides and quantitative study of the amount and timing of secretion. Direct methods are difficult to apply to peptides or their receptors in the CNS, where the cells expressing the peptide are part of a large population of other neurons or endocrine cells.

Peptide agonists and antagonists are becoming available for many peptides, and (as discussed in Chaps. 11–16) these are essential to a successful dissection of the function of peptidergic synapses, as they have been for conventional neurotransmitters.

Ligand-binding assays allow localization and quantification of receptors, using an appropriate tracer ligand. Measurement of receptors may be made in solution, in suspension or by binding to membranes *in situ*. These approaches have the advantage that a physiologically important trait, binding of the ligand to the receptor, is being observed, and they can reveal binding to several related receptors, which are then distinguished by antisera or *in situ* hybridization.

Peptides play a role in the plurichemical coding of neuronal signals

As shown in Figure 18-10, many sets of neurons are chemically coded, giving rise to the concept of plurichemical transmission [21]. In the human lumbar paravertebral ganglion, adrenergic neurons efferent to blood vessels in skin and muscle usually contain NPY along with norepinephrine, while adrenergic neurons innervating hair follicles express primarily norepinephrine. The dual transmission onto blood vessels is important since the catecholamine effects on blood vessels undergo rapid tachyphylaxis, while sustained contraction of the blood vessels is mediated by NPY. In this case, the conventional neurotransmitter norepinephrine and NPY have similar actions on different time scales, leading to rapid but sustained responses of the same

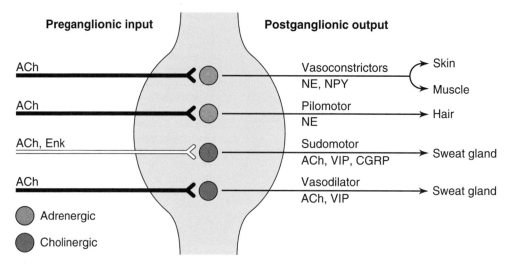

FIGURE 18-10. Plurichemical transmission in a sympathetic ganglion (adapted from [21]). Cholinergic stimulation of distinct ganglionic neurons leads to distinct neurotransmitter release and physiological actions. *ACh*, acetylcholine; *Enk*, enkephalin; *NE*, norepinephrine; *NPY*, neuropeptide Y; *VIP*, vasoactive intestinal peptide; *CGRP*, calcitonin gene-related peptide.

sort. In the sympathetic innervation of sweat glands, another example of plasticity is seen. The sympathetic fibers first express catecholamines as they arrive at the sweat gland, and in a later response to a factor released by the sweat gland, the fibers change to express a cholinergic phenotype. In this later response, a set of peptides is expressed that is different from that expressed when the fibers initially reach the sweat glands. In this way, within a sympathetic ganglion, several functional subgroups of neurons can be identified based upon their content of neuropeptide and conventional neurotransmitter. It is likely that a similar but more complex mixture of phenotypes occurs in the CNS. Peptides are generally released together with classical neurotransmitters, and each transmitter has its own unique effects on target tissues. Neuropeptides have a particularly important role in the integration of incoming and outgoing signals of sympathetic ganglia.

Neuropeptides make a unique contribution to signaling

The release of neuropeptides generally requires a more intense stimulus, resulting in more entry of Ca^{2+} into the presynaptic terminal, than required for release of conventional neurotrans-

mitters, presumably due to the distance the Ca^{2+} must diffuse to reach the LDCVs (Fig. 18-3). As a result, the contribution of peptides to signaling can vary with the pattern of stimulation. For example, in *Aplysia*, several identified motor neurons devote about 10% of their total protein synthesis to their respective peptide neurotransmitters. Peptide release in each case has been shown to require extracellular Ca^{2+}, and release increases with the frequency of action potentials, in the range of frequencies seen in behaving animals. In addition to the peptides, several of the motor neurons secrete ACh. In these motor neurons, the peptide release increases more strongly with action potential frequency than does release of ACh, so the ratio of peptide to ACh is dependent on frequency. In addition, there are unique postsynaptic responses, such as elevation of cAMP concentrations in muscles, which can be mimicked only by application of the peptides and not by the conventional neurotransmitters.

In other examples, the amount of peptide available for release can be depleted by repeated firing of a terminal since new peptide must arrive by axonal transport, while new conventional neurotransmitters are synthesized or recaptured locally and pumped into small synaptic vesicles.

Regulation of neuropeptide expression is exerted at several levels

Control of neuropeptide function is mediated by factors controlling rates of prepropeptide gene transcription, translation, degradation and secretion (Fig. 18-11). On the scale of seconds to minutes, peptide secretion is not always coupled lock-step with classical transmitter release (example above). Peptides are inactivated by diffusion and by proteolysis, so it would be expected that inhibition of specific extracellular proteases could lead to increased effectiveness of their neuropeptide substrates, as has been shown in the cases of CCK and the enkephalins.

On a time scale of minutes to hours, the transcription of prepropeptide mRNA can be controlled, and peptide mRNAs are immediate early genes in many cases, showing extremely rapid responses to stimuli. The rate of translation of existing prepropeptide mRNAs can also change dramatically within a few minutes of stimulation. Since processing enzymes must also be synthesized and inserted into the same LDCVs as the peptide precursors, the rate of production of these enzymes might be expected to show changes under physiological conditions. They do show such changes but usually more slowly than the peptide precursors. As seen above (Figs. 18-4–18-7), the peptide products produced are crucially dependent on the mixture of processing enzymes in the LDCVs.

On a scale of hours to days, dramatic changes can be seen in cells producing peptides that are subjected to chronic stimulation or inhibition. POMC production by intermediate pituitary melanotropes is inhibited by treatment of rats with dopaminergic agonists or exposure of frogs to a light background; POMC production is stimulated by treatment of rats with dopaminergic antagonists or exposure of frogs to a dark background. The expression of processing enzymes, the number of LDCVs and the rate of cell division are also responsive to the treatments. Similarly, the processing of different regions of the pro-TRH precursor responds to thyroid hor-

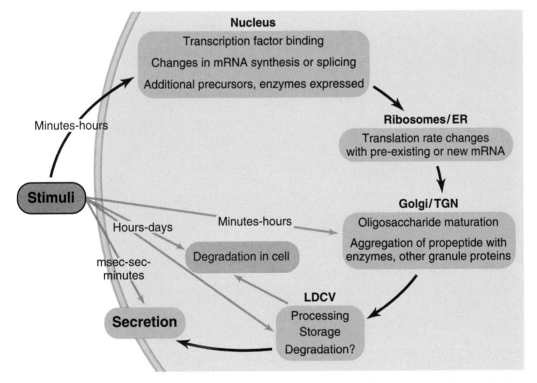

FIGURE 18-11. Regulation of neuropeptide expression is exerted at several levels. *ER*, endoplasmic reticulum; *LDCV*, large dense core vesicle; *TGN*, *trans*-Golgi network.

mone status, and it is possible that the routing of ELH and the BCPs is regulated (Fig. 18-7). In response to changes in steroid hormone concentrations that occur during the estrous cycle in female rats, the concentration of CCK mRNA varies more than twofold in a subset of CCK-producing CNS neurons.

PEPTIDERGIC SYSTEMS IN DISEASE

Diabetes insipidus occurs with loss of vasopressin production in the Brattleboro rat model

In the Brattleboro rat, a single-base deletion in the vasopressin gene alters the COOH terminus of preprovasopressin so that it cannot leave the endoplasmic reticulum; as a result, no neurons make vasopressin [22]. Intriguingly, a frameshift mutation occurs in postmitotic neurons, most often an additional deletion of two nucleotides, so that the neurons regain the ability to produce vasopressin. In the *hpg* mouse, a spontaneous mutation in the gonadotropin hormone-releasing hormone gene results in loss of gonadal function in homozygous animals.

A mutation in the carboxypeptidase E gene causes late-onset diabetes with hyperproinsulinemia

The single-base change in the CPE gene changes Ser[202] to Pro, yielding a CPE molecule that is malfolded, inactive and incapable of exiting from the endoplasmic reticulum [14,23]. The phenotype of late-onset diabetes mellitus is caused by the high concentrations of inactive proinsulin in the blood, with very little mature, functional insulin (Fig. 18-12). In the brains of *fat/fat* mice, there is an excess of immature, biologically inactive neuropeptide fragments, such as neurotensin-Lys-Arg. It is still unclear how the loss of CPE function causes all of the biochemical effects observed, with selective loss of processing of several peptides, while other peptide systems remain relatively quite normal.

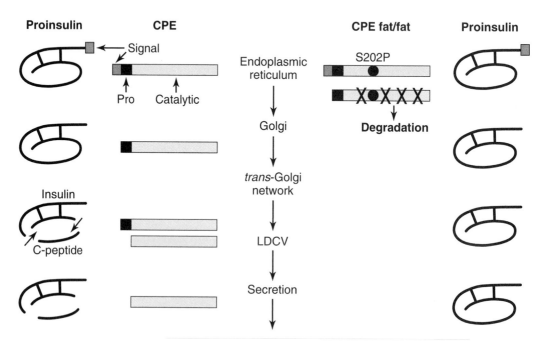

FIGURE 18-12. The *fat/fat* mutation in carboxypeptidase E *(CPE)* leads to secretion of proinsulin, not mature insulin, and results in diabetes. The S202P mutation within CPE results in degradation of the enzyme and defective insulin processing in the *fat/fat* heterozygous mouse. *LDCV,* large dense core vesicle.

Obesity has several central nervous system components

A novel NPY receptor, the Y5 receptor, was recently cloned from rat hypothalamus using an expression cloning approach. The extent to which peptides inhibit adenylyl cyclase through the Y5 receptor correlates well with their ability to stimulate food intake, suggesting that the Y5 receptor may be a feeding receptor. NPY administration into the CNS causes overeating and obesity. A second peptide involved in obesity is leptin, a product of adipocytes. The leptin gene is defective in the *ob/ob* mouse, but in normal mice leptin binds to its receptor in the hypothalamus, causing a decrease in the synthesis and release of hypothalamic NPY.

Cholecystokinin agonists and antagonists yield insights into panic attacks and satiety

There are two CCK receptor subtypes, denoted CCK-A and CCK-B. Protease inhibitors that slow the degradation and inactivation of endogenous CCK promote satiety via CCK-A receptor. By contrast, the CCK-B receptor is important in mediating anxiety and panic attacks, and CCK antagonists are in clinical use to treat anxiety and panic attacks [24].

Enkephalin knockout mice reach adulthood and are healthy

When one of the three endogenous opiate precursor genes was eliminated from the mouse genome by genetic engineering (see Chap. 40), the knockout mice exhibited a normal tail-flick response, but the response was unaltered by foot-shock. Enkephalin knockout mice show a marked increase in supraspinal responses to painful stimuli, such as the response measured with the hot-plate assay. This indicates that enkephalin plays no role in the normal tail-flick response but does play a role in centrally mediated analgesia [25]. Similarly, β-endorphin knockout mice also show a loss in centrally mediated analgesia. Behavioral abnormalities in the enkephalin knockout mice include reduced exploratory activity in an unfamiliar environment and increased offensive aggressiveness in the resident-intruder test. In both enkephalin and β-endorphin knockout mice, there is no compensatory increase in the concentrations of the two remaining endogenous opiate peptides.

REFERENCES

1. Grimmelikhuijzen, C. J. P., Leviev, I., and Carstensen, K. Peptides in the nervous systems of cnidarians: Structure, function and biosynthesis. *Int. Rev. Cytol.* 167:37–89, 1996.
2. Shaw, C. Neuropeptides and their evolution. *Parasitology* 113:S35–S45, 1996.
3. Douglass, J., McKinzie, A. A., and Couceyro, P. PCR differential display identifies a rat brain mRNA that is transcriptionally regulated by cocaine and amphetamine. *J. Neurosci.* 15:2471–2481, 1995.
4. Bloomquist, B. T., Darlington, D. N., Mains, R. E., and Eipper, B. A. RESP18, a novel endocrine secretory protein transcript, and 4 other transcripts are regulated in parallel with POMC in melanotropes. *J. Biol. Chem.* 269:9113–9122, 1994.
5. Nothacker, H. P., Reinscheid, R. K., Mansour, A. et al. Primary structure and tissue distribution of the orphanin FQ receptor. *Proc. Natl. Acad. Sci. USA* 93:8677–8682, 1996.
6. Rouille, Y., Duguay, S. J., Lund, K., et al. Proteolytic processing mechanisms in the biosynthesis of neuroendocrine peptides. *Front. Neuroendocrinol.* 16:322–361, 1995.
7. Seidah, N. G. Molecular strategies for identifying processing enzymes. *Methods Neurosci.* 23:3–15, 1995.
8. Mains, R. E., and Eipper, B. A. The tissue-specific processing of pro-ACTH/endorphin. *Trends Endocrinol. Metab.* 1:388–394, 1990.
9. Liddle, R. A. Cholecystokinin cells. *Annu. Rev. Physiol.* 59:221–242, 1997.
10. Sawada, M., and Dickinson, C. The G cell. *Annu. Rev. Physiol.* 59:273–298, 1997.
11. Reisine, T., and Bell, G. I. Molecular biology of somatostatin receptors. *Endocr. Rev.* 16:427–442, 1995.
12. Loh, Y. P., and Cawley, N. X. Processing enzymes of pepsin family: Yeast aspartic protease 3 and POMC converting enzyme. *Methods Enzymol.* 248:136–146, 1995.
13. Cohen, P., Pierotti, A. R., Chesneau, V., Foulon, T., and Prat, A. *N*-Arginine dibasic convertase. *Methods Enzymol.* 248:703–716, 1995.

14. Fricker, L. D., Berman, Y. L., Leiter, E. H., and Devi, L. A. Carboxypeptidase E activity is deficient in mice with the *fat* mutation; effect on peptide processing. *J. Biol. Chem.* 271:30619–30624, 1996.

15. Eipper, B. A., Milgram, S. L., Husten, E. J., Yun, H. Y., and Mains, R. E. Peptidylglycine alpha-amidating monooxygenase: A multifunctional protein with catalytic, processing and routing domains. *Protein Sci.* 2:489–497, 1993.

16. Srivastava, M. Genomic structure and expression of the human gene encoding cytochrome B_{561}, an integral protein of the chromaffin granule membrane. *J. Biol. Chem.* 270:22714–22720, 1995.

17. Helke, C. J., Krause, J. E., Mantyh, P. W., Couture, R., and Bannon, M. J. Diversity in mammalian tachykinin peptidergic neurons: Multiple peptides, receptors, and regulatory mechanisms. *FASEB J.* 4:1606–1615, 1990.

18. Schwartz, T. W. Locating ligand-binding sites in 7TM receptors by protein engineering. *Curr. Opin. Biotechnol.* 5:434–444, 1994.

19. Cascieri, M. A., Fong, T. M., and Strader, C. D. Molecular characterization of a common binding site for small molecules within the transmembrane domain of G-coupled receptors. *J. Pharmacol. Toxicol. Methods* 33:179–185, 1995.

20. Mansour, A., Fox, C. A., Akil, H., and Watson, S. J. Opioid-receptor mRNA expression in the rat CNS: Anatomical and functional implications. *Trends Neurosci.* 18:22–29, 1995.

21. Benarroch, E. E. Neuropeptides in the sympathetic system: Presence, plasticity, modulation and implications. *Ann. Neurol.* 36:6–13, 1994.

22. Evans, D. A. P., van der Kleij, A. A. M., Sonnemans, M. A. F., Burbach, J. P. H., and van Leeuwen, F. W. Frameshift mutations at two hotspots in vasopressin transcripts in post-mitotic neurons. *Proc. Natl. Acad. Sci. USA* 91:6059–6063, 1994.

23. Naggert, J. K., Fricker, L. D., Varlamov, O., et al. Hyperproinsulinemia in obese fat/fat mice associated with a carboxypeptidase E mutation which reduces enzyme activity. *Nat. Genet.* 10:135–142, 1995.

24. Lydiard, R. B., Brawman-Mintzer, O., and Ballenger, J. C. Recent developments in the psychopharmacology of anxiety disorders. *J. Consult. Clin. Psychol.* 64:660–668, 1996.

25. Konig, M., Zimmer, A. M., Steiner, H., et al. Pain responses, anxiety and aggression in mice deficient in pre-proenkephalin. *Nature* 383:535–538, 1996.

19

Growth Factors

Gary E. Landreth

Basic Neurochemistry: Molecular, Cellular and Medical Aspects, 6th Ed., edited by G. J. Siegel et al. Published by Lippincott–Raven Publishers, Philadelphia, 1999. Correspondence to Gary E. Landreth, Alzheimer's Research Lab, Case Western Reserve University School of Medicine, 10900 Euclid Avenue, Cleveland, Ohio 44106.

GROWTH FACTORS ARE ESSENTIAL FOR NERVOUS SYSTEM DEVELOPMENT AND FUNCTION

Peptide growth factors are proteins that stimulate cellular proliferation and promote cellular survival

This definition has been substantially broadened with the discovery of the diverse and complex roles these molecules play both in the developing animal and in the adult. Historically, the first growth factor to be identified was nerve growth factor (NGF) by Rita Levi-Montalcini [1]. This molecule has been termed a neurotrophic factor since its actions are largely restricted to the nervous system. NGF has an extraordinarily wide array of activities, which has forced a substantial re-evaluation of how growth factors are defined. The nervous system exhibits a remarkable cellular heterogeneity, and one of the major challenges is to elucidate how a relatively small number of growth factors act to direct the development of the nervous system and sustain these cells in the mature animal [2]. Some growth factors act only during restricted periods of development, while others function throughout life. In the past, attempts have been made to distinguish between "neurotrophic factors" and growth factors, but this has not proven to be a useful distinction, given our current appreciation of the broad range of actions of these molecules.

The nervous system is subject to a unique set of constraints during development. Many more neurons are generated during development than are required in the mature nervous system (see Chap. 27). Importantly, after their last mitotic division, neurons are unable to re-enter the cell cycle and can no longer proliferate. As development proceeds there is a period during which as many as half of all neurons die, a process known as normal, or programmed, cell death. Normal cell death occurs at the time that the axonal processes of the innervating neurons arrive at and invade their peripheral target tissues. The selective survival of only a fraction of the initial number of neurons is accomplished by the competition of the innervating processes for a limited amount of trophic factor elaborated by the target tissue. Those neurons which fail to obtain trophic factor then die. This concept forms the basis of what is now known as the "neurotrophic factor hypothesis." This mechanism can account in part for the tailoring of the number of neurons which connect with their targets in the periphery and the size of the target field, resulting in a stable neuronal population whose size is essentially determined at birth. Trophic factors are supplied continuously by the target to those neurons that establish functional connections (Fig. 19-1). While much of the data supporting this hypothesis have been gathered through the study of the PNS, it is clear that analogous mechanisms also operate in the CNS [3].

Trophic factors can also be supplied to neurons and glial cells through less specific mechanisms. Growth factors are synthesized by a wide variety of cell types, including neurons and glial cells. The factors are secreted into the extracellular milieu, where they diffuse and then act in a paracrine fashion on other cells (Fig. 19-1). An analogous process, autocrine stimulation, occurs when a cell synthesizes and secretes a growth factor to which the cell itself is responsive. In this case, the cell provides its own trophic support [4]. These latter mechanisms have been well described in other organ systems, but only recently has evidence been obtained that such processes occur extensively in the nervous system.

Individual neurons and glial cells are responsive to a number of different growth factors. It is likely that the growth factors play both unique and overlapping roles in the development and sustenance of these cells. Perhaps the most dramatic example of this is the elaborate array of trophic factors that have evolved to support the growth and maintenance of spinal motor neurons. There are presently at least 15 different factors known to influence the survival of these cells [5].

Recently, it has been appreciated that some growth factors serve a much wider role. For example, NGF acutely regulates aspects of neurotransmitter synthesis and release, as well as mediating both synaptic plasticity and the stabilization of synaptic contacts. It is likely that in subsequent years we will discover additional novel actions of these molecules.

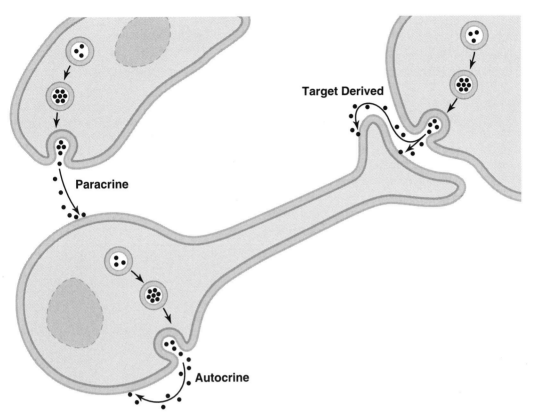

FIGURE 19-1. Mechanisms of growth and trophic factor support. Growth factors can be provided through autocrine mechanisms in which a cell secretes growth factors to which it in turn responds, while paracrine support is mediated by secretion of factors which then act upon neighboring cells. Target-derived support of neurons is mediated by the growth of fibers into their target tissues. The target tissue synthesizes the growth factor and provides it to the innervating neurons.

Cells respond to growth factors as a consequence of their binding to specific cell-surface receptors

The association of growth factors with their receptors leads to activation of extraordinarily complex signal transduction pathways, resulting in intracellular biochemical changes that mediate cellular survival as well as the acquisition and maintenance of the cellular phenotype. The responsiveness of a cell to a particular growth factor is dependent upon expression of specific receptors on the plasma membrane. The regulated expression of such receptors is a well documented feature of development and temporally regulates the sensitivity of cells to growth factors in their environment. It is noteworthy that the receptors for many of the growth factors are themselves protein kinases, whose enzymatic activity is stimulated upon asso-

ciation with their specific ligand, thereby initiating intracellular signaling events [6]. Other growth factor receptors also employ protein kinases to initiate action but do so through the incorporation of these enzymes within large signaling complexes that are assembled subsequent to growth-factor binding. The specificity of growth factor action is governed by the intrinsic structure of the receptor; the extracellular domain imparts ligand binding specificity, while the intracellular domain specifies the intracellular signaling pathways which are activated upon ligand binding.

CLASSES OF GROWTH FACTORS ACTING IN THE NERVOUS SYSTEM

There are several major classes of growth factors which act within the nervous system (Table 19-

1). Some of these, such as the neurotrophins, act almost exclusively in the nervous system, whereas others, for example, fibroblast growth factors and insulin-like growth factor I, act on a number of cell types throughout the body, in addition to the nervous system. Unexpectedly, it has been discovered that a subset of growth factors whose actions were thought to be restricted to the immune system have important actions on both neurons and glial cells. The determination of which molecules can legitimately be termed growth factors thus has become less clear. There are a growing number of factors which act to regulate specific aspects of development and are unlikely to play significant roles or have currently unappreciated roles in the nervous system of the mature animal.

The neurotrophins comprise a family of related molecules which support the survival and phenotypic specificity of subsets of neurons

The neurotrophins (Table 19-2) are small, highly basic proteins of approximately 13 kDa which dimerize to form the biologically active species [7–9]. The neurotrophins have a highly conserved structure. This family includes five distinct members, NGF, brain-derived neurotrophic factor (BDNF), neurotrophin 3 (NT3), neurotrophin 4/5 (NT4/5) and neurotrophin 6 (NT6). NT6 is found only in fish and will not be discussed further.

The neurotrophins interact with two cell-surface receptor species (Fig. 19-2) [10]. The first, termed p75 or the low-affinity neurotrophin receptor, is promiscuous in that it binds all neurotrophin species. The exact function of this molecule is presently unclear. The neurotrophins also bind to the Trk family of receptors. The Trk receptors comprise a small but highly related family of molecules which possess an extracellular ligand-binding domain which selectively interacts with the individual neurotrophin species (Fig. 19-2). Trk A specifically binds NGF, TrkB interacts with BDNF and NT4/5 and Trk C preferentially binds NT3. Importantly, the Trk receptors have an intracellular tyrosine kinase domain which is activated upon neurotrophin binding. The kinase domains of

TABLE 19-1.	GROWTH FACTORS ACTING IN THE NERVOUS SYSTEM
Growth factor	**Receptor**
Neurotrophins	
Nerve growth factor	TrkA
Brain-derived neurotrophic factor	TrkB
Neurotrophin 3	TrkC
Neurotrophin 4/5	TrkB
Neurokines	
Ciliary neurotrophic factor	CNTFRα + LIFRβ + gp130
Leukemia inhibitory factor	LIFRβ + gp130
Interleukin (IL-6)	IL6Rα + gp130
Cardiotrophin 1	LIFRβ + gp130 +?
Fibroblast growth factors	
FGF-1 (acidic FGF)	FGFR1–4
FGF-2 (basic FGF)	FGFR1–3
Transforming growth factor β superfamily	
Transforming growth factors β	TGFβRI and RII
Bone morphogenetic factors	BMPRI and RII
Glial-derived neurotrophic factor	GDNFRα + c-*ret*
Neurturin	?
Epidermal growth factor superfamily	
Epidermal growth factor	EGFR
Transforming growth factor α	EGFR
Neuregulins (GGF, ARIA, SMDF, etc.)	erbB2, 3, 4
Other growth factors	
Platelet-derived growth factor	PDGFRα and β
Insulin-like growth factor I	IGFRI

the Trk family members are highly conserved, and the Trks differ mainly in the structure of their extracellular domains. Trk receptor expression is limited to neurons, and the responsiveness of subpopulations of neurons to the neurotrophins is due to the restricted and selective expression of the individual Trk-receptor species.

The specific actions of the individual neurotrophins have been the subject of intense interest (Table 19-2). It is now evident, through analysis of animals in which the individual neurotrophin genes or their receptors have been knocked out, that each of the family members may act exclusively to support some neuronal subpopulations [11]. However, in some neuronal populations, the actions of several of the

TABLE 19-2.	NEUROTROPHIN TARGETS	
Neurotrophin	**Peripheral**	**Central**
Nerve growth factor		
	Sympathetic neurons, sensory neurons: dorsal root ganglia	Basal forebrain cholinergic neurons, striatal cholinergic neurons, Purkinje cells
Brain-derived neurotrophic factor		
	Sensory neurons: nodose, dorsal root neurons	Spinal motor neurons, basal forebrain cholinergic neurons, substantia nigra dopaminergic neurons, facial motor neurons, retinal ganglion cells
Neurotrophin 3		
	Sympathetic neurons, sensory neurons	Basal forebrain cholinergic neurons, locus ceruleus neurons
Neurotrophin 4/5		
	Sympathetic neurons, sensory neurons: nodose, dorsal root ganglia	Basal forebrain cholinergic neurons, locus ceruleus neurons, motor neurons, retinal ganglion cells

neurotrophins overlap. For example, in the peripheral sensory ganglia, individual neurons are responsive to more than one neurotrophin.

Nerve growth factor is the prototypical member of the neurotrophin family. It was discovered on the basis of its ability to stimulate the dramatic outgrowth of processes from sympathetic ganglia. NGF is absolutely required for the survival of sympathetic neurons and a subset of sensory neurons during development. NGF is synthesized within the tissues that receive innervation

Neurotrophin Receptors

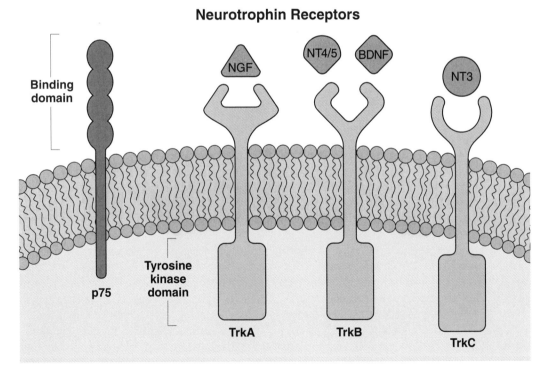

FIGURE 19-2. Neurotrophin receptors. Neurotrophin family members bind specifically to cognate Trk receptors. The low-affinity neurotrophin receptor p75 promiscuously binds all of the neurotrophins. *NT,* neurotrophin; *BDNF,* brain-derived neurotrophic factor, *NGF,* nerve growth factor.

by these neurons and sustains a fraction of the neurons that extend processes into these tissues during the period of development when programmed cell death occurs. The demonstrated ability of the target organs to provide trophic support underlies the neurotrophic hypothesis, and much of the action of NGF and other neurotrophins can be explained on this basis. NGF is required for sympathetic neuron survival not only during development but also throughout life. Sensory neurons are also dependent on NGF during development but become independent of NGF for their survival in the mature animal. It should be pointed out that NGF regulates cell number not by supporting the proliferation of neuronal precursor population but by permitting the selective survival of neurons that are protected from programmed cell death. NGF has not been shown to directly stimulate cell division of neurons or their precursors. NGF, like other classical growth factors, acts to stimulate cellular metabolism by positively regulating a wide array of biosynthetic processes. It stimulates the morphological differentiation of its target cells, promoting extensive outgrowth of axonal and dendritic processes. Indeed, there is evidence that not only does NGF act in a permissive fashion to facilitate the morphological and biochemical differentiation of the neurons and process outgrowth but it is also instructive and plays a role in specifying the phenotype of the neuron [12].

NGF also has actions within the CNS. It is not particularly abundant in the CNS. Its synthesis appears to be largely restricted to the hippocampus and neocortex, and even in these regions it is present at relatively low concentrations compared to the other neurotrophins. The most prominent population of NGF responsive neurons expressing TrkA are the basal forebrain cholinergic neurons. The principal projections of these neurons are to the hippocampus and cortex, which conforms with the concept that NGF acts as a target-derived trophic factor in the CNS, just as it does in the PNS. NGF also acts on a subpopulation of cholinergic neurons within the striatum. These interneurons express the NGF receptor TrkA and respond to NGF. However, they do not appear to rely wholly on NGF for survival, and the specific actions of NGF on this neuronal population have not been clearly

defined. NGF also may have autocrine actions in the CNS as some neuronal populations have been identified which express both TrkA and NGF.

The receptor for NGF is TrkA, a 140-kDa cell surface protein which specifically binds NGF but not other neurotrophins. TrkA is expressed on the neuronal cell body and on neuronal processes. In its action as a target-derived trophic factor, NGF is secreted within the target organ and then binds to TrkA receptors present on the growing neuronal process or synapse. The NGF–TrkA complex is then internalized and subsequently translocated to the cell body by retrograde axonal transport. In cells which respond to NGF through autocrine or paracrine mechanisms, the growth factor can bind to any of the widely distributed TrkA molecules on the neuronal membrane.

NGF has previously unappreciated effects on the physiological responses of mature neurons. It acts as a target-derived trophic factor for pain neurons, which innervate peripheral tissues such as the skin. Inflammation of these peripheral tissues leads to local elevation of NGF synthesis and abundance. Elevated concentrations of NGF are responsible for the enhanced sensitivity to pain that accompanies inflammation. This is due to the ability of NGF to lower the sensory threshold of the pain fibers, leading to hyperalgesia. Nociceptive sensory neurons are wholly dependent upon NGF for their survival as these cells are selectively lost in animals in which either the NGF or TrkA genes have been knocked out. These animals are insensitive to pain and live only a few weeks.

Brain-derived neurotrophic factor was identified on the basis of its ability to stimulate process outgrowth from peripheral sensory neurons. It was isolated from brain and, upon analysis of its structure, discovered to be highly homologous to NGF [7]. BDNF has a different spectrum of targets compared to NGF and acts on both peripheral sensory ganglionic neurons and parasympathetic neurons of the nodose ganglia but not sympathetic neurons. In the CNS, BDNF supports the survival and process outgrowth of basal forebrain cholinergic neurons, dopaminergic neurons in the striatum, retinal ganglion cells and some motor neurons. Analysis of mice in which the BDNF gene was knocked out reveals that the vestibulocochlear neurons are completely lost, accounting for the inability of these mice to maintain balance. BDNF knockout mice die within 1 to 2 weeks of birth. Analysis of the specific actions of BDNF is significantly complicated by the fact that NT4/5 also binds and activates the TrkB receptor. Interestingly, animals in which the TrkB gene has been inactivated die within 1 to 2 days of birth, but the basis of this is not understood given the modest phenotype of the NT4/5 knockout mice.

The discovery that sensory neurons synthesize BDNF has led to the suggestion that its secretion from these neurons results in both its autocrine and its paracrine actions. It is thought that during development, some neurons, for example, sensory neurons of the dorsal root ganglia, may rely on target-derived factors, while during later periods, the neurons synthesize growth factors which support growth through autocrine stimulation and from cells in their immediate environment. These mechanisms serve to lessen the dependence on targets for trophic support. This view is supported by the finding that axotomy, or target removal, has a much diminished effect in older animals. In the PNS, neurotrophins, including BDNF, are also synthesized by glial cells. Glial cells proliferate at later stages of development, largely after all neurons have been born and some have passed through the period of normal cell death. Thus, glia are likely to play a role in providing trophic support in the mature nervous system through paracrine mechanisms. In fact, the data supporting a role for BDNF and NT3 (see below) as target-derived trophic factors are not particularly compelling. It appears that these neurotrophins, in contrast to NGF, may act principally through autocrine and paracrine mechanisms.

Neutrophin 3 is the most abundantly distributed of the neurotrophins and appears to have a wider range of action than other members of this family, particularly in the CNS. It is expressed throughout the CNS. In the mature brain, NT3 is found at high concentrations in the cortex, hippocampus, thalamus and cerebellum.

NT3 also acts on subpopulations of spinal motor neurons and on cochlear neurons. It exerts its actions principally through binding to another member of the Trk family, TrkC.

In the periphery, NT3 uniquely supports proprioceptive neurons in sensory ganglia. These neurons are selectively lost, as are their targets, the muscle sensory organs, in NT3 knockout mice. Mice in which the NT3 receptor TrkC has been knocked out do not live long and have abnormal movements as a consequence of their loss of proprioception.

NT3 plays an earlier role in the development than other neurotrophin family members. It sustains progenitor cells of the neural crest, which then give rise to sympathetic and sensory ganglia, as well as a number of other structures. It is also likely that NT3 functions to regulate the period of time these precursor cells remain mitotically active and, thus, acts indirectly to regulate cell number. In NT3 knockout mice, approximately 70% of neurons within the sensory ganglia are lost, indicating an absolute requirement for NT3 for the survival of neuronal subpopulations. Analysis of the pattern of NT3 expression has shown that it is highly expressed during periods of rapid process extension in regions adjacent to the developing ganglionic neurons. It is therefore likely that these neurons are supported during this period, principally through autocrine and paracrine mechanisms. As the cells differentiate and extend processes to their targets, NT3 expression is found in these end organs. Importantly, there is a coincident, dramatic reduction in NT3 synthesis in the regions within and adjacent to the developing ganglia, rendering the neurons wholly dependent on target-derived trophic support.

NT3 is also critical for glial development. There is good evidence that NT3 acts to stimulate the proliferation of oligodendrocyte precursor cells, probably in concert with platelet-derived growth factor (PDGF) (see below).

Neurotrophin 4/5 is not as well characterized as other members of the neurotrophin family. Much of what is known is derived from analysis of NT4/5 and TrkB knockout mice. Elucidating the actions of NT4/5 is complicated by virtue of the fact that both NT4/5 and BDNF exert their effects via the TrkB receptor. It appears that NT4/5 functions overlap largely with those of the other neurotrophin family members, particularly BDNF. NT4/5 knockout mice are essentially normal, in contrast to BDNF knockout mice, which do not live long. NT4/5 is likely to have unique actions on a subpopulation of neurons in the nodose and geniculate ganglia, which are not supported by BDNF. Like BDNF, NT4/5 acts on sensory neurons and retinal ganglion cells, supporting their survival.

NT4/5 is expressed in muscle and can support facial motor neurons as well as other populations of motor neurons. Interestingly, NT4/5 expression is regulated by the activity of the muscle, and this neurotrophin stimulates axonal sprouting, suggesting that it acts as a muscle-derived trophic factor for motor neurons.

Nerve growth factor and other neurotrophins influence neurotransmission and synaptic plasticity

The discovery that the neurotrophins have acute effects in the mature nervous system and can modulate synaptic efficiency has forced a substantial re-evaluation of the role of these molecules in modulating the dynamic behavior of the nervous system [13,14].

Direct application of neurotrophins to the brain of animals results in the rapid initiation of dramatic seizure activity, reflecting the coordinated discharge of large populations of neurons. The basis of this effect is the result of neurotrophin-stimulated release of neurotransmitters and enhanced synaptic efficiency. This effect has been investigated using cultured neurons in which application of BDNF and NT3 resulted in an increase in neurotransmitter release from presynaptic nerve terminals. An analogous effect in the PNS is the ability of NGF to enhance painful sensations. Thus, neurotrophins can act over short intervals to regulate synaptic transmission, a role not previously attributed to these molecules.

Conversely, synaptic activity can provoke the release of neurotrophins and acutely regulate the synthesis of these factors. It is likely that nor-

mal physiological concentrations of neurotrophins in the CNS are regulated by ongoing neuronal activity in the brain. There are a number of clear examples showing that the synthesis of neurotrophins, most prominently BDNF, is stimulated following neurotransmitter release. In an extreme example, induction of seizure activity in the brain results in the stimulation of NGF and BDNF, but not of NT3, synthesis. A growing body of evidence suggests that there is an intricate interplay between the ability of the neurotrophins to regulate synaptic activity in the brain and the effect of such activity on neurotrophin synthesis and secretion. The enhanced synaptic stimulation of neurons then positively regulates the synthesis of neurotrophins. Insights into these events have come from the examination of complex phenomena like long-term potentiation in the hippocampus (see Chap. 50) using neurotrophin knockout mice.

The ability of neurotrophins to regulate the structural organization of the PNS during development is well documented. The capacity of these molecules to affect the anatomical organization of the CNS is less well studied. Perhaps the most striking example of the ability of neurotrophins to affect neuronal connectivity in the CNS is the development and maturation of the visual cortex. In this system, the axons of lateral geniculate neurons normally invade visual cortex as a broad and diffuse projection. However, as development proceeds, the axonal projection fields of these neurons become progressively smaller and more refined, eventually becoming restricted to the innervation of defined linear arrays of cortical neurons, termed *ocular dominance columns,* that are sensitive to the input from a single eye. Neurotrophins regulate the process by which the restriction and segregation of axonal projections occur. Administration of neurotrophins can block the formation of dominance columns by inhibiting the loss of synapses within the broad projection area. These data suggest that normally the visual neurons compete for a limited supply of neurotrophins elaborated by the cortical neurons and that neurotrophins stabilize synaptic contacts. Thus, neurotrophins appear to play a critical role in the activity-dependent development of cortical connectivity and function.

Neurokines, or neuropoietins, are a small group of molecules which are highly related to cytokines

They share structural similarities and employ common effector mechanisms in their target cells. Neurokines include ciliary neurotrophic factor (CNTF), leukemia inhibitory factor (LIF), cardiotrophin 1 (CT-1), oncostatin-M and interleukin 6 (IL-6) [2]. Some of these molecules act as *bona fide* growth factors while others appear to have more restricted roles and dictate the differentiated phenotype of subpopulations of neurons [15,16]. The cell surface receptors for the neurokines are multisubunit complexes which employ a common receptor subunit, gp130, together with one or more additional subunits that impart ligand-specific binding properties to the receptor (Fig. 19-3). The receptor complex transduces signals through its interaction with cytoplasmic tyrosine kinases of the JAK family. Ligand binding to the receptor leads to the recruitment of JAK kinases to the receptor and activation of their intrinsic tyrosine kinase activity, leading to stimulation of diverse intracellular signaling pathways.

Ciliary neurotrophic factor was discovered through its ability to sustain parasympathetic neurons of the ciliary ganglia. It exhibits an extremely broad range of activity, acting on a number of neuronal populations [8]. CNTF promotes the survival of parasympathetic ganglionic neurons as well as sensory and sympathetic neurons in the PNS. In the CNS, CNTF acts on neurons in the hippocampus, as well as on both cholinergic and GABAergic neurons in the basal forebrain. CNTF, like the neurotrophins, can regulate neurotransmitter release and directly affect ion channel function.

Substantial interest in the biological actions of CNTF has arisen as a result of its action on motor neurons. CNTF is synthesized in muscle and can be actively taken up by motor neurons

Neurokines, Cytokines and Their Receptors

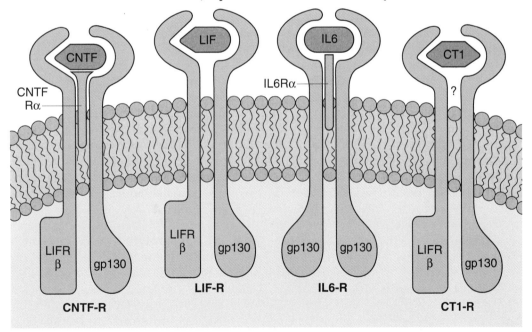

FIGURE 19-3. Neurokines and cytokines related to interleukin (IL-6) bind to cell surface receptor complexes, which share a common structural organization. The four ligands interchangeably employ two distinct receptor subunits, leukemia inhibitory factor receptor β(LIFRβ) and gp130; some employ a ligand-specific α subunit. *CNTF-R*, ciliary neurotrophic factor receptor; *CT1-R*, cardiotrophin 1 receptor; *IL6R*, interleukin-6 receptor; *LIF-R*, leukemia inhibitory factor receptor.

and retrogradely transported to the cell body. Application of CNTF after injury to the nerve will prevent motor neuron death and can partially reverse the progressive loss of motor function in animal models of neuromuscular disease. On this basis, CNTF appears to act as a target-derived trophic factor for these neurons. However, this view is complicated by the fact that CNTF does not possess a secretory signal sequence and it is not known how it is released from its sites of synthesis, primarily in muscle and glial cells in both the CNS and PNS. Of particular interest, injury to the nervous system results in the induction of CNTF synthesis by astrocytes and Schwann cells, suggesting that it plays a role in the response to traumatic injury. In addition to its actions on neurons, it appears that CNTF promotes the differentiation of glial precursor cells into astrocytes and myelin-forming oligodendrocytes.

In humans and mice, mutations in the CNTF gene have no obvious effect, suggesting that other molecules can mediate all of the significant physiological actions of CNTF. Indeed, about 2% of the Japanese population do not have an active CNTF gene. However, knockout of the CNTF receptor gene has dramatic effects, with significant loss of all motor neurons. These data suggest that there must be other as yet undiscovered factors which utilize the CNTF receptor and play a more critical role in development than CNTF itself.

Leukemia inhibitory factor (LIF) is a factor with known actions in the immune system that also acts in the nervous system. Recognition of the action of LIF in the nervous system followed the discovery that it acts on cultured sympathetic neurons to direct a change in neurotransmitter expression from a noradrenergic to a cholinergic phenotype and regulates the expression of neuropeptide transmitters in these cells. LIF exhibits a similar activity toward spinal motor neurons through its ability to stimulate the biosynthesis of acetylcholine. LIF also functions as a trophic factor for peripheral sensory neurons and spinal motor neurons *in vitro,* supporting their survival. *In vivo,* the evidence for a pivotal role for LIF during development is not as strong. LIF-deficient mice demonstrate no anatomical or functional deficits. However, LIF appears to be essential for injury-induced neuropeptide synthesis in the mature nervous system. LIF also acts as a trophic factor for oligodendrocytes and promotes astrocytic survival and differentiation.

Interleukin 6 sustains cultured hippocampal neurons as well as basal forebrain cholinergic and mesencephalic catecholaminergic neurons. IL-6 is likely to be synthesized in the CNS principally by astrocytes, although microglia may also be a source for this cytokine.

Cardiotrophin 1 acts as a survival factor for spinal motor neurons [5]. It is synthesized by both skeletal muscle and cardiac myocytes and is secreted from the latter, suggesting that it acts as a target-derived trophic factor. CT-1 promotes the survival of dopaminergic striatal neurons and ciliary neurons.

Other cytokines, including interleukins 1β, 2, 3, 4, 5, 7, 9, 11 and 12 [2,15,16] have been reported to exhibit neurotrophic actions. Concentrations of these cytokines in nervous tissue are not high, and their effects are not particularly well documented. For many of the cytokines, their significance in nervous system development and function is not clear. These molecules play central roles in immune system function, having many actions following injury to the nervous system, and in disease. In this regard, the microglia are the principal immune effector cells in the brain and function as macrophages. As such, the microglia are a likely source of many of the cytokines reported to be present in the CNS. Astrocytes also synthesize a number of cytokines and are responsive to some of these molecules.

The fibroblast growth factors comprise a gene family of nine members which share substantial sequence homology

While fibroblast growth factors (FGFs) initially were identified on the basis of their ability to stimulate the proliferation of fibroblasts, it was subsequently found that they have an extremely broad distribution in the body and act on a host of different cell types. The FGFs stimulate the proliferation of mesodermally and ectodermally derived cells.

FGFs act on a large number of neuronal populations and all glial cell subtypes [17,18]. In the nervous system, only two members of this family, FGF-1, also termed acidic FGF, and FGF-2, also termed basic FGF, are present at significant concentrations. The FGFs represent the major mitogenic species in the adult nervous system. They are present at significantly higher concentrations than the neurotrophins; FGF-1 and FGF-2 concentrations, respectively, are approximately 500-fold and 50-fold greater than that of NGF [18]. The major FGF translation products do not possess a signal peptide sequence and are found principally within the cytoplasm of cells in which they are expressed. Thus, like several other growth factors, it is not entirely clear how they effect their biological actions.

FGF-1 is expressed at high concentrations in ganglionic sensory neurons in the PNS. In the CNS, FGF-1 is detected at highest concentrations in motor, basal forebrain cholinergic and substantia nigral neurons, as well as in neurons of other subcortical nuclei. FGF-2 is expressed abundantly by astrocytes, although hippocampal pyramidal cells also express it. FGF-1 and FGF-2 do not appear to be highly expressed in the embryonic nervous system and are found at significant concentrations only in the mature nervous system. It is suspected that other members of the FGF family influence development. For example, there is evidence that FGF-8 is involved in axial specification and patterning of limb development. FGFs stimulate the proliferation of neurons in the developing nervous system and glial cells throughout life. FGF-2 stimulates the proliferation of multipotential stem cells, which subsequently give rise to neurons of the cortex [19]. The FGFs also exhibit trophic activity toward mature neurons, promoting the survival of these cells without stimulating DNA synthesis. There is some evidence that the FGFs may play a critical role in facilitating axonal regeneration in the PNS and provide trophic support to neurons following trauma or injury.

The complexity of FGF action is compounded by the existence of at least four receptors for FGF (FGFR1–4). Three FGFRs are expressed in the CNS, where they exist as multiple alternatively spliced products. All of the FGFRs are ligand-activated tyrosine kinases and comprise a distinct subfamily of the receptor tyrosine kinases (see Chap. 25). The interaction of the various FGFs with the four FGFRs and their multiple mRNA splice products is bewilderingly complex and incompletely understood. FGFR1 appears to be expressed exclusively in neurons, while FGFR2 and FGFR3 are expressed principally by glial cells. Interestingly, neurons of the substantia nigra and some motor neurons appear to express both FGF-1 and its receptor, FGFR1, suggesting that FGF-1 may act in an autocrine fashion to support these cells. FGFR1 and FGFR2 appear to play a role in development. Both receptors are expressed prior to the appearance of their ligands, FGF-1 and FGF-2. These data support the view that other FGF family members are more functionally relevant species during embryogenesis. FGFR1 is expressed in the primitive neuroepithelium. A novel aspect of FGF biology is the ability of these growth factors to bind to cell surface proteoglycans, specifically heparan sulfate proteoglycans. Indeed, it appears that these proteoglycans can act as low-affinity receptors for the FGFs. It is thought that FGFs bind to the proteoglycans, which effectively immobilize them and induce or stabilize an active conformation, facilitating binding to the FGFR.

Transforming growth factors β are the prototypical members of a superfamily of related factors which have diverse roles both in development and in the mature animal

There are presently 24 known members of this extended family, which have been assigned to five distinct subfamilies [20]. The actions of most of the transforming growth factor β (TGFβ) superfamily members are best described in organ systems other than brain. However, the TGFβ-related factors have important roles in the nervous system, where they are thought to act principally through autocrine and paracrine mechanisms. This family of growth factors employs a unique receptor complex involving two distinct subunits, both of which are serine/threonine kinases (see Chap. 24). The ligand first binds to the type II subunit, and this dimeric complex then associates with the type I subunit. The hetero-oligomeric receptor complex then initiates intracellular signaling events.

The TGF β subfamily consists of three members in mammals: TGFβ1, TGFβ2 and TGFβ3. TGFβ1 is expressed principally by glial cells and is not present in significant amounts in the mature nervous system. TGFβ1 is thought to function principally following injury to the nervous system, where its expression is dramatically induced in microglial cells. It is synthesized, albeit at lower levels, by astrocytes. In some neurons, TGFβ1 is a component of the response to neurodegeneration or trauma and its synthesis and secretion are elevated in these settings. The synthesis of TGFβ1 following injury in the nervous system is consistent with its effects on inflammatory responses in other organ systems. Although this factor is not particularly well studied in the developing nervous system, it has been reported to play an instructive role in specifying cellular phenotype.

TGFβ2 and TGFβ3 are widely expressed in both the PNS and the CNS. Early in development TGFβ2 is associated with developing fiber tracts, and later in development it is found in astrocytes. TGFβ3 acts as a mitogen for amacrine cells in the developing retina. In the adult, TGFβ2 and TGFβ3 are found in many neuronal populations and in both astrocytes and Schwann cells.

The TGFβ3 family has diverse effects which are likely to be cell type specific and to have as yet unknown functions. TGFβ2, in contrast to many growth factors, can inhibit cellular proliferation and, in some circumstances, is growth-inhibitory toward neurons. It has antimitotic effects on astrocytes and also acts to arrest the proliferation of oligodendrocytes, subsequently promoting their differentiation. TGFβ2 and TGFβ3 also exhibit negative effects on the survival of some neuronal populations, for example, on ciliary ganglionic neurons. In a number of instances, TGFβ2 and TGFβ3 functionally antagonize the action of other growth and trophic factors.

Conversely, there is compelling evidence that TGFβ2 and TGFβ3 act as survival and trophic factors for dopaminergic neurons in the striatum and midbrain [21]. It appears that during development TGFβ2, TGFβ3 and glial-derived neurotrophic factor (GDNF) are expressed locally in regions in which these neurons reside,

while at later times these factors are expressed principally within the projection fields of these neurons. These findings have been interpreted to support the view that members of the TGFβ family act as target-derived trophic factors for dopaminergic neurons. Evaluation of the biological actions of TGFβ has been difficult because in some cases TGFβs appear not to promote neuronal survival or to exhibit direct neurotrophic actions but, rather, may act indirectly by stimulating contaminating non-neuronal cells in culture to secrete neurotrophins or other growth factors.

Bone morphogenetic proteins (BMPs) comprise a TGFβ subfamily of factors which are most highly related to the *Drosophila* decapentaplegic gene product, a critical regulator of morphogenesis and axial specification. As their name indicates, these factors were first identified on the basis of their effect on bone formation. The focus of most studies of these factors has been on their role in inductive events in development. Relatively little is known about their range of actions in the nervous system. Nevertheless, it is clear that these factors have important roles early in the development of the nervous system. BMP2 influences the differentiation of multipotential cells of the neural crest into a neuronal phenotype. The BMPs also have significant roles as trophic factors. BMP2 and BMP6 act as survival factors for neurons of the cerebral cortex and cerebellum. BMP6 is widely expressed in the developing and mature nervous system, and there is a growing literature suggesting that BMP family members act in concert with other factors to regulate neuronal differentiation and survival.

Glial-derived neurotrophic factor (GDNF) shares sequence homology with TGFβ but is a distant member of this family and functions through receptors which are unrelated to those employed by more traditional members of this superfamily. GDNF binds to two receptor species, which oligomerize to form a functionally active receptor complex. GDNF interacts with both the GDNF receptor α subunit and with the c-*ret* proto-oncogene, forming a hetero-oligomeric complex. Ret is a tyrosine kinase which undergoes enzymatic activation and initiates intracellular signaling events upon GDNF binding (see Chap. 25).

GDNF is synthesized in a number of different tissues, and its expression in non-neural tissues is appreciably higher than in the nervous system. As its name suggests, GDNF is synthesized by glial cells, in the CNS by astrocytes and in the PNS by Schwann cells. GDNF was first characterized as a trophic factor which supports the survival and differentiation of dopaminergic cells of the midbrain and striatum [22]. It is this latter cell population that is selectively lost in Parkinson's disease (see Chap. 45). GDNF selectively supports these cells after physical or chemical insults, suggesting that it may have some utility as a therapeutic agent in this disease. GDNF is likely to act as a target-derived trophic factor as it is synthesized in areas receiving dopaminergic innervation and is retrogradely transported to the cell bodies of the dopaminergic neurons.

In the periphery, GDNF acts as a trophic factor for both sympathetic and parasympathetic neurons as well as for several distinct subpopulations of sensory neurons. Consistent with its imputed role as a target-derived trophic factor, it is highly expressed in a variety of tissues with sympathetic and sensory innervation. Importantly, GDNF is a potent trophic factor for spinal motor neurons and can rescue these cells from programmed cell death during development, as well as prevent their death following injury. GDNF is synthesized by skeletal muscle and is retrogradely transported, suggesting that it acts as a target-derived trophic factor for the innervating spinal motor neurons.

A second GDNF-like molecule has been discovered, termed neurturin, which shares substantial structural homology with GDNF. Neurturin acts to support the survival of sympathetic neurons and sensory neurons of the dorsal root ganglia and parasympathetic nodose ganglia. It is not known if this factor can act on CNS neurons.

Epidermal growth factor and related factors have a diverse range of actions in the nervous system

Epidermal growth factor (EGF) is not likely to play a major role in the nervous system, although it has been shown to stimulate the prolif-

eration of populations of multipotential stem cells *in vitro*.

TGFα is structurally related to EGF and is widely expressed throughout the developing embryo, including the nervous system. TGFα binds to and activates EGF receptors and is more likely to be the physiologically relevant ligand for these receptors during development. Little is known about the actions of TGFα in the nervous system, but it is likely to act principally through autocrine or paracrine mechanisms.

Neuregulins are a unique family of growth and differentiation factors which arise from the alternative splicing of mRNAs derived from a single gene [23]. There are currently about a dozen recognized neuregulin isoforms, which include *glial growth factor* (GGF), *heregulin, neu differentiation factor* (NDF), *sensory and motor neuron-derived growth factor* (SMDF) and *acetylcholine receptor-inducing activity* (ARIA). Neuregulins are secreted proteins which contain a region highly homologous to EGF. The neuregulins bind to a family of receptor tyrosine kinases which are homologous to the EGF receptor, termed erbB, or HER in the human [24]. While this complex family of ligands and receptors has been discovered only recently and our knowledge of their action is presently fragmentary, it is already apparent that they play pivotal roles in nervous system growth and differentiation.

Neuregulins are highly expressed in the nervous system and appear to be synthesized principally by neurons. They are expressed in neuroblasts, cortical neurons and peripheral sensory ganglionic cells and spinal motor neurons. An important feature of neuregulin action is that their primary targets are glial cells and muscle. Thus, these molecules are important intermediates subserving neuron–glia interactions. Neuregulins are likely to act principally in a paracrine manner on adjacent glial cells and on non-neuronal target tissues innervated by neuregulin-expression neurons, such as muscle.

Neuregulins act as mitogens and survival factors for the three major glial cell types: astrocytes and oligodendrocytes in the CNS and Schwann cells in the periphery. The neuregulins act on Schwann cells by stimulating their proliferation as well as their motility and migratory activity. It is postulated that this interaction provides a mechanism by which neurons can influence glial metabolism and behavior, which are important both in development and in peripheral nerve regeneration. In mice in which the neuregulin gene has been inactivated, Schwann cells and cranial ganglia fail to develop.

Insight into the function of neuregulins was gained by the observation that they are synthesized by motor neurons and released at the neuromuscular junction, where they interact with the erbB receptors expressed on the muscle cell membrane. Interestingly, in this context, neuregulin was first detected as an activity which stimulated the expression and aggregation of acetylcholine receptors at sites of nerve contact and was dubbed ARIA. Neuregulin/ARIA acts as a synaptic signal which regulates muscle gene expression.

Other growth factors, such as platelet-derived growth factor and insulin-like growth factor, play a role in the nervous system

Platelet-derived growth factor (PDGF) is synthesized by neurons and astrocytes throughout the CNS and by Schwann cells in the PNS. These various cell types also express PDGF receptors, and it is thought that this growth factor acts in an autocrine and paracrine fashion. The best described action of PDGF is on oligodendrocyte progenitor cells, stimulating their proliferation and subsequently promoting their differentiation into mature oligodendrocytes.

Insulin-like growth factor I (IGF-I) has a well-recognized role as a trophic and survival factor for nervous system cells in tissue culture. However, its specific functions in the developing and mature nervous system have been difficult to define largely because its actions as a trophic factor overlap extensively with those of other growth factors. IGF-I is expressed in nervous tissue late in development and is present at highest concentrations in neurons of the olfactory bulb, thalamus, cerebellum and retina [25]. IGF-I and insulin sustain many nervous system-derived cell types in tissue culture. The amount of insulin required to elicit biological effects in most of these

cells is quite high, suggesting that many of the reported effects of insulin on cells of the nervous system *in vitro* are actually mediated by insulin action on the IGF-I receptors. The IGF-I receptor possesses a ligand-stimulated tyrosine kinase domain, the structure of which is quite similar to that of the insulin receptor. The IGF-I receptor is ubiquitously expressed throughout the nervous system and is found at higher concentrations in the developing brain than in the adult, in contrast to IGF-I expression. *In vitro* studies have shown that IGF-I is likely to act principally through autocrine or paracrine mechanisms to promote the proliferation of neuronal and glial precursors and to facilitate their subsequent differentiation and survival.

IGF-I has been the focus of considerable interest due to its actions on motor neurons. It can prevent normal motor neuron cell death during development, reduce the loss of these cells following nerve injury and enhance axonal regeneration. In the adult, injection of IGF-I results in sprouting of motor neuron terminals and an increase in the size of the neuromuscular junction. These and other studies suggest potential therapeutic applications of IGF-I in several neurological diseases, including amyotrophic lateral sclerosis and peripheral neuropathies [26].

GROWTH FACTORS ACT COMBINATORIALLY AND SEQUENTIALLY TO REGULATE NERVOUS SYSTEM DEVELOPMENT

One of the primary outcomes of the investigation of growth factor action has been the recognition that there are a relatively small number of growth factors which must act in concert to orchestrate the survival and differentiation of a diverse population of neuronal and non-neuronal cell types. It is apparent that most cells are dependent upon more than one growth factor both during embryogenesis and after maturation [12]. One of the most significant outcomes from analysis of neurotrophin knockout mice is that they show very modest phenotypic changes in the CNS [11]. This reflects the extensive interconnectivity of neurons in the brain, providing a wide range of cellular contacts from which trophic support may arise. In the PNS, the phenotypes are more dramatic, with significant cell loss, indicating a more restricted source of trophic factors available to these cells. There is ample evidence that both neurons and glial cells express receptors for a number of growth factors which allow the cells to respond to multiple sources of trophic support. Moreover, responsiveness to several factors also serves to broaden cellular sensitivity to changes in the environment during development and in the mature nervous system and may subserve a dynamic response to changing rates of activity or to injury. Also, trophic support for neurons is delivered at different cellular loci. For example, adult sensory neurons express multiple members of the Trk family; however, NGF appears to be delivered to the neurons from their peripheral targets via axonal transport, while BDNF and other factors are supplied to the cell body via paracrine mechanisms.

Motor neurons provide a compelling example of how a single class of neurons can be supported by an extraordinarily wide range of factors. Currently, more than 15 protein factors have been shown to sustain these cells *in vitro* or *in vivo*. Some of these are derived from the muscle target, while others are elaborated by ensheathing Schwann cells and by cells resident within the spinal cord. It is likely that motor neurons rely upon multiple factors for their survival and that different subpopulations of motor neurons may exhibit unique combinations of trophic factor dependence [5].

Detailed study of the actions of growth factors has revealed that they act in concert to mediate developmental events and, further, that they act sequentially [8]. The ability of a neuron to respond to a given trophic factor is frequently dependent on its developmental stage. The complexity of trophic factor dependence exhibited by some populations of neurons is a consequence of both the developmentally regulated expression of growth factor receptors and the spatiotemporal pattern of growth factor expression. For example, pluripotent neural crest cells giving rise to sensory neurons are dependent upon NT3 for proliferation early in development. The cells lose their responsiveness to NT3 and become NGF-dependent during the period when they establish contacts with their peripheral targets. Similarly, neuroblasts of the cortex and hippocampus are stimulated to proliferate in response to FGF-2, and subsequently, they become responsive to NT3, which then promotes their survival and differentiation [19]. These examples illustrate the serial dependence of neurons upon different factors for mitotic expansion, acquisition of a differentiated phenotype and their sustenance in the mature nervous system.

One of the most significant conclusions to be derived from the study of growth factors in the nervous system is that we surely have discovered only a fraction of the growth/trophic factors which are responsible for the generation of the cellular complexity and the specific and extensive interconnections between populations of cells. In the last few years, largely through the power of molecular biology and molecular genetics, we have identified a number of novel factors. This process of discovery will undoubtedly continue at an accelerated pace.

REFERENCES

1. Levi-Montalcini, R., and Angeletti P. Nerve growth factor. *Physiol. Rev.* 48:534–569, 1968.
2. Mehler, M., and Kessler, J. Growth factor regulation of neuronal development. *Dev. Neurosci.* 16:180–195, 1994.
3. Davies, A. The neurotrophic hypothesis: Where does it stand? *Phil. Trans. R. Soc. Lond. B* 351:389–394, 1996.
4. Acheson, A., and Lindsay, R. Non target-derived roles of the neurotrophins. *Phil. Trans. R. Soc. Lond. B* 351:417–422, 1996.
5. Oppenheim, R. Neurotrophic survival molecules for motoneurons: An embarrassment of riches. *Neuron* 17:195–197, 1996.
6. Segal, R., and Greenberg, M. Intracellular signaling pathways activated by neurotrophic factors. *Annu. Rev. Neurosci.* 19:463–489, 1996.
7. Lewin, G., and Barde, Y.-A. Physiology of the neurotrophins. *Annu. Rev. Neurosci.* 19:289–317, 1996.
8. Ip, N., and Yancopoulos, G. The neurotrophins and CNTF: Two families of collaborative neurotrophic factors. *Annu. Rev. Neurosci.* 19:491–515, 1996.

9. McDonald, N., and Chao, M. Structural determinants of neurotrophin action. *J. Biol. Chem.* 270:19669–19672, 1995.

10. Bothwell, M. Functional interactions of neurotrophins and neurotrophin receptors. *Annu. Rev. Neurosci.* 18:223–253, 1995.

11. Snider, W. Functions of the neurotrophins during nervous system development: What the knockouts are telling us. *Cell* 77:627–638, 1994.

12. Lewin, G. Neurotrophins and the specification of neuronal phenotype. *Phil. Trans. R. Soc. Lond. B* 351:405–411, 1996.

13. Lo, D. Neurotrophic factors and synaptic plasticity. *Neuron* 15:979–981, 1995.

14. Thoenen, H. Neurotrophins and neuronal plasticity. *Science* 270:593–598, 1995.

15. Rothwell, N., and Hopkins, S. Cytokines and the nervous system II: Actions and mechanisms of action. *Trends Neurosci.* 18:130–136, 1995.

16. Hopkins, S., and Rothwell, N. Cytokines and the nervous system I: Expression and recognition. *Trends Neurosci.* 18:83–88, 1995.

17. Baird, A. Fibroblast growth factors: Activities and significance of non-neurotrophin neurotrophic growth factors. *Curr. Opin. Neurobiol.* 4:78–86, 1994.

18. Eckenstein, F. Fibroblast growth factors in the nervous system. *J. Neurobiol.* 25:1467–1480, 1994.

19. Temple, S., and Qian, X. bFGF, neurotrophins, and the control of cortical neurogenesis. *Neuron* 15:249–252, 1995.

20. Krieglstein, K., Rufer, M., Suter-Crazzola, C., and Unsicker, K. Neural functions of the transforming growth factor β. *Int. J. Dev. Neurosci.* 13:301–315, 1995.

21. Poulsen, K., Armanini, M., Klein, R., Hynes, M., Phillips, H., and Rosenthal, A. TGFβ2 and TGFβ3 are potent survival factors for midbrain dopaminergic neurons. *Neuron* 13:1245–1252, 1994.

22. Lin, L., Doherty, D., Lile, J., Bektesh, S., and Collins, F. GDNF: A glial cell line derived neurotrophic factor for midbrain dopaminergic neurons. *Science* 260:1130–1132, 1993.

23. Ben-Baruch, N., and Yarden, Y. Neu differentiation factors: A family of alternatively spliced neuronal and mesenchymal factors. *Proc. Soc. Exp. Biol. Med.* 206:221–227, 1994.

24. Carraway, K., and Burden, S. Neuregulins and their receptors. *Curr. Opin. Neurobiol.* 5:606–612, 1995.

25. de Pablo, F., and de la Rosa, E. The developing CNS: A scenario for the action of proinsulin, insulin and insulin-like growth factors. *Trends Neurosci.* 18:143–150, 1995.

26. Lewis, M., Neff, N., Contreras, P., et al. Insulin-like growth factor I: Potential for treatment of motor neuronal disorders. *Exp. Neurol.* 124:73–88, 1993.

Intracellular Signaling

20

G Proteins

Eric J. Nestler and Ronald S. Duman

G proteins comprise several families of diverse cellular proteins that subserve an equally diverse array of cellular functions. These proteins derive their name from the fact that they bind the guanine nucleotides guanosine triphosphate (GTP) and guanosine diphosphate (GDP) and possess intrinsic GTPase activity. G proteins play a central role in signal transduction as well as in a

Basic Neurochemistry: Molecular, Cellular and Medical Aspects, 6th Ed., edited by G. J. Siegel et al. Published by Lippincott–Raven Publishers, Philadelphia, 1999. Correspondence to Eric J. Nestler, Division of Molecular Psychiatry, Departments of Psychiatry and Neurobiology, Yale University School of Medicine and Connecticut Mental Health Center, 34 Park Street, New Haven, Connecticut 06508.

myriad of cellular processes, including membrane vesicle transport, cytoskeletal assembly, cell growth and protein synthesis (see Chaps. 5, 8 and 9).

Mammalian G proteins can be divided into two major categories: heterotrimeric G proteins and small G proteins. This chapter reviews the types of G protein that exist in the nervous system and the ways in which they regulate signal transduction and other processes essential for brain function.

HETEROTRIMERIC G PROTEINS

With the exception of synaptic transmission mediated via receptors that contain intrinsic enzymatic activity, such as tyrosine kinase or guanylyl cyclase, or that form ion channels (see Chap. 10), the family of membrane proteins known as heterotrimeric G proteins may be involved in all other transmembrane signaling in the nervous system. These types of G protein were first identified, named and characterized by Rodbell, Gilman and others close to 20 years ago.

Heterotrimeric G proteins consist of three distinct subunits, α, β and γ. These proteins couple the activation of diverse types of plasma membrane receptor to a variety of intracellular processes. In fact, most types of neurotransmitter and peptide hormone receptor, as well as many cytokine and chemokine receptors, fall into a superfamily of structurally related molecules, termed G protein-coupled receptors. These receptors are named for the role of G proteins in mediating the varied biological effects of the receptors (Chap. 10). Consequently, many types of effector protein are influenced by these heterotrimeric G proteins: ion channels; adenylyl cyclase; phosphodiesterase (PDE); phosphoinositide-specific phospholipase C (PI-PLC), which catalyzes the hydrolysis of phosphatidylinositol 4,5-bisphosphate (PIP_2); and phospholipase A_2 (PLA_2), which catalyzes the hydrolysis of membrane phospholipids to yield arachidonic acid. In addition, these G proteins have been implicated in several other intracellular processes, such as vesicular transport and cytoskeletal assembly.

Multiple forms of heterotrimeric G proteins exist in the nervous system

Three types of heterotrimeric G protein were identified in early studies. G_t, termed transducin, was identified as the G protein that couples rhodopsin to regulation of photoreceptor cell function (see Chap. 47), and G_s and G_i were identified as the G proteins that couple plasma membrane receptors to the stimulation and inhibition, respectively, of adenylyl cyclase, the enzyme that catalyzes the synthesis of cAMP (see Chap. 22).

Since that time, over 35 heterotrimeric G protein subunits have been identified by a combination of biochemical and molecular cloning techniques [1–5]. In addition to G_t, G_s and G_i, the other types of G protein in brain are designated G_o, G_{olf}, G_{gust}, G_z, G_q and G_{11-16}. Moreover, for most of these G proteins, multiple subtypes show unique distributions in the brain and peripheral tissues.

Each G protein is a heterotrimer composed of single α, β and γ subunits

The different types of G protein contain distinct α subunits, which, in part at least, confer the specificity of functional activity. The types of G protein α subunit are listed in Table 20-1, and are categorized based on their structural and functional homologies. Current nomenclature identifies several subfamilies of G protein α subunit: $G_{\alpha s}$, $G_{\alpha i}$, $G_{\alpha q}$ and $G_{\alpha 12}$. The M_r of these proteins varies between 38,000 and 52,000. As a first approximation, these distinct types of α subunit share common β and γ subunits. However, multiple subtypes of β and γ subunits are now known: five β subunits of M_r 35,000 to 36,000 and seven γ subunits of M_r 6,000 to 9,000. These proteins show distinct cellular distributions, and differences in their functional properties are now becoming apparent [1–5].

The functional activity of G proteins involves their dissociation and reassociation in response to extracellular signals

This is shown schematically in Figure 20-1. In the resting state, G proteins exist as hetero-

TABLE 20-1. **HETEROTRIMERIC G PROTEIN α-SUBUNITS IN BRAIN**

Family	$M_r{}^a$	Toxin-mediated ADP-ribosylation	Effector protein(s)
G_s			
$G_{\alpha s1}$	52,000	Cholera	Adenylyl cyclase (activation)
$G_{\alpha s2}$	52,000		
$G_{\alpha s3}$	45,000		
$G_{\alpha s4}$	45,000		
$G_{\alpha olf}$	45,000		
G_i			
$G_{\alpha i1}$	41,000	Pertussis	Adenylyl cyclase (inhibition)
$G_{\alpha i2}$	40,000		?K^+ channel (activation)
$G_{\alpha i3}$	41,000		?Ca^{2+} channel (inhibition)
			?PI-Phospholipase C (activation)
			?Phospholipase A_2
$G_{\alpha o1}$	39,000	Pertussis	K^+ channel (activation)
$G_{\alpha o2}$	39,000		Ca^{2+} channel (inhibition)
$G_{\alpha t1}$	39,000	Cholera and pertussis	Phosphodiesterase (activation) in rods and cones
$G_{\alpha t2}$	40,000		
$G_{\alpha gust}$	41,000	Unknown	Phosphodiesterase (activation) in taste epithelium
$G_{\alpha z}$	41,000	None	?Adenylyl cyclase (inhibition)
G_q	41,000 to 43,000		
$G_{\alpha q}$		None	PI-Phospholipase C (activation)
$G_{\alpha 11}$		Unknown	
$G_{\alpha 14}$			
$G_{\alpha 15}$			
$G_{\alpha 16}$			
G_{12}	44,000	None	Unknown
$G_{\alpha 12}$			
$G_{\alpha 13}$			

a Values shown reflect apparent M_r by gel electrophoresis in most cases. Values shown for $G_{\alpha gust}$, G_z and $G_{\alpha 11-16}$ reflect calculated M_r based on amino acid sequence.
Question marks indicate that the association between the particular G proteins and effector proteins shown in the table remains tentative.

trimers that bind GDP and are associated with extracellular receptors (Fig. 20-1A). When a ligand binds to and activates the receptor, it produces a conformational change in the receptor, which in turn triggers a dramatic conformational change in the α subunit of the G protein (Fig. 20-1B). This conformational change leads to (i) a decrease in the affinity of the α subunit for GDP, which results in the dissociation of GDP from the α subunit and the subsequent binding of GTP as the cellular concentration of GTP is much higher than that of GDP; (ii) dissociation of a βγ subunit complex from the α subunit; and (iii) release of the receptor from the G protein (Fig. 20-1B,C). This process generates a free α subunit bound to GTP as well as a free βγ subunit complex, both of which are biologically active and can regulate the functional activity of effector proteins within the cell [1–5]. The GTP-bound α subunit is also capable of interacting with the receptor and reducing its affinity for ligand. The system returns to its resting state when the ligand is released from the receptor and the GTPase activity that resides in the α subunit hydrolyzes GTP to GDP (Fig. 20-1D). The latter action leads to reassociation of the free α subunit with the βγ subunit complex to restore the original heterotrimers.

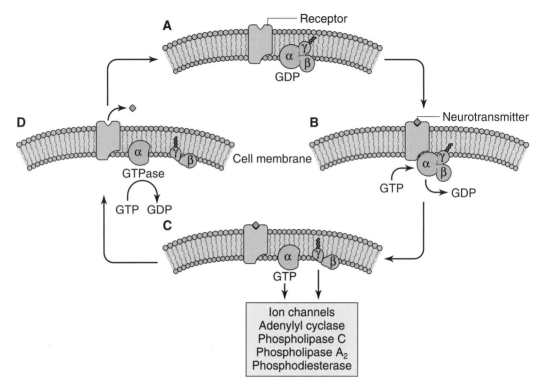

FIGURE 20-1. Functional cycle of heterotrimeric G proteins. **A:** Under basal conditions, G proteins exist in cell membranes as heterotrimers composed of single α, β and γ subunits and are associated only loosely with neurotransmitter receptors. In this situation, GDP is bound to the α subunit. **B:** Upon activation of the receptor by its ligand, such as a neurotransmitter, the receptor physically associates with the α subunit, which leads to the dissociation of GDP from the subunit and the binding of GTP instead. **C:** GTP binding induces the generation of free α subunit by causing the dissociation of the α subunit from its β and γ subunits and the receptor. Free α subunits (bound to GTP) and free βγ subunit dimers are functionally active and directly regulate a number of effector proteins, which, depending on the type of subunit and cell involved, can include ion channels, adenylyl cyclase, phospholipase C, phospholipase A$_2$ and phosphodiesterase. **D:** GTPase activity intrinsic to the α subunit degrades GTP to GDP. This leads to the reassociation of the α and βγ subunits, which, along with the dissociation of ligand from receptor, leads to restoration of the basal state. (From Hyman and Nestler [41] with permission.)

The structural basis of the interactions among the α, β, and γ subunits of G proteins and between the subunits and the associated receptor has become increasingly understood as the crystalline structure of these proteins has been determined [3,6]. Each α subunit has two identifiable domains. One contains the GTPase activity and the GTP-binding site. This domain also appears to be most important in binding βγ subunits as well as various effector proteins. The function of the other domain remains unknown, but it may be involved in the dramatic conformational shift that occurs in the protein upon exchanging GTP for GDP. The ability of the heterotrimeric G protein to bind to a receptor is thought to depend on sites located within all three G protein subunits. Thus, the different α subunits as well as subtypes of β and γ subunits seem to be responsible for targeting a particular type of G protein to a particular type of receptor.

G proteins couple some neurotransmitter receptors directly to ion channels

It is now clearly established that G protein subunits released from the G protein–receptor interaction can directly open or close specific ion channels [2,7]. One of the best examples of this mechanism in brain is the coupling of many types of receptors, including opioid, α_2-adrenergic, D2-dopaminergic, muscarinic cholinergic, $5HT_{1a}$-serotonergic and $GABA_B$ receptors, to the activation of an inward rectifying K^+ channel (GIRK) via pertussis toxin-sensitive G proteins, that is, subtypes of G_o and/or G_i, in many types of neurons. In initial studies, it was controversial as to whether the free α subunit or the free $\beta\gamma$ dimer was responsible for this action. Based on elegant studies in which cloned channel and G protein subunits were expressed in a variety of cell types, it is now the general consensus that the $\beta\gamma$ complex is the more important mechanism [2,7]. In fact, the region of the channel responsible for binding the $\beta\gamma$ complex has been identified [8]. Moreover, it seems that particular combinations of β and γ subtypes are more effective at opening this channel than others. It also appears, however, that subtypes of α_i can open the channel, although not to the same extent as the $\beta\gamma$ subunits.

These same neurotransmitter receptors also are coupled via pertussis toxin-sensitive G proteins to voltage-gated Ca^{2+} channels, although the channels are inhibited by this interaction. In this case, available evidence supports a role for $\beta\gamma$ in mediating this effect, although there is some evidence that α_i and α_o subunits also can be active [2,7]. Binding of the G protein subunits to the Ca^{2+} channels reduces their probability of opening in response to membrane depolarization. This mechanism is best established for L-type Ca^{2+} channels, which are inhibited by the dihydropyridine antihypertensive drugs, such as verapamil, but may also operate for other types of voltage-gated Ca^{2+} channel (see also Chaps. 6 and 23).

Still another example of direct regulation of ion channels by G proteins is the stimulation of L-type Ca^{2+} channels by G_s. In this case, free α subunits appear to bind to the channel and increase their probability of opening in response to membrane depolarization [2].

G proteins regulate intracellular concentrations of second messengers

G proteins control intracellular cAMP concentrations by mediating the ability of neurotrans-

mitters to activate or inhibit adenylyl cyclase. The mechanism by which neurotransmitters stimulate adenylyl cyclase is well known. Activation of those neurotransmitter receptors that couple to G_s results in the generation of free $G_{\alpha s}$ subunits, which bind to and, thereby, directly activate adenylyl cyclase. In addition, free $\beta\gamma$-subunit complexes activate certain subtypes of adenylyl cyclase (see Chap. 22). A similar mechanism appears to be the case for $G_{\alpha olf}$, a type of G protein structurally related to $G_{\alpha s}$ which is enriched in olfactory epithelium and striatum [9].

The mechanism by which neurotransmitters inhibit adenylyl cyclase and decrease neuronal levels of cAMP has eluded definitive identification. By analogy with the action of G_s, it was proposed originally that activation of neurotransmitter receptors that couple to G_i results in the generation of free $G_{\alpha i}$ subunits, which bind to and, thereby, directly inhibit adenylyl cyclase. However, the inhibition of adenylyl cyclase by $G_{\alpha i}$ has been difficult to demonstrate in some cell-free reconstitution experiments. Alternative possibilities are that free $\beta\gamma$-subunit complexes, generated by the release of $G_{\alpha i}$, might directly inhibit certain forms of adenylyl cyclase or bind free $G_{\alpha s}$ subunits in the membrane [10]. Such sequestration of $G_{\alpha s}$ would then decrease basal stimulation of adenylyl cyclase. Indeed, there is now compelling evidence (discussed further in Chap. 22) that $\beta\gamma$ subunits can inhibit certain forms of adenylyl cyclase, whereas other forms of the enzyme are activated by the subunits. In addition to G_i, there is evidence that $G_{\alpha z}$, which can be considered a subtype of the G_i family based on sequence homologies, also can mediate neurotransmitter inhibition of adenylyl cyclase.

The transducin family of G proteins mediate signal transduction in the visual system (see Chap. 47) by regulating specific forms of phosphodiesterase, which catalyze the metabolism of cyclic nucleotides (see Chap. 22) [1–5]. $G_{\alpha t}$ activates PDE via direct binding to the enzyme. Gustducin ($G_{\alpha gust}$) shares a high degree of homology with $G_{\alpha t}$ [4]. It is enriched in taste epithelium and has been speculated to mediate signal transduction in this tissue via the activation of a distinct form of phosphodiesterase.

The ability of neurotransmitter receptors to stimulate the phosphoinositide second-messenger pathway is mediated by the activation of PI-PLC, which, as mentioned above, catalyzes the hydrolysis of PIP_2 to form the second messengers inositol triphosphate (IP_3) and diacylglycerol (DAG) (see Chap. 21). It now appears that neurotransmitter-induced activation of PI-PLC is mediated via G proteins [1–5]. In most cases, G_q is involved, and it is thought that $G_{\alpha q}$ and related α subunits bind to and directly activate certain forms of PI-PLC, particularly the C_β form. In some cell types, it appears that subtypes of G_i and/or G_o may be involved. The mechanism by which G proteins mediate neurotransmitter regulation of arachidonic acid metabolism, via the activation or inhibition of PLA_2, is less well established but also may involve subtypes of G_i or G_o. In each of these cases, possible roles for βγ complexes in the regulation of enzyme activity have been proposed but remain to be established [1,3].

G proteins have been implicated in membrane trafficking

In addition to mediating signal transduction at the plasma membrane, certain heterotrimeric G proteins have been implicated in several processes that involve the trafficking of cell membranes, although the precise mechanisms involved remain obscure. For example, the $G_{\alpha i}$ subunit has been detected at relatively high concentrations in intracellular membranes, including the Golgi complex, transgolgi network and endoplasmic reticulum [11,12]. Experiments that involve activation or inhibition of this subunit with various guanine nucleotides suggest that $G_{\alpha i}$ may regulate the budding of membrane vesicles through these organelles. It also has been suggested that $G_{\alpha i}$ could be involved in the process by which portions of the plasma membrane are vesicularized into the cytoplasm via endocytosis. Synaptic vesicle trafficking is discussed in detail in Chapter 9.

Another example of the involvement of G proteins in membrane trafficking is the proposed role for $G_{\alpha o}$ in the extension of neural processes. $G_{\alpha o}$ is present at very high concentrations in nerve growth cones. Moreover, activation of $G_{\alpha o}$ by guanine nucleotides or overexpression of a constitutively active mutant form of $G_{\alpha o}$ increases nerve outgrowth in cultured

neurons [12]. One interesting possibility is that $G_{\alpha o}$ may interact with growth-associated protein of 43 kDa (GAP-43), another growth cone-enriched protein, to promote the growth of neural processes.

G protein βγ subunits subserve numerous functions in the cell

In early studies, G protein βγ subunits were thought to be inactive proteins that merely sequester active α subunits or anchor them to the plasma membrane. However, it has become clear that βγ subunits, acting as dimers, are highly active biological molecules that play important roles in several cellular functions.

As mentioned above, βγ subunits directly bind to and activate a class of K^+ channels called GIRKs and bind to and modulate the activity of PI-PLC_β and certain classes of adenylyl cyclase. The βγ subunits also bind to several other proteins, including certain protein kinases as well as phosducin and Ras guanine nucleotide exchange factor (see below) [1,3,13]. The ability of such diverse cellular proteins to bind βγ subunits has led to a search for a common structural motif in these various target proteins that is responsible for this binding. One possibility is that these proteins contain a specific amino acid sequence within their primary structures, termed the pleckstrin homology (PH) domain, which binds βγ with high affinity.

One class of protein kinase that binds βγ subunits is called G protein receptor kinases (GRKs). These kinases phosphorylate G protein-coupled receptors that are occupied by ligand and thereby mediate one form of receptor desensitization (see Chap. 24). It now appears that βγ subunits play a key role in this process [13]. As shown in Figure 20-2, the GRK is normally a cytoplasmic protein that does not come into appreciable contact with the plasma membrane receptor under basal conditions. Ligand binding to the receptor activates the associated G protein, which results in the generation of free α and βγ subunits. The βγ subunits, which remain membrane-bound (as will be described below), are now free to bind to the C-terminal domain of the GRK. This draws the GRK into close physical proximity with the receptor and enables receptor phosphorylation. In this way, the βγ sub-

A

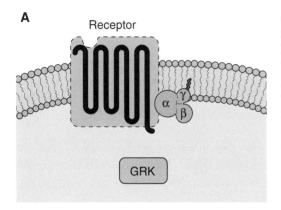

B

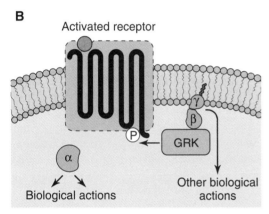

FIGURE 20-2. Schematic illustration of the role of G protein βγ subunits in intracellular targeting of proteins. **A:** Under resting conditions, the receptor is associated loosely with a heterotrimeric G protein and G protein receptor kinases *(GRK)* are cytoplasmic and, therefore, unable to phosphorylate the receptor. **B:** Upon activation of the receptor and G protein, free α subunit is generated, which can lead to a variety of physiological effects. In addition, a free βγ subunit dimer is generated, which can bind to the GRK and draw it toward the membrane, where it can phosphorylate the ligand-occupied receptor. In this way, βγ subunits can target GRKs specifically to those receptor molecules occupied by ligand. Free βγ also produces other physiological effects by interacting with other cellular proteins. The βγ complex is tethered to the membrane by an isoprenyl group on the γ subunit as depicted.

units target GRKs, which have constitutive catalytic activity, to those receptors that are ligand-bound.

Another important role for βγ subunits is regulation of the mitogen-activated protein kinase (MAP-kinase) pathway [14]. MAP-kinases are the major effector pathway for growth factor receptors (see Chaps. 10, 19 and 24). However, signals that act through G protein-coupled re-

ceptors, particularly those coupled to G_i, can modulate growth factor activation of the MAP-kinase pathway. This is mediated via βγ subunits. Activation of the receptors leads to the generation of free βγ subunits, which then activate the MAP-kinase pathway at some early step in the cascade. Some possibilities include direct action of the βγ subunits on Ras (see below) or on one of several "linker" proteins between the growth factor receptor itself and activation of Ras.

The molecular specificity of various subtypes of β and γ subunit is an area of intense research [15]. The five forms of β are highly structurally similar, whereas the seven forms of γ are more divergent. Different forms of β and γ subunits interact with each other with widely varying abilities in *in vitro* expression systems. Identifying which forms of βγ subunit complexes occur *in vivo* and the specificity of these complexes for various target proteins, such as adenylyl cyclases, K^+ channels, GRKs and others, is just beginning.

The functioning of heterotrimeric G proteins is modulated by several other proteins

The function of one major class of modulator protein is to bind to G protein α subunits and to stimulate their intrinsic GTPase activity. These are termed *GTPase-activating proteins* (GAPs) (Fig. 20-3). GAPs had been known to exist for many years for small G proteins (see below), but only recently have analogous proteins been identified for heterotrimeric G proteins [16]. These GAPs, first identified in yeast but subsequently found in mammalian tissues, have been termed *regulators of G protein-signaling* (RGS) proteins. Activation of α subunit GTPase activity hastens the hydrolysis of GTP to GDP and more rapidly restores the inactive heterotrimer; thus, RGS proteins inhibit the biological activity of G proteins.

More than 18 forms of mammalian RGS protein are now known, and most are expressed in brain with highly region-specific patterns [16a]. It is thought that different families of G protein α subunits are likely to be modulated by different forms of RGS protein. Another possibility is that the various forms of RGS protein

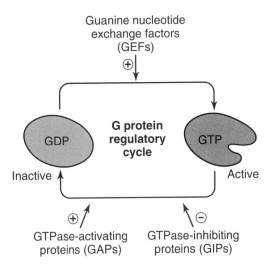

FIGURE 20-3. Schematic illustration of proteins that modulate the functioning of G proteins. The functional activity of G proteins is controlled by cycles of binding GDP versus GTP. This is associated with a major conformational change in the protein as depicted. There are several proteins that regulate this cycle and thereby regulate the functional activity of G proteins. Analogous modulator proteins exist for heterotrimeric G protein α subunits and for small G proteins. There are proteins that facilitate the release of GDP from the G protein and thereby enhance G protein function. Examples of such guanine nucleotide exchange factors *(GEFs)* are receptors for heterotrimeric G proteins or a large number of GEFs specific for various small G proteins. There are proteins, GTPase-activating proteins *(GAPs)*, that activate the GTPase activity intrinsic for the G proteins and thereby inhibit G protein function. Examples are the regulators of G protein-signaling (RGS) proteins for heterotrimeric G proteins and a series of GAPs specific for various small G proteins. There also may be GTPase-inhibitory proteins (GIPs) that exert the opposite effects. Heterotrimeric βγ subunits can be viewed as such; analogous proteins have been proposed for the small G proteins. Phosducin, by binding to βγ subunits, would represent yet another regulatory protein that modulates G protein function.

stimulate α subunit GTPase activity to different extents, which would allow for exquisite fine-tuning of G protein activity in a cell.

The function of RGS proteins in mammalian cells remains poorly understood. One exciting possibility, based on studies in yeast, is that alterations in the activity of specific RGS proteins, for example, via changes in their expression or phosphorylation, could modulate the activity of specific G proteins and, conse-

quently, the sensitivity of specific G protein-coupled receptors.

Phosducin is another protein that modulates G protein function [17,18]. Phosducin is a cytosolic protein enriched in retina and pineal gland but also expressed in brain and other tissues. Phosducin binds to G protein βγ subunits with high affinity. The result is prevention of βγ subunit reassociation with the α subunit. In this way, phosducin may sequester βγ subunits, which initially may prolong the biological activity of the α subunit. However, eventually this may inhibit G protein activity by preventing the direct biological effects of the βγ subunits as well as regeneration of the functional G protein heterotrimer. How phosducin functions in intact cells remains incompletely understood, although the ability of phosducin to bind to βγ subunits is altered upon its phosphorylation by cAMP- or Ca^{2+}-dependent protein kinases [17–19]. This raises the possibility that phosducin may be an important physiological modulator of G protein function.

G proteins are modified covalently by the addition of long-chain fatty acids

Addition of these lipid groups appears to modify the ability of the G proteins to interact with other proteins or with the plasma membrane. Several fatty acid modifications have been demonstrated: myristoyl groups, which consist of 14 carbon chains (C_{14}); farnesyl groups (C_{15}); palmitoyl groups (C_{16}); and geranylgeranyl, or isoprenyl, groups (C_{20}) [20]. Myristoyl groups are added via amide links to N-terminal glycine residues present in certain proteins. Farnesyl and isoprenyl groups are added to cysteine residues of specific C-terminal motifs. Palmitoyl groups also are added to cysteine groups within specific consensus amino acid sequences.

All G protein α subunits are modified in their N-terminal domains by palmitoylation or myristoylation [20–22]. These modifications may regulate the affinity of the α subunit for its βγ subunits and, thereby, the likelihood of dissociation or reassociation of the heterotrimer. The modifications also may help determine whether the α subunit, released upon ligand-receptor interaction, remains associated with the plasma membrane or diffuses into the cytoplasm. This could have important consequences on the types of effector proteins regulated. It is also possible that palmitoylation, but not myristoylation, is regulated dynamically. There is evidence that palmitoylation can be regulated by ligand binding, which makes this a potentially important control point. However, very little is known about palmitoyl transferases and de-palmitoylases, the enzymes responsible for palmitoylation. In contrast, myristoylation appears to be a one-time event in the life cycle of an α subunit.

G protein γ subunits are modified on their C-terminal cysteine residues by isoprenylation [20,23]. There is now strong evidence that this modification plays a key role in anchoring the γ subunit and its associated β subunit to the plasma membrane. The importance of this anchoring is illustrated in Figure 20-2, which shows that the ability of βγ-subunits to target GRKs to ligand-bound receptors depends on this membrane localization.

The functioning of G proteins may be influenced by phosphorylation

G proteins have been reported to undergo phosphorylation by cAMP- and Ca^{2+}-dependent protein kinases and by protein tyrosine kinases. However, the effect of phosphorylation on G protein function and its role in the regulation of physiological processes have been particularly difficult to establish with certainty. This remains an important area of future investigation.

SMALL G PROTEINS

In addition to the heterotrimeric G proteins, other forms of G proteins play important roles in cell function. These proteins belong to a large superfamily often referred to as "small G proteins" based on their low M_r (20,000 to 35,000) [24,25]. The small G proteins, like the heterotrimeric G proteins, bind guanine nucleotides, possess intrinsic GTPase activity and cycle through GDP- and GTP-bound forms (as shown in Fig. 20-1). One unifying feature of the various classes of G protein is that the binding of GTP versus GDP

dramatically alters the affinity of the protein for some target molecule, apparently by inducing a large conformational change. Small G proteins appear to function as molecular switches that control several cellular processes. Examples of small G proteins and their possible functional roles are given in Table 20-2.

The best characterized small G protein is the Ras family, a series of related proteins of ~21 kDa

Ras proteins were identified originally as the oncogene products of Harvey and Kirsten rat sarcoma viruses. Subsequently, normal cellular homologues, also known as proto-oncogenes, of viral Ras were identified. Mammalian Ras proteins are encoded by three homologous genes: the photo-oncogene for Harvey Ras virus (*H-ras*), the proto-oncogene for Kirsten Ras virus (*K-ras*) and neural Ras (*N-ras*), although all three forms of Ras are found in diverse mammalian tissues, including brain. In addition, all three forms of Ras are membrane-associated proteins [24,25].

The activity of Ras is highly regulated by a variety of associated proteins, as shown in Figure 20-3 [24–26]. Guanine nucleotide exchange factors (GEFs) stimulate the release of GDP from inactive Ras, which facilitates the binding of

TABLE 20-2. **EXAMPLES OF SMALL G PROTEINS**

Class[a]	Proposed cellular function
Ras	Signal transduction (control of growth factor and MAP-kinase pathways)
Rac, CDC42	Signal transduction (control of cellular stress responses and MAP-kinase pathways)
Rab	Localized to synaptic vesicles, where it regulates vesicle trafficking and exocytosis
Rho	Assembly of cytoskeletal structures (e.g., actin microfilaments)
ARF	ADP-ribosylation of $G_{\alpha s}$ Assembly and function of Golgi complex
EFTU	Associated with ribosomes, where it regulates protein synthesis
Ran	Nuclear-cytoplasmic trafficking of RNA and protein

[a] ARF, ADP-ribosylation factor; EFTU, eukaryotic elongation factor.

GTP. Thus, GEFs increase the activity of Ras. Multiple forms of GEFs have been identified, some specific for Ras and others for different small G proteins. In contrast, GAPs bind to Ras and activate its intrinsic GTPase activity, thereby reducing the functional activity of Ras. There also may be GTPase-inhibitory proteins (GIPs) that bind Ras and inhibit this GTPase activity, although these remain poorly described.

The analogy between Ras and its related proteins, on the one hand, and heterotrimeric G proteins and their related proteins, on the other, is striking (Fig. 20-3). G protein-coupled receptors essentially function as GEFs for the heterotrimeric G proteins, whereas RGS proteins and βγ subunits function as GTPase-activating and -inhibitory proteins. One major difference between the systems is that the intrinsic GTPase activity of Ras is far lower than that of heterotrimeric G protein α subunits. As a result, GAPs exert a much more profound effect on the functioning of Ras, essentially turning it on and off.

Upon binding GTP, there is a major conformational change in Ras, which is thought to be responsible for its functional activation. Ras has long been known to be a major control point for cell growth. Some of the cellular targets through which Ras produces its myriad effects have been identified. Numerous types of cell signal, including many and perhaps most growth factors, converge on Ras to regulate MAP-kinase pathways and, thereby, produce their diverse effects on cell function (see Chaps. 10 and 24) [24,25]. Briefly, it appears that activation of growth factor receptors results in the activation of a GEF, termed Sos, which in turn activates Ras. Activated Ras then binds to the N-terminal domain of a protein kinase called Raf, the first protein kinase in the MAP-kinase pathway. Ras appears to activate Raf via an indirect mechanism. Ras, which is membrane-bound, draws Raf to the plasma membrane, where it is activated through other means which are not yet completely understood. Anchoring of Ras in the plasma membrane may be mediated by isoprenylation, another point of analogy between Ras and heterotrimeric G proteins (Fig. 20-2). Ras exerts physiological effects via regulation of signaling pathways in addition to the MAP-ki-

nase cascade. Although the mechanisms involved are not as well characterized, Ras has been shown to bind and perhaps regulate phosphatidylinositol-3-kinase, another protein involved in mediating the actions of growth factors, as well as certain isoforms of protein kinase C (see Chap. 21).

Although the major mechanism governing Ras activation is through growth factors, as outlined above, Ras function can be modulated by heterotrimeric G protein and second-messenger pathways [24,25]. The ability of free βγ subunits, particularly those released from G_i, to activate Ras was mentioned earlier. In addition, the cAMP cascade inhibits Ras activity in several systems, although it is unknown whether this occurs via direct phosphorylation by cAMP-dependent protein kinase of Ras or a closely associated protein. The "cross-talk" among these various intracellular cascades emphasizes that the multitude of intracellular messengers do not operate independently of one another but rather are highly integrated to coordinate the response of a cell to a myriad of extracellular signals.

Rab is a family of small G proteins involved in membrane vesicle trafficking

Mammalian tissues contain around 30 forms of Rab, which specifically associate with the various types of membrane vesicles and organelles that exist in cells [27,28]. Rab proteins, named originally as ras-related proteins in brain, are isoprenylated, which directs their association with membranes, as seen with isoprenylation of Ras and G protein γ subunits. However, unlike these other G proteins, the GTP- and GDP-bound forms of Rab appear to regulate association with the membrane compartment.

Subtypes of Rab, particularly Rab3, have been implicated in the regulation of exocytosis and neurotransmitter release at nerve terminals [27–28a]. One possible scheme by which this occurs is shown in Figure 20-4. In its GTP-bound form, Rab is associated with synaptic vesicles, where it interacts with other membrane proteins to create a complex unfavorable for vesicle docking and perhaps fusion. Upon depolarization of the nerve terminal, a Rab GAP is activated, which results in dissociation of the GDP form of

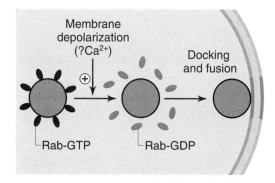

Membrane
depolarization
(?Ca^{2+})

Docking
and fusion

$\oplus$

Rab-GTP   Rab-GDP

FIGURE 20-4. Schematic illustration of the proposed role of Rab in neurotransmitter release. Under basal conditions, GTP is bound to Rab3, which allows Rab3 to associate with other proteins on synaptic vesicles. This creates conditions unfavorable for the docking and fusion of vesicles at the nerve terminal plasma membrane. Membrane depolarization results in hydrolysis of the GTP bound to Rab, possibly via a Ca^{2+}-induced activation of Rab-GTPase activity. Rab then dissociated from the vesicle, which creates a condition more favorable for docking and fusion. A large number of other synaptic vesicle proteins contribute to this process.

Rab from the vesicle membrane. This enables the synaptic vesicle to proceed with docking and fusion. The mechanism by which depolarization leads to activation of a Rab GAP and subsequently to release of Rab from the vesicle remains unknown, but Ca^{2+} is believed to be involved. To complicate matters further, several other proteins are involved in this Rab-synaptic vesicle cycle, including a Rab GDP dissociation inhibitor, which regulates the ability of Rab to bind to synaptic vesicles, and rabphilin, one of several synaptic vesicle proteins which can bind Rab (see Chap. 9).

OTHER FEATURES OF G PROTEINS

Some G proteins can be modified by ADP-ribosylation

Among the tools that facilitated the discovery and characterization of G proteins were the bacterial toxins cholera and pertussis, which were known to influence adenylyl cyclase activity. Subsequently, it was shown that the actions of these toxins are achieved by their ability to catalyze the addition of an ADP-ribose group do-

nated from nicotinamide adenine dinucleotide (NAD) to specific amino acid residues in certain heterotrimeric G protein α subunits [29].

Cholera toxin catalyzes the ADP-ribosylation of a specific arginine residue in G$_{\alpha s}$ and G$_{\alpha t}$ [29,30]. This covalent modification inhibits the intrinsic GTPase activity of these α subunits and thereby "freezes" them in their activated, or free, state (Fig. 20-1C). By this mechanism, cholera toxin stimulates adenylyl cyclase activity and photoreceptor transduction mechanisms. The ability of cholera toxin to ADP-ribosylate G$_{\alpha s}$ may require the presence of a distinct protein, ADP-ribosylation factor (ARF). ARF, which is itself a small G protein (Table 20-2), also is ADP-ribosylated by cholera toxin [30]. ARF has been implicated in controlling membrane vesicle trafficking, perhaps in part through interactions with heterotrimeric G proteins.

In contrast, pertussis toxin catalyzes the ADP-ribosylation of a specific cysteine residue in G$_{\alpha i}$, G$_{\alpha o}$ and G$_{\alpha t}$ [31]. Only α subunits bound to their $\beta\gamma$ subunits can undergo this modification. Pertussis toxin-mediated ADP-ribosylation inactivates these α subunits such that they cannot exchange GTP for GDP in response to receptor activation (Fig. 20-1B). By this mechanism, pertussis toxin blocks the ability of neurotransmitters to inhibit adenylyl cyclase or to influence the gating of K$^+$ and Ca^{2+} channels in target neurons. However, since G$_{\alpha z}$ is not a substrate for pertussis toxin, the toxin may not be able to block neurotransmitter-mediated inhibition of adenylyl cyclase in all cases. The G$_q$ and G$_{11-16}$ types of G-protein α subunit are not known to undergo ADP-ribosylation.

A third type of bacterial toxin, diphtheria toxin, catalyzes the ADP-ribosylation of eukaryotic elongation factor (EFTU), a type of small G protein involved in protein synthesis (Table 20-2) [32]. The functional activity of the elongation factor is inhibited by this reaction. Finally, a botulinum toxin ADP-ribosylates and disrupts the function of the small G protein Rho, which appears to be involved in assembly and rearrangement of the actin cytoskeleton (Table 20-2) [33]. These toxins may be involved in neuropathy (Chap. 36) and membrane trafficking (Chap. 9).

In the absence of bacterial toxins, brain and peripheral tissues contain endogenous ADP-ribosyltransferases, which catalyze the ADP-ribosylation of a relatively small number of cellular proteins [34,35]. Although most of the substrates for such endogenous ADP-ribosylation in brain remain unknown, evidence indicates that $G_{\alpha s}$, ARF and GAP-43 are among them. This has led to the suggestion that ADP-ribosylation may represent a mechanism by which G protein function is regulated *in vivo*. In addition, there is evidence that endogenous ADP-ribosylation of cellular proteins may be regulated by nitric oxide, which functions as a second messenger in the brain and peripheral tissues (see Chaps. 10 and 22).

G proteins may be involved in disease pathophysiology

G proteins are involved in the etiology of several disease states [36,37]. The best characterized examples are endocrinopathies caused by mutations in $G_{\alpha s}$. There are both gain of function and loss of function mutations. Examples of gain of function mutations, which result in increased or constitutive activity of $G_{\alpha s}$, include forms of acromegaly, which involves hypersecretion of growth hormone, and McCune-Albright syndrome, which involves hyperossification of bone, cafe-au-lait skin hyperpigmentation and mixed endocrine hyperfunction. Examples of loss of function mutations include Albright's hereditary osteodystrophy, characterized by abnormal bone formation, as well as forms of pseudohypoparathyroidism, a rare hereditary disease in which target tissues are resistant to the physiological actions of parathyroid hormone despite the existence of a normal number of functionally active hormone receptors. In addition, mutations in $G_{\alpha i}$ have been implicated in certain forms of ovarian and adrenal cortical tumors.

Neurofibromatosis type 1, a familial disorder characterized by multiple benign tumors of certain glial cells, is due to a mutation in the gene that codes for one form of GAP that regulates Ras [38]. The mutation in GAP that leads to neurofibromatosis renders GAP unable to activate GTPase activity of Ras. This means that the GTP-bound form of Ras remains active for abnormally long periods of time and leads, via some unknown mechanism, to abnormal cellular growth.

Of course, the critical importance of Ras and most other small G proteins in cell growth and differentiation is highlighted by the consideration, stated above, that several forms of these proteins are proto-oncogenes. This means that mutations in these proteins that result in alterations in their regulatory properties can lead to oncogenesis. Ras in particular has been implicated in several human cancers [36]. It has been estimated that as many as 30% of all human cancers contain mutations in one of the three Ras genes. While the frequency of Ras mutations in some types of human cancer is very low, others, such as squamous cell carcinoma, lymphatic cancers and colorectal adenocarcinoma, show a very high frequency.

G proteins may be regulated by psychotropic drugs

In addition to their involvement in specific disease states, concentrations of heterotrimeric G protein subunits are altered in specific regions of the central nervous system in response to chronic exposure to many types of psychoactive drug. This has been shown for antidepressant drugs; lithium, which is used in the treatment of mania and depression; and several drugs of abuse [39,40]. Evidence has been presented to suggest that drug-induced alterations in G protein subunit concentrations influence signal-transduction pathways in the brain and thereby contribute to the therapeutic or addictive actions of these drugs.

REFERENCES

1. Neer, E. J. Heterotrimeric G proteins: Organizers of transmembrane signals. *Cell* 80:249–257, 1995.
2. Wickman, K., and Clapham, D. E. Ion channel regulation by G proteins. *Physiol. Rev.* 75:865–885, 1995.
3. Hamm, H. E., and Gilchrist, A. Heterotrimeric G proteins. *Curr. Opin. Cell Biol.* 8:189–196, 1996.
4. Gilman, A. G. G proteins and regulation of adenylyl cyclase. *Biosci. Rep.* 15:65–97, 1995.
5. Fields, T. A., and Casey, P. J. Signalling functions and biochemical properties of pertussis toxin-resistant G proteins. *Biochem. J.* 321:561–571, 1997.

6. Onrust, R., Herzmark, P., Chi, P., et al. Receptor and $\beta\gamma$ binding sites in the α subunit of the retinal G protein transducin. *Science* 275:381–384, 1997.

7. Schneider, T., Igelmund, P., and Hescheler, J. G protein interaction with K^+ and Ca^{2+} channels. *Trends Pharmacol. Sci.* 18:8–11, 1997.

8. Huang, C.-L., Slesinger, P. A., Casey, P. J., Jan, Y. N., and Jan, L. Y. Evidence that direct binding of $G_{\beta\gamma}$ to the GIRK1 G protein-gated inwardly rectifying K^+ channel is important for channel activation. *Neuron* 15:1133–1143, 1995.

9. Herve, D., Levi-Strauss, M., Marey-Semper, I., et al. $G_{(olf)}$ and G_s in rat basal ganglia: Possible involvement of $G_{(olf)}$ in the coupling of dopamine D1 receptor with adenylyl cyclase. *J. Neurosci.* 13:2237–2248, 1993.

10. Sunahara, R. K., Dessauer, C. W., and Gilman, A. G. Complexity and diversity of mammalian adrenylyl cyclases. *Annu. Rev. Pharmacol. Toxicol.* 36:461–480, 1996.

11. Helms, J. B. Role of heterotrimeric GTP binding proteins in vesicular protein transport: Indications for both classical and alternative G protein cycles. *FEBS Lett.* 369:84–88, 1995.

12. Xie, R., Li, L., Goshima, Y., and Strittmater, S. M. An activated mutant of the α subunit of G_o increases neurite outgrowth via protein kinase C. *Dev. Brain Res.* 87:77–86, 1995.

13. Inglese, J., Koch, W. J., Touhara, K., and Lefkowitz, R. $G_{\beta\gamma}$ interactions with PH domains and Ras-MAPK signaling pathways. *Trends Biochem. Sci.* 20:151–155, 1995.

14. Lopez-Ilasaca, M., Crespo, P., Pellici, P., Gutkind, J., and Wetzker, R. Linkage of G protein-coupled receptors to the MAPK signaling pathway through PI 3-kinase. *Science* 275:394–397, 1997.

15. Yan, K., Kalyanaraman, V., and Gautam, N. Differential ability to form the G protein $\beta\gamma$ complex among members of the β and γ subunit families. *J. Biol. Chem.* 271:7141–7146, 1996.

16. Dohlman, H. G., and Thorner, J. RGS proteins and signaling by heterotrimeric G proteins. *J. Biol. Chem.* 272:3871–3874, 1997.

16a. Gold, S. J., Ni, Y. G., Dohlman, H., and Nestler, E. J. Regulators of G protein signaling: Region-specific expression of nine subtypes in brain. *J. Neurosci.* 17:8024–8037, 1997.

17. Xu, J., Wu, D., Slepak, V. Z., and Simon, M. The N terminus of phosducin is involved in binding of $\beta\gamma$ subunits of G protein. *Proc. Natl. Acad. Sci. USA* 92:2086–2090, 1995.

18. Schroder, S., and Lohse, M. J. Inhibition of G protein $\beta\gamma$-subunit functions by phosducin-like protein. *Proc. Natl. Acad. Sci. USA* 93:2100–2104, 1996.

19. Willardson, B. M., Wilkins, J., Yoshida, T., and Bitensky, M. Regulation of phosducin phosphorylation in retinal rods by Ca^{2+}/calmodulin-dependent adenylyl cyclase. *Proc. Natl. Acad. Sci. USA* 93:1475–1479, 1996.

20. Wedegaertner, P., Wilson, P., and Bourne, H. R. Lipid modifications of trimeric G proteins. *J. Biol. Chem.* 270:503–505, 1995.

21. Milligan, G., Parenti, M., and Magee, A. The dynamic role of palmitoylation in signal transduction. *Trends Biochem. Sci.* 20:181–185, 1995.

22. Ross, E. M. Palmitoylation in G protein signaling pathways. *Curr. Biol.* 5:107–109, 1995.

23. Rando, R. R. Chemical biology of protein isoprenylation/methylation. *Biochim. Biophys. Acta* 1330:5–16, 1996.

24. McCormick, F. Ras-related proteins in signal transduction and growth control. *Mol. Reprod. Dev.* 42:500–506, 1995.

25. Marshall, C. J. Ras effectors. *Curr. Opin. Cell Biol.* 8:197–204, 1996.

26. Overbeck, A., Brtva, T., Cox, A., et al. Guanine nucleotide exchange factors: Activators of ras superfamily proteins. *Mol. Reprod. Dev.* 42:468–476, 1995.

27. Liedo, P., Johannes, L., Vernie, P., et al. Ras proteins: Key players in the control of exocytosis. *Trends Neurosci.* 17:426–432, 1994.

28. Pfeffer, S. R., Dirac-Svejstrup, A. B., and Soldati, T. Rab GDP dissociation inhibitor: Putting rab GTPases in their place. *J. Biol. Chem.* 270:17057–17059, 1995.

28a. Sudhof, T. C. Function of Rab3 GDP–GTP exchange. *Neuron* 18:519–522, 1997.

29. Shall, S. ADP-ribosylation reactions. *Biochimie* 77:313–318, 1995.

30. Moss, J., Tsai, S., and Vaughan, M. Activation of cholera toxin by ADP-ribosylation factors. *Methods Enzymol.* 235:640–647, 1994.

31. Locht, C., and Antoine, R. A proposed mechanism of ADP-ribosylation catalyzed by the pertussis toxin S1 subunit. *Biochimie* 77:333–340, 1995.

32. Uchiumi, T., and Kominami, R. A functional site of the GTPase-associated center within 28S ribosomal RNA probed with an anti-RNA autoantibody. *EMBO J.* 13:3389–3394, 1994.

33. Nobes, C. D., and Hall, A. Rho, rac and cdc42 GTPases: Regulators of actin structures, cell adhesion and motility. *Biochem. Soc. Trans.* 23:456–459, 1995.

34. Philibert, K., and Zwiers, H. Evidence for multisite ADP-ribosylation of neuronal phosphoprotein B-50/GAP-43. *Mol. Cell. Biochem.* 149:183–190, 1995.

35. Duman, R. S., Terwilliger, R. Z., and Nestler, E. J. Alterations in nitric oxide-stimulated endogenous ADP-ribosylation associated with long-term potentiation in rat hippocampus. *J. Neurochem.* 61:1542–1545, 1993.

36. Schnabel, P., and Bohm, M. Mutations of signal-transducing G proteins in human disease. *J. Mol. Med.* 73:221–228, 1995.

37. Spiegel, A. M. Genetic basis of endocrine disease. Mutations in G proteins and G protein-coupled receptors in endocrine disease. *J. Clin. Endocrinol. Metab.* 81:2434–2442, 1996.

38. Bernards, A. Neurofibromatosis type I and Ras-mediated signaling: Filling in the GAPs. *Biochim. Biophys. Acta* 1242:43–59, 1995.

39. Milligan, G. Agonist regulation of cellular G protein levels and distribution: Mechanisms and functional implications. *Trends Pharmacol. Sci.* 14:413–418, 1993.

40. Nestler, E. J., and Duman, R. S. Intracellular messenger pathways as mediators of neural plasticity. In: F. E. Bloom and D. J. Kupfer (eds.), *Psychopharmacology: Fourth Generation of Progress.* New York: Raven Press, 1994, pp. 695–704.

41. Hyman, S. E., and Nestler, E. J. Initiation and adaptation: A paradigm to understand psychotropic drug action. *Am. J. Psychiatry* 153:151–162, 1996.

C H A P T E R

21

Phosphoinositides

Stephen K. Fisher and Bernard W. Agranoff

Basic Neurochemistry: Molecular, Cellular and Medical Aspects, 6th Ed., edited by G. J. Siegel et al. Published by Lippincott–Raven Publishers, Philadelphia, 1999. Correspondence to Bernard W. Agranoff, Mental Health Research Institute, Departments of Biological Chemistry and Psychiatry, University of Michigan, 1103 E. Huron, Ann Arbor, Michigan 48104-1687.

BACKGROUND

A large variety of ligands, including neurotransmitters, neuromodulators and hormones, exert their physiological action via an intracellular second-messenger system in which the activated receptor–ligand complex stimulates the turnover of inositol-containing phospholipids. In this chapter, the biochemical and cellular bases of this ubiquitous pathway, as well as its pharmacological significance, are examined in the context of the nervous system. The brief review of the sequence of discoveries that have led to our current view is intended to provide an understanding of the technological and conceptual advances that have made progress possible.

Stimulation of secretion is accompanied by incorporation of inorganic phosphate into phospholipids, revealing a cycle of glycerolipid breakdown and reutilization

In 1953, Hokin and Hokin [1] reported that slices of pancreas incubated with radioactive inorganic phosphate ($^{32}P_i$) exhibited increased phospholipid labeling upon addition of muscarinic agents, such as carbamoylcholine (carbachol), which stimulates amylase secretion. Both lipid labeling and the secretion of amylase were blocked by atropine, a muscarinic receptor antagonist. They had thus discovered a biochemical "handle" with which to begin to investigate the details of receptor action. The observed labeling was confined to two phospholipids, phosphatidate (PA) and phosphatidylinositol (PI).* This demonstration of receptor-stimulated lipid labeling was extended to a number of other ligands, each in the presence of an appropriate tissue. Stimulated lipid labeling in brain homogenates was found to be mediated by a nerve-ending fraction. It later was shown that ligand-stimulated breakdown of phosphoinositides occurred in membrane prepa-

rations if they had been supplemented with guanine nucleotides.

The metabolic relationship between PA and PI lies in the liponucleotide intermediate cytidine diphosphate diacylglycerol (CDP·DAG), which is formed from cytidine triphosphate (CTP) and PA and is the biosynthetic precursor of PI (see Chap. 3); however, under conditions of ligand-stimulated labeling of PA and PI, there is no enhancement of incorporation of labeled glycerol into either of these lipids, indicating that the observed stimulated incorporation of $^{32}P_i$ into PA and PI involves a cycle in which there is degradation and reutilization of the glycerolipid backbone. The initiating step is the breakdown of a phosphorylated derivative of PI, phosphatidylinositol 4,5-bisphosphate [PI(4,5)P$_2$], as discussed below. One reason why the involvement of the polyphosphoinositides was not immediately evident is that they are not easily extracted into lipid solvents under neutral conditions. Acidified lipid extraction solvents, such as chloroform-methanol-HCl, ensure complete extraction of all of the inositol lipids, and thin-layer chromatographic (TLC) systems incorporating oxalate salts in the silica gel matrix have facilitated their separation [2].

Elevation of intracellular Ca^{2+} had been observed in ligand-activated cells in which phospholipid labeling was stimulated [3], but it was unclear whether the elevated intracellular Ca^{2+} was the cause or the result of the stimulated labeling of lipids. This was clarified in 1983 by the demonstration that inositol trisphosphate [I(1,4,5)P$_3$], a cleavage product of PI(4,5)P$_2$, serves as a mediator of intracellular Ca^{2+} release [4]. Thus, lipid breakdown precedes Ca^{2+} release. To better understand the events leading to PI(4,5)P$_2$ breakdown and its resynthesis, it is useful to review the underlying structural chemistry.

CHEMISTRY OF THE INOSITOL LIPIDS AND PHOSPHATES

The three quantitatively major phosphoinositides are structurally and metabolically related

The quantitatively major phosphoinositides consist of PI and the two polyphosphoinositides,

---

*The "Chilton Conference" nomenclature for inositol lipids is used throughout this chapter, for example, PI, PI4P and PI(4,5)P$_2$ for phosphatidylinositol, phosphatidylinositol 4-phosphate and phosphatidylinositol 4,5-bisphosphate, respectively. Note that the IUB recommended nomenclature for these lipids is PtdIns, PtdIns4P and PtdIns(4,5)P$_2$ (see Chap. 3).

phosphatidylinositol 4-phosphate (PI4P) and PI(4,5)P$_2$ (Fig. 21-1A). (See Box 21-1 for discussion of the 3-phosphoinositides.) PI consists of a DAG moiety which is phosphodiesterified to *myo*-inositol, a six-carbon polycyclic alcohol (Fig. 21-1A). *myo*-Inositol, one of nine possible isomers of hexahydroxycyclohexane, has one axial and five equatorial hydroxyls and is by far the most prevalent isomer in nature. Its distinctive configuration can be easily understood by regarding its cyclohexane chair configuration as a turtle in which the axial hydroxyl is the head, while hydroxyls in the five equatorial positions serve as the four limbs and tail (Fig. 21-1A). DAG is affixed to the D-1 hydroxyl, the turtle's right front leg, via a phosphodiester linkage with the *sn*-3 position of glycerol. Using the D (for dextro isomer) numbering convention and looking down at the turtle from above and proceeding counterclockwise, the head is at position D-2, while the left front leg is at D-3, and so on. At present, there are no known brain phosphoinositides containing cyclitols other than *myo*-inositol, nor are there as yet examples of inositol lipids in which the inositol is diesterified to DAG at a position other than D-1.

There exists an unusual uniformity in the fatty acid composition of the inositol lipids of the PI4P series. All three of the major phosphoinositides are enriched in the 1-stearoyl, 2-arachidonoyl ("ST/AR") *sn*-glycerol species (~80% in brain). The polyphosphoinositides PI4P and PI(4,5)P$_2$ are present in much lower amounts than PI and are believed to be localized predominantly, if not exclusively, to the inner leaflet of plasma membranes. The brain is the best known source of the polyphosphoinositides. The total amounts of the three phosphoinositides in brains that had been extracted following focused microwave treatment, to minimize postmortem degradation, were estimated to be 78, 4 and 14 nmol/mg of neostriatal protein for PI, PI4P and PI(4,5)P$_2$, respectively (Van Dongen et al., cited in [2]). Although postmortem breakdown is rapid, a considerable fraction of brain phosphoinositide appears to be in a slowly degraded pool.

The phosphoinositides differ from other phospholipids, such as phosphatidylethanolamine, phosphatidylcholine and phosphatidylserine, in that they contain no nitrogen. They share this property with the phosphatidylglycerol series, which is also formed from the precursor CDP·DAG (see Chap. 3).

PI is phosphorylated to PI4P in a reaction requiring ATP and catalyzed by PI 4-kinase (PI4K) activity. Cloning studies have revealed the presence of three distinct isoforms of PI4K, of 97, 110 and 230 kDa [5–7]. The 97-kDa enzyme is inhibited by adenosine and by the monoclonal antibody 4C5G. In contrast, neither the 110- nor the 230-kDa isoform is markedly inhibited by these agents, but, in contrast to the 97-kDa isozyme, both are sensitive to the fungal metabolite wortmannin. The ability of wortmannin to block the sustained agonist-induced turnover of inositol lipids has led to the suggestion that wortmannin-inhibitable isoforms of PI4K are involved in the regulation of hormone-sensitive pools of phosphoinositides [8]. PI4P is further phosphorylated via PI4P 5-kinase to PI(4,5)P$_2$ (Fig. 21-1B). This enzyme is found in both brain membranes and cytosol and does not phosphorylate PI. At least three isoforms of PIP 5-kinase have been described, types Iα and Iβ of ~68 kDa, and type II, of ~46 kDa [9,10]. There are indications that there is also a PI 5-kinase (PI5K), further adding to the complexity of phosphoinositide metabolism. PI5P can be phosphorylated to PI(4,5)P$_2$ by the type II PIP kinase, the latter acting as a PI5P 4-kinase [11].

Phosphoinositides are cleaved by a family of phosphoinositide-specific phospholipase C isozymes

At least three isoforms, β, γ and δ, of phosphoinositide-specific phospholipase C (PI-PLC) are found in the brain, of approximately 130 to 155, 145 and 85 kDa, respectively (Fig. 21-2). Each is an immunologically distinct entity and the product of a separate gene [12,13]. These have been extensively purified, the cDNA sequences elucidated and antibodies raised to the recombinant proteins. A number of isozymes of each subtype of PI-PLC have been identified, nine in all, identified as β$_1$-β$_4$, γ$_1$-γ$_3$, δ$_1$ and δ$_2$. Isozymes of PI-PLC require the presence of Ca^{2+} for full activation and will hydrolyze the inositol lipids with a selectivity for PI(4,5)P$_2$ over PI, decreasing in the or-

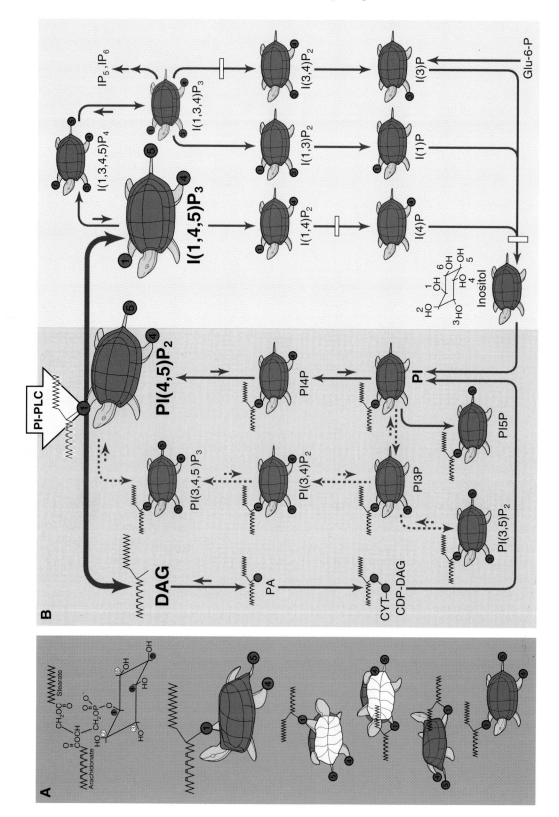

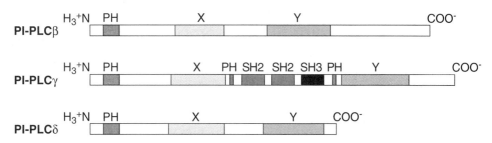

FIGURE 21-2.   Linear representation of the β, γ and δ isoforms of phosphoinositide specific-phospholipase C (PI-PLC). All isoforms contain X and Y domains which are linked to the catalytic activity of the enzyme. The SH2 and SH3 domains are involved in protein–protein interactions. PH, pleckstrin homology domain.

der PI-PLCβ > PI-PLCδ > PI-PLCγ. Despite the similarity of function, only two regions of amino acid homology exist, X and Y, of 150 and 120 amino acid residues, respectively, which are 54 and 42% identical among the isozymes but are differentially localized within each enzyme (Fig. 21-2). A characteristic of the β and δ isoforms is that relatively few, 50 to 70, amino acids separate the X and Y entities, whereas a much larger separation is observed for the γ isoform. In addition, in PI-PLCγ, the region between X and Y contains amino acid sequences that are found in nonreceptor tyrosine kinases, such as src homology 2 and 3 domains (SH2 and SH3), GTPase-activity protein and α-spectrin. All three isoforms possess pleck-strin homology (PH) domains. The latter are considered to enable the enzyme to become tethered to the plasma membrane via an interaction of the PH domain with PI(4,5)P$_2$. The β and δ forms of PI-PLC can be distinguished by the virtual absence of a carboxy-terminal consensus sequence of 400 to 500 amino acids in PI-PLCδ, which is present in PI-PLCβ. Consistent with the absence of putative transmembrane-spanning domains, most PI-PLC activity is localized to the cytoplasm, although a significant amount is associated with membrane fractions.

Three distinct mechanisms of signal transduction are involved in the activation of PI-PLC [14]. As shown in Figure 21-3 (mechanism I), ag-

FIGURE 21-1.   A: Stereochemistry of the inositol lipids. Inositol lipids characteristically contain stearic acid (18:0) and arachidonic acid (20:4 ω6) esterified to the 1 and 2 positions of *sn*-glycerolphosphate, respectively. The phosphate *(red circle)* is diesterified to the 1 position of D-*myo*-inositol. *myo*-Inositol in its favored chair conformation has five equatorial hydroxyls and one axial hydroxyl. Looking at the chair from above and counting counterclockwise, the axial hydroxyl is then in position 2. As indicated by the drawing, the inositol molecule can be conveniently viewed as a turtle in which the diacylglycerol phosphate moiety is attached to the right front leg (position 1), next to the raised head (the axial hydroxyl in position 2). The other equatorial hydroxyls are represented by the remaining limbs and the tail. Phosphatidylinositol *(PI)* can be phosphorylated at position 4 or the rear left leg, as well as at position 5, the tail, to yield phosphatidylinositol 4-phosphate [PI(4)P] and phosphatidylinositol 4,5-bisphosphate [PI(4,5)P$_2$], respectively. Once these relationships are understood, inositol phosphates can be seen from many vantage points without losing sight of their steric configurations, as indicated by the four views of PI(4,5)P$_2$ in the lower portion of the drawing. **B:** Pathways of phosphoinositide degradation and resynthesis. Note that inositol lipids are depicted in the membrane (light gray area), while water-soluble inositol phosphates are depicted in the cytosol (light orange area). Receptor-mediated breakdown *(yellow arrow)* of PI(4,5)P$_2$ via phosphoinositide-specific phospholipase C *(PI-PLC)* leads to the formation of diacylglycerol *(DAG)* and I(1,4,5)P$_3$. The latter is metabolized via either 5-phosphatase or 3-kinase pathways to yield I(1,4)P$_2$ and I(1,3,4,5)P$_4$, respectively. Successive dephosphorylations of these two inositol phosphates result in the formation of I(4)P, I(1)P and I(3)P. I(3)P may also be synthesized from glucose 6-phosphate *(Glu-6-P)*. Inositol monophosphates are then cleaved by monophosphatase to regenerate inositol. Li$^+$ is known to block the dephosphorylation reactions indicated by *yellow bars*. DAG, when released, is metabolized in the plasma membrane to form phosphatidic acid *(PA)* via the action of DAG kinase. PA is subsequently converted to CDP·DAG and, in the presence of inositol, to PI. PI(4,5)P$_2$ is then regenerated by the action of specific kinases on PI and PI(4)P. *Dashed lines* indicate the known reactions in the PI3-kinase pathway (see Box 21-1). In each instance, *short arrows*, in the phospholipid cycle, depict action of a phosphatase. Not shown, possible action of PIP kinase on PI5P to yield PI(4,5)P$_2$. (Reproduced From *Annual Report,* University of Michigan Mental Health Research Institute, 1998 with permission.)

Box 21-1

3-PHOSPHOINOSITIDES

Recent studies have indicated the presence of small amounts of additional inositol lipids that are characterized by the presence of a phosphate group at the D-3 position of the inositol ring, that is, the 3-phosphoinositides. These lipids, principally, PI3P, PI(3,4)P_2 and PI(3,4,5)P_3, are present in both neural and non-neural tissues at concentrations well below those found for either PI4P or PI(4,5)P_2. The structures and metabolic relationships of the 3-phosphoinositides and the quantitatively major inositol lipids are shown in Figure 21-1B. The key enzyme involved in the synthesis of the 3-phosphoinositides is PI 3-kinase (PI3K). Three major classes of PI3K have been described, based on lipid substrate specificity and regulation [1–3]. Class I PI3Ks are able to phosphorylate PI, PI4P and PI(4,5)P_2 to form PI3P, PI(3,4)P_2 and PI(3,4,5)P_3, respectively. The catalytic subunits of this class of PI3K form heterodimeric complexes with adaptor or regulatory proteins that link the enzyme to upstream signaling events. Class I PI3K catalytic subunits can be further subdivided. Type I A catalytic subunits (110 to 130 kDa) interact with PI3K-regulatory proteins (p85) that contain an SH2 domain. The presence of the latter enables the enzyme to more readily associate with phosphorylated tyrosine residues on upstream proteins, thereby linking PI3K to tyrosine kinase-signaling pathways. Type I B catalytic subunits of 110 kDa are stimulated by βγ subunits derived from G proteins. A regulatory protein, p101, that associates tightly with the catalytic subunit has recently been isolated. Both types A and B catalytic subunits of class I PI3K interact with a small-molecular-weight G protein, Ras (see Chap. 20). Class II and class III PI3Ks have a more restricted substrate specificity: class II enzymes are able to phosphorylate PI and PI4P but not PI(4,5)P_2, whereas class III enzymes phosphorylate only PI. Unlike the PI3K-Is, neither PI3K-IIs nor PI3K-IIIs appear to be regulated by extracellular stimuli. Degradation of PI(3,4,5)P_3 and PI(3,4)P_2 is accomplished via phosphatase action at either the 5- or the 4-position to yield PI(3,4)P_2 or PI3P, respectively. It is likely that the latter lipids are dephosphorylated by a 3-phosphatase to yield PI4P and PI. In contrast to their more highly expressed counterparts, the 3-phosphoinositides do not serve as substrates for PI-PLC, the enzyme known to be activated in stimulated phosphoinositide turnover. This observation indicates that the 3-phosphoinositides themselves, rather than their breakdown products, are likely to be the intracellular mediators of biological activity. Although the concentration of PI3P is relatively constant, that of both PI(3,4)P_2 and PI(3,4,5)P_3 can increase dramatically upon receptor activation, a result which suggests that these lipids may play a significant role in cell function [4]. PI(3,4)P_2 and PI(3,4,5)P_3 can bind to specific domains within proteins; both bind to proteins which possess a PH domain, while PI(3,4,5)P_3 can bind and recruit proteins which contain an SH2 domain. Although not yet well defined, roles for 3-phosphoinositides in the regulation of membrane trafficking, PKC activity, cell survival and maintenance of the cytoskeleton have been proposed (see Box 21-2).

—*Stephen K. Fisher and Bernard W. Agranoff*

REFERENCES

1. Kapeller, R., and Cantley, L. C. Phosphatidylinositol 3-kinase. *BioEssays* 16:565–576, 1994.
2. Vanhaesebroeck, B., Leevers, S. J., Panayotou, G., and Waterfield, M. D. Phosphoinositide 3-kinases: A conserved family of signal transducers. *Trends Biochem. Sci.* 22:267–272, 1997.
3. Toker, A., and Cantley, L. C. Signalling through the lipid products of phosphoinositide-3-OH kinase. *Nature* 387:673–676, 1997.
4. Stephens, L. R., Jackson, T. R., and Hawkins, P. T. Agonist-stimulated synthesis of phosphatidylinositol (3,4,5)-trisphosphate: A new intracellular signalling system. *Biochem. Biophys. Acta* 1179:27–75, 1993.

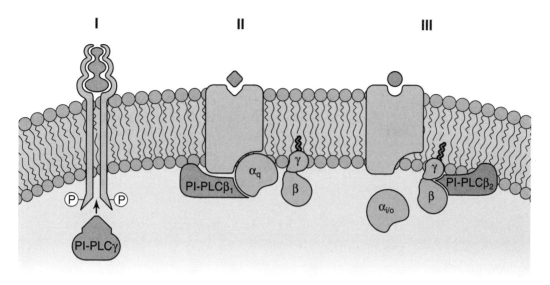

FIGURE 21-3.   Three distinct mechanisms for the activation of phosphoinositide-specific phospholipase C (PI-PLC). In mechanism **I,** the ligand activates a receptor which possesses an intrinsic tyrosine kinase. Following dimerization of the receptor, it becomes autophosphorylated on tyrosine residues present in the cytoplasmic domain of the receptor. PI-PLCγ is then recruited to the plasma membrane via interaction of its SH2 domains with the phosphorylated tyrosine residues on the receptor and activated by phosphorylation. In mechanism **II,** the ligand–receptor interaction results in the dissociation of a pertussis toxin-insensitive G protein (G_q), to liberate α_q. The latter then activates either PI-PLCβ$_1$ or PI-PLCβ$_3$. In mechanism **III,** the ligand–receptor interaction results in the dissociation of a pertussis toxin-sensitive G protein, for example, G_i or G_o, which in turn liberates α_i/α_o and βγ subunits. The latter can then activate either PI-PLCβ$_2$ or PI-PLCβ$_3$. Note that although βγ subunits derived from G_q could also theoretically activate this pathway, this possibility is less likely, given the abundance of G_i or G_o relative to G_q.

onist occupancy of receptors which possess intrinsic tyrosine kinase activity, for example, occupancy of the receptor by platelet-derived growth factor, can result in receptor dimerization and autophosphorylation of the cytoplasmic tails on tyrosine residues. The presence of these phosphorylated tyrosine residues serves to "recruit" proteins, such as PI-PLCγ, which possesses an SH2 domain. In doing so, the cytosolic effector enzyme PI-PLCγ is brought into close proximity to the plasma membrane, the site of its substrate PI(4,5)P$_2$ and of its activation by phosphorylation. Other receptors activate PI-PLC via intervening G proteins (see Chap. 20). Alternatively, the interaction of a ligand with a receptor, for example, a muscarinic cholinergic receptor, results in the activation and dissociation of G_q, a pertussis toxin-insensitive G protein, to liberate α_q (Fig. 21-3, mechanism II). The latter then may activate PI-PLCβ$_1$ and/or PI-PLCβ$_3$. In a third mechanism (Fig. 21-3, mechanism III) the ligand–receptor interaction results in the activation and dissociation

of a pertussis toxin-sensitive G protein, G_i or G_o, which in turn liberates α_i or α_o and βγ subunits. In this case, it is the βγ subunits, but not the α subunit, that can then activate PI-PLCβ$_3$ or, in the case of hematopoietic cells, PI-PLCβ$_2$. Different regions of the PI-PLC molecule appear to be required for α_q or βγ activation. Thus, whereas cleavage of the carboxyl terminal portion of PI-PLCβ$_1$ renders it refractory to α_q regulation, the amino terminal region of the molecule is required for βγ activation.

Cleavage of phosphatidylinositol 4,5-bisphosphate initiates two interlinked cycles: one in which the diacylglycerol backbone is conserved and recycled and another in which inositol is reutilized

As indicated above, it can be inferred that a lipid cycle operates in which existing DAG is conserved. The free DAG is phosphorylated to PA by the enzyme DAG kinase, for which multiple forms, α, β, γ, δ, ε, η, ζ and θ of 64 to 140 kDa, have been identified and characterized. All possess a C-terminal catalytic domain and two or three cysteine-rich repeat sequences [15]. The α, β and γ forms possess EF-hands and, thus, are likely to be regulated by changes in the concentration of cytosolic Ca^{2+}. Expression of the mRNA for the α, β, γ, ζ and θ forms of DAG kinase appears to be highest in brain. DAG kinase converts the DAG released on phosphoinositide cleavage to PA, which can then be converted to PI via CDP·DAG (Fig. 21-1B) (Chap. 3). The synthesis of CDP·DAG is catalyzed by a 51-kDa membrane-bound protein localized to both mitochondria and the endoplasmic reticulum. PI synthase, the enzyme that catalyzes the formation of PI from CDP·DAG and *myo*-inositol, is membrane-associated and primarily localized to the endoplasmic reticulum and Golgi. It is an extremely hydrophobic protein of 24 kDa consisting of 60% hydrophobic, 20% hydrophilic and 20% neutral amino acids [16]. Although these enzymatic steps are seen in the *de novo* biosynthesis of inositol lipids, it is likely that net synthesis and stimulated lipid turnover occur in separate and distinct metabolic compartments: the receptor-stimulated cycle is likely to be confined to the plasma membrane, whereas the various steps in the *de novo* pathway occur in the mitochondrial and/or endoplasmic reticular fractions. The coreleased inositol mono-, bis- and trisphosphates are eventually cleaved by phosphatases to regenerate free inositol, which may then combine with CDP·DAG to form PI via PI synthase. Sequential phosphorylation of PI to $PI(4,5)P_2$ via PI4P closes both loops of this double cycle, as depicted in Figure 21-1B.

THE INOSITOL PHOSPHATES

D-*myo*-Inositol 1,4,5-trisphosphate is a second messenger that liberates Ca^{2+} from the endoplasmic reticulum via intracellular receptors

Of the three inositol phosphates, $I(1)P$, $I(1,4)P_2$ and $I(1,4,5)P_3$, that potentially can be formed upon PI-PLC–activated cleavage of the phosphoinositides, $I(1,4,5)P_3$ is unique in its ability to mobilize Ca^{2+}. This observation is one of the key arguments in support of the hypothesis that $PI(4,5)P_2$ breakdown, rather than that of PI4P or PI, initiates the cellular responses to receptor activation. When directly injected into cells or added to permeabilized cells or membrane fractions, $I(1,4,5)P_3$ elicits increased release of Ca^{2+} from a store that has been associated with the endoplasmic reticulum. That specific receptor sites mediate the action of $I(1,4,5)P_3$ was first inferred from the presence of binding sites in membrane fractions obtained from selected brain regions, notably the cerebellum, the brain region most enriched in these receptors. The purified receptor is a glycoprotein of 260 kDa on sodium dodecyl sulfate-polyacrylamide gel electrophoresis (SDS-PAGE) and is highly selective for $I(1,4,5)P_3$. The $I(1,4,5)P_3$ receptor consists of three distinct regions (Fig. 21-4A): (i) a ligand-binding domain, located at the amino terminal region of the molecule; (ii) a regulatory domain, which contains potential phosphorylation sites for protein kinase A and protein kinase C, as well as two ATP-binding sites, which regulate the affinity with which $I(1,4,5)P_3$ binds to the receptor; and (iii) a six-transmembrane spanning channel domain [17]. The native $I(1,4,5)P_3$ receptor exists as a homotetramer with both amino- and carboxyl-termini facing the cytoplasm. Upon binding of an $I(1,4,5)P_3$ molecule to each of the four subunits, a conformational change in the receptor is presumed to occur which results in opening of the intrinsic Ca^{2+} channel (Fig. 21-4B). At least three distinct forms of the $I(1,4,5)P_3$ receptor are known. Type I predominates in the cerebellum and has been most extensively studied. It is the largest of the three forms of the receptor and, unlike types II and III receptors, the gene possesses a 120-nucleotide insert. Type II $I(1,4,5)P_3$ receptors are found mainly in non-neural tissues, whereas type III receptors occur in both neural and non-neural tissues. Activation of phosphoinositide-linked receptors frequently results in oscillations of the intracellular Ca^{2+} signal. The relationship between $I(1,4,5)P_3$ production and signal oscillations is discussed in Chapter 23.

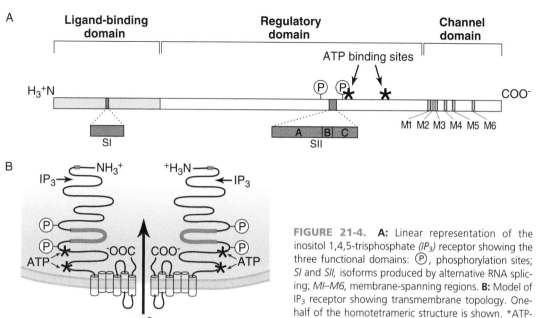

FIGURE 21-4. **A:** Linear representation of the inositol 1,4,5-trisphosphate *(IP₃)* receptor showing the three functional domains: Ⓟ, phosphorylation sites; *SI* and *SII*, isoforms produced by alternative RNA splicing; *MI–M6*, membrane-spanning regions. **B:** Model of IP₃ receptor showing transmembrane topology. One-half of the homotetrameric structure is shown. *ATP-binding sites. (From [17], with permission.)

The metabolism of inositol phosphates leads to regeneration of free inositol

$I(1,4,5)P_3$ can be metabolized either by a 5-phosphatase, a membrane-bound enzyme, to yield inositol 1,4-bisphosphate $[I(1,4)P_2]$ or by a cytosolic 3-kinase to form inositol 1,3,4,5-tetrakisphosphate $[I(1,3,4,5)P_4]$ (Fig. 21-3). Both of these activities may be regarded as "off signals," terminating the action of $I(1,4,5)P_3$. The $I(1,4)P_2$ that results from 5-phosphatase action is dephosphorylated further by an inositol bisphosphatase to inositol 4-monophosphate $[I(4)P]$ and then by the action of inositol monophosphatase to free inositol. $I(1,3,4,5)P_4$, which itself has been suggested to possess a second-messenger function in facilitating the entry of Ca^{2+} into cells, also serves as a substrate for the same 5-phosphatase that acts on $I(1,4,5)P_3$, with the resultant formation, in this instance, of inositol 1,3,4-trisphosphate $[I(1,3,4)P_3]$. Unlike the 1,4,5-trisphosphate isomer, $I(1,3,4)P_3$ is ineffective at mobilizing intracellular Ca^{2+}. $I(1,3,4)P_3$ can be further metabolized to inositol 1,3-bisphosphate $[I(1,3)P_2]$ or inositol 3,4-bisphosphate $[I(3,4)P_2]$ (Fig. 21-1B). These compounds are then dephosphorylated by 3- or 4-phosphatases to yield inositol 1- or 3-monophosphates, respectively.

The inositol polyphosphate 5-phosphatases belong to a family of enzymes that terminate the signals generated by inositol lipid kinases and PI-PLC [18,19]. To date, three types of 5-phosphatase have been identified, all of which share a common "5-phosphatase" domain of approximately 300 amino acids, with several highly conserved motifs. Type I enzymes are 43 to 65 kDa and preferentially hydrolyze $I(1,4,5)P_3$ and $I(1,3,4,5)P_4$, with the attendant formation of $I(1,4)P_2$ and $I(1,3,4)P_3$, but have little or no activity toward membrane-bound phosphoinositides. The prototypic form of a type I 5-phosphatase is a 43-kDa protein that is post-translationally modified by farnesylation of the carboxyl terminus CAAX motif; this modification juxtaposes the enzyme with the membrane. Type II enzymes are larger, 75 to 160 kDa, and will hydrolyze both water-soluble inositol phosphates and lipids that possess a phosphate group at the 5-position of the inositol ring. Three type II 5-phosphatases have been identified. One is a 75-kDa protein, localized to both cytosol and membrane. A second enzyme is most similar to a protein deficient in Lowe's oculocerebrorenal

Box 21-2

PHOSPHOINOSITIDES AND CELL REGULATION

A major focus of studies of the phosphoinositides has centered on the role played by these lipids in transmembrane signaling events, in particular the generation of second messengers linked to Ca^{2+} homeostasis and protein phosphorylation. It is becoming increasingly evident that inositol lipids are also important mediators of other cell functions. One of these is the anchoring of certain cell-surface proteins via a PI-glycan linkage (see Box 3-1). Other putative functions for phosphoinositides include roles in membrane trafficking, maintenance of the cytoskeleton, regulation of PKC activity and cell survival.

Membrane trafficking. There is now ample evidence to implicate both the 3-phosphoinositides and the quantitatively major inositol lipids in membrane-trafficking events within cells. Through its interaction with adaptor protein-2 (AP2), PI3P has been suggested to play a role in the assembly of clathrin-coated pits at the plasma membrane (see Chap. 2). This interaction is noteworthy in that AP2 is the only known protein thus far shown to selectively interact with PI3P, $PI(3,4)P_2$ and $PI(3,4,5)P_3$ being much less effective in this regard [1]. The 3-phosphoinositides also appear to play a role in late endocytic events since inhibition of PI3K with wortmannin prevents the postendosomal sorting of platelet-derived growth factor receptor (PDGF-R). Moreover, mutations of

the PDGF-R that prevent its association with PI3K result in receptors that fail to undergo trafficking from the Golgi to lysosomes. A direct role for the quantitatively major polyphosphoinositides, that is, PI4P and $PI(4,5)P_2$, was first identified by Eberhard et al. [2], who observed that the ATP requirement for Ca^{2+}-regulated exocytosis in chromaffin cells could be attributed to the generation of $PI(4,5)P_2$. Subsequently, three cytosolic proteins, termed *priming of exocytosis proteins* (PEPs), were demonstrated to be prerequisites for exocytosis. PEP1 and PEP3 were identified as PI4P 5-kinase and the PI-transfer protein, respectively, while PEP2 may represent PI4K. Thus, for catecholamine exocytosis to occur, a series of reactions culminating in the synthesis of PI4P and $PI(4,5)P_2$ is required [3]. The need for inositol lipids in membrane-trafficking events could reflect the propensity of these lipids to alter membrane curvature and/or their ability to recruit other proteins necessary for membrane-fusion events. An example of the latter is the finding that $PI(4,5)P_2$ and $PI(3,4,5)P_3$ bind to a synaptic vesicle membrane protein, synaptotagmin (see Chap. 9).

Maintenance of the cytoskeleton. $PI(3,4)P_2$, $PI(3,4,5)P_3$, PI4P and $PI(4,5)P_2$ avidly bind to a group of *capping* proteins that regulate proteins involved in actin assembly, for example, gelsolin and profilin. Upon the binding of

syndrome (OCRL), a human X-chromosome-linked developmental disorder that affects the CNS, kidney and lens. In Lowe's syndrome, $PI(4,5)P_2$ 5-phosphatase activity is most decreased in the Golgi fraction, which has led to the speculation that abnormal $PI(4,5)P_2$ concentrations may lead to altered protein trafficking (see Box 21-2). Synaptojanin (145 kDa) is an additional example of a type II 5-phosphatase; it has been implicated in synaptic vesicle transport (see Chap. 9). A third class of 5-phosphatase has also been identified, consisting of enzymes that associate with tyrosine-phosphorylated receptors (see Chaps. 10 and 25). An example is src homology inositol phosphatase (SHIP) of 145 to 150 kDa, which associates with the adaptor

Box 21-2 *(Continued)*

inositol lipids to these proteins, the barbed ends of the actin filaments become uncapped and the addition of actin monomers is permitted, resulting in the production of filamentous (F-) actin. Because the 3-phosphoinositides are present at relatively low concentrations, it is probable that PI4P and PI(4,5)P$_2$ play the major role in regulation of actin assembly. Direct evidence for phosphoinositide regulation of the actin cytoskeleton has been obtained from experiments with permeabilized platelets. The addition of PI(4,5)P$_2$ [or PI4P, PI(3,4)P$_2$ or PI(3,4,5)P$_3$] to these preparations results in an increase in the number of barbed ends and in the proportion of F-actin. Moreover, the time course of increases in PI(4,5)P$_2$ concentration in stimulated platelets parallels the appearance of F-actin [4].

Regulation of PKC activity. The addition of either PI(3,4)P$_2$ or PI(3,4,5)P$_3$ has been demonstrated to activate the ϵ, η and ζ isoforms of PKC *in vitro*. Consistent with this observation, inhibition of PI3K activity in stimulated platelets prevents phosphorylation of the PKC substrate pleckstrin. It is suggested that a product of PI3K, such as PI(3,4,5)P$_3$, might recruit and localize substrates at the plasma membrane, thereby facilitating their phosphorylation by PKC [5].

Cell survival. An additional role for the 3-phosphoinositides is the promotion of cell survival. PI(3,4)P$_2$ can bind via a PH domain and activate the serine-threonine kinase Akt. In contrast, PI3P, PI(4,5)P$_2$ and PI(3,4,5)P$_3$ are ineffective. Since Akt is a critical mediator of growth factor-induced neuronal survival, the 3-phosphoinositides may play an important role in opposing apoptosis [6].

—*Stephen K. Fisher and Bernard W. Agranoff*

REFERENCES

1. Rapoport, I., Masaya, M., Boll, W., et al. Regulatory interactions in the recognition of endocytic sorting signals by AP-2 complexes. *EMBO J.* 16:2240–2250, 1997.
2. Eberhard, D. A., Cooper, C. L., Low, M. G., and Holz, R. W. Evidence that inositol phospholipids are necessary for exocytosis. *Biochem. J.* 268:15–25, 1990.
3. Martin, T. F. J. Phosphoinositides as spatial regulators of the membrane traffic. *Curr. Opin. Neurobiol.* 7:331–338, 1997.
4. Hartwig, J. H., Bokoch, G. M., Carpenter, C. L., et al. Thrombin receptor ligation and activated Rac uncap actin filament barbed ends through phosphoinositide synthesis in permeabilized human platelets. *Cell* 82:643–653, 1995.
5. Toker, A., and Cantley, L. C. Signalling through the lipid products of phosphoinositide-3-OH kinase. *Nature* 387:673–676, 1997.
6. Franke, T. F., Kaplan, D. R., Cantley, L. C., and Toker, A. Direct regulation of the AKT proto-oncogene product by phosphatidylinositol 3,4-bisphosphate. *Science* 275:665–668, 1997.

molecules src homology collagen-like protein (SHC) or growth factor receptor-binding protein (Grb2) after growth factor receptor activation (see Chaps. 10 and 25). Although the function of this enzyme has still to be defined, it has a unique substrate specificity in that it dephosphorylates only I(1,3,4,5)P$_4$ and PI(3,4,5)P$_3$.

A single enzyme, inositol monophosphatase, leads to loss of the remaining phosphate and the regeneration of free inositol [20]. This enzyme exhibits similar affinities for all five of the equatorial inositol monophosphate hydroxyls. Inositol 2-phosphate, which is not produced in this degradative pathway, is a poor substrate, probably because of its axial configuration. The enzyme is inhibited by Li$^+$ in an uncompetitive manner; that is, the degree of inhibition is a function of substrate concentration. It should be noted that, unlike most other tissues, the brain can synthesize inositol *de novo* by the action of inositol monophosphate synthase, which cyclizes glucose 6-phosphate to form $I(3)P$. The enzyme has been localized immunohistochemically to the brain vasculature [21].

The action of Li^+ on inositol monophosphatase has greatly facilitated the use of [3H] inositol in the study of stimulated phosphoinositide turnover. Berridge and colleagues demonstrated that in the presence of both Li^+ and a phosphoinositide-linked ligand, the amount of labeled intracellular inositol phosphates that accumulate following a preincubation with [3H]inositol can be stimulated as much as 50-fold. In contrast, the presence of either Li^+ or ligand alone has very little effect on [3H]inositol monophosphate accumulation [22]. Although ligand-activated turnover is initiated by $PI(4,5)P_2$ breakdown and the generation of $I(1,4,5)P_3$, this product is quickly degraded. As an index of receptor activation, it is thus more convenient to use an indirect measurement, the accumulation of labeled inositol monophosphates in the presence of Li^+, than to attempt to measure the transient appearance of labeled $I(1,4,5)P_3$ within a few seconds of ligand addition.

Higher inositol phosphates. In contrast to the intracellular roles proposed for $I(1,4,5)P_3$ and $I(1,3,4,5)P_4$, extracellular roles for $I(1,3,4,5,6)P_5$ and IP_6 have been entertained, based on the ability of these inositol phosphates to regulate heart rate and blood pressure when injected into the nucleus of the tractus solitarius [23]. The involvement of $I(1,3,4,5,6)P_5$ in the allosteric regulation of avian hemoglobin in a fashion analagous to that of 2,3-diphosphoglyceric acid in mammals has long been known. IP_6 (phytate) is a well-known component of plant seeds and, while seeds form part of a bird's diet, $I(1,3,4,5,6)P_5$ appears to be synthesized in avian erythrocytes from inositol. Demonstration of specific IP_6-binding sites in brain and anterior pituitary gland supports the possibility of a role for these inositol polyphosphates in mammalian brain [24].

Cyclic inositol phosphates. When PI is cleaved by PI-PLC, two inositol monophosphates are released in relatively equal amounts: D-*myo*-inositol 1-phosphate [$I(1)P$] and D-*myo*-inositol 1:2 cyclic phosphate [$I(c1:2)P$]. Similarly, there is evidence that $PI(4,5)P_2$ breakdown results in the production of $I(cl:2,4,5)P_3$, the cyclic analog of $I(1,4,5)P_3$. A cyclase which cleaves $I(c1:2)P_1$ to $I(1)P$ is inactive against the higher analogs, a result suggesting that the latter are degraded by phosphatases to the cyclic monophosphate prior to cleavage of the cyclic phosphate ring. Although $I(cl:2,4,5)P_3$ is able to mobilize intracellular Ca^{2+}, it is less effective than $I(1,4,5)P_3$. It is also less well cleaved by the 5-phosphatase, potentially extending its lifetime as a second messenger. A physiological role for the cyclic inositol phosphates is, however, not yet documented.

DIACYLGLYCEROL

Protein kinase C is activated by diacylglycerol

The formation of DAG can result in activation of protein kinase C (PKC), an enzyme that was first described in the late 1970s. At least ten isoforms of PKC, 70 to 80 kDa, may exist in mammalian tissues [25,26]. Four conserved (C) and five variable (V) regions can be discerned (Fig. 21-5). The C1 region contains two cysteine-rich repeats and represents the site at which DAG regulates the enzyme. A "pseudosubstrate" sequence is also present in this region of the molecule; it blocks kinase activity until the enzyme becomes activated by DAG. The C2 region confers the Ca^{2+} sensitivity of PKC, whereas the C3 and C4 domains are, respectively, the ATP- and substrate-binding sites. PKC isoforms can be distinguished by their Ca^{2+} sensitivity. The conventional isoforms of PKC, α, β and γ, are Ca^{2+}-sensitive, whereas the "novel" isoforms, δ, ϵ, η, σ and μ, lack the C2 region and are accordingly Ca^{2+}-insensitive. An additional variation in PKC structures is observed for the ζ and λ isoforms, which possess only one cysteine-rich repeat. These isoforms are not regulated by DAG and are constitutively active. The V3 "hinge" re-

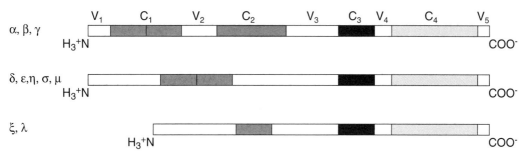

FIGURE 21-5. Linear representation of protein kinase C (PKC) isozymes. All isozymes contain constant *(C)* and variable *(V)* regions. The "conventional" PKC isozymes possess two C1 domains and one C2 domain. Note the absence of a C2 domain in the δ, ε, η, σ and μ (novel) isoforms and the presence of only one C1 domain in the constitutively active ζ and λ (atypical) isoforms.

gion of the molecule is susceptible to proteolysis following persistent activation of PKC.

Although many cellular proteins are potential targets for phosphorylation by PKC, the myristoylated, alanine-rich protein kinase C substrate (MARCKS) appears to be the major *in vivo* substrate. MARCKS is an acidic, filamentous, actin cross-linking protein that is found in high concentrations at presynaptic junctions and that is targeted to the plasma membrane via a myristoylated amino-terminal, membrane-binding domain. This interaction keeps MARCKS in close proximity to PKC, thereby facilitating efficient phosphorylation. Upon phosphorylation, MARCKS undergoes a translocation from the membrane to the cytoplasm and its ability to cross-link actin filaments is lost. Other PKC substrates include vinculin, talin, the adducins and the annexins. Since each of these proteins is involved in linking plasma or intracellular membranes to cytoskeletal structures, an important aspect of PKC signaling appears to be the regulation of membrane-cytoskeletal interactions. A summary of early events involved in inositol lipid signaling is shown in Figure 21-6.

From overexpression studies, it can be inferred that individual isoforms of PKC are targeted to distinct subcellular locations, for example, PKCα to the endoplasmic reticulum and PKCδ to the Golgi. Targeting of PKC isozymes to subcellular loci appears to occur via interaction of the enzyme with localized intracellular binding proteins. Such proteins may or may not be substrates for PKC. An example of the latter category would be receptors for activated C kinase (RACK 1). RACKS are thought to interact only with activated PKCs and to target translocated PKCs.

Diacylglycerols can be derived from phosphoinositides and other lipids

The phorbol esters are useful for studying the function of PKC since they mimic the stimulatory effects of DAG on the enzyme. These tumor-promoting plant products and their synthetic derivatives are able to penetrate intact cells. Many inferences regarding the intracellular actions of PKC are based on results of studies on whole-cell preparations with the phorbol esters. These substances, like DAG, may produce feedback inhibition of signal transduction at a number of metabolic levels. Results of experiments using phorbol esters in whole cells thus are often complex and must be interpreted cautiously. Notwithstanding this consideration, based on experiments with phorbol esters, there is now ample evidence to implicate PKC in a number of complex processes, including long-term potentiation (see Chap. 50) [27].

Since $I(1,4,5)P_3$ production leads to increased intracellular Ca^{2+}, which in turn stimulates PKC action, the two messengers DAG and $I(1,4,5)P_3$ generally act in concert. DAG can, however, arise in cells from sources other than the phosphoinositides. For example, it can be generated from the action of a phosphatidylcholine (PC)-specific PLC or from the transfer of phosphorylcholine from PC to ceramide in

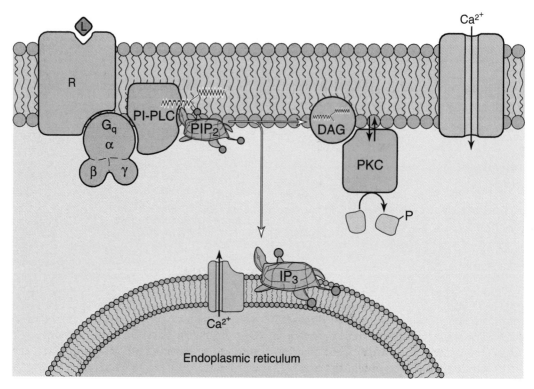

FIGURE 21-6.   Linkage between receptor activation, phosphoinositide hydrolysis, Ca^{2+} signaling and activation of protein kinase C *(PKC)*. Agonist occupancy of a cell-surface receptor results in the activation of phosphoinositide-specific phospholipase C *(PI-PLC)*, which in this example is mediated through an intervening G protein, G_q. Phosphatidylinositol 4,5-bisphosphate *(PIP₂)* is phosphodiesteratically cleaved by PI-PLC to yield diacylglycerol *(DAG)* and inositol 1,4,5-trisphosphate *(IP₃)*. DAG activates PKC, following its translocation (↓↑) from cytosol to plasma membrane. Activation of PKC results in the phosphorylation of many cellular proteins, for example, the myristoylated, alanine-rich PKC substrate (MARCKS). When released, four molecules of IP₃ interact with a specific IP₃ receptor present in the endoplasmic reticulum and Ca^{2+} is liberated, raising its concentration in the cytosol. Depletion of the intracellular pool of Ca^{2+} results in the opening of a plasma membrane Ca^{2+} channel.

the synthesis of sphingomyelin (see Chap. 3). If the DAG released from stimulated phosphoinositide turnover specifically activates cellular PKC, one might expect ST/AR DAG to be a particularly effective activator of the enzyme. It turns out to be only marginally better than other long-chain fatty acyl DAGs; however, chemical analysis indicates that brain DAG is enriched in the ST/AR species. It would therefore seem that ST/AR DAG is *de facto* the principal activator of PKC *in vivo*, even though the enzyme shows little specificity for it. Useful synthetic DAG analogs for experiments on PKC include the relatively soluble species 1-oleoyl, 2-acetyl *sn*-glycerol (OAG).

If DAG is an intracellular messenger that

activates PKC, what then is the "off signal" that terminates its action? Phosphorylation of DAG to PA in the lipid-labeling cycle could serve this purpose. Additional possibilities include the action of DAG lipase, which can cleave DAG to fatty acid and monoacylglycerol (MAG). Although this hydrolytic activity can be demonstrated readily, it should be noted that for the labeling cycle to remain truly regenerative, it would be necessary to reacylate MAG to DAG. Such deacylation–reacylation reactions could be of importance in the generation of arachidonate for prostanoid synthesis from inositide intermediates. Also of interest, *de novo* synthesized PI is enriched in 16:0 and 18:1 fatty acids. Conversion of the *de novo* product to ST/AR PI undoubtedly relies on such deacylation–reacylation reactions.

FUNCTIONAL CORRELATES OF PHOSPHOINOSITIDE-LINKED RECEPTORS IN THE NERVOUS SYSTEM

The complexity of the brain is reflected by a diverse array of receptors coupled to stimulation of phosphoinositide turnover

A large number of pharmacologically distinct receptors are linked to the activation of PI-PLC.

TABLE 21-1. PHARMACOLOGICAL PROFILE OF RECEPTOR-ACTIVATED PHOSPHOINOSITIDE HYDROLYSIS IN NEURAL TISSUES	
Receptor	**Subtype(s)**
Muscarinic	m_1 and m_3
Adrenergic	α_{1A} and α_{1B}
Histaminergic	H_1
Serotonergic	5-HT$_2$ and 5-HT$_{1c}$
Glutamatergic	Metabotropic
Endothelin	
Purinergic	P_2
Thromboxane	A_2
Prostaglandin	E_2
Bradykinin	B_2
Vasopressin	V_1
Nerve growth factor	
Cholecystokinin	
Neuropeptide Y	
Neurotensin	
Gastrin-releasing peptide	
Bombesin	
Substance P	
Oxytocin	
Eledoisin	
Neurokinin	
Vasointestinal peptide	
Angiotensin	
Gonadotropin-releasing hormone	
Platelet-activating factor	
Thyrotropin-releasing hormone	

Table 21-1 summarizes the presently known extent of this diversity [28]. Phosphoinositide hydrolysis elicited by the activation of muscarinic, adrenergic, histaminergic, serotonergic, glutamatergic and endothelin receptors is reliably observed in brain slices, primary cultures of neurons and glia and cultured neurotumor cells. For the other receptors listed, much of the evidence linking them to phosphoinositide hydrolysis is limited to studies performed with either neurotumor cells or other neurally derived tissues. In some instances, the same transmitter may be linked to multiple mechanisms of signal transduction. For example, acetylcholine interacts with two subtypes of muscarinic receptors to stimulate phosphoinositide hydrolysis. Other subtypes of muscarinic receptors are linked to inhibition of adenylyl cyclase activity, while nicotinic cholinergic receptors act as ligand-gated ion channels.

What is the physiological significance of stimulated phosphoinositide turnover in the nervous system?

Because the nervous system is so enriched in the components of the phosphoinositide-signaling system, it is rarely ideal for examining the signal transduction of a single ligand in detail. There is, in addition, likely to be convergence of several receptors on any given brain cell type. Hence, the best-understood models of signal transduction via stimulated phosphoinositide turnover are extraneural, for example, secretion by the salivary or pancreatic glands and activation of platelets by thrombin or of leukocytes by chemotactic peptides. It is probable that there are diverse roles for the phosphoinositides and derived messengers in the nervous system, ranging from mediating the primary signal of neurotransmission to modulating neuronal signals, secretion, membrane trafficking and perhaps contraction (see Box 21-2).

Does the sharing of a single system by multiple cell-surface receptors lead to degeneracy of the signal?

Given the ability of the brain to recognize a wide variety of extracellular signals, such as neurotransmitters and hormones, it would seem that the sharing of an intracellular second-messenger system would lead to degradation of signal and degeneration of information. In the case of the nervous system, it may be that there are anatomically discrete second-messenger domains within a single cell. Video-enhanced microscopic methods for studying Ca^{2+} signaling [29] have offered an experimental approach to address this possibility, and results indicate that each phosphoinositide-linked receptor may possess its own specific "Ca^{2+} signature" [30]. It is also possible that the sharing of second-messenger systems has useful physiological value, for example, in heterologous desensitization. Thus, if the loss of response to a given receptor can lead to loss of response to another receptor, this suggests the sharing of one or more steps in the transduction process. Such sharing could be part of a physiological process whereby various neuronal inputs are integrated intracellularly.

Does the action of Li$^+$ on the phosphoinositide-labeling cycle explain the therapeutic action of Li$^+$ in manic-depressive psychosis?

Given the striking effect of Li$^+$ on the metabolism of the inositol phosphates (see above) and the clinical effectiveness of Li$^+$ in bipolar mental illness (see Chap. 52), it is tempting to speculate that the therapeutic effects of Li$^+$ are mediated via a regulation of inositol lipid turnover. It has been suggested that the uncompetitive inhibition of inositol monophosphatase by Li$^+$ mediates its therapeutic action in affective disorders [31]. The inositol-depletion hypothesis proposes that monophosphatase inhibition *in vivo* lowers inositol concentrations in cells that are most actively producing inositol monophosphate, that is, those that have maximally activated their phosphoinositide-linked receptors. This selectivity is a result of the uncompetitive nature of the Li$^+$ inhibition since the degree of inhibition is proportional to the amount of the substrate, that is, inositol monophosphate. Thus, PI synthase is proposed to be slowed by a lack of inositol substrate and overactive cells are thought to be selectively inhibited. Although clinically therapeutic doses of Li$^+$ do achieve sufficiently high concentrations of Li$^+$ in

the brain (about 1 mM) to inhibit the monophosphatase, experiments in rats with even higher doses show only a 25% lowering of brain inositol. This degree of lowering of brain inositol would not appear to be sufficiently near the K_m of PI synthase to slow PI synthesis. It has also been observed that Li$^+$ must be administered for many days before a therapeutic effect is seen. This suggests that delayed effects of Li$^+$, such as regulation of enzymes, might better correlate with the clinical effect. While the inositol-depletion hypothesis (see also Chap. 52) appears attractive in many respects, its validity remains to be demonstrated. A number of other biochemical sites of Li$^+$ action have been reported [32].

ACKNOWLEDGMENTS

This work was supported by NS 23831 (S. K. F.) and MH 46252 (S. K. F. and B. W. A.).

REFERENCES

1. Hokin, L. E., and Hokin, M. R. Enzyme secretion and the incorporation of P^{32} into phospholipides of pancreas slices. *J. Biol. Chem.* 203:967–977, 1953.
2. Hajra, A. K., Fisher, S. K., and Agranoff, B. W. Isolation, separation and analysis of phosphoinositides from biological sources. In A. A. Boulton, G. B. Baker and L. A. Horrocks (eds.), *Neuromethods (Neurochemistry). Vol. 8, Lipids and Related Compounds.* Clifton, NJ: Humana Press, pp. 211–255, 1988.
3. Michell, R. H. Inositol phospholipids and cell surface receptor function. *Biochim. Biophys. Acta* 415:81–147, 1975.
4. Streb, H., Irvine, R. F., Berridge, M. J., and Schulz, I. Release of Ca^{2+} from a nonmitochondrial intracellular store in pancreatic acinar cells by inositol-1,4,5-trisphosphate. *Nature* 306:67–69, 1983.
5. Wong, K., and Cantley, L. C. Cloning and characterization of a human phosphatidylinositol 4-kinase. *J. Biol. Chem.* 269:28878–28884, 1994.
6. Nakagawa, T., Goto, K., and Kondo, H. Cloning, expression and localization of 230-kDa phosphatidylinositol 4-kinase. *J. Biol. Chem.* 271: 12088–12094, 1996.
7. Meyers, R., and Cantley, L. C. Cloning and characterization of a wortmannin-sensitive human

phosphatidylinositol 4-kinase. *J. Biol. Chem.* 272:3284–4390, 1997.

8. Nakanishi, S., Catt, K. J., and Balla, T. A wortmannin-sensitive phosphatidylinositol 4-kinase that regulates hormone-sensitive pools of inositol lipids. *Proc. Natl. Acad. Sci. USA* 92:5317–5321, 1995.

9. Loijens, J. C., Boronenkov, I. V., Parker, G. J., and Anderson, R. A. The phosphatidylinositol 4-phosphate 5-kinase family. *Adv. Enzyme Regul.* 36:115–140, 1996.

10. Divecha, N., Truong, O., Hsuan, J. J., Hinchliffe, K. A., and Irvine, R. F. The cloning and sequence of the C isoform of PtdIns4P 5-kinase. *Biochem. J.* 309:715–719, 1995.

11. Rameh, L. E., Tolias, K. F., Duckworth, B. C., and Cantley, L. C. A new pathway for the synthesis of phosphatidylinositol 4,5-bisphosphate. *Nature* 390:192–196, 1997.

12. Rhee, S. G., Suh, P.-G., Ryu, S.-H., and Lee, S. Y. Studies of inositol phospholipid-specific phospholipase C. *Science* 255:546–550, 1989.

13. Williams, R. L., and Katan, M. Structural views of phosphoinositide-specific phospholipase C: Signalling the way ahead. *Structure* 4:1387–1394, 1996.

14. Fisher, S. K. Homologous and heterologous regulation of receptor-stimulated phosphoinositide hydrolysis. *Eur. J. Pharmacol.* 288:231–250, 1995.

15. Hodgkin, M. N., Pettitt, T. R., Martin, A., and Wakelam, M. J. O. Regulation of "signalling diacylglycerol" in cells: The importance of diacylglycerol kinase. *Biochem. Soc. Trans.* 24:991–994, 1996.

16. Tanaka, S., Nikawa, J., Hideaki, I., Yamashita, S., and Hosaka, K. Molecular cloning of rat phosphatidylinositol synthase cDNA by functional complementation of the yeast *Saccharomyces cerevisiae* pis mutation. *FEBS Lett.* 393:89–92, 1996.

17. Mikoshiba, K. Inositol 1,4,5-triphosphate receptors. *Trends Pharmacol. Sci.* 14:86–89, 1993.

18. Mitchell, C. A., Brown, S., Campbell, J. K., Munday, A. D., and Speed, C. J. Regulation of second messengers by the inositol polyphosphate 5-phosphatases. *Biochem. Soc. Trans.* 24:994–1000, 1996.

19. Drayer, A. L., Pesesse, X., DeSmedt, F., Communi, D., Moreau, C., and Erneaux, C. The family of inositol and phosphatidylinositol polyphosphate 5-phosphatases. *Biochem. Soc. Trans.* 24:1001–1005, 1996.

20. Atack, J. R. Inositol monophosphatase, the putative therapeutic target for lithium. *Brain Res. Rev.* 22:183–190, 1996.

21. Wong, Y.-H. H., Kalmbach, S. J., Hartman, B. K., and Sherman, W. R. Immunohistochemical staining and enzyme activity measurements show *myo*-inositol-1-phosphate synthase to be localized in the vasculature of brain. *J. Neurochem.* 48:1434–1442, 1987.

22. Berridge, M. J., Downes, C. P., and Hanley, M. R. Lithium amplifies agonist-dependent phosphatidylinositol responses in brain and salivary glands. *Biochem. J.* 206:587–595, 1982.

23. Vallejo, M., Jackson, T., Lightman, S., and Hanley, M. R. Occurrence and extracellular actions of inositol pentakis- and hexakisphosphate in mammalian brain. *Nature* 330:656–658, 1987.

24. Nicoletti, F., Bruno, V., Cavallaro, S., Copani, A., Sortino, M. A., and Canonico, P. L. Specific binding sites for inositolhexakisphosphate in brain and anterior pituitary. *Mol. Pharmacol.* 37:689–693, 1990.

25. Nishizuka, Y. Protein kinase C and lipid signaling for sustained cellular responses. *FASEB J.* 9:484–496, 1995.

26. Jaken, S. Protein kinase C isozymes and substrates. *Curr. Opin. Cell Biol.* 8:168–173, 1996.

27. Angenstein, F., and Staak, S. Receptor-mediated activation of protein kinase C in hippocampal long-term potentiation: Facts, problems and implications. *Prog. Neuropsychopharmacol. Biol. Psychiatry* 21:427–454, 1997.

28. Fisher, S. K., Heacock, A. M., and Agranoff, B. W. Inositol lipids and signal transduction in the nervous system. An update. *J. Neurochem.* 58:18–38, 1992.

29. Tsien, R. Y., and Poenie, M. Fluorescence ratio imaging: A new window into intracellular ionic signaling. *Trends Biochem. Sci.* 11:450–455, 1986.

30. Palmer, R. K., Yule, D. I., McEwen, E. L., Williams, J. A. and Fisher, S. K. Agonist-specific calcium signaling and phosphoinositide hydrolysis in human SK-N-MCIXC neuroepithelioma cells. *J. Neurochem.* 63:2099–2107, 1994.

31. Berridge, M. J., Downes, C. P., and Hanley, M. R. Neural and developmental actions of lithium: A unifying hypothesis. *Cell* 59:411–419, 1989.

32. Jope, R. S., and Williams, M. B. Lithium and brain signal transduction systems. *Biochem. Pharmacol.* 47:429–441, 1994.

22

Cyclic Nucleotides

Ronald S. Duman and Eric J. Nestler

Basic Neurochemistry: Molecular, Cellular and Medical Aspects, 6th Ed., edited by G. J. Siegel et al. Published by
Lippincott–Raven Publishers, Philadelphia, 1999. Correspondence to Ronald S. Duman, Laboratory of Molecular Psychiatry,
Department of Psychiatry, Yale University School of Medicine and Connecticut Mental Health Center, 34 Park Street, New
Haven, Connecticut 06508.

THE SECOND-MESSENGER HYPOTHESIS

The mechanisms by which extracellular agents that act on plasma membrane receptors, such as neurotransmitters and circulating hormones, produce alterations in intracellular processes have been one of the most intensely investigated areas in the biomedical sciences for several decades. One of the seminal advances in this field came in the late 1950s when Earl Sutherland and his colleagues demonstrated that epinephrine induces glycogenolysis in the liver by stimulating the synthesis of an intracellular second messenger, 3′,5′-cyclic adenosine monophosphate (cAMP). Since that time, cAMP and other small molecules, such as 3′,5′-cyclic guanosine monophosphate (cGMP), Ca^{2+}, nitric oxide and the metabolites of phosphatidylinositol and of arachidonic acid, have been shown to serve a myriad of second-messenger roles in the nervous system; these messengers mediate many of the actions of most types of extracellular signal on diverse aspects of neuronal function (Fig. 22-1). This chapter reviews the proteins involved in the synthesis and metabolism of the cyclic nucleotide second messengers cAMP and cGMP in the nervous system.

ADENYLYL CYCLASES

Regulation of cAMP formation by neurotransmitter receptors and intracellular messenger pathways is determined by the activity of the synthetic enzyme adenylyl cyclase, also termed adenylate cyclase. Adenylyl cyclase can be activated directly by forskolin, a plant diterpene which has been useful in studies of enzyme regulation and purification. The substrate for adenylyl cyclase is a complex of Mg^{2+} and ATP. In addition, free divalent cation, such as free Mg^{2+}, in excess of ATP is a requisite cofactor for enzyme activity. As shown in Figure 22-2, adenylyl cyclase forms cAMP by creating a cyclic phosphodiester bond with the α-phosphate group of ATP, with the concomitant release of pyrophosphate, which provides energy for the reaction.

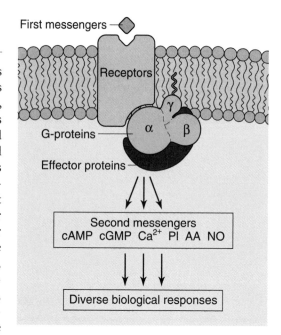

FIGURE 22-1. Schematic illustration of the second-messenger hypothesis. This hypothesis, supported by decades of research, states that many types of first messenger in the brain, through the activation of specific plasma membrane receptors and G proteins, stimulate the formation of intracellular second messengers, which mediate many of the biological responses of the first messengers in target neurons. Prominent second messengers in the brain include cAMP; cGMP; Ca^{2+}; the metabolites of phosphatidylinositol *(PI)*, such as inositol trisphosphate and diacylglycerol; and of arachidonic acid *(AA)*, such as prostaglandins, prostacyclins, thromboxanes and leukotrienes; and nitric oxide *(NO)*.

Biochemical and molecular cloning studies indicate the existence of several forms of adenylyl cyclase which comprise a distinct enzyme family [1,2]. To date, nine forms of the enzyme, referred to as types I through IX, have been identified, although type IX has not been fully characterized. Additional forms may be found when discrete brain regions and tissue types are examined. All of the enzyme forms that have been identified are membrane-bound and stimulated by $G_{\alpha s}$ and forskolin. However, the different forms of adenylyl cyclase exhibit distinct patterns of expression in brain and peripheral tissues and are regulated differentially by Ca^{2+}/calmodulin, by the G protein subunits $G_{\alpha i}$ and $G_{\beta\gamma}$ and by phosphorylation.

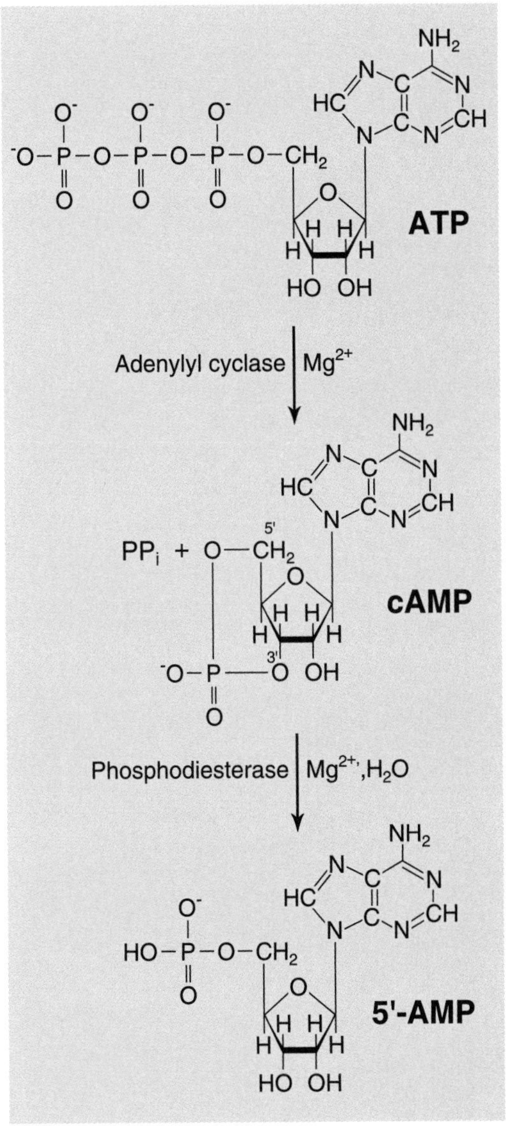

FIGURE 22-2. Chemical pathways for the synthesis and degradation of cAMP. cAMP is synthesized from ATP by the enzyme adenylyl cyclase with the release of pyrophosphate and hydrolyzed into 5′-AMP by the enzyme phosphodiesterase. Both reactions require Mg^{2+}. Analogous reactions underlie the synthesis and degradation of cGMP (not shown).

Multiple forms of adenylyl cyclase exist in the nervous system

As mentioned earlier, these enzymes show considerable variability in the levels and region-specific patterns of expression in the brain. Types I and VIII appear to be expressed exclusively in the brain, adrenal gland and retina [3–5]. In the brain, these enzymes are expressed at highest levels in the hippocampus and neocortex. The catalytic activities of types I and VIII are stimulated by Ca^{2+}/calmodulin (see below) and thereby could be regulated by activation of *N*-methyl-D-aspartate (NMDA) glutamate receptors that flux Ca^{2+} into neurons and have been implicated in several forms of neural plasticity. Further evidence for a role of type I adenylyl cyclase in synaptic plasticity is the finding that mice lacking this form of the enzyme have deficits in spatial memory as well as long-term potentiation [6], a cellular model of learning and memory seen in hippocampus and other brain regions (see Chap. 50).

Type II adenylyl cyclase is expressed at high concentrations in many brain regions but is also found at lower concentrations in lung and olfactory tissue [3,5]. The highest concentrations are found in hippocampus, hypothalamus and cerebellum, with moderate concentrations in neocortex, piriform cortex and amygdala. Type III adenylyl cyclase is highly enriched in olfactory epithelium and is expressed at lower concentrations in other brain regions, as well as in lung and heart [7]. Type IV adenylyl cyclase is widely distributed and has been found in all tissues and cell types tested to date [8].

Type V adenylyl cyclase is highly enriched in brain and is localized largely to the striatum and related structures, such as the nucleus accumbens and olfactory tubercle, which are innervated by dopamine. As a result, it often is referred to as "striatal adenylyl cyclase" [9,10]. The type V enzyme is also expressed in heart and kidney, where it is associated with blood vessels; the anterior lobe of the pituitary; and the retina. All of these tissues share the common feature of having dopamine innervation, and it has been suggested that type V adenylyl cyclase is associated uniquely with dopamine actions [9]. Type VI adenylyl cyclase is structurally similar to the type V enzyme, and both are inhibited by free Ca^{2+} at physiological concentrations (0.1 to 1.0 μM) [11]. Type VI adenylyl cyclase is enriched in brain and heart, with low expression in other tissues, such as testes, muscle, kidney and lung.

Type VII adenylyl cyclase is found in several tissues; concentrations are highest in lung and spleen, moderate in heart and low in brain, kidney and skeletal muscle [12,13]. In the brain, concentrations are highest in cerebellar granule cells and lower in hippocampus, neocortex and striatum. Less is known about the type IX enzyme, which to date has not been characterized extensively.

The different forms of adenylyl cyclase are similar in structure

Hydropathicity profiles of amino acid sequences indicate that adenylyl cyclases contain two regions (M_1 and M_2), each of which consists of six putative membrane-spanning hydrophobic domains [1,2] (Fig. 22-3). This is preceded by a short, variable amino terminus. In addition, there are two large cytoplasmic domains (C_1 and C_2), one between the two hydrophobic regions and the other at the carboxy terminus of the protein. The predicted molecular weight of type I adenylyl cyclase is 124,000 [14], although other types of analysis indicate a native molecular mass of over 200 kDa. This suggests that adenylyl cyclases may exist as a dimer or as a complex with other regulatory proteins.

The two cytoplasmic domains are the most highly conserved portions of the known forms of adenylyl cyclase and are similar to each other within a given enzyme molecule. C_1 is larger, with 360 to 390 amino acids, than C_2, with 255 to 330 amino acids. These cytoplasmic regions have been subdivided into *a* and *b* domains (Fig. 22-3). C_{1a} and C_{2a} are similar to each other and to certain sequences of both membrane-bound and soluble guanylyl cyclases, which catalyze the synthesis of cGMP (see below). These are thought to be the catalytic domains of the enzyme and to contain nucleotide-binding sites. Both C_1 and C_2 appear to be necessary for catalytic activity: there is no enzymatic activity when only one of the domains is expressed, but activity is reinstated when the two halves are coexpressed [8]. It is still unknown whether C_{1a} and C_{2a} act in concert as catalytic domains or if one is catalytic and the other regulatory. The smaller C_{1b} and C_{2b} regions appear to be involved in regulation of catalytic activity (see below). Adenylyl cyclases also are glycosylated and show several potential sites for phosphorylation, as will be discussed below. All known forms of adenylyl cyclase are inhibited by P-site inhibitors, which are adenosine analogues that probably act at the catalytic site of the enzyme.

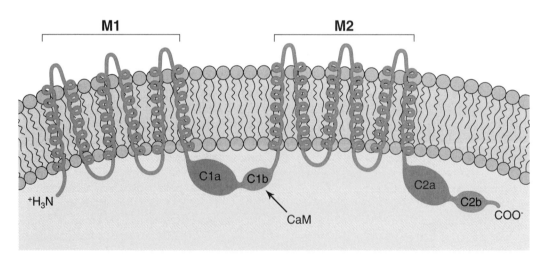

FIGURE 22-3. Schematic illustration of the proposed topographical structure of adenylyl cyclases. Hydropathicity profiles predict that adenylyl cyclases contain two hydrophobic regions *(M1 and M2)*, each of which contains six membrane-spanning regions and two relatively less hydrophobic regions *(C1 and C2)*, which are thought to be located in the cytoplasm. The catalytic domains may be located within C1 and C2, and both are necessary for functional activity of the enzyme. The carboxy *(COO⁻)* portion of the C1 and C2 domains determines whether βγ subunit complexes inhibit (type I) or stimulate (types II and IV) adenylyl cyclases. The C1b domain contains a calmodulin *(CaM)*-binding site and is thought to mediate Ca²⁺/calmodulin activation of certain forms of the enzyme.

The topographical structure of adenylyl cyclases is similar to that of membrane transporters and ion channels. However, there is currently no convincing evidence of a transporter or channel function for mammalian adenylyl cyclases. The structural similarity may indicate that these functionally divergent protein families are derived in an evolutionary sense from related proteins.

Adenylyl cyclases are regulated by $G_{\alpha s}$ and $G_{\alpha i}$

Each of the different forms of adenylyl cyclase is stimulated by activated $G_{\alpha s}$, that is, $G_{\alpha s}$ bound to guanosine triphosphate (GTP). As described in Chapter 20, activation by G protein-coupled receptors occurs when ligand binds to the receptor and catalyzes the exchange of guanosine diphosphate (GDP) for GTP at the α subunit. This promotes the dissociation of the α and βγ subunits, which allows for activated $G_{\alpha s}$ to interact with and stimulate adenylyl cyclase. GTPase activity contained within the α subunit hydrolyzes GTP to GDP and thereby leads to reassociation with the βγ complex.

It is also notable that adenylyl cyclase types I and VIII are activated synergistically by $G_{\alpha s}$ and Ca^{2+}/calmodulin. This finding suggests that these forms of the enzyme are capable of responding to receptors coupled to $G_{\alpha s}$ as well as to those that increase intracellular Ca^{2+} levels. This may be of particular importance to the function of these proteins in integrating the consequences of multiple extracellular stimuli as well as in synaptic plasticity.

In contrast to $G_{\alpha s}$, several forms of $G_{\alpha i}$ can inhibit the catalytic activity of adenylyl cyclase when the enzyme is activated by either $G_{\alpha s}$ or forskolin. This includes the $G_{\alpha i1}$, $G_{\alpha i2}$, $G_{\alpha i3}$ and $G_{\alpha z}$ subtypes. $G_{\alpha i}$-mediated inhibition of adenylyl cyclase is most dramatic for the type V and type VI enzymes. Type I adenylyl cyclase also can be inhibited by these $G_{\alpha i}$ subtypes, as well as by $G_{\alpha o}$, but this inhibition is observed more readily when the type I enzyme is activated by Ca^{2+}/calmodulin than by $G_{\alpha s}$. Type VIII adenylyl cyclase differs from the type I enzyme in this respect since it does not appear to be inhibited appreciably by $G_{\alpha i}$ [15].

Adenylyl cyclase subtypes also are regulated by βγ subunits

The type of regulation seen varies dramatically with the different forms of adenylyl cyclase [1,2,16]. In the presence of $G_{\alpha s}$, addition of βγ complexes inhibits type I but stimulates types II and IV adenylyl cyclases. The type III, V and VI enzymes do not appear to be influenced by βγ subunits. The concentration of βγ required for its inhibitory effect on type I adenylyl cyclase is much higher than that of free $G_{\alpha s}$ required to activate this enzyme. This implies that dissociation of βγ from other, more abundant G proteins, such as $G_{\alpha i}$ and $G_{\alpha o}$, would be the primary source of βγ for this type of inhibition to occur *in vivo*. βγ also inhibits Ca^{2+}/calmodulin-stimulated type I adenylyl cyclase and acts as a better inhibitor of this enzyme than either $G_{\alpha i}$ or $G_{\alpha o}$.

Activation of types II and IV adenylyl cyclase by βγ complexes not only is dependent on the presence of $G_{\alpha s}$ but the enzymes are activated synergistically by these G protein subunits. As is the case for inhibition of type I adenylyl cyclase, the concentration of βγ for activation of the types II and IV enzymes is higher than that for $G_{\alpha s}$. This implies that activation of receptors coupled to $G_{\alpha s}$ and $G_{\alpha i}/G_{\alpha o}$ may be able to activate types II and IV adenylyl cyclase, and these responses could be synergistic under certain conditions. Studies on chimeras of the different enzymes indicate that the stimulatory effect of βγ resides in the carboxy half of the adenylyl cyclase molecule [8]. These studies involved "noncovalent" chimeras, where the amino half of the type I enzyme, containing the first membrane-spanning and cytoplasmic domains, is co-expressed in cultured cells with the carboxy half of either the type I or type II enzyme, containing the second membrane-spanning and cytoplasmic domains. Depending on whether the carboxy portion is from type I or II, the coexpressed chimera is either inhibited or stimulated, respectively, by βγ complexes.

In addition to the selective responses of adenylyl cyclases to βγ subunits, it is likely that different forms of β and γ subunits influence the various forms of adenylyl cyclase in different ways [17]. There are five known forms of β and seven known forms of γ. Differential expression and regulation of these subunits could provide additional mechanisms for selectively controlling adenylyl cyclase catalytic activity in specific neuronal cell types.

Adenylyl cyclases show differential regulation by Ca^{2+}

This regulation [1,2] suggests an important series of mechanisms by which various forms of adenylyl cyclase may be regulated *in vivo* by receptors that influence ligand- or voltage-gated Ca^{2+} channels or receptors that influence intracellular Ca^{2+} levels via coupling to $G_{\alpha o}$ and release of inositol trisphosphate (IP_3) (see Chap. 21). Types I, III and VIII adenylyl cyclase are activated by Ca^{2+}/calmodulin, and this effect is synergistic with $G_{\alpha s}$. In contrast, types II, IV, V and VI adenylyl cyclase are insensitive to Ca^{2+}/calmodulin. The C_{1b} domain of adenylyl cyclase appears to mediate activation of the enzyme by Ca^{2+}/calmodulin (Fig. 22-3). This is established best for the type I enzyme. Activation of this form of adenylyl cyclase by Ca^{2+}/calmodulin can be blocked by a peptide fragment of the C_{1b} portion. This peptide is also capable of binding Ca^{2+}/calmodulin itself. Current mutagenesis studies are defining the precise amino acid sequence required for Ca^{2+}/calmodulin binding and activation of catalytic activity.

Although types V and VI adenylyl cyclase are not influenced by Ca^{2+}/calmodulin, these two forms are inhibited by free Ca^{2+}. The concentrations of Ca^{2+} required for this inhibition are in the physiological range (0.1 to 1.0 μM). It has been suggested that types V and VI adenylyl cyclase may be inhibited by entry of Ca^{2+} into neurons via voltage-gated channels [1].

Adenylyl cyclases are regulated upon phosphorylation

In addition to direct regulation by binding G protein subunits and Ca^{2+}, certain forms of adenylyl cyclase are regulated upon their phosphorylation by second messenger-dependent protein kinases (see Chap. 21). Activation of cAMP-dependent protein kinase is reported to inhibit types V and VI adenylyl cyclase, and both of these enzymes contain consensus sequences

for this kinase [18]. In contrast, types II and V adenylyl cyclase are phosphorylated and activated by protein kinase C (PKC). Although these initial observations are exciting, much further work is needed to define the physiological role played in adenylyl cyclase phosphorylation by second messenger-dependent protein kinases and perhaps by other protein kinases.

Three general categories of adenylyl cyclase can be delineated based on their regulatory properties

These include the following: (i) adenylyl cyclases (types I, III and VIII) that are activated synergistically by $G_{\alpha s}$ and Ca^{2+}/calmodulin and inhibited, in at least some cases, by βγ subunits; (ii) adenylyl cyclases (types II, IV and perhaps VII) that are activated synergistically by $G_{\alpha s}$ and βγ; and (iii) adenylyl cyclases (types V and VI) that are inhibited by $G_{\alpha i}$ and free Ca^{2+} [1,2]. The differential sensitivity of adenylyl cyclase types I through VIII to G protein α and βγ subunits and to Ca^{2+} provides potentially complex mechanisms for the regulation of cAMP formation.

These pathways are illustrated schematically in Figure 22-4. While many features of the schemes remain hypothetical, they do suggest different patterns of regulation of cAMP formation in cells that contain various forms of adenylyl cyclase. For example, in cells that contain types I, III or VIII adenylyl cyclase (Fig. 22-4A), cAMP formation would be stimulated by extracellular signals that activate receptors coupled to $G_{\alpha s}$ as well as by those signals that increase Ca^{2+} entry into the cells. Neurons expressing type I adenylyl cyclase may have inherently high rates of cAMP formation due to basal stimulation by Ca^{2+}/calmodulin. In fact, the high adenylyl cyclase enzyme activity known to be present in the brain may be partly explained in this way. This high rate of enzyme activity could underlie the requirement for additional mechanisms by which this type of adenylyl cyclase is inhibited: cAMP formation would be inhibited in these cells not only by signals that activate receptors coupled to $G_{\alpha i}$ but also by additional signals that activate receptors coupled to other G proteins, such as $G_{\alpha o}$ and $G_{\alpha q}$, via the release of βγ subunits. This could provide a mechanism for keep-

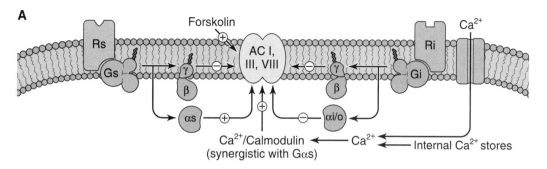

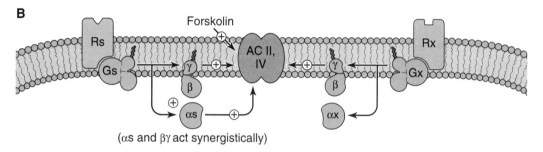

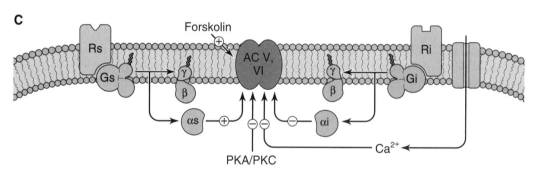

FIGURE 22-4. Schematic illustration of the mechanisms by which the activity of adenylyl cyclases *(AC)* may be regulated. Whereas all forms of adenylyl cyclase are activated by $G_{\alpha s}$ *(αs)* and forskolin, different types of the enzyme can be distinguished by their regulation by Ca^{2+} and G protein subunits. **A:** Since adenylyl cyclase types I, III and VIII are stimulated by Ca^{2+}/calmodulin, an increase in cellular Ca^{2+}, which can result from either increased entry of Ca^{2+} into the cell or increased release of Ca^{2+} from internal stores, would be expected to activate these enzymes. The actions of Ca^{2+}/calmodulin are synergistic with $G_{\alpha s}$. In addition, in the presence of activated $G_{\alpha s}$, type I adenylyl cyclase is inhibited by βγ subunits. The effect of βγ on the type III and VIII enzymes remains unknown. The potency of $G_{\alpha s}$ to activate the enzyme is some ten- to 20-fold higher than that of βγ complexes to inhibit it so that activation of the enzyme is the predominant effect when only stimulatory receptors and G_s are activated. $G_i(\alpha i)$ mediates neurotransmitter inhibition of these adenylyl cyclases. This has been established particularly well for the type I enzyme. **B:** Adenylyl cyclase types II and IV are not sensitive to Ca^{2+}/calmodulin and, in the presence of activated $G_{\alpha s}$, are stimulated by βγ complexes. The receptors *(Rx)* and G protein α subunits that provide the βγ subunits with this type of regulation could involve receptors coupled to several types of G protein, such as G_i, G_o, G_q and others. Activation by βγ is synergistic with $G_{\alpha s}$. While the same βγ complexes are shown for all of the G proteins listed, there are several known subtypes of β and γ subunits, which may well influence the various types of adenylyl cyclase in different ways. **C:** Adenylyl cyclase types V and VI are inhibited by free Ca^{2+}. In addition, these enzymes are inhibited upon phosphorylation by cAMP-dependent protein kinase *(PKA)* or protein kinase C *(PKC)*. Types V and VI adenylyl cyclases also are inhibited by $G_{\alpha i}$, but are not influenced by βγ subunits.

ing "in check" the high cAMP synthetic capacity present in the brain, as well as multiple mechanisms for the regulation of cAMP formation by a variety of extracellular signals.

A very different situation would exist in cells that express types II, IV and perhaps VII adenylyl cyclase (Fig. 22-4B). In these cells, enzyme activity would not be stimulated by Ca^{2+}/calmodulin but would be increased by signals that activate receptors coupled to $G_{\alpha s}$, as well as by additional signals that activate receptors coupled to other G proteins through the generation of free $\beta\gamma$ subunit complexes. This would provide a mechanism by which cAMP formation is regulated in an integrated manner by multiple extracellular stimuli. In fact, there are several examples in brain of interactions between receptors coupled to $G_{\alpha s}$ and those coupled to other G proteins. For example, stimulation of adenylyl cyclase activity in cerebral cortex by activation of β-adrenergic receptors, which are coupled to $G_{\alpha s}$, can be potentiated by activation of α_1-adrenergic or $GABA_B$ receptors, which are coupled to other G proteins. In these same cells, stimulation of α_1-adrenergic or $GABA_B$ receptors alone has little or no effect on cAMP formation [19]. This potentiation could result from the release of free $\beta\gamma$ complexes from the G proteins coupled to the α_1-adrenergic or $GABA_B$ receptors, such as $G_{\alpha o}$ and/or $G_{\alpha q}$. However, these potentiating effects are dependent on extracellular Ca^{2+} and, therefore, could be mediated by activation of Ca^{2+}-dependent intracellular pathways.

The third situation would be cells that express types V and VI adenylyl cyclase. In these cells, these adenylyl cyclases would be activated potently by $G_{\alpha s}$ (Fig. 22-4C). However, this activation would be tightly controlled since the same signals would lead to activation of cAMP-dependent protein kinase, causing feedback inhibition through phosphorylation and inhibition of the adenylyl cyclases. Activation of the adenylyl cyclases would be controlled further by receptors coupled to $G_{\alpha i}$ and those that increase levels of free Ca^{2+} since both $G_{\alpha i}$ and free Ca^{2+} exert an inhibitory effect on these enzymes. In addition, receptors coupled to $G_{\alpha q}$, which lead to activation of PKC, also would be expected to inhibit types V and VI adenylyl cyclase. These types of mechanisms may be of particular relevance to psychotropic drugs that act on dopamine-rich brain regions, such as neostriatum and nucleus accumbens, including drugs of abuse and antipsychotic drugs, since type V adenylyl cyclase is highly enriched in these brain areas.

Adenylyl cyclase is subject to long-term regulation in the nervous system

Prolonged exposure of cells to a receptor agonist typically leads to desensitization of receptor function, whereas prolonged exposure to antagonist can lead to sensitization of receptor function. Increasing evidence suggests that such desensitization and sensitization can be achieved, depending on the receptor and cell type involved, through alterations in the receptors themselves as well as through alterations in the series of proteins downstream of the receptor that mediate receptor function, including adenylyl cyclase. Investigation of the possible mechanisms underlying adaptations in adenylyl cyclase that are involved in desensitization and sensitization of receptor function have only begun; one such mechanism could be phosphorylation of the enzyme or alterations in its expression at transcriptional, translational and post-translational levels.

Processes of receptor desensitization and sensitization are understood best for receptors coupled positively or negatively to the cAMP system. Agonist- and antagonist-dependent changes in these receptors are discussed elsewhere (see Chaps. 10 and 12). However, research has indicated that adaptations in postreceptor signaling proteins also play an important role in controlling receptor sensitivity under a variety of physiological and pathological conditions. One example where adaptations in adenylyl cyclase have been related to long-term adaptations in receptor function is opiate tolerance and dependence. In this case, chronic exposure to opiates leads to coordinate upregulation in the activity of the cAMP cascade in specific opiate-responsive brain regions, including higher levels of adenylyl cyclase and cAMP-dependent protein kinase and, in some cases, lower levels of inhibitory G proteins [20]. Upregulation of the cAMP cascade contributes to opiate tolerance and dependence by opposing the acute actions of opiates, which stimulate receptors coupled to $G_{\alpha i}$. Increased expression of adenylyl cyclase, which in some brain regions is seen selectively for the type I and VIII enzymes, may be achieved at the level of gene expression since higher levels of enzyme mRNA are observed as well [21,22] (see Box 53-1).

In addition to drug regulation of adenylyl cyclase mediated through agonist or antagonist effects on receptors, some drugs produce direct effects on the adenylyl cyclase protein. One example is forskolin, which directly stimulates the catalytic activity of all known forms of the enzyme, as mentioned earlier. Another example is lithium, which has been the drug of choice in the treatment of bipolar disorder. Lithium acutely inhibits adenylyl cyclase, apparently by interfering with the Mg^{2+}-binding sites of the enzyme. This accounts for some of the side effects of lithium, such as inhibition of thyroid hormone production, which is dependent on the cAMP cascade. However, chronic lithium administration, which is required for its beneficial clinical effects, leads to increases in adenylyl cyclase expression in the brain [23], which may represent a compensatory response to acute inhibition of the enzyme. Whether this upregulation of adenylyl cyclase contributes to the clinical effects of lithium remains unknown.

GUANYLYL CYCLASE

Guanylyl cyclase, also termed guanylate cyclase, catalyzes the synthesis of cGMP from GTP in a reaction analogous to that shown in Figure 22-2 for adenylyl cyclase. Two major classes of guanylyl cyclase are known to exist, identified originally on the basis of their subcellular distribution: membrane-bound and soluble [24–27]. The general mechanisms by which these types of guanylyl cyclase are thought to be regulated by extracellular signals are shown in Figure 22-5.

Membrane-bound forms of guanylyl cyclase are plasma membrane receptors

These transmembrane proteins possess cell-surface domains that function as neuropeptide receptors, a single transmembrane domain and intracellular domains that contain guanylyl cyclase catalytic activity. The binding of ligand to the receptor and its consequent activation of the receptor domain leads to activation of the catalytic domain.

These enzymes also contain another domain, termed the protein-kinase domain, based on its structural homology to protein kinases. It is thought that this domain contains an ATP-binding site which is required for guanylyl-cyclase activity. Indeed, the binding of ATP to the site may play a role in transducing the binding of ligand at the receptor domain to the activation of enzyme in the catalytic domain. This would be functionally homologous to the role of GTP-binding to G proteins in transducing the binding of ligand to G protein-coupled receptors in the regulation of adenylyl cyclase.

Three forms of membrane-bound guanylyl cyclase, with M_r of ~120,000, have been identified to date in mammalian tissues by molecular cloning. Two of these are plasma membrane receptors for atrial natriuretic peptide (ANP) and related peptides. ANP is a 28-amino-acid peptide isolated originally from cardiac atria as an important factor in the regulation of sodium excretion and blood pressure. Guanylyl cyclase A binds ANP, as well as brain natriuretic peptide (BNP), and is located primarily in the heart. Guanylyl cyclase B is expressed in neuronal tissue and binds C-type natriuretic peptide (CNP). Increasing evidence suggests that these peptides play important roles as extracellular signals in diverse tissues, including brain. It appears that activation of guanylyl cyclase, and the subsequent increase in cellular cGMP levels, mediates some of the cellular actions of these peptides on target tissues. The third form, guanylyl cyclase C, is localized to the intestine. Guanylyl cyclase C binds the endogenous peptide guanylin and can be activated by a bacterial enterotoxin.

Membrane-bound forms of guanylyl cyclase can be viewed as signal-transducing enzymes. They are structurally homologous to other signal-transducing enzymes, such as certain protein tyrosine kinases and phosphatases, which also possess receptor moieties in their

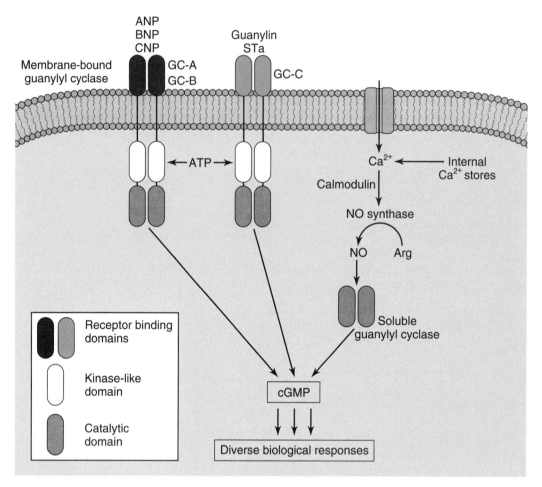

FIGURE 22-5. Schematic illustration of the mechanisms by which primary messengers stimulate guanylyl cyclase. Two major classes of guanylyl cyclase (GC) are known: membrane-bound and soluble. The membrane-bound forms *(GC-A, GC-B* and *GC-C)* contain extracellular receptor domains that recognize specific peptide ligands, atrial natriuretic peptide *(ANP)* and related peptides: GC-A binds ANP and brain natriuretic peptide *(BNP)* and GC-B binds C-type natriuretic peptide *(CNP)*. GC-C binds the endogenous peptide guanylin, as well as a heat-stable bacterial enterotoxin *(STa)*. The membrane-bound receptors contain an intracellular kinase-like domain that binds ATP and a catalytic domain that synthesizes cGMP from GTP. The soluble forms contain the catalytic domains only, α and β subunits, and are activated by nitric oxide *(NO)*. Catalytic activity of soluble guanylyl cyclase is dependent on the presence of both α and β subunits. Primary messengers lead to activation of NO synthesis by increasing cellular levels of Ca^{2+}, which in conjunction with calmodulin activates NO synthase. Primary messengers increase cellular Ca^{2+} levels in most cases by depolarizing neuronal membranes and thereby activating voltage-dependent Ca^{2+} channels and increasing the flux of Ca^{2+} into the cell via nerve impulses, glutamate, acetylcholine or substance P. In some cases, Ca^{2+} can enter the cell directly via ligand-gated ion channels, as with NMDA glutamate receptors. Primary messengers also can regulate cellular Ca^{2+} by stimulating Ca^{2+} release from intracellular stores.

extracellular amino terminus and enzyme catalytic activity in their intracellular domain (see Chap. 25). Activation of many of these receptors occurs upon ligand-induced dimerization of the receptors, and a similar mechanism may occur for the membrane-bound forms of guanylyl cyclase.

Soluble forms of guanylyl cyclase are activated by nitric oxide

These enzymes are homologous to the catalytic domains of the membrane-bound forms of guanylyl cyclase. They are considered heterodimers because they appear to exist, under physiological conditions, as complexes of α and β subunits, each with M_r of 70,000 to 80,000. Both types of subunit contain catalytic and heme-binding domains, although the latter is not required for basal catalytic activity. The αβ heterodimer is required for enzyme activity. This is similar to the situation for adenylyl cyclase, which contains two catalytic entities within a single polypeptide chain (Fig. 22-5).

Multiple isoforms of the α and β subunits of guanylyl cyclase have been cloned and shown to exhibit distinct tissue and cellular distributions. Most of the isoforms are expressed in the brain, including $α_{1–3}$, $β_1$ and $β_3$. The $β_2$ subunit is found primarily in the lung. This isoform also contains a consensus sequence at its carboxy terminus for isoprenylation or carboxymethylation, which could anchor the protein to the plasma membrane. It has been proposed that specific isoforms of the α and β subunits of guanylyl cyclase may form heterodimers with distinct functional and regulatory properties, although this remains to be established with certainty.

A major advance in our understanding of the regulation of soluble guanylyl cyclase was the demonstration that these enzymes are activated potently by nitric oxide (NO) [28,29]. It is thought that NO activates these enzymes via interactions with their heme prosthetic groups. This conclusion is supported by the finding that removal of the heme group results in an enzyme that cannot be activated by NO. However, there are additional sites. Vicinal thiols, known to be regulated by NO, also could contribute to the actions of NO. It is through the generation of NO that numerous types of neurotransmitter, including glutamate, acetylcholine, substance P, histamine and bradykinin, are thought to activate guanylyl cyclase and to increase cellular levels of cGMP in the brain and elsewhere. Similarly, all organic nitrate drugs, including nitroglycerin and nitroprusside, which are used in the treatment of ischemic heart disease, induce vasodilation via the activation of soluble guanylyl cyclase and increased levels of cGMP.

Nitric oxide functions as a second messenger

The synthesis of NO is catalyzed by the enzyme NO synthase (NOS). This enzyme converts arginine into free NO and citrulline in a reaction that requires a tetrahydrobiopterin cofactor and NADPH [28,29]. Three types of NOS have been identified by molecular cloning [27,30]. Type I NOS, also referred to as neuronal NOS, is found at high concentrations in nervous tissue. Ca^{2+}/calmodulin binds to neuronal NOS and increases its catalytic activity (Fig. 22-5). Thus, neurotransmitters that increase cellular Ca^{2+} levels would be expected to stimulate guanylyl cyclase activity in neurons that contain this form of NOS. Type II NOS is referred to as macrophage NOS or inducible NOS. It is expressed at low levels under basal conditions but is induced in response to immunological challenge. Type III NOS is referred to as endothelial NOS and is activated by Ca^{2+}/calmodulin. In addition, this form of NOS is associated with the plasma membrane and the production of endothelium-derived relaxing factor. Despite this nomenclature, there is evidence that types II and III NOS, in addition to type I, contribute to signal transduction in the brain.

It also has been hypothesized that NO might serve as an intercellular messenger (see Chap. 10). According to this scheme, NO, generated in response to an increase in intracellular Ca^{2+} in one neuronal cell type, might diffuse out of the cell and into a second neuron, where it would stimulate guanylyl cyclase activity and produce specific physiological effects. Such a role for NO has been proposed for long-term potentiation [31].

It is important to note that, in addition to guanylyl cyclase, certain ADP-ribosyltransferases may be NO-stimulated enzymes. This means that some of the physiological actions of NO might be mediated through the ADP-ribosylation of specific G proteins or other cellular proteins (see Chap. 20).

CYCLIC NUCLEOTIDE PHOSPHODIESTERASES

Given the significant role of cyclic nucleotides in signal-transduction pathways, it is not surprising that their metabolism and synthesis is highly regulated. Such metabolism is achieved by a large number of enzymes, the phosphodiesterases (PDE), which catalyze the conversion of cAMP and cGMP into 5'-AMP and 5'-GMP, respectively, via hydrolysis of the 3'-phosphoester bonds (Fig. 22-2).

There are multiple forms of phosphodiesterase in brain

Seven major families of PDE, listed in Table 22-1, have been delineated based primarily on two criteria: (i) the kinetic properties of each enzyme for hydrolyzing cAMP and cGMP and (ii) the mechanisms for regulation of PDE activity [32,33] (Fig. 22-6). The kinetic properties are characterized according to the affinity of each enzyme for cAMP or cGMP. The affinity is derived from the K_m values: a low K_m signifies that the enzyme has a high affinity for substrate. For example, a low-K_m PDE typically has a K_m of <5 μM.

The PDE1 family consists of several soluble subtypes in the brain and peripheral tissues, which are stimulated by Ca^{2+}/calmodulin. Two isozymes of PDE1, with M_r of 61,000 and 63,000, account for more than 90% of total brain PDE activity. Separate genes for each of these isozymes have been identified and are referred to as PDE1A (61,000) and PDE1B (63,000). Both enzymes exhibit relatively low affinity for cGMP and cAMP. PDE1A is expressed at highest concentrations in cerebral cortex and hippocampus and at moderate concentrations in amygdala [34]. Expression of PDE1B is high in brain regions innervated by dopamine, including striatum, nucleus accumbens and olfactory tubercle, with moderate expression in hippocampus and cerebral cortex [35]. An additional isozyme, PDE1C, with an M_r of 73,000, also encoded by a distinct gene, has been identified in brain and testes. Interestingly, PDE1C has a high affinity for cAMP, in contrast to the low affinity that PDE1A and PDE1B exhibit for cyclic nucleotides.

TABLE 22-1. **CLASSIFICATION AND SELECTED PROPERTIES OF CYCLIC NUCLEOTIDE PHOSPHODIESTERASES**

Family	Regulatory and kinetic characteristics	Genes described	Selective inhibitors[a]
I	Ca^{2+}/calmodulin-stimulated, regulated by Ca^{2+}/calmodulin and phosphorylation, low affinity for cAMP and cGMP except PDE1C gene product, which has high affinity for cAMP	PDE1A (59–61 kDa) PDE1B (63 kDa) PDE1C (67 kDa, 75 kDa in brain)	Trifluoperazine, vinpocetine, 8-methoxymethyl-3-isobutyl-1-methylxanthine
II	cGMP-stimulated, regulated by cGMP, low affinity for cAMP and cGMP	PDE2 (105 kDa, soluble and particulate)	Erytho-9-(2-hydroxy-3-nonyl) adenine
III	cGMP-inhibited, regulated by phosphorylation and cGMP, high affinity, cGMP > cAMP	PDE3A PDE3B (110–135 kDa)	Milrinone, enoximone, amrinome[b]
IV	cAMP-specific, regulated by phosphorylation and cAMP, high affinity, cAMP >>> cGMP	PDE4A PDE4B PDE4C PDE4D (short and long forms of each gene product)	Rolipram, Ro20-1724
V	cGMP-binding, cGMP-specific; regulated by phosphorylation, cGMP; high affinity, cGMP >>> cAMP	PDE5A (smooth muscle)	Sildenafil, zaprinast
VI	Retina cGMP-specific, regulated by transducin, high affinity, cGMP >>> cAMP	PDE6A (α subtype) PDE6B (rod β subtype) PDE6C (cone β subtype)	—
VII	cAMP-specific, rolipram-insensitive	PDE7A	—

[a] In addition to the relatively specific inhibitors listed, there are a number of compounds, particularly the methylxanthines (for example, theophylline, isobutylmethylxanthine, caffeine), which inhibit most major forms.
[b] The compounds listed here are among a large number that have been developed as specific inhibitors of PDE III.

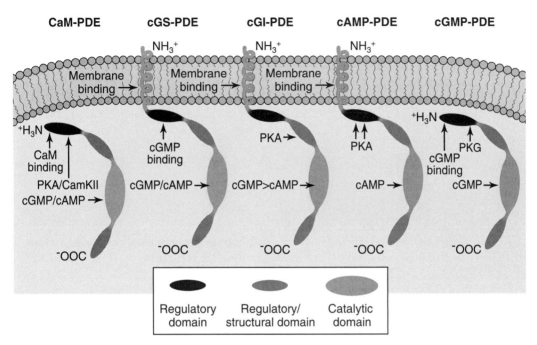

FIGURE 22-6. Schematic illustration of the overall structure and regulatory sites of representative phosphodiesterase *(PDE)* subtypes. The catalytic domain of the PDEs is relatively conserved, and the preferred substrate(s) for each type is shown. The regulatory domains are more variable and contain the sites for binding of Ca^{2+}/calmodulin *(CaM)* and cGMP. The regulatory domains also contain sites of phosphorylation by cAMP-dependent protein kinase *(PKA)*, protein kinase C *(PKC)* and cGMP-dependent protein kinase *(PKG)*. In addition, the amino terminus contains a hydrophobic sequence in certain forms of cGS-PDE (PDE2), cGI-PDE (PDE3) and cAMP-PDE (PDE4) that could anchor the enzyme to the membrane. *CaM-PDE,* calmodulin-stimulated PDE; *cGS-PDE,* cGMP-stimulated PDE; *cGI-PDE,* cGMP-inhibited PDE; *cAMP-PDE,* cAMP-specific PDE; *cGMP-PDE,* cGMP-specific PDE. NH_3^+, amino terminus; ^-OOH, carboxy terminus.

The activity of PDE1 isozymes can be regulated under physiological conditions by those extracellular signals that influence intracellular Ca^{2+} levels. This may be particularly relevant, in a physiological sense, for PDE1C, given its high affinity for cAMP. There is also evidence that these enzymes are regulated by protein phosphorylation [36,37]. The 61,000 and 63,000 isozymes are good substrates for cAMP-dependent and Ca^{2+}/calmodulin-dependent protein kinase, respectively. Such phosphorylation decreases the functional capacity of the enzymes by decreasing their affinity for Ca^{2+}/calmodulin complexes.

There are two PDE families that are regulated by cGMP: PDE2 is stimulated and PDE3 is inhibited. Both of these PDE types are found in soluble and membrane-associated forms. cGMP-stimulated PDE2 has low affinity for cAMP and cGMP. There are at least two cyclic

nucleotide-binding sites on PDE2 isozymes: one is presumably the catalytic site and the other is possibly the high-affinity site which allosterically regulates the catalytic activity of the enzyme. PDE2 can be activated 10- to 50-fold by the concentrations of cGMP found in cells. However, stimulation is transient since cGMP is also a substrate for the enzyme and, therefore, is metabolized rapidly. Localization studies demonstrate that PDE2 expression is restricted largely to the brain and adrenal gland [38]. Within the brain, highest concentrations of the enzyme are seen in the cerebral cortex, striatum and hippocampus. PDE2 may be a primary effector for the physiological actions of cGMP in cells that do not express appreciable amounts of cGMP-dependent protein kinase. In contrast to PDE2, there is currently no evidence for the presence of cGMP-inhibited PDE3 in the brain. Instead, PDE3, which has a low K_m for cAMP, is enriched in heart and vascular tissues, where it regulates cardiac and smooth muscle contraction.

The PDE4 isozymes are cAMP-specific, high-affinity PDEs. Members of this family are found in many tissues in both soluble and membrane-associated forms and are abundant in the central nervous system. PDE4A and PDE4B are expressed at relatively high concentrations in hippocampus, cerebral cortex and striatum and represent the majority of the membrane-bound form of PDE4 in these brain regions [39]. PDE4D represents the majority of the soluble PDE4 in the brain. Expression of PDE4C is relatively low in nervous tissue. Multiple isozymes have been identified, and at least four separate genes exist, which are highly conserved across several mammalian species [32]. The PDE4 isozymes are regulated by phosphorylation and by binding cAMP. In addition, expression of certain PDE4 genes is regulated significantly by activation of the cAMP intracellular pathway. Indeed, this is considered a primary mechanism for enhancing the function of these isozymes in some cell types.

Soluble PDE isozymes that hydolyze cGMP with high affinity are grouped into two families: PDE5 is expressed in smooth muscle, including lung and penis, and PDE6 in retina. The PDE5 and PDE6 isozymes are referred to also as the cGMP-specific PDEs, which display a 50-fold selectivity for cGMP relative to cAMP. Although both of these PDE types have high affinity for cGMP, they are distinct structurally. There are several members of the PDE6 family, all of which are light-activated photoreceptor isozymes. Activation of photoreceptor PDE6 in rod and cone outer segments is mediated by transducin, a G protein specific to retina (see Chaps. 20 and 47). These PDEs are multimeric enzymes, composed of α, β and γ subunits. They are inactive in the dark; light results in their activation via a complex biochemical cascade analogous to mechanisms for activation of G protein-coupled receptors. Briefly, light induces a conformational change in the retinal protein rhodopsin, which is structurally and functionally homologous to a G protein-coupled receptor. This leads to activation of transducin, which is structurally and functionally homologous to $G_{\alpha s}$. Free transducin α subunits then directly bind to and acti-

vate PDE6. The rapid resulting hydrolysis of cGMP leads to changes in specific ionic currents in the photoreceptors and thereby mediates the physiological effects of light.

A seventh type of PDE has been cloned based on homology screening. This PDE, like PDE4 isozymes, hydrolyzes cAMP with high affinity. However, it is not inhibited by rolipram, a specific inhibitor of PDE4. PDE7 is expressed at high levels in skeletal muscle. Although relatively low levels of PDE7 are expressed in whole brain, it is possible that certain regions express higher levels of this or a related form of PDE.

Phosphodiesterases show a distinctive molecular structure

Members of each of the seven PDE families have been characterized by molecular cloning techniques [32,33]. All of the enzymes thus far identified in mammalian tissues contain a highly conserved region of approximately 300 amino acids toward the carboxy terminus. Deletion studies have confirmed that this region represents the catalytic domain. Within this region, there are a number of conserved histidine residues that appear to play a role in folding of the proteins and are required for their catalytic activity, based on mutational analyses. The histidine residues may bind zinc, given the structural similarities of the PDEs to zinc hydrolases.

The regions outside the catalytic domain, particularly the amino terminus, are much more variable across the different PDE families. These regions contain many of the regulatory sites that control PDE activity. For example, the amino terminus contains the Ca^{2+} calmodulin-binding site on PDE1. Similarly, those PDEs that possess high-affinity cGMP-binding sites that apparently serve an allosteric function, such as PDE2 and PDE6, share a distinct conserved site within this region. There are also several phosphorylation sites within this region in PDE1, PDE3, PDE4 and PDE6. There is evidence for an additional phosphorylation site in the carboxy terminus of certain PDE4 isozymes.

The association of PDE isozymes with the cell membrane is mediated by a conserved, hydrophobic sequence in the amino terminus of the proteins. This has been demonstrated most

convincingly for PDE4A: when the amino terminus is removed, PDE4A is no longer localized to
the membrane fraction. A similar amino-terminal sequence is found in the membrane-bound
forms of PDE2, and it may mediate the membrane association of certain PDE3 isozymes.

In addition to the numbers of distinct genes
that encode the seven described families of
PDEs, there is evidence that multiple protein
products can be derived from individual genes.
This has been established for the PDE1, PDE2
and PDE4 gene families. These multiple forms
provide yet another mechanism to increase the
diversity of PDEs expressed in different tissues
or under different biological conditions. For example, the four PDE4 genes give rise to at least
17 variants as a result of alternative splicing or
the presence of multiple promoter start sites
within the gene [32]. Many of these variants are
conserved across species, which suggests that
they may have functional importance.

While the physiological significance of
most of these PDE4 variants has not been appreciated fully, certain variants have been shown to
differ dramatically with respect to their regulatory properties. Short and long forms of *PDE4D*
are generated by alternative splicing. Expression
of the short forms, D1 and D2 (67-72 kDa), results from activation of an intronic promoter,
whereas expression of the long form, D3 (93
kDa), results from activation of another promoter located further upstream. The long form,
but not the short forms, contains a site for phosphorylation and is regulated by cAMP-dependent protein kinase [40]. Although the short
forms are not regulated by phosphorylation,
their expression is increased at the transcriptional level by cAMP [41]. The *PDE4A–C* genes
also appear to be capable of giving rise to short
and long forms that may be regulated in a similar manner. The activity of the long, but not the
short, form is enhanced by phosphatidic acid
and phosphatidylserine.

Phosphorylation is a primary mechanism for regulation of phosphodiesterase activity

PDE1 is phosphorylated by Ca^{2+}/calmodulin-
dependent protein kinase II (CaM-kinase II),
which results in decreased affinity of this enzyme
for Ca^{2+}/calmodulin and an increase in the concentration of Ca^{2+} needed for its activation.
PDE1 also is phosphorylated by cAMP-dependent protein kinase, which also decreases the
binding of Ca^{2+}/calmodulin. The inhibition of
PDE1 by cAMP-dependent protein kinase could
sustain intracellular cAMP concentrations under certain physiological conditions.

cAMP-dependent protein kinase also phosphorylates PDE2, PDE3 and PDE4, although the
effects of phosphorylation are different for each
of these enzymes. Only the particulate form of
PDE2 is phosphorylated by the protein kinase,
but this does not influence enzyme activity.
Phosphorylation of PDE3 by cAMP-dependent
protein kinase in rat adipocytes stimulates the
catalytic activity of the enzyme. PDE3 in these
cells also is phosphorylated and activated by an
insulin-activated kinase, which has not yet been
identified with certainty.

PDE4 is activated similarly upon phosphorylation by cAMP-dependent protein kinase. As
discussed above, only the long form of PDE4 is
phosphorylated; the short forms lack the amino
terminus that contains the phosphorylation site.
This provides a mechanism for a rapid and readily reversible activation of PDE4 by phosphorylation, as well as more long-term and sustained regulation of PDE4 by gene expression.
Certain PDE4 isozymes are phosphorylated by
PKC, by mitogen-activated protein kinase
(MAP-kinase) and in response to insulin. These
phosphorylation reactions are characterized incompletely and their functional consequences
are not yet established.

Phosphodiesterase inhibitors show promise as pharmacotherapeutic agents

This may not be surprising given the
widespread role of cyclic nucleotides in the regulation of cell function [32,33]. The best examples of drugs that influence PDEs are the
methylxanthines; these drugs are used therapeutically in the treatment of obstructive pulmonary disease and are the mild stimulants
present in coffee, tea and related substances. Inhibition of PDE contributes to some of the clinical effects of these drugs.

Other examples of PDE inhibitors with possible clinical usefulness are inhibitors of PDE3 or PDE4 (Table 22-1). Based on the localization of PDE3 to heart and vascular tissue and the role of cAMP in mediating heart muscle contraction and smooth muscle relaxation, a large number of PDE3 inhibitors have been developed for possible clinical applications to cardiovascular medicine. Sildenafil, an inhibitor of PDE5, which is enriched in vascular smooth muscle, has been found to be effective for the treatment of male impotence.

Inhibitors of PDE4 have been developed as possible antidepressants. The rationale for this application comes from the observation that many types of antidepressant treatment appear to increase cAMP function in the brain. Persistent increases in cAMP function may lead to some of the long-term adaptive changes in the brain thought to underlie the antidepressant effects of these agents [42]. Although early clinical trials demonstrated that PDE4-specific inhibitors have antidepressant efficacy, these drugs also produce unwanted side effects that have limited their use. The presence of multiple PDE4 subtypes in the brain raises the possibility that more selective inhibitors may be developed that retain antidepressant actions without unwanted side effects.

Further evidence for the importance of PDE4 isozymes in neuronal function comes from the *dunce* mutation in *Drosophila*. This mutation, which results in learning and memory deficits, involves loss of function of a cAMP-specific PDE that is functionally homologous to PDE4. Of course, this observation would appear primarily to highlight the importance of cAMP in neuronal function, as opposed to any specific role for PDE in the nervous system.

FUNCTIONAL ROLES FOR cAMP AND cGMP

cAMP serves as an intracellular second messenger for numerous extracellular signals in the nervous system. In fact, the number of functional processes regulated by cAMP is too large to enumerate here in detail. It is important, however, to review the general types of effect that cAMP exerts in neurons.

cAMP can be viewed as subserving two major functions in the nervous system

First, cAMP mediates some short-term aspects of synaptic transmission: some rapid actions of certain neurotransmitters on ion channels that do not involve ligand-gated channels are mediated through cAMP. Second, cAMP, along with other intracellular messengers, plays a central role in mediating other aspects of synaptic transmission: virtually all other effects of neurotransmitters on target neuron functioning, both short-term and long-term, are achieved through intracellular messengers. This includes regulation of the general metabolic state of the target neurons, as well as modulatory effects on neurotransmitter synthesis, storage, release and receptor sensitivity; cytoskeletal organization and structure; and neuronal growth and differentiation. This also includes those long-term actions of neurotransmitters that are mediated through alterations in neuronal gene expression.

It is important to emphasize that such a role for cAMP and other intracellular messengers is not limited to actions of neurotransmitters mediated via G protein-coupled receptors. Thus, although activation of ligand-gated ion channels leads to initial changes in membrane potential independent of intracellular messengers, it also leads to numerous additional, albeit slower, effects that are mediated via intracellular messengers. For example, activation of certain glutamate receptors, which are ligand-gated ion channels, leads rapidly to membrane depolarization and more slowly to increases in cellular levels of cAMP by activation of Ca^{2+}/calmodulin-sensitive forms of adenylyl cyclase. cAMP then mediates several other effects of glutamate on the neurons. By virtue of numerous interactions between cAMP and other intracellular messenger pathways, these pathways play the central role in coordinating a myriad neuronal processes and adjusting neuronal function to environmental cues [43].

Most of the effects of cAMP on cell function are mediated via protein phosphorylation

By far the most important mechanism by which cAMP exerts its myriad physiological effects is through the specific activation of cAMP-dependent protein kinase. This was demonstrated first by Krebs and coworkers for cAMP regulation of glycogenolysis, and shortly thereafter it was shown to be a widespread mechanism by Paul Greengard and his colleagues. Indeed, cAMP-dependent protein kinase is now known to phosphorylate virtually every major class of neural protein; this accounts for the ability of cAMP to influence so many diverse aspects of neuronal function. The ability of cAMP to activate protein kinases and the role of protein phosphorylation in the regulation of neuronal function are covered in greater detail in Chapter 24.

How do a wide variety of neurotransmitters and hormones produce tissue- and cell-specific biological responses if many such responses are mediated by the same intracellular messengers, cAMP and cAMP-dependent protein kinase? Specificity is achieved at two levels: at the level of tissue-specific receptors for the neurotransmitter or hormone and at the level of tissue-specific substrate proteins for the protein kinase. Only tissues which possess specific receptors will respond to a certain neurotransmitter or hormone. Moreover, since all cells contain very similar catalytic subunits of cAMP-dependent protein kinase (see Chap. 24), the nature of the proteins that are phosphorylated in a given tissue depends on the types and amounts of protein expressed in that tissue and on their accessibility to the protein kinase.

There are a small number of known exceptions to the rule that the physiological effects of cAMP in mammals are achieved via the activation of cAMP-dependent protein kinase. The best established exception is certain cation channels in olfactory epithelium and other tissues, which directly bind and are gated by cAMP.

The mechanisms by which cGMP produces its physiological effects are more varied

It has been more difficult to identify second-messenger actions of cGMP compared to cAMP. This probably reflects the lower concentrations of cGMP in most tissues and the likelihood that cGMP plays a less widespread role in cell function.

Nevertheless, physiological actions of cGMP are being identified. The best studied action is in the retina (see above), where cGMP mediates the effects of light on cation channels in rod outer segments apparently by directly binding to and gating the channels. In addition, cGMP activates and inhibits specific forms of PDE, also through direct binding to the enzymes.

In addition to such direct actions of cGMP on effector proteins, many physiological effects of cGMP probably are mediated via the activation of cGMP-dependent protein kinase and the subsequent phosphorylation of specific substrate proteins (see Chap. 24). For example, the ability of neurotransmitters to influence certain ion channels in target neurons is mediated through increased cellular cGMP, activation of cGMP-dependent protein kinase and the subsequent phosphorylation of the channels, or some associated protein, by the protein kinase. As another example, in certain neuronal cell types, neurotransmitters that increase cGMP through the activation of cGMP-dependent protein kinase and the phosphorylation and activation of DARPP-32, an inhibitor of protein phosphatase 1, would alter the phosphorylation state of the numerous proteins dephosphorylated by this protein phosphatase (see Chap. 24).

FUTURE PERSPECTIVES

Although tremendous progress has been made in characterizing the enzymes that control the synthesis and metabolism of cyclic nucleotides in the nervous system, our understanding of the regulation and interaction of these systems is far from complete. It is likely that additional subtypes of these enzymes exist, each with a unique distribution in the brain and distinct functional and regulatory properties. One area that requires further investigation concerns the interactions between cyclic nucleotide-mediated signal-transduction pathways and growth factor-regulated pathways, for example, the MAP-kinase-signaling cascades.

Future studies of cyclic nucleotide-mediated and other signal-transduction pathways in the brain will utilize recent advances in molecular and cellular neurobiology to determine the role of these pathways in the coordinate functioning of individual neurons and of synaptic connections among neurons. These approaches combined with gene mutation technology will allow a more complete investigation of the function of specific signal-transduction proteins in neuronal function and complex behavior. Characterization of these signal-transduction pathways will elucidate how dysfunction of these systems contributes to psychiatric and neurological disorders.

REFERENCES

1. Cooper, D. M. F., Mons, N., and Karpen, J. W. Adenylyl cyclases and the interaction between calcium and cAMP signaling. *Nature* 374:421–424, 1995.
2. Sunahara, R. K., Dessauaer, C. W., and Gilman, A. G. Complexity and diversity of mammalian adenylyl cyclases. *Annu. Rev. Pharmacol. Toxicol.* 36:461–480, 1996.
3. Feinstein, P., Schrader, K., Bakalyar, H., et al. Molecular cloning and characterization of a Ca^{2+}/calmodulin-insensitive adenylyl cyclase from rat brain. *Proc. Natl. Acad. Sci. USA* 88:10173–10177, 1991.
4. Cali, J. J., Zwaagstra, J. C., Mons, N., Cooper, D. M. F., and Krupinski, J. Type VIII adenylyl cyclase—A Ca^{2+} calmodulin-stimulated enzyme expressed in discrete regions of rat brain. *J. Biol. Chem.* 269:12190–12195, 1994.
5. Mons, N., Yoshimura, M., and Cooper, D. Discrete expression of Ca^{2+}/calmodulin-sensitive and Ca^{2+}-insensitive adenylyl cyclases in the rat brain. *Synapse* 14:51–59, 1993.
6. Wu, Z. I., Thomas, S. A., Villacres, E., et al. Altered behavior and long-term potentiation in type I adenylyl cyclase mutant mice. *Proc. Natl. Acad. Sci. USA* 92:220–224, 1995.
7. Bakalyar, H. A., and Reed, R. R. Identification of a specialized adenylyl cyclase that may mediate odorant detection. *Science* 250:1403–1406, 1990.
8. Gao, B., and Gilman, A. G. Cloning and expression of a widely distributed (type IV) adenylyl cyclase. *Proc. Natl. Acad. Sci. USA* 88:10178–10182, 1991.
9. Glatt, C. F., and Snyder, S. H. Cloning and expression of an adenylyl cyclase localized to the corpus striatum. *Nature* 361:536–538, 1993.
10. Pieroni, J. P., Miller, D., Premont, R. T., and Lyengar, R. Type-5 adenylyl cyclase distribution. *Nature* 363:679, 1993.
11. Krupinski, J., Lehman, T. C., Frankenfield, C. D., Zwaagstra, J. C., and Watson, P. A. Molecular diversity in the adenylyl cyclase family. Evidence for 8 forms of the enzyme and cloning of type VI. *J. Biol. Chem.* 267:24858–24862, 1992.
12. Watson, P. A., Krupinski, J., Kempinski, A. M., and Frankenfield, C. D. Molecular cloning and characterization of the type VII isoform of mammalian adenylyl cyclase expressed widely in mouse tissues and in S49 lymphoma cells. *J. Biol. Chem.* 269:28893–28898, 1994.
13. Hellevuo, K., Yoshimura, M., Mons, N., Hoffman, P. L., Cooper, D. M. F., and Tabakoff, B. The characterization of a novel human adenylyl cyclase which is present in brain and other tissues. *J. Biol. Chem.* 270:11581–11589, 1995.
14. Krupinski, J., Caissonn, F., Bakalyar, H., et al. Adenylyl cyclase amino acid sequence: Possible channel- or transporter-like structure. *Science* 244:1558–1564, 1989.
15. Nielsen, M. D., Chan, G., Poser, S., and Storm, D. R. Differential regulation of type I and type VIII Ca^{2+}-stimulated adenylyl cyclases by G_i-coupled receptors *in vivo*. *J. Biol. Chem.* 271:33308–33316, 1996.
16. Tang, W., and Gilman, A. G. Type-specific regulation of adenylyl cyclase by protein $\beta\gamma$ subunits. *Science* 254:1500–1503, 1991.
17. Wickman, K., and Clapham, D. E. Ion channel regulation by G proteins. *Physiol. Rev.* 75:865–885, 1995.
18. Premont, R. T., Jacobowitz, O., and Iyengar, R. Lowered responsiveness of the catalyst of adenylyl cyclase to stimulation by G_s in heterologous desensitization: A role for cAMP dependent phosphorylation. *Endocrinology* 131:2774–2783, 1992.
19. Duman, R. S., and Enna, S. J. Modulation of receptor-mediated cyclic AMP production in brain. *Neuropharmacology* 26:981–986, 1987.
20. Nestler, E. J., and Aghajanian, G. Molecular and cellular basis of addiction. *Science* 278:58–63, 1997.
21. Matsuoka, I., Maldonado, R., Defer, N., Noel, F., Hanoune, J., and Roques, B. Chronic morphine administration causes region-specific increase of brain type VIII adenylyl cyclase mRNA. *Eur. J. Pharmacol.* 268:215–216, 1994.
22. Lane-Ladd, S. B., Pineda, J., Boundy, V., Aghajanian, G. K., and Nestler, E. J. CREB in the locus coeruleus: Biochemical, physiological and behavioral evidence for a role in opiate dependence. *J. Neurosci.* 17:7890–7901, 1997.

23. Colin, S., Chang, H., Mollner, S., et al. Chronic lithium regulates the expression of adenylate cyclase and G$_i$-protein α-subunit in rat cerebral cortex. *Proc. Natl. Acad. Sci. USA* 88:10634–10637, 1991.

24. Koesling, D., Bohme, E., and Schultz, G. Guanylyl cyclases, a growing family of signal-transducing enzymes. *FASEB J.* 5:2785–2792, 1991.

25. Yuen, P. S. T., and Garbers, D. L. Guanylyl cyclase-linked receptors. *Physiol. Rev.* 75:865–885, 1995.

26. Nakane, M., and Murad, F. Cloning of guanylyl cyclase isoforms. *Adv. Pharmacol.* 26:7–18, 1994.

27. McDonald, L. J., and Murad, F. Nitric oxide and cyclic GMP signaling. *Proc. Soc. Exp. Biol. Med.* 211:1–6, 1996.

28. Hope, B. T., Michael, G. J., Knigge, K. M., and Vincent, S. R. Neuronal NADPH diaphorase is a nitric oxide synthase. *Proc. Natl. Acad. Sci. USA* 88:2811–2814, 1991.

29. Bredt, D. S., and Snyder, S. H. Nitric oxide, a novel neuronal messenger. *Neuron* 8:3–11, 1992.

30. Marletta, M. A. Nitric oxide synthase: Aspects concerning structure and catalysts. *Cell* 78:927–930, 1994.

31. Garthwaite, J., and Boulton, C. Nitric oxide signaling in the central nervous system. *Annu. Rev. Physiol.* 57:683–706, 1995.

32. Conti, M., Nemoz, G., Sette, C., and Vicini, E. Recent progress in understanding the hormonal regulation of phosphodiesterases. *Endocr. Rev.* 16:370–389, 1995.

33. Beavo, J. Cyclic nucleotide phosphodiesterases: Functional implications of multiple isoforms. *Physiol. Rev.* 75:725–748, 1996.

34. Yan, C., Bentley, J. K., Sonnenburg, W. K., and Beavo, J. A. Differential expression of the 61 kDa and 63 kDa calmodulin-dependent phosphodiesterases in the mouse brain. *J. Neurosci.* 14:973–984, 1994.

35. Polli, J. W., and Kincaid, R. L. Molecular cloning of DNA encoding a calmodulin-dependent phosphodiesterase enriched in striatum. *Proc. Natl. Acad. Sci. USA* 89:11079–11083, 1992.

36. Sharma, R. K., and Wang, J. H. Differential regulation of bovine brain calmodulin-dependent cyclic nucleotide phosphodiesterase isozymes by cyclic AMP-dependent protein kinase and calmodulin-dependent protein phosphatase. *Proc. Natl. Acad. Sci. USA* 82:2603–2607, 1986.

37. Hashimoto, Y., Sharma, R. K., and Soderling, T. R. Regulation of Ca^{2+} calmodulin-dependent cyclic nucleotide phosphodiesterase by the autophosphorylated form Ca^{2+} calmodulin-dependent protein kinase II. *J. Biol. Chem.* 264:10884–10887, 1989.

38. Repaske, D. R., Corbin, J. G., Conti, M., and Goy, M. F. A cyclic GMP-stimulated cyclic nucleotide phosphodiesterase gene is highly expressed in the limbic system of the rat brain. *Neuroscience* 56:673–686, 1993.

39. McPhee, I., Pooley, L., Lobban, M., Bolger, G., and Houslay, M. D. Identification, characterization and regional distribution in brain of RPDE-6 (RNPDE4A5), a novel splice variant of the PDE4A cyclic AMP phosphodiesterase family. *Biochem. J.* 310:965–974, 1995.

40. Sette, C., Vicini, E., and Conti, M. The rat PDE3/IVd phosphodiesterase gene codes for multiple proteins differentially activated by cAMP-dependent protein kinase. *J. Biol. Chem.* 269:18271–18274, 1994.

41. Swinnen, J. V., Tsikalas, K. E., and Conti, M. Properties and hormonal regulation of two structurally related cAMP phosphodiesterases from the rat Sertoli cell. *J. Biol. Chem.* 266:18370–18377, 1991.

42. Duman, R. S., Heninger, G. R., and Nestler, E. J. A molecular and cellular theory of depression. *Arch. Gen. Psychiatry* 54:597–606, 1997.

43. Hyman, S. E., and Nestler, E. J. *The Molecular Basis of Psychiatry.* Washington, DC: American Psychiatric Press, 1993.

23

Calcium

James W. Putney, Jr.

Basic Neurochemistry: Molecular, Cellular and Medical Aspects, 6th ed., edited by G. J. Siegel et al. Published by Lippincott–Raven Publishers, Philadelphia, 1999. Correspondence to James W. Putney, Jr., Calcium Regulation Section, Laboratory of Signal Transduction, National Institute of Environmental Health Sciences–National Institutes of Health, P.O. Box 12233, Research Triangle Park, North Carolina 27709-2203.

THE CONCEPT OF Ca^{2+} AS A CELLULAR SIGNAL

In most eukaryotic cells, a large electrochemical gradient for Ca^{2+} exists across the plasma membrane. The transmembrane potential across the membrane is 70 to 90 mV. The interior of the cell is the more negative, yet the cytoplasmic concentration of Ca^{2+} ([Ca^{2+}]$_i$) is less than one-ten thousandth of that in the extracellular milieu. There are also intracellular organelles, such as the endoplasmic reticulum (ER) and secretory granules, that contain one- to ten thousand fold greater concentrations of Ca^{2+} than the cytoplasm. It is likely that these gradients for Ca^{2+} evolved because of the difficulty in carrying out a phosphate-based energy economy in the high Ca^{2+} concentrations in seawater. Nonetheless, the system that has evolved provides opportunities for rapid changes in [Ca^{2+}]$_i$, and indeed, cells have developed mechanisms to produce such changes and to sense them very rapidly, thus using changes in [Ca^{2+}]$_i$ as a cellular signaling mechanism. This chapter focuses on the mechanisms of Ca^{2+} storage and compartmentalization in cells and the mechanisms by which cellular Ca^{2+} signaling occurs in neurons and other cell types.

MEASUREMENT OF CELLULAR Ca^{2+} CONCENTRATIONS AND MOVEMENTS

From the earliest measurements of tissue calcium, it was clear that total calcium gives largely a measure of stored calcium. Through the years, scientists have used a variety of indirect measures of [Ca^{2+}]$_i$. These include shortening or tension in muscles; secretion from secretory cells; the activity of Ca^{2+}-dependent enzymes, most notably glycogen phosphorylase; and flux of K$^+$, or K$^+$ current, as a reflection of Ca^{2+}-activated K$^+$ channels. In addition, investigators often use the radioactive calcium ion [^{45}Ca^{2+}] as an indirect indicator of Ca^{2+} concentrations and Ca^{2+} movements.

From the 1980s until the present, more direct methods have been used to estimate cytoplasmic calcium and calcium ion movements in cells. Beginning as far back as the 1970s, a few laboratories began to develop technology to utilize the calcium-activated photoprotein aequorin to measure intracellular calcium. While this method is an extremely sensitive one, it has the disadvantage of requiring difficult microinjection, cell permeabilization or cellular transfection procedures to introduce the protein into the cytoplasm. The invention of fluorescent Ca^{2+} indicators that can be introduced easily into almost any vertebrate cell revolutionized research in the calcium signaling field (Fig. 23-1) [1]. The majority of these compounds are derivatives of the calcium ion chelator 1,2-bis(o-aminophenoxy)ethane-N-N-N'-N'-tetraacetic acid (BAPTA), including 1-[2-(5-carboxyoxazol-2-yl)-6-aminobenzofuran-5-oxy]2-(2'-amino-5'-methylphenoxy)-ethane-N,N,N',N-tetraacetic acid (fura-2) and its cousin 1-[2-amino-5-(6-carboxyindol-2-yl) phenoxy]-2-(2-amino-5'-methylphenoxy) ethane N,N,N',N'-tetraacetic acid (indo-1).

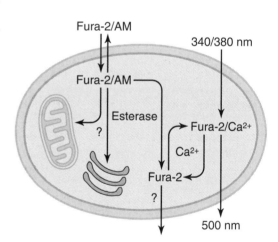

FIGURE 23-1. Introduction of esterified fluorescent Ca^{2+} indicators into cells. The fluorescent indicator, in this example fura-2, is presented to cells as the acetoxymethyl ester *(Fura-2/AM)*. This relatively lipid-soluble chemical permeates into the cytoplasm of cells, where esterases cleave the acetoxymethylester groups, liberating the Ca^{2+}-binding moiety *(Fura-2)*. Fura-2 then reversibly combines with Ca^{2+} and, when excited alternatively with light of wavelengths 340 and 380 nm, gives rise to fluorescence at 500 nm, which can be used for quantitation of [Ca^{2+}]$_i$. Potential complications with the use of these fluorescent dyes, indicated in this figure by *?*, are uptake into intracellular organelles and leak of dye from the cells. (Redrawn and modified from [3] with permission.)

Their major advantage is that their fluorescence spectra are shifted upon binding of calcium ions. For fura-2, the excitation spectrum is shifted; for indo-1, the emission spectrum is shifted. This allows one to utilize these indicators in fluorescence microscope systems, either with photomultiplier detectors or intensified cameras, and to obtain reasonable calibration of intracellular calcium ion concentrations. A family of such indicators, each of which has properties applicable to special experimental situations, has been developed.

Yet another method of assessing calcium ion movements in cells is by direct measurements of the current that such movement generates. Such currents were detected originally by impaling cells with microelectrodes, but most of the understanding of Ca^{2+} channel functions has come from more recent work utilizing the powerful patch-clamp technique (see Chap. 6). In the whole-cell configuration, the investigator is afforded the opportunity of measuring calcium currents while manipulating both the intracellular and extracellular milieus. With excised patches, the behavior of single calcium channels can be investigated while similarly controlling their environments. This approach, which is described in Chapter 6, has been very useful for describing voltage-activated Ca^{2+} channels [2].

Ca^{2+} REGULATION AT THE PLASMA MEMBRANE

Although there are a number of mechanisms in cells for buffering or sequestering Ca^{2+} and thereby preventing untoward or inappropriate rises in $[Ca^{2+}]_i$, in the long term, it is the activity of plasma membrane transport processes that determines the steady-state concentration of $[Ca^{2+}]_i$. This is because the plasma membrane acts as a Ca^{2+} buffer of infinite capacity. In *in vitro* experiments, this results from incubation volumes very much larger than the cell volume. *In vivo* this results from clamping of the extracellular concentration of Ca^{2+} by dietary and endocrine mechanisms.

Two distinct mechanisms for controlling $[Ca^{2+}]_i$ at the plasma membrane are a Ca^{2+}–ATPase pump and a Na^+–Ca^{2+} exchanger

The basic properties of both the pump and the exchanger have been discussed in Chapter 5. Of the two mechanisms, the plasma membrane Ca^{2+} pump is the more common and is believed to be ubiquitous in eukaryotic cells. The Na^+–Ca^{2+} exchanger is present only in some cell types; it is found most commonly in excitable cells, such as nerve and muscle. As its name implies, the exchanger can, at least in theory, drive extrusion of Ca^{2+} from the cell by a process coupled to the inward movement of Na^+ down its concentration gradient. However, because in resting cells the outward electrochemical gradient is so very large, there is debate as to the extent to which the exchanger actually contributes to the lowering of $[Ca^{2+}]_i$ at least under resting conditions. This debate hinges on assumptions about the stoichiometry and driving forces for the exchanger in intact cells. However, it is clear that turnover of Ca^{2+} through the exchanger can be substantial, and this may be important in the minute-to-minute control of $[Ca^{2+}]_i$ during activity. The exchanger is of pharmacological interest because of the possibility that digitalis glycosides, which disturb the normal transmembrane Na^+ gradient, augment cardiac contraction by facilitating Ca^{2+} entry or delaying Ca^{2+} exit via the exchanger (see Chap. 5). It also has been suggested that the exchanger provides a rapidly responding buffer that can allow inward movement of Ca^{2+} under conditions requiring restoration of Ca^{2+} to intracellular storage organelles [3].

The plasma membrane Ca^{2+}–ATPase pump effects outward transport of Ca^{2+} against a large electrochemical gradient for Ca^{2+}. The mechanism of the pump involves its phosphorylation by ATP and the formation of a high-energy intermediate. This basic mechanism is similar for both the plasma membrane and the ER pumps; however, the structures of these distinct gene products are substantially different. As discussed below, the ER pump, sometimes called a sarcoendoplasmic reticulum Ca^{2+}–ATPase (SERCA) pump, is inhibited potently by certain natural and synthetic toxins that do not affect the plasma membrane pump. The plasma membrane pump, but not the SERCA pump, is controlled in part by Ca^{2+} calmodulin, allowing for rapid activation when cytoplasmic Ca^{2+} rises.

Ca^{2+} STORES AND Ca^{2+} POOLS

Within cells, the major calcium storing, buffering and signaling organelle appears to be the ER or, as discussed below, a specialized compartment of it. Other specialized structures that may be involved in calcium storage include the mitochondria and the nucleus. There was, for a time, a rather widely held belief that mitochondria represented the major source of signaling calcium that was released by hormone or neurotransmitter receptor activation. Perhaps the most convincing demonstration that mitochondria were not involved primarily in hormonal responses came with the discovery of inositol 1,4,5-trisphosphate (IP_3, or $I(1,4,5)P_3$ to distinguish it from other positional isomers), as the mediator of intracellular release of Ca^{2+} (reviewed in [4] and discussed below; see also Chap. 21). IP_3 was clearly shown to act only on nonmitochondrial stores. As the default for nonmitochondrial calcium storage was thought to be the ER, this was taken as evidence that the ER was the critical storage site for signaling calcium. Whether this is a property of the generic ER or a more specialized component of it is a matter of some debate. This is discussed in more detail in a subsequent section.

The only known mechanism for accumulation of Ca^{2+} by the endoplasmic reticulum is through the actions of SERCA pumps

Inside the lumen of the ER, the Ca^{2+} storage capacity is enhanced substantially by one or more low-affinity calcium-binding proteins. In muscle, this protein is calsequestrin, while in most other cells the major protein is calreticulin. Each molecule of calreticulin has multiple Ca^{2+}-binding sites with an affinity in the high micromolar range and one high-affinity site with a binding constant in the nanomolar range. The signifi-

cance of this high-affinity site is not known.

The function of the calcium-storage capacity of the ER is at least threefold. The rapid rate of Ca^{2+} uptake by endoplasmic pumps provides a short-term cytoplasmic Ca^{2+} buffer to resist untoward and transient changes in $[Ca^{2+}]_i$. In other instances, signaling pathways may call upon this Ca^{2+} to be released to provide an elevation of $[Ca^{2+}]_i$ to activate cellular enzymes or other appropriate processes. This release is, in some instances, coupled to an activation of Ca^{2+} entry across the plasma membrane, a process known as capacitative calcium entry, which is discussed in a subsequent section of this chapter. Finally, the association of Ca^{2+} with Ca^{2+}-binding proteins in the ER fulfills a chaperone function that is essential for normal protein synthesis.

Mitochondria may accumulate Ca^{2+} by an energy-dependent process

This does not involve a specific ATPase transporter, as for the ER, but rather, Ca^{2+} is accumulated via an electrogenic Ca^{2+} channel. The energy for driving accumulation of Ca^{2+} comes from the substantial mitochondrial membrane potential. This potential is generated by the large proton gradient that is established by the electron transport chain and necessary for the coupling of respiration to the synthesis of ATP. Experimentally, mitochondrial accumulation of Ca^{2+} can be driven either by a substrate for oxidative metabolism or by ATP. In the latter case, the hydrolysis of ATP drives H^+ accumulation and generates membrane potential through reversal of the H^+–ATPase. Drugs that either interfere with electron transport, such as antimycin, or collapse the proton gradient, such as protonophore uncouplers, block mitochondrial uptake of Ca^{2+}. Careful experiments with either subcellular fractions, permeable cells or *in situ* imaging of sequestered Ca^{2+} have demonstrated that the kinetics of Ca^{2+} uptake by mitochondria are inconsistent with significant accumulation of Ca^{2+} by this organelle under resting conditions (Fig. 23-2). However, once the threshold for uptake is reached, the driving force for Ca^{2+} accumulation is substantial, and when $[Ca^{2+}]_i$ is elevated for a prolonged period of time, mito-

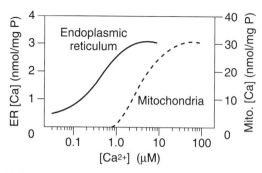

FIGURE 23-2. ATP-dependent uptake of calcium into endoplasmic reticulum and mitochondria as a function of extraorganellar Ca^{2+} concentration. Stylized data taken from results originally reported in Burgess et al. [23]. As $[Ca^{2+}]$ was raised, ATP-dependent Ca^{2+} uptake into the endoplasmic reticulum *(ER)* and mitochondrial pools increased. Data for ER uptake were determined as the amount of Ca^{2+} [$^{45}Ca^{2+}$] taken up by saponin-permeabilized hepatocytes after addition of ATP and in the presence of mitochondrial inhibitors. The curve for mitochondrial (Mito.) uptake was obtained by subtracting the ATP-dependent uptake in the presence of these inhibitors from that in the absence of inhibitors. For additional details consult Burgess et al. [23]. (Redrawn and modified from [3] with permission.)

chondria can accumulate Ca^{2+} to remarkable concentrations. This uptake of Ca^{2+} may serve as a protection for the cell from the deleterious effects of prolonged $[Ca^{2+}]_i$ elevation. While the uptake of Ca^{2+} by mitochondria is an electrogenic process, the efflux is neutral, either a Ca^{2+} for $2H^+$ or $2Na^+$ exchange, and proceeds more slowly than cytoplasmic and plasma membrane buffering. Thus, Ca^{2+} accumulated during periods of prolonged stress is released to the cytoplasm at a sufficiently slow rate such that the excess can be removed from the cell without elevating the concentration of Ca^{2+} in the cytoplasm.

Calcium is stored at other significant sites in the cell

These include secretory granules and the nucleus. The Ca^{2+} in secretory granules generally has been considered to be relatively inert and to function largely in a structural capacity. However, evidence has suggested that this Ca^{2+} can be released during cell stimulation and can participate in the control of secretion. The nuclear pores generally prevent the development of substantial gradients of Ca^{2+} between the nucleoplasm and cytoplasm. However, the nuclear envelope can store Ca^{2+} as it is an extension of the endoplasmic reticulum. There is evidence that cell stimulation can lead to discharge of this Ca^{2+} directly into the nucleoplasm, where it may play a role in regulating functions of the nucleus.

Ca^{2+} SIGNALING

The process of calcium signaling comprises a series of molecular and biophysical events that link an external stimulus to the expression of some appropriate intracellular response through an increase in cytoplasmic Ca^{2+} as a signal. The external signal is most commonly a neurotransmitter, hormone or growth factor; but in the case of excitable cells, the initial chemical stimulus may bring about membrane excitation, which in turn activates a calcium-signaling pathway.

Release of intracellular Ca^{2+} is mediated primarily via inositol 1,4,5-trisphosphate receptors and ryanodine receptors

The calcium ions that give rise to a $[Ca^{2+}]_i$ signal can come from one or two sources: intracellular Ca^{2+} stores and external Ca^{2+} entering across the plasma membrane. Typically, both sources are utilized. The most ubiquitous of the intracellular Ca^{2+} release mechanisms involves the phosphoinositide specific phospholipase C (PI-PLC)-derived second messenger IP_3, which acts by binding to a specific receptor on the endoplasmic reticulum or to a specialized component of the endoplasmic reticulum. The functional IP_3 receptor/channel appears to be a homotetramer containing four binding sites for IP_3. Distinct subtypes of the receptor exist, representing products of at least three distinct genes, and additional forms arise as a result of alternative splicing of mRNA. The origin of IP_3 and the characteristics of IP_3 receptors are discussed in Chapter 21.

The interaction of IP_3 with its receptor involves complex and poorly understood regulatory interactions among the receptor, IP_3 and

Ca^{2+}, the latter exerting influence from both the cytoplasmic and luminal aspects of the receptor. Ca^{2+} in the lumen of the ER appears to sensitize the receptor to IP_3. On the cytoplasmic surface, low concentrations of Ca^{2+} sensitize the receptor while higher concentrations are inhibitory. These actions may contribute to the "all-or-none" oscillatory behavior of $[Ca^{2+}]_i$ signals seen in some cell types. This phenomenon will be discussed in more detail below.

The other major type of intracellular Ca^{2+}-mobilizing receptor is the ryanodine receptor. The ryanodine receptor is named for a toxin that binds to the molecule with high affinity and which led to its purification and characterization. It is also a homotetramer, and the IP_3 and ryanodine receptors share considerable structural homology [5]. In its most specialized setting, in skeletal muscle, the ryanodine receptor is gated by a direct conformational interaction with a dihydropyridine receptor in the *t*-tubule membrane (see Chap. 43). This coupling allows for rapid release of stored Ca^{2+} when an action potential invades the *t*-tubule system. However, the physiological ligand for the ryanodine receptor is usually Ca^{2+} itself; that is, it is considered to be a *Calcium-Induced Calcium Release* (CICR) receptor–Ca^{2+} channel. Because Ca^{2+} can sensitize the IP_3 receptor to IP_3, the IP_3 receptor also can exhibit CICR behavior. However, some IP_3 is always required for its action, while the ryanodine receptor can function as a "pure" CICR receptor. Although the ryanodine receptor is thought to be regulated primarily by CICR, there is also a small water-soluble molecule that can function as a regulatory ligand for at least some forms of the ryanodine receptor. Cyclic adenosine diphosphate ribose (cADPr) [6] functions in a manner somewhat similar to IP_3: it increases the probability of the ryanodine receptor channel opening by increasing its sensitivity to Ca^{2+}. It is tempting to speculate that Ca^{2+} signaling in neurons may be regulated by changing concentrations of cADPr, and there is limited evidence for this suggestion. In at least one cell type, the sea urchin oocyte, both the IP_3 receptor and a cADPr-sensitive ryanodine receptor seem to function in a somewhat redundant, or perhaps cooperative, manner to produce a regenerative intracellular Ca^{2+} signal.

Ca^{2+} enters cells either via voltage- or ligand-dependent channels or by means of capacitative entry

There are at least three fundamental mechanisms of regulated calcium ion entry across the plasma membrane. These involve the actions of voltage-dependent Ca^{2+} channels, ligand-gated channels and the process of capacitative calcium ion entry.

Voltage-dependent Ca^{2+} channels are found in a variety of excitable cell types, including neurons, muscles and endocrine and neuroendocrine cells [2]. They are almost never found in classical "nonexcitable" cells, such as epithelial cells, leukocytes and fibroblasts. By definition, these channels can be activated by membrane depolarization and are subject to the complex combinations of voltage-dependent activation and voltage-dependent or calcium-mediated inactivation mechanisms similar to the voltage-dependent regulation of Na^+ channels described by Hodgkin and Huxley (see Chap. 6). These are the Ca^{2+} channels that provide activator Ca^{2+} for cardiac contractility, for contraction of some smooth muscle types and, generally, for discharge of neurotransmitters. In most instances, their activation is initiated by membrane depolarization, whether by a propagated action potential or by the opening of other ligand-gated channels. In some cases, the channels are activated by removing an inhibitory influence, such as a decrease in a hyperpolarizing K^+ conductance, or by sensitizing the channels to activation at resting membrane potential through phosphorylation.

There are at least five different molecular types of voltage-dependent Ca^{2+} channel, differing in their gating kinetics, modes of inactivation and regulation by Ca^{2+} and sensitivity to specific marine toxins [7] (see Box 23-1). The distinctions between the types of channel are of considerable interest because the different subtypes are believed to subserve different cellular functions. For example, the control of neurotransmitter release in peripheral sympathetic neurons appears to be under the predominant control of N-type calcium channels.

Ligand-gated ion channels are numerous, and some permit sufficient entry of Ca^{2+} to provide for cellular activation. Here, receptor-gated channels denote channels that are gated directly by binding of agonist, not through the generation of second messengers, generally because the ligand-binding site is located on the channel protein. These are invariably nonspecific cation channels; there are as yet no clearly identified receptor-gated channels that are specific for Ca^{2+} ions. These channels are discussed in detail in other chapters in this volume (see Chaps. 10, 11, 13, 15–17).

Capacitative Ca^{2+} entry is by far the predominant mode of regulated Ca^{2+} entry in nonexcitable cells, but it also occurs in a number of excitable cell types. This is the pathway of Ca^{2+} entry usually associated with the activation of PLC and the formation of IP_3 (see Chap. 21). Intracellular application of IP_3 mimics the ability of hormones and neurotransmitters to activate calcium ion entry, and activation of calcium ion entry by hormones and neurotransmitters can be blocked by intracellular application of low-molecular-weight heparin, a potent antagonist of IP_3 binding to its receptor. There is considerable evidence for the presence of an IP_3 receptor, or a protein similar to it, in the plasma membrane of some cell types. $I(1,3,4,5)P_4$, a product of IP_3 phosphorylation, has been shown in some cases to augment the action of IP_3 in activating calcium ion entry, but in others, IP_3 alone is clearly sufficient.

However, the current view of the regulation of calcium ion entry by PLC-linked stimuli holds that activation occurs not as a direct result of the action of IP_3 on the plasma membrane but, rather, as a result of the depletion of calcium ions from an intracellular store by IP_3 [8]. In the context of this capacitative model, the actions of intracellularly applied IP_3 and heparin reflect the effects of these maneuvers on the intracellular release process, rather than directly on the plasma membrane. The reported actions of $I(1,3,4,5)P_4$, if in fact they do represent physiological control mechanisms, may reflect its ability of $I(1,3,4,5)P_4$ to augment the calcium-releasing ability of IP_3, rather than a distinct and specific action at the plasma membrane. The ca-

pacitative model for calcium ion entry originally was proposed on the basis of circumstantial evidence from the relative rates of emptying and refilling of intracellular stores of calcium, but more direct tests of the model have arisen from the discovery of reagents, such as thapsigargin and cyclopiazonic acid, that inhibit the Ca^{2+}–ATPase responsible for storing intracellular calcium in the IP_3-sensitive pool (Fig. 23-3). These reagents make it possible to deplete this pool of its Ca^{2+} without stimulating the formation of any inositol phosphates. Thus, numerous reports have demonstrated that in cells treated with such agents, Ca^{2+} entry across the plasma membrane is activated [9]. Importantly, this Ca^{2+} entry is not facilitated by concomitant stimulation of inositol phosphate production.

Two general mechanisms by which a depleted intracellular Ca^{2+} pool might communi-

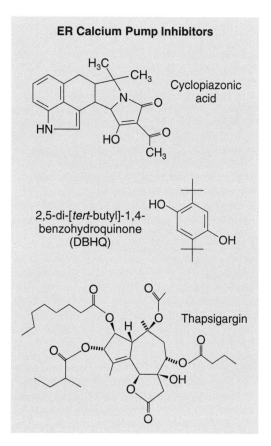

FIGURE 23-3. Structures of compounds that inhibit sarcoendoplasmic reticulum Ca^{2+}–ATPase (SERCA) calcium pumps.

Box 23-1

VOLTAGE-GATED CALCIUM ION CHANNELS

Voltage-gated Ca^{2+} channels are heterogeneous in structure and regulation. Multiple types of voltage-dependent Ca^{2+} channels have been characterized physiologically [1] and multiple Ca^{2+}-channel subunits have been cloned [2]. Differential regional expression of specific subunit isoforms and cellular localization of Ca^{2+}-channel types are well documented. These differences and the existence of multiple types of Ca^{2+} channels in individual neurons have been postulated to be important in controlling many Ca^{2+}-dependent cellular processes including neurotransmitter release, gene expression and neurite outgrowth.

Ca^{2+} channels have been classified pharmacologically and biophysically. The channels are designated L-, T-, N-, P-, Q- and R-type. Each channel has different voltage ranges and rates for activation and inactivation [3]. Low-voltage-activated (LVA) T-type currents are distinguished from high-voltage-activated (HVA) L-, N-, P-, Q- and R-type currents based on the relatively hyperpolarized potential at which they are activated. T-type channels, believed to function as a pacemaker, typically are activated slowly and inactivated rapidly, whereas the HVA channels are activated much more rapidly and vary in the extent and rate of their inactivation. The N-type typically are inactivated more rapidly then the L-, P- and Q-types. The HVA channels can be distinguished by their pharmacological sensitivities to specific blockers and toxins [4]. The L-type channels are found in skeletal as well as neuronal tissue and are sensitive to dihydropyridines such as the agonist BayK-2844 and the antagonist nifedipine [5]. The N-type channels are irreversibly blocked by the snail toxin ω-conotoxin GVIA and are thought to be responsible for neurotransmitter release at synaptic junctions. Another snail toxin, ω-conotoxin MVIIC, inhibits N-, P- and Q-type currents. Preferential block by the spider toxin ω-agatoxin-IVA can be used to isolate the P-type channels, which were initially identified in Purkinje cells due to the high level of expression in those cells. Insensitivity to all these compounds defines the R-

---

cate with the plasma membrane have been considered [3]. There is evidence from a number of studies that the IP_3 receptor is associated with the cytoskeleton, and this association might result in tethering of the IP_3 receptor to the plasma membrane. Depletion of intracellular calcium stores causes a conformational change in the IP_3 receptor, which could be conveyed to the plasma membrane via the cytoskeleton or by a more direct protein–protein interaction. Alternatively, signaling could occur through the action of a diffusible messenger released by the depleted intracellular calcium store and acting on calcium channels in the plasma membrane. Proposed candidates for this signaling messenger are cGMP (Chap. 22), a metabolite of cytochrome P450, and the poorly

characterized calcium influx factor (CIF) (reviewed in [3,9]). However, subsequent studies have cast doubt on each of these proposals. There is pharmacological evidence that a GTP-dependent step is involved as well as a tyrosine kinase (see Chaps. 20 and 25). These latter findings have led to the proposal that vesicle transport may be involved, in that preformed and active calcium channels may be inserted into the membrane by vesicle fusion. There is little direct evidence for this suggestion, however.

In contrast to the case for voltage-dependent and receptor-gated channels, the channels associated with capacitative calcium ion entry only recently have been characterized electrophysiologically. In leukocytes, the current asso-

---

Box 23-1 *(Continued)*

type channel that may actually be comprised of multiple channel types. The T-type channels and the recombinant "R-type" currents have a higher sensitivity to blockade by Ni^{2+}.

Each channel type has been cloned and is composed of a large α_1 subunit in combination with one or more smaller accessory subunits [6]. At least six α_1, four β, one α_2 and one δ subunits have been cloned [2]. The large α_1 subunit has four domains, each with six transmembrane segments, which form the ion pore of the channel. Five neuronal α_1 subunits (denoted A-E) have been described to date. Heterologous expression of the α_1 subunits in recombinant systems has pharmacological properties similar to those of native Ca^{2+} channel types (L-type: α_{1C}, α_{1D}; N-type: α_{1B}; Q/P-type: α_{1A}; R-type: α_{1E}). The pairing of molecular clones with functional channel types is, however, incomplete and may be affected by the coordinate expression of one or more auxiliary subunits. The subunit composition of native Ca^{2+} channels is further complicated by the diversity of the auxiliary subunits $\alpha_{2(A-E)}/\delta$, β_{1-4} and γ described to date.

The functional roles of all these subunits are not fully understood.

—Torben R. Neelands and Robert L. Macdonald

REFERENCES

1. Tsien, R. W., Lipscombe, D., Madison, D. V., Bley, R. K, and Fox, A. P. Multiple types of neuronal calcium channels and their selective modulation. *Trends Neurosci.* 11:431–438, 1988.
2. Perez-Reyes, E., and Schneider, T. Molecular biology of calcium channels. *Kidney Int* 48:1111–1124, 1995.
3. Catterall, W. A. Molecular properties of sodium and calcium channels. *J. Bioenerg. Biomembr.* 28:219–230, 1996.
4. Adams, M. E., and Olivera, B. M. Neurotoxins: Overview of an emerging research technology. *Trends Neurosci.* 17:151–155, 1994.
5. Hockerman, G. H., Peterson B. Z., Johnson, B. D., and Catterall, W. A. Molecular determinants of drug binding and action on L-type calcium channels. *Annu. Rev. Pharmacol. Toxicol.* 37:361–396, 1997.
6. De Waard, M., Gurnett, C. A., and Campbell, K. P. Structural and functional diversity of voltage-activated calcium channels. *Ion Channels* 4:41–87, 1996.

---

ciated with the depletion of intracellular Ca^{2+} stores is highly Ca^{2+}-selective, even over Ba^{2+}, in contrast to other known Ca^{2+} channels, and, on the basis of noise analysis, is believed to involve minute single channels [10] (see Chap. 6). This is the calcium release-activated calcium current (I_{CRAC}). However, in other cell types, the current is more akin to "conventional" Ca^{2+} channels in being similarly permeable to Ca^{2+} and Ba^{2+} and showing readily identifiable single channels with conductances in the picosiemens range. These marked electrophysiological distinctions may be indicative of distinct channel types mediating capacitative calcium ion entry in different cell types.

While the molecular identity of the capacitative Ca^{2+} entry channel is not known, a candidate is a homolog of the *Drosophila* mutant *trp*. This photoreceptor mutant is incapable of maintaining a sustained photoreceptor potential. This phenotype is mimicked by the calcium ion entry blocker lanthanum, suggesting that the deficit is related to a failure of calcium ion entry. The photoreceptor signaling mechanism in insects involves an IP$_3$-signaling system, and it may be that the normally sustained photoreceptor potential depends on capacitative calcium ion entry [11]. When *trp* was cloned and sequenced, homology was detected between this protein and the α_1 subunit of the voltage-sensitive calcium channel, also termed the dihydropyridine receptor, which is believed to contain the ion channel region of the protein. As might be expected, *trp* does not contain the charged residues in the S4 transmembrane segment which are believed to provide the voltage-sensing capabilities of the voltage-sensitive channel. Six distinct mammalian homologs of *Drosphila trp* have been cloned at least partially from human material and designated *Htrp*-1 through -6 [12]. Some of these proteins have been expressed in mammalian cells and have been shown to augment capacitative calcium ion entry.

The major function of capacitative calcium ion entry is to provide for sustained Ca^{2+} signaling. However, it is also important in providing a means for rapid replenishment of intracellular stores following their release by IP_3 and the cessation of agonist activation. How is this accomplished in those excitable cells which do not express capacitative calcium ion entry? The answer may be that excitable cells generally do, while nonexcitable cells generally do not, express a rapidly turning over sodium–calcium exchange transporter. This transporter could provide an energy-efficient route for rapidly adjusting cytoplasmic Ca^{2+} in response to rapid uptake demands of a depleted intracellular Ca^{2+} store. Because the resting turnover of this exchanger is relatively fast, it may be that such a pathway replenishes intracellular stores in the absence of any store-dependent regulation.

Periodic temporal and spatial patterns of Ca^{2+} signaling give rise to calcium oscillations and waves

As discussed above, the IP_3 receptor is subject to complex and only partially understood regulation by both IP_3 and calcium. The complicated kinetic behavior of the IP_3 receptor is believed to underlie calcium oscillations and waves. In excitable cells, oscillations in $[Ca^{2+}]_i$ which reflect periodic fluctuations in membrane electrical activity have been known for some time, the clearest example being the rhythmic cardiac action potentials that drive bursts of Ca^{2+} release, entry and extrusion and thereby maintain the pumping activity of the heart. However, $[Ca^{2+}]_i$ often will oscillate in nonexcitable cells or in excitable cells through mechanisms which have nothing to do with the excitable nature of the surface membrane. Much effort has been devoted to understanding the control mechanisms giving rise to $[Ca^{2+}]_i$ waves and oscillations [13].

Intracellular calcium oscillations generally fall into one of two categories involving different mechanisms. The two major kinds of $[Ca^{2+}]_i$ oscillation are baseline transients, or spikes, and sinusoidal oscillations. Figure 23-4 illustrates these two oscillatory patterns. Baseline spikes are characterized by rapidly-rising transient increases in $[Ca^{2+}]_i$ rising from a baseline of $[Ca^{2+}]_i$ which is generally quite close to the resting concentration. In contrast, sinusoidal oscillations more closely resemble true sine-wave oscillations; they are generally of a higher frequency than baseline spikes, >1/min as opposed to frequencies of <1/min for baseline spikes. They also generally appear as symmetrical oscillations superimposed on a sustained concentration of $[Ca^{2+}]_i$ somewhat above the prestimulus baseline. Another notable difference between the two types of oscillation is that baseline spikes may, at least in some instances, continue throughout prolonged periods of stimulation, while sinusoidal oscillations tend to diminish with time, generally lasting for only a few minutes. However, the most significant and characteristic distinction between the two types of oscillation is the relationship of the oscillation amplitude and frequency to stimulus strength, or agonist concentration. For baseline spikes, increasing the agonist concentration increases the frequency with little effect on the amplitude, while for sinusoidal oscillations, increasing the agonist concentration increases the average $[Ca^{2+}]_i$ without affecting the frequency of the oscillations. Furthermore, for baseline spikes, but not for sinusoidal oscillations, the latency before the first $[Ca^{2+}]_i$ spike is inversely related to the agonist concentration. The same mechanism underlying the varying frequency of spiking also may be responsible for the varying latency for the first spike, but this is not necessarily so. The persistent, constant amplitude baseline spikes require a positive feedback mechanism, sometimes called *feed-forward,* to generate the spikes, with either a negative feedback or some capacity limitation, such as full depletion of an

A

Baseline spikes

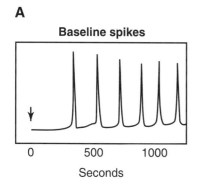

Seconds

Spikes due to positive feedback on calcium release

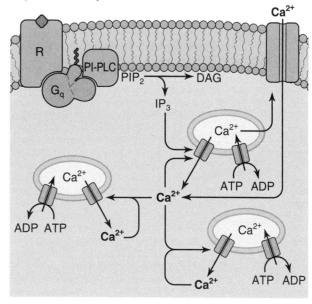

B

Sinusoidal oscillations

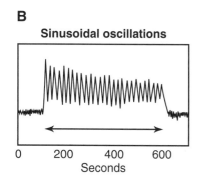

Seconds

Negative feedback by protein kinase C

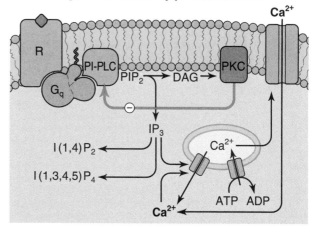

FIGURE 23-4. Patterns and mechanisms for major types of [Ca^{2+}]$_i$ oscillation. **A, Left:** A single rat hepatocyte treated with vasopressin exhibits low-frequency baseline spikes of [Ca^{2+}]$_i$. **A, Right:** The mechanism for baseline [Ca^{2+}]$_i$ spiking is seen as being initiated by a small release of Ca^{2+} from a "calciosome" by IP$_3$, and then, in the presence of a sensitizing concentration of IP$_3$, Ca^{2+} regeneratively activates release at neighboring release sites, leading to an all-or-none [Ca^{2+}]$_i$ wave propagating through the cell. **B, Left:** A single mouse lacrimal acinar cell treated with methacholine exhibits higher frequency sinusoidal oscillations superimposed on an elevated baseline. **B, Right:** The mechanism underlying sinusoidal oscillations is suggested to occur as follows: phosphoinositide-specific phospholipase C *(PI-PLC)* activation leads to production of IP$_3$ and mobilization of Ca^{2+}, but also to protein kinase C *(PKC)* activation. With some delay, the latter inhibits PI-PLC, causing a fall in IP$_3$ and an attenuation of the [Ca^{2+}]$_i$ signal. The inhibition of PI-PLC also attenuates the PKC signal, leading to a cyclical increase in [Ca^{2+}]$_i$. Continuing cycling of this feedback loop gives rise to sinusoidal oscillations. *R*, receptor; *DAG*, diacylglycerol. (Redrawn and modified from [3] with permission.)

intracellular pool, to terminate each spike. However, negative feedback alone is sufficient to explain the behavior of constant-frequency sinusoidal oscillations.

In most instances, baseline spiking will continue for at least a few cycles in the absence of extracellular Ca^{2+}, and thus, it is generally agreed that they represent cycles of discharge and reuptake of Ca^{2+} by intracellular stores. Although other models have been proposed, the currently favored mechanism of baseline $[Ca^{2+}]_i$ spiking involves fluctuations in $[Ca^{2+}]_i$ while cellular concentrations of IP_3 are constant (Fig. 23-4). Models along this theme require that Ca^{2+} itself provide both positive and negative regulation of the $[Ca^{2+}]_i$ signal. An important piece of evidence for such regulation would be the demonstration of $[Ca^{2+}]_i$ spiking induced by direct intracellular application of IP_3. This has been demonstrated in oocytes and, in a few cases, in small, mammalian cells by intracellular introduction of IP_3 through whole-cell patch pipette perfusion. These findings suggest a mechanism that operates distally to the production of IP_3 exists for generating $[Ca^{2+}]_i$ spikes.

As discussed above, biphasic regulation of IP_3-induced Ca^{2+} release by Ca^{2+} is reminiscent of the behavior of the CICR channel from skeletal muscle. In addition, the inhibitory action of Ca^{2+} on IP_3-induced Ca^{2+} release develops more slowly than the activation, with a time constant of about 0.5 sec. There is obvious similarity between this scheme, which involves a rapid Ca^{2+} activation of release followed by a more slowly developing Ca^{2+} inhibition, and the feed-forward and feedback regulation of action potentials by depolarization. As discussed above, changes in ER luminal $[Ca^{2+}]$ also may regulate the sensitivity of the IP_3 receptor. Thus, these kinetically distinct modes of regulation of the IP_3 receptor by both cytoplasmic and luminal Ca^{2+} may provide the ingredients for production of regenerative spikes and waves of $[Ca^{2+}]_i$.

Much less attention has been paid to sinusoidal oscillations of intracellular Ca^{2+}, although strictly speaking, they may represent the only instance in which the term "oscillations" is applied correctly. These are roughly symmetrical fluctuations usually superimposed on a raised basal level of $[Ca^{2+}]_i$. The most significant characteristic of these oscillations is their constant frequency at different agonist concentrations. These sinusoidal oscillations are considerably simpler than the baseline spike type of $[Ca^{2+}]_i$ oscillation and can be explained most simply by a single negative feedback on the $[Ca^{2+}]_i$-signaling mechanism. Although this may not apply in all cases, it appears that the negative feedback responsible for the sinusoidal oscillations is often due to protein kinase C (PKC). The site of negative inhibition appears to be on or proximal to PI-PLC. Activation of PI-PLC increases diacylglycerol (DAG), which in turn activates PKC. The latter feeds back and inhibits PI-PLC (see Chap. 21). This leads to a diminution in DAG production, diminished PKC activity and relief of the inhibition of PI-PLC. Continuous cycling of this delayed feedback loop generates oscillations in PI-PLC activity, which, in the absence of some feed-forward input, gradually damp down to a sustained level under tonic control by the opposing forces of receptor activation and PKC inhibition. It is important to point out that in this particular scheme $[Ca^{2+}]_i$ is simply a passive follower of the oscillating IP_3 production and plays no obvious active role in generating or modulating the oscillations. Thus, this particular type might more appropriately be called "DAG oscillations" or "PI-PLC/PKC oscillations" (Fig. 23-4).

Release of intracellular Ca^{2+} may occur from "calciosomes," a subfraction of the endoplasmic reticulum

There is considerable evidence placing the major site of calcium sequestration and the source of intracellular calcium for signaling in the ER. In addition to the points already made, early subcellular fractionation studies reported good correlations between classical enzymatic markers for ER and ATP-dependent Ca^{2+} accumulation, or IP_3-mediated Ca^{2+} release. Calcium uptake into the IP_3-sensitive store is augmented by oxalate, a property generally associated with the ER.

However, there are some inconsistencies with the idea that the IP_3-sensitive calcium store and the ER are entirely coincident. For one, there is really no correlation between the quantity of ER present in a given cell type and its sensitivity to calcium signaling through IP_3. In contrast to the studies cited above, there are at least an equal number of subcellular fractionation studies in which a separation of IP_3-induced Ca^{2+} release or IP_3 binding from enzymatic markers for the ER has been observed. Perhaps the sarcoplasmic reticulum of muscle presents the best characterized paradigm for an organelle distinct from generic ER and specialized for storing and releasing calcium (see Chap. 43). A biochemical characteristic of sarcoplasmic reticulum that distinguishes it from ER is the presence of high concentrations of a high-capacity, low-affinity calcium-binding protein, calsequestrin. A similar protein is found in nonmuscle cells, calreticulin, a protein structurally and functionally homologous to calsequestrin. On the basis of such findings, it was proposed that an organelle specialized for storing and releasing calcium existed and that this organelle was distinct from generic ER. It has been proposed that this organelle be designated "calciosome" [14].

With the exception of skeletal muscle, perhaps the most extensively characterized cell with respect to its Ca^{2+}-releasing and -sequestering organelles is the Purkinje cell of the cerebellum. The Purkinje cells of birds are especially amenable to immunocytochemical studies because they contain much higher concentrations of IP_3 receptors than any other cell type and unusually high concentrations of SERCA pumps and ryanodine receptors. In addition, the major calcium-storage protein is almost identical to mammalian calsequestrin, which facilitates immunocytochemistry because of the availability of high-affinity antibodies. In these cells, IP_3 receptors are not linked tightly to SERCA pumps or even calsequestrin. However, a population of vacuoles that were positive for calsequestrin as well as for either the IP_3 receptor or the ryanodine receptor was found. This could qualify these structures as calciosomes since presumably they are involved in storing as well as releasing calcium [15]. Specialized stacks of ER, rich in IP_3 receptor but without substantial quantities of SERCA pumps or calsequestrin, were suggested to act as either reservoirs of receptor or buffers of cytoplasmic IP_3. Interestingly, overexpression of IP_3 receptors in fibroblasts leads to the formation of structures similar to the IP_3 receptor-containing ER stacks of Purkinje cells.

Although the nature of the calciosome as a specialized subcompartment of the ER is widely accepted [15], the term "calciosome" has not gained universal acceptance. This may be due to the fact that in many systems the distinction between the calciosome and the ER is still not established clearly [16].

Although distinct, Ca^{2+}-signaling events in excitable and nonexcitable cells share some common characteristics

Traditionally, calcium-signaling research has been divided into two separate categories: studies focusing on excitable cells, like nerve and muscle, and studies focusing on electrically nonexcitable cells, such as epithelial or blood cells. Although both electrically excitable and nonexcitable cells utilize the release of intracellular Ca^{2+} as one means of generating cytoplasmic calcium signals, excitable cells often accomplish this by CICR while for nonexcitable cells the predominant mechanism involves IP_3 [17]. Also, signaling in both cell types depends to a large degree on plasma membrane Ca^{2+} channels; but the Ca^{2+} channels in the plasma membranes of nonexcitable cells do not appear to be regulated by membrane potential, and their pharmacology is quite distinct from that of the channels in excitable cells. However, calcium-signaling mechanisms in excitable and nonexcitable cells may be much more alike than is generally appreciated. A general paradigm for Ca^{2+} signaling in virtually all cell types has evolved. This paradigm involves a coordinated regulation of intracellular calcium ion release and calcium ion entry across the plasma membrane of the cell [17]. For reasons probably having to do with the distinct functions subserved by excitable and nonexcitable cells, interesting distinctions as well as similarities in basic mechanisms have evolved in these two general cell types.

In electrically nonexcitable cells, Ca^{2+} signaling is typically a biphasic process. Neurotransmitters and hormones cause a release of calcium ions to the cytoplasm from an intracellular organelle, and this is followed by entry of calcium ions into the cytoplasm across the plasma membrane. The intracellular-release phase of the calcium signal is attributable to IP_3, while the second phase of the response is attributed to capacitative calcium ion entry, a process of retrograde signaling such that the empty calcium-storage organelle produces a signal for calcium ion entry across the plasma membrane.

In many instances, neurons and other electrically excitable cells also may utilize the IP_3-signaling system. For example, there are smooth muscle types which function in the IP_3 mode, the voltage-dependent calcium channel and CICR mode or even combinations of the two. In some instances, when intracellular calcium ions are released by IP_3 in excitable cells, this may be coupled to capacitative calcium ion entry, but there are clear examples where this is not the case. Rather, virtually all excitable cells have plasma membrane Ca^{2+} channels that are activated by membrane depolarization. In addition, excitable cells frequently express another intracellular Ca^{2+} release channel, the ryanodine receptor (discussed above). The physiological activator of the ryanodine receptor is believed to be Ca^{2+} itself; the channel opens when the Ca^{2+} concentration in its vicinity increases rapidly, generating CICR, and this can give rise to the re-generative "all-or-none" calcium ion release behavior for which muscle and nerve cells are noted. In heart cells, for example, Ca^{2+} signaling is initiated by membrane depolarization, which activates surface membrane voltage-gated Ca^{2+} channels. A rapid entry of calcium ions serves as a "trigger" for activating the ryanodine receptor and, subsequently, a much larger release of intracellular calcium ions [17].

The common conceptual feature of these two calcium-signaling motifs (Fig. 23-5) is that they provide tight coordination of calcium ion entry and intracellular calcium ion release. They also provide amplification for the calcium signal but in functionally distinct ways. In excitable cells, the process of CICR amplifies the *magnitude* and *spatial distribution* of the momentary calcium signal, assuring, in the case of the heart for example, sufficient Ca^{2+} for catalyzing rapid cross-bridge formation and force development. In nonexcitable cells, the retrograde signaling provided by capacitative calcium ion entry amplifies the duration of the calcium signal, providing sustained, tonic responses of, for example, exocrine gland cells.

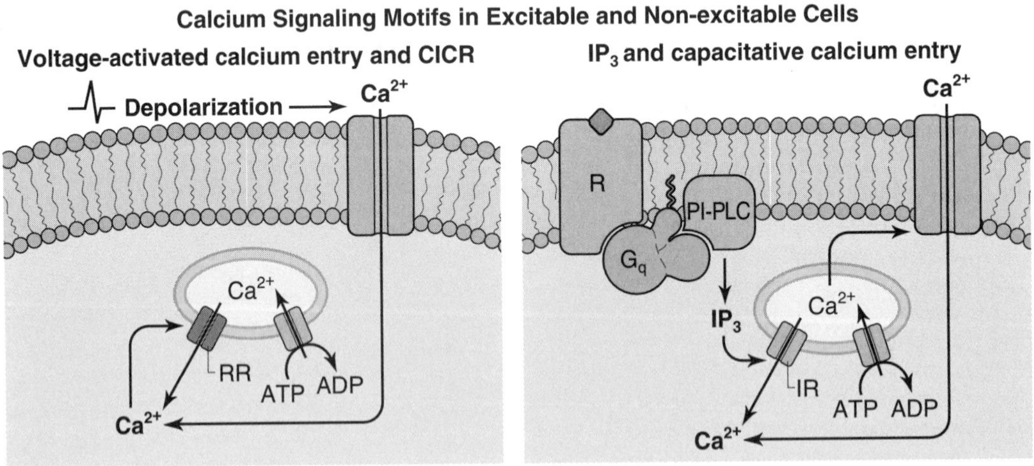

Calcium Signaling Motifs in Excitable and Non-excitable Cells

FIGURE 23-5. Motifs of $[Ca^{2+}]_i$ signaling. In electrically excitable cells **(left)**, Ca^{2+} may enter when voltage-dependent Ca^{2+} channels are activated by the depolarization associated with action potentials. This Ca^{2+} can cause further release of intracellularly stored Ca^{2+} by activating a Ca^{2+}-induced Ca^{2+} release (*CICR*) mechanism associated with the ryanodine receptor (*RR*) Ca^{2+} channel. In electrically nonexcitable cells **(right)**, signaling generally is initiated when an agonist activates a surface membrane receptor (*R*), which, usually through a G protein (G_q or G_i), activates phosphoinositide-specific phospholipase C (*PI-PLC*), which degrades phosphatidylinositol 4,5-bisphosphate, releasing the soluble messenger, inositol 1,4,5-trisphosphate (*IP$_3$*). IP_3 activates an IP_3 receptor (*IR*) and, thus, releases Ca^{2+} from an intracellular organelle to the cytoplasm. The release of Ca^{2+} from the organelle causes a signal to be generated, which activates a plasma membrane Ca^{2+} entry pathway: capacitative Ca^{2+} entry. (Modified from [17] with permission.)

These characteristics of excitable and nonexcitable cells are not as distinct as once believed. For example, capacitative calcium ion entry contributes to calcium signaling in a number of excitable cell types [9]. Also, as discussed in the preceding section, the all-or-none regenerative calcium signals which occur in nerves and muscles now are known to occur in nonexcitable cells. Thus, it is interesting that while the term nonexcitable appropriately describes the electrophysiological behavior of their surface membranes, the regenerative intracellular Ca^{2+} spikes that often are exhibited by so-called nonexcitable cells constitute a clear example of excitable behavior of their intracellular milieu. This occurs because the IP_3 receptor functions as a CICR receptor whose sensitivity to Ca^{2+} is regulated by the binding of IP_3 and *vice versa*. Perhaps this is not so surprising given the considerable homology between the amino acid sequences of the IP_3 and ryanodine receptors. Electrically nonexcitable cells generally contain only a single, rather homogeneous intracellular pool of calcium, which is sensitive to IP_3, while electrically excitable cells may have a more complex arrangement of intracellular calcium pools regulated by distinct mechanisms.

Thus, there may be substantially greater similarity between Ca^{2+}-signaling systems in excitable and nonexcitable cells than is generally thought. Cognizance of variations in calcium-signaling motifs becomes especially important given the relationship between patterns of gene expression and specific calcium-signaling pathways. It may be useful for neuroscientists and others traditionally focusing on excitable cells to take note of developments in the rapidly evolving field of calcium signaling and calcium channels in nonexcitable cells [17].

Ca^{2+}-REGULATED PROCESSES

Ca^{2+} is required for acute cellular responses, such as contraction or secretion

Sydney Ringer is credited with the first appreciation of the role of calcium as a regulator of cell function. He discovered that frog hearts beat longer *in vitro* if the saline solutions are made from "hard" water rather than from distilled water, and with this observation the role of Ca^{2+} in excitation–contraction coupling was discovered (see Chap. 43). Subsequently, Ca^{2+} was found to act as a signal for a myriad cellular responses, for example, secretion and changes in cell metabolism. Ca^{2+} is the major component of the signaling pathways that regulate epithelial cell secretion, including both discharge of proteins and regulation of transepithelial secretion of salts and water, and carbohydrate metabolism in the liver, including both glycogenolysis and gluconeogenesis (see Chaps. 31 and 42). In blood cells, various functions are subtended by PI-PLC-dependent $[Ca^{2+}]_i$ signaling, including secretion and chemotaxis. Ca^{2+} mediates the shortening of muscle by interacting with specific calcium-binding proteins; in fast skeletal muscle, this is troponin, leading to disinhibition of the myosin ATPase (see Chap. 43). In other muscle types, regulation of the phosphorylation of myosin light chain is mediated by calcium. In virtually all cases, the initial target of calcium is a specific calcium-binding protein, the most extensively characterized of which is calmodulin (see Chap. 22) [18]. Calmodulin was discovered as a Ca^{2+}-dependent regulator of cyclic nucleotide phosphodiesterase [18]. This protein now is recognized to be the most ubiquitous Ca^{2+}-sensing protein, found in all eukaryotic organisms including yeasts. Calmodulin has four binding sites for Ca^{2+} with dissociation constants in the 1 to 10 μM range. The binding of Ca^{2+} induces a conformational change which imparts signaling information to a number of different molecules, including protein kinases and phosphatases.

Ca^{2+} also plays a role in more prolonged cellular events, such as mitogenesis and apoptosis

Throughout the life span of organisms, cells make decisions about growth, division, function and death. Following mitosis, a cell must either commit to re-enter the cell cycle or exit into G_o, a quiescent state in which a differentiated function is maintained (see Chap. 27). In many, but not all, cell types, such cells may at a later time and with an appropriate stimulus re-enter the cell cycle to divide further. In circumstances in which a particular cell function is no longer needed, as in the case of the thymus, systemic signals may instruct cells to undergo a complex process of self-digestion and packaging, termed apoptosis [19]. Mutations in key genes that control mitogenesis can lead to inappropriate cell division or cancers; these are proto-oncogenes, and the transforming forms of the genes are oncogenes. It is noteworthy, although perhaps not unexpected, that the vast majority of proto-oncogenes code for proteins involved in signal-transduction pathways. One proto-oncogene, *Bcl-2*, acts as a suppressor of apoptosis such that if it is expressed in excess, cancerous growth can result.

Ca^{2+} signaling is believed to play an important role in the regulation of cell growth and differentiation [20] as well as in apoptosis [19] (discussed below). Ca^{2+} generally is required in the incubation medium for activation of mitogenesis, and in many instances, documented increases in $[Ca^{2+}]_i$ are associated with the actions of mitogenic agents. Calcium ionophores or thapsigargin can stimulate DNA synthesis, especially if combined with a PKC activator such as an active phorbol ester. This action of phorbol esters may explain their well-known tumor-promoting activity, but this has not been proven.

In addition to cytoplasmic Ca^{2+} serving as a regulator of mitogenesis, there is evidence for a role of intracellular Ca^{2+} stores, perhaps implicating a role for capacitative calcium ion entry. Interestingly, in various cell lines, depletion of intracellular stores by thapsigargin has been shown to induce mitogenesis; a quiescent, or G_o, state; or apoptosis. These differential effects could result from thapsigargin-induced Ca^{2+} signals or from inhibition of protein synthesis due to the diminished concentrations of stored Ca^{2+}. The concentration of ER Ca^{2+} plays an important role at various steps involved in protein synthesis. In those instances in which prolonged treatment with thapsigargin induces apoptosis, inhibition of protein synthesis could contribute to this process as well.

Sustained increases in intracellular Ca^{2+} have toxic effects on cells [21]. However, in the case of thapsigargin, it appears that the cells are killed by the specific, genetically programmed process known as apoptosis. When cells die due to toxic insult, the process is often one of necrosis; this is a relatively nonspecific process involving cell lysis, the release of cellular contents, which subsequently must be "cleaned up" by the immune system, involving an inflammatory reaction. However, complex organisms also have the need for cells to die at appropriate times in development and in maintenance of normal organ function. In such instances, a more orderly, noninflammatory process of programmed cell death, or apoptosis, occurs. This involves degradation of nuclear DNA by specific endonucleases, resulting in the characteristic DNA ladders which are diagnostic of apoptosis; cellular shrinkage; and ultimately the packaging of cellular constituents in membrane-delimited structures, known as apoptotic bodies, for disposition by leukocytes [19].

There is considerable evidence for a role of Ca^{2+} signaling in apoptosis [19]. For example, studies of glucocorticoid-induced apoptosis have identified a Ca^{2+} influx associated with lymphoid cell death. In addition, the action of glucocorticoids to induce apoptosis could be mimicked by Ca^{2+} ionophores. Similarly, thapsigargin triggers a full apoptotic response. Chelation of Ca^{2+} by intracellular chelators, extracellular EGTA, or overexpression of the Ca^{2+}-binding protein calbindin inhibits apoptosis due to glucocorticoids and other agents. Finally, calmodulin antagonists have been reported to disrupt apoptosis in a variety of systems. Together these data suggest a central role for Ca^{2+} in apoptosis in response to glucocorticoids and other agents [19]. However, there is also evidence that in addition to changes in cytoplasmic calcium serving as a signal or modulator for apoptosis, a fall in the concentration of Ca^{2+} in the ER can signal a full apoptotic response, independently of the associated rise in cytoplasmic Ca^{2+} [22]. It is not clear at this time whether this involves the same signaling pathway involved in capacitative calcium ion entry.

REFERENCES

1. Tsien, R. Y., Rink, T. J., and Poenie, M. Measurement of cytosolic free Ca^{2+} in individual small cells using fluorescence microscopy with dual excitation wavelengths. *Cell Calcium* 6:145–157, 1985.

2. Miller, R. J. Voltage-sensitive Ca^{2+} channels. *J. Biol. Chem.* 267:1403–1406, 1992.

3. Putney, J. W., Jr. *Capacitative Calcium Entry.* Austin, TX: Landes Biomedical Publishing, 1997.

4. Berridge, M. J. Discovery of the $InsP_3$-Ca^{2+} pathway. A personal reflection. *Adv. Second Messenger Phosphoprotein Res.* 26:1–7, 1992.

5. Furuichi, T., Kohda, K., Miyawaki, A., and Mikoshiba, K. Intracellular channels. *Curr. Biol.* 4:294–303, 1994.

6. Lee, H. C., Walseth, T. F., Bratt, G. T., Hayes, R. N., and Clapper, D. L. Structural determination of a cyclic metabolite of NAD^+ with intracellular Ca^{2+}-mobilizing activity. *J. Biol. Chem.* 264:1608–1615, 1989.

7. Dunlap, K., Luebke, J. I., and Turner, T. J. Exocytotic Ca^{2+} channels in mammalian central neurons. *Trends Neurol. Sci.* 18:89–98, 1995.

8. Putney, J. W., Jr. A model for receptor-regulated calcium entry. *Cell Calcium* 7:1–12, 1986.

9. Putney, J. W., Jr., and Bird, G. S. J. The inositol phosphate-calcium signalling system in non-excitable cells. *Endocr. Rev.* 14:610–631, 1993.

10. Penner, R., Fasolato, C., and Hoth, M. Calcium influx and its control by calcium release. *Curr. Opin. Neurobiol.* 3:368–374, 1993.

11. Hardie, R. C., and Minke, B. Phosphoinositide-mediated phototransduction in *Drosophila* photoreceptors: The role of Ca^{2+} and *trp*. *Cell Calcium* 18:256–274, 1995.

12. Zhu, X., Jiang, M., Peyton, M., et al. *trp*, a novel mammalian gene family essential for agonist-activated capacitative Ca^{2+} entry. *Cell* 85:661–671, 1996.

13. Thomas, A. P., Bird, G. S. J., Hajnóczky, G., Robb-Gaspers, L. D., and Putney, J. W., Jr. Spatial and temporal aspects of cellular calcium signalling. *FASEB J.* 10:1505–1517, 1996.

14. Volpe, P., Krause, K.-H., Hashimoto, S., et al. "Calcioisome," a cytoplasmic organelle: The inositol 1,4,5-trisphosphate-sensitive Ca^{2+} store of nonmuscle cells? *Proc. Natl. Acad. Sci. USA* 85:1091–1095, 1988.

15. Pozzan, T., Rizzuto, R., Volpe, P., and Meldolesi, J. Molecular and cellular physiology of intracellular calcium stores. *Physiol. Rev.* 74:595–636, 1994.

16. Rossier, M. F., and Putney, J. W., Jr. The identity of the calcium storing inositol 1,4,5-trisphosphate-sensitive organelle in non-muscle cells: Calciosome, endoplasmic reticulum . . . or both? *Trends Neurosci.* 14:310–314, 1991.

17. Putney, J. W., Jr. Excitement about calcium signaling in inexcitable cells. *Science* 262:676–678, 1993.

18. Klee, C. B., and Newton, D. L. Calmodulin: An overview. In J. R. Parratt (ed), *Control and Manipulation of Calcium Movement.* New York: Raven Press, 1985, pp. 131–145.

19. Schwartzman, R. A., and Cidlowski, J. A. Apoptosis: The biochemistry and molecular biology of programmed cell death. *Endocr. Rev.* 14:133–151, 1993.

20. Berridge, M. J. Control of cell division: A unifying hypothesis. *J. Cyclic Nucleotide Res.* 1:305–320, 1975.

21. Orrenius, S., and Nicotera, P. The calcium ion and cell death. *J. Neural Transm.* 43:1–11, 1994.

22. Bian, X., Hughes, F. M., Jr., Huang, Y., Cidlowski, J. A., and Putney, J. W., Jr. Roles of cytoplasmic Ca^{2+} and intracellular Ca^{2+} stores in induction and suppression of apoptosis in S49 cells. *Am. J. Physiol.* 272:C1241–C1249, 1997.

23. Burgess, G. M., McKinney, J. S., Fabiato, A., Leslie, B. A., and Putney, J. W., Jr. Calcium pools in saponin-permeabilized guinea-pig hepatocytes. *J. Biol. Chem.* 258:15336–15345, 1983.

24

Serine and Threonine Phosphorylation

Eric J. Nestler and Paul Greengard

Basic Neurochemistry: Molecular, Cellular and Medical Aspects, 6th Ed., edited by G. J. Siegel et al. Published by Lippincott–Raven Publishers, Philadelphia, 1999. Correspondence to Eric J. Nestler, Laboratory of Molecular Psychiatry, Departments of Psychiatry and Neurobiology, Yale University School of Medicine and Connecticut Mental Health Center, 34 Park Street, New Haven, Connecticut 06508.

PROTEIN PHOSPHORYLATION IS OF FUNDAMENTAL IMPORTANCE IN BIOLOGICAL REGULATION

Protein phosphorylation is the major molecular mechanism through which protein function is regulated in response to extracellular stimuli both inside and outside the nervous system. Virtually all types of extracellular signals, including neurotransmitters, hormones, light, neurotrophic factors and cytokines, produce most of their diverse physiological effects by regulating phosphorylation of specific phosphoproteins in their target cells. Virtually every class of neuronal protein is regulated by phosphorylation. Although proteins are known to be covalently modified in many other ways, including ADP-ribosylation, acylation (acetylation, myristoylation, isoprenylation), carboxymethylation, tyrosine sulfation and glycosylation, none of these mechanisms is nearly as widespread and readily subject to regulation by physiological stimuli as is phosphorylation. Thus, protein phosphorylation is by far the most prominent mechanism of neural plasticity. In this chapter, we present an overview of the vital role played by protein phosphorylation in the regulation of neuronal function.

Regulation of protein phosphorylation involves a protein kinase, a protein phosphatase and a substrate protein

These components interact according to the scheme shown in Figure 24-1. A substrate protein is converted from the dephospho form to the phospho form by a protein kinase, and the phospho form is converted back to the dephospho form by a protein phosphatase [1].

Protein kinases are classified as protein serine-threonine kinases, which phosphorylate substrate proteins on serine or threonine residues, or as protein tyrosine kinases, which phosphorylate substrate proteins on tyrosine residues. A small number of protein kinases, as will be seen below, are referred to as "dual-function" kinases because they phosphorylate substrate proteins on serine-threonine and tyrosine residues. Over 95% of protein phosphorylation occurs on serine residues, 3 to 4% on threonine

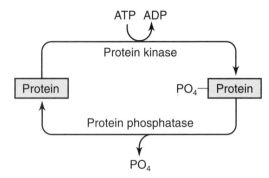

FIGURE 24-1. Schematic diagram of the conversion of a dephosphoprotein to a phosphoprotein by a protein kinase and the reversal of this reaction by a protein phosphatase.

residues and less than 1% on tyrosine residues. In all cases, the kinases catalyze the transfer of the terminal (γ) phosphate group of ATP to the hydroxyl moiety in the respective amino acid residue; Mg^{2+} is required for this reaction. Protein phosphatases catalyze the cleavage of this phosphoester bond through hydrolysis.

Because phosphate groups are highly negatively charged, phosphorylation of a protein alters its charge, which can then alter the conformation of the protein and ultimately its functional activity. A change in the state of protein phosphorylation can be achieved physiologically through increases or decreases in the activity of either a protein kinase or a protein phosphatase. Examples of each of these mechanisms are known to occur in the nervous system, often in concert with one another, to elicit complex temporal patterns of protein phosphorylation.

A general scheme of the diverse pathways through which extracellular signals regulate neuronal function through protein phosphorylation is illustrated in Figure 24-2. Two major mechanisms are involved. In one, the extracellular signals, or first messengers, regulate protein kinases or protein phosphatases indirectly by acting on plasma membrane receptors, thereby regulating the intracellular concentration of a second messenger in target neurons [1]. This is the case for first messengers that act through G protein-coupled receptors, including receptors for many neurotrans-

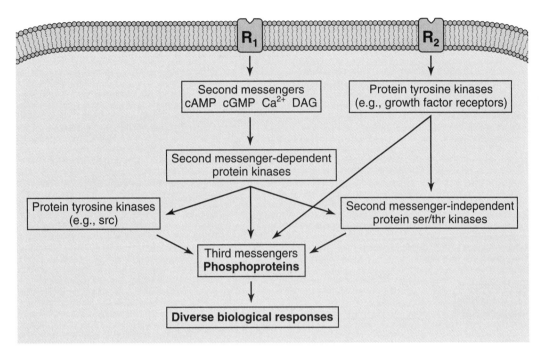

FIGURE 24-2. Signals in the brain. Extracellular signals, termed first messengers, produce specific biological responses in target neurons via a series of intracellular signals, termed second or third messengers. Second messengers in the brain include cAMP, cGMP, Ca^{2+} and diacylglycerol *(DAG)*. cAMP and cGMP produce most of their second-messenger actions through the activation of cAMP-dependent and cGMP-dependent protein kinases, respectively. Ca^{2+} exerts many of its second-messenger actions through the activation of Ca^{2+}-dependent protein kinases, as well as through a variety of physiological effectors other than protein kinases. Not illustrated in the figure is that some protein phosphatases can also be regulated directly by second messengers, for example, calcineurin, which is activated by Ca^{2+}. The brain also contains a large number of other protein serine-threonine kinases (see Table 24-1) that are not activated directly by second-messenger pathways or by protein tyrosine kinases. The brain and other tissues contain two major classes of protein tyrosine kinases. Some of these enzymes are physically associated with plasma membrane receptors, such as most growth factor receptors, and become activated upon ligand binding to the receptors. Others, such as src, are not physically associated with receptors but are influenced indirectly by both second-messenger pathways and receptor protein tyrosine kinases.

mitters, hormones, cytokines and sensory stimuli such as odorants. It also holds for first messengers that act through receptors containing intrinsic ion channels, for example, some glutamate, GABA and acetylcholine receptors, and thereby regulate second-messenger concentrations. Prominent second messengers in the nervous system that directly activate protein kinases include cAMP, cGMP, Ca^{2+} and diacylglycerol (DAG). The next steps in these pathways are the activation of specific classes of protein serine-threonine kinases or protein phosphatases by these second messengers and the subsequent phosphorylation or dephosphorylation of specific substrate proteins,

leading, through one or more steps, to specific biological responses.

In the other major mechanism, first messengers directly regulate protein kinase and phosphatase activities by acting on plasma membrane receptors that possess the enzyme activity within their cytoplasmic domains [2] (see Chap. 25). This is the case for most types of neurotrophic factors as well as many cytokines. The intrinsic protein kinase and phosphatase activities are stimulated upon ligand binding, which leads to changes in the phosphorylation state of specific substrate proteins and to the generation of specific biological responses.

PROTEIN SERINE-THREONINE KINASES

Protein kinases differ in their cellular and subcellular distribution, substrate specificity and regulation

These properties determine the functional roles played by the more than 70 types of protein kinases that have been found in mammalian tissues, most of which are known to be expressed in neurons [2,3]. The major classes of protein serine-threonine kinases in the brain, listed in Table 24-1, are covered in this chapter. The ma-

TABLE 24-1. MAJOR CLASSES OF PROTEIN SERINE-THREONINE KINASES

Second messenger-dependent protein kinases
  cAMP kinase
  cGMP kinase
  Ca^{2+}/calmodulin kinases
  Protein kinase C

MAP kinases
  ERKs
  JNKs or SAPKs

MAPKinase-regulating kinases
  MEKs
  SEKs
  Raf
  MEK kinases

CDKs
  Cdc-2

CDK-regulating kinases
  CAK
  CAK kinase

GRKs

Others
  RSKs
  Casein kinases

This list is not intended to be comprehensive. The protein kinases listed are present in many cell types in addition to neurons and are included here because of their multiple functions in the nervous system, including regulation of neuron-specific phenomena. Not included are other protein kinases present in diverse tissues, including brain, that play a role in generalized cellular processes, such as intermediary metabolism, and that may not play a role in neuron-specific phenomena. MAP kinase, mitogen activated protein kinase; ERK, extracellular signal-regulated kinase; JNK, Jun kinase; SAPK, stress-activated protein kinase; MEK, MAP kinase and ERK kinases; SEK, SAPK kinase; CDK, cyclin-dependent kinase; Cdc, cell division cycle; CAK, CDK-activating kinase; GRK, G protein receptor kinase; RSK, ribosomal S6 kinase.

jor classes of protein tyrosine kinases in the brain are discussed in Chapter 25. Among the best studied protein kinases in the brain are those activated by the second messengers cAMP, cGMP, Ca^{2+} and DAG [1,2].

cAMP-dependent protein kinase (protein kinase A; PKA) is composed of catalytic and regulatory subunits. The holoenzyme of the kinase, which consists of a tetramer of two catalytic (C) and two regulatory (R) subunits, is inactive. cAMP activates the holoenzyme by binding to the regulatory subunits, thereby causing dissociation of the holoenzyme into free regulatory and free active catalytic subunits [1]. Three isoforms of the C subunit, each of about 40 kDa, and four isoforms of the R subunit, each of 50 to 55 kDa, have been cloned from mammalian tissues. The three C subunits, designated Cα, Cβ and Cγ, exhibit a very similar and broad substrate specificity, that is, they phosphorylate a large number of physiological substrate proteins, and can generally be considered isoforms of one another. The four R subunits consist of two forms each of type I and type II proteins. RIIα and RIIβ, but not RIα and RIβ, undergo autophosphorylation, as described below. Most of these R and C subunits of the protein kinase show a wide cellular distribution in the brain.

PKA activity is present throughout the cell, associated with the plasma membrane and the cytoplasmic and nuclear fractions. The kinase is highly compartmentalized within the cell, in large part via a series of anchoring proteins, termed A kinase anchor proteins (AKAPs) [4]. Several forms of AKAPs are known, many of about 75 to 79 kDa. AKAPs bind specifically with the RIIα and RIIβ subunits of the protein kinase and thereby tether these regulatory subunits and their bound catalytic subunits to specific subcellular sites, for example, postsynaptic densities. Postsynaptic densities are specializations in distal dendrites that appose presynaptic nerve terminals and are believed to contain some of the neurotransmitter receptors and other proteins required for synaptic transmission. In this way, AKAPs keep the protein kinase in close proximity to the cascade of signal-transduction proteins it phosphorylates to regulate synaptic transmission. The important role played by AKAPs under physiological conditions is indicated by experiments in which synthetic polypeptides that disrupt AKAP–RII interactions have been shown to disrupt specific physiological effects of PKA [4].

cGMP-dependent protein kinase (PKG) is a dimer of two identical subunits. Each subunit, with an M_r of ~75,000, contains a regulatory domain, which binds cGMP, and a catalytic domain [1,4a]. As with the cAMP-dependent enzyme, cGMP activates the inactive holoenzyme by binding to the regulatory domain of the molecule; however, unlike the cAMP-dependent enzyme, activation of the cGMP-dependent holoenzyme is not accompanied by dissociation of the subunits. PKG shows a much more limited cellular distribution and substrate specificity than PKA. This reflects the smaller number of second-messenger actions of cGMP in the regulation of cell function.

Calcium/calmodulin-dependent protein kinases (CaM kinases; CaMKs) are one of two major classes of calcium-dependent kinases in the nervous system. The brain contains at least six major types of CaMK, each with very different properties. CaMK II, like the cAMP-dependent enzyme, exhibits a broad cellular distribution and substrate specificity and can be considered a "multifunctional protein kinase" in that it probably mediates many of the second-messenger actions of Ca^{2+} in many types of neurons [1,5]. By analogy to PKG, CaMK II contains a regulatory domain, which, in the resting state, binds to and inhibits a catalytic domain; this inhibition is relieved when Ca^{2+}/calmodulin binds to the regulatory domain. Several isoforms of this enzyme have been cloned, including multiple α and β subunits of ~50 and 60 kDa, respectively. The enzyme exists under physiological conditions as large multimeric complexes of identical or distinct isoforms.

CaMKs I and IV also appear to play important roles in mediating many of the second-messenger actions of Ca^{2+} in the nervous system, although their precise substrate specificity remains only partially known [6]. One interesting feature of CaMK I and IV is that both appear to be activated not only by Ca^{2+}/calmodulin-binding but also upon their phosphorylation by other protein kinases, which have been termed CaMK I kinase and CaMK IV kinase, respectively [6]. These CaMK kinases may also be Ca^{2+}/calmodulin-dependent enzymes. The CaMK IV kinase enzyme has been cloned. Interestingly, this kinase is itself phosphorylated and inhibited by PKA, thereby providing a prominent mechanism by which the cAMP and Ca^{2+} cascades interact, as will be covered in greater detail below.

The remaining three types of CaMK are phosphorylase kinase, myosin light chain kinase and CaMK III [1,7]. These enzymes appear to phosphorylate fewer substrate proteins, and in some cases only one type, under physiological conditions, and each may therefore mediate relatively fewer actions of Ca^{2+} in the nervous system.

Protein kinase C (PKC) comprises the other major class of Ca^{2+}-dependent protein kinases and is activated by Ca^{2+} in conjunction with DAG and phosphatidylserine [8]. Multiple forms of PKC have been cloned, and the brain is known to contain at least seven species of the enzyme. The variant forms of PKC exhibit different cellular distributions in the brain and different regulatory properties. For example, they differ in the relative ability of Ca^{2+} and DAG to activate them: some require both Ca^{2+} and DAG, whereas others can be activated by DAG alone, apparently without an increase in cellular Ca^{2+} concentrations. However, these enzymes show similar substrate specificities and, as a result, are often considered isoforms.

PKC exists under physiological conditions as single polypeptide chains of about 80 kDa. Each polypeptide contains a regulatory domain, which, in the resting state, binds to and inhibits a catalytic domain. This inhibition is relieved when Ca^{2+} and/or DAG binds to the regulatory domain. PKC exhibits a broad substrate specificity and mediates numerous second-messenger functions of Ca^{2+} in target neurons.

Under basal conditions, PKC is predominantly a cytoplasmic protein. Upon activation by Ca^{2+} or DAG, the enzyme associates with the plasma membrane, the site of many of its known physiological substrates, including receptors and ion channels. In fact, the translocation of PKC from the cytoplasm to the membrane has long been used as an experimental measure of enzyme activation. Such translocation has often been assayed by phorbol ester binding; phorbol esters are tumor-promoting agents that selectively bind to and activate PKC. Recently, the molecular basis of the translocation of PKC from the cytoplasm to the plasma membrane has been solved. Activated PKC, but not the inactive form of the enzyme, binds with high affinity to a series of membrane-associated proteins, termed receptors for activated C kinase (RACK) [9]. RACKs thereby function by analogy with the AKAPs for PKA to direct or recruit these widely expressed enzymes to subcellular sites where their activity is required.

Diverse actions of extracellular signals are mediated by second messenger-dependent protein kinases. The intracellular application by microinjection or transfection of PKA, PKG, CaMK II or PKC into particular types of neurons has been shown to mimic specific physiological responses (regulation of ion channels, neurotransmitter release and gene transcription) to specific first messengers (neurotransmitters or nerve impulses) for those neurons [1,5,10–12]. Where specific inhibitors of the kinases are available, their application has been shown to block the ability of the neurotransmitters to elicit those responses. Taken together, these findings demonstrate that activation of these second messenger-dependent protein kinases is both a necessary and sufficient step in the sequence of events by which certain first messengers produce some of their physiological effects.

Transgenic methodologies have provided further evidence for the importance of second messenger-dependent protein kinases in the regulation of brain signal transduction. The best example to date is provided by mice lacking subunits of CaMK II. These animals show deficiencies in a form of synaptic plasticity, long-term potentiation, in the hippocampus as well as abnormal spatial learning, a form of learning dependent on hippocampal function (see also Chap. 50).

The mitogen-activated protein kinase cascade is second messenger-independent

Although the second messenger-dependent protein kinases were identified first as playing an important role in neuronal function, we now know that many other types of protein serine-threonine kinases are also essential (see Table 24-1). Indeed, one of the most critical discoveries of the 1990s has been the delineation of the mitogen-activated protein kinase (MAPK) cascades.

MAPK were first described as "mitogen-activated protein-kinases" and shown to play an important role in cell growth. The same enzymes were described in brain as "microtubule-associated protein kinases" for their phosphorylation of microtubule-associated proteins and other neuronal cytoskeletal proteins. However, the mechanisms by which the activity of the enzymes were controlled by extracellular signals remained a mystery until recent years, when these mechanisms were elucidated based largely on advances in yeast signal transduction and the subsequent identification of homologous signaling proteins in mammalian cells [3,13,14].

The basic scheme for MAPK cascades is shown in Figure 24-3. MAPK, inactive under basal conditions, is activated by phosphorylation by another protein kinase, termed MAPK kinase. MAPK kinase itself is activated by phosphorylation by still another protein kinase, termed MAPK kinase kinase. MAPK kinase kinase is activated upon interaction with a member of the Ras superfamily of small G proteins, which are bound to the plasma membrane (see Chap. 20). The exact mechanism of activation remains unknown, but it is believed that Ras and related proteins, in the activated GTP-bound form, can bind MAPK kinase kinase and thereby draw the kinase to the plasma membrane, where it is activated by as yet unknown factors, perhaps even an additional kinase, MAPK kinase kinase kinase. The mechanism governing the activation of Ras and related proteins by extracellular signals is quite complex and involves numerous "linker" proteins, for example, Shc, Grb and Sos, that couple Ras to a variety of plasma membrane-associated growth factor-protein tyrosine kinase receptors (see Chaps. 19, 20 and 25).

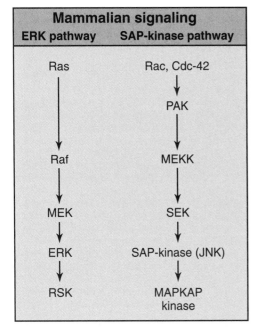
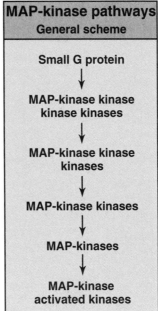
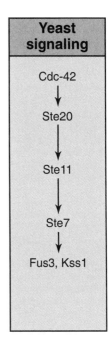

FIGURE 24-3. Schematic diagram of mitogen-activated protein kinase *(MAP-kinase)* pathways. To the **right** is shown the original pathway delineated in yeast. To the **left** are shown the homologous pathways more recently identified in mammalian cells, including brain. *MEKK,* MEK kinase; *MEK,* MAPK and ERK kinase; *ERK,* extracellular signal-regulated kinase; *RSK,* ribosomal S6 kinase; *SEK,* SAP-kinase kinase; *SAP-kinase,* stress-activated protein kinase; *JNK,* Jun kinase; *MAPKAP kinase,* MAP-kinase-activated protein kinase; *PAK,* p21-activated kinase.

The best characterized family of MAPK in the brain are the extracellular signal-regulated protein kinases (ERKs) that are activated by the neurotrophins and related growth factors (Fig. 24-3) [3,13,14]. The MAPK kinases responsible for phosphorylation and activation of the ERKs are referred to as ERK kinases II (MEKs). MEK phosphorylates ERK on a threonine and tyrosine residue, both of which are required for ERK activation. MEK is, therefore, an example of a dual-function protein kinase that can phosphorylate a substrate protein on these two types of residue. The phosphorylated threonine and tyrosine residues in all known forms of ERK are separated by a single amino acid, giving rise to the conserved threonine–amino acid–tyrosine sequence (T-X-Y). The MAPK kinase kinases responsible for MEK activation include a group of protein serine-threonine kinases termed Raf. Raf, in turn, is activated in part by one of three known forms of Ras, which is activated in response to the binding of many types of growth factors to their receptors. Thus, the neu-

rotrophins, such as nerve growth factor (NGF), brain-derived neurotrophic factor (BDNF) and related growth factors, such as epidermal growth factor and insulin, bind to plasma membrane receptors that possess intrinsic protein tyrosine kinase activity in their cytoplasmic domains. Activation of this activity upon growth factor binding leads to Ras activation via a cascade of linker proteins, as mentioned above (see Chap. 19).

The brain contains numerous forms of ERK, MEK and Raf (designated ERK1, 2, 3; MEK1, 2; Raf 1, 2, 3; and so on), which are expressed in distinct populations of neurons. Given that the major activators of the ERK cascade are growth factors, it is not surprising that these enzymes have been implicated in neuronal growth, differentiation and survival. Moreover, it has become apparent that these enzymes also are likely to play a role in synaptic transmission in the adult nervous system.

A second family of MAPK is referred to as stress-activated protein kinases (SAPKs)

[3,13,14]. This includes JNKs, or Jun kinases, named originally for their phosphorylation of the transcription factor c-Jun. SAPKs were first identified in peripheral tissues based on their activation in response to cellular forms of stress, which include X-ray irradiation and osmotic stress. More recently, they have been demonstrated to be activated in brain by several cytokines as well as synaptic activity. As shown in Figure 24-3, SAPKs are activated by SAPK kinases (SEKs), which are in turn activated by MEK kinases. The Ras-like small G proteins implicated in MEK kinase activation are Rac and Cdc-42. In this case, it appears that Rac/Cdc-42 triggers activation of MEK kinase by stimulating its phosphorylation by still another protein kinase termed p21 activated kinase (PAK). Thus, PAK can be considered a MAPK kinase kinase kinase, which is analogous to the cascade of protein kinases found in yeast (Fig. 24-3).

A dramatic feature of MAPK cascades is the series of successive protein kinases involved. While the evolutionary basis of such cascades remains unknown, they clearly evolved very early and could provide the basis for explosive amplification of an initiating extracellular signal that acts on very rare plasma membrane receptors. One of the major challenges in current research is to define the precise mechanisms for the myriad effects of MAPK by identifying their physiological substrate proteins. Among the best-characterized substrate proteins are transcription factors [3,13,14] (See Chap. 26). Phosphorylation of c-Jun by JNK is thought to increase transcriptional activity of c-Jun. Elk-1, also a transcription factor, is phosphorylated and activated by ERK. Upon phosphorylation, Elk-1 complexes with other proteins to form serum response factor, which binds to the serum response element present in the promoters of numerous genes, including c-Fos, another transcription factor.

Other types of proteins are also known to be physiological substrates for the MAPKs. Tyrosine hydroxylase, the rate-limiting enzyme in the synthesis of catecholamine neurotransmitters, is phosphorylated by ERK, which appears to increase the activity of the enzyme in response to other activating stimuli (see below and Chap. 12). Phospholipase A_2, the first enzyme in the generation of prostaglandin and related metabolites of arachidonic acid, is phosphorylated and activated by ERK. Cytoskeletal proteins, such as microtubule-associated proteins and tau, are also prominent substrates, although the precise effect phosphorylation has on the physiological activity of these proteins remains poorly understood. Finally, among the substrates for the MAPK are still other protein kinases. Thus, one important effector mechanism for ERK is phosphorylation and activation of ribosomal S6 kinase (RSK), a protein serine-threonine kinase first identified for its phosphorylation and regulation of ribosomal proteins but now known to phosphorylate other types of substrates, including the transcription factor cAMP response element-binding protein (CREB) [12]. An analogous motif is seen for the SAPKs, which also appear to produce some of their biological effects via the phosphorylation and activation of other serine-threonine kinases, such as MAPK-activated protein kinase (MAPKAP) [14].

The brain contains many other types of second messenger-independent protein kinases

Examples of second messenger-independent protein kinases are listed in Table 24-1. Many of these include enzymes that were identified originally in association with a particular substrate protein but shown later to play a more widespread role in brain signal transduction [1–3]. The functional role of one of these, β-adrenergic receptor kinase (βARK), a type of G protein receptor kinase (GRK), is discussed further below.

Other examples of protein serine-threonine kinases are the cyclin-dependent kinases (CDKs), identified originally for their role in the control of the cell cycle [3]. Such kinases, again identified originally in yeast, are among a large number of proteins termed cell division cycle (Cdc) proteins. The prototypical CDK is Cdc-2, which is phosphorylated and activated by another protein kinase termed CDK-activating kinase (CAK). This phosphorylation depends on the presence of a protein, termed cyclin, which is required for Cdc-2 activity. CAK activity requires still another protein kinase, termed CAK-activating kinase (CAKAK), although the details of these cascades remain preliminary. While the function of Cdc-2 is best understood within the context of cell-cycle control, as stated above, the enzyme has been shown to phosphorylate neuron-specific proteins, which raises the possibility that CDKs, expressed at high concentrations in nondividing adult neurons, modulate aspects of synaptic transmission.

Most protein serine-threonine kinases undergo autophosphorylation

The autophosphorylation of most protein kinases is associated with an increase in kinase activity [1,5]. In some instances, such as with the RII subunit of PKA, autophosphorylation appears to represent a positive feedback mechanism for kinase activation, in this case by enhancing the rate of dissociation of the RII and C subunits. In the case of CaMK II, autophosphorylation causes the catalytic activity of the enzyme to become independent of Ca^{2+} and calmodulin. This means that the enzyme, activated originally in response to elevated cellular Ca^{2+}, remains active after Ca^{2+} concentrations have returned to baseline. By this mechanism, neurotransmitters that activate CaMK II can produce relatively long-lived alterations in neuronal function. In other instances, such as with the receptor-associated protein tyrosine kinases (discussed in Chap. 25), autophosphorylation is an obligatory step in the sequence of molecular events through which those kinases are activated and produce physiological effects.

PROTEIN SERINE-THREONINE PHOSPHATASES

For many years, much less was known about protein phosphatases than protein kinases. This reflected the general inclination to concentrate on "turn-on" processes as opposed to "turn-off" processes as well as the greater technical difficulties associated with the study of protein phosphatases. However, a systematic characterization of protein phosphatases in the nervous system and peripheral tissues has been initiated in more recent years. This work has indicated that mammalian cells contain numerous forms of protein phosphatases and that many first messengers elicit physiological responses in the brain

through the specific regulation of these enzymes. Protein phosphatases, like protein kinases, are classified as protein serine-threonine phosphatases or protein tyrosine phosphatases, based on the amino acid residues they dephosphorylate.

The brain contains multiple forms of protein serine-threonine phosphatases

These differ in their regional distribution, substrate specificity and regulation by cellular messengers. The original classification of protein serine-threonine phosphatases as protein phosphatase 1 or 2 (PP1 or PP2) was based on their preferred dephosphorylation of, respectively, the β or α subunit of phosphorylase kinase. PP2 was later subdivided into three subtypes, termed PP2A through C, based on differential biochemical and regulatory properties. Each of these enzymes, including several subtypes, has now been cloned along with several additional protein serine-threonine phosphatases [3,15,16]. The current classification of these various enzymes, listed in Table 24-2, has retained their historical nomenclature, despite the fact that we now know that such classification does not follow particular structural or functional properties. For example, PP1 and PP2A are closely related structurally and functionally, whereas PP2C is more distantly related based on amino acid homology.

Protein phosphatase 1. Four subtypes of PP1, derived from three genes, are known. These enzymes, listed in Table 24-2, are highly homologous and exhibit similar substrate specificities; therefore, they can be considered isoforms. However, the proteins exhibit very distinct patterns of distribution in the brain. PP1 appears to be the most prevalent serine-threonine protein phosphatase in mammalian cells. It also phosphorylates a wide array of substrate proteins. Its activity is highly regulated by a series of proteins, known as PP1 inhibitor proteins, as will be discussed below.

The subcellular localization of PP1 appears to be determined by a series of other proteins, which are now considered to be integral subunits of the enzyme [3,15,16]. For example, the M subunit targets PP1 to myofibrils in smooth

TABLE 24-2.   CLASSES OF PROTEIN SERINE-THREONINE PHOSPHATASES

Protein phosphatases	Inhibitor proteins
PP1	
α, β, γ₁, γ₂	Inhibitor 1, inhibitor 2, DARPP-32, NIPP1
PP2A	Inhibitor 1²ᴬ, inhibitor 2²ᴬ
PP2B (calcineurin)	Immunophilins
	Cyclosporin A–cyclophilin, FK506–FK506-binding pro-
tein	
PP2C	
PP4	
PP5	
Others?	
Dual-function phosphatases (VH1 family)	
MKP (MAPK phosphatases), Cdc25	

PP, protein phosphatase; VH1, vaccinia virus; MAPK, mitogen-activated protein kinase; Cdc, cell division cycle; DARPP-32, dopamine and cAMP-regulated phosphoprotein of 32 kDa; NIPP1, nuclear inhibitor of PP1.

muscle. In addition, the several known isoforms of PP1 show region-specific expression in the brain. Certain forms, PP1α and PP1γ1, are highly enriched in dendritic spines of certain neurons, which presumably reflects the important role played by the enzyme in synaptic transmission. The subunit responsible for this dendritic localization may be a protein termed spinophilin [16a]. The cell nucleus also contains high concentrations of PP1, where it is believed to play an important role in the dephosphorylation of transcription factors critical to the control of gene transcription.

Protein phospatase 2A is a multisubunit enzyme composed of three subunits: a catalytic, or C, subunit; an A subunit, which is believed to provide structural support to the C subunit; and a B subunit, which is believed to determine the subcellular localization and substrate specificity of the C subunit (Table 24-2) [3,15,16]. There are two known forms of the C subunit, but these are very similar functionally and are considered to be isoforms of each other. In contrast, there appear to be multiple forms of the B subunit, which are expressed differentially in mammalian tissues. While the precise functions of individual B subunits remain incompletely understood, it appears that B subunits expressed in a particular cell specify the cell type-specific functions of the phosphatase. PP2A is largely a cytosolic enzyme but also exists in the cell nucleus.

Protein phosphatase 2B, also called calcineurin, is a Ca^{2+}/calmodulin-activated enzyme composed of two major subunits: the A subunit contains the catalytic activity and is highly homologous to PP1 and the B subunit contains two calmodulin-like domains and is thought to be responsible for binding Ca^{2+}/calmodulin [3,15,16]. PP2B is expressed in a region-specific manner in the brain, enriched particularly in striatal regions. PP2B, like PP1, exhibits a broad substrate specificity. Moreover, based on its regulation by Ca^{2+}, it is believed to mediate many physiological responses to neurotransmitters and nerve impulses. PP2B binds with high affinity to AKAPs, which localize the enzyme to subcellular sites also enriched in PKA, such as postsynaptic densities [4,9]. As will be seen below, this is presumably one molecular basis for the complex interactions found between PP2B, the protein kinase and other regulatory proteins.

The activity of PP2B is also regulated by a series of proteins termed immunophilins [16,17]. These proteins, the prototypical example of which is cyclophilin, were first identified as the targets of potent immunosuppressive drugs, such as cyclosporin and FK-506. It is now known that immunophilins bind to PP2B and inhibit its catalytic activity and that immunosuppressive drugs promote this action. Both the A and B subunits of PP2B are involved in the binding of immunophilins. The immunosuppressive/immunophilin-mediated reduction in PP2B activity results in loss of the ability of Ca^{2+} to activate T lymphocytes, which mediates the immunosuppressive effects of the drugs. Although first described in the immune system, immunophilins are expressed in the brain in a region-specific manner and have been implicated in the regulation of synaptic transmission [18]. It will be interesting in future studies to further elaborate the functional importance of PP2B–immunophilin interactions in the regulation of neuronal function.

Protein serine-threonine phosphatases play a critical role in the control of cell function

This is demonstrated by a variety of naturally occurring toxins that inhibit cellular protein phosphatase activity [15,16]. Some of these are potent tumor-promoting agents. Examples of such toxins are okadaic acid and microcystin, which are potent inhibitors of PP1 and PP2A. In addition to demonstrating the critical balance maintained in cells between protein phosphorylation and dephosphorylation, these protein phosphatase inhibitors have been used as tools to elaborate the specific role of protein phosphatases in the nervous system. One of the best-characterized examples of neural plasticity in which protein phosphatases have been shown to play a critical role is long-term depression in hippocampus, a phenomenon wherein low-frequency stimulation of presynaptic nerve activity reduces the ability of the postsynaptic neuron to respond to subsequent stimulation [5,10].

Protein phosphatase 1 and protein phosphatase 2A are regulated by protein phosphatase inhibitor proteins

This is best established for PP1, which is inhibited by at least four such proteins: inhibitor 1, inhibitor 2, dopamine- and cAMP-regulated phosphoprotein of 32 kDa (DARPP-32) and nuclear inhibitor of PP1 (NIPP1) (see Table 24-2) [17]. Inhibitor 1 is a substrate for PKA; inhibitor 2 is a substrate for glycogen synthase kinase-3; DARPP-32 and NIPP1 are substrates for PKA and casein kinases. Phosphorylation of inhibitor 1 and DARPP-32 leads to activation of their phosphatase-inhibitory activity, whereas phosphorylation of inhibitor 2 and NIPP1 leads to inactivation of their phosphatase-inhibitory activity. All four inhibitors are low-molecular-weight, acid-soluble, heat-stable proteins and exhibit some homology in their amino acid composition.

Whereas inhibitors 1 and 2 and NIPP1 appear to be widely distributed in mammalian tissues, including brain, DARPP-32 shows a much more restricted distribution. The protein is enriched in discrete populations of neurons in the brain, most prominently those that express D1-dopamine receptors. Some neuronal cell types thus appear to contain unique species of phosphatase inhibitor proteins. The critical role played by these various proteins in neuronal function is illustrated below.

In contrast to inhibitor 1, DARPP-32 and NIPP1, which regulate signal transduction, the function of inhibitor 2 appears to be different. There is increasing evidence that inhibitor 2 associates with PP1 as the phosphatase is newly synthesized and contributes to the proper folding of the enzyme [17]. Inhibitor 2 can thus be considered a chaperone protein. The inactive PP1–inhibitor 2 complex can then be activated upon phosphorylation of inhibitor 2 by glycogen synthase kinase-3. Whether this process is regulated in neurons in association with synaptic activity remains unknown.

Inhibitor proteins have more recently been identified for PP2A [16,17]. These proteins have been designated inhibitor 1^{2A} and inhibitor 2^{2A} to distinguish them from inhibitors 1 and 2 of PP1. The structural and functional properties of these PP2A inhibitors remain poorly characterized. In addition to regulation by these inhibitors, there is evidence that PP2A may be directly inhibited upon its phosphorylation by as yet unidentified protein serine-threonine and tyrosine protein kinases. The role of PP2A in the brain is less well understood compared to PP1 and PP2B. In peripheral tissues, PP2A is implicated in the control of cell growth via the dephosphorylation of some of the components of the MAPK cascades as well as of Cdc-2 and related CDKs.

Mitogen-activated protein kinase phosphatases are dual-function protein phosphatases

Just as the MAPK kinases are unique as dual-functioning kinases in that they phosphorylate MAPK on threonine and tyrosine residues, there are unique dual-functioning protein phosphatases that reverse the phosphorylation and activation of MAPK [19]. Such MAPK phosphatases (MKPs) were first identified as a product of vaccinia virus (VH1) and later found in all eukaryotic cells. There are now numerous members of this VH1 family of dual-functioning protein phosphatases. These enzymes are more closely related, in terms of their amino acid sequences, to protein tyrosine phosphatases than to protein serine-threonine phosphatases.

Some members of this family have been shown to mediate the dephosphorylation of MAPKs under physiological conditions. Others dephosphorylate Cdc-2 and related CDKs. However, relatively little is known to date about the regional distribution of these dual-functioning phosphatases in the brain and the specific role these enzymes play in the regulation of neuronal signal transduction. Considerable interest has focused on one particular MAPK phosphatase, which can be induced very rapidly, at the level of gene transcription, in target cells in response to cellular activation [20].

NEURONAL PHOSPHOPROTEINS

Virtually all types of neuronal proteins are regulated by phosphorylation

Examples of neuronal phosphoproteins are given in Table 24-3. Regulation of these proteins by phosphorylation is reviewed in detail elsewhere [1,5,7,12,21–24]. Phosphorylation of these many types of proteins is involved in carrying out or regulating virtually every process in the nervous system. Indeed, it is difficult to identify a neural process, including an example of neural plasticity, in which phosphorylation of specific phosphoproteins is not integrally involved.

Phosphorylation of enzymes that synthesize neurotransmitters regulates the capacity of a neuron for synaptic transmission. Phosphorylation of ion channels regulates the ability of these channels to open or close and thereby mediates synaptic potentials of neurotransmitters as well as more general changes in neuronal excitability.

Phosphorylation of receptors and other signaling proteins regulates the ability of neurotransmitters and other first messengers to produce their physiological effects. Phosphorylation of synaptic vesicle-associated proteins regulates neurotransmitter release in response to subsequent stimuli. Phosphorylation of cytoskeletal and related proteins regulates axoplasmic transport as well as neuronal growth, shape, survival and elaboration and retraction of dendritic and axonal processes. Phosphorylation of transcription factors and ribosomal proteins regulates the expression of specific genes in target neurons, the ultimate form of signal transduction and neural plasticity.

Protein phosphorylation is an important mechanism of memory

Phosphorylation of any of the aforementioned types of proteins can be viewed as "molecular memory": a change in the structure and function of a protein that reflects perturbation of a specific signal-transduction pathway in a specific neuronal cell type. Presumably, learning and memory manifested at a behavioral level are established through the accumulation of many types of phosphorylation events that alter the functioning of individual neurons and the neural circuits in which they operate. Short-term memory may involve the phosphorylation of presynaptic or postsynaptic proteins in response to synaptic activity, which would result in transient facilitation or inhibition of synaptic transmission. Long-term memory may involve the phosphorylation of proteins that play a part in the regulation of gene expression, which would result in more permanent modifications of synaptic transmission [1]. For example, long-term potentiation (LTP), one of the most extensively studied models of memory at the cellular level, seems to be initiated through short-term changes in calcium-dependent protein phosphorylation and maintained by longer-term changes in gene expression [6,10,25]. Although the specific presynaptic and postsynaptic proteins regulated in this manner have not yet been identified with certainty, one model proposes that the phosphorylation of glutamate receptors may be involved [10,21,22].

TABLE 24-3. CLASSES OF NEURONAL PROTEINS REGULATED BY PHOSPHORYLATION

Enzymes involved in neurotransmitter biosynthesis and degradation
  Tyrosine hydroxylase
  Tryptophan hydroxylase

Neurotransmitter receptors
  β-Adrenergic receptors
  α_2-Adrenergic receptors
  Muscarinic cholinergic receptors
  Opioid receptors
  $GABA_A$ receptor subunits
  NMDA glutamate receptor subunits
  Non-NMDA glutamate receptor subunits
  Nicotinic acetylcholine receptor subunits

Neurotransmitter transporters
  Monoamine-reuptake transporters
  Monoamine vesicle transporters (VAT)

Ion channels
  Voltage-dependent Na^+, K^+, Ca^{2+} channels
  Ligand-gated channels
  Ca^{2+}-dependent potassium channels

Enzymes and other proteins involved in the regulation of second messenger
  G proteins
  Phospholipases
  Adenylyl cyclases
  Guanylyl cyclases
  Phosphodiesterases
  IP_3 receptor

Protein kinases
  Autophosphorylated protein kinases (protein kinases phosphorylating themselves)
  Protein kinases phosphorylated by other protein kinases (many examples)

Protein phosphatase inhibitors
  DARPP-32
  Inhibitors 1 and 2

Cytoskeletal proteins involved in neuronal growth, shape and motility
  Actin
  Tubulin
  Neurofilaments (and other intermediate filament proteins)
  Myosin
  Microtubule-associated proteins
  Actin-binding proteins

Synaptic vesicle proteins involved in neurotransmitter release
  Synapsins I and II
  Clathrin
  Synaptophysin
  Synaptobrevin

Transcription factors
  CREB family members
  Fos and Jun family members
  STATs
  Steroid and thyroid hormone receptors
  NFκB-IKB family

Other proteins involved in DNA transcription or mRNA translation
  RNA polymerase
  Topoisomerase
  Histones and nonhistone nuclear proteins
  Ribosomal protein S6
  eIF (eukaryotic initiation factor)
  eEF (eukaryotic elongation factor)
  Other ribosomal proteins

Miscellaneous
  Myelin basic protein
  Rhodopsin
  Neural cell adhesion proteins
  MARCKS
  GAP-43

This list is not intended to be comprehensive but, instead, to indicate the wide array of neuronal proteins regulated by phosphorylation. Some of the proteins are specific to neurons, but most are present in many cell types in addition to neurons and are included because their multiple functions in the nervous system include the regulation of neuron-specific phenomena. Not included are the many phosphoproteins present in diverse tissues, including brain, that play a role in generalized cellular processes, such as intermediary metabolism, and that do not appear to play a role in neuron-specific phenomena. NMDA, *N*-methyl-D-aspartate; CREB, cAMP response element-binding proteins; STAT, signal-transducing activators of transcription; GAP-43, growth-associated protein of 43 kDa; MARCKS, myristoylated alanine-rich C kinase substrate; IP_3, inositol trisphosphate; DARPP-32, dopamine and cAMP-regulated phosphoprotein of 32 kDa.

Neuronal phosphoproteins differ considerably in the number and types of amino acid residues phosphorylated

The complexity of intracellular regulation is underscored by the now well-established observation that many, perhaps even most, proteins are phosphorylated on more than one amino acid residue by more than one type of protein kinase. Depending on the protein, phosphorylation of different residues can lead to similar or opposite changes in the function of that protein. It may take, for example, phosphorylation of multiple nearby residues to produce a change in the charge of the protein sufficient to result in some critical change in function. This appears to be the case for MAPKs, activation of which requires the phosphorylation of nearby threonine and tyrosine residues. In contrast, phosphorylation of one residue may activate a protein, whereas phosphorylation of another might inhibit it; this is the case for CREB, as will be described below. In still other cases, interactions among the sites of phosphorylation of a protein can be more complex: phosphorylation of one residue can influence the ability of the other residues to undergo phosphorylation. An example of this situation is DARPP-32 (discussed below). Phosphorylation of neuronal proteins by more than one protein kinase can integrate the activities of multiple intracellular pathways to achieve coordinated regulation of cell function.

The phosphorylation of a protein can influence its functional activity in several ways

For many proteins, a change in charge and conformation, due to the addition of phosphate groups to the primary structure, results in alterations in their intrinsic functional activity. For example, the catalytic activity of an enzyme can be switched on or off, or an ion channel can open or close upon such a change in charge and conformation. For many other proteins, phosphorylation-induced changes in charge and conformation result in alterations in the affinity of the proteins for other molecules. For example, phosphorylation alters the affinity of numerous enzymes for their cofactors and end-product inhibitors, phosphorylation of receptors can alter their affinity for G proteins and phosphorylation of some transcription factors alters their DNA-binding properties.

Phosphorylation can provide the primary mechanism by which a protein is regulated physiologically, or it can exert a modulatory influence on protein function. This point is illustrated by consideration of ion channels. Phosphorylation of some ion channels represents the primary mechanism by which the channels are gated, that is, whether they are open or closed. This appears to be the case, for exam-

ple, for a nonspecific cation channel in noradrenergic neurons of the locus ceruleus, which is activated by the phosphorylation of the channel or a closely associated protein by PKA (see later discussion of opiate addiction). In contrast, phosphorylation of most other channels, for example, voltage-gated Na^+, K^+ and Ca^{2+} channels, plays a modulatory role by altering the probability of the channels to open or close in response to a change in membrane potential (see Chap. 6).

To illustrate some of the roles played by protein phosphorylation in the regulation of nervous system function, five well-characterized neuronal phosphoproteins are discussed in detail.

Tyrosine hydroxylase is the rate-limiting enzyme in the biosynthesis of the catecholamine neurotransmitters dopamine, norepinephrine and epinephrine. A number of extracellular signals have been shown to stimulate catecholamine biosynthesis *in vivo,* effects mediated at least in part through increases in the catalytic activity of tyrosine hydroxylase (see also Chap. 12). We now know that such changes in the catalytic activity of tyrosine hydroxylase are achieved largely through cAMP-dependent and Ca^{2+}-dependent phosphorylation of the enzyme [26,27].

Tyrosine hydroxylase is a tetramer of identical 60-kDa subunits. The enzyme is an effective substrate for at least three protein kinases: PKA, CaMK II and PKC. One site, serine 40, of tyrosine hydroxylase is phosphorylated by all three kinases, whereas a second site, serine 19, is phosphorylated only by CaMK II. Phosphorylation of either site by CaMK II is reported to require the presence of an "activator" protein, termed 14-3-3, which has been cloned. Phosphorylation appears to increase the catalytic activity of tyrosine hydroxylase by increasing the V_{max} of the enzyme and the affinity of the enzyme for its pterin cofactor and by decreasing the affinity of the enzyme for its end-product inhibitor. Tyrosine hydroxylase also contains additional serine residues that are phosphorylated by other protein kinases. For example, the enzyme is phosphorylated on serine 31 by ERK, which is also thought to increase the catalytic activity of the enzyme.

Tyrosine hydroxylase is present in neurons

in the CNS and PNS that synthesize cate-cholamines. The enzyme is also present at high concentrations in cells that are developmentally related to catecholaminergic neurons, such as adrenal chromaffin cells and pheochromocytoma cells. Tyrosine hydroxylase is predominantly a cytosolic protein and is present in high concentrations in catecholaminergic nerve terminals.

The regulation of phosphorylation of tyrosine hydroxylase is effected by stimuli that increase Ca^{2+} or cAMP concentrations in neurons, including nerve impulse conduction and certain neurotransmitters in well-defined regions of the nervous system, in the adrenal medulla and in cultured pheochromocytoma cells. In addition, tyrosine hydroxylase phosphorylation is stimulated by nerve growth factor in certain cell types, possibly via the activation of ERKs. These changes in the phosphorylation of tyrosine hydroxylase have been shown to correlate with changes in the catalytic activity of the enzyme and in the rate of catecholamine biosynthesis.

Several key questions remain with regard to the regulation of tyrosine hydroxylase by phosphorylation. What is the precise effect of the phosphorylation of each of these serine residues on the catalytic activity of the enzyme? How does the phosphorylation of multiple residues affect enzyme activity? Does the phosphorylation of one residue affect the ability of the others to be phosphorylated? Tyrosine hydroxylase provides a striking example as to how multiple intracellular messengers and protein kinases converge functionally through the phosphorylation of a single substrate protein. Phosphorylation of tyrosine hydroxylase by cAMP-dependent and Ca^{2+}-dependent protein kinases and by MAPK casades enables a catecholaminergic cell to adjust its rate of neurotransmitter biosynthesis to a host of external stimuli and to changing physiological needs.

β-Adrenergic receptors, of which three subtypes have been cloned, mediate many of the effects of norepinephrine and epinephrine in the brain and peripheral tissues. One of the dramatic features of β-adrenergic receptor function is its rapid desensitization in response to agonist stimulation. It is now known that one important mechanism for this desensitization is phospho-rylation of the receptor both by PKA and by a receptor-associated protein kinase, βARK (Fig. 24-4).

Activation of the β-adrenergic receptor leads, via coupling with G_s, to activation of adenylyl cyclase and increased concentrations of cAMP and of activated PKA. The activated kinase then leads to the many physiological effects of β-adrenergic receptor stimulation via the phosphorylation of numerous substrate proteins. However, among those proteins phosphorylated by the kinase is the receptor itself, which is phosphorylated on several serine residues in its cytoplasmic domains. This phosphorylation reduces subsequent activation of the receptor, although the precise mechanism for desensitization remains unknown. One possibility is that phosphorylation of the receptor triggers internalization of the receptor from the plasma membrane, rendering it inaccessible to further agonist stimulation. Internalized receptor can either be returned to the plasma membrane upon its dephosphorylation or undergo proteolysis during periods of prolonged agonist exposure.

Phosphorylation of the β-adrenergic receptor by PKA can be viewed as a classical example of negative feedback: activation of the receptor stimulates intracellular cascades that feed back to reduce further receptor activation. Phosphorylation of the receptor by PKA could also mediate heterologous desensitization of the receptor: any neurotransmitter–receptor system that works through cAMP would be expected to stimulate β-adrenergic receptor phosphorylation via PKA and lead to receptor desensitization. This is one mechanism by which one neurotransmitter–receptor system can affect another.

The β-adrenergic receptor is also phosphorylated on several distinct serine residues by βARK, a protein serine-threonine kinase which is constitutively active and not regulated by second messengers (Fig. 24-3). Rather, this kinase can phosphorylate the receptor only when the receptor is bound to ligand; that is, the binding of ligand to the receptor alters the conformation of the receptor such that it is rendered a good substrate for the receptor kinase. Upon phosphorylation by βARK, the receptor is then able to bind an additional protein, called βarrestin,

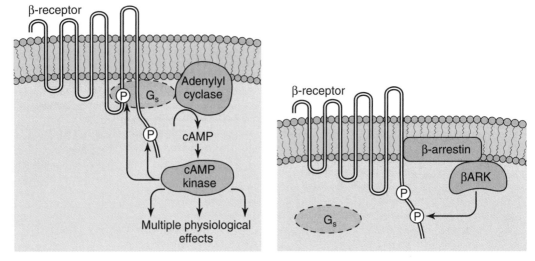

FIGURE 24-4.   Scheme illustrating desensitization of the β-adrenergic receptor mediated by receptor phosphorylation. **A:** Activation of the β-adrenergic receptor by its ligand results, via coupling with G_s, in stimulation of adenylyl cyclase, increased concentrations of cAMP and stimulation of cAMP-dependent protein kinase, which mediates the physiological effects of β-receptor activation through the phosphorylation of numerous cellular proteins. The protein kinase also phosphorylates several serine residues in cytoplasmic domains of the receptor, which results in receptor desensitization. **B:** Activation of the β-adrenergic receptor also results in a conformational change in the receptor, which renders it an effective substrate for β-adrenergic receptor kinase *(βARK)*. βARK phosphorylates the receptor at distinct serine residues, which leads to the functional "uncoupling" of the receptor from G_s, thereby resulting in receptor desensitization. This uncoupling requires the action of an additional protein, termed βarrestin, which interacts preferentially with the phosphorylated receptor to prevent its activation of G_s.

which in a sense sequesters the receptor and renders it unable to interact further with ligand or G protein. Recent work (described in Chap. 20) has shown that the βγ subunits of G proteins are required to bring βARK, predominantly a cytosolic enzyme, into close association with those plasma membrane-associated receptors that are occupied by ligand.

Phosphorylation of the β-adrenergic receptor by βARK, like its phosphorylation by the cAMP-dependent enzyme, would represent an example of negative feedback. However, unlike phosphorylation by cAMP-dependent protein kinase, phosphorylation by βARK represents an example of homologous desensitization: only the β-adrenergic receptor would be affected in this process and, moreover, only those receptor molecules occupied by ligand would be affected.

This model of receptor desensitization appears to be a general mechanism by which many G protein-coupled receptors are desensitized upon persistent ligand binding [28]. Thus, there are at least six forms of βARK-like kinases

cloned to date, which are referred to as GRKs. The GRKs are differentially expressed in the nervous system, and each GRK appears to phosphorylate a distinct subset of G protein-coupled receptors. To date, GRKs have been shown to phosphorylate and desensitize several G protein-coupled receptors, which, in addition to the β-adrenergic receptor, include the α_2-adrenergic receptor and the δ-opioid receptor. In addition, several forms of arrestins are known which are believed to contribute to the specific desensitization of G protein-coupled receptor function by the various GRKs.

Synapsins regulate the release of neurotransmitter from nerve endings. They represent a family of four synaptic vesicle-associated phosphoproteins [29]. They are expressed primarily in neurons, where they are associated with small synaptic vesicles in virtually all nerve terminals throughout the CNS and PNS. Synapsins Ia and Ib, which are referred to collectively as synapsin I, are derived from a single gene by alternative splicing and exhibit M_r of 86,000 and 80,000, respectively. Synapsins IIa and IIb, also derived from a single gene, are, respectively, 55- and 74-kDa proteins.

Synapsin I phosphorylation regulates neurotransmitter release. Synapsin I possesses a head, or globular, domain, which is phosphorylated on one serine residue by PKA and by CaMK I. It also possesses a tail, or filamentous, domain, which is phosphorylated on two other serine residues by CaMK II. It appears that dephosphosynapsin I binds both to vesicles and to actin. Synapsin I thereby "cages" the vesicles; that is, it inhibits their availability for release (Fig. 24-5) (see Chap. 9).

Phosphorylation of synapsin I on its tail domain by CaMK II decreases its affinity for synaptic vesicles. The subsequent dissociation of the

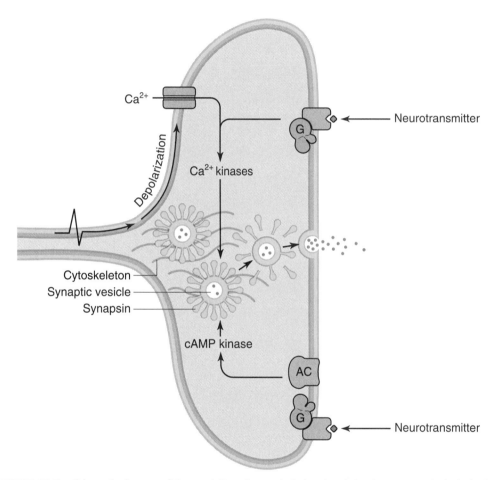

FIGURE 24-5. Schematic diagram of the regulation of synapsin I phosphorylation in nerve terminals. In the basal state, dephosphorylated synapsin I is bound to synaptic vesicles, which anchors the vesicles to the nerve terminal cytoskeleton. Upon phosphorylation, synapsin I is released from the vesicles, which frees the vesicles from the cytoskeleton and makes them available for exocytosis and neurotransmitter release. Nerve impulse conduction stimulates synapsin I phosphorylation through depolarization of the nerve terminal plasma membrane, an increase in free Ca^{2+} concentrations and activation of Ca^{2+}/calmodulin-dependent protein kinases (CaMKs). Such phosphorylation of synapsin I is involved in various Ca^{2+}-dependent mechanisms of regulation of neurotransmitter release, including the phenomenon of post-tetanic potentiation. Some neurotransmitters stimulate, or inhibit, synapsin I phosphorylation by binding to presynaptic receptors and thereby altering concentrations of Ca^{2+} and CaMK activity or concentrations of adenylyl cyclase (AC) and cAMP-dependent protein kinase activity. Such phosphorylation, or dephosphorylation, of synapsin I may be part of the mechanisms by which certain neurotransmitters acting on presynaptic receptors of axon terminals regulate neurotransmitter release.

protein from the vesicles "decages" them and thereby enables a greater number of vesicles to be poised for fusion and neurotransmitter release in response to the next nerve impulse [29]. This scheme is supported by a series of experiments with several neuronal preparations, in which the intracellular application of dephosphosynapsin I, but not phosphosynapsin I, into nerve terminals inhibits spontaneous and impulse-evoked neurotransmitter release, whereas application of CaMK II facilitates neurotransmitter release. Phosphorylation of synapsin I on its tail domain also decreases its affinity for actin; this may contribute further to the phosphorylation-induced decaging of vesicles within the nerve terminal cytoplasm and to the subsequent facilitation of neurotransmitter release. The precise function of phosphorylation of the head domain of synapsin I remains less clearly understood, but it may regulate the tethering of synaptic vesicles to the nerve terminal cytoskeleton.

Synapsin I phosphorylation has been shown to be highly regulated by nerve impulses as well as several neurotransmitters [1]. There is now compelling evidence that such regulation of synapsin phosphorylation is responsible for physiologically important modulation of neurotransmitter release by these first messengers. For example, recent work has demonstrated clearly that synapsin phosphorylation underlies post-tetanic potentiation, one of the best-described phenomena of activity-dependent neural plasticity. Post-tetanic potentiation refers to an enhancement in neurotransmitter release that occurs in many nerve cells following a *tetanus* (a series of closely spaced stimuli). Synapsin I phosphorylation, which occurs in response to the influx of Ca^{2+} during a tetanus, would be expected to enhance the amount of neurotransmitter released by a subsequent stimulus by triggering the release of synapsin I from synaptic vesicles and thereby enabling a larger number of vesicles to dock at the nerve terminal plasma membrane for exocytosis, as mentioned above (see Fig. 24-5). Indeed, recently developed mutant mice that lack synapsin I are deficient in post-tetanic potentiation [30]. Similarly, neurotransmitter receptors that increase or decrease concentrations of Ca^{2+} or cAMP would similarly be expected to modulate neurotransmitter release via regulation of synapsin phosphorylation.

More recent studies have shown that synapsin I is also phosphorylated by the MAPK cascades on distinct serine residues in the molecule [31]. This phosphorylation has also been found to alter the affinity of synapsin I for certain cytoskeletal elements within the nerve terminal cytoplasm. Phosphorylation of synapsin I by MAPK cascades thereby provides a putative mechanism by which neurotrophic factors may regulate neurotransmitter release in the brain.

The synapsins also play a role in the regulation of synaptogenesis. The introduction of synapsin I or synapsin II into several neuronal preparations has been shown to promote the maturation of synapses. This action is associated with the appearance of a number of other synaptic vesicle-associated proteins. In fact, axonal development and synaptogenesis are impaired in mice deficient in synapsin I. The mechanisms by which the synapsins influence the expression of other proteins and promote the differentiation of synaptic nerve terminals have not yet been established. Nevertheless, these results indicate that in addition to regulating neurotransmitter release at fully functional synapses, the synapsins may participate in the functional maturation of synapses during development and possibly even synaptogenesis in the adult nervous system. The results thereby highlight a general theme in biology: a protein that subserves a particular function in adult cells may function very differently within the same cells during development.

Dopamine- and cAMP-regulated phosphoprotein of 32 kDa (DARPP-32) is a protein phosphatase inhibitor enriched in dopaminoceptive neurons. It was discovered during a study of the regional distribution of neuronal phosphoproteins in rat brain. It is one of several substrates for PKA that are highly concentrated in the basal ganglia. DARPP-32 has an apparent M_r of 32,000 by sodium dodecyl sulfate (SDS)-polyacrylamide gel electrophoresis, but its actual molecular mass based on sequencing data is ~23,000. It is phosphorylated *in vitro* on a single threonine residue by PKA or PKG. Phospho-DARPP-32, but not the dephospho form of the protein, inhibits PP1 with a K_i of about 1 nM.

In contrast, it is not an effective inhibitor of protein phosphatases 2A, 2B or 2C. DARPP-32 is also phosphorylated on serine residues by casein kinases I and II; such phosphorylation influences the ability of the threonine residue to be phosphorylated by PKA.

DARPP-32 is highly enriched in neurons in the brain that possess D1-dopamine receptors, and it appears to be present in all such neurons. It is also present in renal tubular epithelial cells, parathyroid hormone-producing cells in the parathyroid gland and tanocytes, all of which are known to express the D1 receptor. However, DARPP-32 is not selective for cells that express the D1 receptor: it is expressed at physiologically important levels by many cell types in the brain that lack this receptor, such as choroid epithelial cells.

The state of phosphorylation of DARPP-32 is regulated in D1-dopaminoceptive neurons by the neurotransmitter dopamine, which acts through increases in cAMP concentrations and activation of PKA. DARPP-32 phosphorylation can also be stimulated in these, as well as in other, cell types by other types of hormones and neurotransmitters that activate the cAMP and cGMP pathways. Moreover, in cell types that lack D1 receptors but express DARPP-32, DARPP-32 phosphorylation is regulated by several neurotransmitters and hormones that affect the cAMP and cGMP cascades. Changes in the phosphorylation state of DARPP-32, through activation of its phosphatase-inhibitory activity, indirectly influence the phosphorylation state of other proteins and thereby mediate some of the effects of dopamine and of these other first messengers on cell function.

The full spectrum of proteins regulated in this way by DARPP-32 phosphorylation has not yet been identified, although the Na^+,K^+-ATPase and voltage-gated Ca^{2+} channels represent examples of well-characterized target proteins [32,33]. Regulation of these proteins by DARPP-32 provides a mechanism by which alterations in DARPP-32 phosphorylation lead, under physiological conditions, to changes in the electrical excitability of neurons as well as in the ion-transport properties of nonexcitable peripheral tissues.

Several types of physiological actions for DARPP-32 can be envisioned. First, DARPP-32 phosphorylated and activated in response to dopamine or another first messenger and cAMP or cGMP can act as a positive-feedback signal for these messengers by reducing the dephosphorylation of other substrates for the same protein kinase. Second, DARPP-32 can reduce the dephosphorylation of substrate proteins for other protein kinases and, in so doing, mediate the effects of first- and second-messenger systems on one another. Third, DARPP-32, through its phosphorylation by PKA or PKG and its dephosphorylation by PP2B (calcineurin), can integrate certain physiological effects of first messengers that influence the cAMP and Ca^{2+} systems.

An example of this latter mechanism is illustrated in Figure 24-6. In this scheme, extracellular signals that activate the cAMP pathway would phosphorylate and activate DARPP-32, whereas extracellular signals that activate the Ca^{2+} pathway would dephosphorylate and inactivate DARPP-32. Changes in DARPP-32 activity would then lead to altered activity of PP1 and, as a result, to altered dephosphorylation of Na^+,K^+-ATPase, a prominent substrate for this enzyme. Changes in the phosphorylation state of the Na^+, K^+-ATPase would result in altered sodium transport across the cell membrane and, in excitable cells, to altered membrane potential. Considerable evidence has been obtained to support this scheme in several cell types [32]. Analogous mechanisms appear to operate for regulation of Ca^{2+} channel activity [33]. Moreover, the scheme can account for some of the antagonistic actions of dopamine, acting through cAMP, and glutamate, acting through Ca^{2+}, on excitability in striatal neurons.

Recently, the physiological importance of DARPP-32 has been demonstrated clearly by phenotypic abnormalities seen in mice that lack this protein. The mice show deficient electrophysiological, transcriptional, neurochemical and behavioral responses to D1-receptor stimulation. These findings support the scheme, outlined above, wherein DARPP-32 exerts a feedforward action by facilitating the diverse physiological effects of D1-receptor stimulation and, presumably, of the stimulation of other receptors coupled positively to the cAMP pathway that also phosphorylate DARPP-32.

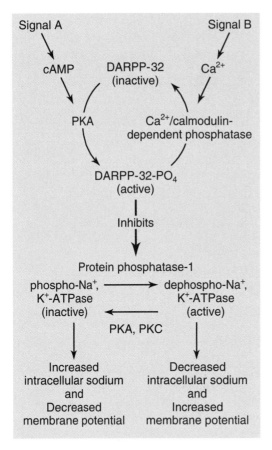

FIGURE 24-6. Scheme illustrating hypothetical role of dopamine and cAMP-regulated phosphoprotein of 32 kDa (*DARPP-32*) in mediating the effects of first messengers with opposing physiological actions and in regulating Na$^+$,K$^+$-ATPase activity. This scheme, involving bidirectional control of Na$^+$,K$^+$-ATPase activity, appears to be applicable to several tissues, including brain and kidney. In addition, similar schemes operate for other phosphoproteins, for example, voltage-gated Ca^{2+} channels. *PKA*, cAMP-dependent protein kinase; *PKC*, protein kinase C.

Cyclic AMP response element binding protein (CREB) is a prototypical example of a transcription factor whose physiological activity is regulated by phosphorylation. It is one of a family of proteins that mediates some of the effects of cAMP on gene expression [34]. CREB binds to a specific sequence of DNA, termed a cAMP response element (CRE), in the promoter (regulatory) regions of genes and thereby increases or decreases the rate at which those genes are transcribed (see Chap. 26).

The details of the mechanism by which CREB influences gene expression are becoming increasingly understood (Fig. 24-7) [11,34]. In the basal, or unstimulated, state, CREB is bound to its CREs but does not alter transcriptional rates under most circumstances. Stimulation of a cell by a variety of first messengers leads to the phosphorylation and activation of CREB, which then leads to the regulation of gene transcription. Such phosphorylation of CREB occurs on a single serine residue, serine 133, and can be mediated by one of several protein kinases.

The detailed mechanisms involved in CREB phosphorylation were first established for the cAMP pathway. A first messenger that increases cAMP concentrations leads to activation of PKA and to translocation of the free catalytic subunit of the protein kinase into the nucleus, where it phosphorylates CREB on serine 133. Such phosphorylation then promotes the binding of CREB to a CREB-binding protein (CBP). CBP, upon binding CREB, interacts directly with the RNA polymerase II complex, which mediates the initiation of transcription. In most cases, such interactions lead to the activation of transcription, although it is possible that the expression of some genes may be repressed.

Stimulation of a cell by first messengers that increase cellular Ca^{2+} concentrations similarly activates CREB (Fig. 24-7). This appears to occur via the phosphorylation of CREB on serine 133 by a CaMK, probably CaMK IV as well as, possibly, CaMK I. It remains to be established whether the activated kinase translocates to the nucleus, by analogy with the catalytic subunit of the cAMP kinase, or whether elevated Ca^{2+} signals enter the nucleus and activate the kinase already there. Interestingly, phosphorylation of CREB on a distinct serine residue, serine 142, by CaMK II appears to inhibit the transcriptional activity of CREB *in vitro*, although whether this inhibitory effect occurs *in vivo* is unknown.

CREB is also phosphorylated on serine 133 by stimulation of growth factor-signaling cascades [11]. This apparently occurs via a complex pathway involving MAPK cascades (Fig. 24-7). Thus, as outlined earlier, nerve growth factor and related neurotrophins that act on receptor tyrosine kinases lead to the successive activation of Ras, Raf, MEK and ERK. Activated ERK then

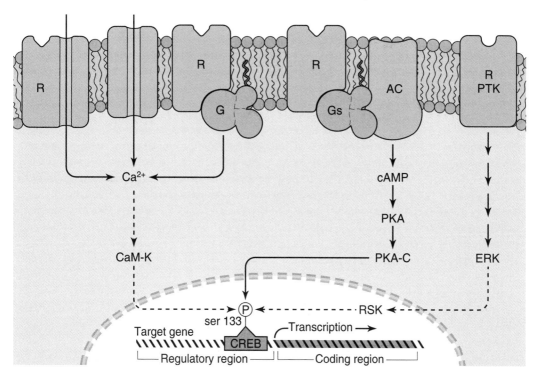

FIGURE 24-7. Schematic illustration of the mechanism by which diverse types of first messengers converge on the phosphorylation of serine 133 of cAMP response element-binding protein *(CREB)*. Some first messengers do this by increasing cAMP concentrations by activation of G protein-coupled receptors *(R)*, G_s, adenylyl cyclase *(AC)* and cAMP-dependent protein kinase *(PKA)*, which then phosphorylates CREB on ser 133. Others do so by increasing Ca^{2+} concentrations by activation of ionotropic receptors *(R)* that flux Ca^{2+}, by activation of voltage-gated Ca^{2+} channels through membrane depolarization or by activation of G protein-coupled receptors that elevate intracellular Ca^{2+} concentrations, for example, via the phospholipase C pathway. Increased concentrations of Ca^{2+} then lead to activation of Ca^{2+}/calmodulin-dependent protein kinases (type IV and, possibly, I) *(CaM-K)*, which also phosphorylate CREB on ser 133. Still others do so by activating ERK: by activation of receptor-associated protein tyrosine kinases *(R-PTK)* and the mitogen-activated protein kinase cascade (see Fig. 24-3). Activation of extracellular signal-regulated kinase *(ERK)* then phosphorylates and activates ribosomal S6 kinase *(RSK)*, which also phosphorylates CREB on ser 133. The step at which the cytoplasmic signal is transduced to the nucleus is well established for PKA: activation of the kinase leads to its dissociation and generation of the free catalytic subunit *(PKA-C)*, which then translocates to the nucleus and phosphorylates CREB. The process is less well established for the CaMKs and ERK, as indicated by the *dashed lines*. Phosphorylation of CREB on ser 133 activates its transcriptional activity and leads to changes in the rate of transcription of target genes.

phosphorylates and activates a serine-threonine kinase, RSK, which appears to directly activate CREB via the phosphorylation of serine 133. Other MAPK-activated kinases may also phosphorylate and activate CREB.

There is evidence that the dephosphorylation of CREB is catalyzed by PP1 and, perhaps, PP2A [16,17]. Phosphorylation of NIPP-1 (a protein phosphatase inhibitor protein described above) may contribute to the tightly timed pulse of phospho-CREB induced in the nucleus following cell stimulation. According to this scheme, the catalytic subunit of PKA, for example, would rapidly phosphorylate CREB, resulting in a change in transcription, and, with a slightly slower time course, phosphorylate and reduce the phosphatase-inhibitory activity of NIPP1. This would release PP1 from its tonic inhibition and result in CREB dephosphorylation.

The number of neural genes known to contain CREs is growing as more and more genes are cloned. Prominent examples are tyrosine hydroxylase, c-fos, proenkephalin, prodynorphin, somatostatin and vasoactive intestinal polypeptide (VIP). Expression of these genes has been shown to be regulated at their CREs by the phosphorylation of CREB or a CREB-like protein. In fact, for some genes, for example, tyrosine hydroxylase, activation of CREB appears to be the critical transcriptional mechanism controlling both the basal level of gene expression and the induction of expression seen in response to cellular stimulation.

Consideration of CREB highlights the view, mentioned earlier in this chapter, that among the many cellular processes regulated by protein phosphorylation is gene transcription. This view is further underscored by the knowledge that virtually all classes of transcription factors undergo phosphorylation by numerous types of protein kinases. Even transcription factors that are regulated primarily through alterations in their own transcription, such as c-Fos and other immediate early gene-transcription factors, are influenced by phosphorylation. For example, c-Fos is heavily phosphorylated on a series of serine residues in the C-terminal domain of the protein by several types of protein kinases. The likely functional importance of these phosphorylation sites is indicated by the fact that the difference between c-Fos (the normal cellular form of the protein) and v-Fos (the viral oncogene product) is a frameshift mutation in the v-Fos protein, which obliterates the phosphorylated serine residues. It is speculated that the loss of these phosphorylation sites removes one mechanism by which the cell can regulate the protein, thereby leading to cellular transformation.

CELLULAR SIGNALS CONVERGE AT THE LEVEL OF PROTEIN PHOSPHORYLATION PATHWAYS

Individual intracellular messenger pathways, such as cAMP, Ca^{2+} and MAPK pathways, are often drawn as distinct biochemical cascades that operate in parallel in the control of cell function. While this is useful for didactic purposes, it is now well established that these various pathways function as complex webs, with virtually every conceivable type of interaction seen among them.

This can be illustrated by known interactions between the cAMP and Ca^{2+} pathways. A first messenger that initially activates the cAMP pathway would be expected to exert secondary effects on the Ca^{2+} pathway at many levels via phosphorylation by PKA. First, Ca^{2+} channels and the inositol trisphosphate (IP_3) receptor will be phosphorylated by PKA to modulate intracellular concentrations of Ca^{2+}. Second, phospholipase C (PLC) is a substrate for PKA, and its phosphorylation modulates intracellular calcium concentrations, via the generation of IP_3, as well as the activity of PKC, via the generation of DAG, and several types of CAMK. Similarly, the Ca^{2+} pathway exerts potent effects on the cAMP pathway, for example, by activating or inhibiting the various forms of adenylyl cyclase expressed in mammalian tissues (see Chap. 22).

The cAMP and Ca^{2+} pathways also interact at the level of protein kinases and protein phosphatases. This is illustrated by DARPP-32, which is phosphorylated and activated by PKA and then inhibits PP1, which can dephosphorylate numerous substrates for Ca^{2+}-dependent protein kinases. Another example is the physical association between PKA and PP2B (a Ca^{2+}/calmodulin-activated enzyme) via the AKAP-anchoring proteins.

Multiple interactions are also being demonstrated between the traditional second-messenger pathways and the MAPK cascades. Free $\beta\gamma$ G protein subunits, generated upon activation of receptors coupled to the G_i family, lead to activation of the ERK pathway. The mechanism by which this occurs, which may involve an interaction between the $\beta\gamma$ subunits and Ras or Raf, is a subject of intensive research (see Chap. 20). In addition, increases in cellular Ca^{2+} concentrations lead to stimulation of the ERK pathway, apparently via phosphorylation by CaMKs of proteins, for example, Shc and Grb, that link growth factor receptor tyrosine kinases to Ras. Activation of the cAMP pathway exerts the opposite effect in most cells: it results in inhibition of the ERK pathway, possibly via the phosphorylation and inhibition of Raf by PKA.

Another major way by which intracellular messenger pathways interact is via phosphorylation of the same substrate proteins. There are numerous examples of this, some discussed earlier in this chapter. Perhaps the most striking example is provided by CREB, which is phosphorylated on the same single serine residue by PKA, CaMK and RSK, activated by the MAPK cascade.

The above discussion suggests that a single extracellular signal may elicit changes in virtually every intracellular signaling cascade, which would raise questions as to how specific biological responses are achieved in a cell. In reality, such specificity is achieved because not all of the aforementioned interactions occur in every cell type. Specific interactions depend on the strength and persistence of the original extracellular signal, the subcellular location where the signal acts and the specific subtypes of individual signaling proteins that are expressed in a cell at the relevant subcellular sites. In addition, regulation of intracellular messenger pathways does not depend on the actions of a single extracellular signal but, rather, on the integration of multiple signals that impinge on cells at any given point in time.

Nevertheless, rather than being generated through a single molecular pathway, most physiological responses should be viewed as the complex product of the coordinated actions of multiple cellular messengers involving multiple molecular pathways. This extraordinary complexity underscores the difficulty in determining the precise molecular basis of a given physiological process. The central role of protein phosphorylation as a regulatory mechanism that mediates the actions of many individual cellular messengers and the interactions among them imbues the study of protein phosphorylation with a unique potential: to provide an experimental framework within which the layers of molecular steps that underlie and regulate cell function may be unraveled.

PROTEIN PHOSPHORYLATION MECHANISMS IN DISEASE

The study of protein phosphorylation has helped to clarify the mechanisms involved in the causes and manifestation of disorders of the nervous system. Two illustrative examples are given here: Alzheimer's disease and opiate addiction.

Abnormal phosphorylation of specific neural proteins may contribute to the development of Alzheimer's disease

Alzheimer's disease is a serious dementing illness of enormous medical and societal importance (see Chap. 46). It involves the degeneration of specific types of neurons in the brain. An invariable feature of Alzheimer's disease is the appearance of amyloid plaques. These plaques contain the β/A4 amyloid protein, and there is some evidence to suggest that the accumulation of β/A4 contributes to neuronal degeneration and that mutations in the gene that codes for this protein are involved in a small number of cases of familial Alzheimer's disease.

β/A4 is derived from amyloid precursor protein (APP) through proteolytic processing. In normal cells, APP is processed into fragments that are not associated with disease states. It is not yet known why APP is cleaved anomalously to yield β/A4 to a greater extent in Alzheimer's disease. However, increasing evidence indicates that signal-transduction pathways involving protein phosphorylation are potent regulators of APP cleavage and can alter the rates of cleavage both at normal sites and at sites yielding putative amyloidogenic fragments [35].

The role of PKC in this process has received the most attention. Activators of PKC, or inhibitors of PP1, such as okadaic acid, dramatically stimulate APP proteolysis, whereas PKC inhibitors diminish cleavage of the protein. The finding that PKC regulates APP processing raises the possibility that agents that regulate this protein kinase, or specific protein phosphatases, might prove to be useful in the clinical management of Alzheimer's disease. Further support for the potential clinical utility of drugs that influence protein kinases or protein phosphatases in Alzheimer's disease is the evidence that aberrant phosphorylation mechanisms, that is, excessive phosphorylation of neurofilament and microtubule-associated proteins, may contribute to the formation of neurofibrillary tangles, another component of the structural pathology of Alzheimer's disease [35].

Upregulation of the cAMP pathway is one mechanism underlying opiate addiction

The mechanisms by which opiates induce tolerance, dependence and withdrawal in specific target neurons has been a major focus of research for many years. The inability to account for prominent aspects of opiate addiction on the basis of alterations in endogenous opioid peptides or in opiate receptors has shifted attention to postreceptor mechanisms [36].

The noradrenergic neurons of the locus ceruleus have provided a useful model system for the study of opiate addiction (see Box 53-1). Acutely, opiates inhibit these neurons, in part by inhibiting the cAMP pathway via inhibition of adenylyl cyclase. Chronically, these neurons become tolerant to opiates; that is, their firing rates recover toward normal levels with continued exposure to the drug. Furthermore, they become dependent on opiates; that is, their firing rates increase far above control levels upon removal of the drug. These changes in the electrical excitability of locus ceruleus neurons mediate many of the physical signs and symptoms associated with opiate-withdrawal syndromes.

Increasing evidence indicates that a chronic opiate-induced upregulation of the cAMP pathway, manifested by increased concentrations of adenylyl cyclase, PKA and several phosphoprotein substrates for the protein kinase, contributes to opiate tolerance, dependence and withdrawal exhibited by locus ceruleus neurons [35]. This upregulated cAMP pathway can be viewed as a homeostatic response of the neurons to persistent opiate inhibition of the cells. In the chronic opiate-treated state, the upregulated cAMP pathway helps return neuronal firing rates to control levels, that is, tolerance. Upon abrupt removal of the opiate via the administration of an opiate receptor antagonist, the upregulated cAMP accounts for part of the withdrawal activation of the cells.

Chronic opiate-induced upregulation of the cAMP pathway appears to be mediated in part by CREB: chronic opiate administration increases CREB expression; mice deficient in CREB show attenuated physical opiate dependence and withdrawal; and selective reductions of CREB in the locus ceruleus prevent upregulation of specific components of the cAMP pathway in response to chronic opiate administration [36]. This latter action is associated with attenuation of the electrical excitability of locus ceruleus neurons and of physical opiate dependence and withdrawal.

Upregulation of the cAMP pathway may be a common mechanism by which a number of neuronal cell types respond to chronic opiates and develop tolerance and dependence (see Chap. 53). There is also evidence that similar mechanisms involving alterations in the cAMP second-messenger and protein phosphoryation pathway may mediate aspects of addiction to other types of drugs of abuse, for example, cocaine and alcohol [36].

REFERENCES

1. Nestler, E. J., and Greengard, P. *Protein Phosphorylation in the Nervous System.* New York: Wiley, 1984.
2. Hunter, T., and Sefton, B. M. (eds.) *Protein Phosphorylation. Part A. Methods in Enzymology,* vol. 200. New York: Academic Press, 1991.
3. Hunter, T. Protein kinases and phosphatases: The yin and yang of protein phosphorylation and signaling. *Cell* 80:225–236, 1995.
4. Coghlan, V., Hausken, Z., and Scott, J. Subcellular targeting of kinases and phosphatases by association with bifunctional anchoring proteins. *Biochem. Soc. Trans.* 23:592–596, 1995.
4a. Lohmann, S. M., Vaandrager, A. B., Smolenski, A., Walter, U., and De Jonge, H. R. Distinct and specific functions of cGMP-dependent protein kinases. *Trends Biochem. Sci.* 22:307–312, 1997.
5. Schulman, H. Protein phosphorylation in neuronal plasticity and gene expression. *Curr. Opin. Neurobiol.* 5:375–381, 1995.
6. Picciotto, M., Nastiuk, K., and Nairn, A. Structure, regulation, and function of calcium/calmodulin-dependent protein kinase I. *Adv. Pharmacol.* 36:251–275, 1996.
7. Palfrey, H. C., and Nairn, A. C. Calcium-dependent regulation of protein synthesis. *Adv. Second Messenger Phosphoprotein Res.* 30:191–223, 1995.
8. Nakamura, S., and Nishizuka, Y. Lipid mediators and protein kinase C activation for the intracellular signaling network. *J. Biochem.* 15:1029–1034, 1994.

9. Mochly-Rosen, D. Localization of protein kinases by anchoring proteins: A theme in signal transduction. *Science* 268:247–251, 1995.

10. Nicoll, R. A., and Malenka, R. C. Contrasting properties of two forms of long-term potentiation in the hippocampus. *Nature* 377:115–118, 1995.

11. Xing, J., Ginty, D., and Greenberg, M. Coupling of the RAS-MAPK pathway to gene activation by RSK2, a growth factor-regulated CREB kinase. *Science* 273:959–963, 1996.

12. Hemmings, H. C., Jr., Nairn, A. C., McGuinness, T. L., Huganir, R. L., and Greengard, P. Role of protein phosphorylation in neuronal signal transduction. *FASEB J.* 3:1583–1592, 1989.

13. Kortenjann, M., and Shaw, P. The growing family of MAP kinases: Regulation and specificity. *Crit. Rev. Oncog.* 6:99–115, 1995.

14. Block, C., and Wittinghofer, A. Switching to Rac and Rho. *Structure* 3:1281–1284, 1995.

15. Barford, D. Protein phosphatases. *Curr. Opin. Struct. Biol.* 5:728–734, 1995.

16. Wera, S., and Hemmings, B. Serine/threonine protein phosphatases. *Biochem. J.* 311:17–29, 1995.

16a. Allen, P. B., Ouimet, C. C., and Greengard, P. Spinophilin, a novel protein phosphatase 1 binding protein localized to dendritic spines. *Proc. Natl. Acad. Sci. USA* 94:9956–9961, 1997.

17. Shenolikar, S. Protein phosphatase regulation by endogenous inhibitors. *Cancer Biol.* 6:219–227, 1995.

18. Steiner, J. P., Dawson, T. M., Fotuhi, M., and Snyder, S. H. Immunophilin regulation of neurotransmitter release. *Mol. Med.* 2:325–333, 1996.

19. Keyse, S. An emerging family of dual specificity MAP kinase phosphatases. *Biochim. Biophys. Acta* 1265:152–160, 1995.

20. Nebreda, A. R. Inactivation of MAP kinases. *Trends Biochem. Sci.* 19:1–2, 1994.

21. Soderling, T. R. Modulation of glutamate receptors by calcium/calmodulin-dependent protein kinase II. *Neurochem. Int.* 28:359–361, 1996.

22. Roche, K., O'Brien, R., Mammen, A., Bernhardt, J., and Huganir, R. Characterization of multiple phosphorylation sites on the AMPA receptor GluR1 subunit. *Neuron* 16:1179–1188, 1996.

23. Levitan, B. Modulation of ion channels by protein phosphorylation and dephosphorylation. *Annu. Rev. Physiol.* 56:193–212, 1994.

24. Catterall, W. A. Structure and function of voltage-gated ion channels. *Annu. Rev. Biochem.* 64:493–531, 1995.

25. Martin, K. C., and Kandel, E. R. Cell adhesion molecules, CREB, and the formation of new synaptic connections. *Neuron* 17:567–570, 1996.

26. Mallet, J. Catecholamines: From gene regulation to neuropsychiatric disorders. *Trends Pharmacol. Sci.* 17:129–135, 1996.

27. Kumer, S., and Vrana, K. Intricate regulation of tyrosine hydroxylase activity and gene expression. *J. Neurochem.* 67:443–462, 1996.

28. Freedman, N., and Lefkowitz, R. Desensitization of G protein-coupled receptors. *Recent Prog. Horm. Res.* 51:319–351, 1996.

29. Greengard, P., Valtorta, F., Czernik, A. J., and Benfenati, F. Synaptic vesicle phosphoproteins and regulation of synaptic function. *Science* 259:780–785, 1993.

30. Li, L., Chin, L., Shuypliakov, O., et al. Impairment of synaptic vesicle clustering and of synaptic transmission, and increased seizure propensity, in synapsin I-deficient mice. *Proc. Natl. Acad. Sci. USA* 92:9235–9239, 1995.

31. Jovanovic, J., Benfenati, F., Siow, Y., et al. Neurotrophins stimulate phosphorylation of synapsin I by MAP kinase and regulate synapsin I–actin interactions. *Proc. Natl. Acad. Sci. USA* 93:3679–3683, 1996.

32. Li, D., Aperia, A., Celsi, G., da Cruz e Silva, E., Greengard, P., and Meister, B. Protein phosphatase-1 in the kidney: Evidence for a role in the regulation of medullary $Na(+)$-$K(+)$-ATPase. *Am. J. Physiol.* 269:673–680, 1995.

33. Surmeier, D., Bargas, J., Hemmings, H. C., Jr., Nairn, A., and Greengard, P. Modulation of calcium currents by a D1 dopaminergic protein kinase/phosphatase cascade in rat neostriatal neurons. *Neuron* 14:385–397, 1995.

34. Frank, D., and Greenberg, M. CREB: A mediator of long-term memory from mollusks to mammals. *Cell* 79:5–8, 1994.

35. Gandy, S., and Greengard, P. Processing of Alzheimer Aβ-amyloid precursor protein: cell biology, regulation, and role in Alzheimer disease. *Int. Rev. Neurobiol.* 35:29–50, 1994.

36. Nestler, E. J., and Aghajanian, G. K. Molecular and cellular basis of addiction. *Science* 278:58–63, 1997.

Tyrosine Phosphorylation

Lit-fui Lau and Richard L. Huganir

TYROSINE PHOSPHORYLATION IN THE NERVOUS SYSTEM

Protein phosphorylation is one of the most important mechanisms in the regulation of cellular functions. Proteins can be phosphorylated on serine, threonine or tyrosine residues. Most phosphorylation occurs on serine and threonine, with less than 1% on tyrosine. This perhaps accounts for the late discovery of tyrosine phosphorylation, which was found first on polyoma virus middle T antigen in 1979 by Hunter and colleagues [1]. Since then, a growing number of proteins have been shown to be tyrosine-phosphorylated. Originally, tyrosine phosphorylation was believed to be involved primarily in reg-

Basic Neurochemistry: Molecular, Cellular and Medical Aspects, 6th Ed., edited by G. J. Siegel et al. Published by Lippincott–Raven Publishers, Philadelphia, 1999. Correspondence to Richard L. Huganir, Johns Hopkins University School of Medicine, 725 N. Wolfe Street, 904A PCTB, Baltimore, Maryland 21205.

ulating cell proliferation since many oncogene products and growth factor receptors are protein tyrosine kinases (PTKs) [2]. However, it is clear that tyrosine phosphorylation is involved in regulating a variety of cellular processes. In fact, the nervous system contains large amounts of PTKs and protein tyrosine phosphatases (PTPs) [3], and some of these are exclusively expressed in neuronal tissues. For example, Figure 25-1 shows the immunocytochemical staining of a cultured hippocampal neuron with an antiphosphotyro-sine antibody [4]. It reveals the presence of tyrosine-phosphorylated proteins in the cell body as well as synapses and suggests that tyrosine phosphorylation plays a role in neuronal function. Furthermore, many neuronal processes are affected by PTK or PTP inhibitors and by deletion of genes encoding for PTKs and PTPs.

Tyrosine phosphorylation is controlled by a balance of the activity between PTKs and PTPs (Fig. 25-2). PTKs catalyze the transfer of the γ-phosphate from ATP to its substrate, while PTPs

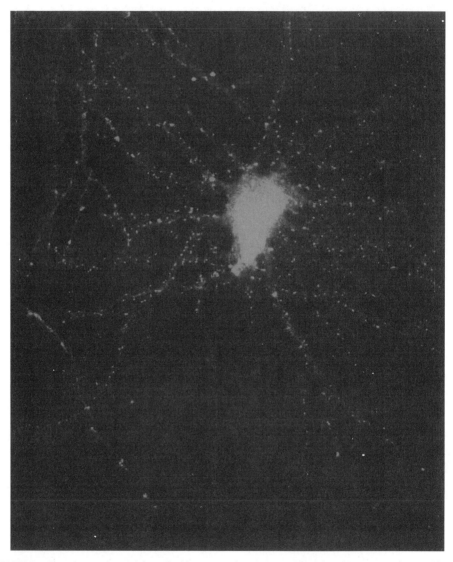

FIGURE 25-1.   Phosphotyrosine staining of a hippocampal neuron. A cultured rat hippocampal pyramidal neuron is stained with an antiphosphotyrosine antibody and detected by a secondary antibody conjugated to rhodamine. The staining reflects the presence of tyrosine-phosphorylated proteins throughout the neuron, including the cell body and synaptic regions.

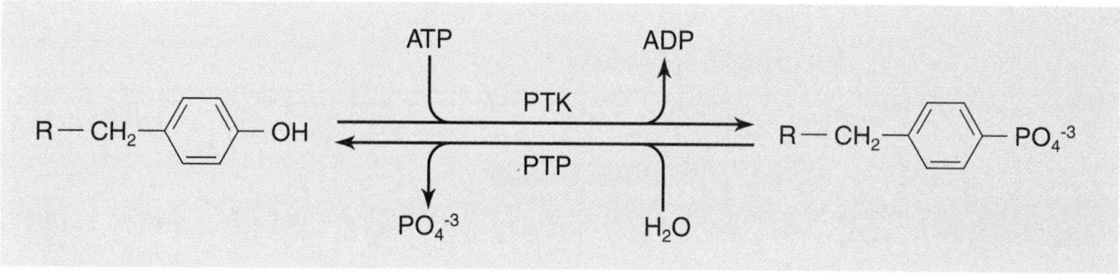

FIGURE 25-2. Tyrosine phosphorylation and dephosphorylation. Protein tyrosine kinases *(PTKs)* catalyze the transfer of the γ-phosphate group from ATP to the hydroxyl group of tyrosine residues, whereas protein tyrosine phosphatases *(PTPs)* remove the phosphate group from phosphotyrosine. *R,* protein.

remove phosphate from phosphotyrosine (Fig. 25-2). Phosphorylation of a tyrosine residue changes a polar environment to a negatively charged one. It also increases the size of the tyrosine side chain. These changes consequently elicit a change in the structure of the substrate protein, altering its function. Alternatively, the phosphotyrosine sequence becomes a molecular adhesive which can change the subcellular distribution of the tyrosine-phosphorylated protein or interacting proteins, initiating assembly of signal-transduction complexes.

PROTEIN TYROSINE KINASES

PTKs can be divided into receptor protein tyrosine kinases (RPTKs) and nonreceptor protein tyrosine kinases (NRPTKs). RPTKs are integral membrane proteins, while NRPTKs lack a transmembrane domain and are distributed in different intracellular compartments. The catalytic activity of each type may be influenced by extracellular stimuli.

Nonreceptor protein tyrosine kinases contain a catalytic domain, as well as various regulatory domains important for proper functioning of the enzyme

NRPTKs are found in the inner leaflet of the plasma membrane, cytosol, endosomal membranes and nucleus. These include the Src, Jak, Abl, Tec and focal adhesion kinase (Fak) families (Fig. 25-3). Since a great deal is known about the structural features of the Src tyrosine kinase family, we will use it as an example to illustrate

the principles in NRPTK signaling and to indicate differences found in other families when appropriate. The catalytic domain is about 250 amino acids in length and is by itself a functional enzyme. However, most, if not all, PTKs are larger and contain regulatory domains that maintain a low basal tyrosine kinase activity. The regulatory domains also can target the protein to a particular subcellular localization, interact with potential substrates and bind to other signaling molecules. The structural domains of the Src kinase family are, in order from the N-terminus: the SH4 (Src homology 4), SH3, SH2 and SH1 domains. SH1 is the catalytic domain. SH2 and SH3 are both molecular adhesives important for protein–protein interaction. SH4 resides at the very N-terminus and plays a role in membrane attachment. Between the SH4 and the SH3 domains is a region whose sequence varies considerably among different members of the Src family.

The SH4 domain is at the very N-terminus of the Src family kinases and contains a myristoylation site critical for membrane localization. *N*-myristoylation is catalyzed cotranslationally by *N*-myristoyl transferase. Following removal of the N-terminal methionine, myristate is transferred from myristoyl coenzyme A (CoA) to the glycine residue at the second position. Myristoylation is necessary but not sufficient for membrane localization. The basic residues in the SH4 domain in Src and Blk interact with the negatively charged head groups of phospholipids and help to anchor these kinases to the membrane. Other Src family members contain a cysteine residue in the SH4 domain necessary for palmitoylation. This

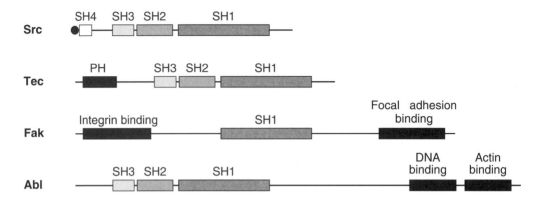

FIGURE 25-3. Examples of nonreceptor protein tyrosine kinase (NRPTK) families. Four families of NRPTKs are shown with different structural features. Src, Tec and Fak families can be localized to the membrane by their myristoylated moiety, pleckstrin homology *(PH)* domain and integrin-binding domain, respectively. Abl family members lack these membrane interaction domains and are found in the nucleus, where they regulate gene transcription. SH1 is the catalytic domain, while the other domains play important regulatory functions. The black circle indicates a myristic acid moiety.

extra lipid moiety inserts into the lipid bilayer and stabilizes interaction with the membrane. While myristoylation is irreversible, the electrostatic interaction and palmitoylation are reversible. For example, Ser17 in Src can be phosphorylated by protein kinase A (PKA). Phosphorylation decreases the local positive charge and consequently dissociates Src from the negatively charged membrane. Similarly, palmitate can be removed from the cysteine residue to translocate Src family kinases to the cytosol. An N-terminal pleckstrin homology (PH) domain in the Tec family tyrosine kinases affects the anchoring of these kinases to membrane by binding specifically to phosphatidylinositol-3,4,5-trisphosphate (PI-3,4,5-P_3).

The unique domain of Src. Following the SH4 domain from the N-terminus is a unique region with considerable variation in the amino acid sequences among different Src family members. This unique domain may be involved in protein–protein interactions. For example, the unique region of Lck is linked to CD4 and CD8, while those of Fyn and Lyn may be associated with the T- and B-cell antigen receptors. This region also contains a number of protein phosphorylation sites. As discussed above, phosphorylation of Ser17 in Src may disrupt its association with the membrane.

The SH3 domain is C-terminal to the unique domain and interacts with proline-rich sequences [5]. This domain is about 60 amino acid residues in length and is composed of five β strands. It forms a globular structure by having the N- and C-termini come close together. SH3 domains mediate intermolecular protein–protein interactions between Src-like kinases and other proteins and intracellular interactions as well. SH3 domains interact with short amino acid sequences within proteins that consist of specific proline-rich motifs in a left-handed helix.

There are two types of SH3 domain ligand. Type I ligands have a consensus sequence of RPLPPLP. Type II ligands adopt an inverted orientation and have a consensus sequence of ØPPLPXR, where Ø represents a hydrophobic amino acid. Small peptide ligands have a low affinity for the SH3 domain (5 to 50 μM) and a low sequence specificity. Interaction between SH3 domains and proteins has higher affinity and specificity. SH3 domains from different members of the Src family tyrosine kinases also have slightly different specificities for their proline-rich ligands.

The neuronal form of Src contains a six-amino-acid insert within the SH3 domain [6]. This insertion decreases the affinity of the SH3 domain for known ligands since most of the SH3 binding proteins fail to interact with the neuronal form of Src. This insertion may change the specificity of the Src SH3 domain to neuronal targets and increase its activity by reducing intramolecular interaction (see below). The Src SH3 domain also can be tyrosine-phosphorylated by the platelet-derived growth factor receptor (PDGFR), resulting in a decreased affinity of the SH3 domain for its ligand. Since the SH3 domain helps to keep Src in the inactive state (see below), its phosphorylation may regulate Src activity.

The SH2 domain is about 100 amino acid residues in length and lies between the SH3 and SH1 domains. This domain interacts with phosphotyrosine in a sequence-specific manner [5], binding to tyrosine phosphorylation sites of proteins only when they are phosphorylated, thus regulating intra- and intermolecular protein–protein interactions. SH2–phosphotyrosine interactions are sequence-specific for different SH2 domains. SH2 domains contain two binding pockets for their target peptides. One of these pockets contains a positively charged arginine residue, which interacts with the negatively charged phosphate group on the tyrosine residue. The other pocket interacts with three to five amino acids C-terminal to the phosphotyrosine and plays a major role in determining substrate specificity. However, amino acids N-terminal to the phosphotyrosine also may contribute to SH2 domain binding. The affinity of an SH2 domain for its interacting phosphotyrosine peptide is in the nanomolar range. Removal of the phosphate group from the peptide reduces the affinity for the peptide by about three orders of magnitude. Like the SH3 domain, the N- and C-termini of the SH2 domain come together, allowing the domain to form a protruding globular structure so that it can be inserted into a protein without significant disruption of the protein structure. However, there is less sequence homology among different SH2 ligands than among SH3 ligands (Table 25-1). Cooperativity is found between the SH2 and SH3 domains in ligand binding such that a ligand capable of interacting with both domains associates with Src more tightly than a ligand that binds to only one of them. SH3 and SH2 do-

| TABLE 25-1. | SPECIFICITY AND AFFINITY OF SH2, PHOSPHOTYROSINE BINDING (PTB) AND SH3 DOMAINS |

Domains	Consensus sequence of ligands	K_D
SH2	pYR$_1$R$_2$R$_3$	1–10 nM
PTB	Ø NPXpY	25–100 nM
SH3	RPLPPLP, Ø PPLPXR	5–50 μM

The consensus sequences of the ligands interacting with SH2, PTB and SH3 domains are listed with their dissociation constants. Both SH2 and PTB domains bind to phosphotyrosine in a sequence-specific manner. Tyrosine dephosphorylation can reduce the affinity of the SH2 domain to its ligand by 1,000-fold. R_1, R_2 and R_3 represent variable amino acids depending on the specific SH2 domain involved. X represents any amino acid. Ø represents a hydrophobic amino acid; pY represents phosphotyrosine.

mains are found in a variety of signaling molecules, as depicted in Figure 25-4.

The SH1 domain is the catalytic domain. The crystal structure of the Src-family tyrosine kinase hck has been solved [7]. Its catalytic (SH1) domain has an overall bilobal structure, with a small ATP-binding N-terminal lobe and a large peptide-binding C-terminal lobe. The N-lobe contains a glycine-rich sequence, GXGXXGXV, and an invariable downstream lysine for ATP binding. Mutation of this lysine often leads to loss of catalytic activity. The C-lobe contains a glutamate residue which catalyzes transfer of the phosphate group from ATP to tyrosine. ATP fits in the cleft between the two lobes with its γ-phosphate pointing outward, while the protein substrate interacts at the cleft opening. There is considerable flexibility in the relative orientation of these two lobes. The active conformation of the kinase allows the proper alignment of the ATP terminal phosphate with the substrate. However, the two lobes of an inactive kinase are swung apart so that the ATP terminal phosphate is not aligned with the substrate. Figure 25-5A shows the X-ray crystallographic analysis of hck.

The consensus substrate sequences for PTKs are less distinct than those for serine/threonine protein kinases, such as PKA and protein kinase C (PKC). In general, tyrosine residues neighbored by glutamic acid residues are pre-

Group 1: Enzymes

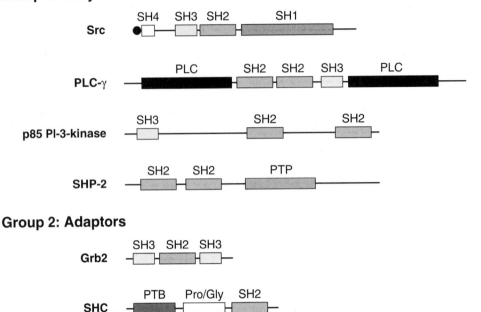

Group 2: Adaptors

FIGURE 25-4.   SH2, SH3 and phosphotyrosine binding *(PTB)* domain-containing signaling proteins. SH2, SH3 and PTB domains are important molecular "adhesives." These domains are found in enzymes and play important roles in the regulation of enzyme function. They also are found in proteins lacking any apparent catalytic domain, in which case they may serve as adaptor proteins, assembling signal-transduction complexes. The PTB domain of insulin receptor substrate-1 *(IRS-1)* shares a low degree of homology with the one on SHC. The black circle indicates a myristic acid moiety. *PLC,* phospholipase C; *PI3-kinase,* phosphatidylinositol-3-kinase; *PTP,* protein tyrosine phosphatase; *PH,* pleckstrin homology; *SHP,* SH2-containing PTP; *Grb,* growth factor receptor-binding protein.

FIGURE 25-5.   A: Crystal structure of the Src family kinase hck. The catalytic domain of Src family tyrosine kinases consists of an N-terminal ATP-binding lobe and a C-terminal substrate-binding lobe. There is considerable flexibility in the relative orientation of these two lobes. The active conformation allows the proper alignment of the ATP terminal phosphate, the substrate and a catalytic glutamate residue (Glu310). However, the two lobes of an inactive kinase are swung apart, disrupting proper alignment (From [7], with permission). **B:** Regulation of Src activity. Src activity can be regulated in a number of ways. In the inactive state, phosphorylated Y527 interacts with the SH2 domain. In addition, the SH3 domain binds the linker region between the SH1 and SH2 domains. These two intramolecular interactions pull the two lobes of the catalytic domain apart and inactivate the kinase. Therefore, dephosphorylation of Y527 by protein tyrosine phosphatases, for example, CD45 and SHP-2, activates the kinase. Phosphorylation of Y527 by Csk inactivates the kinase. Inactivation is also achieved by dephosphorylating the autophosphorylation site Y416 by SHP-1. Alternatively, Src can be activated by binding to an autophosphorylated receptor protein tyrosine kinase *(RPTK),* such as the platelet-derived growth factor receptor. The RPTK autophosphorylation site binds to the src SH2 domain and thus disrupts the inhibitory intramolecular interactions and activates the kinase. Association of Src with tyrosine-phosphorylated Fak activates the kinase in a similar fashion.

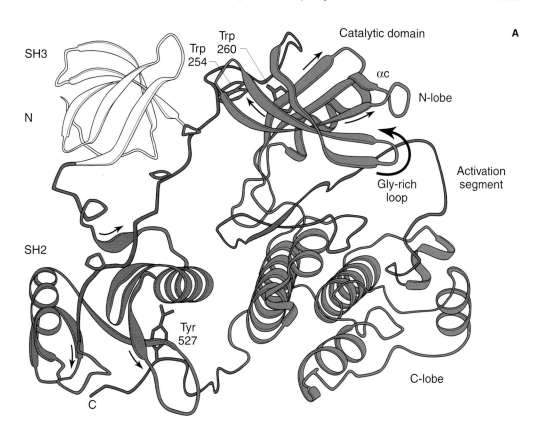

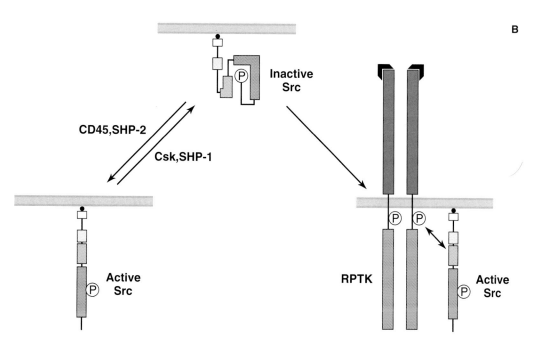

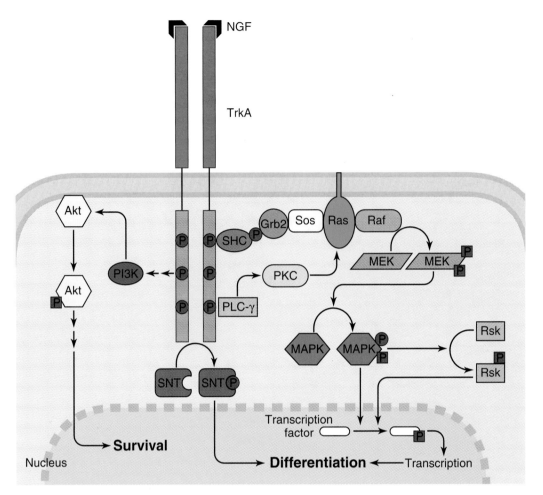

FIGURE 25-9.   Signal-transduction mechanisms in nerve growth factor (NGF)-mediated neuronal survival and differentiation. NGF binds to TrkA and induces autophosphorylation on three different sites in the intracellular domain. One site interacts with SHC, which eventually leads to the activation of mitogen-activated protein kinase (MAPK) and transcription. TrkA also induces tyrosine phosphorylation of suc-associated neurotrophic factor-induced target (SNT) via a mechanism independent of all known signaling mechanisms. MAPK-induced transcription and SNT tyrosine phosphorylation are believed to be important in neuronal differentiation. TrkA autophosphorylation also activates phosphatidylinositol-3-kinase (PI3K) by recruiting it to the membrane. PI3K generates PI-3,4,5-trisphosphate from PI-4,5-bisphosphate. PI-3,4,5-trisphosphate is hydrolyzed to yield PI-3,4-bisphosphate, which activates Akt by translocating it to the membrane. Activated Akt can promote neuronal survival. PLC, phospholipase C; SOS, son of sevenless; MEK, MAPK/Erk kinase; Grb2, growth factor receptor binding protein; SHC, SH2-containing protein.

ferred. Some PTKs phosphorylate not only the tyrosine residue but also serine/threonine residues. These are called the dual-specificity protein kinases. For example, MAPK/Erk kinase (MEK) phosphorylates mitogen-activated protein kinase (MAPK) on both threonine and tyrosine residues in the activation loop. Phosphorylation on both amino acid residues is necessary for the activation of MAPK (see Chap. 24).

The regulatory domain. The region C-terminal of the SH1 domain is called the regulatory domain because it contains a tyrosine residue (Y527 in Src) critical for modulating kinase activity. Under basal conditions, Y527 is phosphorylated by another NRPTK, C-terminal Src kinase (Csk), and is bound to the Src SH2 domain. Formation of this intramolecular bridge favors the interaction of Src SH3 domain with the polyproline helix in the linker region between SH1 and SH2 domains. These intramolecular interactions push a critical acidic residue away from the active site, resulting in inhibition of Src kinase activity. Activation of Src is achieved by the dephosphorylation of Y527 by a PTP, which destabilizes the two intramolecular interactions, allowing the catalytic acidic residue to approach the active site. Subsequently, autophosphorylation of Y416 in the activation loop of Src relieves some more constraints on the active site and increases phosphorylation of Src tyrosine kinase substrates.

This model nicely accounts for a number of observations. For example, v-Src, the tumorigenic form of Src, lacks the negative regulatory domain containing Y527 and, thus, has very high basal activity. Mutation of Y527 to phenylalanine also increases Src activity. In addition, dephosphorylation of Src regulates its activity in two ways. Dephosphorylation of Y527 catalyzed by the leukocyte common antigen (CD45) or an SH2 domain-containing PTP (SHP-2) leads to activation, while dephosphorylation of Y416 by another phosphatase (SHP-1) inactivates Src. Figure 25-5B shows the regulatory mechanisms for Src family tyrosine kinases.

Tyrosine-phosphorylated membrane proteins or intracellular second messengers also can activate NRPTKs. Although NRPTKs do not possess an extracellular domain from which they can communicate with the outside world, they are able to associate specifically with transmembrane proteins and to "borrow" extracellular domains to respond to the appropriate ligands. For example, activation of the PDGFR results in autophosphorylation of a number of tyrosine residues, including Y579 in the juxtamembrane region. This phosphotyrosine-containing peptide sequence interacts with the Src SH2 domain and displaces the negative regulatory domain, resulting in Src activation. The displaced Src C-terminal tail is now accessible for PTPs, allowing prolonged activation of Src despite a transient autophosphorylation of the PDGFR. A similar mechanism applies to the activation of Src by autophosphorylated Fak (Fig. 25-5B).

Many PTKs can be activated by autophosphorylation, which occurs only if two PTK molecules are in close proximity. The Jak/Tyk tyrosine kinases are NRPTKs, constitutively associated with transmembrane proteins, which act as receptors for extracellular ligands, such as gp130 and leukemia-inhibitory factor receptor β (LIFRβ). For example, the binding of ciliary neurotrophic factor (CNTF) to gp130 and LIFRβ and a third membrane-bound component, CNTFRα, results in the formation of a quaternary complex, allowing the transphosphorylation and activation of Jak/Tyk.

Other NRPTKs are activated not by association with membrane proteins but indirectly by second messengers produced in the cytoplasm in response to extracellular stimuli. For instance, proline-rich tyrosine kinase 2 (PYK2) is a member of the Fak family [8]. It is highly expressed in the nervous system and can be activated by calcium and PKC. Activation of PYK2 regulates ion-channel function and activates the MAPK cascade. Therefore, it has both acute and chronic effects on the nervous system and may be the molecule linking G proteins and MAPK activation.

Receptor protein tyrosine kinases consist of an extracellular domain, a single transmembrane domain and a cytoplasmic domain

The cytoplasmic domain is composed of a juxtamembrane domain, one or two catalytic do-

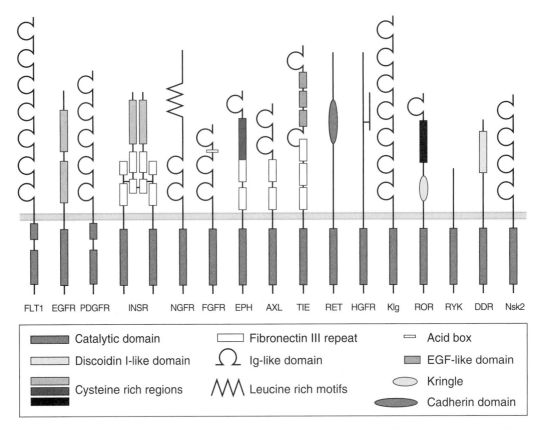

FIGURE 25-6. Schematic structures of receptor protein tyrosine kinase (RPTK) families. RPTKs can be divided into different families according to the structural features in the extracellular domain. Following the extracellular domain are the transmembrane and intracellular domains, the latter containing the catalytic domain. (From [2], with permission).

mains and a C-terminal tail. Like the NRPTKs, the additional structures besides the catalytic domain are important for the proper functioning of these enzymes. RPTKs can be classified into at least 14 families, including the epidermal growth factor receptor (EGFR), PDGFR, fibroblast growth factor receptor (FGFR), nerve growth factor receptor (NGFR), insulin receptor (INSR) and erythropoietin-producing hepatocellular receptor (EphR) found in the nervous system (Fig. 25-6). Additional aspects of growth factor receptors are discussed in Chapter 19.

The extracellular region of different PTKs is composed of different domains. For instance, the EGFR extracellular domain contains two cysteine-rich regions. The PDGFR extracellular domain consists of five immunoglobulin-like repeats. Other domains found in the extracellular

region of RPTKs include fibronectin III repeats, kringle domains and leucine-rich motifs. The extracellular domain contains the binding site for RPTK ligands, which can range from soluble factors and extracellular matrix proteins to surface proteins expressed on other cells. The extracellular domain also may be involved in the dimerization of RPTKs, a process critical for the activation of intrinsic tyrosine kinase activity.

The transmembrane domain in the RPTK is a hydrophobic segment of 22 to 26 amino acids situated in the cell membrane. It is flanked by a proline-rich region in the N-terminus and a cluster of basic amino acids in the C-terminus. This combination of structures secures the transmembrane domain within the lipid bilayer. There is a low degree of homology in the transmembrane domain, even between two closely

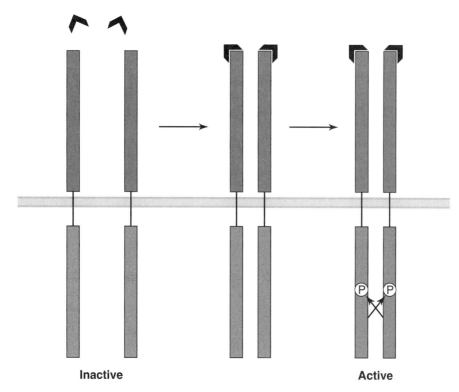

Inactive   **Active**

FIGURE 25-7.   Activation of receptor protein tyrosine kinase (RPTK) by dimerization and transphosphorylation. Autophosphorylation is a key step in the activation of PTKs. To achieve autophosphorylation, some PTKs dimerize and transphosphorylate each other. Ligand binding induces dimerization of RPTKs so that the catalytic domains are in close proximity for transphosphorylation. The autophosphorylated RPTK, thus, is activated. Some nonreceptor protein tyrosine kinases (NRPTKs) can be activated without dimerization (see Fig. 25-5B). However, others, such as Jak/Tyk kinases, are activated by transphosphorylation. Jak/Tyk tyrosine kinases are associated constitutively with transmembrane proteins gp130 and leukemia-inhibitory factor receptor β (LIFRβ). Extracellular ciliary neurotrophic factor (CNTF) induces the formation of a quaternary complex consisting of CNTF, LIFRβ, gp130 and another membrane protein known as CNTF receptor α. Consequently, the associated Jak/Tyk are dimerized, allowing transphosphorylation and activation.

related RPTKs, suggesting that the primary sequence does not contain important information for signal transduction.

The cytoplasmic domain. The intracellular domain primarily consists of the catalytic domain and various autophosphorylation sites that regulate catalytic function and serve as docking sites for proteins that contain SH2 domains. The protein kinase catalytic domains of RPTKs are highly conserved and similar in structure to the NRPTK catalytic domains. Please refer to the section on the SH1 domain in NRPTKs for details on the structure and function of the catalytic domain of the tyrosine kinase.

RPTK activation. Ligand binding to RPTKs induces receptor dimerization, which allows transphosphorylation between the two subunits. Transphosphorylation or autophosphorylation of RPTKs in many cases increases intrinsic catalytic activity (Fig. 25-7). Different RPTKs use slightly different mechanisms to induce dimerization and transphosphorylation. PDGF is a dimer consisting of subunits A and B in different combinations (AA, BB and AB). Its receptor also consists of two subunits (α and β). PDGF dimers can cross-link two PDGFRs because of their bivalency and, thus, can induce transphosphorylation. The INSR consists of two catalytic domains cross-linked by intermolecular disulfide bonds even in its basal state. However, ligand binding is required to activate the transphosphorylation reaction. Finally, since each EGFR binds to only one EGF molecule, its dimerization is not dependent on ligand-induced cross-linking. Instead, the extracellular domains of EGFRs probably interact with each other as a consequence of the conformational change induced by EGF binding.

RPTK inactivation. Once activated by their ligands, surface RPTKs with their bound ligands are rapidly internalized and degraded. These processes quickly terminate the action of the ligands. The intrinsic tyrosine-kinase activity appears to be important for both internalization and degradation. For example, mutant EGFR without the lysine for ATP binding is neither internalized nor degraded in NIH3T3 cells. A positive role has been assigned to internalization of RPTKs. In neurons, internalized TrkA is trans-

ported from the axon terminal to the cell body where it influences signal-transduction cascades that affect gene expression.

Tyrosine phosphorylation of RPTKs. Phosphorylation of specific tyrosine residues on the RPTKs can recruit SH2 domain-containing signaling molecules to the site of action. These signaling molecules include phospholipase C-γ1 (PLC-γ1), phosphatidylinositol-3-kinase (PI-3-kinase), growth factor receptor-binding protein 2 (Grb2), SH2-containing protein (SHC) and Src. Each signaling molecule recognizes a specific tyrosine phosphorylation site on the RPTK, as indicated in Figure 25-8. Recruitment of PLC-γ1 and PI-3-kinase to the membrane brings the enzymes to their substrates in the lipid bilayer. PLC-γ1 is phosphorylated and activated by RPTKs, whereas association of PI-3-kinase with the autophosphorylated RPTKs in-

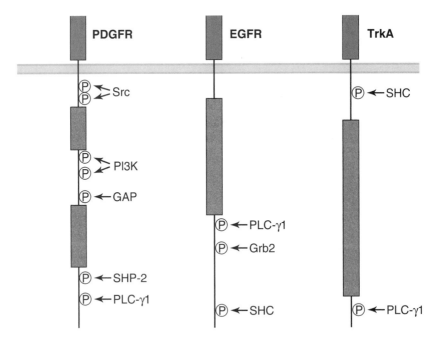

FIGURE 25-8.   Recruitment of different signaling molecules to different tyrosine-phosphorylation sites on receptor protein tyrosine kinases (RPTKs). RPTKs usually are autophosphorylated on several different sites. Each tyrosine-phosphorylation site has a unique sequence for interaction with specific signaling molecules containing SH2 or phosphotyrosine binding (PTB) domains. This provides specificity and diversity for RPTK signaling. *PDGFR,* platelet-derived growth factor receptor; *EGFR,* epidermal growth factor receptor; *PLC,* phospholipase C; *GAP,* GTPase-activating protein; *Grb2,* growth factor receptor binding protein; *PI3K,* phosphatidylinositol-3-kinase; *SHC,* SH2-containing protein; *SHP,* SH-domain containing tyrosine phosphatase.

duces its activity allosterically. PLC-γ1 catalyzes formation of diacylglycerol and inositol trisphosphate (IP$_3$) from phosphatidylinositol-4,5-bisphosphate (PIP$_2$) (see also Chap. 21). Diacylglycerol activates PKC, while IP$_3$ triggers calcium release from intracellular stores. PI-3-kinase incorporates a phosphate group in the 3′ position on the inositol ring of phosphatidylinositol phospholipids. One of the products, PI-3,4-P$_2$, activates Akt kinase to promote neuronal survival [9].

Recruitment of Grb2 to the membrane activates the MAPK pathway. Grb2 is an adaptor molecule carrying one SH2 and two SH3 domains (Fig. 25-4). The Grb2 SH2 domain recognizes the tyrosine-phosphorylated moiety on certain RPTKs, such as EGFR (Fig. 25-8), and anchors Grb2 to these membrane-spanning proteins. The Grb2 SH3 domains interact with son of sevenless (SOS), a guanine nucleotide exchange protein. SOS stimulates the release of GDP and subsequent binding of GTP to the membrane-bound, low-molecular-weight, GTP-binding protein ras (see Chap. 20). GTP-bound ras interacts with and translocates the serine/threonine protein kinase raf to the plasma membrane, where raf becomes activated. Activated raf phosphorylates MEK, which in turn stimulates MAPK. One of the substrates of MAPK is p90Rsk. Both MAPK and p90Rsk translocate to the nucleus after phosphorylation, where they phosphorylate and activate transcription factors such as, serum-responsive factor (SRF), T-cell-specific transcription factor and cAMP responsive element-binding protein and, thus, alter gene expression.

Some RPTKs cannot interact directly with Grb. They activate the MAPK pathway with the help of an adaptor molecule, such as SHC or insulin receptor substrate-1 (IRS-1). SHC contains a 160-amino-acid-long phosphotyrosine-binding domain (PTB) which recognizes an autophosphorylation site on some RPTKs. Unlike the SH2 domain, which recognizes the sequence C-terminal of the phosphotyrosine, PTB domains recognize amino acid residues upstream of the phosphotyrosine. The consensus sequence for interaction with the PTB domain of SHC is ØNPXpY, where Ø is a hydrophobic amino acid and X is any amino acid. IRS-1 contains a putative PTB domain which shares a low degree of homology with the PTB domain in SHC. Both IRS-1 and SHC are phosphorylated by the RPTKs with which they interact. Tyrosine phosphorylation of these adaptor molecules leads to interaction with the SH2 domain of Grb2 and activation of the MAPK cascade. A PTP, SHP-2, plays a role similar to that of IRS-1 and SHC and links the RPTK to the MAPK pathway (see below). RPTKs that interact with a PTB-binding domain-containing adaptor molecule include the nerve growth factor receptor (TrkA), EGFR, INSR and insulin-like growth factor 1 (IGF-1) receptor. Figure 25-9 (see p. 504) shows the role of IRS-1, SHC and SHP-2 in RPTK-mediated gene expression.

PROTEIN TYROSINE PHOSPHATASES

The low level of tyrosine phosphorylation in cells is probably due to the high specific activity of PTPs, which is about 10 to 1,000 times that of PTKs. PTP1B from human placenta was the first PTP purified [10]. Based on the sequence of PTP1B, many PTPs were isolated very rapidly using molecular biological techniques, including the polymerase chain reaction and low-stringency hybridization. Like PTKs, PTPs can be divided into RPTPs and NRPTPs and further subdivided into different families according to structural features (Fig. 25-10).

Nonreceptor protein tyrosine phosphatases are structurally different from serine/threonine phosphatases and contain a cysteine residue in their active sites

Although the catalytic domains of PTKs and serine/threonine kinases are highly conserved, the catalytic domains of PTPs are unrelated to that of the serine/threonine phosphatases. The catalytic domain of PTPs is approximately 200 to 300 amino acids in length and is composed of a

Nonreceptor Protein-tyrosine Phosphatases

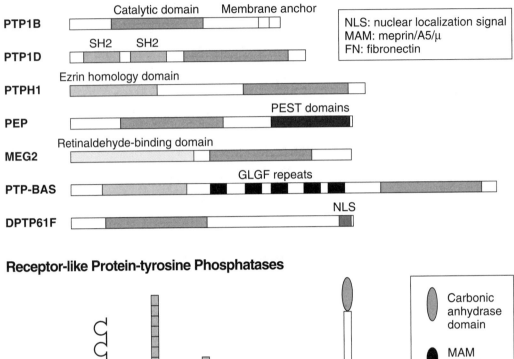

Receptor-like Protein-tyrosine Phosphatases

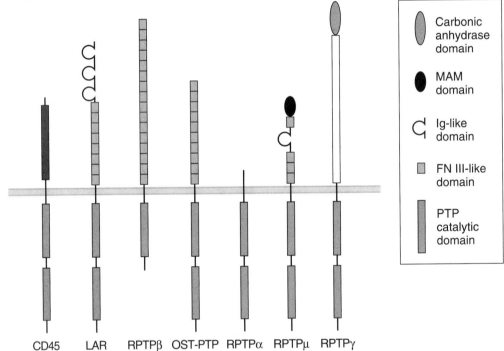

FIGURE 25-10. Schematic structures of nonreceptor protein tyrosine phosphatases (NRPTPs) and receptor protein tyrosine phosphatases *(RPTPs)*. NRPTPs contain a catalytic domain and various regulatory domains. RPTPs are composed of an extracellular domain, a transmembrane domain and an intracellular domain with one or two catalytic domains. Like receptor protein tyrosine kinases, the structural features of the extracellular domains divide the RPTPs into different families. (From [35], with permission).

central β sheet enclosed by α helices. The highly conserved motif, (I/V)HCXXGXGRS/TG, forms the base of the active-site cleft. The catalytic reaction mechanism is composed of two different steps. First, the nucleophilic thiolate anion of the active-site cysteine residue, Cys215 of PTP1B, attacks the phosphotyrosine on the substrate. A thiophosphate intermediate is then formed, accompanied by release of the dephosphorylated product. The second step involves hydrolysis of the thioester bond by an aspartate residue, Asp181 of PTP1B, to regenerate the free cysteine residue and phosphate. Vanadate and pervanadate are widely used PTP inhibitors. Vanadate reversibly inhibits PTPs by competing with phosphotyrosine for the active site. Pervanadate irreversibly inhibits PTPs by binding to the active site and oxidizing the catalytic cysteine to cysteic acid ($-SO_3H$).

The phosphotyrosine-recognition subdomain, confers substrate specificity of PTPs by creating a deep pocket (9 Å) so that only the phosphotyrosine moiety is long enough to reach the cysteine nucleophile located at the base of this pocket. Dual-specificity PTPs lack the phosphotyrosine-recognition subdomain and have a shallow catalytic-site cleft (6 Å). Therefore, the active site is accessible to all three phosphorylated hydroxyamino acids. An example of a dual-specificity protein phosphatase is MKP-1, which inactivates MAPK by removing phosphate from both the threonine and tyrosine residues in the activation loop.

SH2 domains are found in the PTPs SHP-1 and SHP-2 and play an important role in their function. These PTPs, respectively, are also known as SHPTP1, PTP1C and HCP and SHPTP2, PTP1D and Syp [11]. Each of these PTPs contains two SH2 domains in the N-terminus, followed by the catalytic domain (Fig. 25-4). SHP-1 is expressed most highly in hemopoietic cells and is involved in their development and function. SHP-2 is expressed ubiquitously. Despite considerable sequence homology, these two PTPs are thought to serve quite different functions. SHP-1 negatively regulates RPTK activity by dephosphorylating autophosphorylation sites. In contrast,

SHP-2 has a positive role in the tyrosine-phosphorylation pathway. It recruits Grb2 to RPTKs and activates the subsequent steps in the MAPK pathway. For example, PDGF induces autophosphorylation of the PDGFR, which binds to the SH2 domain of SHP-2 (Fig. 25-8). The PDGFR then phosphorylates SHP-2 and creates a binding site on SHP-2 for Grb2. Furthermore, SHP-2 can activate the Src-family tyrosine kinases by dephosphorylating the negative-regulatory, tyrosine-phosphorylation site at the C-terminus.

The SH2-containing PTPs are normally inactive in the basal state under the influence of the SH2 domains. Binding of SHP-2 to autophosphorylated RPTKs increases its activity by changing the conformation of the enzyme and allowing access of substrates to its active site.

Receptor protein tyrosine phosphatases consist of an extracellular domain, a transmembrane domain and one or two intracellular catalytic domains

RPTPs can be divided into different classes by the structural features of the extracellular domain (Fig. 25-10), which includes the immunoglobulin-like, fibronectin III-like, MAM and carbonic anhydrase domains. The immunoglobulin-like domains contain intramolecular disulfide bonds and a homophilic binding site for cell–cell adhesion molecules, such as neural cell adhesion molecule (NCAM). The fibronectin III-like domains originally were identified in the extracellular matrix protein fibronectin. They consist of conserved hydrophobic residues and may interact with integrins. The MAM domains are named because of their presence in *m*eprins, *A*5 glycoprotein and PTPμ. These domains contain four conserved cysteine residues. The carbonic anhydrase domains contain only one of the three histidine residues required for catalyzing the hydration of carbon dioxide and are unlikely to be catalytically active. Both the MAM and carbonic anhydrase domains have been suggested to play a role in cell adhesion.

The **catalytic domains** of RPTPs are in the intracellular region of the protein. All RPTP families, except RPTPβ, contain two tandem catalytic domains. Mutational studies have demonstrated that the first catalytic domain of CD45, which is proximal to the membrane, contains all of the enzymatic activity and is necessary and sufficient for its biological activity. The second catalytic domain of CD45, which is distal to the membrane, appears to be inactive. However, the second catalytic domain carries all of the phosphorylation sites and, therefore, may be important for the regulation of phosphatase activity and specificity.

Dimerization and subcellular localization. Once, it was believed that PTP activity was constitutive and that tyrosine phosphorylation was regulated solely by activating the PTKs. However, it has since been shown that PTPs play a more active role in the regulation of tyrosine phosphorylation in cells. This was suggested first by the discovery of RPTPs, such as CD45, that have a large extracellular domain, reminiscent of RPTKs, whose activity is regulated by ligand binding to its extracellular domain. Chimeric studies fusing the intracellular domain of CD45 with the extracellular and transmembrane domains of the EGFR show that the CD45 intracellular catalytic domain is constitutively active [12]. Addition of EGF suppresses the PTP activity of the chimera, suggesting that dimerization may negatively regulate RPTP activity. Indeed, X-ray crystallographic analysis has indicated that dimerization of the RPTPα membrane proximal catalytic domain may inactivate it by preventing it from interacting with its substrates. Therefore, a potential regulatory mechanism of RPTP would be inhibition by ligand-induced dimerization, in contrast to activation by dimerization in RPTKs.

Alternatively, RPTPs can be targeted to specific subcellular microenvironments, where their potential substrates reside. PTP targeting can be achieved through interaction with intracellular- or extracellular-adaptor molecules. One such adaptor molecule is lymphocyte-phosphatase associated phosphoprotein (LPAP; CD45-AP), which binds to CD45. It is a 32-kDa transmembrane protein with a very short extracellular domain. The transmembrane domain of CD45 is critical for its interaction with LPAP. A cytoskeletal protein, fodrin, has been implicated in the interaction with the cytoplasmic tail of CD45.

ROLE OF TYROSINE PHOSPHORYLATION IN THE NERVOUS SYSTEM

Tyrosine phosphorylation plays a role in virtually every step in the development and function of a neuron, including survival and differentiation, the extension of axons to their targets and synapse formation and function (Fig. 25-11). Due to the large number of topics involved, the following is by no means a complete account of all of the functions of tyrosine phosphorylation in the nervous system. However, these examples demonstrate the significance of tyrosine phosphorylation in neuronal function (Fig. 25-11).

Tyrosine phosphorylation is involved in every stage of neuronal development

Neuronal survival and differentiation are promoted by neurotrophins and the Trk family of RPTKs. NGF promotes the survival of neurons during a period of programmed cell death in embryonic and early postnatal developmental stages. It is a target-derived neurotrophic factor that modulates the functions of the innervating axon terminals as well as gene expression in the distant cell body (see Chap. 19).

NGF was discovered over 40 years ago. Its action on neuronal survival and differentiation has long been recognized. However, its signal-transduction mechanism had remained unknown until the identification of a 140-kDa protein, TrkA RPTK, as the NGFR in 1991 [13]. Since then, other members of the Trk family have been discovered as receptors for other neurotrophins. For example, brain-derived neurotrophic factor (BDNF) has the highest affinity toward TrkB, while neutrophin-3 (NT-3) is the preferred ligand for TrkC. A 75-kDa transmembrane protein, p75, also termed the low-affinity NGFR, has been identified as a neurotrophin receptor. All neurotrophins can bind to p75 with a low affinity. Although not a PTK itself, p75 can interact with other Trk proteins and may modify the ligand-binding affinity, dose responsiveness and PTK activity. For instance, it increases the affinity of TrkA for NGF while decreasing its re-

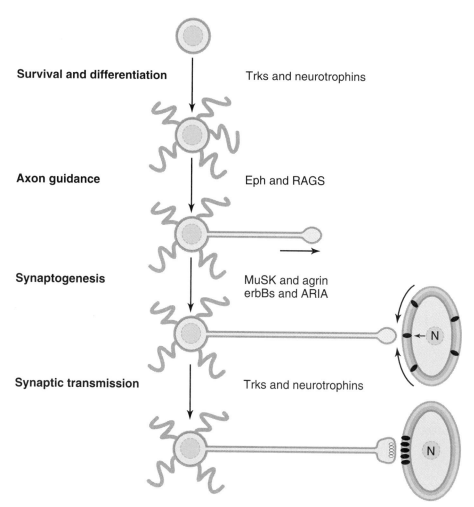

Survival and differentiation   Trks and neurotrophins

Axon guidance   Eph and RAGS

Synaptogenesis   MuSK and agrin
erbBs and ARIA

Synaptic transmission   Trks and neurotrophins

FIGURE 25-11.   Examples of the role of protein tyrosine kinases and protein tyrosine phosphatases in the lifetime of a neuron *(N)*. Tyrosine phosphorylation appears to be an important signal-transduction mechanism in every step in the development of a neuron, starting from the survival and differentiation of stem cells, to axon guidance and synaptogenesis and to synaptic transmission at a mature synapse. Examples of each step are given on the right, indicating the receptors and their ligands. *Eph*, erythropoietin-producing hepatocellular factor; *RAGS*, repulsive axon guidance signal; *MuSK*, muscle specific kinase; *ARIA*, acetylcholine receptor inducing activity.

sponse to NT-3. The tyrosine-kinase activity of TrkA is enhanced by p75. Transgenic mice that do not express p75 survive through adult life but with significant loss of certain sensory and sympathetic neurons, suggesting a significant role for p75 in neuronal survival in the peripheral nervous system.

NGF induces differentiation of rat pheochromocytoma PC12 cells into cells with many characteristics of mature sympathetic neurons (Fig. 25-9). This is a well-characterized model system that has been used extensively to study mechanisms of the action of NGF. Studies with PC12 cells show that NGF induces autophosphorylation of at least four different tyrosine residues on human TrkA. These are Y490 in the juxtamembrane region, Y674, Y675 in the catalytic domain and Y785 in the C-terminal tail. Each phosphotyrosine serves a different function in the NGF signaling pathway (Fig. 25-8). Y674 and Y675 are the first tyrosine residues phosphorylated and are important for subsequent activation of the intrinsic kinase activity. Phosphorylation of Y490 and Y785 creates SH2-binding sites for SHC and PLC-γ1, respectively. Recruitment of PI-3 kinase to TrkA possibly involves an adaptor molecule. These three signaling molecules are in turn activated by tyrosine phosphorylation by TrkA, eventually leading to the biological effects of NGF. Independent of any of the known signaling pathways used by TrkA, a novel protein, suc-associated neurotrophic factor-induced tyrosine-phosphorylated target (SNT), is tyrosine-phosphorylated upon NGF treatment of PC12 cells. SNT is specifically activated in response to differentiation but not in response to mitogenic factors. This suggests the existence of yet another unknown signaling pathway used by TrkA to induce differentiation of neurons.

Neurotrophins acting on the same Trk tyrosine kinase can induce either cellular proliferation or differentiation depending on the cell type, suggesting that cell context determines the response to Trk activation. This may partly be related to the duration of MAPK activation. Transient activation of the MAPK pathway is associated with mitogenic response while prolonged activation induces differentiation of PC12 cells. While many aspects of TrkA signaling have been discovered, it remains unclear how TrkA promotes survival and differentiation of neurons.

Axon guidance. In many cases, the growth cone at the leading end of an axon navigates a trajectory over a long distance before it finds its target. Various extracellular cues help the growth cone navigate through different terrains to reach its destination. Growth cones often travel in segments, such that the whole journey is subdivided into shorter stretches which the growth cone will travel one at a time, detecting cues along the way until it finds its final target. Furthermore, axons may stick together and form fascicles, which can serve as a "highway" for future traveling growth cones. Extracellular cues that influence axon guidance can be attractive or repulsive and diffusible or immobilized to the cell surface or the extracellular matrix (see Chaps. 7, 27 and 28).

One of the best studied model systems of axon guidance in vertebrates is the retinotectal system. Anterior and posterior retinal axons project to the posterior and anterior tectum, respectively. Similarly, the dorsal and ventral retinal axons innervate the ventral and dorsal tectum, respectively. This reversal of projection is important for the rectification of the upside-down and back-to-front retinal image. Using membrane stripe and growth cone collapse assays, Bonhoeffer and colleagues have identified a 25-kDa protein called repulsive axon guidance signal (RAGS) as an important axon guidance molecule in this system [14]. It is expressed most highly in the posterior tectum and repels the posterior retinal axons from this region.

The receptor for RAGS is the Eph RPTK, discovered in the human erythropoietin-producing hepatocellular carcinoma cell line [15]. The ligands for Eph family RPTK are either glycophosphatidylinositol (GPI)-anchored or transmembrane proteins (see Box 3–1). Their biological activity is lost if they are detached from the membrane. This implies that Eph-mediated axon guidance is limited to short-range contact-dependent activity. Accordingly, the Eph family of receptors can be divided into those interacting with GPI-linked ligands, including the epithelial cell kinase (Eck) subgroup, and transmembrane ligands, including the Eph-like kinase (Elk) subgroup. Activated, the Eck family binds PI-3-kinase, whereas the Elk family binds Src, Yes and p120-GTPase-activating protein (GAP). The Elk family ligands are also tyrosine phosphorylated upon binding their receptors, suggesting a bidirectional flow of information. However, the exact signal-transduction mechanism leading to the repulsion of growth cones is largely unknown. It is known that repulsion of growth cones from the signal requires a local depolymerization of F-actin, while steering of the growth cone toward the signal requires an accumulation of F-actin, leading to the recruitment of microtubules. There is evidence that small G proteins, Rho and Rac, may play a role in axon guidance by regulating actin polymerization (see Chaps. 8, 27 and 29).

The Eph receptor family may have a role in the fasciculation of axons of cortical neurons growing on astrocytes in culture. The interacting proteins in this case are the Eph receptor Rek7, expressed on the axons, and the Eph ligand AL-1, found on the astrocyte surface. It is postulated that the axons clump together in a bundle because of the repulsive interaction with the astrocytes.

Another RPTK found in *Drosophila*, derailed, also plays a role in axon guidance as a small subset of embryonic interneurons fail to find their targets in the derailed mutant. Basic fibroblast growth factor (bFGF) present in the optic tract may activate FGFR in the growth cone of retinal ganglion cells. Addition of bFGF to the developing retinotectal tract impairs the correct innervation of tectum from the retinal ganglion cells. Expression of dominant negative FGFR in retinal ganglion cells also prevents axons from entering their target. NRPTKs appear to have a role in axon guidance. For instance, although deletion of the Abl gene in *Drosophila* does not yield gross morphological defects, a double mutant of Abl and fasciclin I causes major defects in axon guidance and fasciculation. Several RPTPs are expressed predominantly in the growth cones and axons in *Drosophila* and are likely to regulate the fasciculation of axons. For instance, in *Drosophila* mutants that lack *Drosophila* leukocyte antigen-related proteins (DLAR) or *Drosophila* protein-tyrosine-phosphate phosphohydrolase (DPTP), motor neurons fail to defasciculate and consequently bypass their targets.

Synapse formation. Not only is tyrosine phosphorylation involved in guiding axons to their target, once the growth cone reaches its target, tyrosine phosphorylation also plays a role in the formation of a proper synaptic structure. For instance, the acetylcholine receptor (AChR) is concentrated at the postsynaptic membrane of the neuromuscular junction at a density of 10,000 receptors/μm^2, which is about three orders of magnitude higher than that of the extrasynaptic region. The high concentration of AChR at the neuromuscular junction allows rapid, reliable and efficient synaptic transmission. In fact, transmission across a synapse is so rapid that the idea of a chemical synapse was not readily accepted at the turn of the century. The strategic positioning of the AChR right on the crest of junctional folds at the neuromuscular synapse reduces the distance (30 to 50 nm) for the neurotransmitter to travel before reaching its receptor. Furthermore, the high concentration of AChR at the neuromuscular junction makes it more likely that a depolarization is higher than the threshold to trigger muscular contraction. The significance of this is demonstrated by the pathological condition myasthenia gravis, in which there is muscle weakness due to a reduction of AChR present at the neuromuscular junction. Two mechanisms contribute to the enrichment of AChR at the neuromuscular junction: (i) clustering of pre-existing, diffusely distributed surface AChR and (ii) local synthesis of the receptor by subsynaptic nuclei. Both mechanisms are mediated by tyrosine phosphorylation, as discussed below.

Agrin induces clustering of the AChR at the neuromuscular junction by activating the muscle-specific kinase (MuSK) RPTK. The clustering of pre-existing AChR at the postsynaptic membrane is triggered by a neuronally derived extracellular matrix protein discovered by McMahan's [16] laboratory in the 1980s called agrin, from the Greek word *ageirein* meaning "to assemble." Since then, the agrin hypothesis [16] has been supported by a number of experiments from various laboratories and confirmed by the agrin knockout mutant mouse [17]. These mice are stillborn and never move, probably due to lack of neuronal transmission across the neuromuscular junction. Microscopic analysis reveals the absence of AChR clusters at the neuromuscular junction.

The molar ratio of agrin to AChR at the neuromuscular junction is 1:50 to 100, suggesting that agrin induces AChR clustering through some intracellular signal-transduction mechanism rather than via any structural constraints. Tyrosine phosphorylation of the AChR may play a role in its clustering at the neuromuscular junction. First, agrin induces tyrosine phosphorylation of the AChR prior to clustering of the receptor in muscle [18]. All agents which induce AChR clustering in muscle cells in culture also induce tyrosine phosphorylation of the AChR.

These include agrin, rapsyn, electrical fields and latex beads. However, PTK inhibitors which inhibit AChR tyrosine phosphorylation also inhibit AChR clustering. Although tyrosine phosphorylation appears to be important to the action of agrin on muscle, a causal relationship between AChR tyrosine phosphorylation and clustering has not been established.

The putative receptor for agrin is an RPTK known as MuSK [19]. The extracellular domain of MuSK resembles that of the ROR family RPTKs, while the kinase domain is similar to that of the Trk neurotrophic receptor (Fig. 25-6). MuSK is expressed at low concentrations in proliferating myoblasts and is induced upon differentiation and fusion. It is downregulated dramatically in mature muscle except at the neuromuscular junction. These properties are consistent with the role of MuSK in muscle development and the function of neuromuscular junction.

MuSK knockout mice show disruption of AChR clusters at the neuromuscular junction [19] similar to that seen with the agrin knockout mice [17]. Furthermore, muscle cells in culture from these mutant mice do not respond to agrin. Expression of MuSK in immature myotubes stimulates agrin binding. These data strongly indicate that MuSK is necessary for the response to agrin. It is postulated that MuSK is part of the agrin receptor, and a myotube-associated specificity component (MASC) is required to form the agrin receptor. This is similar to the CNTF receptor, in which more than one component is required for the assembly of the intact receptor.

Synapses in the central nervous system share a similar structural architecture with the neuromuscular junction. Proteins important for the organization of the neuromuscular junction are also found in the central nervous system. For instance, agrin is expressed in the brain during periods of intense synaptogenesis. Therefore, it is possible that similar mechanisms are employed for clustering neurotransmitter receptors in the central nervous system.

Acetylcholine receptor-inducing activity (ARIA) increases the expression of AChR subunits by subsynaptic nuclei through activation of the erbB RPTKs. In addition to clustering of pre-existing AChRs, neuronal innervation increases the transcription of AChR subunits in nuclei near the synapse despite the downregulation of AChR synthesis in extrasynaptic regions. This transcriptional regulation results in a local concentration of AChR subunit mRNAs in the subsynaptic cytoplasm. Innervation also switches the AChR subunit composition from $\alpha_2\beta\gamma\delta$ to $\alpha_2\beta\epsilon\delta$ since transcription of the ϵ subunit is most sensitive to neuronal input. The switchover from γ to ϵ in the AChR complex increases the conductance of the channel but decreases the duration of its opening.

Transcriptional control of the AChR is regulated by ARIA, which was first identified in the late 1970s by Fischbach's laboratory as the trophic factor for the expression of AChR in muscle present in chick brain and spinal cord [20]. It is a member of the neuregulin family, which also includes neu differentiation factor, heregulin and glial growth factor. The precursor of ARIA is a 67-kDa transmembrane glycoprotein which is proteolysed to the 42-kDa mature ARIA before its release from the motor neuron. Similar to agrin, the released ARIA is deposited on the basal lamina in the synaptic cleft. The interaction is so stable that even after denervation the ARIA deposited on the basal lamina can be recognized by regenerated muscle fiber as the site for active synthesis of AChR, even in the absence of neuronal innervation. Besides its action on the AChR, ARIA can increase the synthesis of voltage-gated Na^+ channels, which are concentrated at the depths of junctional folds of the neuromuscular junction at a concentration of $5,000/\mu m^2$. The synthesis of two other synaptic proteins, AChE and rapsyn, is unaffected by ARIA.

The effect of ARIA on gene expression is dependent on tyrosine phosphorylation, as evidenced by its inhibition by PTK inhibitors and potentiation by a PTP inhibitor. In fact, ARIA induces tyrosine phosphorylation of 185-kDa proteins in the muscle [21]. The 185-kDa proteins turn out to be the components of the ARIA receptor, which are members of the EGFR tyrosine kinase family. This family contains four known members: erbB1 (EGFR), erbB2, erbB3 and erbB4. The last three members are found in the muscle and can respond to ARIA. However, erbB3 does not possess intrinsic tyrosine kinase activity, so it has to couple with another erbB protein to respond to ARIA. erbB3 and erbB4 are present at the neuromuscular junction and can interact directly with ARIA [22]. Like many other RPTK pathways, activation of AChR gene expression depends on the MAPK signaling pathway.

Tyrosine phosphorylation plays an important role in synaptic transmission

A number of synaptic molecules, such as neurotransmitter receptors, voltage-gated ion channels, enzymes and proteins involved in neurotransmitter release, are tyrosine-phosphorylated. The importance of tyrosine phosphorylation on animal behavior has been demonstrated using genetic techniques. For example, mutant mice missing PTKs show diminished long-term potentiation (LTP) and/or learning and memory [23] (see Chap. 50).

Tyrosine phosphorylation of neurotransmitter receptors, including the AChR, *N*-methyl-D-aspartate (NMDA) receptor and

GABA$_A$R, plays a pivotal role in modulating synaptic efficacy and plasticity. Several neurotransmitter receptors and voltage-gated ion channels in both the peripheral and central nervous systems are tyrosine-phosphorylated (Table 25-2). Furthermore, tyrosine phosphorylation of these surface signal-transducing molecules significantly modulates their electrophysiological properties, producing a prominent effect on neuronal signal propagation.

Acetylcholine receptors. Due to its enrichment and easy access in the *Torpedo* electric organ, the AChR is one of the best studied neurotransmitter receptors (see Chap. 11). It sits on the postsynaptic side of the mammalian neuromuscular junction. Upon binding acetylcholine, this ligand-and-gated ion channel depolarizes the sarcolemma and triggers muscle contraction. The AChR is composed of five subunits, $\alpha_2\beta\gamma\delta$ (embryonic) or $\alpha_2\beta\epsilon\delta$ (adult). Each subunit has four transmembrane domains, with both the N- and C-termini in the extracellular space. Between the third and fourth transmembrane domains is a large cytoplasmic region in which there are a number of consensus phosphorylation sites (Fig.

TABLE 25-2. **REGULATION OF ION CHANNEL FUNCTION BY TYROSINE PHOSPHORYLATION**

Ion channel	Tyrosine-phosphorylated subunits	PTK/PTP	Effect
mAChR	β, γ, δ	PTKs in electric organ	Inhibition
		Agrin/MuSK	?
		Fyn, Fyk, Src	?
		MuSK	?
NMDAR	NR2A/B	Src	Potentiation
		INSR	Potentiation
GABA$_A$R	β, γ	Src	Potentiation
Voltage-gated potassium channel	Kv1.5	Src, PYK2	Inhibition
Delayed rectifier potassium channel (RAK)		PTK activated by mAChR1 (PYK2?)	Inhibition
Voltage-gated cationic channel		PKA-activated PTP	Potentiation

Various ion channels are listed with their tyrosine-phosphorylated subunits, protein tyrosine kinases and protein tyrosine phosphatases (PTK/PTP) specific for them and the effect of tyrosine phosphorylation on their electrophysiological activity. The G protein-coupled muscarinic acetylcholine receptor (mAChR1) appears to activate tyrosine phosphorylation indirectly by the activation of phospholipase C (PLC)-β, which raises intracellular calcium concentrations and generates diacylglycerol, a protein kinase C (PKC) activator. The elevated calcium concentration and activated PKC may activate PYK2 and lead to the tyrosine phosphorylation and inhibition of RAK. NMDAR, *N*-methyl-D-aspartate receptor; INSR, insulin receptor; MuSK, muscle specific kinase; PKA, protein kinase A.

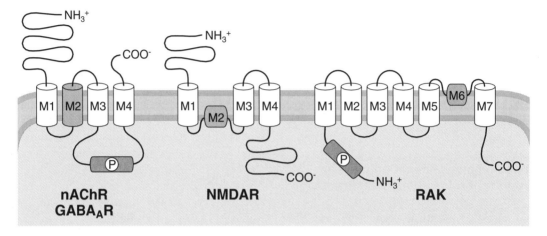

FIGURE 25-12. Transmembrane topology of three ligand-gated ion channel subunits and their potential domains for tyrosine phosphorylation. Both the acetylcholine receptor *(AChR)* and GABA_A receptor *(GABA_AR)* subunits have four transmembrane domains with both the N- and C-termini on the outside. Tyrosine phosphorylation sites are present within the large intracellular loop between the third and fourth transmembrane domains. *N*-Methyl-ᴅ-aspartate *(NMDA)* receptor subunits have a somewhat different topology. They have three transmembrane domains and a membrane-spanning domain. Tyrosine-phosphorylation sites for this ion channel have not been resolved but most likely are present in the large intracellular C-terminal tail. The delayed rectifier potassium channel *(RAK)* has six transmembrane domains and a membrane-spanning domain. Mutagenesis studies have revealed the intracellular N-terminus as the tyrosine-phosphorylation site-bearing region, although other studies have suggested the presence of other tyrosine-phosphorylation sites.

25-12). A single conserved tyrosine residue in the cytoplasmic loop of each of the β, γ and δ subunits is phosphorylated by PTKs in the postsynaptic membrane [24]. Tyrosine phosphorylation, like serine phosphorylation, of the AChR regulates its rate of desensitization [25].

The AChR is highly tyrosine-phosphorylated in intact electric organ and muscle, in contrast to its low tyrosine phosphorylation in cultured rat myotubes, <0.001 mol phosphate/mol subunit. This raises the possibility that innervation increases the tyrosine phosphorylation of the AChR. In fact, tyrosine phosphorylation of the AChR increases as muscle is innervated during development or in culture [18]. However, denervation results in loss of phosphotyrosine on the AChR. In light of the similar subunit and site specificity of agrin- and neuron-induced tyrosine phosphorylation of the AChR, agrin probably mediates the regulation of AChR tyrosine phosphorylation by the motor neuron.

The physiological PTK responsible for phosphorylating the AChR is unknown. Since MuSK RPTK is the putative agrin receptor, it is a candidate kinase for phosphorylating the AChR. Indeed, coexpression of MuSK and AChR together with rapsyn in quail fibroblasts induces tyrosine phosphorylation of the AChR. The AChR also has been shown to bind to Fyn, Fyk and Src NRPTKs and can be phosphorylated by these enzymes. Although agrin regulates tyrosine phosphorylation of the AChR, the exact physiological role of this phosphorylation remains to be elucidated.

***N*-Methyl-ᴅ-aspartate receptors.** Glutamate is the major excitatory neurotransmitter in the central nervous system (see Chap. 15). Its receptors can be divided into three types: AMPA/kainate, NMDA and metabotropic receptors. The first two types are ligand-gated ion channels, while the metabotropic receptors are G protein-linked. The AMPA/kainate receptors mediate fast excitatory synaptic transmission, while the NMDA receptors play a critical role in the induction of synaptic plasticity and excitotoxicity. The NMDA receptors are composed of two different types of subunit: NR1 and NR2.

The activity of NMDA receptors is enhanced by tyrosine phosphorylation. In spinal cord dorsal horn neurons, PTK inhibitors diminish NMDA receptor activity. However, intracellular perfusion of Src or a PTP inhibitor potentiates the NMDA current. Although it is still unknown whether direct tyrosine phosphorylation of the NMDA receptor regulates its activity, accumulating evidence has suggested that tyrosine phosphorylation of the NR2 subunits regulates NMDA function. For instance, the NR2A and 2B subunits are tyrosine-phosphorylated *in vivo* [4,26]. Heterologous cells expressing NMDA receptors composed of the NR1 and NR2A subunits exhibited increased NMDA-induced current in the presence of v-Src, while NMDA receptors consisting of NR1 with other NR2 subunits are not potentiated by v-Src. Furthermore, NMDA receptor conductance in excised patches can be potentiated by tyrosine phosphorylation, suggesting that the NMDA receptor itself or some tightly associated tyrosine-phosphorylated proteins are mediating the increase. In fact, Src has been suggested to interact with the NMDA receptor *in vivo* via its unique N-terminal domain [27]. Another NRPTK, Fyn, phosphorylates the NR2 subunits *in vitro*. Identification of tyrosine-phosphorylation sites and analysis of their effect on the electrophysiology of the NMDA receptor will be the next step in the elucidation of the direct involvement of NMDA receptors in regulation by tyrosine phosphorylation. The NR2B subunit from the dentate gyrus has increased tyrosine phosphorylation during the maintenance phase of LTP, suggesting a role for tyrosine phosphorylation in synaptic plasticity. However, the NMDA receptor also can be inhibited indirectly by PDGFR in cultured hippocampal neurons. The PDGFR activates PLC-γ1 to produce IP$_3$, a calcium-elevating agent. The increase in intracellular calcium in turn inhibits NMDA receptor activity. Therefore, tyrosine phosphorylation directly or indirectly influences the NMDA receptors in both the positive and negative directions.

GABA receptors. GABA is one of the major inhibitory neurotransmitters in the central ner- vous system (see Chap. 16). The subunits from the GABA$_A$ receptor (GABA$_A$R) include α, β, γ and δ. The GABA$_A$R complex is believed to be pentameric and similar in structure to the AChR, with each subunit spanning the membrane four times. Similar to the AChR, the intracellular region between the third and fourth transmembrane domains contains a number of consensus protein-phosphorylation sites (Fig. 25-12). Coexpression of GABA$_A$R subunits α1, β1 and γ2L with v-Src induces tyrosine phosphorylation on both the β and γ subunits. GABA-mediated whole-cell current is also potentiated [28]. Mutation of a tyrosine residue on the γ subunit abolished the potentiating effect of v-Src, suggesting that direct tyrosine phosphorylation of GABA$_A$R increases its activity.

Activation of the PDGFR inhibits GABA$_A$R in hippocampal neurons. Similar to its effect on the NMDA receptor, the PDGFR can activate PLC-γ1, generate IP$_3$ and increase intracellular calcium, which inhibits the GABA$_A$R. GABAergic transmission is inhibited by NT-3, the ligand for the RPTK TrkC. Therefore, direct tyrosine phosphorylation of the GABA$_A$R potentiates its activity, while release of intracellular calcium from RPTK activation appears to inhibit its function.

Voltage-gated ion channels. Besides the neurotransmitter-gated ion channels, some voltage-gated ion channels are targets of PTKs. These include a delayed rectifier potassium channel (RAK), hKv1.5 and a voltage-gated cation channel in *Aplysia* bag cell neurons. Tyrosine phosphorylation inhibits these voltage-gated ion channels.

Voltage-gated potassium channels maintain resting potential, regulate excitability and repolarize the membrane after an action potential. Modulation of potassium channels by tyrosine phosphorylation will influence these membrane properties. Delayed rectifier potassium channels (RAK) coexpressed with the m1 muscarinic AChR in *Xenopus* oocytes are inhibited by carbachol, a nonmetabolizable analog of acetylcholine [29]. Activation of the m1 muscarinic receptor releases diacylglycerol and IP$_3$ from the hydrolysis of PIP$_2$. Diacylglycerol activates PKC and IP$_3$ releases calcium from intracellular stores. Possibly by their action on a PYK2-related tyrosine kinase, calcium and PKC eventually lead to tyrosine phosphorylation of RAK on Y132 in the cytoplasmic domain near the N-terminus, resulting in an impaired RAK response. Similarly, the human potassium channel hKv1.5 is tyrosine-phosphorylated and suppressed when coexpressed with v-Src in transfected cells [30]. *In vivo* association between hKv1.5 and Src is mediated by proline-rich sequences on the potassium channel and Src SH3 domain.

The voltage-gated cation channel displays two modes of activity patterns in *Aplysia* bag cell neurons. In the bursting mode, the channel rapidly switches between the open and closed states for a brief period of time, followed by a longer period of inactivity. In the nonbursting mode, the channel opens and closes briefly. Treatment of the inside-out patch with a purified PTP switches the channel from the bursting to the nonbursting mode, thus increasing the channel opening time [31]. Apparently, an endogenous PTP can be activated by PKA to induce a similar mode switching in the cationic channel. However, it is unknown whether these effects are mediated by direct tyrosine dephosphorylation of the channel or some closely associated protein.

Synaptic transmission. Neurotrophins are known for their long-term effects on survival and differentiation of neuronal stem cells. However, accumulating evidence has suggested that neurotrophins also can have an acute effect on synaptic transmission in both the peripheral and central nervous systems. At the frog neuromuscular junction, BDNF and NT-3 can potentiate both the evoked synaptic transmission and spontaneous miniature synaptic response [32]. Similarly, at the hippocampal Schaffer collateral-CA1 synapse, these two neurotrophins, but not NGF, increase synaptic transmission by 200 to 300% [33].

Long-term potentiation (LTP) also is affected by neurotrophins. Mutant mice lacking BDNF show diminished LTP. Treatment with TrkB-IgG fusion protein, which adsorbs endogenous BDNF, also reduces LTP induced in the hippocampus [34]. However, addition of exogenous BDNF promotes the induction of LTP. Although both neurotrophins and LTP can potentiate synaptic transmission at the same synapse, they use at least partially distinct mechanisms since (i) unlike their effect on LTP, NMDA-receptor antagonists do not block the action of neurotrophins [33] and (ii) LTP does not completely occlude neurotrophin-mediated potentiation and *vice versa* [33].

Exactly how the neurotrophins enhance synaptic transmission is still unclear, but both pre- and postsynaptic mechanisms appear to be involved. At the frog neuromuscular junction and the Schaffer collateral-CA1 synapse, neurotrophin potentiation of synaptic transmission appears to increase neurotransmitter release at the presynaptic nerve terminal [32,33]. Since potassium channels are inhibited by tyrosine phosphorylation (see above, under Voltage-gated ion channel), it is possible that the action of neurotrophins can be mediated by tyrosine phosphorylation of these channels, which results in prolonged depolarization and, consequently, enhanced neurotransmitter release from the presynaptic terminal. Another protein that has the potential to alter neurotransmitter release is synaptophysin, a neurotransmitter vesicle protein that is tyrosine-phosphorylated.

A postsynaptic mechanism has been suggested at the Schaffer collateral-CA1 synapse. The high-affinity BDNF receptor TrkB has been found in the postsynaptic density. Furthermore, injection of a Trk tyrosine kinase inhibitor, K252a, into the postsynaptic neuron inhibits the facilitatory response of BDNF. Finally, the NT-3-induced increase in the frequency of neuronal impulse activity in cultured cortical neurons has been attributed to a third mechanism, such as reduction of the inhibitory GABA$_A$R activity.

A number of studies have shown that neuronal activity can increase neurotrophin expression. This strengthens the notion that the action of neurotrophins is closely linked to neuronal activity. For instance, induction of LTP at the perforant path-dentate granule cell synapses increases the expression of NGF and BDNF mRNA. Furthermore, LTP induction at the Schaffer collateral-CA1 synapse results in an increased expression of BDNF and NT-3.

ACKNOWLEDGMENTS

We would like to thank Drs. David Ginty and Alexander Kolodkin for their suggestions in this chapter.

REFERENCES

1. Eckhart, W., Hutchinson, M. A., and Hunter, T. An activity phosphorylating tyrosine in polyoma T antigen immunoprecipitates. *Cell* 18:925–933, 1979.
2. Vandergeer, P., Hunter, T., and Lindberg, R. A. Receptor protein-tyrosine kinases and their signal transduction pathways [Review]. *Annu. Rev. Cell Biol.* 10:251–337, 1994.
3. Wagner, K. R., Mei, L., and Huganir, R. L. Protein tyrosine kinases and phosphatases in the nervous system [Review]. *Curr. Opin. Neurobiol.* 1:65–73, 1991.
4. Lau, L. F., and Huganir, R. L. Differential tyrosine phosphorylation of *N*-methyl-D-aspartate receptor subunits. *J. Biol. Chem.* 270:20036–20041, 1995.
5. Pawson, T. Protein modules and signalling networks [Review]. *Nature* 373:573–580, 1995.
6. Brugge, J. S., Cotton, P. C., Queral, A. E., Barrett, J. N., Nonner, D., and Keane, R. W. Neurones express high levels of a structurally modified, activated form of pp60c-Src. *Nature* 316:554–557, 1985.
7. Sicheri, F., Moarefi, I., and Kuriyan, J. Crystal structure of the Src family tyrosine kinase hck. *Nature* 385:602–609, 1997.
8. Lev, S., Moreno, H., Martinez, R., et al. Protein tyrosine kinase PYK2 involved in Ca^{2+}-induced regulation of ion channel and MAP kinase functions. *Nature* 376:737–745, 1995.
9. Dudek, H., Sandeep, R. D., Franke, T. F., et al. Regulation of neuronal survival by the serine-threonine protein kinase Akt. *Science* 275:661–665, 1997.
10. Tonks, N. K., Diltz, C. D., and Fischer, E. H. Purification of the major protein-tyrosine-phosphatases of human placenta. *J. Biol. Chem.* 263:6722–6730, 1988.
11. Tonks, N. K., and Neel, B. G. From form to function—signaling by protein tyrosine phosphatases [Review]. *Cell* 87:365–368, 1996.
12. Desai, D. M., Sap, J., Schlessinger, J., and Weiss, A. Ligand-mediated negative regulation of a chimeric transmembrane receptor tyrosine phosphatase. *Cell* 73:541–554, 1993.
13. Klein, R., Jing, S. Q., Nanduri, V., O'Rourke, E., and Barbacid, M. The Trk proto-oncogene encodes a receptor for nerve growth factor. *Cell* 65:189–197, 1991.
14. Drescher, U., Kremoser, C., Handwerker, C., Loschinger, J., Noda, M., and Bonhoeffer, F. *In vitro* guidance of retinal ganglion cell axons by RAGS, a 25 kDa tectal protein related to ligands for eph receptor tyrosine kinases. *Cell* 82:359–370, 1995.
15. Hirai, H., Maru, Y., Hagiwara, K., Nishida, J., and Takaku, F. A novel putative tyrosine kinase receptor encoded by the Eph gene. *Science* 238:1717–1720, 1987.
16. McMahan, U. J. The agrin hypothesis [Review]. *Cold Spring Harb. Symp. Quant. Biol.* 55:407–418, 1990.
17. Gautam, M., Noakes, P. G., Moscoso, L., et al. Defective neuromuscular synaptogenesis in agrin-deficient mutant mice. *Cell* 85:525–535, 1996.
18. Wallace, B. G., Qu, Z., and Huganir, R. L. Agrin induces phosphorylation of the nicotinic acetylcholine receptor. *Neuron* 6:869–878, 1991.
19. Dechiara, T. M., Bowen, D. C., Valenzuela, D. M., et al. The receptor tyrosine kinase MuSK is required for neuromuscular junction formation *in vivo*. *Cell* 85:501–512, 1996.
20. Harris, D. A., Falls, D. L., Dill-Devor, R. M., and Fischbach, G. D. Acetylcholine receptor-inducing factor from chicken brain increases the level of mRNA encoding the receptor alpha subunit. *Proc. Natl. Acad. Sci. USA* 85:1983–1987, 1988.
21. Corfas, G., Falls, D. L., and Fischbach, G. D. ARIA, a protein that stimulates acetylcholine receptor synthesis, also induces tyrosine phosphorylation of a 185-kDa muscle transmembrane protein. *Proc. Natl. Acad. Sci. USA* 90:1624–1628, 1993.
22. Zhu, X. J., Lai, C., Thomas, S., and Burden, S. J. Neuregulin receptors, erbB3 and erbB4, are localized at neuromuscular synapses. *EMBO J.* 14:5842–5848, 1995.
23. Grant, S. G., O'Dell, T. J., Karl, K. A., Stein, P. L., Soriano, P., and Kandel, E. R. Impaired long-term potentiation, spatial learning, and hippocampal development in Fyn mutant mice. *Science* 258:1903–1910, 1992.
24. Huganir, R. L., Miles, K., and Greengard, P. Phosphorylation of the nicotinic acetylcholine receptor by an endogenous tyrosine-specific protein kinase. *Proc. Natl. Acad. Sci. USA* 81:6968–6972, 1984.

25. Hopfield, J. F., Tank, D. W., Greengard, P., and Huganir, R. L. Functional modulation of the nicotinic acetylcholine receptor by tyrosine phosphorylation. *Nature* 336:677–680, 1988.

26. Moon, I. S., Apperson, M. L., and Kennedy, M. B. The major tyrosine-phosphorylated protein in the postsynaptic density fraction is *N*-methyl-D-aspartate receptor subunit 2B. *Proc. Natl. Acad. Sci. USA* 91:3954–3958, 1994.

27. Yu, X. M., Askalan, R., Keil, G. J., and Salter, M. W. NMDA channel regulation by channel-associated protein tyrosine kinase Src. *Science* 275:674–678, 1997.

28. Moss, S. J., Gorrie, G. H., Amato, A., and Smart, T. G. Modulation of GABA$_A$ receptors by tyrosine phosphorylation. *Nature* 377:344–348, 1995.

29. Huang, X. Y., Morielli, A. D., and Peralta, E. G. Tyrosine kinase-dependent suppression of a potassium channel by the G protein-coupled m1 muscarinic acetylcholine receptor. *Cell* 75:1145–1156, 1993.

30. Holmes, T. C., Fadool, D. A., Ren, R. B., and Levitan, I. B. Association of Src tyrosine kinase with a human potassium channel mediated by SH3 domain. *Science* 274:2089–2091, 1996.

31. Wilson, G. F., and Kaczmarek, L. K. Mode-switching of a voltage-gated cation channel is mediated by a protein kinase A-regulated tyrosine phosphatase. *Nature* 366:433–438, 1993.

32. Lohof, A. M., Ip, N. Y., and Poo, M. M. Potentiation of developing neuromuscular synapses by the neurotrophins NT-3 and BDNF. *Nature* 363:350–353, 1993.

33. Kang, H. J., and Schuman, E. M. Long-lasting neurotrophin-induced enhancement of synaptic transmission in the adult hippocampus. *Science* 267:1658–1662, 1995.

34. Figurov, A., Pozzo-Miller, L. D., Olafsson, P., Wang, T., and Lu, B. Regulation of synaptic responses to high-frequency stimulation and LTP by neurotrophins in the hippocampus. *Nature* 381:706–709, 1996.

35. Hunter, T. Tyrosine phosphorylation—past, present and future. *Biochem. Soc. Trans.* 24:307–327, 1996.

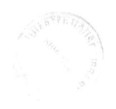

26

Transcription Factors in the Central Nervous System

James Eberwine

The functioning of the CNS requires regulated communication between neurons that are in contact with one another. Generally, this can be viewed as presynaptic neurons modulating the activity of postsynaptic neurons. While the propagation of action potentials is the most rapid form of neuron–neuron communication, there is a slower form of communication where the neurotransmitters and neuromodulators re-leased into the synaptic cleft from presynaptic axons bind to postsynaptic neuronal membranes, inducing the postsynaptic cell to respond. This postsynaptic response can be a cascade of events, often resulting in regulation of the production of mRNA and proteins within cells. This direct cell–cell communication can be modulated by factors which diffuse over long distances and, consequently, do not require spe-

Basic Neurochemistry: Molecular, Cellular and Medical Aspects, 6th Ed., edited by G. J. Siegel et al. Published by Lippincott–Raven Publishers Philadelphia, 1999. Correspondence to James Eberwine, Department of Pharmacology, University of Pennsylvania Medical Center, 36th and Hamilton Walk, Philadelphia, Pennsylvania 19104.

cific secretion into the synaptic cleft, yet it can also function in selected cell types to again alter transcription and post-transcriptional events. In this chapter, the regulation of transcription in neurons will be discussed first by presenting some basic background concerning transcription and then by highlighting two important classes of modulators of transcription, namely, those associated with glucocorticoid and cAMP regulation of transcription. Finally, given the complexities of transcriptional regulation, a brief discussion of possible sites for pharmacological intervention in the transcriptional process will be presented.

THE TRANSCRIPTIONAL PROCESS

To understand regulation of transcription, it is necessary to categorize the molecules involved. Transcription is the process by which RNA is made from genomic DNA. DNA is a linear polymer composed of four nucleotides, deoxyadenosine, deoxyguanosine, deoxycytosine and thymidine, which are linked in a linear sequence via phosphate linkages. Genomic DNA is double-stranded DNA, oriented in an anti-parallel arrangement such that base pairing of adenosine with thymidine and of guanosine with cytosine will stabilize the structure. The linear sequence of the nucleotides contains sequences known as genes which are the regions of genomic DNA that can be copied into RNA. This arrangement suggests that the functional structure of the DNA sequences giving rise to RNAs is modular, with an RNA-encoding region as well as functional regions of sequence both 5' and 3' to the transcription unit (Fig. 26-1). The transcription process giving rise to mRNA requires the binding of proteins responsible for RNA synthesis to the DNA template immediately 5' to the start of transcription. The protein which synthesizes mRNA is

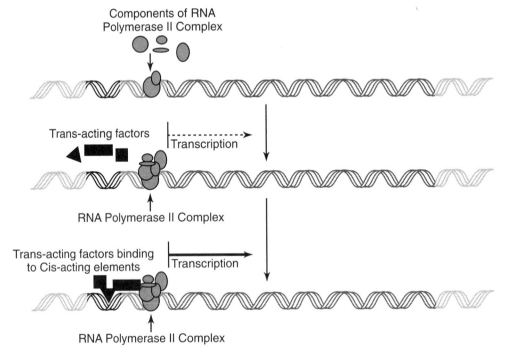

FIGURE 26-1. Formation and regulation of the transcriptional complex. The transcribed region of a gene is indicated in *black*. Immediately to the **right** of this box, on the 5'-side, is an *orange helix*, indicating the TATA box sequence. These are *cis*-regulatory sequences. The transcription complex binds to the TATA box and can initiate transcription when stimulated. Transcription can be regulated by binding of various *trans*-acting factors to the enhancers *(black shapes)* adjacent to the TATA box. The positioning of these sequences permits a direct interaction between *trans*-acting factors and the RNA polymerase II complex.

known as RNA polymerase II. RNA polymerase II is a large protein complex composed of multiple subunits. This protein binds to a DNA sequence, which is known as the TATA box because of the linear arrangement of the DNA sequence and its proximity to the start of transcription. However, RNA polymerase II does not bind to the TATA box without the prior association of several other proteins, including transcription factors TFIID, TFIIA and others, with this DNA region [1]. These proteins interact with one another, forming a complex to which RNA polymerase II can bind. This scaffolding of protein interactions at the TATA box forms the transcriptional complex. This basic transcriptional complex is likely the same for all genes in all eukaryotic cells, yet it is clear that transcription of selective genes can be on or off, as well as differentially regulated, in distinct cell types to yield different amounts of mRNA. This process of transcriptional regulation is complex and involves the association of several other proteins in particular arrangements with the transcribed genes. The arrangement and identity of transcriptional accesory proteins, also called transcription factors, can be unique for individual genes.

Finally, and perhaps most importantly, transcription is the starting point for a series of biological amplifications necessary for cellular functioning. To illustrate this point, a single gene can be transcribed into multiple mRNAs, in some cases, giving rise to thousands of mRNA molecules (Fig. 26-2). Next, each of these mRNAs may be translated into hundreds of protein molecules, hence providing the quantities required for cellular viability. Cells could not function without this amplification of genetic information. The involvement of transcription factors in regulating the first biological amplification step is the subject of the remainder of this chapter.

REGULATION OF TRANSCRIPTION BY TRANSCRIPTION FACTORS

Transcription factors are categorized as *trans*-acting factors because they are regulatory agents which are not part of the regulated gene(s). These *trans*-acting factors regulate gene transcription by binding directly or through an intermediate protein to the gene at a particular DNA sequence, called a *cis*-regulatory region. This *cis*-regulatory region is usually located in the 5'-flanking promoter region of the gene and is composed of a specific nucleotide sequence, for example, the cAMP response element (consensus sequence TGACGTCA). There is also a class of *cis*-regulatory elements called enhancers, which can be positioned anywhere in a gene and, consequently, are not restricted to the promoter region, which bind, for example, the glucocorticoid receptor. Binding of the *trans*-acting factor to the *cis*-regulatory region alters the intiation of transcription, probably through a direct interaction of the *trans*-acting factor with the RNA–polymerase complex. This binding likely occurs through the secondary and tertiary structures of the genomic DNA–protein complexes. Usually, transcription factors bind as dimers to the DNA, suggesting that there are dimerization sites on transcription factors, as well as DNA-binding sites. There are several types of transcription factors, which are grouped by virtue of sequence similarities in their protein interaction and/or DNA-binding domains (Fig. 26-3). Similarities in protein–protein interaction sites suggest that monomers of different transcription factors can interact to form heterodimers. An individual heterodimer may bind to multiple *cis*-acting elements or, alternatively, interact with differing affinity for the same *cis*-acting element as compared with the homodimer. Indeed, these types of protein interactions do occur and provide a major source of regulatory complexity.

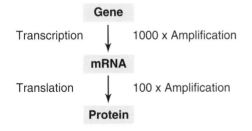

FIGURE 26-2. Gene expression as a biological amplifier. Transcription is an amplification step, giving rise to thousands of mRNA molecules from a single gene. Translation is a second amplification process, producing hundreds of protein molecules from a single mRNA molecule.

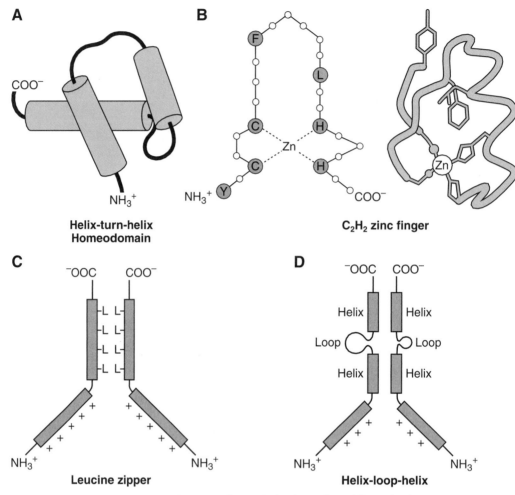

FIGURE 26-3. Structure of transcription factors from different families.

A particular *cis*-acting element may be present in multiple genes so that activation of a single transcription factor has potential for altering the expression of multiple target genes. Furthermore, an individual transcription factor may increase transcription of one gene while decreasing the transcription of another gene. This difference is partly due to the positioning of the *cis*-acting element relative to the start of transcription as well as to the identity of the protein partners in the heterodimer complex. It is important to note that, with the increase in sequence information being generated by the Human Genome Project, *cis*-acting elements can be found in genes, suggesting potential gene regulatory mechanisms without any biological information. While *cis*-acting element sequence identification in a gene is indeed predictive and necessary, this is often not sufficient to fully characterize the transcriptional regulation of that gene. *cis*-Acting elements for a particular gene are commonly nonfunctional in all tissues and, even more often, silent in one tissue and active in another due to the differential distribution of transcription factors.

GLUCOCORTICOID AND MINERALOCORTICOID RECEPTORS AS TRANSCRIPTION FACTORS

The steroid hormones known as mineralocorticoids and glucocorticoids are synthesized in the adrenal cortex of mammals [2]. The physiological mineralocorticoid is aldosterone, and it is involved in regulating unidirectional Na^+ transport across the epithelium. The physiological glucocorticoid in most mammalian species is cortisol; however, in rats and mice, it is corticosterone (CORT). Initially, glucocorticoids were characterized by their ability to stimulate glycogen deposition and by their release into the circulation in response to stress. Glucocorticoids regulate a wide range of responses, including aspects of immunosuppression and inflammation (Chap. 49). Glucocorticoids are released in response to increases in circulating adrenocorticotrophic hormone.

Two distinct classes of mineralocorticoid-binding sites were first described in the rat kidney. High-affinity cytosolic aldosterone-binding sites are termed mineralocorticoid receptors [3]. Lower-affinity aldosterone-binding sites are termed glucocorticoid receptors. Glucocorticoid receptors are the same as dexamethasone-binding receptors [4].

While the affinity of mineralocorticoid receptors for aldosterone is higher than that for CORT, circulating concentrations of CORT are several orders of magnitude higher than aldosterone. CORT is effectively blocked from binding to the mineralocorticoid receptors by plasma proteins such as transcortin, which bind preferentially to CORT. Another mechanism that serves to alter the balance of CORT and aldosterone binding to receptors is the activity of 11β-hydroxysteroid dehydrogenase, which, in the rat kidney, rapidly oxidizes CORT to inactive metabolites. This facilitates binding of aldosterone to mineralocorticoid receptors in the presence of high concentrations of CORT [5].

Corticosteroid receptors regulate transcription in the nervous system

Intracellular binding sites selective for [³H]-CORT were first identified in various brain regions, in particular the hippocampus, of adrenalectomized rats. A similar autoradiographic pattern was obtained using [³H]-aldosterone as a ligand, suggesting that these receptors were mineralocorticoid receptors. The [³H]-dexamethasone-binding pattern shows selective differences in the pattern of binding compared to the CORT and aldosterone patterns, suggesting the existence of multiple corticosteroid receptors. [³H]-CORT binding performed in the presence of unlabeled dexamethasone or aldosterone reveals that CORT binds to at least two receptor types in the brain.

Two high-affinity intracellular corticosteroid receptors have been characterized and are distinguished on the basis of binding properties, amino acid sequence, neuroanatomical distribution and physiological function. The type I corticosteroid receptor, or mineralocorticoid receptor, is localized in various brain regions, including the septum and hippocampus [6]. The type I receptor binds CORT and aldosterone with high affinity, ~0.5 nM. The relative steroid binding affinity of the type I receptor for CORT is greater than or equal to that for aldosterone, which is greater than that for dexamethasone. The type I receptor is present in all subregions of the hippocampus, namely, in the CA1, CA2, CA3 and the granular cells of the dentate gyrus (Fig. 26-4).

The type II corticosteroid receptor, also called the glucocorticoid receptor, is widely distributed in the brain and exhibits high-affinity binding to dexamethasone. The type II receptor binds with ten-fold lower affinity to corticosterone, 5 nM, as compared with the type I receptor. The relative binding affinities for steroid interaction with the glucocorticoid receptor are such that dexamethasone binding is greater than corticosterone binding, which is much greater than aldosterone binding. Glucocorticoids are present at high concentrations in all regions of the hippocampus, with the exception of the CA3 region, where concentrations are exceedingly low [7].

Mineralocorticoid and glucocoticoid receptors can coexist in the same neurons as evident from their demonstrated colocalization in the CA1 region of the hippocampus [8]. These CA1 neurons are exquisitely sensitive to the whole range of glucocorticoid concentrations. Because of their high affinity for corticosteroids, the type I receptors are approximately 80% occupied, suggesting that the number of type I receptors is likely to be the rate-limiting factor in mineralocorticoid receptor functioning. However, glucocorticoid receptor functions are most

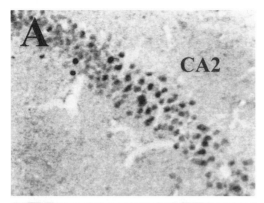

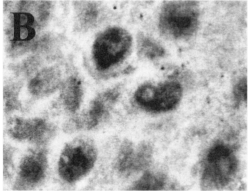

FIGURE 26-4. Immunohistochemical localization of type I corticosteroid receptor (mineralocorticoid receptor) in the rat hippocampus. **A:** Mineralocorticoid immunoreactivity is concentrated in pyramidal cell fields of the cornu ammons *(CA2)*. **B:** High-power photomicrograph shows that steroid-bound mineralocorticoid receptors are primarily localized to neuronal cell nuclei. (Photomicrographs courtesy of Dr. James P. Herman, Department of Anatomy and Neurobiology, University of Kentucky.)

dependent on the extent of glucocorticoid receptor occupancy and are likely to be regulated by the concentration of the available steroid. The presence of multiple binding sites for corticosteroids as well as their differing concentrations in different cell types form the molecular basis for their differential actions in the rat brain [9].

The mechanisms of corticosteroid receptor regulation of transcription have been elucidated

Both type I and type II corticosteroid receptors are members of a superfamily of ligand-activated transcription factors defined by protein se-

quence similarity. Included in this superfamily are various other steroid receptors, such as the estrogen receptor, as well as members of the retinoic acid receptor family and thyroid hormone receptors. The ligand-activated transcription factor superfamily is estimated to contain several hundred members. Mineralocorticoid and glucocorticoid receptors are each composed of four distinct protein regions, including an N-terminal region, a DNA-binding domain, a nuclear localization signal and a C-terminal hormone-binding region. The N-terminal region is associated with activation of transcription through an as yet unknown mechanism. The DNA-binding domain is a charged protein sequence, known as a zinc-finger. In this case, there are two fingers, each composed of the sequence Cys-X2-Cys-X13-Cys-X2-Cys. The C-terminal region binds glucocorticoids, which, when bound, initiate the conformational change of the receptor which facilitates its translocation.

In the cytoplasm, the mineralocorticoid and glucocorticoid receptors are associated with a large multiprotein complex which contains the heat shock proteins (HSP) HSP70 and HSP90 (Fig. 26-5). This complex maintains unbound corticosteroid receptors in a ligand-accessible but inactive protein conformation. Binding of ligand causes dissociation of receptors from the heat shock proteins, followed by translocation of the activated receptors to the nucleus. In the nucleus, ligand-bound corticosteroid receptors bind to a *cis*-acting element called glucocorticoid response element (GRE). The GRE is a 20-base palindromic sequence, TGGTACAAATGTTCT, and is also called an enhancer element because it generally functions to enhance transcription. The GRE can be positioned anywhere within the gene, not just in the promoter region. Modulation of corticosteroid-responsive genes occurs through interactions of the type I or II receptors, bound to the enhancer sequence, with the transcriptional complex.

Ligand-bound corticosteroid receptors have been shown to interact to form heterodimers with other transcription factors, such as the jun protein. Such interactions are responsible for transactivation of the *cis*-regulatory sites known as AP-1 sites and for the glucocorticoid-mediated suppression of transcription, such as

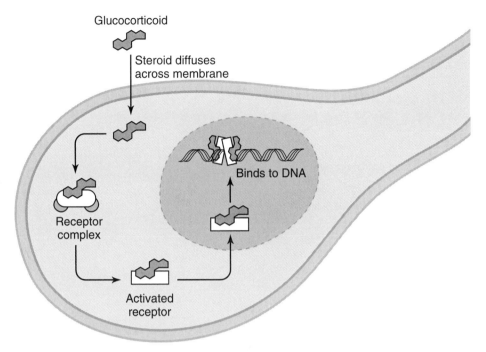

FIGURE 26-5. Activation of glucocorticoid receptors. Glucocorticoids ( ) diffuse across the plasma membrane and bind to the glucocorticoid receptor. Upon glucocorticoid receptor binding to the steroid, the receptor undergoes a conformational change which permits it to dissociate from the chaperone heat shock proteins *(light orange circles)*. The activated glucocorticoid receptor translocates across the nuclear membrane and binds as a homo- or heterodimer to glucocorticoid response element sequences to regulate gene transcription.

that seen in the pro-opiomelanocortin gene. A number of such specific protein interactions have been reported; these interactions and their locations relative to other transcription factors transform a ubiquitous steroid hormone signal into a tissue-specific, graded cellular response.

cAMP REGULATION OF TRANSCRIPTION

cAMP controls phosphorylation of the cAMP response element–binding protein

Activation of a transcription factor known as the cAMP response element (CRE) is the final step in a signal-transduction pathway which is intiated by the binding of a specific class of cell-surface receptors (Fig. 26-6) [10]. Binding of a ligand to a G_s protein-coupled receptor, such as the D1 dopamine receptor or the 5-hydroxytryptamine-1 receptor, liberates G_s protein from the G-protein complex (Chap. 20). Subsequently, G_s activates adenylyl cyclase, which in turn stimulates cAMP production. The increase in intracellular cAMP induces the dissociation of protein kinase A (PKA) catalytic subunits from their regulatory subunits (Chap. 22). The catalytic subunits move into the nucleus, where they phosphorylate a number of proteins, including the CREB transcription factor. This phosphorylation event activates CREB protein and transcription is stimulated [11]. The genes which are activated by CREB are those which have the *cis*-acting palindromic CRE consensus sequence (TGACGTCA) in the promoter region. This is distinct from the enhancer activity of the previously discussed GREs, which can function at sites distinct from the promoter region of a given gene. CREB protein appears to be ubiquitously expressed in the brain, with high concentrations in the hippocampus (Fig. 26-7) and cortex. As seen in Figure 26-7, it is apparent that much of the CREB immunoreactivity is present in the nucleus of CA1 pyramidal cells.

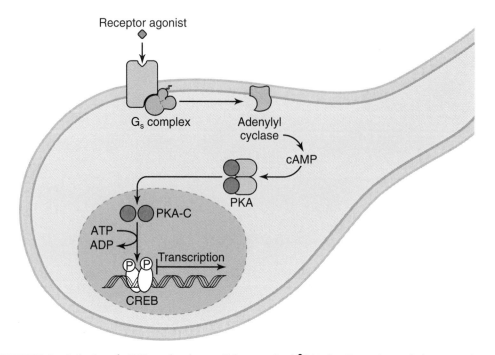

FIGURE 26-6. Activation of cAMP-regulated genes. When agonists (◆) bind to G protein-coupled receptors that activate dissociation of G_s from the G_s complex, G_s will interact with the enzyme adenylyl cyclase, resulting in synthesis and increase of intracellular cAMP. cAMP binds to the regulatory subunits *(orange ovals)* of protein kinase A *(PKA)*. This binding facilitates the dissociation of the catalytic subunits *(gray circles)* from the PKA complex, which then translocate across the nuclear membrane and phosphorylate cAMP response element–binding protein *(CREB)* and CREB-related proteins. Phosphorylated CREB increases gene transcription *(right arrow)*.

The critical feature of CREB protein activation is phosphorylation of CREB, which is required for CREB-mediated stimulation of transcription [12]. PKA phosphorylates CREB on a serine amino acid positioned at amino acid 133 in the CREB protein sequence. How phosphorylation activates CREB-mediated transcription is unclear. Some investigators believe that phospho-CREB has a slightly higher affinity for CRE binding and others believe that transcription factor interaction with the transcriptional complex is stimulated by phosphorylation. The time course for CREB stimulation of transcription is relatively rapid, peaking at approximately 30 min after cAMP stimulation, followed by a gradual decrease to basal levels of activation over the course of several hours. This decrease in activation occurs through the activity of protein phosphatase 1 and other phosphatases, which remove the phosphate group from CREB protein. It is important to note that there is increasing evidence that CREB phosphorylation can be induced by factors other than an increase in intracellular cAMP concentrations. The relative contribution of these other stimulators, including an increase in intracellular Ca^{2+}, to the transcriptional activation exhibited by phospho-CREB is under active investigation.

In large part, the modulation of CREB-regulated genes represents the intracellular balance of active kinases and phosphatases, which is a reflection of cellular activation. This is one of the major differences between CREB and glucocorticoid receptor-regulated transcription: CREB is an integrator of intracellular homeostasis, while the glucocorticoid receptor integrates whole-body homeostasis.

The cAMP response element–binding protein is a member of a family containing interacting proteins

After the mRNA encoding CREB protein was cloned and sequenced, several other members of

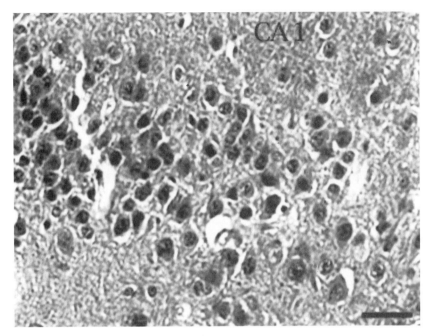

FIGURE 26-7. Immunohistochemical localization of cAMP response element–binding protein *(CREB)* in rat hippocampal neurons. Using a polyclonal antibody which recognizes both CREB and phospho-CREB protein, it is apparent that CREB protein is enriched in the nucleus of pyramidal cells of the CA1 region of the hippocampus. Scale bar is 30 μm. (Photomicrograph courtesy of Dr. Stephen Ginsberg, Department of Pathology, University of Pennsylvania.)

the CREB family of transcription factors were identified. Using homology screens, the polymerase chain reaction and interaction screening assays, a protein called cAMP response element modulator (CREM) was isolated. CREM can both stimulate and inhibit cAMP-mediated gene transcription. Transcriptional inhibition can occur as a result of generation of modified CREM proteins because of alternative splicing of the CREM gene (Fig. 26-8). Among these different proteins are the α, β and γ forms of CREM, which lack the glutamine-rich region present in the activator forms of both CREM and CREB that is required for stimulation of transcription [13]. Inhibition occurs due to heterodimer formation between this inactivating form of CREM and either CREM or CREB [14]. The alternatively spliced forms of CREM as well as those recently discovered for CREB, which can also act as transcriptional inhibitors, occur in a tissue- and cell type-specific manner. Additionally, recent data have shown that CREB can interact with other leucine zipper-containing transcription factors to produce heterodimers which can

interact with *cis*-acting elements distinct from the CRE, as previously discussed with regard to the corticosteroid receptors. These findings provide a mechanism for generation of tissue- and cell-type differences in cAMP responsiveness [15].

The function of the cAMP response element–binding protein has been modeled in transgenic organisms

The observation that serotonin stimulates learning and memory in the *Aplysia* system with the subsequent discovery that cAMP will mimic this effect suggested that cAMP was involved in this physiological process (see Chap. 50). Recently, direct evidence for the involvement of CREB in learning and memory was presented in the *Drosophila* system (see below). *Drosophila* as an experimental system has several advantages over mammalian systems, including the ease of generation of mutant as well as transgenic flies.

The role of CREB in learning and memory was first anticipated by screening *Drosophila*

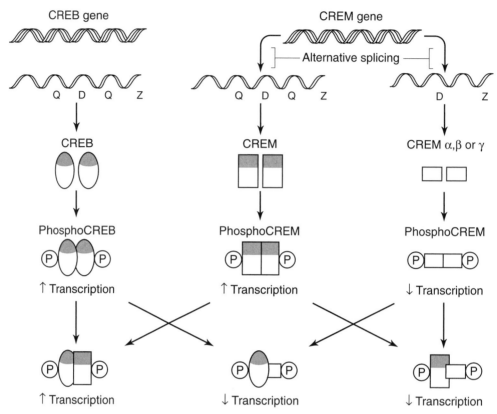

FIGURE 26-8.   Mechanism for generation of activators and repressors of cAMP-stimulated transcription. The cAMP response element binding protein *(CREB)* and the cAMP response element modulator *(CREM)* genes can give rise to alternatively spliced mRNAs, which give rise to distinct protein products. While CREB and CREM can stimulate CRE-mediated gene expression, generation of the α, β or γ forms of CREM will produce proteins which can heterodimer-ize with activated CREB and CREM subunits inhibiting their stimulatory capacity. The symbols used to highlight functional regions of CREB and CREM protein are *Q* for the polyglutamine tract, which stimulates transcription; *D* for the DNA-binding region; and *Z* for the leucine-zipper region, which is involved in dimerization.

mutants in a learning and memory task in which flies were behaviorally tested in an odorant-association task, where an odorant was paired with an electric shock. Flies with "normal" phenotype learn that the odorant is associated with an electric shock and will learn to avoid the odorant. Two fly mutants were discovered that could not learn this association: *dunce* and *rutabaga*. The *dunce* mutant was deficient in cAMP phosphodiesterase, which breaks down cAMP, and the *rutabaga* mutant had a mutation in adenylyl cyclase, which synthesizes cAMP. These data combined with the prior *Aplysia* work suggested that CREB was involved in acquisition of learning and memory [16].

More recently, with the same odorant-association behavioral test, the specific role of CREB in learning and memory was assessed by using a dominant-negative CREB (dCREB) protein expressed in transgenic flies [17]. This dCREB complexes with normal CREB through a functional leucine-zipper region, yet inhibits the transcriptional activation mediated by normal CREB protein. The experiment was designed so that dCREB was controlled by a heat shock promoter and could be activated in the adult animal. This experimental paradigm allows for the assessment of the role of CREB in the adult animal, by using heat shock to induce dCREB expression, rather than by examining the behavioral consequences of CREB deficiency during development. Heat shock, in and of itself, does not alter learning and memory [18]. Data from these experiments show that the form of memory requiring protein synthesis, called long-term memory (Chap. 50), was inhibited by expression of dCREB. This inhibition was not observed when a mutant dCREB, in which the leucine zipper was inactivated by site-directed mutagenesis, was expressed in flies. This leucine-zipper mutant precludes dCREB dimerization with normal CREB. These data show that the relative concentrations of activating and inhibiting CREB monomers are critical to the development of long-term memory.

The dissection of CREB involvement in various physiological or behavioral paradigms in the mammalian system has been much slower than in *Drosophila*. In the mammalian system, targeted gene disruption has been used in attempts to inhibit CREB function. In one set of experiments, the exon of the gene containing the initiator methionine was deleted in hopes of blocking CREB production. However, the targeting of this region facilitated an alternative splicing event so that a previously undiscovered spliced variant mRNA of the CREB gene was produced, and was, in fact, upregulated. In the other targeted disruption experiments, the DNA-binding region was disrupted and, indeed, CREB protein production inhibited. Unfortunately, this disruption resulted in perinatal lethality, so no adult animals could be generated. The problem with the design of these experiments is that targeted disruption of CREB production would result in a developmental deficit, making it difficult to attribute any particular modification of behavior in the adult to a direct deficiency of CREB.

What is needed to directly assess the involvement of CREB in adult mammalian neurons is the production of a conditional knockout mouse in which the knockout could be activated in the adult animal in a tissue-specific manner. This mutant could be similar to the production of a dominant-negative mutant, as was done in the *Drosophila* system or potentially through induction of genetic recombination in adult neurons using an inducible system similar to that being used to produce conditional knockouts for

other genes (see Chap. 40). Such a model system would be very useful in understanding the potential involvement of CREB in long-term memory in the mammalian system as well as in other physiological conditions associated with CREB functioning, such as opiate tolerance and withdrawal (Chap. 53) or aspects of behavioral aggressiveness (Chap. 49).

TRANSCRIPTION AS A TARGET FOR DRUG DEVELOPMENT

It should be clear from this brief discussion of transcription factors that disruption of transcription factor function may have dire consequences for neuronal functioning. Because of their pivotal role in the regulation of multiple genes, they are potential targets for pharmacological intervention in the control of disease processes. The problem with development of drugs targeted to transcription factors is that there are several hundred estimated *trans*-acting factors in the nucleus, many of which can heterodimerize to produce distinct transcriptional responses. The strategies being investigated to modulate transcription factor function focus on antisense knockout of expression and modulators targeted toward post-translational modifiers of transcription factors. Such modifiers include protein kinases and phosphatases.

Often, it is desirable to block expression of particular genes which are activated by transcription factors. The antisense knockout experiments are directed toward this end and require the addition of an antisense oligonucleotide, which will anneal to the *cis*-acting regulatory element for a particular transcription factor in a specific gene. The hope is that a triple helical structure will form around this oligonucleotide-binding site, inhibiting the expression of the downstream gene.

This same strategy can be attempted at the mRNA level, to inhibit the translation of individual mRNAs. These experiments are almost never 100% efficient; hence, the problem becomes how much neutralization is necessary to elicit the desired effect. If the antisense oligonculeotide is targeted toward the mRNA for a particular transcription factor or splice form of a transcription factor, then it may be possible to knock down or reduce the expression of that particular protein. The result of such a knockdown will be a new balance of transcription factor subunits in the cell, likely resulting in alteration of the relative amounts of particular homo- and heterodimers.

Finally, development of drugs targeted toward modification of kinases and phosphatases required for activation or inhibition of particular transcription factors is a promising therapeutic approach. The problem with this paradigm is the specificity of the kinases and phosphatases since they will often act enzymatically on multiple proteins (Chaps. 24 and 25). Furthermore, such drugs often lack specificity and may interact with multiple kinases or phosphatases.

Clearly, transcription is a critical regulatory nexus in neuronal function. More information is being generated about the biology of transcription factors, including how many transcription factor genes exist, which proteins dimerize, identification of the *cis*-acting elements to which they bind and how transcription is modulated by these proteins. From these studies, significant insight into the mechanisms of transcriptional responses to the local environment and to pharmacological agents in the normal and abnormal nervous system will be gained.

REFERENCES

1. Hori, R., and Carey, M. The role of activators in assembly of RNA polymerase II transcription complexes. *Curr. Opin. Gen. Dev.* 4:236–244, 1994.
2. Funder, J. Adrenal steroids: New answers, new questions. *Science* 237:236–237, 1987.
3. Arriza, J. L., Weinberger, C., Cerelli, G., et al. Cloning of the human mineralocorticoid receptor complementary DNA: Structural and functional kinship with the glucocorticoid receptor. *Science* 237:268–275, 1987.
4. Hollenberg, S., Weinberger, C., Ong, E., et al. Primary structure and expression of a functional human glucocorticoid receptor cDNA. *Nature* 318:635–641, 1985.
5. Reul, J., and deKloet, E. Two receptor systems for corticosterone in rat brain: Microdistribution

6. Arriza, J., Simerly, R., Swanson, L., and Evans, R. The neuronal mineralocorticoid receptor as mediator of glucocorticoid response. *Neuron* 1:887–896, 1988.
7. Chao, H., Choo, P., and McEwen, B. Glucocorticoid and mineralocorticoid receptor mRNA expression in rat brain. *Neuroendocrinology* 50:365–371, 1989.
8. deKloet, E., Wallach, G., and McEwen, B. Differences in corticosterone and dexamethasone binding in rat brain and pituitary. *Endocrinology* 96:598–609, 1975.
9. Herman, J., Patel, P., Akil, H., and Watson, S. Localization and regulation of glucocorticoid and mineralocorticoid receptor messenger RNAs in the hippocampal formation of the rat. *Mol. Endocrinol.* 3:1886–1894, 1989.
10. Habener, J. Cyclic AMP response element binding proteins: A cornucopia of transcription factors. *Mol. Endocrinol.* 4:1087–1094, 1990.
11. Montminy, M., Gonzalex, G., and Yamamoto, K. Regulation of cAMP-inducible genes by CREB. *Trends Neurosci.* 13:184–188, 1990.
12. Yamamoto, K., Gonzalez, G., Biggs, W., and Montminy, M. Phosphorylation-induced binding and transcriptional efficacy of nuclear factor CREB. *Nature* 334:494–498, 1988.
13. deGroot, R., and Sassone-Corsi, P. Hormonal control of gene expression: Multiplicity and versatility of cyclic adenosine 3',5'-monophosphate-responsive nuclear regulators. *Mol. Endocrinol.* 8:145–153, 1993.
14. Foulkes, N., and Sassone-Corsi, P. More is better: Activators and repressors from the same gene. *Cell* 68:411–414, 1992.
15. Hai, T., and Curran, T. Cross-family dimerization of transcription factors Fos/Jun and ATF/CREB alters DNA binding specificity. *Proc. Natl. Acad. Sci. USA* 88:3720–3724, 1991.
16. Tully, T., Preat, T., Boynton, S., and Del Vecchio, M. Genetic dissection of consolidated memory in *Drosophila*. *Cell* 79:59–67, 1994.
17. Yin, J., Del Vecchio, M., Zhou, H., and Tully, T. CREB as a memory modulator: Induced expression of a dCREB2 activator isoform enhances long-term memory in *Drosophila*. *Cell* 81:107–115, 1995.
18. Yin, J., Wallach, J., Del Vecchio, M., et al. Induction of a dominant negative CREB transgene specifically blocks long-term memory in *Drosophila*. *Cell* 79:49–58, 1994.

and differential occupation. *Endocrinology* 117:2505–2511, 1985.

Growth, Development and Differentiation

27

Development

Jean de Vellis and Ellen Carpenter

Basic Neurochemistry: Molecular, Cellular and Medical Aspects, 6th Ed., edited by G. J. Siegel et al. Published by Lippincott–Raven Publishers, Philadelphia, 1999. Correspondence to Jean de Vellis, Neurochemistry Group, 68225 MRRC, University of California Los Angeles Medical School, 760 Westwood Plaza, Los Angeles, California 90024.

FUNDAMENTAL CONCEPTS UNIFYING DEVELOPMENTAL DIVERSITY

Development is the study of the principles and processes that underlie growth and evolution of a biological organism. Most developmental research has been devoted to studying the early periods of intense and extensive transformations that are associated with the unfolding of an organism from a single fertilized egg through embryogenesis to postnatal maturation. During this period, the immense diversity of neural phenotypes emerges [1,2]. What are the mechanisms that regulate the systematic and highly coherent series of events that fashion the vast neural circuitry? In this chapter, we examine the molecular and cellular processes that give rise to the enormous phenotypic diversity of the brain during these developmental periods in neural tissue.

Two fundamental concepts mold our perspective of how the nervous system develops and functions: the dynamic interdependence of genes and the environment and that of neuronal and neuroglial cells. During development, the systematic expression of the genetic blueprint creates and continuously molds the environment at all levels of its hierarchical organization, extending from the level of the single cell to the surroundings of the organism. The genetic machinery, in turn, relies on feedback from the environment to function properly. This interaction creates a highly integrated, self-referential process that links the genetic information with the multitude of influences existing at all of the different layers of the environment [3]. Great progress has been made in the systematic dissection of individual linear pathways of environmental–genetic connections. For example, a growth factor and its receptor activate an intracellular signaling pathway to induce the expression of a specific gene. In this way, many environmental signals and numerous cell processes have been correlated with the appearance of different neural phenotypes.

The presumption behind these studies is that knowledge of these single linear paths of environmental–genetic linkage will provide an understanding of the basis of phenotypic diversity. As we have discovered and examined the function of more and more extracellular factors, receptors and signaling pathways impinging upon an extensive genetic network functioning in a highly complex, combinatorial fashion, our research perspective is being transformed from a simple linear to a more realistic and integrated parallel model (Fig. 27-1). Multiple families of extracellular factors influence many receptors and intracellular signaling pathways which exhibit considerable interaction, or "cross-talk." In addition, a network of transcription factors is being elucidated. This network is characterized by extensive inter- and intrafamily interactions contributing to multiple levels of control over the expression and functional activity of transcription factors responsible for differential gene expression. Thus, in contrast to the linear model, neural phenotypic diversity arises from highly integrated networks of intracellular processes linked to environmental signals.

Biological interdependence in neural development is also dramatically displayed in the relationship of neuronal and glial cells [3–6]. The intimate coupling of these two types of cells is a major locus of genetic and epigenetic interaction in determining the functioning and the morphological, chemical and electrical development of the nervous system. Students have traditionally been taught that the neuronal cell represents the structural unit of the nervous system, relegating glia to the status of passive packaging. This narrow perspective has now been replaced by the accumulated evidence for glial cell regulation of nearly every aspect of neuronal development and function, supporting the premise that the fundamental functional unit of the nervous system is the dynamic interaction of neuronal and glial cells.

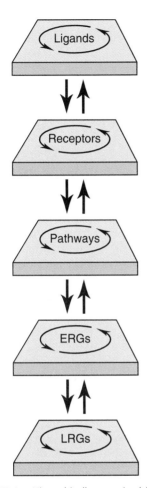

FIGURE 27-1. Hierarchically organized levels of information processing underlying the generation of neural phenotypic diversity. The enormous phenotypic diversity of the nervous system requires a mechanism that can generate increasing degrees of restriction in cell phenotype, such as cell shape and neurotransmitter expression. The original, simple linear perspective of an extracellular factor acting through its receptor to direct the expression of phenotypic characteristics is now being replaced by the recognition that each level of information processing is itself a complex domain of interacting components. In this view, many families of signaling molecules, or factors, bind to a growing number of interacting receptors, with overlapping specificity and component makeup, to activate many different, interacting intracellular signaling pathways, leading to the complex expression pattern of early response genes (*ERGs*). These ERGs, many of which function as transcription factors, in turn interact to regulate the final expression of late response genes (*LRGs*), encoding proteins that are phenotypic determinants. Thus, from this perspective, the developmental fate of each cell is determined by the sum total of the multiple signals and combinatorial intracellular processes.

GENERAL DEVELOPMENT OF THE NERVOUS SYSTEM

During animal development, a single fertilized egg cell divides and differentiates to produce all of the cells and tissues of the mature organism. Genetic information contained in the fertilized egg provides all of the instructions to produce these tissues. The initial divisions of a fertilized egg produce a blastula. The blastula undergoes gastrulation to produce the three primary germ layers of the developing embryo. During gastrulation, cells migrate inward between the upper and lower layers of the blastula through the primitive streak, resulting in a trilaminar "sandwich." The initial point of inward migration is established by the organizer, which in *Xenopus* is the dorsal lip of the blastopore and in birds and mammals is the node. The resulting gastrula has three layers, the ectoderm, the endoderm and the mesoderm. The nervous system develops from the ectoderm following an inductive signal from the mesoderm. The initial mesodermal cells condense to form the notochord, which elongates under the primitive streak along the anterior–posterior axis of the developing embryo. Signals are released from the notochord which induce the ectoderm to thicken into neural ectoderm in the area immediately overlying the notochord (Fig. 27-2). This neural ectoderm is now committed to develop into neural tissue, as can be demonstrated by transplantation experiments in which neural ectoderm surgically placed into other areas of the developing embryo produces auxiliary neural tissue. In addition, neural ectoderm arising in different places along the anterior–posterior axis of the developing embryo is predestined to develop into specific brain regions. Three proteins secreted by the organizer can induce production of anterior neural plate markers in undifferentiated ectodermal cells. These three proteins, noggin, follistatin and chordin, may establish anterior neural domains by inactivating two neural inhibitors, bone morphogenetic protein 2 (BMP2) and BMP4. The establishment of posterior domains within the neural plate may stem from signaling by basic fibroblast growth factor (bFGF) or by retinoic acid. Neither of these molecules is by itself sufficient to generate regional posterior identity, but

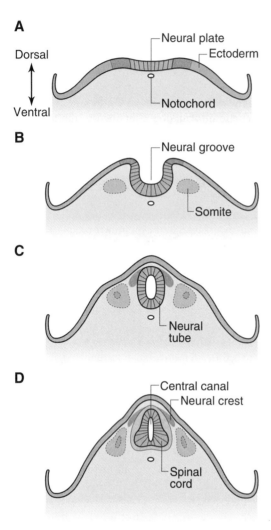

A

Dorsal

Ventral

Neural plate
Ectoderm
Notochord

B

Neural groove
Somite

C

Neural tube

D

Central canal
Neural crest
Spinal cord

FIGURE 27-2. Four stages in the development of the neural tube. **A:** After gastrulation, the mesodermally derived notochord induces the overlying ectoderm to form the neural plate. The most lateral portions of the neural plate will give rise to the neural crest (*dark orange areas*). **B:** The neural plate invaginates to form the neural groove. **C:** The neural tube fuses at its dorsal margin and separates from the overlying ectoderm. Neural crest cells (*dark orange*) separate from the neural tube and begin to migrate into the periphery. **D:** At trunk levels, the neural tube forms the spinal cord surrounding a central canal. (Modified from Cowan [7], with permission.)

both may mediate signals established by some other mechanism. An additional mechanism used to regionalize the neural plate may be the expression of head-specific genes. Deletion of several of these genes, notably *Lim-1* and *Otx-I*, deletes all head structures, suggesting a role for

these genes in establishing the most anterior portion of a developing animal. Cerberus, a secreted protein expressed in the gastrulating endomesoderm, also has forebrain-inducing activity.

Once the neural plate has been induced by the underlying mesoderm, it begins to differentiate into the neural tube, the primary rudiment of the developing CNS [7]. The center of the neural plate develops a groove in the direction of the anterior–posterior axis, and the edges of the plate rise up, forming the neural folds (Fig. 27-2). The neural folds fuse together along the dorsal edge of the animal, and the neural tube separates from the overlying dorsal ectoderm. During neural tube formation, the adjacent mesoderm is segmented into blocks of tissue called somites. The somites provide precursor cells for axial and appendicular skeletal elements and attached musculature. During neural tube closure, a population of cells separates from the neural folds and migrates into the periphery (Fig. 27-2). These cells are the neural crest (NC), which provides a progenitor population for the developing PNS. The NC migrates away from the neural tube along defined pathways through the anterior half of each adjacent somite and along a dorsal pathway under the ectoderm. NC cells which migrate through the somites populate the dorsal root ganglia as neurons and glia, contribute Schwann cells to the peripheral nerves and provide neurons and glia for the sympathetic ganglia. NC cells which migrate along the dorsal pathway develop into melanocytes.

The neural tube is a pseudostratified epithelium with cells extending between the apical and basal surfaces of the epithelial wall. The neuroepithelium initially contains only one undifferentiated population of stem cells. With time, these cells give rise to the two main lineages, neuronal and glial stem cells, and subsequently many different sublineages. After the final mitotic division, neurons migrate away from the ventricular surface of the neural tube to form the mantle zone. This outward migration is guided by radial glial fibers, which provide a scaffold extending from the ventricular zone to the surface of the developing brain. The accumulation of postmitotic neuronal cells results in the progressive thickening of the neural tube to produce expansions of the CNS, brain and spinal cord.

DEVELOPMENTAL PROCESSES: ENVIRONMENTAL FORCES MOLDING GENETIC POTENTIAL

Developing cells of the nervous system are embedded in complex fields of mechanical tension, biochemical signals and electrical current. This constantly changing pattern of spatial and temporal information for each cell is created, in large part, by the chemistry of the nerve cells themselves and represents the major environmental forces that drive the sequence of developmental processes. The dynamic interaction between these environmental influences and the machinery of nerve cells forces the cells to undergo considerable transformation during periods of growth and survival, migration and sorting and morphological and biochemical differentiation [8,9].

Selective cell survival and proliferation determine the number of each type of nerve cell

A basic tactic in creating complex biological systems is to generate an excess of elements and then, through a set of selective processes, to determine which elements will remain to participate in the final organizational pattern. This strategy is widely used in the construction of the vertebrate nervous system. During development, the interaction between genetic and epigenetic forces is expressed, in part, as the balance between cell survival and cell death [10]. Intimately linked to this balance is the control of cell proliferation.

For invertebrate development, genetic instructions are the prime controller of population size and diversity. Because of the short life span and the relatively simple nervous system necessary to control the organism in a relatively constant ecological niche, the most reliable and economical approach is to rapidly generate simple, preprogrammed neuronal/glial circuitry. The development of the nematode *Caenorhabditis elegans* is an example of a cell lineage that is generated independently of the environment. Precursor cells undergo cycles of stereotyped divisions, creating a number of restricted, preprogrammed cellular lineages. Even the small amount of cell death appears to be due to intrinsic instructions that select specific pathways to terminate in senescence.

Vertebrate development reflects the other extreme of the genetic/epigenetic continuum: unlike invertebrates, numerous environmental cues are employed to direct lineage decisions, including the decisions for survival, division and death. Prolonged gestation and the plasticity inherent in allowing outside influences to guide developmental decisions permit the construction of large-scale, highly interconnected, activity-dependent circuitries.

Early experiments demonstrated that the presence and size of the target tissue are critical in determining the number and functions of the surviving neuronal cells [11]. Removal of limb buds or transplantation of an extra limb bud results in a predictable decrease or increase, respectively, of the innervating motor and sensory neurons. Each set of neuronal cells exhibits a characteristic degree of target-dependent cell death during development: some groups remain quite stable in number, while others lose up to two-thirds of the cell progeny. What are the factors that influence the balance between cellular survival and death? The nature of the microenvironment of the cell soma as well as the environment into which the cell process grows are both important. Critical factors produced in the innervated target tissue contribute to the regulation of cell survival: limited amounts of soluble factor(s) released by target cells lead to competition among cells dependent on the factor. Thus, during specific periods of early cell development, trophic factors are necessary for survival (Chap. 19).

Specific paths of cell migration to final target environments are controlled by gradients of diffusible and substrate-bound neurochemical signals

Migration of cells plays a significant role in brain morphogenesis. Most neurons travel long distances through the complex extracellular terrain of the developing embryo to reach their final position. What mechanisms are used by neurons to move along the path, and what signals are used to guide them? The most common mechanism for cell translocation is a combination of (i) the extension of a cell process and its attachment to the substratum, followed by (ii) the pulling of the entire cell toward the point of attachment by means of contractile proteins associated with an intracellular network of microfilaments (see Chaps. 7, 8 and 29).

Directional control of cell movement appears to be of two types: (i) cells moving along other "guide" cells arranged as scaffolding and (ii) cells moving across a multicellular terrain guided by a concentration gradient. For example, small molecules diffusing through or attached to the extracellular matrix can alter the behavior of a cell (see Chap. 7). In the complex neuropil of the cerebral cortex, molecular signals undoubtedly permit neurons to distinguish radial glial processes along which they travel from the other neuronal, glial and endothelial surfaces.

NC cell movement is another model of molecular control of cell migration and contrasts with that seen in cortical systems. Since there are no glial cells to create highways for the crest cells, the migration of these cells into the spaces surrounding the neural tube depends on the nature of the extracellular matrix. In order to migrate to specific destinations, a number of signals must be regulated in a coordinated fashion both temporally and spatially. Nearly all of the major components of the matrix, collagen, fibronectin, laminin, proteoglycans and hyaluronic acid, regulate NC cell migration. For example, NC cell migration correlates with the appearance of high amounts of hyaluronic acid.

A variety of substrate- and cell-attached factors influence neural development by regulating adhesion properties of cells (Chap. 7). Interactions occur directly between cells or between a cell and the extracellular matrix. The molecules mediating these interactions have been implicated in regulating the specificity and timing of cell–cell adhesion and the consequences on cell morphology and physiology. Hence, they influence the ability of cells not only to migrate but to sort themselves out and to stabilize spatial relationships considered important for the process of differentiation.

Cell process outgrowth determines the cytoarchitecture and circuitry of the nervous system

Cell process elongation and branching determine the final morphological phenotype of the cell and its participation in the local and global neural circuitries [12–14]. On average, each of the billions of neuronal cells forms more than 10,000 specific interconnections. This process of morphological differentiation requires the directed growth of a considerable number of cell processes to multiple specific targets, often at great distances from the cell body. Control over the active elongation of a cell process creates the final size and geometry of the neuronal axon and dendritic tree. What are the molecular mechanisms that control the progressive elongation of a cell process? What environmental signals are present to guide the processes through a complex, three-dimensional, multicellular terrain? What are the processes that determine the time and place of branching? Are the molecules implicated in regulating cellular migration involved in controlling neurite outgrowth? In general, many of the same soluble and matrix components that regulate cell proliferation, survival and migration have been shown to also mediate process outgrowth *in vivo* and *in vitro*.

Growth cones are located at the leading edge of a neurite and display two types of motile structures: long spike-like structures called filopodia and thin, broad sheets of membrane called lamellipodia. These delicate structures are important in pathfinding and outgrowth branching (see Chap. 8). Growth cone movement can be influenced by small soluble factors. Local concentration gradients of nerve growth factor (NGF) and/or FGF can initiate and direct growth and movement. Specific neurotransmitters, such as serotonin and dopamine, can also alter neurite elongation and growth cone movement. For example, serotonin inhibits neuronal outgrowth of specific subsets of neurons. Inhibition of neurite outgrowth can also be suppressed by electrical activity.

Adhesion molecules [15], either on the cell or in the extracellular matrix, may also play an important role in neurite outgrowth since they mediate neurite–neurite and neurite–glia interactions. The probability of outgrowth initiation, rate of elongation and degree of branching of neurites is strongly influenced by the adhesive quality of the substrate. Adhesion of growth cone structures may stabilize extensions. Growth cones may follow the path of greatest adhesiveness, leading to directional control over neurite outgrowth. The glycoprotein laminin, found in the extracellular matrix and on the surface of Schwann cells, can accelerate neurite outgrowth.

Neuron–glia interaction may also be involved in outgrowth. Sympathetic neurons grown in the absence of Schwann cells extend unbranched, axon-like neurites; in the presence of glial cells, however, process outgrowth is extensively branched and dendrite-like in form. In CNS preparations, this interaction is further characterized by the specificity of the astrocytic environment: glia from local homotypic regions give rise to branched neurites and glia from heterotopic regions induce unbranched neurites.

Intracellular pathways are involved in the regulation of neurite outgrowth. cAMP and inositol phospholipids have been implicated as intracellular regulators, and work on the control of Ca^{2+} influx has helped to establish a causal relationship with neurite outgrowth: Ca^{2+} influx can regulate both neurite elongation and growth cone movements. Studies of invertebrate neurons and isolated growth cones suggest that in the presence of various agents that inhibit neurite outgrowth, for example, serotonin and electrical activity, the amount of free cytoplasmic Ca^{2+} is closely correlated with neurite outgrowth. Further support of Ca^{2+}-mediated control of neurite growth has been obtained from studies under conditions in which neurite outgrowth and Ca^{2+} influx could be directly manipulated. Data suggest that specific levels of Ca^{2+} influx promote normal neurite elongation and growth cone movements.

The basic cytoarchitecture of the cortex is the result of a plastic process of neurite outgrowth, as discussed above, relying on adhesion factors and control of terminal arborization, which can be dependent on neuronal activity. The final lattice-like pattern of complex cortical circuitry and its computational capacity arise from a combination of selective and nonselective process outgrowth and synapse formation events coupled to regressive events, including selective cell death, process elimination and synapse elimination. These events can be activity-dependent and/or -independent processes. For example, the vertical connections in the cortex arise with little dependence on neuronal activity during development, whereas the horizontal connecting outgrowth is clearly regulated by evoked or spontaneous neural activity. Thus, the formation of cortical clusters is dependent on patterned visual activity; binocular deprivation can eliminate the clustered organization of the horizontal connections. In the case of cortical cluster organization, selective elimination of collaterals, and not cell death, is the essential molding parameter.

In summary, a number of parameters of outgrowth initiation, elongation, branching and cessation combine to generate axonal or dendritic geometry. These components can be modulated *in vitro* by a variety of soluble and substrate-bound factors, suggesting that, *in vivo*, control over morphological differentiation is multifactorial.

MOLECULAR MECHANISMS OF DEVELOPMENT

Environmental factors control developmental decisions made by cells of each lineage

Diffusible growth factors (see Chap. 19) control the processes of proliferation and differentiation [6,16]. The discovery of NGF in the early 1950s began an era of remarkable success in developmental neurochemistry. Physiological effects of NGF can be classified as (i) an essential neurotrophic or nourishing influence during early development, resulting in selective neuronal survival; (ii) a potent influence on neuronal differentiation; or (iii) a strong neurotropic or guiding influence on direction of neurite growth. The main experimental strategy employed over the years to demonstrate the presence of the different activities of NGF has been to either block, via specific antibodies or drugs, or enhance, via addition of exogenous NGF, its actions. The survival and differentiation influences of neurotrophins are not unique. Since the mid-1980s, the existence of many other such factors has been reported (see Chap. 19). The sections of this chapter on cell lineages illustrate the rapidly growing importance of growth factors and cytokines in neural cell development.

Genetic networks function in neural development

One of the most fascinating and rapidly growing fields of research is the elucidation of the complex network of genetic information that controls development. The immense phenotypic diversity of the nervous system reflects the coordination of the numerous genetic programs that regulate cell type-specific gene expression. How does a cell become responsive to a given set of environmental signals, encode this information into specific channels of intracellular transduction and regulate differential gene expression? The answer lies, in part, in the complex world of transcriptional regulators. It is estimated that 5% of the mammalian genome, about 5,000 genes, encode for transcription factors (Fig. 27-3). Of these, up to one-half are anticipated to have expression restricted to the nervous system. The large number of transcription factors can be subdivided into families whose members share a conserved amino acid sequence responsible for DNA-binding and dimerization. At present, 12 distinct motifs have been identified. Four classes are illustrated in Figure 27-4. Research demonstrates that members of these and other classes can function as transcriptional regulators exerting control over the developmental processes of proliferation and differentiation [17] (see also Chap. 26).

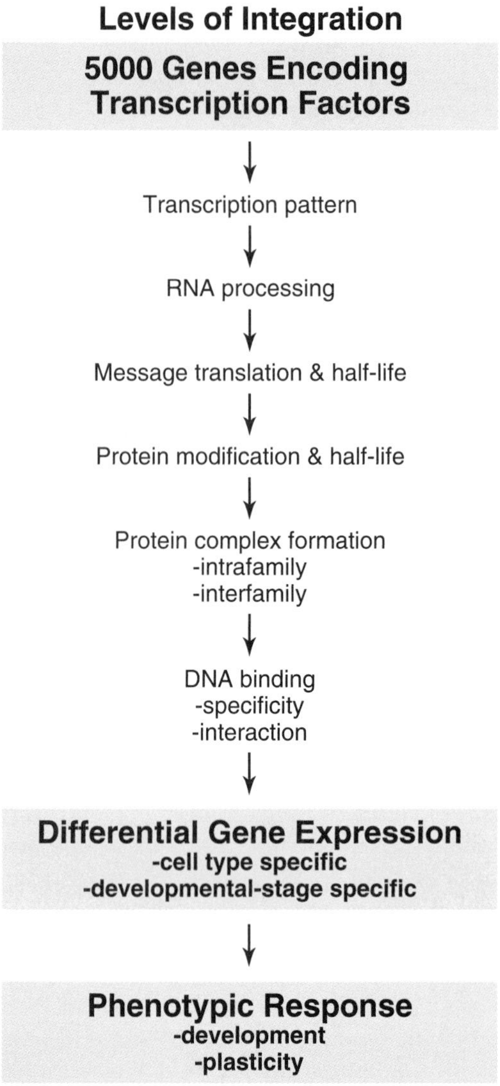

There are multiple levels of integration within the transcriptional regulator network

Part of the complexity of control lies in the large number of different factors available to generate cell type-specific transcriptional regulation. More importantly, control over the expression and functional state of these numerous transcription factors is a source of considerable complexity and opportunity for combinatorial integration. Figure 27-3 illustrates the many points or levels of control that can be exerted over these developmental regulators. For example, the ability to alter the transcriptional expression of these factors is an initial and key point of control. As shown, other classical points of control, such as translation, are expected to add levels of complexity. Because the activity of most of these transcriptional regulators can be controlled by phosphorylation and dimerization, the number of permutations of interactive modes increases rapidly. Heterodimer formation can determine whether a transcriptional regulator is functionally active or not.

Levels of Integration

5000 Genes Encoding Transcription Factors

↓

Transcription pattern

↓

RNA processing

↓

Message translation & half-life

↓

Protein modification & half-life

↓

Protein complex formation
-intrafamily
-interfamily

↓

DNA binding
-specificity
-interaction

↓

Differential Gene Expression
-cell type specific
-developmental-stage specific

↓

Phenotypic Response
-development
-plasticity

FIGURE 27-3. Levels of integration within the transcription factor network. Of the estimated 5,000 genes in the human genome encoding for transcription factors, perhaps half will exhibit expression specific to the nervous system. This predicted restriction in expression is considered to reflect the need to generate the combinatorial control mechanisms necessary to create the enormous phenotypic diversity unique to neural development. Listed are the various levels of processing whereby complex interactions among many factors and many events are integrated to carry out the critical task of differential gene expression that determines the unique phenotypic response during development and adult plasticity.

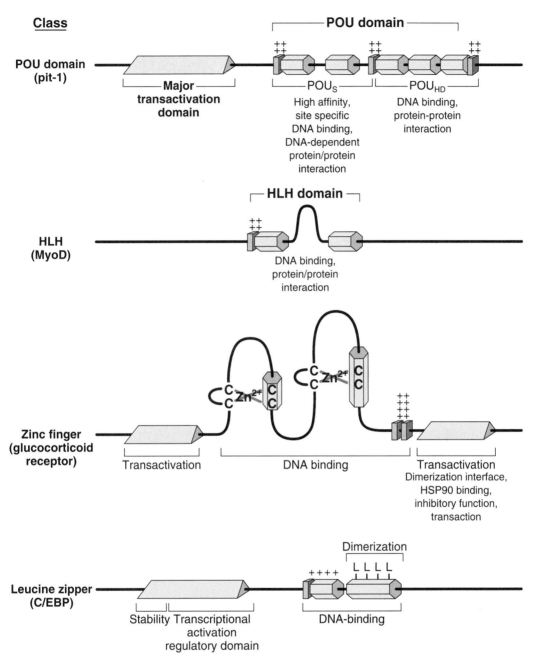

FIGURE 27-4. Major classes of transcription factors. Twelve distinct families of transcription factors have been classified by their DNA-binding motifs. Four examples of these transcription factors implicated in the control of cell proliferation and differentiation are depicted here. Conserved regions unique to each family include regions of basic amino acids functioning as DNA-binding sites (*solid rectangles*) and putative helical regions associated with DNA binding or dimerization (*cylinders*) are shown. Transcriptional activation domains (*solid triangles*) are generally not conserved even within a family, generating considerable diversity of functional transactivation among interacting family members. Each family has at present more than half a dozen members. The classes shown possess a POU domain (Pituitary-1, pit-1), a basic helix-loop-helix domain (*HLH, MyoD*), a nuclear receptor type of zinc-finger domain (glucocorticoid receptors), or the basic region/leucine zipper domain (*bZIP;* CCAAT/enhancer binding proteins, *C/EBP*). (Modified from He and Rosenfeld [20], with permission.)

Thus, at any point of time in the life of a given cell, the sum total of activity at all levels of integration will be reflected by the nature of the genetic program that is read. This program not only creates the new cell phenotype but also sets the stage for the next round of developmental decisions, in part due to the alteration in the pattern of expression of transcriptional regulators now unleashed to reverberate in the cell physiology.

Early response genes function as development-control signals

How do epigenetic influences participate in decision making? Environmental influences come in the form of growth factors, neurotransmitters and other ligands that are linked to changes in membrane receptors and intracellular signaling pathways, as well as agents or fields capable of altering membrane electrical properties. Most extracellular signals trigger a change in cell physi-

ology that can last for several days. How do these changes come about? In particular, how can environmental factors "start the ball rolling" and trigger a new wave of genomic activity? Researchers have found that ligand-induced changes result in a very rapid gene expression that is independent of any protein synthesis [18]. This large class of genes can be expressed within minutes of cell activation. Because of the very rapid onset of expression, these genes are referred to as early response genes (ERGs), or primary response genes (Fig. 27-5).

Ligand-activated intracellular signaling pathways induce the transcription of ERGs that encode for four categories of cell proteins: (i) transcription factors, (ii) cytoplasm enzymes and structural components, (iii) secreted cytokines and (iv) membrane proteins. Each category represents developmentally important factors, such as interleukin 6 (IL-6) and the NGF receptors. Most of the known transcription factors, including members of the families illus-

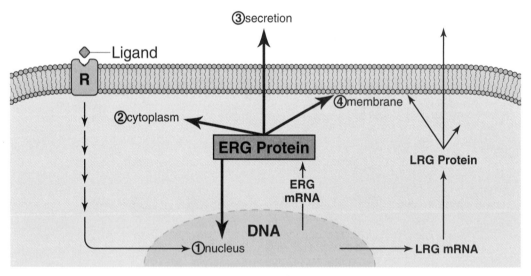

FIGURE 27-5. Early response genes. This figure illustrates the four major classes of early response gene (*ERG*) products serving as either ① nuclear transcription factors, such as Fos and Jun; ② cytoplasmic enzymes, such as nitric oxide synthetase and prostaglandin synthetase II or structural components, such as actin; ③ secreted factors, such as interleukin 6 and other cytokines; or ④ membrane receptors such as nerve growth factor receptor. All of these ligand-inducible ERGs are considered to play a role in regulating developmental events. Of particular importance are the ERGs encoding transcription factors, which have the ability to regulate the genomic response of neural cells to extracellular signals. The characteristic rapid and transient induction of this class of ERG mRNAs and proteins represents a self-referral loop of genetic control, whereby genetic information is rapidly expressed only to return to the nucleus and directly participate in the subsequent combinatorial control of late response gene (*LRG*) transcription and phenotypic alterations. Thus, the cell type-specific, differential control of ERG and LRG expression may be closely coupled. (Modified from [34], with permission.)

trated in Figure 27-4, are ERGs. Therefore, transcriptional regulation of many transcriptional regulators is under tight and rapid control by environmental agents. In addition, since a developing cell is normally exposed to many different signals at a given movement, the ligand-mediated, rapid and transient induction of ERGs represents a tightly controllable, complex mode of encoding environmental information to carry out developmental decisions (Fig. 27-6).

A number of ERG transcription factors have already been shown to play important roles in regulating cell proliferation and differentiation. For example, combinatorial activity of the leucine zipper transcription factors superfamily,

including members of the *fos* and *jun* families, is necessary for a cell to respond to a mitogen and enter the cell cycle. Thus, neural phenotypic diversity can be explained in terms of the history of expression of transcriptional regulators, some members changing rapidly (ERGs), some slowly. Together, they exert a combinatorial hold on the genetic programs and physiology of the cell and determine cell fate.

Transcriptional regulator networks function in invertebrate development

Our understanding of the genetic network orchestrating neural development in mammals is rapidly

ERGs and Differential Gene Regulation

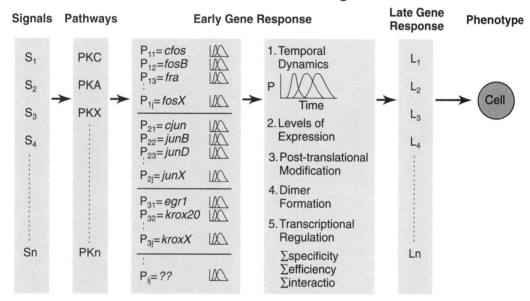

FIGURE 27-6. The early response gene (*ERG*) network and phenotypic diversity. This figure emphasizes the complexity of ERG transcription factor interaction during neural development. The level and kinetics of expression of ERG mRNAs and the subsequent dynamics of interaction among ERG proteins are shown. A wide range of environmental signals ($S_1, S_2 \ldots Sn$) can influence a cell by activating intracellular pathways, indicated here by specific protein kinases (*PKs*), such as protein kinases C (*PKC*) and A (*PKA*), . . . (*PKn*). These kinases are considered to activate target transcription factors capable of inducing the expression of a constellation of ERG families ($P_1, P_2 \ldots P_i$) with family members such as *cfos* (P_{11}), *fosB* (P_{12}), *fra1* (P_{13}) . . . *fosX* (P_{1j}, hypothetical). The total number of ERGs is equal to (i) $\times$ (j) $= P_{ij}$, estimated to be several hundred. Each pathway induces a largely overlapping subset of ERGs, displaying its own characteristic kinetics and levels of mRNA accumulation, denoted by the small generic graphic symbol inserted to the right of each ERG. The next level of potential complexity is evident in the five main properties summarized for ERG protein synthesis, modification and interaction, which together orchestrate the late gene response ($L_1 \ldots Ln$). The concept of combinatorial control suggests that, in addition to the complexity of both ligand–receptor coupling and interaction among signaling pathways responsible for transcriptional activation, the various members of different families of ERG transcription factors extensively interact during the process of transcriptional control of late response genes, exerting a primary role in determining phenotypic diversity. (Modified from [33], with permission.)

increasing, due in large part to the considerable advancement in developmental research of the fly. As part of the genetic network in *Drosophila*, a large number of genes encoding transcription factors and proteins for cell–cell communication help define cell lineages. Most transcription factors perform more than one function during development. For example, many participate during early segmental processes as well as in the later development of the neural, sexual and bristle components. Figure 27-7 illustrates how four major groups of genes interact during development to create the primary body axis and segmentation pattern of the embryo. For example, four maternal-effect proteins, such as bicoid and dorsal, are active in the

unfertilized egg. Upon fertilization, these genes establish anterior–posterior concentration gradients that lead to differential effects on the expression of a variety of other genes encoding transcription factors, such as gap genes, which in turn organize the anterior–posterior axis of the embryo. Thus, a maternal-effect mutant has no head and two caudal regions. Gap genes, for example, *Krüppel*, help to define the middle segment and to activate the expression of pair-rule genes including *hairy* and *fushi tarazu*, segment polarity genes such as *engrailed* and homeotic genes (see below). Mutations of gap genes produce embryos with deleted middle segments. Homeotic genes, named for the homeobox DNA-binding sequence, specify the identity of each segment. For example, mutation of the *Antennapedia* gene results in the antenna on the head being replaced by a leg! A similar regulatory cascade of transcription factors organizes the dorsal–ventral axis (Fig. 27-8).

Our understanding of gene regulation of neural development in *Drosophila* is most complete for the embryonic sensory nervous system [19]. The entire sensory system appears within 5 to 9 hr after fertilization and is known in detail. Five sets of genes have been described that progressively determine the structure and function of this system. The first set of genes are known as prepattern genes, described above, that set up the anterior–posterior and dorsal–ventral body axis and segmentation. Many of these genes contain homeodomains and serve multiple roles during different developmental events, for example, the pair-rule gene *fushi tarazu*, later controls the development of the fly CNS. Following the establishment of the body coordinates, proneural gene expression makes cells competent to become neural precursors. All of the proneural genes encode helix–loop–helix (HLH) transcriptional regulators. The *achaete-scute* complex (AS-C) is a set of four proneural genes required for sensory organ formation. Mutations lead to no or very few neuronal precursors. *Daughterless (da)* expression is necessary for sensory organ precursors to appear. Because *AS-C* and *da* genes code for basic HLH transcription factors, these two gene products can interact to form heterodimers capable of regulating specific target genes. Two additional HLH proteins interact to expand and further refine the complexity of combinatorial control exerted by

Genetic Network Cascade in *Drosophila* Segment Development

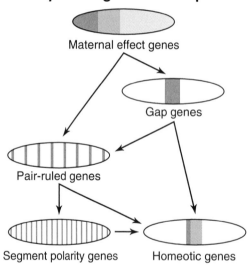

FIGURE 27-7. Genetic network cascade in early *Drosophila* development. Body segmentation in the *Drosophila* embryo results from the sequential and spatially localized expression of specific genes. During early development, maternal-effect genes set up the anterior–posterior orientation of the oblong embryo. Within a very short time, four different groups of genes, depicted here, that encode for transcription factors are expressed and function to regulate not only each other's expression but also many other genes whose products are necessary for proper sequential transformation of linear positional information into a periodic pattern. Note the alternating patterns of gene expression (*orange* vs. *white* areas) that establish boundaries necessary for proper segmentation. (Modified from [33], with permission.)

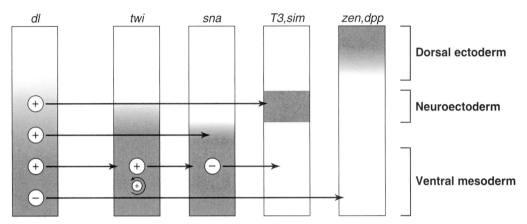

FIGURE 27-8. Dorsal–ventral morphogenesis in *Drosophila*: transcription factor regulatory cascade. The generation of the dorsal–ventral axis is dependent upon a network of transcription factors. The key nuclear morphogen is
dorsal (*dl*), a member of the *rel/NFκB* family, whose shallow gradient in early embryo nuclei (**left box:** a schematic
side view section representation of the embryo, dorsal is at top, ventral at bottom) is based upon a gradient in nuclear translocation: nuclear localization of transcription factors in ventral nuclei (*dark orange*), both nuclear and cytoplasmic localization in lateral regions (*light orange*) and only cytoplasmic localization in dorsal regions (*white*), where
it remains inactive. *dl* creates, in turn, the expression gradient of at least six other transcription factors (see **four boxes
to right**). *dl* activates the expression of *twist* (*twi*), a helix-loop-helix (HLH) transcription factor, and *snail* (*sna*), a zinc-
finger transcription factor. The combined expression of *twi* and *sna* leads to induction of the ventral mesoderm. In
addition, the combination of *twi*-positive autoregulation (*small circular arrow*) and the ability of *dl* to activate *sna*
along with *twi* creates a relatively steep gradient of *sna* expression that creates, in turn, a sharply bound domain of
inhibition of *T3,* one of the members of the *AS-C* HLH transcription factor family and *single-minded (sim)*, an HLH.
Thus, the activation of *T3* and *sim* by *dl* (*top long arrow*) is limited to a narrow lateral band of nuclei that become cells
of the neuroectoderm that form the nervous system. The dorsal ectoderm cells arise from the control of *zerknült (zen)*
and *decapentaplegic (dpp)*, both homeobox transcription factors. Since *dl* exerts a strong inhibitory influence over *zen*
and *dpp* (*bottom long arrow*), the gradient of these (**last box**) is the inverse of *dl*.

these transcription factors. *Hairy (h)*, named for
mutants with ectopic bristles, and *extra-
macrochaete (emc)* can interact to form heterodimers with *AS-C* and *da*, but since h and emc
are HLH proteins lacking functional basic DNA-
binding domains, the heterodimers formed are
inactive. In this way, *h* and *emc* negatively regulate
AS-C and *da* with the resulting loss of neural tissue. Neuronal precursors then express the third
set of genes, neurogenic genes, represented by
HLH transcription factors like the *enhancer of
split (E[spl])* complex and membrane proteins
such as *mastermind (mam)*. This set of genes mediate lateral inhibition among cells in proneural
cell clusters. Mutations lead to lack of suppression, causing all cells in a cluster to enter the neural lineage. The fourth set are neuronal type-selec-
tor genes, controlling the type of sensory neurons
that a precursor becomes and, hence, the type of
sensory organ that forms. The *cut* gene product is
a homeodomain transcription factor that controls
cell type-specific gene expression and organ type.

Finally, cells express cell lineage genes that determine the phenotypic makeup of the cells in the
sensory organ. Two genes in particular decide the
identity of the final cell phenotypes and, hence,
how many neurons and glia will be in each organ.
In *numb* mutations, involving loss of a zinc-finger
transcription factor, all progeny become socket or
hair cells with the loss of neuronal and glial cells.
Another gene, *oversensitive*, has the opposite effect: all neurons and glia and no socket or hair
cells. Thus, PNS development relies on the sequential expression of HLH, homeobox and zinc-
finger classes of transcription factors that participate in a complex combinatorial network to
progressively determine neural cell fate.

Transcriptional regulator networks determine vertebrate development

The remarkably similar mechanisms of genetic
and developmental control between invertebrates and vertebrates stand in contrast to the

timing and form of development in phylogenetically distant species. Similarities include the existence of highly conserved families of HLH and homeobox transcriptional regulators specifying cell fate. In mammalian development, a genetic regulatory network analogous to that described for *Drosophila* seems to function [20]. It has been demonstrated that in the developing mammalian CNS homologous sets of genes are expressed, representing a genetic network regulating the development of the hindbrain segments, termed rhombomeres. Additional studies have implicated other transcriptional regulators in regional pattern formation in more anterior parts of the CNS and in the spinal cord.

The developing mammalian hindbrain is transiently divided into a set of morphologically identifiable rhombomeres. Rhombomeres appear in the floor of the fourth ventricle during early development and may be analogous to segments used to develop the body plan of invertebrates. Rhombomeres are cell lineage-restriction units and express a number of genes in accord with their boundaries. Figure 27-9 shows the expression pattern of several classes of genes in the vertebrate hindbrain, including early expressed transcription factors such as *kreisler* and *Krox-20*, Eph family tyrosine kinase receptors including *Sek* and *Ebk* genes, Eph receptor ligands including *Elk* and *Elf* genes, *Hox* genes and genes coding for signaling molecules such as *Fgf-3*. All of these genes are expressed during the development of the hindbrain and may be responsible for creating positional values along the length of the hindbrain and establishing the position and identity of hindbrain segments [21]. Expression of the *hox* genes in particular is tied to the development of positional value in the hindbrain. Expression of *hox* genes precedes the formation of the rhombomeres, and the ordered expression of these genes within the different rhombomeres creates a set of nested expression domains with a two-segment periodicity. Rhombomere-specific expression of the different genes further refines the pattern and may establish the segmental identity of individual rhombomeres. *Hox* gene expression may be activated by other transcriptional regulators, including *Krox-20* and *kreisler*, which are expressed prior to *hox* gene expression. Disruption of *Krox-20* and *kreisler* activity

also disrupts the pattern of *hox* gene expression and rhombomere formation, suggesting that these two genes act upstream of the *hox* genes.

The development of other regions of the CNS is not likely to rely on an overt pattern of

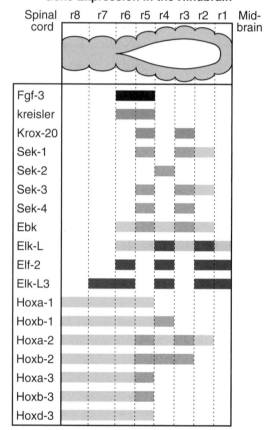

FIGURE 27-9. Segmental restricted hindbrain gene expression. Vertebrate rhombomeres (*r1–8*) are analogous to the *Drosophila* segments and are shown in this schematic of the anterior neural tube and forebrain expansion. Below the neural tube is shown the expression pattern of individual genes (*dark orange or black,* strong expression; *light orange or gray,* weak expression; *no bar,* no expression). These genes include signaling molecules, such as *fibroblast growth factor 3 (Fgf-3);* transcription factors, such as *kreisler* and *Krox-20;* Eph family tyrosine kinase receptors, such as *Sek* and *Ebk* genes; and the Hox homeobox genes *Hox-a* and *Hox-b.* Note that each of the genes is expressed in a spatially restricted manner. These overlapping expression domains create unique combinations of transcription factors within each rhombomere which are considered, in turn, to regulate the phenotype of the cells in each hindbrain region.

segmentation such as is seen in the hindbrain. Pattern and spatial position in the midbrain may stem from signals provided by the isthmic region. Signals from the isthmic region regulate the expression of two genes, *engrailed-1* and *engrailed-2*, which are expressed in a gradient which decreases anteriorly and posteriorly from the isthmic region. This graded expression may establish the overall pattern of the midbrain. Graded *engrailed* expression may be regulated by molecules secreted from the posterior border of the mesencephalic field. Two possible secreted signaling molecules are Wnt-1 and FGF8. Ectopic expression of FGF8 induces ectopic expression of Wnt-I and *engrailed,* as well as production of cells with characteristics of the midbrain.

In the forebrain, a number of transcriptional regulators are expressed in specific domains. These genes include the *Emx, Otx, Dlx* and *Nkx* homeobox genes; *Pax-6,* a paired box gene; *BF-1* and *BF-2 winged helix* genes; and *Tbr-1.* Descriptive expression studies using these genes have suggested that segmentation may act in developing the diencephalon, although the segments identified by gene expression patterns are not restricted lineage units as seen in the hindbrain. The nested expression pattern shown by the *Otx* and *Emx* genes is similar to the pattern created by *hox* gene expression, but the lack of linkage between the four members of this family suggests that a different mechanism is used to establish domains within the forebrain. Some of these genes are expressed in the ventricular zone, suggesting a role in initial patterning of the neuraxis, while others are expressed in the mantle layer, suggesting a role in differentiation. Spinal cord development and regionalization may also be under the control of transcriptional regulators [22]. Regional diversity may be imparted by expression of more distal *hox* genes, which continue to be expressed in accord with "segmental" boundaries within the spinal cord. One inherent difference is that the segmentation visible in the spinal cord is imparted by the periodicity of the surrounding mesoderm and not by intrinsic factors within the spinal cord. Surgical manipulation of this mesoderm disrupts spinal cord segmentation; removal of the adjacent somites can completely eliminate spinal cord segmentation. The dorsal–ventral axis of the spinal cord is likely to form through the concurrent action of two signaling systems. A ventralizing signal initially comes from the notochord; transplantation of a second notochord adjacent to the spinal cord results in differentiation of ventral spinal cord cells. This signal may be carried by a molecule called *sonic hedgehog,* which is produced by the notochord during early development. The neuroepithelium responds to this signal by developing the floorplate, the most ventral portion of the spinal cord. Once floorplate formation has been induced, the floorplate itself begins to produce sonic hedgehog. This signal in turn induces the production of cells appropriate for the ventral part of the spinal cord, in particular, the motor neurons. The dorsalizing influence may stem from the action of the BMP signaling system. The differentiation of dorsal cell types arises by contact-mediated induction from the overlying ectoderm. BMPs produced by this ectoderm elevate the levels of *Pax* and *Msx* genes within the spinal cord. These same genes are repressed by sonic hedgehog signaling and may be required, though are insufficient by themselves, to induce formation of dorsal cell types.

CELL LINEAGES OF THE NERVOUS SYSTEM

The neural crest lineage is progressively restricted to specific sublineages

The developmental fate of most cells is not fixed initially but becomes progressively restricted by epigenetic and genetic interactions. Work on molecular mechanisms in CNS neuronal lineage development is just beginning [9]. In contrast, we have considerable information about the multipotent NC cells and how they become progressively restricted to specific sublineages [21,23,24]. NC cells migrate from the neural tube along specific pathways to their peripheral destinations. At these target sites, they differentiate into a diverse number of cell types, including Schwann cells and neuronal cells of the PNS, pigment cells, endocrine cells and cells forming connective tissue of the face and neck (Fig. 27-10). Although the

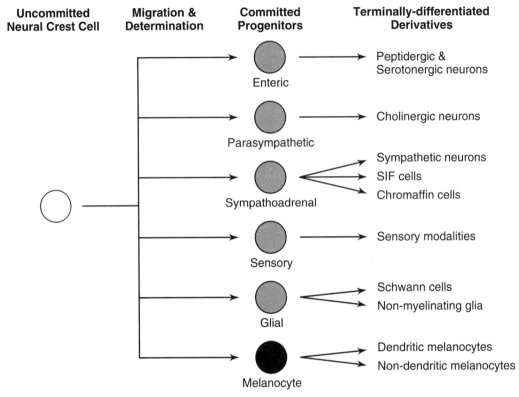

Uncommitted Neural Crest Cell	Migration & Determination	Committed Progenitors	Terminally-differentiated Derivatives

FIGURE 27-10. Neuropoietic model of neural crest cell lineage. Analogous to the process of hemopoiesis, early multipotent neuropoietic stem cells undergo extensive migration along complex pathways to different embryonic environments. Committed progenitor cells, including enteric, parasympathetic and others as listed, generate restricted sublineages under the influence of environmental growth factors. These cell populations expand in number and undergo terminal differentiation to the final adult phenotypes. *SIF,* small, intensely fluorescent cells. (Modified from [35], with permission.)

anatomical and temporal developmental pathways have been extensively described, the molecular mechanisms responsible for the progressive restriction are just now being discovered.

A basic property of differentiated neuronal cells is the expression of one classical neurotransmitter and several neuropeptides. *In vivo* studies with NC cells first demonstrated that the choice of neurotransmitter phenotype could be altered by the environment. In these studies, NC cells were examined by means of chimera transplantation. Two of the final NC cell phenotypes are sympathetic, mainly adrenergic cells, and parasympathetic, cholinergic cells. Presumptive adrenergic neurons transferred to the presumptive cholinergic region of young embryos migrated along the path of vagal NC cells and became cholinergic instead of sympathetic. The nature of the environment could thus switch

neurotransmitter phenotype. The inverse experiment also worked: presumptive cholinergic cells become adrenergic when transferred to the adrenergic region. Thus, premigratory NC cells from different axial levels share some common developmental potential and differentiate in a manner appropriate for their final position. These transplantation experiments using heterogeneous cell populations, however, could be interpreted as evidence for selective or instructive processes: selective cell elimination of an inappropriate phenotype or environmental instructions of appropriate cell phenotype.

Environmental factors control lineage decisions of neural crest cells

Several experimental approaches have shown that environmental factors are critical in determining neurotransmitter phenotype by altering existing cell properties and not by selecting different hypothetical subpopulations of NC cells. For example, during normal postnatal development, the innervation of the sweat glands of the foot pads of cats and rats switches from noradrenergic to cholinergic. Research shows that environmental cues of the target tissue specify both early and late neurotransmitter phenotypes. Cross-innervation studies provide further evidence that the target can retrogradely specify neurotransmitter properties of the neuron that innervates it. Neurons that ordinarily provide noradrenergic innervation of hairy skin become cholinergic and peptidergic when induced to innervate sweat glands. Converse experiments give expected results.

The cellular and molecular mechanisms that specify neurotransmitter phenotype have been described by culture experiments (Fig. 27-11). Polypeptide growth factors such as NGF, bFGF and IL-6 appear to be the primary controllers of neuronal differentiation of the sympathoadrenal progenitor cells. Research findings demonstrate that bFGF promotes the prolifera-

tion and initial differentiation of the sympathoadrenal precursor. For example, bFGF leads to increased neurite outgrowth and upregulation of neuron-specific genes. The survival of these committed neuronal precursor cells, however, ultimately depends upon NGF responsiveness and availability. bFGF can upregulate the low-affinity neurotrophin as receptor ($p75^{NT}$), and cell depolarization induces *trk* genes, which together can produce high-affinity, functional NGF receptors, providing trophic responsiveness.

A number of cytokines appear to control the final stage of differentiation of the sympathetic neuronal lineage. Long ago, it was found that individual sympathetic neurons grown on heart cell monolayers modify their biochemical, pharmacological and electrical properties and shift from adrenergic to cholinergic phenotypes. Growing the neurons in heart cell conditioned medium produces similar results, suggesting that non-neuronal cells, for example, heart myoblasts or glial cells, release a soluble factor, now termed cholinergic differentiation factor (CDF), also known as leukemia inhibitory factor (LIF),

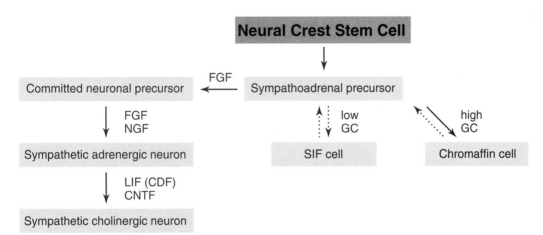

FIGURE 27-11. Growth factor control of neural crest lineage decisions. Regional and temporal differences in environmental factors influence the final phenotype of neural crest progeny. A number of environmental factors influence the committed precursors that give rise to the final four mature phenotypes of the sympathoadrenal lineage. Under conditions of low or high concentrations of glucocorticoids *(GC)*, the sympathoadrenal precursors become either small, intensely fluorescent *(SIF)* cells of the sympathetic ganglia or chromaffin cells of the adrenal medulla, respectively. In environments containing high concentrations of fibroblast growth factor *(FGF)* and nerve growth factor *(NGF)* and little or no glucocorticoid, committed neuronal precursors appear, which terminally differentiate into either sympathetic adrenergic neuronal cells or, under the influence of cholinergic differentiation factor *(CDF)*, also known as leukemia inhibitory factor, *(LIF)* and ciliary neurotrophic factor *(CNTF)* switch neurotransmitter phenotype and become sympathetic cholinergic neuronal cells.

that is responsible for the developmental switch. Ciliary neurotrophic factor (CNTF), belonging to the same cytokine subfamily as IL-6 and CDF, also increases cholinergic and decreases nor-adrenergic properties. While promoting the cholinergic phenotype, CNTF and CDF also inhibit sympathetic neuroblast proliferation. Thus, non-neuronal cells are a source of many molecules that can influence the choice of neurotransmitter and neuropeptide in cultured sympathetic neurons, suggesting that the spatiotemporal differential expression of a variety of cytokines helps determine the diversity of cell fate.

One more key player is known to participate in sympathoadrenal lineage fate. The presence and concentrations of glucocorticoid strongly influence lineage decisions. Since sympathetic ganglia cells normally grow *in vivo* in the presence of glial cells and become predominantly adrenergic, a second factor was sought in order to explain the discrepancy with the *in vitro* switch studies that showed the appearance of the cholinergic phenotype. Studies showed that physiological levels of glucocorticoid can modulate biochemical differentiation by blocking the shift from adrenergic to cholinergic phenotype. CDF effects can also be blocked by conditions that mimic neuronal activity, such as elevated potassium concentrations. In addition, the concentration of glucocorticoid is an important determinant of the path of the sympathoadrenal precursor: low concentrations generate small, intensely fluorescent (SIF) cells and high concentrations generate chromaffin cells.

Research has begun to identify the intracellular signaling pathways activated by environmental factors that lead to the induction of developmental control genes in NC cells and their derivatives. For example, developmental restriction of melanogenesis normally occurs before embryonic day 5 in the quail. This process can be altered by treating embryonic day 9 dorsal root ganglion cells with phorbol ester, which activates protein kinase C (PKC). Schwann cell precursors, which normally lack melanogenic activity, undergo a metaplastic transformation into melanocytes when PKC activity is reduced. This suggests that environmental signals capable of altering levels of PKC regulate lineage decisions in NC cells.

Neural crest lineage is transcriptionally regulated

A number of candidate control genes have been characterized that could give rise to progressive restriction in migrating behavior and control over proliferation and differentiation. Several newly discovered genes appear to underlie cell lineage commitment, while other genes appear important as mediators of the ligand-dependent switch of neurotransmitter phenotype in committed neuronal cells. In mammalian development, a gene analogous with the *AS-C* genes in *Drosophila*, which determine whether a cell becomes a neuronal precursor, has been described. The *mammalian achaete-scute homolog-1 (MASH1)* gene is transiently expressed by spatially restricted subsets of early CNS neuroepithelial and PNS NC cells. The precursors of sympathetic and enteric neurons express this bHLH transcription factor just prior to the onset of cell type-specific gene expression, such as tyrosine hydroxylase (TH), suggesting that *MASH1* is a marker of cells as they enter the sympathoadrenal lineage. It is likely that *MASH1* is an NC control gene determining the commitment step of lineage development. It is expected that *MASH1*, like the activity of *AS-C* genes, will be regulated by a number of other HLH gene families homologous to *da* (E12), *emc* (Id) or *h* (HES) by way of alternative HLH pairing, or heterodimerization, leading to either enhanced or inhibited function in the differentiating mammalian NC cells and CNS.

Once the cells are committed to the sympathoadrenal lineage, a choice of neurotransmitter phenotype must take place. The developmental switch between chromaffin and neuronal phenotype is associated with changes in cell type-specific gene expression, which require the differential control of NC genetic programs. The molecular mechanism integrating the influences of these two types of environmental signals, peptide growth factors and glucocorticoids, involves, in part, the antagonistic interaction of transcription factors (see Chap. 26). Culture work demonstrates that FGF and NGF are antagonistic to glucocorticoid in their ability to upregulate chromaffin-specific genes. The opposite control is also true. Two classes of transcription factors, FOS, as part of the peptide-inducible AP-1 complex, and glucocorticoid receptors (see Fig. 27-4), have been shown to interact in a similar, reciprocal inhibitory fashion. This suggests that, as part of the combinatorial control process, interaction between these different families of transcription factors represents a probable molecular mechanism of reciprocal inhibition exerted by environmental factors.

Glial cell development is critical to nervous system development

Our understanding of glial cell development in the CNS has advanced rapidly since the mid-1980s [22]. The discovery and initial characterization of the oligodendrocyte-type 2 astrocyte (O-2A) cell lineage now represents the most extensively characterized cell lineage system available to study nervous system development. A variety of cellular and molecular approaches have provided us with a preliminary understanding of the environmental signals and the phenotypic responses that are of importance *in vitro*. The current success in cell identification, using antibodies against glia-specific antigens and molecular probes for detecting cell type-specific mRNAs, has led to a rapid increase in our understanding of the key environmental agents that regulate the rate and direction of glial cell differentiation along specific lineage pathways.

The oligodendrocyte lineage has been studied *in vitro*

Oligodendrocytes (OLs) are generated postnatally and pass through a series of cell phenotypes from undifferentiated stem cells to mature myelin-forming cells. This sequential process of maturation of OLs can be reproduced in culture (Fig. 27-12). In the rat, four main stages of development *in vitro* have been delineated. The oligodendroblast, also referred to as the O-2A bipotential progenitor cell, is a proliferating, bipolar cell. These cells, when cultured in chemically defined medium containing 0.5% (low) serum to enhance survival, rapidly differentiate in a relatively synchronous manner into mature oligodendrocytes over a 3- to 5-day period. In contrast, under high serum conditions, many cells become positive for glial fibrillary acidic protein (GFAP) and negative for the O4 marker. These GFAP$^+$/O4$^-$ cells are called type 2

astrocytes (AIIs). This cell type is controversial, perhaps being an artifact of tissue culture [25] or a "reactive" OL. Bipolar oligodendroblast cells become multipolar, O4$^+$ "pre-OL" cells. These O4$^+$/galactocerebroside glycolipid$^-$ cells become "immature OLs" with the appearance of galactocerebroside glycolipid expression. The "mature OL" phenotype is identified by the sequential appearance of additional myelin-specific antigens, proteolipid protein (PLP) and then myelin basic protein (MBP). Thus, immunostaining with glia-specific markers defines seven phenotypically distinct cell types *in vitro*, six of which compose the OL lineage: OL precursors, oligodendroblast cells, pre-OL cells, immature OL cells, mature OL cells, multipolar AII cells (A2B5$^+$/GFAP$^+$) and flat AI cells (A2B5$^-$/GFAP$^+$). This classification scheme can be used to monitor the rate, direction and extent of OL cell differentiation.

Oligodendrocyte lineage *in vivo* resembles that seen *in vitro*

Preliminary descriptions of the patterns of gliogenesis in the forebrain subcortical white matter using immunocytochemical probes are available and closely resemble the *in vitro* data. Similar findings have been reported for the cerebellum. The subventricular zones (SVZ) covering portions of the lateral ventricles are considered to be the origin of progenitor cells that multiply and eventually migrate to and differentiate within the overlying white and gray matter. The separation of OL and AI lineage is considered to occur during embryonic development based on retroviral studies and double labeling, ultrastructural localization and cell morphology.

A number of glial markers provide static yet overlapping information concerning OL lineage development. Small, proliferating, ganglioside GD3$^+$, undifferentiated "neuroectodermal" cells are densely packed in the embryonic SVZ. Starting at embryonic day 16 and continuing to 7 to 10 postnatal days, larger GD3$^+$/carbonic anhydrase$^+$ "progenitor" cells appear in the SVZ, many of which are A2B5$^+$ and may be similar to the oligodendroblasts described *in vitro* above. These cells migrate into the overlying subcortical white matter. By the end of the first postnatal week, the GD3$^+$/carbonic anhydrase$^+$ cells diminish in

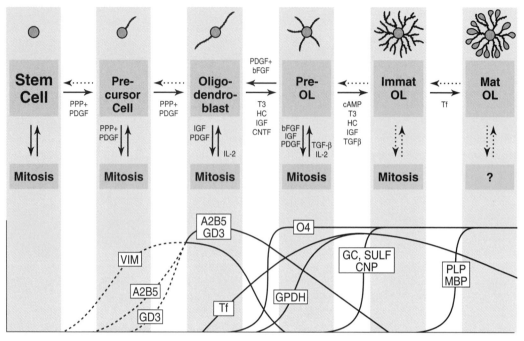

FIGURE 27-12. The oligodendrocyte *(OL)* lineage. The figure illustrates the characteristics that accompany the sequential differentiation within the oligodendrocyte lineage beginning from very early stem cells to the mature oligodendrocyte. This version depicts six cell phenotypes based on morphology, proliferative regulation and immunological determinants defined primarily from *in vitro* data. The various growth factors listed have been shown to regulate cell proliferation and/or differentiation. *Dashed arrows* indicate a possible particular direction, though without clear experimental support. The time course of expression of cell type-specific markers is shown at the bottom. Note that each main stage of lineage development displays not only a different morphology but also a unique antigen profile. Growth factors include basic fibroblast growth factor *(bFGF)*, cAMP, ciliary neurotrophic factor *(CNTF)*, hydrocortisone *(HC)*, insulin-like growth factor *(IGF)*, interleukin 2 *(IL-2)*, platelet-poor plasma *(PPP)*, platelet-derived growth factor *(PDGF)*, transferrin *(Tf)*, transforming growth factor β *(TGFβ)* and triiodothyronine *(T3)*. Cell markers (dotted lines indicate unresolved expression pattern): ganglioside *(A2B5)*, 2,3-cyclic nucleotide-3-phosphohydrolase *(CNP)*, ganglioside *(GD3)*, glycerolphosphate dehydrogenase *(GPDH)*, galactocerebroside glycolipid *(GC)*, ganglioside *(O4)*, proteolipid protein *(PLP)*, myelin basic protein *(MBP)*, sulfatide *(SULF)* and vimentin *(VIM)*.

number while O4$^+$ and galactocerebroside glycolipid$^+$/carbonic anhydrase$^+$ cells rapidly increase in number in the white matter rats. Thus, early stages of OL differentiation appear to occur in the SVZ, which contains a heterogeneous population of "progenitor" phenotypes. The subsequent development of O4$^+$ progenitors into galactocerebroside glycolipid$^+$ "immature" OLs and MBP$^+$ "mature" OLs occurs in the white and gray matter and not the SVZ or neighboring subcortical regions.

Growth factors regulate oligodendrocyte development

The OL cell lineage culture is an excellent system to study the influence of growth factors on cell lineage development. Each of the four main stages of

OL lineage progression can be identified by its characteristic markers, and through the use of growth factors, experiments can be designed to increase or decrease the degree of proliferation and/or block, delay or accelerate maturation of developing precursor cells. Although research shows that OL differentiation is a "default" pathway, occurring in serum-free medium, in the absence of environmental signals, a number of studies demonstrate that OL development is more complex and is responsive to numerous environmental signals. For example, OL lineage cells continue to proliferate for extended periods *in vivo,* in contrast to *in vitro.* In addition, treatment of OL progenitor cells with growth factors known to be present in the developing CNS yields a complex set of ligand-dependent, phenotypic responses.

bFGF and platelet-derived growth factor (PDGF) are two of the key molecular signals controlling OL cell development (Fig. 27-13). In the presence of PDGF, OL progenitor cells are stimulated to divide with a short cell cycle length of 18 hr; are highly motile and bipolar; and differentiate in a synchronous, symmetrical, clonal fashion with a time course similar to that *in vivo*. In the presence of bFGF, however, progenitor cells are stimulated to divide with a longer cell cycle length of 45 hr; become nonmotile pre-OLs with a multipolar shape; and are inhibited

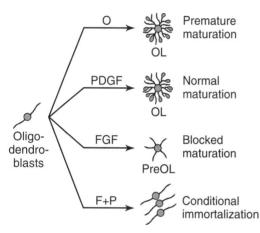

FIGURE 27-13. Growth factor control of oligoden-drocyte *(OL)* lineage decisions. *In vitro* studies have demonstrated that the developmental fate of O-2A progenitor cells in culture can be regulated by environmental factors. Progenitor cells cultured in the absence of either basic fibroblast growth factor *(FGF)* or platelet-derived growth factor *(PDGF)* develop to mature OLs but do so on a timetable more rapid than *in vivo*. The addition of PDGF stimulates several rounds of cell division, slowing/delaying the time of development to mature OLs so that it more closely resembles the normal *in vivo* time course. In contrast, FGF stimulates continual proliferation while blocking phenotypic development at the pre-OL (04$^+$/galactocerebroside glycolipid$^-$) cell stage. Evidence suggests that FGF can lead to downregulation of cell surface galactocerebroside glycolipid and simplification of morphology indicating possible "dedifferentiation" or plasticity of the galactocerebroside glycolipid$^+$ cell phenotype. The combination of both factors leads to a stable condition of the immature O-2A phenotype exhibiting continual proliferation. Upon removal of either FGF or both factors, cells leave the state of "conditional" immortalization and proceed to differentiate normally.

from expressing galactocerebroside glycolipid, PLP or MBP. Progenitor cells treated with both bFGF and PDGF exhibit a third phenotypic response, remaining motile, bipolar progenitor cells that divide indefinitely and do not differentiate. This ligand-dependent, conditional "immortalization" can greatly expand the OL progenitor cell population over extended periods of time. Upon removal of bFGF or both mitogens, the progenitor cells differentiate along the OL lineage.

The source of PDGF *in vitro* appears to be AI cells, but *in vivo* PDGF is produced by neurons [26]. From *in situ* hybridization data, the PDGF α receptor is expressed only in galactocerebroside glycolipid$^-$/OL lineage cells and not in identifiable astrocytes or neuronal cells. In addition, bFGF appears to upregulate the PDGFα receptor in OL progenitor cells. By altering the responsiveness of these cells to PDGF, bFGF and PDGF together maintain the "proliferative" state. These studies indicate that (i) there is no obligatory relationship between cell proliferation and differentiation, (ii) different environmental signals lead to different behavioral responses and (iii) cooperation between extracellular signals can generate additional, unique phenotypes. In addition, both diffusible (CNTF) and nondiffusible, that is, extracellular matrix-bound, components act directly on OL progenitor cells to inhibit OL differentiation and/or induce the AII phenotype. Thus, cell–cell interaction in the developing CNS in the form of diffusible and nondiffusible factors modulates normal OL development, including commitment to OL (or AII) cell fate, the extent of cell division and the timing and rate of cell differentiation.

Transferrin is an iron carrier protein that acts as a trophic factor for neurons, astrocytes and OLs [27]. As the blood–brain barrier gets established during development, neural cells become dependent on transferrin produced by OLs and choroid plexus epithelial cells (Fig. 27-14). OLs are the major source of transferrin in the CNS. This suggests an important function for OLs in addition to myelination of axonal tracts. Transferrin concentration in CSF is highest at the time of peak myelination. Oligodendrocytes, myelin and several areas of the brain contain higher concentrations of iron than the liver, presumably in the form of ferritin-bound iron.

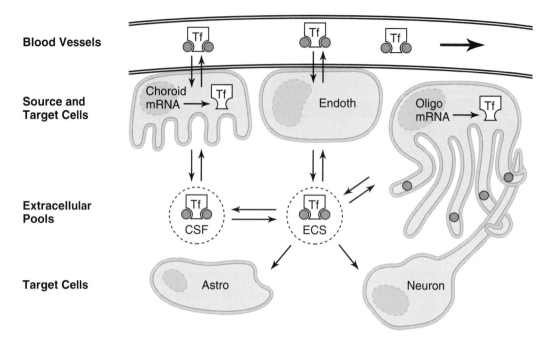

Blood Vessels

Source and Target Cells

Choroid mRNA

Endoth

Oligo mRNA

Extracellular Pools

CSF

ECS

Target Cells

Astro

Neuron

FIGURE 27-14. Regulation of transferrin *(Tf)* in the CNS. Tf is an important molecule regulating the movement and storage of iron in the nervous system. Although blood-borne Tf is exchanged by choroid epithelial cells and the endothelial cells of the capillary beds in the brain, only the oligodendrocytes and choroid cells in the brain can produce Tf *in vivo*. Each Tf molecule can bind two atoms of iron *(dark orange balls)* that in the brain are distributed between the two large pools, the cerebrospinal fluid *(CSF)* and the extracellular space *(ECS)*. Astrocytes and neurons are considered to be completely dependent upon these pools and, in turn, upon the oligodendrocytes, choroidal cells and the body for Tf.

The Schwann cell lineage is also characterized by sequential and overlapping expression of many stage-specific markers

Expression patterns of antigens allow delineation of at least six developmental stages, both *in vivo* and *in vitro,* that give rise to two types of Schwann cells in the adult (Fig. 27-15). The appearance of S100 and O4 proteins defines the immature Schwann cell stage. Then, a nonmyelinating Schwann cell type can be defined by the appearance of galactocerebroside and association with axons. These cells also express neural cell adhesion molecule (NCAM) and L1 recognition molecule. Note the curious combination of antigens in the nonmyelinating Schwann cell: O4 and galactocerebroside glycolipid indicative of the CNS OL phenotype, and GFAP and S100 found in CNS astrocytes. From this stage, cells move along one of two possible paths. In the PNS, the ensheathing glial cells, depending upon the size of the axons with which they are associated, either remain at the nonmyelinating stage (small axons) or begin to produce myelin-associated proteins and the sheath (large axons) (Fig. 27-16). The latter developmental path involves the appearance of proliferative, premyelinating Schwann cells that express myelin genes, such as P_0, MBP and MAG. These cells then lose GFAP, NGF receptor, N-CAM and L1, while producing myelin membrane as myelinating Schwann cells.

cAMP in culture can mimic most of the effects of axons, including expression of early progenitor antigens, suggesting that a cAMP trigger drives most Schwann cell development *in vivo*. For example, cell proliferation by bFGF or PDGF requires the presence of high concentrations of intracellular cAMP. The role of cAMP may be to upregulate mitogen membrane recep-

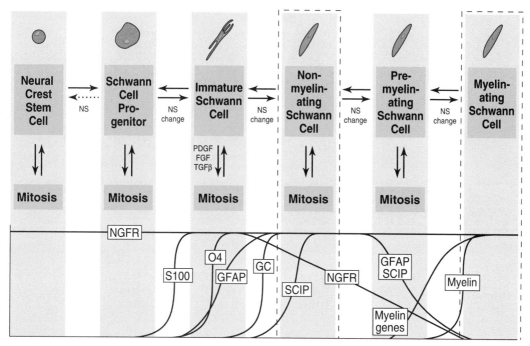

FIGURE 27-15. The Schwann cell lineage. The Schwann cell is the axon-ensheathing cell of the PNS and, thus, displays many properties and developmental processes similar to CNS oligodendrocytes. The figure illustrates the sequential differentiation of Schwann cells from early, unchacacterized neural crest stem cells to the final two mature phenotypes, surrounded by *dashed boxes:* the nonmyelinating and the myelinating Schwann cells of the adult, based on the size of the axons they ensheath. See Figure 27-16 for the developmental anatomy of these two mature phenotypes. Unlike CNS oligodendrocytes, the vast majority of Schwann cells do not become myelin-producing. This six-stage version of Schwann cell development is based upon cell morphology, proliferative potential and, most importantly, the expression of stage-specific antigens, that is, the appearance and/or disappearance of specific markers (**bottom**), derived from both *in vivo* and *in vitro* data. It appears that upon reaching the nonmyelinating phenotype (**box 4 from left**), cells are fated either to remain in this state and represent the adult population of nonmyelinating cells or to differentiate further, expressing myelin-associated genes. The premyelinating phenotypes then become myelinating cells of the PNS (stage 6). Growth factors are fibroblast growth factor *(FGF)*, platelet-derived growth factor *(PDGF)* and transforming growth factor β *(TGFβ)*. Cell markers include nerve growth factor receptor *(NGFR)*, monoclonal antibody against a soluble cytoplasmic protein *(S100)*, glial fibrillary acidic protein *(GFAP)* and suppressed cAMP-inducible POU domain transcription factor *(SCIP)*.

tors. Thus, in the developing nerve, axon-associated factors elevate cAMP, which is responsible for inducing two key events. The first event is the expression of O4 antigen and the responsiveness to mitogens in immature progenitors and non-myelinating Schwann cells. The second event is the further differentiation into premyelinating and myelinating Schwann cells, if the suppression of proliferation takes place owing to some secondary permissive signal associated with the ensheathed large caliber axons.

Of great interest is the expression pattern of suppressed cAMP-inducible POU domain pro-

tein (SCIP). SCIP is a member of the POU family of transcription factors with characteristics of an early response gene, originally defined by the presence of a homology domain between the four transcription factors, Pit-1, Oct-1, Oct-2 and Unc-86. POU proteins are usually considered to function as transcriptional activators of cell type-specific genes and determine cell fate. In CNS and PNS myelinating cells, SCIP is expressed at high levels only during a very narrow window of development and acts as a repressor of myelin-specific genes. In Schwann cells, SCIP is expressed in the progenitors but not in the

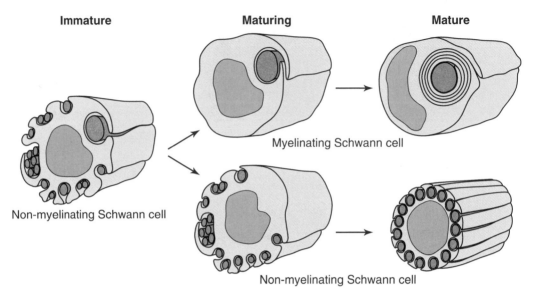

Immature   **Maturing**   **Mature**

Myelinating Schwann cell

Non-myelinating Schwann cell

Non-myelinating Schwann cell

FIGURE 27-16.   Schwann cell development and axonal sorting. Immature O4-positive Schwann cells can be found to take one of two paths of differentiation. Initially, both large- and small-caliber axons, usually <1 μm diameter, are found embedded in furrows along the surface of a chain of immature Schwann cells. This illustration shows a cross-section through a single cell. During the period of cell proliferation and axonal sorting, large axons that require myelin laminar ensheathment separate, by some undefined process of axonal/Schwann cell interaction, from smaller-caliber axons that require only a simple, nonmyelin ensheathment. In maturing, myelinating Schwann cells, single axons are enveloped by the lips of the trough on the cell surface, one of which elongates to create the myelin wrapping as the number of turns of membrane increase, and the lamellae become more compact as the cytoplasmic content is lost. In maturing, nonmyelinating Schwann cells, no myelin membrane is formed but many small-caliber axons remain completely embedded within separate furrows in each cell. Thus, the adult nerve contains two Schwann cell pheno-types, nonmyelinating and myelinating. (Modified from [36], with permission.)

more mature, myelinating Schwann cells (Fig. 27-15). In these proliferating nonmyelinating and premyelinating Schwann cells, SCIP acts on promoters of myelin-associated genes, such as P_0 and MBP, as a repressor. Thus, SCIP expression is found in cells with elevated concentrations of cAMP to be correlated with rapid downregulation of the ERG *c-jun* transcription factor and the onset of rapid proliferation and repression of myelin genes. In response to denervation, SCIP is rapidly and transiently re-expressed during the period of rapid cell proliferation of premye-linating Schwann cells and is considered to an-tagonize the expression of myelin-specific genes.

CONCLUSIONS

Most development focuses on the formation of the complexity of neural tissue during embry-onic and postnatal development. These changes provide a basis for later juvenile and adult stages of growth, in which the dynamic interaction be-tween the genes and the environment contin-ues. Although development is now less dra-matic, environmental signals continue to produce lasting changes in neural structure and function in the adult nervous system. Ge-netic–epigenetic interaction is now associated with physiological and behavioral learning (Chap. 50). It is likely that the main elements employed during early development that allow a cell to "learn" to participate in the system are the same elements used during the continual process of learning and corresponding plastic modification of the nervous system across the life span of the organism. Learning during the life of the organism is correlated with changes at every level of the hierarchy of information flow (Fig. 27-1) leading to the continued expression and refinement of neuronal/glial networks. Ex-ternal and internal events continue to regulate gene expression, and neuronal and glial cells continue to interact metabolically. In its broadest sense, development continues during adulthood [28]. Since neural plasticity can be defined as the long-lasting changes in neural structure and function following environmental perturbation, the term is applicable to adult development. The molecular and cellular basis of adult neural plasticity has focused on environment-induced changes in neurotransmitter metabolism, synaptic structure and function and local circuits. Three experimental models have proven to be most successful in helping to delineate the molecular basis of plasticity: environmental control over catecholamine biosynthesis, long-term potentiation [29] and experience-dependent alterations in brain structure and function. In this summary, we will highlight the first research area.

Neurotransmitters transduce electrical information from one cell to another, participating in the pattern of information flow in the nervous system. States of altered neurotransmitter metabolism can lead to changes in neuronal processing and physiological and behavioral control. Since the concentration of neurotransmitters in synaptic terminals is partly determined by the activity of rate-limiting synthesizing enzymes, which in turn depends on appropriate activation of signal pathways, transcription factors and mRNA transcription, environmental change of short duration can lead to significant, long-lasting alterations in brain function [30,31]. For example, brief, excitatory perturbation of sympathetic neurons via electrical, pharmacological or behavioral input can lead to long-term changes in the concentrations of neurotransmitters. These perturbing signals all lead to cell depolarization, which may be linked to the later events of enhanced transcriptional rates of TH, the rate-limiting enzyme in the synthesis of catecholamines, and decreased transcriptional rates for the polypeptide precursor for substance P, a small putative peptide neurotransmitter colocalized with catecholamines. Thus, not only do neurotransmitter concentrations undergo long-lasting alterations following brief environmental stimulation, but neurotransmitters are also differentially regulated by the same external stimuli.

CNS neurons show similar responsiveness, suggesting that the phenomenon is widespread and of fundamental importance in the control of adult function. *In vivo* and *in vitro* experiments demonstrate that a single, brief stimulation of the locus ceruleus (LC), leading to cell depolarization, results in increased amounts of mRNA and TH activity. Increases in TH can still be observed for several weeks. It has been suggested that another, more subtle consequence of environmental perturbation could be detected based on the unique, extensive axonal domain of the LC. Since TH is synthesized in the cell body, the influence of induced amounts of TH will be determined in part by the distance traversed by TH to reach the synaptic terminal and thus influence synaptic function. Because of the variable axonal path length and the constant rate of axoplasmic flow, the initial environmental stimulation will result in maximal elevations of TH activity in the LC by 2 days; neurotransmitter activity, however, will peak in the cerebellum at 4 days and in the frontal cortex at 12 days. In this way, the genomic activation in a single location is expressed in an anatomically dispersed temporal sequence. Since the LC has extensive and diffuse axonal projections that are involved in controlling shifts in states of arousal, vigilance and attention, brief environmental stimulation of PNS and CNS neurons in the adult nervous system can lead to gene activation and long-lasting patterns of altered synaptic function.

In the future, rapid advances in molecular biology, cell culture and grafting will further our understanding of how the abstract genetic intelligence becomes progressively and continually transformed into the hierarchically organized dynamic networks of information and structure. Throughout the life span of an organism, environmental perturbation leads to alterations in neural structure and function. Therefore, development can be viewed as a continual process of short- and long-term information storage whereby genetic and epigenetic interaction, at every step of development, is represented in the evolving structural and functional design of the nervous system. The nervous system is always adapting and we are always learning.

ACKNOWLEDGMENTS

The authors thank Sharon Belkin and Carol Gray of the Mental Retardation Research Center for help in preparing the illustrations. The author's research was supported by NICHD Grant 2P01-HD06576 and National Multiple Sclerosis Society Grant RG-2751.

REFERENCES

1. Purves, D., and Lichtman, J. W. *Principles of Neural Development.* Sunderland, MA: Sinauer Associates, 1985.
2. Smythies, J. R., and Bradley, R. J. (eds.). *International Review of Neurobiology.* New York: Academic Press, 1992.
3. Arenander, A. T., and de Vellis, J. Frontiers of glial physiology. In R. Rosenberg (ed.), *The Clinical Neurosciences.* New York: Churchill Livingstone, 1983, pp. 53–91.
4. Fedoroff, S., and Vernadakis, A. (eds.). *Astrocytes,* Vol. 2. Orlando, FL: Academic Press, 1987.
5. Lauder, J., and McCarthy, K. Neuronal–glial interactions. In S. Federoff and A. Vernadakis (eds.), *Astrocytes,* Vol. 2. Orlando, FL: Academic Press, 1987, pp. 295–314.
6. Jacobson, M. *Developmental Neurobiology,* 3rd ed. New York: Plenum Press, 1991.
7. Cowan, W. M. The development of the brain. *Sci. Am.* 241:12–133, 1979.
8. Patterson, P. H. Process outgrowth and the specificity of connections. In Z. W. Hall (ed.), *An Introduction to Molecular Neurobiology.* Sunderland, MA: Sinauer Associates, 1992, pp. 388–427.
9. McConnell, S. K. The generation of neuronal diversity in the developing central nervous system. *J. Neurosci.* 15:6987–6998, 1995.
10. Oppenheim, R. W. Cell death during development of the nervous system. *Annu. Rev. Neurosci.* 14:453–501, 1991.
11. Hynes, R. O. Integrins: Versatility, modulation, and signaling in cell adhesion. *Cell* 69:11–25, 1992.
12. Shankland, M., and Macagno, E. R. (eds.). *Determinants of Neuronal Identity.* New York: Academic Press, 1992.
13. Mattson, M. P. Cellular signaling mechanisms common to the development and degeneration of neuroarchitecture. A review. *Mech. Ageing Dev.* 50:103–157, 1989.
14. Katz, L. C., and Callaway, E. M. Development of local circuits in mammalian visual cortex. *Annu. Rev. Neurosci.* 14:31–56, 1992.
15. Tessier-Lavigne, M., and Goodman, C. S. The molecular biology of axon guidance. *Science* 274:1123–1133, 1996.
16. Patterson, P. H. Neuron–target interactions. In Z. W. Hall (ed.). *An Introduction to Molecular Neurobiology.* Sunderland, MA: Sinauer Associates, 1992, pp. 428–459.
17. He, X., and Rosenfeld, M. G. Mechanisms of complex transcriptional regulation: Implications for brain development. *Neuron* 7:183–196, 1991.
18. Arenander, A. T., and Herschman, H. R. Primary response gene expression in the nervous system. In S. Loughlin and J. Fallon (eds.). *Neurotrophic Factors.* New York: Academic Press, 1992, pp. 89–128.
19. Jan, Y. N., and Jan, L. Y. Genes required for specifying cell fates in *Drosophila* embryonic sensory nervous system. *Trends Neurosci.* 13:493–498, 1990.
20. Lumsden, A., and Krumlauf, R. Patterning the vertebrate neuraxis. *Science* 274:1109–1115, 1996.
21. Hatten, M. E., Kettenmann, H., and Ransom, B. R. Glial cell lineage. *Glia* 4:124–243, 1991.
22. Tanabe, Y., and Jessell, T. M. Diversity and pattern in the developing spinal cord. *Science* 274:1115–1123, 1996.
23. Anderson, D. J. Cellular and molecular biology of neural crest cell lineage determination. *Trends Genet.* 13:276–280, 1997.
24. Anderson, D. J. Molecular control of cell fate in the neural crest: The sympathoadrenal lineage. *Annu. Rev. Neurosci.* 116:129–158, 1993.
25. Espinosa de los Monteros, A., Zhang, M., and de Vellis, J. O2A progenitor cells transplanted into the neonatal rat brain develop into oligodendrocytes but not astrocytes. *Proc. Natl. Acad. Sci. USA* 90:50–54, 1993.
26. Ellison, J. A., Scully, S. A., and de Vellis, J. Evidence for neuronal regulation of oligodendrocyte development: Cellular localization of platelet-derived growth factor receptor and A-chain mRNA during cerebral cortex development in the rat. *J. Neurosci. Res.* 44:28–39, 1996.
27. Espinosa de los Monteros, A., Pena, L. A., and de Vellis, J. Does transferrin have a special nervous system? *J. Neurosci. Res.* 24:125–136, 1989.
28. Kaas, J. H. Plasticity of sensory and motor maps in adult mammals. *Annu. Rev. Neurosci.* 14:137–167, 1991.
29. Teyler, T. J., and DiScenna, P. Long-term potentiation. *Annu. Rev. Neurosci.* 10:131–161, 1987.

30. Black, I. B., Adler, J. E., Dreyfus, C. F., Friedman, W. F., LaGamma, E. F., and Roach, A. H. Biochemistry of information storage in the nervous system. *Science* 236:1263–1268, 1987.

31. Black, E. B., Adler, J. E., Dreyfus, C. F., et al. Neurotransmitter plasticity at the molecular level. *Science* 225:1266–1279, 1984.

32. Arenander, A. A., and de Vellis, J. Early response gene expression signifying functional coupling of neuroligand receptor systems in astrocytes. In S. Murphy (ed.). *Astrocytes.* New York: Academic Press, 1993, pp. 109–136.

33. Wilkinson, D. G., and Krumlauf, R. Molecular approaches to the segmentation of the hind brain. *Trends Neurosci.* 13:335–339, 1990.

34. Arenander, A., and de Vellis, J. Early response gene induction in astrocytes as a mechanism for encoding and integrating neuronal signals. *Prog. Brain Res.* 94:177–188, 1992.

35. Anderson, D. J. The neural crest cell lineage problem: neuropoiesis? *Neuron* 3:1–12, 1989.

36. Peters, A., Palay, S. L., and F. Webster, H. (eds.). *The Fine Structure of the Nervous System: The Neurons and Supporting Cells.* Philadelphia: W.B. Saunders Company, 1976.

28

Axonal Transport

David L. Stenoien and Scott T. Brady

Basic Neurochemistry: Molecular, Cellular and Medical Aspects, 6th Ed., edited by G. J. Siegel et al. Published by Lippincott–Raven Publishers, Philadelphia, 1999. Correspondence to Scott T. Brady, Department of Cell Biology and Neuroscience, University of Texas Southwestern Medical Center, 5323 Harry Hines Boulevard, Dallas, Texas 75235-9111.

NEURONAL ORGANELLES IN MOTION

The axon comprises a major portion of the total volume and surface area in most neurons and may extend several thousand cell body diameters. Since the genetic material and effectively all of the protein synthesis machinery are localized to the cell body, a supply line is maintained to provide structural and functional materials to sites all along the length of the axon. Insights as to how neurons accomplish this task can be obtained by viewing living axons with video-enhanced light microscopy [1] (Fig. 28-1).

Such video images reveal an array of organelles moving down the axon toward the nerve terminal, termed anterograde direction, as well as returning to the cell body, termed retrograde di-

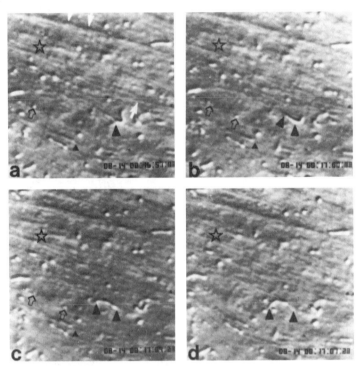

FIGURE 28-1.   Sequential video images of fast axonal transport in isolated axoplasm from the squid giant axon. In this preparation, anterograde axonal transport proceeds in the direction from **upper left** to **lower right**, or from 10 o'clock toward 4 o'clock. The field of view is approximately 20 μm, and the images were recorded in real time on videotape. The large, sausage-shaped structures *(filled triangles)* are mitochondria. Medium-sized particles *(open arrows)* most often move in the retrograde, that is, right to left, direction. Most structures of this size are lysosomal or prelysosomal organelles. The majority of moving particles in these images are faint and moving rapidly, 2 μm/sec, so they are difficult to catch in still images; however, in the region above the *star,* a number of these organelles can be visualized in each panel. The entire field contains faint parallel striations, like those indicated by the *white arrows* in panel **a,** that correspond to the cytoskeleton of the axoplasm, primarily microtubules. The movement of membranous organelles is along these structures, although organelles can occasionally be seen to switch tracks as they move, like the mitochondrion indicated by *large triangles*. (From [44], with permission.)

rection. The movements create patterns as engrossing as the ant farms of our childhood and initially appear as chaotic. Some organelles glide smoothly, while others move in fits and starts. On closer examination, an underlying order emerges: the organelles moving in the anterograde direction are typically fainter and smaller but more numerous than those moving in the retrograde direction, and all appear to travel along gently curving fibrils. Occasionally, two organelles are seen travelling in opposite directions along the same fibril, appearing destined for a head-on collision but seeming to pass through each other; other organelles hop from one fibril to another. The images imply, and other studies confirm, that the organelles represent membrane-bound packets of materials en route to a variety of intraneuronal destinations. The structural elements of the axon, the cytoskeleton, are equally dynamic, though they are unseen in these images because they move and change more slowly, by several orders of magnitude.

The life cycle of these organelles, their kinetics and molecular cargo, the molecular motors driving their transport and the substrates along which these movements track constitute interrelated aspects of what is broadly termed axonal transport. A primary aim of this chapter is to provide an understanding of this form of intraneuronal traffic. Achieving this goal requires an appreciation of the dynamics and structure of the relevant neuronal components and structures. Studies of how cellular structures and components move from where they are synthesized to where they are utilized comprise an area of intensive research in cellular and molecular neurobiology. To encompass this topic, we examine how our concepts of axonal transport evolved to the present understanding of this complex and dynamic field.

DISCOVERY AND CONCEPTUAL DEVELOPMENT OF FAST AND SLOW AXONAL TRANSPORT

The size and extent of many neurons presents a special set of challenges

Since protein synthesis for the entire neuron takes place in the cell body, which may represent only 0.1% of the total cell volume, growth and maintenance of neuronal processes require timely, efficient delivery of material to axonal and dendritic domains. The idea that materials must be transferred from the cell body to the axon was suggested by Ramon y Cajal and other pioneers during the early part of this century. For many years, the existence of such transport processes could only be inferred.

The first experimental evidence for axonal transport resulted from studies on peripheral nerve regeneration, which were stimulated by the desire to improve treatment of limb injuries sustained during World War II. In the classic work of Weiss and Hiscoe [2], surgical constriction of a sciatic nerve branch led to morphological changes in the nerve that directly implicated the cell body as the source of materials for axonal regrowth. After several weeks, the axon appeared swollen proximal to the constriction but shriveled on the distal side. Following removal of the constriction, a bolus of accumulated axoplasm slowly moved down the nerve at 1 to 2 mm per day, very nearly the rate observed for outgrowth of a regenerating nerve. Weiss and Hiscoe concluded that the cell body supplies a bulk flow of material to the axon. This view dominated the field for two decades, but the characteristics of this slow "flow" of material did not seem adequate to explain some aspects of nerve growth and function.

Cell biologists subsequently provided convincing arguments for the necessity of this intracellular transport. Neuronal protein synthesis was almost completely restricted to the cytoplasm surrounding the nucleus, termed translational cytoplasm, which includes polysomes, the rough endoplasmic reticulum and the Golgi complex; and ribosomes were undetectable in the axon [3]. If proteins cannot be synthesized in the axon, then materials necessary for axonal function have to be supplied by transport from the cell body. Axonal transport must be a normal, ongoing process in neurons. By the mid-1960s, the use of radioactive tracers confirmed the existence of a slow "bulk flow" component of transport. Using autoradiography, Droz and Leblond [4] elegantly showed that systemically injected [³H]amino acids were incorporated into nerve cell proteins and transported along the sciatic nerve as a wavefront of radioactivity. These methods demonstrated that newly synthesized proteins were transported, but some re-

TABLE 28-1.	MAJOR RATE COMPONENTS OF AXONAL TRANSPORTS	
Rate component	Rate (mm/day)	Structure and composition
Fast transport		
Anterograde	200–400	Small vesiculotubular structures, neurotransmitters, membrane proteins and lipids
Mitochondria	50–100	Mitochondria
Retrograde	200–300	Lysosomal vesicles and enzymes
Slow transport[a]		
SCb	2–8	Microfilaments, metabolic enzymes, clathrin complex
SCa	0.2–1	Neurofilaments and microtubules

[a]SCb, slow component b; SCa, slow component a.

sponses of the neuron occurred too rapidly to be explained solely by a slow "flow."

Shortly thereafter, radiolabeling and histochemical studies demonstrated that faster rates of transport occur [5]. Unlike slow transport, the faster components move material bidirectionally, toward and away from the cell body. Both endogenous proteins and exogenously applied labels were detected moving at fast transport rates. These findings expanded the concept of axonal transport: materials move in both anterograde and retrograde directions and rates vary by as much as three orders of magnitude (Table 28-1).

At first, emphasis was placed on the characterization of fast and slow axonal transport. The kinetics of axonal transport were analyzed by injection of radiolabeled amino acids into

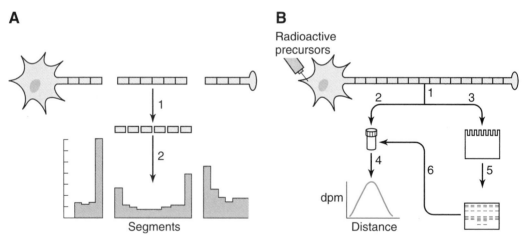

FIGURE 28-2. Schematic diagram of two common methods for analyzing the component rates of axonal transport. **A:** Accumulation of transported material can be studied at a focal block of axonal transport caused by a cut, a crush, a cold block or a ligature. This approach is a variation of that employed by Weiss and Hiscoe [2] and has been used often in studies of fast axonal transport. In this example, two cuts have been made in order to detect both anterograde and retrograde transport. After time for accumulation at the ends, the nerve segments are cut into uniform segments for analysis (step 1). Each segment is analyzed either for radioactivity in labeled nerves or for enzyme activity, and the rate of accumulation is estimated (step 2). **B:** With segmental analysis, the nerve must be pulse-labeled, usually with radioactive precursors. After an appropriate injection–sacrifice interval to label the rate component of interest, the nerve is also cut into segments (step 1). In some cases, only a single segment is used as a "window" onto the transport process. Each segment is analyzed both by counting the radioactivity in an aliquot (step 2) and by gel electrophoresis (step 3), where each lane corresponds to a different segment. The amount of radioactivity in different polypeptides can be visualized with fluorography (step 5) and individual bands cut out of the gel (step 6) for analysis by liquid scintillation counting. The distribution of either total radioactivity or radioactivity associated with a specific polypeptide can then be plotted (step 4). *dpm,* disintegrations per minute. (Adapted from [6], with permission.)

the vitreous of the eye or the dorsal root ganglia, to "label" sensory neurons, or into the ventral spinal cord, to label motor neurons. In the case of fast transport, a wavefront of labeled protein was detected traveling away from the cell body at 250 to 400 mm per day in mammals. Using this same approach, slow transport rates were shown to approximate 1 mm per day. Rates for fast transport were also determined by measuring the amount of a transported substance such as acetylcholinesterase or norepinephrine accumulating at a nerve constriction over a few hours, well before bulk accumulation of axoplasm is detectable. These two approaches for studying axonal transport, locating a radiolabeled wavefront by analysis of successive nerve segments and monitoring the accumulation of materials at a constriction with time (Fig. 28-2), generated considerable information on the kinetics and the metabolic and ionic requirements of axonal transport [5]. Such findings formed the basis for more detailed characterization of axonally transported materials and for studies of the underlying molecular mechanisms.

Fast and slow components of axonal transport differ in both their constituents and their rates

Fast transport is bidirectional: many proteins that are distributed by fast anterograde transport also return in the retrograde direction. In contrast, proteins transported at slow rates are degraded when they reach their destination and are not detected in the retrograde component. Axoplasmic fractionation studies have shown that proteins moved by fast anterograde and retrograde transport are predominantly membrane-associated, while most slowly transported materials are recovered in soluble fractions.

When labeled polypeptides traveling down the axon are analyzed by sodium dodecyl sulfate (SDS) polyacrylamide gel electrophoresis, materials traveling in the axon can be grouped into five distinct rate components [6]. Each rate component is characterized by a unique set of polypeptides moving coherently down the axon (Fig. 28-3). As polypeptides associated with each rate class were identified,

most were seen to move only with a single rate component. Moreover, proteins that have common functions or interact with each other tend to move together. These observations led to a new view of axonal transport, the structural hypothesis [3]. This model can be stated simply: proteins and other molecules move down the axon as component parts of discrete subcellular structures rather than as individual molecules (Table 28-1).

The structural hypothesis was formulated in response to observations that axonal transport rate components move as discrete waves, each with a characteristic rate and a distinctive composition. It can explain the coherent transport of functionally related proteins and is consistent with the relatively small numbers of motor molecules in neurons. The only assumption is that the number of elements which can interact with transport motor complexes is limited and this requires appropriate packaging of the transported material. Different rate components result from packaging of transported material into different cytologically identifiable structures. In fact, the faster rates reflect the transport of proteins preassembled as membranous organelles, including vesicles and mitochondria, or of proteins contained in the lumen of these organelles (Fig. 28-4), whereas slower rates reflect the transport of cytoskeletal proteins. Thus, tubulin and the microtubule-associated proteins (MAPs) move as microtubules (MTs) and neurofilaments (NFs) move as neurofilaments. Cytoplasmic proteins that are not integral components of a cytoskeletal element may be linked to those structures (Fig. 28-5). While disputes continue regarding the size and composition of the transported package for cytoskeletal and cytoplasmic proteins (polymers, oligomers, macromolecular complexes and others), the idea that complexes of proteins, rather than individual polypeptides, are moved has gained general currency.

Although five distinct major rate components have been identified, the original categories of fast and slow transport remain useful. All membrane-associated proteins move in one of the fast rate components, while cytoplasmic proteins move as part of the slow com-

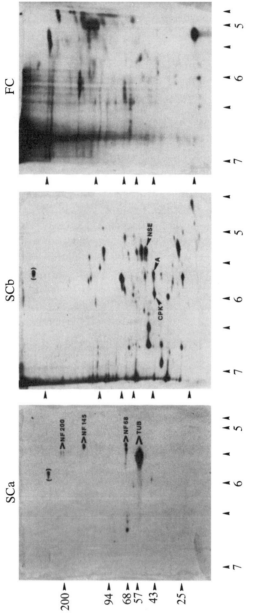

FIGURE 28-3.   Two-dimensional fluorographs showing the [^{35}S]methionine-labeled polypeptides in the three major anterograde rate components of axonal transport: *SCa*, slow component a; *SCb*, slow component b; *FC*, fast component. Note that each rate component has not only a characteristic rate but also a characteristic polypeptide composition. The discovery that each rate component has a different polypeptide composition led to the structural hypothesis. (From [45], with permission.)

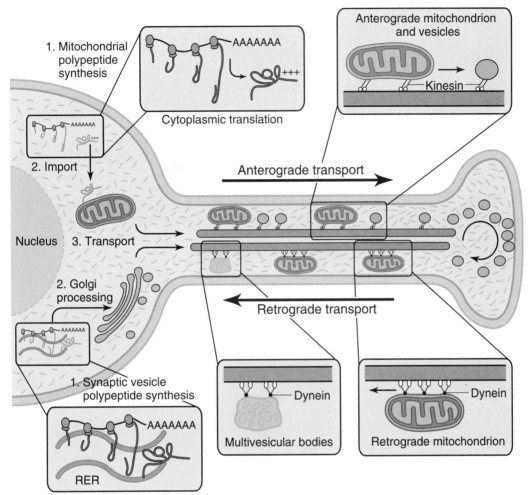

FIGURE 28-4. Schematic illustration of the movement of membrane-associated material in fast axonal transport. Fast axonal transport represents the movement of membrane-bound organelles along axonal microtubules in both the anterograde and the retrograde directions. Two major classes of membrane-bound organelles that are synthesized and packaged by different pathways are depicted. Synaptic vesicle polypeptides are translated on endoplasmic reticulum-bound ribosomes, at which time membrane proteins become properly oriented within the lipid bilayer and secretory polypeptides enter into the lumen of the endoplasmic reticulum. These polypeptides are further processed within the Golgi apparatus, where the appropriate post-translational modifications and sorting of polypeptides destined for the axon occur. Once these polypeptides are packaged into vesicular organelles, and the appropriate motor molecules are present, the organelles are transported down the axon utilizing axonal microtubules as "tracks" at rates of 200 to 400 mm per day. Movement in the anterograde direction is believed to be mediated by the molecular motor kinesin, while the force necessary to move retrograde organelles is thought to be generated by cytoplasmic dynein. Unlike the synthesis of vesicular polypeptides, mitochondrial polypeptides that are supplied by the host cell are synthesized on cytoplasmic ribosomes and contain a targeting sequence that directs the polypeptides to the mitochondria. Following assembly and the association of motor molecules, the mitochondria move down the axon at rates of 50 to 100 mm per day. Mitochondria can also be detected moving back toward the cell body in the retrograde direction. The morphology of retrogradely transported mitochondria is distinctly different from that of mitochondria moving in the anterograde direction and is believed to represent degenerating organelles that are not metabolically active. *RER,* rough endoplasmic reticulum.

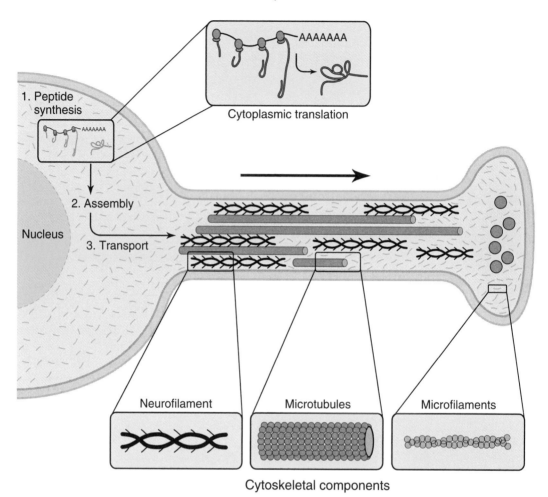

Cytoskeletal components

FIGURE 28-5.   Schematic illustration of the movement of cytoskeletal elements in slow axonal transport. Slow axonal transport represents the movement of cytoplasmic constituents including cytoskeletal elements and soluble enzymes of intermediary metabolism at rates of 0.2 to 2 mm per day, which are at least two orders of magnitude slower
than those observed in fast axonal transport. As proposed in the structural hypothesis and supported by experimental evidence, cytoskeletal components are believed to be transported down the axon in their polymeric forms, not as
individual subunit polypeptides. Cytoskeletal polypeptides are translated on cytoplasmic polysomes and then assembled into polymers prior to transport down the axon in the anterograde direction. In contrast to fast axonal transport,
no constituents of slow transport appear to be transported in the retrograde direction. Although the polypeptide
composition of slow axonal transport has been extensively characterized, the motor molecule(s) responsible for the
movement of these cytoplasmic constituents has not yet been identified.

ponents. Current studies indicate that the various organelles transported anterogradely are
moved along the axon by one or more motor
molecules (see below). The differing rates of
fast anterograde transport appear to result
from the varying sizes of organelles, with increased drag on larger structures resulting in a
slower net movement (Fig. 28-1). Less is
known about molecular mechanisms of slow
transport.

**Features of fast axonal transport,
demonstrated by biochemical and
pharmacological approaches, are
apparent from video images**

Video microscopy of axoplasm [1], as described
briefly at the beginning of this chapter, directly
confirmed the bidirectionality of fast transport
that had been inferred from accumulation of radiolabeled materials on both sides of a crush and

established that populations of organelles moving in each direction are different. Observations that transport is inhibited by agents that disrupt MTs are consistent with the movement of organelles along fibrils that have been identified as MTs by correlated video and electron microscopy. Video microscopy reveals that organelle movement can continue in an apparently normal fashion in axons isolated from their cell bodies and divested of plasma membrane. The implication is that transport must be driven by local energy-generating mechanisms, as predicted from observations that application of a cold block or metabolic poison (dinitrophenol or cyanide) to a discrete region of a nerve inhibits transport locally [5].

FAST AXONAL TRANSPORT

Newly synthesized membrane and secretory proteins destined for the axon travel by fast anterograde transport

However, not all membrane-bounded organelles (MBOs) are destined for the axon. As a result, the first stage of transport must be synthesis, sorting and packaging of organelles. Once assembled, the organelle must be committed to the transport machinery and moved down the axon. Finally, organelles must be targeted and delivered to specific domains in the axon, such as presynaptic terminals, axolemma and nodes of Ranvier. Axonal constituents include integral membrane proteins, secretory products, membrane phospholipids, cholesterol and gangliosides. As predicted by the structural hypothesis and apparent in video microscopy, rapid transport is achieved by packaging materials into MBOs (Figs. 28-4 and 28-6). Clearly, an understanding of how MBOs are formed in the cell body and routed to the fast-transport system in axons is essential [7].

Passage through the Golgi apparatus is obligatory for most proteins destined for fast transport

In all cell types, secretory and integral membrane proteins are synthesized on polysomes bound to the endoplasmic reticulum. Secretory proteins enter the lumen of the reticulum, whereas membrane proteins become oriented within the bilayer of the membranes (Fig. 28-6). In contrast, components of the cytoskeleton and enzymes of intermediary metabolism are synthesized on so-called free polysomes, which are actually associated with the cytoskeleton. Newly formed membrane-associated proteins must be transferred to the Golgi apparatus for processing and post-translational modification, including glycosylation, sulfation and proteolytic cleavage, as well as for sorting. Pathways for transfer between Golgi and endoplasmic reticulum involve both an MT-dependent step and sorting events mediated by G proteins [8]. After progressing through the Golgi, coated vesicles bud off from the *trans*-Golgi membrane. Transport to their various destinations is typically mediated by MTs and motor molecules. Membrane and secretory proteins become associated with membranes either during or immediately following their synthesis, then maintain this association throughout their lifetime in the cell. For example, inhibiting synthesis of either protein or phospholipid leads to a proportional decrease in the amount of both protein and phospholipid in fast transport, whereas application of these inhibitors to axons has no effect on transport. This suggests that fast axonal transport depends on *de novo* synthesis and assembly of membrane components.

Fast-transport proteins leave the endoplasmic reticulum in association with transfer vesicles that bud off and undergo Ca^{2+}-dependent fusion with the Golgi apparatus. Drug studies have demonstrated a requirement that most proteins destined for fast axonal transport traverse the Golgi stacks, where membrane proteins are post-translationally modified, sorted and packaged [9] (see Fig. 2-9). This suggests that proteins in fast axonal transport must either pass through the Golgi complex or associate with proteins that do. Transfer from the Golgi apparatus to the fast-transport system appears to be mediated by clathrin-coated vesicles [8] (see Fig. 2-8). Coated vesicles, however, are rarely observed in axons, and clathrin, the major coat protein, is primarily a slow-transport protein [3]. Thus, Golgi-derived coated vesicles shed their coats prior to undergoing fast transport

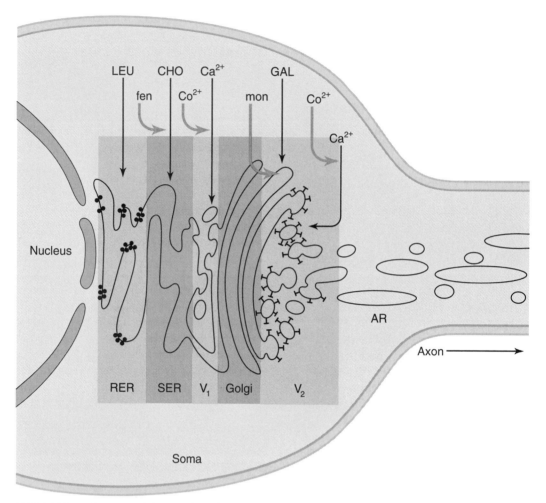

FIGURE 28-6.   Summary of pharmacological evidence indicating that newly synthesized membrane and secretory proteins in neurons reach the axons by a pathway similar to that utilized for intracellular transport in non-neuronal cells. Incorporation sites are indicated for several precursors of materials in fast axonal transport: *LEU,* leucine for proteins; *CHO,* choline for phospholipids; *GAL,* galactose for glycoproteins and glycolipids. Sites of action for several inhibitors are also indicated, including fenfluramine *(fen),* monensin *(mon)* and Co^{2+}. One possible site for Ca^{2+}-mediated vesicle fusion is at the transition from rough endoplasmic reticulum *(RER)* and smooth endoplasmic reticulum *(SER)* to the Golgi apparatus via one type of transition vesicle *(V1).* The subsequent budding of vesicles *(V2)* off the Golgi apparatus, presumably mediated by clathrin-coated vesicles, is a second site for Ca^{2+} involvement. The microtubule guides for the axonal vesiculotubular structures in transport and the axoplasmic reticulum *(AR)* are not shown.

and travel down the axon as either individual uncoated vesicles or other membrane-bound structures (Fig. 28-6).

Anterograde transport moves synaptic vesicles, axolemmal precursors and mitochondria down the axon

Fast anterograde transport represents movement of MBOs along MTs away from the cell body at rates ranging in mammals from 200 to 400 mm per day or from 2 to 5 µm per second [3,10]. Anterograde transport provides newly synthesized components essential for neuronal membrane function and maintenance. Ultrastructural studies have demonstrated that the material moving in fast anterograde transport includes many small vesicles and tubulovesicular structures as well as mitochondria and dense core vesicles [11,12]. Material in fast anterograde transport is needed for supply and turnover of intracellular membrane compartments (mitochondria and endoplasmic reticulum), secretory products and proteins required for the maintenance of axonal metabolism. The net rate appears to be largely determined by size, with the smallest MBOs in almost constant motion, while mitochondria and larger structures frequently pause, giving a lower average rate [13].

A variety of materials move in fast anterograde transport, including membrane-associated enzymes, neurotransmitters, neuropeptides and membrane lipids. Most are synthesized in the cell body and transported intact, but some processing events occur in transit. For example, neuropeptides may be generated by proteolytic degradation of propeptides (see Chap. 18). This biochemical heterogeneity extends to the MBOs themselves. The small organelles are particularly varied in function and composition: some correspond to synaptic vesicle precursors and contain neurotransmitters and associated proteins, while others may contain channel proteins or other materials destined for the axolemma. Biochemical and morphological studies have provided a description of the materials transported in fast transport but are not as well suited for identifying the underlying molecular mechanisms involved in translocation.

Video microscopy allows study of molecular mechanisms through direct observation of organelle movements while precise control of experimental conditions is maintained. Fast axonal transport continues unabated in isolated axoplasm from giant axons of the squid *Loligo pealeii* for hours [1,13]. Video microscopy applied to isolated axoplasm permits a more rigorous dissection of the molecular mechanisms for fast axonal transport through biochemical and pharmacological approaches because isolated axoplasm has no plasma membrane or other permeability barriers. Such studies have extended earlier observations on the properties of fast anterograde transport and demonstrated the existence of new motor proteins that are responsible for movement of MBOs in the axon (see below).

Retrograde transport returns trophic factors, exogenous material and old membrane constituents to the cell body

MBOs moving in retrograde transport are structurally heterogeneous and, on average, larger than the structures observed in anterograde

transport, which are commonly tubulovesicular [11,12]. Multivesicular or multilamellar bodies are common in retrograde transport, and these are thought to represent materials to be delivered to lysosomes in the cell body. The larger size of these retrograde vectors affects the rate of transport by increasing drag due to interactions with cytoplasmic structures [1,13].

Both morphological and biochemical studies indicate that MBOs returning in retrograde transport differ from those in anterograde transport. Repackaging of membrane components apparently accompanies turnaround, or conversion from anterograde to retrograde transport. The mechanisms of repackaging are incompletely understood, but certain protease inhibitors and neurotoxic agents will inhibit turnaround without affecting either anterograde or retrograde movement. The specificities of effective protease inhibitors implicate a thiol protease, but the identity of the responsible enzyme is unknown [14]. Consistent with this proposal, protease treatment of purified synaptic vesicles affects directionality of their movements in the axoplasm and presynaptic terminals. Fluorescent synaptic vesicles normally move in the anterograde direction, but protease pretreatment of these vesicles results in retrograde transport [10].

Uptake of exogenous materials by endocytosis in distal regions of the axon results in the return of trophic substances and growth factors to the cell body [15]. These factors assure survival of the neuron and modulate neuronal gene expression. Changes in the return of trophic substances play critical roles during development and regeneration of neurites (see Chaps. 27 and 29). Retrograde transport of exogenous substances also provides a pathway for viral agents to enter the CNS. Once retrogradely transported material reaches the cell body, the cargo may be delivered to the lysosomal system for degradation, to nuclear compartments for regulation of gene expression or to the Golgi complex for repackaging.

Molecular sorting mechanisms ensure delivery of proteins to discrete membrane compartments

While pathways by which selected membrane-associated proteins are delivered to the correct destination have been established in general terms, many intriguing questions regarding the selection process itself remain [16]. How is it that certain membrane proteins remain in the cell body, for example, glycosyltransferases of the Golgi, while others are packaged for delivery to the axon? Among transported proteins, how do some, such as sodium and potassium ion channels, reach the axolemma while others, such as presynaptic receptors, synaptic vesicles or secreted neuropeptides, travel the length of the axon to the nerve terminal or enter the synaptic cleft? Finally, how are organelles such as the synaptic vesicle directed toward axons and presynaptic terminals but not into dendritic arbors? This question becomes particularly compelling for dorsal root ganglion sensory neurons, where the central branch of the single axon has presynaptic terminals while the peripheral branch of that same axon has none.

The answers to these questions remain incomplete, but some mechanisms have begun to emerge [16]. Some information comes from studies on polarized epithelial cells, where the identity of molecular destination signals for delivery of newly synthesized proteins to basolateral or apical membranes can be assayed. These mechanisms are relevant to the neuron because viral proteins which normally go to epithelial basolateral membranes end up in neuronal dendritic compartments, while those targeted to apical compartments may be moved into the axon [17]. However, the underlying mechanisms appear to be complex. Signals may be "added on," as post-translational modifications including glycosylation, acylation or phosphorylation [18], or "built in," in the form of discrete amino acid sequences [19]. Both mechanisms appear to operate in cells. For example, addition of mannose-6-phosphate to proteins directs them to lysosomes, while amino acid sequences have been identified that direct proteins into the nucleus or into mitochondria. In general, the targeting signals are likely to direct proteins to specific organelles, whereas other mechanisms direct organelles to appropriate final destinations.

Specific membrane components must be delivered to their sites of utilization and not left at inappropriate sites [3]. A synaptic vesicle should go to presynaptic terminals because they serve no function in an axon or cell body. The problem is compounded because many presynaptic terminals are not at the end of an axon. Often, numerous terminals occur sequentially along a single axon, making *en passant* contacts with multiple targets. Thus, synaptic vesicles cannot merely move to the end of axonal MTs and targeting of synaptic vesicles becomes a more complex problem. Similar complexities arise with membrane proteins destined for the axolemma or a nodal membrane.

One proposed mechanism for targeting of organelles to terminals may have general implications. The synapsin family of phosphoproteins [20], which is concentrated in the presynaptic terminal, may be involved in targeting synaptic vesicles. Dephosphorylated synapsin binds tightly to both synaptic vesicles and actin microfilaments (MFs), while phosphorylation releases both of them. Dephosphorylated synapsin inhibits axonal transport of MBOs in isolated axoplasm, while phosphorylated synapsin at similar concentrations has no effect [21]. When a synaptic vesicle passes through a region rich in dephosphorylated synapsin, it may be crosslinked to the available MF matrix by synapsin. Such cross-linked vesicles would be removed from fast axonal transport and are effectively targeted to a synapsin- and MF-rich domain, the presynaptic terminal. Calcium-activated kinases subsequently mobilize targeted vesicles for transfer to active zones for neurotransmitter release [20] (see Chap. 9). This suggests a general mechanism that with variations, might target MBOs to other specific domains [3].

Finally, this chapter has focused almost entirely on axonal transport, but dendritic transport also exists. Since dendrites usually include postsynaptic regions while most axons terminate in presynaptic elements, dendritic and axonal transport each receives a number of unique proteins. Evidence for sorting mechanisms comes from studies in cultured hippocampal neurons using two different viral proteins. Basolaterally targeted viral glycoproteins were transported exclusively to the dendritic processes of cultured neurons, whereas glycoproteins of the apically budding virus were found in axons [17]. An added level of complexity for intraneuronal transport phenomena is the intriguing observation that mRNA is routed into dendrites, where it is implicated in local protein synthesis at post-synaptic sites, but that ribosomal components and mRNA are largely excluded from axonal domains [22]. Similar processes of mRNA transport have been described in glial cells [23].

SLOW AXONAL TRANSPORT

Cytoplasmic and cytoskeletal elements move coherently at slow transport rates

Two major rate components have been described for slow axonal transport, representing movement of cytoplasmic constituents including cytoskeletal elements and soluble enzymes of intermediary metabolism [3]. Cytoplasmic and cytoskeletal elements in axonal transport move with rates at least two orders of magnitude slower than fast transport. In favorable systems, the coherent movement of NFs and MT proteins provides strong evidence for the structural hypothesis [24]. Particularly striking evidence was provided by pulse-labeling experiments in which NF proteins moved over periods of weeks as a bell-shaped wave with little or no trailing of NF protein. Similarly, coordinated transport of tubulin and MAPs makes sense only if MTs are being moved since MAPs do not interact with unpolymerized tubulin.

Slow component a (SCa) comprises largely the cytoskeletal proteins that form NFs and MTs. Rates of transport for SCa proteins in mammalian nerve range from 0.2 to 0.5 mm per day in optic axons to 1 mm per day in motor neurons of the sciatic nerve and can be even slower in poikilotherms such as goldfish. Although the polypeptide composition of SCa is relatively simple, the contribution of SCa to slow transport varies considerably. For large axons, such as α motor neurons in the sciatic nerve, SCa is a large fraction of the total protein in slow transport, while the amount of material in SCa is relatively reduced for smaller axons, such as optic axons [25]. The amount and the phosphorylation state of SCa protein in axons are the major determinants of axonal diameter.

Slow component b (SCb) represents a complex and heterogeneous rate component, including hundreds of distinct polypeptides ranging from cytoskeletal proteins like actin and, in some nerves, tubulin [25] to soluble enzymes of intermediary metabolism, such as the glycolytic enzymes [3]. The structural correlate of SCb is not as easily identified as the MTs and NFs of SCa. The actin is presumed to form MFs, but actin represents only 5% to 10% of the protein in SCb. Most proteins in SCb may be assembled into labile aggregates that can interact transiently with the cytoskeleton. Polypeptides such as HSC70, a constitutively expressed member of the heat shock family, may organize these complexes during transport [3].

While these two rate components can be identified in all nerves examined to date, the rates and the precise compositions vary among nerve populations. For example, SCa and SCb are readily resolved as discrete waves moving down optic axons, but differences in rate are smaller in the motor axons of sciatic nerve, so the two peaks overlap. Moreover, virtually all tubulin moves with SCa in the optic axons, while a significant fraction of axonal tubulin moves at SCb rates in sciatic nerve axons [25]. In each nerve, certain polypeptides may be used to define the kinetics for a given slow component of axonal transport. For SCa, these signature polypeptides are the NF triplet proteins, while actin, clathrin and calmodulin serve a similar role for SCb.

Axonal growth and regeneration are limited by rates of slow axonal transport

The rate of axonal growth during development and regeneration of a nerve is roughly equivalent to the rate of SCb in that neuron [3]. This suggests that critical roles are played by the slow axonal transport proteins in growth and regeneration. During development, SCb proteins are prominent and relatively little NF protein is detectable. Tubulin can be detected moving at both SCb and SCa rates. Once an appropriate target is reached, synaptogenesis and myelination begin; there is upregulation of NF protein synthesis and a gradual slowing of slow transport.

Axonal regeneration involves a complex set of cell body and axonal responses to a lesion [3] (Chap. 29). Downregulation of NF triplet and upregulation of specific tubulin isotypes are hallmarks of cell body responses to a lesion. In CNS neurons which fail to regenerate, changes in NF and tubulin expression are reduced or absent. Since changes in protein expression do not alter axonal cytoskeletal composition until after a regenerating growth cone has formed and extended for some distance, such changes in expression do not affect neurite growth but may reflect activation of a cellular program for neurite growth. Axonal MTs must be disassembled as part of the reorganization of the cytoskeleton for growth, then reassembled for neurite extension. During axonal growth, specific tubulin genes are upregulated; during development and regeneration, MAPs are differentially expressed. Finally, in growth and regeneration, there are characteristic changes in the axonal transport of tubulin, with an increase in the fraction of tubulin moving at SCb rates.

Properties of slow transport suggest molecular mechanisms

Information about mechanisms of slow axonal transport is relatively limited. They are energy-dependent and require an intact axonal cytoskeleton. Indirect evidence suggests that MTs play a critical role because transport of NFs can be pharmacologically uncoupled from MT transport without eliminating slow transport [26]. In contrast, all agents which disrupt MTs appear to block slow transport of all components. While this does not rule out a role for the MF cytoskeleton in slow transport movements, MTs appear to provide motive force for other elements of the cytoskeleton.

The macroscopic rates measured by radiolabel experiments should not be taken to reflect maximum rates of the motors involved. As with mitochondrial transport, the net rate of slow-component proteins reflects both the rate of actual movement and the fraction of a time interval that a structure is moving [24]. The elongate shape of cytoskeletal structures and their potential for many interactions mean that net displacements are discontinuous. If a structure is

moving at a speed of 2 μm per sec, but on average moves at that rate only for 1 sec out of every 100 sec, then the average rate for the structure will translate to only 0.02 μm per sec.

MT movements in growing neurites have been visualized directly in an elegant series of studies from Kirschner and colleagues [27]. Tubulin may be tagged with a caged fluorescein, which is visualized only when uncaged by photoactivation. Labeled tubulins may be injected into a *Xenopus* oocyte and the oocyte allowed to develop into an embryo. In early embryos, much of the tubulin remains tagged because protein synthesis is limited. If caged fluorescent tubulin is locally photoactivated in a neurite, patches of fluorescent tubulin move down the axon. Fluorescent patches remain discrete during movements in the anterograde direction at slow transport rates, as predicted by the structural hypothesis. Observations of moving MTs can also be made using rhodamine-labeled tubulin. Under favorable conditions, individual fluorescent MTs can be detected moving in neurites and growth cones. These MTs translocate as intact structures. In the growth cone, they appear to be pulled and even bent in conjunction with growth cone movements. Recent studies have permitted visualization of MTs nucleated at the microtubule-organizing center and being translocated toward the cell periphery. When combined with studies of axonal transport using radiolabels and direct observations of individual MTs with video microscopy, there is little doubt that MTs and NFs can and do move in the axon as intact cytoskeletal structures [24], although optimal conditions may be needed to see these movements.

As with membrane proteins, cytoplasmic and cytoskeletal proteins are differentially distributed in neurons and glia. Progress has been made toward identification of targeting mechanisms, and some general principles have begun to emerge. Since cytoplasmic constituents move only in the anterograde direction, a key mechanism for targeting of cytoplasmic and cytoskeletal proteins appears to be differential metabolism [3]. The concentration of actin and other proteins in presynaptic terminals can be explained by slower turnover in the presynaptic terminal relative to NF proteins and tubulin.

Proteins with slow degradative rates in the terminal accumulate and reach a higher steady-state concentration. Alteration of degradation rates for a protein can change the rate of accumulation for that protein. For example, some protease inhibitors cause the appearance of NF rings in affected presynaptic terminals.

While slow transport of cytoskeletal proteins has received the most attention, all other cytoplasmic proteins must be delivered to distal regions of the neuron as well. Many of these are classical proteins of the "cytosol" that are readily solubilized during extractions. These include the enzymes of glycolysis and regulatory proteins like calmodulin and HSC70 [3]. However, in pulse chase radiolabel studies, soluble proteins move down the axon as regularly and systematically as cytoskeletal proteins. This coherent transport of hundreds of different polypeptides indicates a higher level of organization of cytoplasmic proteins than has been traditionally assumed. Such organization is likely necessary to facilitate interactions with motor proteins and targeting mechanisms and to assure a reliable delivery of all required proteins to the axon.

MOLECULAR MOTORS: KINESIN, DYNEIN AND MYOSIN

Prior to 1985, the only molecular motors characterized in vertebrate cells were muscle myosins and flagellar dyneins. Myosins had been purified from nervous tissue, but no clear functions were established. Given evidence that fast axonal transport was microtubule-based, many investigators looked for dynein in the cytoplasm, with equivocal success. Moreover, the biochemical properties of fast transport were inconsistent with both myosin and dynein [10]. The pharmacology and biochemistry of fast axonal transport created a picture of organelle transport distinct from muscle contraction or flagellar beating.

The characteristic properties of different molecular motors aid in their identification

One striking difference between fast axonal transport and myosin- or dynein-based motility

emerged from studies with ATP analogues. Adenylyl-imidodiphosphate (AMP-PNP), a nonhydrolyzable analogue of ATP, is a weak competitive inhibitor of both myosin and dynein. However, when AMP-PNP is perfused into axoplasm, bidirectional transport stops within minutes [1,28]. Both anterograde and retrograde moving organelles freeze in place on MTs. Inhibition of fast axonal transport by AMP-PNP indicated that fast axonal transport involved a new class of motors [1,28] and suggested that this new motor should have a high affinity for MTs in the presence of AMP-PNP. The polypeptide composition of this new motor molecule was soon defined and it was christened kinesin [29,30]. This discovery raised the possibility of other novel motor molecules, and soon additional classes of molecular motor began to be identified. The proliferation of motor types has transformed our understanding of cellular motility.

All three classes of molecular motor proteins are now known to be large protein families with diverse cellular functions [10]. Both the kinesin family [31,32] and the myosin family [33] have been defined and their proteins grouped into subfamilies. Finally, the elusive cytoplasmic version of dynein was identified and a multigene family of flagellar and cytoplasmic dyneins defined. Members of a given motor protein family share significant homology in their motor domains with the defining member, kinesin, dynein or myosin; but they also contain unique protein domains that are specialized for interaction with different cargoes. This large number of motor proteins may reflect the number of cellular functions that require force generation or movement, ranging from mitosis to morphogenesis to transport of vesicles. Here, we focus on motor proteins that are thought to be important for axonal transport or neuronal function, starting with kinesin.

Kinesins mediate anterograde transport in a variety of organisms and tissues

Since its discovery, much has been learned about the biochemical, pharmacological and molecular properties of kinesin [34]. Kinesin is the most abundant member of the kinesin family in vertebrates and is widely distributed in neuronal and non-neuronal cells. The holoenzyme is a heterotetramer comprising two heavy chains of 115 to 130 kDa and two light chains of 62 to 70 kDa. Structural studies have shown that kinesin is a rod-shaped protein approximately 80 nm in length with two globular heads connected to a fan-like tail by a long stalk. High-resolution electron microscopic immunolocalization of kinesin subunits and molecular genetic studies both indicate that kinesin heavy chains are arranged in parallel with their amino termini, forming the heads and much of the stalk. The kinesin heavy chain heads comprise the motor domains, containing both ATP- and MT-binding motifs. This motor domain is the most highly conserved region within the kinesin family. Binding of kinesin to MTs is stabilized by AMP-PNP, and this property remains a hallmark of kinesins. Kinesin light chains localize to the fan-like tail and may con-

tribute to part of the stalk. The stalk itself is formed by α-helical coiled coil domains that are present in both heavy and light chains. Kinesin light chains appear to be unique to conventional kinesin but are highly conserved across species. Light chains are thought to be involved in organelle binding and may play a role in targeting of kinesin isoforms to different types of MBO [35].

Considerable evidence implicates kinesin as a motor molecule for fast axonal transport. Kinesin is an MT-activated ATPase with minimal basal activity [34]. MTs will glide across kinesin-coated glass surfaces with motor movement toward the plus end [10,30]. Since axonal MTs have a uniform polarity with their plus ends distal, the directionality of kinesin is consistent with an anterograde transport motor. Immunofluorescence and electron microscopy have shown that kinesin is associated with MBOs that are, in turn, associated with MTs [36,37] (Fig. 28-7).

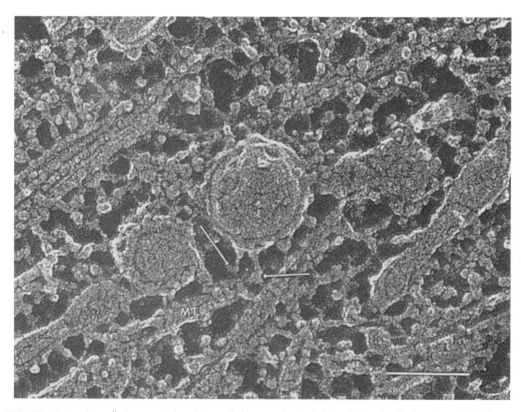

FIGURE 28-7. Axonally transported vesicles and the axonal cytoskeleton in longitudinal section. Quick-freeze, deep-etch electron micrograph of a region of rat spinal cord neurite rich in membrane-bound organelles and microtubules. *Arrows* point to rod-shaped structures that appear as cross bridges between organelles and microtubules. The bar at the **lower right** indicates 100 nm. (From [37], with permission.)

While these properties of kinesin were consistent with a role in axonal transport of MBOs, they were insufficient to prove the hypothesis that kinesin was the fast axonal transport motor. Such proof came from inhibition of kinesin function by antibodies against both heavy and light chains of kinesin [10,35]. Since kinesin light chains are associated only with conventional kinesin, the ability of kinesin light chain antibodies to inhibit transport is compelling evidence that kinesin is involved in fast axonal transport. Finally, reduction of kinesin levels using antisense oligonucleotides and gene deletion also implicates kinesin in axonal transport processes [31].

In neurons and non-neuronal cells, kinesin is associated with a variety of MBOs, ranging from synaptic vesicles to mitochondria to lysosomes. In addition to its role in fast axonal transport and related phenomena in non-neuronal cells, kinesin appears to be involved in constitutive cycling of membranes between the Golgi complex and endoplasmic reticulum [38]. However, kinesin is not associated with all cellular membranes. For example, the nucleus, membranes of the Golgi complex and the plasma membrane appear to lack kinesin. Kinesin interactions with membranes are thought to involve the light chains and carboxyl termini of heavy chains. However, neither this selectivity nor the molecular basis for binding of kinesin and other motors to membranes is well understood.

Cloning and immunochemical studies of kinesin subunits have demonstrated that multiple isoforms of kinesin heavy and light chains exist in the brain. At least two heavy chain genes are expressed in mammals, a ubiquitous kinesin heavy chain gene expressed in all tissues and a neuron-specific heavy chain gene that is expressed only in brain [34]. At least two different genes exist for the kinesin light chains as well, and differential splicing for one of these light chain genes generates three different light chain polypeptides. These different kinesin isoforms are differentially expressed in tissues. Heterogeneity in kinesin heavy and light chains may regulate the transport of different MBO types and ensure that organelles reach their correct destinations in the axon. Radiolabeled isoforms of the kinesin heavy chains move down the axon at different net rates that correlate with different MBO types, such as synaptic vesicles and mitochondria [39]. These observations suggest that kinesin isoforms exist to transport different types of organelles.

Multiple members of the kinesin superfamily are expressed in the nervous system

Kinesin has been purified and then cloned from many species, including *Drosophila*, squid, sea urchin, chicken, rat and human. Conventional kinesin is highly conserved. Once the sequence of the kinesin motor domain was available, related proteins with homology only in the motor domain began to be identified. Kinesin-related proteins (KRPs) were first identified in yeast and fungal mutants with defective cell division, but many others are now known [31,32].

All of the members of the large kinesin family of proteins have well-conserved motor domains, but KRPs are highly variable in sequence and structure. Even the position of the motor domain varies. Kinesin and many other family members have amino-terminal motor domains, but other KRPs have motor domains at the carboxyl terminus and some have centrally located motor domains. This variation in structure has functional significance. To date, all tested amino and central motor domain proteins move toward the MT plus end, while carboxyl motor domain proteins move toward the MT minus end. Many KRPs are known only from their sequences and expression, but a few have been examined for function. A number of KRPs are involved in various steps of cell division, but precise cellular functions are still being defined for most of these new motors.

Systematic cloning strategies based on the conserved motor domain sequences have identified a remarkable number of KRPs expressed in the brain [32]. Members of several KRP families expressed in the brain have been implicated in forms of MBO transport. Kinesin-inhibiting factor 3 (KIF3) and its homologue $KRP_{85/95}$ have been implicated in membrane trafficking in mouse brain and sea urchin, respectively. This KRP has been purified from sea urchin and found to be a heterotrimer with two related KRP motor subunits and a larger accessory subunit that may serve a purpose analogous to that of ki-nesin light chains. The *unc-104* gene product in the nematode *Caenorhabditis elegans* was origi-nally proposed as a synaptic vesicle motor be-cause *unc-104* mutants had defects in synaptic vesicle localization. Subsequently, two related proteins, KIF1A and KIF1B, were cloned from mouse brain and their distributions examined. KIF1A was neuron-specific and appeared to be associated with synaptic vesicles, while KIF1B was ubiquitously expressed and reported to be associated with mitochondria. Since kinesin has also been localized on mitochondria, some MBOs may have multiple motor types or there may be subsets of MBOs with specific motors. Several other KRPs expressed in nervous tissue have been implicated in the transport of MBO types that were previously shown to have con-ventional kinesin. The extent to which these KRPs reflect unique transport mechanisms rather than functional redundancy within the ki-nesin family is not known.

Curiously, functions proposed for some brain KRPs [32] are very different from func-tions proposed for similar or identical KRPs in non-neuronal cells. For example, members of the MCAK/KIF2 family have been implicated in both mitotic spindle function and axonal mem-brane transport. Similarly, mouse KIF4 was re-ported to associate with unidentified MBOs in neurites, but its chicken homologue chromoki-nesin was shown to bind to chromosomal DNA and to mediate chromosomal movements in the mitotic spindle. Finally, CHO1 was originally found to have a role in mitotic spindle function, but members of the CHO1 family were subse-quently implicated in the transport of MTs into dendrites [40]. Transfection of insect cells with CHO1 fusion proteins induced formation of ta-pering dendrite-like processes containing MTs with both plus- and minus-end distal MTs. This suggests that CHO1 or a related KRP may par-ticipate in organizing the unique MT cytoskele-ton of dendrites.

Although the last to be discovered, the ki-nesin family of motor proteins has proven to be remarkably diverse. So far, there are at least 14 distinct subfamilies in the kinesin family, and more are likely to emerge, all with homology in the motor domain. Within a subfamily, how-ever, the more extensive sequence similarities are presumed to reflect related functions. At pre-sent, many questions remain about the function of these various motors in the nervous system.

Cytoplasmic dyneins may have multiple roles in the neuron

The identification of kinesin as a plus-end-di-rected microtubule motor suggested that it is in-volved in anterograde transport but left the identity of the retrograde motor an open ques-tion. Since flagellar dynein was known to be a minus-end-directed motor, interest in cytoplas-mic dyneins was renewed. Identification of the cytoplasmic form of dynein in nervous tissue was an indirect result of the discovery of kinesin.

Although dynein binding to MTs is not sta-bilized by AMP-PNP, both cytoplasmic dynein and kinesin associate with MTs in nucleotide-depleted extracts and both are released by addi-tion of ATP. Early studies with ATP-free MT ex-tracts showed that they are substantially enriched in a minor high-molecular-weight MAP, MAP1c. Biochemical analysis showed that MAP1c was not in fact related to MAP1a and -1b but, instead, was closely related to flagellar dynein heavy chains. This discovery led to the purification and characterization of brain cyto-plasmic dynein [41]. Like flagellar dyneins, cyto-plasmic dynein is a high-molecular-weight pro-tein complex comprising two heavy chains and multiple light and intermediate chains that form a complex of more than 1,200 kDa.

As with the kinesins, dynein heavy chains are a multigene family with multiple flagellar and cytoplasmic dynein genes [32]. The 530-kDa dynein heavy chain contains the ATPase ac-tivity and MT-binding domains. There may be 10 to 15 dynein heavy chain genes in an organ-ism, but the size of the dynein heavy chain has slowed genetic analyses. At present, dynein genes are grouped as members of either flagellar or cy-toplasmic dynein subfamilies. The three inter-mediate, 74 kDa; four light-intermediate, 55 kDa; and variable number of light chains present in dyneins may also have flagellar and cytoplas-mic forms.

The two or more cytoplasmic dynein heavy chain genes could be involved in different cellular functions, but much dynein functional diversity may be due to its many associated polypeptides. The intermediate and light chains of cytoplasmic dynein are thought to be important for both regulation and interactions of dynein with other cellular structures. In addition, a second protein complex, known as dynactin, copurifies with cytoplasmic dynein under some conditions. The dynactin complex is similar in size to dynein and contains ten subunits that include p150^{Glued}; dynamitin, an actin-related protein; and two actin-capping polypeptides, among others [32]. The p150^{Glued} polypeptide interacts with both dynein intermediate chains and the actin-related subunits. Dynamitin may play a role in the binding of cytoplasmic dynein to different types of cargo. Finally, actin-related protein (Arp1) forms a short filament that may include actin as well as the capping proteins. This short filament may interact with both p150^{Glued} and components of the membrane cytoskeleton like spectrin. Dynactin may mediate cytoplasmic dynein binding to selected cargoes, including the Golgi complex and the membrane cytoskeleton. The wide range of functions associated with cytoplasmic dynein is matched by its complexity and its ability to interact with accessory factors. Additional proposed functions include a role in mitosis and in anchoring and localizing the Golgi complex.

A number of studies have implicated cytoplasmic dynein as playing a role in retrograde axonal transport [10,32]. *In vitro* motility studies demonstrate that cytoplasmic dynein generates force toward the minus end of MTs, consistent with a retrograde motor. Dynein immunoreactivities have been associated with MBOs, and cytoplasmic dynein accumulates on the distal side of a nerve ligation coincidentally with retrogradely transported MBOs. Finally, retrograde transport has been reported to be more sensitive than anterograde transport to ultraviolet light (UV)-vanadate treatment. Since exposure of dynein to UV irradiation in the presence of vanadate and ADP cleaves the dynein heavy chain, this has been a signature of dyneins, although other ATP-binding proteins may be affected as well.

In the nervous system, the most frequent role proposed for dynein is as a motor for retrograde axonal transport, but its properties are also consistent with a motor for slow axonal transport [10]. Consistent with this possibility, a study on the axonal transport of radiolabeled cytoplasmic dynein indicated that most cytoplasmic dynein and dynactin moved with SCb [42]. The ability of dynactin to interact with both cytoplasmic dynein and the membrane cytoskeleton suggests a model in which dynactin links dynein to the membrane cytoskeleton, providing an anchor for dynein-mediated movement of axonal MTs. Some role for the membrane cytoskeleton in the mechanisms of slow axonal transport is likely since neurons require interaction with a solid substrate for neurite growth. Taken together, these studies suggest that cytoplasmic dynein has a wide variety of functions in the nervous system, from anchoring the Golgi to retrograde transport to transport of MTs. Cytoplasmic dynein appears to have adapted to fulfill many cellular functions that require minus-end-directed MT movements.

Different classes of myosin are important for neuronal function

Myosins are remarkably diverse in structure and function. To date, 14 subfamilies of myosin have been defined by sequence homologies [33]. The brain is an abundant source of nonmuscle myosins and one of the earliest studied. Despite their abundance and variety, the roles of myosins in neural tissues have only recently begun to be defined.

Myosin II is in the same subfamily as myosins in muscle thick filaments, and it forms large, two-headed myosins with two light chains per heavy chain. Although myosin II is abundantly expressed in the brain, little is known about its function in the nervous system. In other nonmuscle cells, myosin II has been implicated in many types of cellular contractility and may serve a similar function in developing neurons. However, myosin II remains abundant in the mature nervous system, where examples of cell contractility are less common.

The second myosin type identified in nervous tissue was the myosin I family. Myosin I was first described in protists and subsequently purified from brain. Myosin I is a single-headed myosin with a short tail that uses calmodulin as a light chain [33]. Myosin I in many cell types has been implicated in both endocytosis and exocytosis, so it may play an important role in delivery and recycling of receptors. Myosin I is enriched in microvilli and may be involved in some aspects of growth cone motility, along with myosins from other subfamilies. In both cases, it may link MF bundles to the plasma membrane through a membrane-binding domain. Recently, the myosin I family has been implicated in mechanotransduction by the stereocilia of hair cells in the inner ear and vestibular apparatus. A myosin I isoform, myosin Iβ, has been localized to the tips of stereocilia, where it appears to mediate sensory adaptation by opening and closing the stretch-activated calcium ion channel (see Box 47-1).

Two other myosin types have been implicated in hearing and vestibular function [33]. The defect in the Snell's *waltzer* mouse was found to be a mutation in a myosin VI gene which produces degeneration of the cochlea and vestibular apparatus. Myosin VI is localized to the cuticular plate of the hair cell under stereocilia. Similarly, mutations in a myosin VII gene are responsible for the *shaker-1* mouse and several human genetic deafness disorders. This myosin, myosin VIIa, is found in a band near the base of the stereocilia, distinct from distributions of myosin Iβ and myosin VI.

Another myosin type that plays a role in nervous tissue is myosin V [33]. Of the myosins identified in brain, myosin I and myosin V are the strongest candidates to act as an organelle motor and myosin V has been reported in association with vesicles purified from squid axoplasm. Myosin V is the product of the mouse *dilute* locus. Mice carrying the mutant *dilute* allele show defects in pigment granule movement that result in a dilution of the coat color. These mice also exhibit complex neurological defects that may be due to altered endoplasmic reticulum localization in dendrites. Curiously, a mutation in a form of myosin V found in yeast is suppressed by a KRP gene, suggesting an interaction between these two motor molecules. Finally, there is evidence that myosin V plays a role in growth cone motility, where it is enriched in filopodia.

Matching motors to physiological functions may be difficult

The three classes of motors are similar in their biochemical and pharmacological sensitivities in many respects [10]. However, some hallmark features can be used to identify a motor. In the case of kinesin, the most distinctive characteristic is stabilization of binding to MTs by AMP-PNP. The affinity of myosin for MFs and of dynein for MTs is weakened by treatment with either ATP or AMP-PNP. As a result, if a process is frozen in place by AMP-PNP, kinesins are likely to be involved. If kinesin is not involved in a process which requires MTs, dyneins are likely to be involved. Similarly, processes requiring MFs suggest that myosins are required. In the case of fast axonal transport, we know that MTs are required, and this process is completely inhibited by AMP-PNP, implicating the kinesin family. The development of new pharmacological and immunochemical probes specific for different motors will facilitate future studies.

While many motor proteins are found in nervous tissue, there are few instances in which we fully understand their cellular functions. The proliferation of different motor molecules and the existence of numerous isoforms raise the possibility that some physiological activities require multiple motors. There may be cases in which motors serve a redundant role to ensure that the physiological activity is maintained in the event of a loss of one motor protein. Finally, the existence of so many different types of motor molecules suggests that novel physiological activities requiring molecular motors may be as yet unrecognized.

AXONAL TRANSPORT AND NEUROPATHOLOGY

Inhibition of axonal transport leads rapidly to loss of function in the distal axon, and dying back neuropathies are frequently associated with chronic exposure to neurotoxins that inhibit axonal transport. Some of these neurotoxins may act directly on the motor molecules that underlie axonal transport. For example, acrylamide has been found to inhibit kinesin function. Others may indirectly affect the delivery of materials by transport through effects on energy metabolism or by blocking conversion from anterograde to retrograde transport.

A variety of neurological diseases are also thought to involve axonal transport. For example, motor neuron diseases like amyotrophic lateral sclerosis (ALS) appear to interfere with both fast and slow axonal transport. Analysis of axonal transport in an animal model of ALS documented deficits in both the slow transport of NFs and the fast transport of mitochondria to the axon [43]. While ALS-like diseases may be caused by a number of different pathogenic mechanisms, all forms feature accumulations of NFs and a dying back neuropathy in motor neurons characteristic of axonal transport deficits (see Chap. 18). Similar arguments can be made for a variety of neurodegenerative diseases, including diabetic neuropathies and Alzheimer's disease. Even when the primary pathogenic pathway has only indirect effects on transport, anything that compromises the timely and efficient delivery of material by axonal transport processes is likely to produce neuronal degeneration.

CONCLUSIONS

The functional architecture of neurons is comprised of many specializations in cytoskeletal and membranous components. Each of these specializations is dynamic, constantly changing and being renewed at a rate determined by the local environment and cellular metabolism. The processes of axonal transport represent the key to neuronal dynamics. Recent advances have provided important insights into the molecular mechanisms underlying axonal transport, although many questions remain. Continued exploration of these phenomena will provide a basis for understanding neuronal dynamics in development, regeneration and neuropathology.

ACKNOWLEDGMENTS

The authors thank Janet Cyr and Richard Hammerschlag for their efforts on related chapters in earlier editions. Preparation of this chapter was supported in part by grants from the National Institute of Neurological Disease and Stroke (NS23868 and NS23320), from the Welch Foundation (1237) and from the Muscular Dystrophy Association and a joint grant from NASA and the National Institute of Aging (NAG2-962/AG12646).

REFERENCES

1. Brady, S. T., Pfister, K. K., Leopold, P. L., et al. Fast axonal transport in isolated axoplasm. *Cell Motil. Cytoskeleton* 17 (Video Suppl. 2):22, 1990.
2. Weiss, P., and Hiscoe, H. Experiments in the mechanism of nerve growth. *J. Exp. Zool.* 107:315–395, 1948.
3. Brady, S. T. Axonal dynamics and regeneration. In A. Gorio (ed.), *Neuroregeneration.* New York: Raven Press, 1993, pp. 7–36.
4. Droz, B., and Leblond, C. P. Migration of proteins along the axons of the sciatic nerve. *Science* 137:1047–1048, 1962.
5. Grafstein, B., and Forman, D. S. Intracellular transport in neurons. *Physiol. Rev.* 60:1167–1283, 1980.
6. Brady, S. Axonal transport methods and applications. In A. Boulton and G. Baker (eds.), *Neuromethods, General Neurochemical Techniques.* Clifton, NJ: Humana Press, 1985, pp. 419–476.
7. Calakos, N., and Scheller, R. H. Synaptic vesicle biogenesis, docking, and fusion: A molecular description. *Physiol. Rev.* 76:1–29, 1996.
8. Rothman, J. E., and Wieland, F. T. Protein sorting by transport vesicles. *Science* 272:227–234, 1996.
9. Hammerschlag, R., Stone, G. C., Bolen, F. A., et al. Evidence that all newly synthesized proteins destined for fast axonal transport pass through the Golgi apparatus. *J. Cell Biol.* 93:568–575, 1982.
10. Brady, S. T. Molecular motors in the nervous system. *Neuron* 7:521–533, 1991.
11. Smith, R. S. The short term accumulation of axonally transported organelles in the region of localized lesions of single myelinated axons. *J. Neurocytol.* 9:39–65, 1980.
12. Tsukita, S., and Ishikawa, H. The movement of membranous organelles in axons. Electron microscopic identification of anterogradely and retrogradely transported organelles. *J. Cell Biol.* 84:513–530, 1980.

13. Brady, S. T., Lasek, R. J., and Allen, R. D. Video microscopy of fast axonal transport in isolated axoplasm: A new model for study of molecular mechanisms. *Cell Motil.* 5:81–101, 1985.

14. Sahenk, Z., and Lasek, R. J. Inhibition of proteolysis blocks anterograde–retrograde conversion of axonally transported vesicles. *Brain Res.* 460:199–203, 1988.

15. Kristensson, K. Retrograde transport of macromolecules in axons. *Annu. Rev. Pharmacol. Toxicol.* 18:97–110, 1987.

16. Kelly, R. B., and Grote, E. Protein targeting in the neuron. *Annu. Rev. Neurosci.* 16:95–127, 1993.

17. Simons, K., Dupree, P., Fiedler, K., et al. Biogenesis of cell-surface polarity in epithelial cells and neurons. *Cold Spring Harb. Symp. Quant. Biol.* 57:611–619, 1992.

18. Blenis, J., and Resh, M. D. Subcellular localization specified by protein acylation and phosphorylation. *Curr. Opin. Cell Biol.* 5:984–989, 1993.

19. Schatz, G., and Dobberstein, B. Common principles of protein translocation across membranes. *Science* 271:1519–1526, 1996.

20. Greengard, P., Benfenati, F., and Valtorta, F. Synapsin I, an actin-binding protein regulating synaptic vesicle traffic in the nerve terminal. *Adv. Second Messenger Phosphoprotein Res.* 29:31–45, 1994.

21. McGuinness, T. L., Brady, S. T., Gruner, J., et al. Phosphorylation-dependent inhibition by synapsin I of organelle movement in squid axoplasm. *J. Neurosci.* 9:4138–4149, 1989.

22. Steward, O. Targeting of mRNAs to subsynaptic microdomains in dendrites. *Curr. Opin. Neurobiol.* 5:55–61, 1995.

23. Kalwy, S. A., and Smith, R. Mechanisms of myelin basic protein and proteolipid protein targeting in oligodendrocytes. *Mol. Membr. Biol.* 11:67–78, 1994.

24. Baas, P. W., and Brown, A. Slow axonal transport: The polymer transport model. *Trends Cell Biol.* 7:380–384, 1997.

25. Oblinger, M. M., Brady, S. T., McQuarrie, I. G., et al. Differences in the protein composition of the axonally transported cytoskeleton in peripheral and central mammalian neurons. *J. Neurosci.* 7:453–462, 1987.

26. Griffin, J. W., George, E. B., Hsieh, S., et al. Axonal degeneration and disorders of the axonal cytoskeleton. In S. G. Waxman, J. D. Kocsis and P. K. Stys (eds.), *The Axon: Structure, Function and Pathophysiology.* New York: Oxford University Press, 1995, pp. 375–390.

27. Reinsch, S. S., Mitchison, T. J., and Kirschner, M. Microtubule polymer assembly and transport during axonal elongation. *J. Cell Biol.* 115:365–380, 1991.

28. Lasek, R. J., and Brady, S. T. Adenylyl imidodiphosphate (AMPPNP), a nonhydrolyzable analogue of ATP, produces a stable intermediate in the motility cycle of fast axonal transport. *Biol. Bull.* 167:503, 1984.

29. Brady, S. T. A novel brain ATPase with properties expected for the fast axonal transport motor. *Nature* 317:73–75, 1985.

30. Vale, R. D., Reese, T. S., and Sheetz, M. P. Identification of a novel force-generating protein, kinesin, involved in microtubule-based motility. *Cell* 42:39–50, 1985.

31. Bloom, G. S., and Endow, S. A. Motor proteins 1: Kinesins. *Protein Profile* 2:1109–1171, 1995.

32. Hirokawa, N. Kinesin and dynein superfamily proteins and the mechanism of organelle transport. *Science* 279:519–526, 1998.

33. Mermall, V., Post, P. L., and Mooseker, M. S. Unconventional myosins in cell movement, membrane traffic and signal transduction. *Science* 279:527–533, 1998.

34. Brady, S. T. A kinesin medley: Biochemical and functional heterogeneity. *Trends Cell Biol.* 5:159–164, 1995.

35. Stenoien, D. S., and Brady, S. T. Immunochemical analysis of kinesin light chain function. *Mol. Biol. Cell* 8:675–689, 1997.

36. Pfister, K. K., Wagner, M. C., Stenoien, D., et al. Monoclonal antibodies to kinesin heavy and light chains stain vesicle-like structures, but not microtubules, in cultured cells. *J. Cell Biol.* 108:1453–1463, 1989.

37. Hirokawa, N., Pfister, K. K., Yorifuji, H., et al. Submolecular domains of bovine brain kinesin identified by electron microscopy and monoclonal antibody decoration. *Cell* 56:867–878, 1989.

38. Lippincott-Schwartz, J., Cole, N., Marotta, A., et al. Kinesin is the motor for microtubule-mediated Golgi-to-ER membrane traffic. *J. Cell Biol.* 128:293–306, 1995.

39. Elluru, R., Bloom, G. S., and Brady, S. T. Fast axonal transport of kinesin in the rat visual system: Functionality of the kinesin heavy chain isoforms. *Mol. Biol. Cell* 6:21–40, 1995.

40. Sharp, D. J., Kuriyama, R., and Baas, P. W. Expression of a kinesin-related motor protein induces Sf9 cells to form dendrite-like processes with a nonuniform microtubule polarity orientation. *J. Neurosci.* 16:4370–4382, 1996.

41. Paschal, B. M., Shpetner, H. S., and Vallee, R. B. MAP1C is a microtubule-activated ATPase which translocates microtubules *in vitro* and has dynein-like properties. *J. Cell Biol.* 105:1273–1282, 1987.

42. Dillman, J. F., Dabney, L. P., Karki, S., et al. Functional analysis of dynactin and cytoplasmic dynein in slow axonal transport. *J. Neurosci.* 16:6742–6752, 1996.

43. Collard, J.-F., Côté, F., and Julien, J.-P. Defective axonal transport in a transgenic mouse model of amyotrophic lateral sclerosis. *Nature* 375:61–64, 1995.

44. Brady, S. T., Lasek, R. J., and Allen, R. D. Fast axonal transport in extruded axoplasm from giant squid axon. *Science* 218:1129–1131, 1982.

45. Tytell, M., Black, M. M., Garner, J. A., and Lasek, R. J. Axonal transport: Each of the major rate components consist of distinct macromolecular complexes. *Science* 214:179–181, 1981.

CHAPTER

29

Axon Sprouting and Regeneration

Carl W. Cotman

Basic Neurochemistry: Molecular, Cellular and Medical Aspects, 6th Ed., edited by G. J. Siegel et al. Published by Lippincott–Raven Publishers, Philadelphia, 1999. Correspondence to Carl W. Cotman, Institute for Brain Aging & Dementia, University of California, Irvine, California 92697-4550.

INTRODUCTION

Once formed, the circuitry of the nervous system must be maintained and even modified to maintain optimal function. In the course of a lifetime, some neurons can become damaged due to ischemia, trauma and disease. Because mature neurons do not divide, they require repair, often including process regeneration and connectivity restoration. Research examining regeneration in the nervous system is one of the exciting frontiers in neurochemistry. In this chapter, the innate capacity of CNS neurons to repair and regenerate connections is described in relationship to the extrinsic signals that the cells encounter. Furthermore, recent data indicating that the nervous system has an ability to incorporate transplanted neurons and other cells are discussed. Such paradigms provide new strategies of research to investigate the mechanisms regulating functional plasticity, circuitry repair and restoration of function after injury.

Recent research has shown that the brain has a remarkable capacity for plastic responses throughout life; immediate functional plasticity is coupled with long-lasting structural change (Chap. 50). In the last few years, it has been shown that the healthy nervous system exhibits subtle and specific neural plasticity in response to activity such as learning a new task. In addition, the brain has the capability to repair itself after cell loss due to injury or neurodegenerative disease. The study of plasticity in animal models, coupled with current methods, has advanced to the point where it is realistic to examine the principles learned from basic research and to apply them to the human brain and clinical interventions. In fact, several experimental paradigms that have emerged have proven to be excellent models in which to test possible therapies. Tissue transplantation and manipulation of neurotrophic factors, either by themselves or in combination, are therapeutic strategies now be-

ing evaluated for disorders such as Parkinson's disease (see Chap. 45).

From a structural viewpoint, the CNS is a complex of specialized neurons organized in groups and interconnected by synapses. Although general principles of plasticity exist, it is becoming increasingly clear that each population of neurons responds in a distinct manner to experience and damage. Neurons are, in turn, supported by astrocytes, oligodendrocytes and microglia (see Fig. 1-1). The system is fed by a microvascular system that is isolated from the rest of the body by the blood–brain barrier (Chap. 32). The separate parts of the CNS operate in concert to produce coordinated responses. Thus, the consequences of damage generally extend beyond the immediate site of injury and impact other parts of a larger neuronal network.

Figure 29-1 illustrates the type of responses and the possible outcomes after damage to a simple circuit. If the axon of neuron A is severed, then contact with neuron B is lost. The ideal response would be for the axon to regenerate. This does not occur naturally in the adult mammalian CNS; rather, a compensatory response is mobilized, including the sprouting of new fibers from undamaged neurons. If the sprouting is from homologous neurons, the outcome is likely to maintain or improve the rate of recovery. The sprouts can also come from heterologous neurons. However, in this case the outcome is difficult to predict. In some cases, function appears to be restored, but in other cases, it is possible that functional recovery is hindered. Furthermore, if the axon is severed very close to the soma, the neuron will die. If the neuron is left with sufficient sustaining axon collaterals and external support, however, it will survive and increase its innervation of remaining targets. In all cases, synapses are reformed and the remaining circuitry reaches a new functional state as a result of new synapse formation and the modification of existing networks.

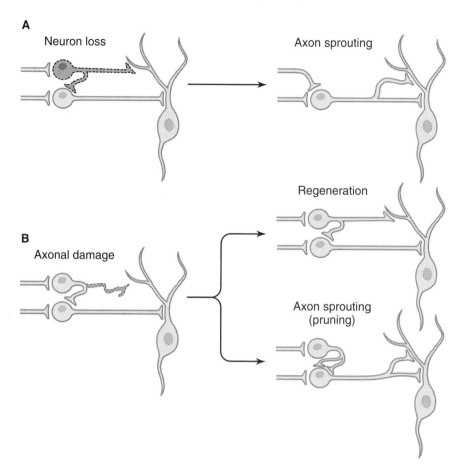

FIGURE 29-1. After injury, the CNS can mobilize a number of responses. **A:** If neurons degenerate, the natural response is that the axons of healthy neurons sprout and form new connections to replace those of the lost neurons, a process referred to as axon sprouting. This process includes the branching and growth of axons and formation of new synapses in reaction to an abnormal stimulus such as an injury, termed reactive synaptogenesis. **B:** When an axon is severed, the ideal response would be for the axon to regenerate, but this does not occur successfully in the absence of interventions. The damaged cell can and often does, however, mobilize a growth response, such as increased collateralization on available target cells, termed pruning. Thus, in either case, the circuitry can be rebuilt, particularly when homologous cells are available. In other cases, the incorrect inputs can be formed and only regeneration will restore function. Current research is directed at understanding these neuronal responses and directing them toward successful recovery of lost functions.

Generally, when damaged axons regrow and re-establish their original connections, the process is known as *regeneration*. *Axon sprouting* refers to the process whereby axons from undamaged neurons form new branches. Synapse formation that occurs in reaction to a stimulus, for example, entorhinal cortex lesions, not normal development, is called *reactive synaptogenesis*. The term reactive synaptogenesis applies only to situations in which synapses have been formed and makes no assumptions as to the driving stimulus or the type of sprouting involved [1,2].

AXON SPROUTING AND REACTIVE SYNAPTOGENESIS

If a peripheral nerve is partially damaged, function is restored before the severed fibers regenerate. In 1885, Exner recognized this fact and proposed that the mechanism was due to collateral sprouting [3].

Classically, it was recognized that the PNS has the capacity to sprout and regenerate, while it was generally accepted that the CNS circuitry is fixed and that once damaged, growth and repair cannot occur (Chap. 36). This assumption was challenged in a series of studies, and it was discovered that the spinal cord and brain can support sprouting and circuitry remodeling (for review, see [3]).

The response of the hippocampus to the unilateral removal of the entorhinal cortex provides an illustration of the general principles of reactive synaptogenesis

One of the best illustrations of the general principles and mechanisms of reactive synaptogenesis is represented by the response of the hippocampus to the unilateral removal of the entorhinal cortex input [4]. Fibers of the entorhinal cortex represent a major input to the dentate gyrus and terminate in the outer two-thirds of the dentate gyrus molecular layer. This

circuitry is of particular interest because of its critical role in higher cognitive functions, such as learning and memory, and its vulnerability to degeneration in Alzheimer's disease and, to a lesser degree, during the course of aging (see Chaps. 30, 46 and 50). Thus, this system is an excellent model not only for minor cell loss but also for changes triggered by significant injury to the brain. These studies also provide insight into the mechanisms underlying more subtle events, such as learning, that occur over much longer time periods.

Following unilateral ablation of the entorhinal cortex, over 80% of the synapses degenerate and are subsequently replaced by sprouting and new synapse formation from remaining fibers, including cholinergic projections from the medial septum, the commissural-associational pathway of CA4 neurons and projections from the contralateral entorhinal cortex. The

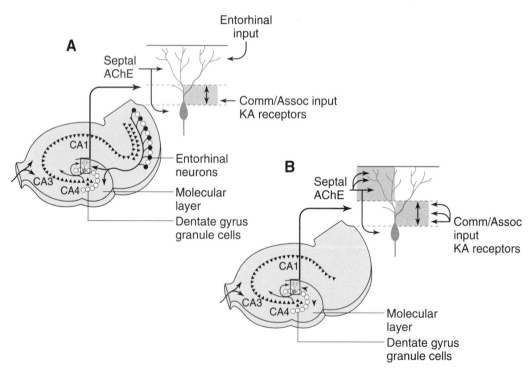

FIGURE 29-2. Changes in the dentate gyrus molecular layer following a unilateral entorhinal lesion. **A:** Normal distribution of entorhinal inputs to the outer two-thirds of the molecular layer and commissural/associational *(Comm/Assoc)* inputs and kainic acid *(KA)* receptors in the inner third of the molecular layer. Cholinergic inputs, visualized with acetylcholinesterase *(AChE)* histochemistry, occupy the outer molecular layer as well as a thin band of fibers in the supragranular zone. **B:** Following an entorhinal ablation, the cholinergic afferents sprout and AChE staining intensifies in the outer molecular layer. Comm/Assoc afferents sprout and expand outward into the denervated zone. This is accompanied by an expansion of KA receptor distribution. (From [54], with permission.)

projections from the ipsilateral and contralateral CA4 neurons normally terminate in the inner one-third of the dentate gyrus molecular layer. Following entorhinal lesions, these fibers sprout into the denervated zone, eventually occupying the inner half of the molecular layer (Fig. 29-2).

Fibers from the contralateral entorhinal cortex, normally sparse in the molecular layer, sprout extensively in the denervated zone after a unilateral lesion. The behavior of single fibers can be traced using anterograde labeling methods with the lectin tracer *Phaseolus vulgaris* leucoagglutinin (PHAL), a marker that is transported via axoplasmic flow throughout the axon and its branches. Single neurons in the entorhinal cortex are injected with the tracer, and after a few days the tissues are processed histochemically to trace the fibers. In control animals, these fibers exhibit sparse branching and form primarily *en passant,* bouton-type synapses. In lesioned animals, the fiber density increases and single axons exhibit more branch points (Fig. 29-3). Some axons exhibit high-density, localized sprouting, and in some, but not all animals, tangle-like structures are observed in the denervated outer molecular layer. The number of synapses increases approximately 100-fold.

Because contralateral entorhinal input is essentially homologous to the lost entorhinal input, the sprouted fibers likely participate in the recovery of function following unilateral entorhinal ablation. Consistent with this idea, studies show that a unilateral entorhinal lesion causes temporary deficits in spontaneous or reinforced alternation tasks and that the rate of behavioral recovery corresponds to the rate of sprouting of the homologous contralateral fibers [5–7]. This response of the brain may maintain function in the same manner as the early recovery after partial transection of the sciatic nerve in the PNS. Remaining fibers are known to sprout and restore function prior to regeneration.

To some extent, remodeling in the normal, healthy brain may involve processes that parallel those involved in remodeling that occurs after injury [3,8]. It appears that the brain has some intrinsic capabilities for plasticity and that these are enhanced when the homeostasis of the brain is challenged. It is interesting, in this respect, that, following injury, regions not primarily associated with the lesion also exhibit synaptic density changes and subsequent recovery of control levels over a long period of time. The synaptic changes occur despite the absence of degenerating terminals within these zones. Thus, pronounced transneuronal changes may occur after major trauma to the CNS, suggesting that reactive synaptogenesis may adjust the functional integrity of complex circuitry in areas with and without a primary lesion [9].

Sprouting in the adult brain results in an increase in the inputs already present without new pathway formation

The capacity for extensive remodeling and growth must be restrained when such remodeling is not required. Because the anatomy of the hippocampal formation is very well defined, examination of synaptic plasticity in the entorhinal/dentate circuit allows the establishment of a set of principles regulating axon sprouting. All new synapses appear to originate from fiber systems normally present in the circuit. The spatial arrangements of inputs, termed the lamination pattern, reorganizes so that CA4 synapses terminate further distally on the granule cell dendritic tree and septal cholinergic synapses reduce their domain to the reduced entorhinal zone. Relamination of inputs in the dentate gyrus may be due to (i) an invasion of CA4 fibers into regions previously occupied by entorhinal inputs or (ii) an outward growth of the dendritic tree, which carries CA4 synapses and fibers more distal from the cell body. If the dendrites grow, then the first-order branch points would be located farther from the soma. Indeed, the first-order stem appears to lengthen by 35 μm, which is exactly the increase in the width of the CA4 termination zone. Apparently, the outward growth of the dendritic tree causes the migration of CA4 fibers toward the outer molecular layer and a new lamination pattern [10,11].

Thus, although no new circuits are formed, fiber connections assume new spatial relationships on their normal target cells. Clearly, restraints are placed on the extent of axon growth and synapse formation in the mature brain. This is not the case in the developing brain, in which entire new pathways may develop (Chap. 27).

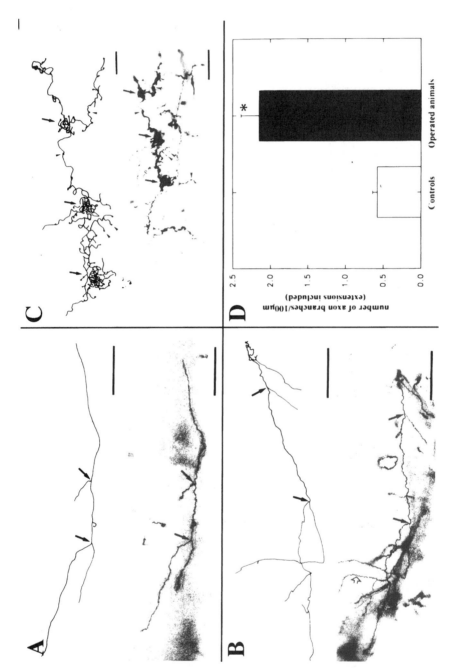

FIGURE 29-3. After a unilateral entorhinal lesion, the entorhinal–dentate pathway originating from the opposite entorhinal cortex shows extensive axon sprouting. **A:** Control; **B, C:** two examples of the behavior of single fibers after lesion. **D:** Quantitative data show the extent and change in fiber sprouting (From [52], with permission.)

The restraints operational in the mature brain may involve myelin-based or other types of growth inhibitors in neuronal pathways, such as has been defined in the spinal cord (see below).

Collateral sprouting and reactive synaptogenesis occur in discrete stages

During development, a specific sequence of events occurs that results in the formation of specific connections and neuronal circuits. When an injury occurs in the mature brain, the growth process must be executed in the context of a damaged system. The old system must be cleared and coordinated with the initiation of growth and the formation of new synapses.

The interaction of a growing axon and its environment involves several key factors and stages. Over the past several years, studies in cell culture have shown that neuronal growth requires a minimum of two extrinsic conditions: a supply of select neurotrophic factors (Chap. 19) and a proper substrate or set of cell-adhesion molecules (Chap. 7). These are also critical conditions for axon sprouting and regeneration *in vivo*. Thus, as illustrated in Figure 29-4, the key cells and molecular events required *in vivo* are (i) glial involvement in clearing degeneration, (ii) neurite outgrowth-promoting factors, (iii) composition of the extracellular matrix and expression of cell-adhesion molecules, (iv) events specifying targeting and (v) synapse formation and the expression of molecular systems regulating neurotransmitter release and proper postsynaptic receptors.

Glial cells set the pace for reactive synaptogenesis

Microglia are reactive and increase in number within the denervated zone by the first day, peak by postlesion day 3 and return to normal conditions by about 8 days. Astrocyte reactivity appears to follow the microglial response, peaking at approximately postlesion day 4 and remaining reactive for approximately 2 weeks. Microglia, in particular, engage in a robust phagocytotic reaction and engulf degenerating terminals, myelin and debris. Astrocytes also appear to be involved primarily in the removal of degenerating termi-

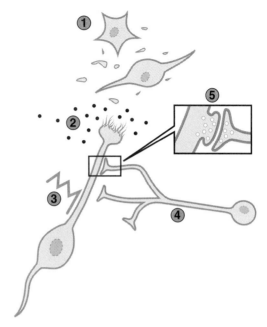

FIGURE 29-4. Stages in the mechanisms of axon sprouting and reactive synaptogenesis. The CNS has to face the complex problem of clearing the damage as the circuitry is being rebuilt and remodeled. ①Microglia and astrocytes clear the products of degeneration. ②Neurite sprouting factors are needed. ③Cell adhesion molecules and extracellular matrix support growth. ④Mechanisms must operate to specify the target. ⑤ The appropriate machinery to create new functional synapses needs to be mobilized. Many of these mechanisms are similar to those essential for normal development.

nals and the stripping of them from postsynaptic densities.

The rate of synapse formation appears to be inversely related to the rate at which degenerating terminals are cleared. Thus, the clearance reaction appears to be critical to subsequent synapse formation. To determine if the glial response and the removal of degenerating material paces the re-innervation process, it is necessary to delay degeneration and to determine if there is a corresponding delay in sprouting. The "Ola" mouse exhibits delayed axonal degeneration, and in this strain, the glial reaction and sprouting response are similarly delayed [12].

Cellular lipids also appear to follow a process of degradation and recycling involving the induction of apolipoprotein E (ApoE) within astrocytes in the outer molecular layer. Lipids released from degenerating axons and dendrites are salvaged by astrocytes, released in the form of an ApoE–cholesterol lipoprotein complex and accumulated in neurons via the low-density lipoprotein receptor pathway [13]. These lipids are thus reused in the processes of dendritic re-modeling and synapse formation.

Cytokines and neurotrophic factors are induced after lesions of the entorhinal cortex

In response to entorhinal cell loss, increased syntheses of nerve growth factor (NGF), brain-derived neurotrophic factor (BDNF), ciliary neurotrophic factor (CNTF), interleukin 1B (IL-1B), basic fibroblast growth factor (FGF-2) and transforming growth factor (TGF-β1) have been described. The list will probably continue to grow as additional factors are recognized and analyzed in this model. Some of these factors regulate glial responses and others are directed at neurons and their growth responses (see Chap. 19).

It is generally believed that most of these changes are involved in the evolution of the growth process. Detailed studies, however, have suggested that another mechanism may complicate the analysis. After entorhinal lesions, there is a surge of glutamate release, which can and does induce a transient neurotrophin increase; for example, NGF increases briefly after the lesion. If this increase is blocked by an NMDA antagonist, the growth response is not suppressed, indicating that the initial induction is not an essential part of the growth response. NGF, however, does appear to be necessary for cholinergic sprouting.

Over a period of several days, NGF protein concentrations appear to increase after entorhinal lesions, reaching a maximum 8 days postlesion and returning to control values by 30 days. To determine if this increase is essential for cholinergic sprouting, an antibody to NGF was given for 8 days prior to an entorhinal lesion. The antiserum blocked the collateral sprouting of cholinergic fibers, suggesting that a supply of NGF and its action on these cells are important parts of the growth response [14,15].

Cell adhesion molecules influence neuronal growth

There are several cell adhesion molecules that can support and stimulate neuronal growth. Isoforms of the neural cell adhesion molecule (NCAM) have been shown to mediate axonal outgrowth after peripheral nerve injury and during reinnervation through interactions with other cell-surface molecules (see Chap. 7). After entorhinal cortex lesions, the embryonic form of NCAM is expressed on dendrites and axons within the denervated outer molecular layer by 24 hr. Astrocytes express NCAM at a later time, between 2 and 4 days, which may support and guide the sprouting reaction [16].

The adhesion molecule L1 can also enhance neuronal growth and may participate in the reinnervation process. L1 has been reported to mediate neuritic outgrowth, axon fasciculation and regeneration. Two to twelve days after entorhinal lesions, L1 immunoreactivity decreases but then increases again as synapses reform. The time course and reappearance of L1 parallel the maturation phase of synapse formation, which suggests that L1 is involved in the maturation and stabilization of synapses after they have made contact [17,18]. Thus, after entorhinal lesions, neurotrophic factors and cell adhesion molecules appear to participate in the process of reactive synaptogenesis.

Cytoskeletal protein concentrations increase after lesions

Sprouting in the CNS may involve a reactivation of mechanisms that operate primarily during development. There are many examples of developmentally regulated genes, including those encoding cytoskeletal proteins normally expressed during development. For example, the fetal form of α-tubulin, referred to as Tα1 in the rat, is expressed at high levels in the fetal brain during development of neuronal processes, and its expression is normally greatly reduced in the mature brain. Other examples are tau protein and microtubule-associated protein 2 (MAP2), two of the major microtubule-associated proteins that form the cytoskeleton of neurons in the vertebrate nervous system (see Chap. 8). MAP2 and tau proteins promote the assembly and integrity of microtubules in axons and dendrites, suggesting a major role in the determination of neuronal morphology.

In mature neurons, altered gene expression and increased synthesis of both microtubules and associated proteins are observed during periods of neurite outgrowth. For example, following axonal injury to the mature nervous system, $T\alpha 1$ is rapidly reinduced and maintained at high concentrations during axon outgrowth [19]. Other mRNAs induced include tau, α-tubulin, β-tubulin and β-actin. These results support the idea that the neuronal cytoskeleton is dynamically modified in response to lesions, which may involve the re-expression of mechanisms normally activated during development. Furthermore, following entorhinal cortex lesions in adult rats, MAP2 protein, which is expressed primarily in the inner molecular layer, is redistributed from the inner layer to the outer layer in the processes of sprouting neurons [20].

Synaptic proteins are produced in response to lesions

Synaptic proteins and growth-associated proteins increase in response to entorhinal lesions. The neuronal growth-associated phosphoprotein GAP-43 is expressed on growth cone membranes during periods of axonal growth. GAP-43 is decreased in the outer molecular layer for the first few days after entorhinal cortex lesions and then returns to normal by 2 to 3 weeks with an increase of approximately 300% in the number of labeled terminals. Many of these also exhibit an increase in synaptophysin, indicating that new terminals are being formed [21]. Because the new synapses are functional, it can be assumed that the essential molecules are regenerated. The exact mechanistic sequence for reinnervation and assembly of components is as yet undefined.

Molecular cascades involving cytokines appear to regulate the growth response

Increasing evidence indicates that the biological role of growth factors exceeds that of simply promoting cell growth, and indeed, they have major roles as physiological regulators. Even though growth factors generally promote growth, depending on interactions with other molecules, they can also inhibit growth. Recent studies *in vitro* and *in vivo* demonstrate that there are physiological interactions between various growth factors, consistent with the idea that multiple growth factors coordinate their actions in molecular cascades.

Following brain injury, several cellular and molecular events occur near the injury site that determine the physiological response of the remaining cells and appear to be associated with the action of growth factors. After injury, one of the earliest cellular responses appears to involve microglia. This is followed by increases in astrocytic reactivity. This cellular sequence has led to various investigations examining possible cascades of growth factors involving these cells. Indeed, glial cells such as microglia and astrocytes are common sources of growth factors and have a determining role in the injury response. One such cascade is illustrated in Figure 29-5. Microglia release cytokines, such as IL-1, that induce reactive astrocytes. In this process, IL-1 promotes the release of other growth factors, such as IL-6 and NGF, by astrocytes. Reactive astrocytes also secrete CNTF and FGF-2, which may have an autocrine role for astrocytes [22]. In the normal brain, CNTF is low, but it and its receptor (CNTFRα) are induced in astrocytes within 3 days. The receptor is also induced on neurons between 7 and 10 days, which correlates with the remodeling process, suggesting that CNTF plays a role in the overall response. Microglia also release TGFβ1, which regulates the action of FGFs on cells and protects and strengthens the extracellular matrix. Extracellular matrix components such as proteoglycans, in turn, potentiate the action of growth factors such as FGF-2 (see above). As growth factors are released into the extracellular fluid, they become available to other cells, such as neurons, which also produce growth factors, such as NGF. Not only do these growth factors work in concert to regulate growth factor production, but some also increase the responsiveness of cells to other growth factors. For example, studies have shown

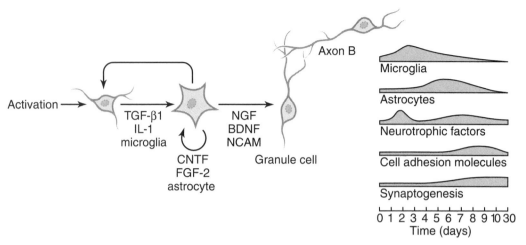

FIGURE 29-5.   Simplified mechanism by which growth factors may regulate neuronal plasticity following injury to the CNS. Primed by the original insult, microglia, astroglia and neurons interact with each other by releasing growth factors to the extracellular space. The actions of growth factors are organized in molecular cascades in which one growth factor affects the release or action of another growth factor. This generally results in increased cell survival and/or sprouting. *IL-1*, interleukin-1; *TGF-β1*, transforming growth factor β1; *FGF-2*, basic fibroblast growth factor 2; *NGF*, nerve growth factor; *CNTF*, ciliary neurotrophic factor; *BDNF*, brain-derived neurotrophic factor; *NCAM*, neural cell adhesion molecule.

that cells in culture cannot respond to NGF until they are primed with FGF-2 [23]. In this case, FGF-2 induces receptors for NGF in cells, preparing them for the action of NGF. Thus, it is highly likely that growth factors are organized in molecular cascades to act as major regulators of cell development and plasticity.

The hippocampus in Alzheimer's disease shows plasticity similar to that observed in the rodent brain after entorhinal lesions

One of the goals of modern neurochemistry is to employ the findings from basic research and animal models to predict and evaluate mechanisms in human disease. Alzheimer's disease causes extensive neuronal degeneration in select brain areas, including the entorhinal cortex, the origin of the major excitatory projection to the hippocampus. The course of degeneration is such that the neurons of the entorhinal cortex in layers II and III projecting into the hippocampus are among the first affected. However, while degeneration is a prominent feature of Alzheimer's disease, reactive growth in both neurons and glial cells is exhibited in this disease as well (Chap. 46).

In the dentate gyrus of the normal brain, there is a light cholinergic input, whereas in the Alzheimer brain, the cholinergic input is increased in the denervated zone, as predicted from the animal models discussed earlier [24]. The fetal forms of several cytoskeletal proteins are also re-expressed in the Alzheimer brain. As predicted from entorhinal cortex lesion models, the message for Tα1 is present in the Alzheimer brain at high levels [19]. These results suggest that as neurons are lost in the early period of the disease, the remaining cells sprout and form new synapses to compensate for lost connections and to maintain neuronal circuitry.

In Alzheimer's disease, plasticity may become pathological and result in plaque biogenesis

One of the neuropathological hallmarks of Alzheimer's disease is the presence of senile plaques in select brain areas. Plaques are extracellular deposits that consist primarily of a polypeptide product called amyloid. Plaques also have certain neuritic and cellular involvement, such as with astrocytes and microglia. In the dentate gyrus, plaques appear to form along the areas of interface between degeneration and neuronal sprouting and are a locus of concentrated sprouted axons, such as has been observed in some animals after entorhinal lesions (see Fig. 29-3). It has been suggested that there is an abortive turning of the sprouting reaction into plaque formation [25]. In fact, Ramon y Cajal in 1928 [26] had suggested that sprouting fibers were attracted to plaques by some neurotrophic factor, which was a remarkable insight considering that at the time there was little knowledge regarding the role of neurotrophic factors in the brain.

Plaques located along the sprouting zone in the dentate gyrus accumulate a variety of neurotrophic factors and cell adhesion molecules, which probably attract neuronal growth responses [27]. Once in the area, the processes become dystrophic, degenerate and then regenerate again because of the favorable growth-stimulating environment. Further, the process of degeneration causes an inflammatory response, which continues to drive the evolution of the cycle. In this proposed mechanism, β-amyloid binds neurotrophic factors and cell adhesion molecules and stimulates inflammatory responses and degeneration. Because β-amyloid persists in the tissue, it may convert a reversible acute phase response that would usually increase and decrease, as described above for an acute injury, into a chronic response [28].

It is ironic that the initial and/or subsequent mechanisms that promote growth and slow degeneration may in certain circumstances contribute to the disorganization of the environment and the evolution of disease. This mechanism may abort the compensation process of axon sprouting. That is, as entorhinal neurons degenerate, other entorhinal neurons form connections to replace those lost and to delay functional decline; however, some of the growth response is misdirected into plaques and drives decline.

REGENERATION

Peripheral nerve and Schwann cells promote regeneration

Axons will sprout local branches but when a fiber tract within the CNS is damaged and continuity is lost, regeneration does not occur. Motor neurons, which have processes that reside in both the CNS and the PNS, do regenerate, however. In the absence of intervention, motor neurons are one of the only CNS neurons to regenerate following axotomy. This ability appears to be a function of the environment of the peripheral nerve and an intrinsic capacity of motor neurons for regrowth (Chap. 36). What is the nature of the essential difference?

Using mRNA differential display, an extracellular signaling molecule, Reg-2, has been identified; it is uniquely expressed in regenerating and developing rat motor or sensory neurons [29]. Reg-2 is a secreted 16-kDa protein that belongs to a family of proteins found in the pancreas and gastrointestinal tract. It is not normally expressed in the CNS or PNS but is increased within 24 hr after sciatic nerve crush. It is transported orthogradely along growing sensory and motor neurons and accumulates at the site of nerve ligation or damage. To test the possibility that Reg-2 participates in motor neuron regeneration, an anti-Reg-2 polyclonal antiserum was injected into the area of nerve injury and the axons that had regenerated 3 mm past the injection were counted 4 days after injection. The treatment was found to reduce the number of regenerated axons to approximately one-third (Fig. 29-6). This demonstrates that secreted Reg-2 serves as a stimulus to promote regeneration. More recent studies have investigated the site of action of Reg-2.

Schwann cell differentiation and proliferation are essential for establishing the environment for motor neuron regeneration. For example, inhibition of Schwann cell mitosis interferes with regeneration in the mature PNS. Thus, Reg-2 may serve as a signal from the nerve to Schwann cells to proliferate. To test this hypothesis, Reg-2 was added to cultured Schwann cells and their rate of proliferation monitored. Indeed, Reg-2 acts as a Schwann cell mitogen. Once activated, Schwann cells appear to provide an appropriate extracellular matrix and neurotrophic factors to neurons. The nature of the initial signal causing an induction of Reg-2 in neurons is unknown at present. It may be damage to the nerve itself or another manifestation of the injury process, such as the production of cytokines. Cytokines are produced as a conse-

A

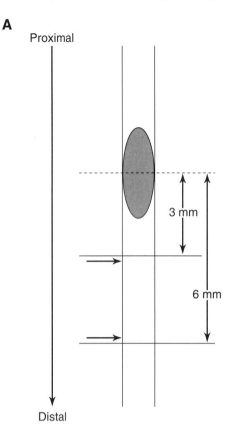

quence of the inflammatory responses by cells of the immune system as well as glia in the CNS. Studies examining the control of Reg-2 transcription in the pancreas have identified two IL-6 response elements in the promoter region of the rat Reg-2 gene. Thus, a number of multicellular signaling steps appear to allow motor neurons to regenerate. Transcriptional regulation and communication between the cell membrane and the nucleus are discussed in Chapter 26.

Peripheral nerve and Schwann cells will induce brain and spinal cord neurons to regenerate

Taken together, these data suggest that if CNS neurons encounter a PNS-type environment, they may be induced to regenerate. Will inducers such as peripheral nerve or Schwann cells induce CNS neurons other than motor neurons to regenerate? A simple experiment is to place a section of peripheral nerve in the CNS and determine if it will induce axons to enter the nerve and regenerate.

Sometimes in science, the use of new techniques combined with old strategies enables completion of experiments, which reinforces ideas that have been recognized for a long time. In 1911, Tello first showed that CNS neurons can regenerate in the presence of peripheral nerve transplants. A few weeks after transplantation of pieces of peripheral nerve, silver staining techniques demonstrated that bundles of nerve fibers regenerated into the peripheral nerves. Interestingly, use of denervated peripheral nerves had a greater effect than did use of fresh nerves. These findings were largely neglected until Aguayo and coworkers began a systematic and elegant series of studies to examine regeneration in the spinal cord and optic nerve [30,31].

B

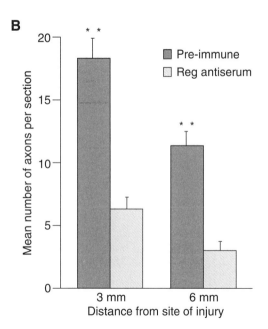

FIGURE 29-6.   Inhibition of the factor Reg-2 secreted by the axons of motor neurons retards regeneration. **A:** The sciatic nerve was crushed, an antiserum against Reg-2 was injected into the nerve and the axons which regenerated 3 and 6 mm from the crush were counted at 6 days. **B:** There is a reduction in the antiserum-treated axons compared to preimmune sera controls. (From [29], with permission.)

Peripheral nerves placed in the medulla oblongata and thoracic spinal cord of adult rats initiated the growth of several hundred fibers into the graft. Some of the bridges were up to 30 to 40 mm long, indicating the potential of fibers to grow beyond their normal lengths. As the fibers re-entered the CNS at the level of the thoracic cord, however, they stopped growing within 1 to 2 mm of the end of the graft. Thus, the regenerated fibers did not recreate inputs to the segments of the spinal cord. Similar experiments examining different regions of the CNS have since been conducted, demonstrating equally impressive regeneration. These results indicate that many CNS neurons have the capacity to regrow over long distances.

A key question is whether or not the fibers are capable of forming synapses in their target areas. Such a capability appears to be limited in the spinal cord, probably because few fibers exit the graft due to the attractive conditions in the graft relative to the more inhibitory conditions in the external environment. In the optic system, however, some fibers are able to regenerate and re-establish functional contacts. Transection of the mammalian optic nerve results in the death of retinal ganglion cells and in the failure of the surviving cut axons to regenerate. When a cut optic nerve is sutured to a portion of autologous peripheral nerve, fewer retinal ganglion cells degenerate and optic nerve axons grow into the peripheral nerve graft (Fig. 29-7A). As many as one-fifth of the surviving retinal ganglion neurons will grow axons into the graft. The regenerating fibers can grow for distances of up to 4 cm, which is double that of the normal retinotectal projection, at rates of 1 to 2 mm per day [32]. As fibers regenerate, axonal transport of cytoskeletal proteins such as tubulin, neurofilament and actin changes to resemble transport of these proteins in the developing optic nerve [33]. Analysis of the constituents of the peripheral nerve graft revealed that the presence of Schwann cells or their extracellular matrix in the graft promotes CNS fiber regeneration. Adhesion molecules on the surface of Schwann cells and specific extracellular matrix proteins, such as laminin, influence axonal outgrowth. If these molecules are bound with antibodies that inhibit their function, fiber regeneration is also inhibited.

The optic nerve normally sends projections to the superior colliculus. If the free end of a peripheral nerve graft to the optic nerve is placed in the superior colliculus of the host, the regenerated axons will arborize in the superior colliculus, penetrate it for short distances and form functional synapses on neuronal elements within the superior colliculus. The newly formed synapses are well differentiated in both morphology and function. Illumination of specific regions of the retina produces either excitatory or inhibitory responses in postsynaptic superior

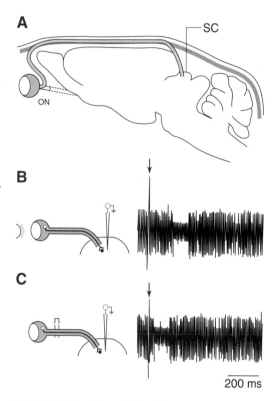

FIGURE 29-7. Transected optic nerve can regenerate through a peripheral nerve graft and form functional synapses within the superior colliculus (SC). **A:** Diagram of adult rat brain in sagittal section showing peripheral nerve grafts ◑ used to replace the transected optic nerve (ON). One end of an autologous peroneal nerve graft was attached to the orbital stump of the ON transected close to the eye. The distal end of the graft was inserted into the SC. **B:** Inhibition of ongoing activity of an SC neuron by light flash. **C:** Inhibition of spontaneous activity of the same neuron after electrical stimulation of the peripheral nerve graft. Each trace represents 25 superimposed sweeps. Stimuli were delivered at *arrows*. (Adapted from Vidal-Sanz et al., *J. Neuroscience* 7:2894, 1987 and Kierstad et al., *Science* 246:255, 1989, with permission.)

collicular neurons similar to the "on" and "off" cells described in the normal superior colliculus (Fig. 29-7B,C). The number of synapses formed, however, is small relative to normal. Nonetheless, the capacity appears to be present in this system, suggesting that further improvements using additional interventions may be possible.

Axons can be induced to regenerate after spinal cord injury and can mediate functional recovery if myelin-associated inhibitory molecules are blocked

Two factors have greatly stimulated progress on the recovery from spinal cord injury: fundamental advances in the field of regeneration [34] and the surge of popular interest and mobilization of resources due to well known individuals such as Christopher Reeve becoming victims of spinal cord injury. In patients, spinal cord injuries are classified according to their segmental level and categorized as complete or incomplete, depending on the sparing of sensory or motor function and on the nature of the mechanisms that generated the injury. Fractures of vertebral bodies or luxation of vertebrae lead to concussion, contusion or laceration of the spinal cord. Concussion signifies a transient depression of spinal cord function without anatomical damage, while contusion involves direct anatomical damage and the probability of permanent damage. Most cases of human spinal cord injury result in acute contusion due to displacement of fragments of bone or intervertebral disc into the spinal cord during fracture dislocation or burst fracture of the spine. Cases of complete spinal cord transection are rare but can arise from injuries such as gunshot wounds. Christopher Reeve, for example, suffered a contusion injury, which led to the disruption of nerve impulses across the injury site.

At the site of injury after a contusion injury, there is a rapid alteration of the microvascular system leading to multifocal hemorrhages. At 4 to 8 hr after injury, aneurysmal dilations and ruptures of the arteries are observed. Both neurons and glia are affected. Neurons show necrotic alterations that include the appearance of ghost cells, swelling of the endoplasmic reticulum and replacement of the cytoplasmic reticulum by fine granularity. Necrosis of axons in

the white matter is associated with the development of a space between the myelin sheath and axon and, in some cases, the loss of oligodendrocytes. By 4 hr after injury, numerous axons within the central white matter show swelling and accumulation of organelles. These changes evolve in a centrifugal manner over the next several days. After the first few hours, a massive gliosis evolves.

Reactive gliosis is a response that follows after nearly every type of injury and involves reactive microglia and astrocytes. Microglia take on an activated phenotype; increase the number of processes; upregulate cell surface molecules, including the complement C3 receptor; and become active phagocytes. This is compounded by the further invasion of macrophages and the generation of inflammatory responses. Astrocytes become hypertrophied and undergo limited proliferation within 1 to 2 days after the injury. Within the first week, astrocytes begin to accumulate at the margins of the injury and delineate the boundaries of a cavity that will form at the later chronic phase. In severe spinal cord injury, a large cavity develops at the injury site. After removal of debris, astrocytic processes with end feet that are rich in glial fibrillary acid protein (GFAP) form multilayered interfaces between necrotic and intact tissues. This border between cavities of microcysts and intact tissues is known as the astrocytic or glial scar. An inhibitory role of scar tissue for regenerating axons was originally postulated by Ramon y Cajal and has been confirmed by the results of subsequent experiments.

When CNS axons are severed, local connectivity may be re-established by the growth of damaged cell processes or the extension of collateral sprouts from adjacent undamaged neurons. Whereas cut axons will regrow for long distances in the PNS or the CNS of fish and invertebrates, mammalian CNS axons rarely grow for more than a few millimeters through the injured area. The failure of CNS axons to regrow for long distances has been attributed to several factors. One example is proteoglycan growth inhibitors associated with glial scars [35]. A growth inhibitor associated with glial scars is thought to include the carbohydrate component of putative heparan-sulfate proteoglycans.

Recent studies have shown that the CNS contains various growth-inhibitory molecules. Another factor is myelin-associated neurite growth inhibitors produced by oligodendrocytes [36]. Cell culture studies have shown that growing neurites normally avoid rat oligodendrocytes and myelin, but the mechanism remains unclear. Similarly, in different areas of the adult brain and spinal cord, the growth-associated protein GAP-43, a marker for the plastic potential of neurons, is generally absent in heavily myelinated regions. Myelin appears to be associated with growth arrest. It appears that associated with oligodendrocytes there are inhibitory factors that are not metabolites of these cells but are part of the cellular membranes because oligodendrocyte membranes also inhibit neurite growth.

Recent studies show that oligodendrocytes express two cell surface proteins, of 35 kDa (NI-35) and 250 kDa (NI-250), and two glycoproteins of the J1 family, of 160 kDa and 180 kDa, all of which inhibit neurite outgrowth. Neurites will not normally grow over oligodendrocytes or over preparations of these factors. For example, dorsal root ganglion neurons growing on laminin and in the presence of NGF show long-lasting growth cone collapse and growth arrest when they encounter NI-35/250. Preceding collapse, intracellular Ca^{2+} increases. If calcium is depleted or the mobilization of intracellular Ca^{2+} is blocked by compounds such as dantrolene, growth cone collapse is prevented. Pertussis toxin also prevents collapse, whereas mastoparan, an activator of G proteins, induces collapse by itself. Thus, it appears that Ca^{2+} and G proteins represent components of the intracellular second-messenger cascade leading to the rapid retraction of growth cones and long-lasting growth arrest. If the interaction of these proteins with growing axons could be prevented, it is possible that regeneration would be more successful.

To test the hypothesis that these proteins restrain regeneration in the mammalian CNS, antibodies have been prepared that bind to the parent molecule and mask it from axonal contact. In culture, nerve fibers will grow over oligodendrocytes in the presence of antibodies against oligodendrocyte-associated growth-inhibitory proteins (Fig. 29-8).

The next key question is whether these antibodies are sufficiently efficient to stimulate regeneration *in vivo* and lead to behavioral recovery after spinal cord injury. Rats with a hemisection of the spinal cord were implanted with hybridoma cells that produced monoclonal antibodies to myelin-associated neurite growth proteins (IN-1) at the time of the injury. The IN-1 monoclonal antibody treatment resulted in the growth of corticospinal axons around the lesion site and into the spinal cord caudal to the lesion. Some of these axons regenerated up to distances of 1 cm within 2 weeks. The number of fibers regenerating such long distances, however, is low and represents only about 5 to 10% of corticospinal axons. In the absence of IN-1, growth around the lesion site and into the spinal cord caudal to the injury was restricted to within 1 mm.

Quantitative and qualitative analyses of reflex and locomotor function in these animals showed that the intervention produced functionally significant results (Fig. 29-9). Contact placing, a reflex known to be dependent on the integrity of the corticospinal pathway, was significantly improved. Stride length was further improved and reached values similar to controls in the treated animals. In spite of remarkable improvement in some aspects of motor function, the error rate of foot placement on grid runways was not improved. Apparently, this requires more complete regeneration and greater remodeling of ascending projections.

The success of the intervention illustrates that the suppression of myelin-associated neurite inhibitors in adult spinal cord–lesioned rats can enhance regeneration and anatomical plasticity of corticospinal and brainstem pathways and mediate improvements in locomotor function. These results are exciting because they indicate that interventions may reverse what would otherwise be permanent losses. They are also consistent with data obtained from experiments in animals and humans with subtotal spinal cord lesions, indicating that substantial recovery may be mediated by relatively small numbers of fibers. In the intact nervous system, these proteins may have a critical role in the normal development of circuitry by directing the growth of developing projections into the proper areas [34].

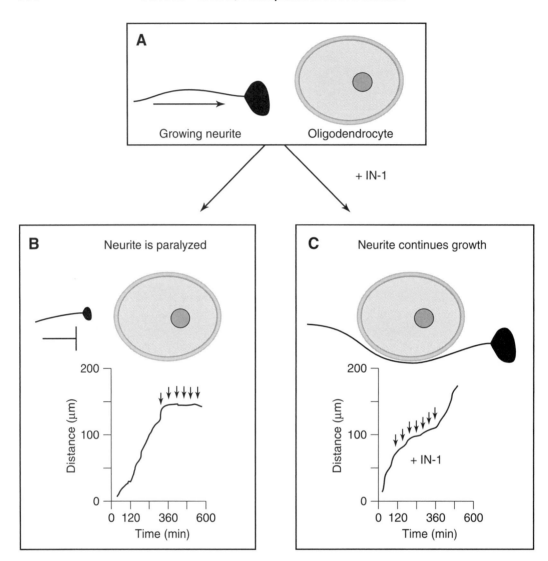

FIGURE 29-8. Neutralization of growth-inhibitor proteins associated with oligodendrocytes promotes the growth of neurites near oligodendrocytes. **A:** Dorsal root ganglion neuronal process with growth cone *(black area)* growing on laminin in the presence of nerve growth factor makes contact with an oligodendrocyte. **B:** Growth cone subsequently collapses (60 min later) and remains paralyzed. Velocity plot shows arrest of growth cone upon encounter with oligodendrocyte. Contact is indicated by *arrows*. **C:** No growth arrest occurs in the presence of antibodies neutralizing NI-35/250. Velocity plot shows continued growth despite contact with oligodendrocyte *(arrows)*. (From [34], with permission.)

Thus, mammalian CNS axons have the ability to elongate for surprising distances when presented with the appropriate cellular milieu. Severed CNS axons will grow for long distances when provided with a stimulating and noninhibitory environment, suggesting that axonal regeneration depends more on the non-neuronal environment of the growing fibers than on the origin of the parent cell bodies. This observation illustrates the influence of extrinsic conditions, such as growth factors, inhibitory factors and basal lamina, on the developing or regenerating axon. A variety of other growth-inhibiting molecules have been identified, such as the collapsin/semaphorin family and the repulsive axon guidance signal (RAGS), a molecule with

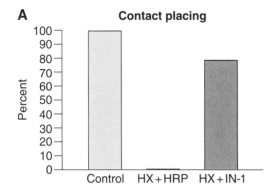

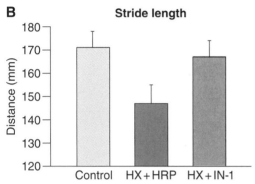

FIGURE 29-9. Treatment with an antibody against an inhibitory factor (IN-1) improves reflex and locomotor function in rats after hemisection *(Hx)* of the spinal cord. **A:** Contact placing is improved in IN-1-treated animals and returns to near that in unlesioned control animals. **B:** Stride length also improves, indicating that the treatment can improve locomotor activity. (From [53], with permission.)

homology to a family of recently cloned tyrosine receptor kinase ligands of the Eph family. In fact, accumulating evidence suggests the operation of multiple factors in CNS regeneration.

BRAIN AND SPINAL CORD TRANSPLANTS

The cell-replacement strategy of transplantation has been developed in an attempt to overcome the intrinsic limitation of neurons to divide and replace lost cells. Through successful cell replacement, the damaged brain can be reconstructed, to a certain extent, to compensate for neuronal loss. Partial survival of brain tissue implants in rats was first reported by Elizabeth Dunn in 1917 [37]. There has been great

progress in this area primarily because of the advancement of cellular and molecular approaches. Poor integration of the implanted tissue with the host tissue and lack of control of the activity of host cells vs. implanted cells has restrained advancement in this field. Progress in the field corresponds to a better understanding of the optimal conditions for survival and integration of the implanted cells. Two critical variables that have been defined are the types of cells used and the developmental stage of those cells. In general, brain tissue implants can be performed with three different objectives: (i) to restore a cell population and its connectivity that has been damaged, (ii) to provide a new or additional source of the product of a particular cell population that is needed to regain function and/or (iii) to test hypotheses by manipulating the normal CNS environment.

Regeneration of adult axons can occur in white matter tracts if the astrocytic reaction is absent

As discussed above, astrocytes form a scar around the injury site, which has been proposed to interfere with regeneration of mature axons. This may serve as a physical barrier and/or generate attractant or inhibitory molecules that prevent the growth of fibers through the scar. Although inactivation of myelin-associated neurite molecules may allow regeneration, the scar may prevent the full expression of potential benefits. To evaluate the contribution of the glial scar and its role in retarding regeneration, a method is needed to implant mature neurons into white matter tracts and to determine if, in the absence of scarring, regeneration proceeds. It is possible that adult white matter is an inherently conducive highway for axonal regeneration from an adult neuron in the absence of glial scarring.

One approach is to insert small numbers of adult neurons into white matter tracts by using a microinjection technique that displaces but does not damage the white matter [38]. Accordingly, adult dorsal root ganglia neurons were dissociated and placed into a suspension, and 0.5 μl of the suspension was very slowly and carefully injected into the corpus callosum of adult hosts. As discussed above, dorsal root ganglia neuron regeneration has been shown previously to be inhibited by mature oligodendrocytes or CNS myelin components. Within 2 to 4 days, however, axons from dorsal root ganglia neurons had exited from the transplant and entered into the host tract in continuity with host-tract glial structures. Once out of graft territory, donor axons did not appear to fasciculate with each other, branch or otherwise wander from the host tract. The regenerating axons formed "bullet-shaped" growth cones with a single leading filopodium similar to that in developing CNS pathways. At 6 days, the fibers entered the host gray matter, where they branched, suggesting a switch of growth signals. Approximately 35% of the transplanted neurons survived and 80% of these had axons that reached the midline of the corpus callosum.

In most transplantation protocols, immature neurons survive and regenerate better than adult neurons; however, in this minimal trauma protocol, no differences were observed between survival and regeneration of immature and adult donor neurons. This further indicates that the nature of the intervention is critical.

In some experiments, regeneration was less robust, and it appeared that the injection had disrupted the host tissue to varying degrees. A number of proteoglycans, some of which are of astrocytic origin, are known to inhibit axon growth *in vitro*, and their upregulation *in vivo* coincides with the age at which the CNS fails to support regeneration. Transplants exhibiting robust regeneration had very low concentrations of chrondroitin-6-sulfate proteoglycan in the matrix at the graft–host interface. In contrast, transplanted cells with axons that failed to enter the adjacent host white matter showed intense staining for this proteoglycan. The orientation and reactivity of astrocytes appeared to be similar in cases with successful and unsuccessful regeneration. Taken together, these findings suggest that the production of a reactive extracellular matrix is associated with the failure of regeneration in the mature CNS. At the border of this apparent "molecular scar," there may be many inhibitory matrix proteins, and these need to be further identified and evaluated. The molecules that trigger upregulation of the pro-

teoglycan-rich matrix may be derived from a breakdown of the blood–brain barrier and the generation of an inflammatory response.

Thus, axons can regenerate along myelin pathways if trauma is minimal and inhibitory proteoglycans and other possible products are not generated. However, oligodendrocytes and myelin-inhibitory proteins block axonal outgrowth. At one level, these results may appear contradictory. The key concept is that there is a basic difference in the intrinsic restraints on regeneration in the normal adult nervous system vs. the traumatized or injured CNS. That is, in a nondisturbed state, it appears that oligodendrocytes cannot mask the growth-promoting potential of other cell types, such as astrocytes. The balance favors growth; however, when disturbed, various reactions are engaged that can inhibit regeneration. One explanation is that a breakdown in the integrity of the blood–brain barrier initiates the increased production of inhibitory molecules. The CNS must be resealed from inflammatory attack, but in the process of restoring the blood–brain barrier, the activated mechanism retards regeneration in this postulated mechanism. Thus, the normal, healthy CNS is more permissive to neuronal regeneration and remodeling than is the traumatized CNS, in which external interventions are required to facilitate regeneration and overcome inhibitory processes.

At one level, these data appear very convincing, but the donor cells are not mature CNS neurons. Further, the analysis is correlative and many molecules and cellular properties not analyzed may account for the observation. An *in vitro* experiment in slice cultures has tested in another way the relative importance of neuronal properties vs. those of the environment. Immature neurons regenerate and can restore function. However, as the nervous system matures, the ability to regenerate is lost. Is this loss due to the neurons or the maturing environment?

Simple systems are very important in research as they afford the potential to dissect variables inherent in complex mechanisms (Fig. 29-10). Slice cultures maintain the structural characteristics of the CNS and can be manipulated so that the age of the target vs. source can be varied. A hippocampus, for example,

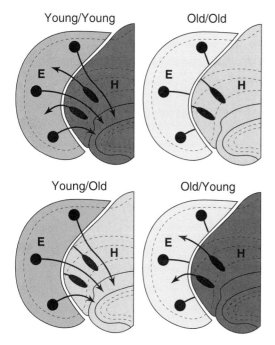

Young/Young Old/Old

Young/Old Old/Young

FIGURE 29-10. Cocultured slices were prepared in which the ages of the target and regenerating cell sources were varied. Axons from younger tissues regenerate across the coculture interface, whereas those from older tissues do not, regardless of the age of the target. Thus, in this preparation, failure of regeneration by entorhinal cortex axons is due to maturation of the axon and not the pathway or target. (From [39], with permission.)

ated inflammatory responses are absent. This demonstrates that the most critical variable is the developmental program of the neurons, not the environment [39]. Thus, it is essential to rejuvenate the program in neurons.

Transplants of olfactory ensheathing cells can mediate repair of the adult corticospinal tract

In some areas of the CNS, such as the adult olfactory system, neurosensory cells are continuously replaced and their newly formed axons grow and form functional connections. The olfactory pathway is lined with specialized ensheathing cells that share both Schwann cell and astrocytic characteristics. These cells are unusual, however, in that they accompany axons into the CNS and, thus, appear to provide a regenerative environment in the adult CNS. Will these cells support regeneration in other parts of the CNS, such as the spinal cord? This is an important issue for two reasons. First, it addresses the idea that extrinsic inducers can facilitate regeneration in an otherwise hostile environment. Second, olfactory ensheathing cells can be derived from adult human donors, raising the possibility of their clinical use.

As discussed above, transplants of peripheral nerve or Schwann cells can enhance the growth of cut corticospinal axons, but the axons fail to enter host pathways. This is not the case with the use of olfactory ensheathing cells [40]. The corticospinal tract was destroyed unilaterally by a focal electrolytic lesion in the medial ventral part of the dorsal columns between the first and second cervical segments. A suspension of ensheathing cells from the adult olfactory bulb was injected into the lesion site. Over 2 to 3 weeks, the ensheathing cells established a one-to-one relationship with individual corticospinal axons and induced them to regenerate through the transplant and into the denervated caudal host tract. After re-entry into the caudal part of the host corticospinal tract, the axons became myelinated by oligodendrocytes.

To determine if these regenerated fibers were capable of mediating functional recovery, the rats were tested to determine if they were capable of executing a forepaw-reaching task in

can be cultured with an entorhinal cortex and the entorhinal axons project to the correct terminal fields. In order to investigate the effect of age vs. environment on regeneration, a young entorhinal cortex can be opposed to a young target, an old combined with old or other combinations of old and young tissues. Young–young cocultures regenerate; old–old cocultures do not. However, if a young hippocampus is cocultured with an old entorhinal cortex, the mature neurons do not regenerate, though the younger cells will innervate the older tissues. General tissue factors such as the formation of a glial scar or the onset of myelination appear to be noncritical in this model since in the young–old and old–young combinations the projection failed in one direction but succeeded in the opposite direction across the same interface. Further, peripherally medi-

which the animals reach through an aperture to obtain a food reward. Fourteen of 21 animals tested were able to perform forepaw reaching on the lesioned side. These animals showed successful transplants and regeneration, whereas those animals unable to accomplish the task had the corticospinal tract completely destroyed by the lesion, suggesting that the recovery depended on the presence of intact fibers in the corticospinal tract. In one animal, function was regained even though the rat had only 698 out of a normal total of approximately 50,000 corticospinal axons [40]!

Transplants integrate into central nervous system circuitry and may restore some function in Parkinson's disease

Parkinson's disease is characterized by a chronic and progressive deterioration of voluntary movements and the development of tremor, rigidity and bradykinesia. It is well established that the symptoms of Parkinson's disease are the result of an almost complete loss of the striatal neurotransmitter dopamine, which is normally provided by neurons in the substantia nigra. Therapeutic replacement of striatal dopamine, for example, administration of levodopa (L-DOPA), reverses some of the symptoms of parkinsonism; however, long-term drug treatment has not been successful for diverse reasons. Thus, a large body of research has been devoted to finding ways to replace the cells which no longer release dopamine in the striatum.

Current research strategies are focused on three areas: (i) techniques to increase dopamine neuron survival and the density and extent of dopamine reinnervation in the striatum, (ii) addition of dopamine neurons in the denervated areas which can reconstruct the function of the normal pathway and (iii) identification and use of appropriate sources of cells which will re-establish function. Some studies have emphasized the use of adrenal cell transplants, which normally produce dopamine but increase their production when implanted into the rat brain. Other studies have used fetal human cell grafts. In animal studies, embryonic mescencephalic tissue grafting in mammalian models of Parkinson's disease has been shown to restore dopaminergic transmission and to reverse sensorimotor deficits [41–43]. These results have prompted the use of similar approaches in clinical trials in human subjects affected by Parkinson's disease.

Following tissue grafting, some patients have shown improvement of motor symptoms. More than 200 patients have received intrastriatal grafts of dopamine neurons, which survive and can innervate the human striatum. The results have been very encouraging and, in general, have followed the predictions from animal research (Chap. 45).

In clinical studies, there is recovery as evidenced by a reduction in the therapeutic doses of L-DOPA and by the performance on motor tasks. In several patient studies, improvement is related to the nature and size of the transplant. For example, in a double-blinded study where standard measures of motor performance were assessed, those individuals with large-volume transplants of human fetal tissues excelled over those with small-volume transplants when evaluated 6 months after surgery [44]. In fact, several studies have shown that transplants of human neurons will survive and improve function [44–47], although, as might be expected, variable outcomes are experienced in such studies. Adrenal grafts survive very poorly following transplantation into the striatum, although they are capable of inducing sprouting of host-derived fibers within the caudate. In contrast, robust survival of fetal nigral implants can be achieved within the human striatum, and this is associated with extensive reinnervation of the striatum, as predicted from animal studies. The first autopsy studies have been published and are quite remarkable (Fig. 29-11). These studies show extensive reinnervation and growth, as predicted from animal studies.

A potential limitation of tissue-grafting approaches is that, because Parkinson's disease is a progressive disorder, any long-term positive effect due to the graft is counteracted by further degeneration of endogenous dopaminergic neurons. Fortunately, this has not proven to be a problem since fetal tissue grafts have survived for several years, as long as the patients are immunosuppressed. The source of the cells is a problem since

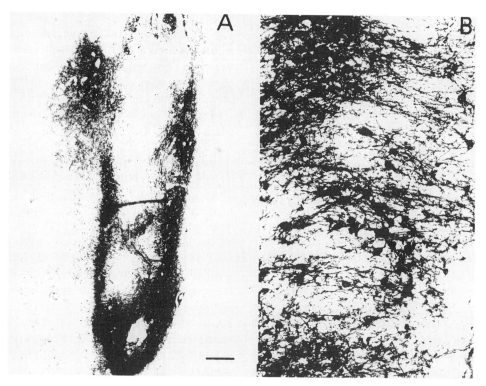

FIGURE 29-11. Fetal grafts placed into the brain of patients with Parkinson's disease show extensive growth within the human striatum. (From [45], with permission.) **A:** Low power photomicrograph illustrates the survival of grafted neurons. **B:** Medium power photomicrograph illustrates the extensive growth of grafted neurons into the host striatum. *Scale bar:* A, 1000 μm; B, 100 μm.

immunosuppression is undesirable and the use of human fetal cells creates issues regarding the reliability and source of the cells and medical ethics.

Central nervous system stem cells provide an opportunity to improve the prospects for successful transplantation

Perhaps the greatest unsolved problem facing the field of transplantation is identifying a source of cells which is ethically acceptable and which cells can integrate into the nervous system and serve the essential needs of the system. As illustrated above, the most successful strategies are those which most closely approximate the natural solution to the problem. Most neurons in the adult CNS are terminally differentiated and survive the lifespan of the animal. In other tissues, like bone, skin and intestinal epithelium, a population of stem cells self-renew and generate new progeny in response to select signals. It has been contended over the years that the CNS does not contain stem cells.

Recently, it has become clear that the CNS has the capacity to regenerate all neural cell types: neurons, astrocytes and oligodendroglia [48,49]. In the adult CNS, a rapidly dividing population of stem cells in the subventricular zone of the lateral ventricle and certain other regions is capable of at least limited cell replacement. These cells can form neurons or glia, depending on the region and signals present. Stem cells can be cultured, expanded and, in the presence of select neurotrophic factors such as FGF or epidermal growth factor, maintained in a proliferative or differentiated state (Fig. 29-12). Thus, stem cells provide an exciting potential for rebuilding function. Stem cells generated in specific loci have the capacity to migrate over long distances and integrate into existing cell populations. The basic paradigm to illustrate the presence and migratory ability of stem cells is to inject bromodeoxyuridine to identify proliferating cells. In parallel, cell cultures developed from specific regions of the adult brain contain multi-

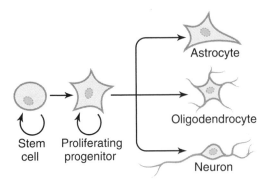

FIGURE 29-12. Self-renewing stem cells will give rise to progenitor cells, which can be terminally differentiated into neurons or glial cells. The exact pathway can be regulated *in vitro* by specific factors or *in vivo* by the local environment. (Modified from [49], with permission.)

potent cells which can differentiate into neurons. Such studies have shown that the subependymal zone generates cells which migrate into the olfactory bulb and become neurons and that hippocampal stem cells can, for example, migrate into the dentate gyrus granule cell layer and assume the properties of neurons. The striatum and other areas, such as the raphe nucleus, may also generate new neurons.

Stem cells can be cultured, genetically engineered to express various genes and maintained almost indefinitely. Various studies have shown that these immortalized progenitor cells can integrate into the brain and participate in the recovery of function [50]. For example, introduction of a cell line expressing NGF can reverse the cholinergic deficit and ameliorate learning and memory deficits in cognitively impaired aged rats [51]. The transplants caused fiber sprouting toward the implantation site, increased expression of p75 and hypertrophy of cholinergic neurons. Experiments on animal models of Parkinson's disease have shown improvements with progenitor cell transplants. The transplanted cells do not disrupt the normal brain cytoarchitecture and are well integrated into the brain.

Immortalized progenitor cells offer an exciting new approach for most transplant experiments. They are safe in that there are no current data indicating adverse events such as the formation of tumors or development of immune responses. The development and application of a gene-transfer procedure is an ethical concern with respect to research activity and clinical application. Immortalized cells can be generated in large numbers for general use under fully acceptable and controlled conditions. These cells may also eliminate the need for fetal primary tissue in clinical application yet allow scientists to take advantage of advances in the field.

SUMMARY AND CONCLUSIONS

Research over the past decade has shown that the brain is highly plastic at the level of its circuitry. The brain has a remarkable potential to rebuild circuitry in response to injury or neurodegenerative disease. Characterization of the neurochemistry and molecular regulation of sprouting and reactive synaptogenesis will provide an opportunity not only to understand normal brain plasticity mechanisms but also to develop strategies to regulate these mechanisms, to help prevent brain injury and to stimulate recovery.

REFERENCES

1. Cotman, C. W., and Nadler, J. V. Reactive synaptogenesis in the hippocampus. In C. W. Cotman (ed.), *Neuronal Plasticity.* New York: Raven Press, 1978, pp. 227–271.
2. Nieto-Sampedro, M., and Cotman, C. W. Synaptic plasticity. In G. Adleman (ed.), *Encyclopedia of Neuroscience.* Boston: Birkhauser, 1987, pp. 1166–1167.
3. Cotman, C. W., Nieto-Sampedro, M., and Harris, E. W. Synapse replacement in the nervous system of adult vertebrates. *Physiol. Rev.* 61:684–782, 1981.
4. Deller, T., and Frotscher, M. Lesion-induced plasticity of central neurons: Sprouting of single fibres in the rat hippocampus after unilateral entorhinal cortex lesion. *Prog. Neurobiol.* 53:687–727, 1997.
5. Reeves, T. M., and Smith, D. C. Reinnervation of the dentate gyrus and recovery of alternation behavior following entorhinal lesions. *Behav. Neurosci.* 101:179–186, 1987.
6. Reeves, T. M., and Steward, O. Changes in the firing properties of neurons in the dentate gyrus with denervation and reinnervation: Implications for behavioral recovery. *Exp. Neurol.* 102:37–49, 1988.

7. Scheff, S. W., and Cotman, C. W. Recovery of spontaneous alternation following lesions of the entorhinal cotrex in adult rats: Possible correlation to axon sprouting. *Behav. Biol.* 21:286–293, 1977.

8. Purves, D., Hadley, R. D., and Voyvodic, J. T. Dynamic changes in the dendritic geometry of individual neurons visualized over periods of up to three months in the superior cervical ganglion of living mice. *J. Neurosci.* 6:1051–1060, 1986.

9. Hoff, S. F., Scheff, S. W., Kwan, A. Y., and Cotman, C. W. A new type of lesion induced synaptogenesis: I. Synaptic turnover in non-denervated zones of the dentate gyrus in young adult rats. *Brain Res.* 222:1–13, 1981.

10. Caceres, A., and Steward, O. Dendritic reorganization in the denervated dentate gyrus of the rat following entorhinal cortical lesions: A Golgi and electron microscope analysis. *J. Comp. Neurol.* 214:387–403, 1983.

11. Steward, O. Synapse replacement on cortical neurons following denervation. *Cereb. Cortex* 9:81–132, 1991.

12. Steward, O. Signals that induce sprouting in the central nervous system: Sprouting is delayed in a strain of mouse exhibiting delayed axonal degeneration. *Exp. Neurol.* 118:340–351, 1992.

13. Poirier, J., Baccichet, A., Dea, D., and Gauthier, S. Cholesterol synthesis and lipoprotein reuptake during synaptic remodelling in hippocampus in adult rats. *Neuroscience* 55:81–90, 1993.

14. van der Zee, C. E. E. M., Fawcett, J., and Diamond, J. Antibody to NGF inhibits collateral sprouting of septohippocampal fibers following entorhinal cortex lesion in adults rats. *J. Comp. Neurol.* 326:91–100, 1992.

15. Varon, S. S., Conner, J. M., and Kuang, R.-Z. Neurotrophic factors: Repair and regeneration in the central nervous system. *Rest. Neurol. Neurosci.* 8:85–94, 1995.

16. Stryen, S. D., Lagenaur, C. F., Miller, P. D., and DeKosky, S. T. Rapid expression and transport of embryonic N-CAM in dentate gyrus following entorhinal cortex lesions: Ultrastructural analysis. *J. Comp. Neurol.* 349:486–492, 1994.

17. Jucker, M., D'Amator, F., Mondadori, C., et al. Expression of the neural adhesion molecule L1 in the deafferented dentate gyrus. *Neuroscience* 75:703–715, 1996.

18. Stryen, S. D., Miller, P. D., Lagenaur, C. F., and DeKosky, S. T. Alternative strategies in lesion-induced reactive synaptogenesis: Differential expression of L1 in two populations of sprouting axons. *Exp. Neurol.* 131:165–173, 1995.

19. Cotman, C. W., Geddes, J. W., and Kahle, J. S. Axon sprouting in the rodent and Alzheimer's disease brain: A reactivation of developmental mechanisms? In J. Storm-Mathisen, J. Zimmer, and O. P. Ottersen (eds.), *Progress in Brain Research.* Amsterdam: Elsevier, 1990, vol. 83, pp. 427–434.

20. Dow, K., Mirski, S., Roder, J., and Riopelle, R. Neuronal proteogylcans: Biosynthesis and functional interaction with neurons *in vitro*. *J Neurosci.* 8:3278–3289, 1988.

21. Masliah, E., Fagan, A. M., Terry, R. D., DeTerese, R., Mallory, M., and Gage, F. H. Reactive synaptogenesis assessed by synaptophysin immunoreactivity is associated with GAP-43 in the dentate gyrus of the adult rat. *Exp. Neurol.* 113:131–142, 1991.

22. Yoshida, K., and Gage, F. H. Fibroblast growth factors stimulate nerve growth factor synthesis and secretion by astrocytes. *Brain Res.* 538:118–126, 1991.

23. Cattaneo, E., and McKay, R. Proliferation and differentiation of neuronal stem cells regulated by nerve growth factor. *Nature* 347:762–765, 1990.

24. Geddes, J. W., Monaghan, D. T., Cotman, C. W., Lott, I. T., Kim, R. C., and Chui, H. C. Plasticity of hippocampal circuitry in Alzheimer's disease. *Science* 230:1179–1181, 1985.

25. Damon, D., D'Amore, P., and Wagner, J. Sulfated glycosaminogylcans modify growth factor-induced neurite outgrowth in PC12 cells. *J. Cell Physiol.* 135:293–300, 1988.

26. Ramon y Cajal, S. *Degeneration and Regeneration of the Nervous System*, R. M. May (trans.). London: Oxford University Press, 1928.

27. Cotman, C. W., and Cummings, B. J. Trophic factors and cell adhesion molecules can drive dysfunctional plasticity and senile plaque formation in Alzheimer's disease through a breakdown in spatial and temporal regulation. In: M. Tuszynski, K. Bankiewicz, and J. Kordower (eds.) *CNS Regeneration: Basic Sciences and Clinical Advances.* San Diego: Academic Press (in press).

28. Cotman, C. W., Tenner, A. J., and Cummings, B. J. β-Amyloid converts an acute phase injury response to chronic injury responses. *Neurobiol. Aging* 15:723–731, 1996.

29. Livesey, F. J., O'Brien, J. A., Li, M., Smith, A. G., Murphy, L. J., and Hunt, S. P. A Schwann cell mitogen accompanying regeneration of motor neurons. *Nature* 390:614–618, 1997.

30. Aguayo, A. J., Clarke, D. B., Jelsma, T. N., Kittlerova, P., Friedman, H. C., and Bray, G. M. Effects of neurotrophins on the survival and regrowth of injured retinal neurons. *Ciba Found. Symp.* 196:135–148, 1996.

31. Carter, D. A., Bray, G. M., and Aguayo, A. J. Long-term growth and remodeling of regenerated retino-collicular connections in adult hamsters. *Neuroscience* 14:590–598, 1994.

32. Aguayo, A. J., Raminsky, M., Bray, G. M., et al. Degenerative and regenerative responses of injured neurons in the central nervous system of adult mammals. *Philos. Trans. R. Soc. Lond. B Biol. Sci.* 331:337–343, 1991.

33. McKerracher, L., Vidal-Sanz, M., and Aguayo, A. J. Slow transport rates of cytoskeletal proteins change during regeneration of axotomized retinal neurons in adult rats. *Neuroscience* 10:641–648, 1990.

34. Schwab, M. E., and Bartholdi, D. Degeneration and regeneration of axons in the lesioned spinal cord. *Physiol. Rev.* 76:319–370, 1996.

35. Bovolenta, P., Wandosell, F., and Nieto-Sampedro, M. CNS glial scar tissue: A source of molecules which inhibit central neurite outgrowth. In A. C. H. Yu, L. Hertz, M. D. Norenberg, E. Sykova, and S. G. Waxman (eds.), *Progress in Brain Research*. Amsterdam: Elsevier, 1992, pp. 367–379.

36. Schwab, M. E. Myelin-associated inhibitors of neurite growth and regeneration in the CNS. *Trends Neurosci.* 13:452–456, 1990.

37. Bjorklund, A. Brain implants, transplants. In G. Adelman (ed.), *Encyclopedia of Neuroscience*. Boston: Birkhauser, 1987, pp. 165–167.

38. Davies, S. J. A., Fitch, M. T., Memberg, S. P., Hall, A. K., Raisman, G., and Silver, J. Regeneration of adult axons in white matter tracts of the central nervous system. *Nature* 390:680–683, 1997.

39. Li, Y., and Raisman, G. Sprouts from cut corticospinal axons persist in the presence of astrocytic scarring in long-term lesions of the adult rat spinal cord. *Exp. Neurol.* 134:102–111, 1995.

40. Li, Y., Field, P. M., and Raisman, G. Repair of adult rat corticospinal tract by transplant of olfactory ensheathing cells. *Science* 277:2000–2002, 1997.

41. Dunnett, S. B. Transplantation of embryonic dopamine neurons: What we know from rats. *J. Neurol.* 238:65–74, 1991.

42. Hoffer, B., and Olson, L. Treatment strategies for neurodegenerative diseases based on trophic factors and cell transplantation techniques. *J. Neural Transm. Suppl.* 49:1–10, 1997.

43. Lindvall, O. Neural transplantation: A hope for patients with Parkinson's disease. *Neuroreport* 8:iii–x, 1997.

44. Kopyov, O. V., Jacques, D. S., Lieberman, A., Duman, C. M., and Rogers, R. L. Outcome following intrastrial fetal mesencephalic grafts for Parkinson's patients is directly related to the volume of grafted tissue. *Exp. Neurol.* 146:526–545, 1997.

45. Kordower, J. H., Goetz, C. G., Freeman, T. B., and Olanow, C. W. Dopaminergic transplants in patients with Pakinson's disease: Neuroanatomical correlates of clinical recovery. *Exp. Neurol.* 144:41–46, 1997.

46. López-Lozano, J. J., Bravo, G., Brera, B., et al. Long-term improvement in patients with severe Parkinson's disease after implantation of fetal ventral mesencephalic tissue in cavity of caudate nucleus: 5-year follow up in 10 patients. Clinica Puerta de Hierro Neural Transplantation Group. *J. Neurosurg.* 86:931–942, 1997.

47. Wenning, G. K., Odin, P., Morrish, P., et al. Short- and long-term survival and function of unilateral intrastriatal dopaminergic grafts in Parkinson's disease. *Ann. Neurol.* 42:95–107, 1997.

48. Palmer, T. D., Takahashi, J., and Gage, F. H. The adult rat hippocampus contains primordial neural stem cells. *Mol. Cell. Neurosci.* 8:389–404, 1997.

49. Sah, D. W. Y., Ray, J., and Gage, F. H. Bipotent progenitor cell lines from human CNS. *Nat. Biotechnol.* 15:574–580, 1997.

50. Martínez-Serrano, A., and Björklund, A. Immortalized neural progenitor cells of CNS gene transfer and repair. *Trends Neurosci.* 20:530–538, 1997.

51. Martínez-Serrano, A., Fischer, W., Söderstrom, S. Ebendal, T., and Bjorkland, A. Long-term functional recovery from age-induced spatial impairments by nerve growth factor gene transfer to the rat basal forebrain. *Proc. Natl. Acad. Sci. USA* 93:6355–6360, 1996.

52. Deller, T., Frotscher, M., and Nitsch, R. Sprouting of crossed entorhinal-dentate fibers after an entorhinal lesion: Anterograde tracing of fiber reorganization with Phaseolus vulgar-leucoagglutin (PHAL). *J. Comp. Neurol.* 365:42–55, 1996.

53. Bregman, B. S., Kunkel-Bagden, E., Schnell, L., Dai, H. N., Gao, D., and Schwab, M. E. Recovery from spinal cord injury mediated by antibodies to neurite growth inhibitors. *Nature* 378:498–501, 1995.

54. Cotman, C. W., and Anderson, K. J. Synaptic plasticity and functional stabilization in the hippocampal formation: Possible role in Alzheimer's disease. In: S. Waxman (ed.), *Physiological Basis for Functional Recovery in Neurological Disease*. New York: Raven Press, 1988, pp. 313–336.

30

Biochemistry of Aging

Caleb E. Finch and George S. Roth

Basic Neurochemistry: Molecular, Cellular and Medical Aspects, 6th Ed., edited by G. J. Siegel et al. Published by Lippincott–Raven Publishers, Philadelphia, 1999. Correspondence to Caleb E. Finch, Neurogerontology Division, Andrus Gerontology Center and Department of Biological Sciences, University of Southern California, Los Angeles, California 90089-0191.

OVERVIEW ON AGING

Despite taxonomic diversity, general aging changes can be shown in short- and long-lived mammals

Most mammalian species share a canonical pattern of aging in the brain and other organs [1,2], which implies strong similarities in the putative genes that regulate the rates of aging. Although we focus on aging in mammals, other animal models are discussed below. These general features of aging emerge on a schedule that is scaled with the life span, which implies a genetic basis for molecular and cellular mechanisms in aging shared among mammals that has persisted during the last 100 million years of evolution. Nonetheless, individuals in each species and genotype show major differences in the outcomes of aging as a function of diet and other environmental factors.

Among general aging changes of mammalian brains are atrophy of pyramidal neurons, synaptic diminution, decrease of striatal dopamine (DA) receptors, accumulation of oxidation products and of pigments and increase of astrocyte and microglial activity (Tables 30-1 to 30-3). Moreover, nearly all mammals examined, with the notable exception of laboratory rodents, accumulate the amyloid β-peptide (Aβ) as extracellular deposits in the neuropil and cerebrovasculature (see Chap. 46), which constitute one of the diagnostic criteria for Alzheimer's disease (AD) in humans. Neurofibrillary tangles generally are not found outside of aging in humans, although aging rodents do show neurocytoskeletal abnormalities. A major goal in the study of the neurochemistry of aging is to identify mechanisms which are independent of Aβ. Because wild-type laboratory rodents do not accumulate Aβ in the brain during aging, we may conclude provisionally that neuronal atrophy and increased glial activities can arise from causes other than the accumulation of Aβ in the brain.

Extents of aging in species with different life spans often are compared in proportion to maximal life spans, not absolute ages, which implies assumptions about "the rate of aging." One might suppose that the threefold greater rates of glucose oxidation and protein synthesis per gram of brain tissue in rats compared to humans and macaques (p. 260 in [1]) are due to greater neuronal metabolism and, thereby, cause faster neuronal aging. However, oxygen consumption per neuron differs by <10% between rat and human. Thus, species differences in whole-brain metabolism may reflect neuronal density more than biosynthesis rates. Moreover, the general correlations between brain size, basal metabolism and life span in different orders of mammals encompass many exceptions and cannot be considered as arising from strict constraints (see pp. 251, 276–278 in [1]).

Aging changes involve gene–environment interactions

Aging processes are difficult to resolve into tractable hypotheses that can be tested experi-

TABLE 30-1. **COMPARATIVE BRAIN AGING IN MAMMALS: GENERAL CHARACTERISTICS**[a]

	Age-related changes of mammals scaled on a unit life span: a sampling	
	Midlife	Senescence
Reproduction	Menopause or total infertility in women, in association with imminent depletion of ovarian oocytes (C, D, Hm, H, P, M, Op, R, Wh)	Decreased male fertility (H, P, M, R)
Tumors	Many endocrine-related tumors of reproductive organs (H, P, M, R, D)	
Growth hormone		Decreased frequency of pulses: smaller amplitude (H, P, R)
Thermoregulation		Impaired response to cold (H, M, R), impaired febrile response (H, P)
Coronary and cerebral arteries	Early atherosclerotic lesions (H, M, R)	Widespread atherosclerosis (H, P, D, R, Rb, M)
Immune functions	Slow decline in humoral antibody production (H, P, R, M)	
Bone	Onset of osteoporosis (H, P, R, Rb, M)	Female osteoporosis > male (H, P, R, Rb, M)
Joints		Arthritic changes very common (C, D, H, M, R)
Reaction times		Generally slowed (H, R)
Vision		Universally decreased accommodation of eye (presbyopia) (H, P)
Hearing		Sporadic loss (H)
Striatal dopaminergic neurons	Onset of D2 receptor decline (H, M, P, R, Rb)	Dopamine conc. decline (H, M, R, Rb)
Large neurons		Heterogeneous changes; some show increased size and dendritic complexity; others show atrophy and dendritic withering (H, R, M)
Cerebrovascular β/A4		Widespread in absence of Alzheimer's disease (H, P, D)

[a] Onset of senescence in population (usual age, in years): C, cattle 15 to 25; D, dog 10 to 15; H, human 60 to 80; Hm, golden hamster 2 to 3; M, mouse 2 to 3; Op, opossum >2; P, (rhesus) monkey 20 to 30; R, rat 2 to 3; Rb, rabbit 4 to 6; Wh, pilot whale >40, uncertain.
Excerpted with permission of University of Chicago Press, from Finch [1], pp. 154–155 and [2].

TABLE 30-2. **NEURONAL ATROPHY AND NEUROPATHOLOGY**

Age-related change	Laboratory rodents	Dog	Primate	Normal human
Cholinergic forebrain neuron				
Atrophy	++/−	—	0	+
Hypertrophy	+/−	—	+	+
Hyperactivity of astrocytes/microglia	+	+	+	+
Neurofibrillary tangles (NFT) in cholinergic forebrain neurons	0	0	0	+
Senile plaques with β/A4 amyloid	0	+	+	+
Cerebrovascular amyloid	0	+	++	++
Cerebrovascular arteriosclerosis	+/−	+	++	+++

TABLE 30-3. AGE CHANGES IN RODENT STRIATUM, HIPPOCAMPUS AND NEUROMUSCULAR JUNCTION[a]

	Region		
	Striatum (ST)	Hippocampus (HC)	Neuromuscular junction (NMJ) (diaphragm)
Neuronal loss			
Intrinsic neurons	−20% Acetylcholinergic	−20% pyramidal (cholinoceptive)	Negligible
Afferent projections	−35 to 0% Nigrostriatal	−20 to 0% forebrain Acetylcholinergic	Negligible
Dopamine (DA) system			
Dopamine concentration	0 to −20%	—	—
D2 receptor mRNA	−20%	—	—
D2 receptor	−10 to −50%	—	—
DA uptake	−25 to 0%	—	—
DA release			
K$^+$ induced	0	—	—
Muscarinic (M$_2$)	Less sensitive	—	—
D2	0	—	—
Cholinergic system			
Choline acetyltransferase	—	−50 to +35%	—
Acetylcholinesterase	—	−25 to 0%	+35%
Muscarinic receptor			
M$_1$	0	0	—
M$_2$	−40%	−50%	—
M$_1$ mRNA	0	0	—
Nicotinic receptor	−40%	−50%	+35%[b]
Choline uptake	−20 to 0%	−20 to 0%	+35%
Acetylcholine release, basal depolarization	0	0	—
by K$^+$	−30%	−30%	—
Nicotinic	—	Less sensitive	—
M$_2$ autoreceptor	More sensitive	Less sensitive	—
MEPP[c]	—	—	0

[a] Data from literature compare changes in 24- to 30-month-old (life span) vs. 3- to 6-month-old (young adult) male rats and mice.
[b] α-Bungarotoxin binding.
[c] Miniature end plate potentials.

mentally. The nervous system, like other organs, displays complex age-related changes that arise from environmental interactions across the life span. For example, humans show increased risk of depression and mortality after death of a spouse; the impact from death of long-term cage mates in multiply housed rodents is unknown. Therefore, it is important to account for individual changes during aging in the experimental design. However, some brain aging processes show trends that are general enough for molecular and genetic analyses. Overall, the nervous system shows a remarkable ability to compensate for minor changes or even major injury throughout life.

CELL NUMBERS

The distinction between neuronal loss and neuronal atrophy during aging is a major issue

Most brain neurons in mammals are postmitotic and, thus, at risk for irreversible damage that will be more long-lasting to functionality than damage in organs with cell replacement, such as liver or skin. The old tenet of massive neocortical and hippocampal neuronal loss during aging is not supported by rigorous analyses of individuals without stroke or other neurodegenerative diseases by the optical dissector method [3,3a]. Many early studies on brain aging changes were confounded by unrecognized pathological lesions. The distinction between aging and disease in the brain, as in other organs, is often subtle. Figure 30-1 shows neuron counts in the hippocampus of humans and rats, species which have minimal loss during aging; however, the subiculum shows a trend for neuronal loss in humans but not in rodents. Another example is that the gonadotropin-releasing hormone (GnRH)-containing neurons in the hypothalamus, which drive ovulatory surges of gonadotropins, show no evidence of being lost during the loss of estrous cycle in reproductive aging (see p. 184 in [1]).

Because cell counts are easily biased toward larger neurons, atrophy has been misinterpreted as cell loss [2]. Neuronal atrophy during aging generally is reported as a decrease of mean perikaryal area. However, a few studies have shown that the mean perikaryal area decrease is the result of an increase of small neurons at the expense of the large [2,4]. By microspectrophotometry, brains from normal, elderly individuals and from individuals with AD often show nucleolar shrinkage or loss of cell body RNA in large neurons [2]. Nucleolar shrinkage probably represents reduced ribosomal RNA synthesis. In some specimens, the losses may represent early stages of AD and other diseases, which were not severe enough to be diagnosed. However, some neurons, human basal forebrain cholinergic neurons, show hypertrophy during normal aging, which contrasts with atrophy of these neurons in rodents [2].

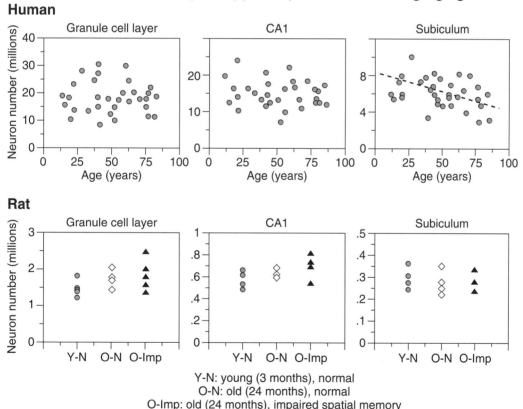

FIGURE 30-1. Neuron number during aging. At least some hippocampal neuronal populations show no loss during normal aging in humans and rats, as analyzed by the rigorous morphometric technique optical dissection. Subicular neurons in humans, however, show a trend of age-related loss. Old rats classified behaviorally as having normal or impaired spatial memory did not differ in hippocampal number. (Redrawn from West [3] and Rasmussen et al. [3a] with permission.)

Very long-term responses to 6-hydroxydopamine are a model for neuronal atrophy during aging and in Parkinson's disease

During Parkinson's disease (PD), nucleoli shrink in the surviving neurons of the substantia nigra compacta (SNC) and dopaminergic activity is decreased [2]. In contrast, in a lesion model, increased synthesis and release of DA and increased tyrosine hydroxylase (TH) activity are seen, indicating DA hyperactivity. In this model, adult rats were given unilateral injections of the neurotoxin 6-hydroxydopamine (6-OHDA) and sacrificed 9 months later. Striatal DA initially was depleted on the lesioned side, with increased 3,4-dihydroxyphenylacetic acid (DOPAC):DA ratios; this latter change indicates increased DA release at the surviving striatal terminals. SNC dopaminergic cell bodies that survived the 6-OHDA lesion showed cell atrophy, with 30% shrinkage of cell bodies, nuclei and nucleoli of TH-immunoreactive neurons compared to the contralateral (nonlesioned) side; similar atrophy occurs during PD. The nucleolar shrinkage implies decreased synthesis of ribosomes, which would be consistent with loss of neuronal RNA in the substantia nigra during PD. Moreover, the striatum is the only major brain region to show a loss of bulk RNA during normal aging [2]. By *in situ* hybridization, TH mRNA decreased to a deficit of >80% on the lesioned side. The SNC of PD shows a similar loss of TH mRNA [2]. Despite the 80% loss of nigral TH mRNA 9 months after lesioning, the striatum showed complete recovery of TH protein and activity. These slowly developing changes suggest a need for prolonged studies to model human neurological diseases spanning a decade or more.

Glial hyperactivity generally is observed during aging but not always with irreversible neurodegeneration

Astrocytic hyperactivity in aging is seen in healthy humans and laboratory rodents, with 10 to 30% increases in astrocyte volume occurring during aging, in association with increased cellular expression of the intermediate filament glial fibrillary acidic protein (GFAP) and GFAP mRNA [4,5]. While astrocytes in the adult brain may proliferate as well as migrate from other brain regions, in the hippocampus of aging rats the numbers of astrocytes change much less than the increases in GFAP. It is unlikely that the astrocytic hyperactivity is caused by neurodegenerative events, since in rodents astrocytic hyperactivity starts by middle age [3,3a,5], when there is little evidence for neurodegeneration.

Microglia are of interest because of their similarity to bone marrow-derived macrophages, their presence in degenerating brain regions during PD and AD and their capacity to produce reactive oxygen species and cytokines, which have important influences on neighboring neurons and astrocytes. In AD brains, microglia, like astrocytes, are clustered around the amyloid-containing senile plaques, which suggests their participation in inflammatory processes [6]. Moreover, resident microglia contain mRNA for C1q, a complement protein [6]. Microglial numbers appear to increase during normal aging [5], although the data are relatively limited.

The molecular mechanisms of glial hyperactivity may include oxidative damage since age changes in astrocytes and microglia are slowed by diet restriction [5]. As discussed below, diet restriction slows some oxidative aspects of aging that could be factors in AD-related changes and other age-related neurodegenerations with more anatomical specificity. Other astrocytic changes may be related to elevations of glucocorticoids [7,8].

Transgenic mice provide models of age-related neurodegeneration

A major new focus of transgenic technology includes attempts to develop a murine model of AD that shows age-related increases of the Aβ peptide in the brain in association with neuronal dysfunction. After many frustrations, several transgenic murine models show pertinent features as a function of increased age. For example, overexpression of mutant human amyloid precursor protein (APP695) induced Aβ deposits in cortical and limbic structures and behavioral deficits in spatial and alternation tasks [9,9a]. Other transgenes with normal human APP751, but not

APP695, showed Aβ deposits and abnormalities in the microtubule-associated protein tau (Alz50 immunoreactivity) in association with behavioral impairments [10]. Transgenic mice that express the normal human APP695 and mutant presenilin-1 (PS1), which is a familial risk factor (see Chap. 46), also show increased hippocampal Aβ [11]. The extensive inflammatory proteins and other proteins found in senile plaques [6] have not been reported in these transgenic animals. Transgenic mice that express up to sevenfold increased levels of S100β, a calcium-binding protein which can affect survival of neurons, had no detectable effect on APP transcription [12].

Transgenic mice that overexpress the bcl-2 proto-oncogene are protected against apoptotic neuronal death [13]. The increase of apoptotic neurons in the rat striatum during aging [14] may be pertinent to the loss of dopamine-2 receptor (D2R)-containing neurons during aging since exposure of primary striatal neuronal cultures to DA also induced apoptotic death [15]. Death is prevented by antioxidants, such as *N*-acetylcysteine and catalase, which is consistent with the production of free radicals by the spontaneous auto-oxidation of DA. Mice transgenic for the human Cu-Zn superoxide dismutase have less 4-hydroxy-2-nonenol at 25 months than normal mice, suggesting increased protection against free radical-induced lipid peroxidation [16]. In addition, similar mice showed protection against age-related neurotensin receptor loss in selected brain regions [17]. Thus, free radical damage may be critical in the degeneration and death of various neuronal populations (see also Chaps. 34 and 45).

PLASTICITY AND AGING

How aging impairs neuronal plasticity is one of the major themes in neurogerontology

This question is pertinent both to changes in memory during normal aging and to the extreme deficits in AD. Sprouting is one measure of plasticity. Some neurons retain considerable capacity for sprouting, as shown by aberrant sprouting responses during AD, wherein abnormal looking neurites appear in senile plaques and neurons sprout in response to the loss of afferents (see Chaps. 29 and 46). At the electrophysiological level, frequency and post-tetanic potentiation show consistent impairment in aging rat hippocampus [18].

Responses to deafferenting lesions may show age changes that are specific for brain regions and genotype or species. Aging male rats show slower responses in collateral sprouting after lesions of the entorhinal cortex or septum that deafferented the hippocampus [18a], which has heterotypic and homotypic reinnervation, with marked impairment in the induction of growth-associated protein of 43 kDa (GAP-43) mRNA [19]. In general, 2-year-old rats eventually recovered as many synapses as the young after 3 to 6 months (see Chap. 29). Larger impairments of plasticity are shown by the superior cervical ganglia (SCG), in which explants from young rats showed fivefold increases of substance P, whereas 2-year-old rats showed no elevations [20]. Extensive heterogeneity in sprouting responses among individual old rats could be a consequence of differences in age-related pathological lesions, such as pituitary tumors and kidney lesions [1,2].

Many adaptive hormonal and cellular responses are slowed during aging

These include the slower induction of liver enzymes during metabolic stresses [1]. Several genes have altered expression in liver because of age changes in hormonal regulation, rather than fundamental impairments in the genomic apparatus. By analogy, we may consider age changes in circulating hormones as well as locally acting paracrine and autocrine growth factors as involved in slowed sprouting responses. One candidate in slowed synaptic sprouting responses is corticosterone, which slows the rate of synaptic replacement [8,21]. Most rat strains show a strong trend for increased blood corticosterone during aging [7,8] in contrast to little or no change in C57BL/6J mice [8]. Gonadal steroids have complex effects on sprouting, with gender differences and interactions with adrenal steroids [21]. Deficits of testosterone, which are common in old rats with testicular tumors, may explain the loss of vasopressin fibers in many limbic regions, which was reversed in limbic regions by testosterone implants within 1 month [22]. See Chapter 49 for details of adrenal and gonadal steroids in the brain.

The supersensitization, or upregulation, of receptors in response to chronic treatment with antagonists is partially impaired

Impairment is observed in three neural systems of aging rodents: striatal D2R, in response to haloperidol [23], pineal β-adrenergic receptors in response to reserpine or constant light [23] and cortical muscarinic receptors in response to oxotremorine [24]. In contrast to impaired supersensitization, receptor downregulation by agonists generally shows no age changes. Effects of aging on the regulation of receptor gene expression by agonists and antagonists have not been examined in detail.

NEUROTRANSMITTERS AND RECEPTORS

The loss of cholinergic markers during Alzheimer's disease and aging has led to the cholinergic hypothesis of memory deficits

Cholinergic functions, which are quantitatively minor among other brain neurotransmitters, are studied intensively because of this hypothesis [25]. In general, aging changes in neurotransmitters and receptors are selective in rodents and neurologically normal humans. Many changes are not consistent even in the same species, for example, whether cholinergic forebrain neurons atrophy or hypertrophy at different times during aging [2]. The largest age changes, however, are relatively modest by comparison with the major (>90%) loss of basal ganglia DA during PD (see Chap. 45) and the variable (25 to 90%) loss of choline acetyltransferase (ChAT) and other cholinergic markers during AD (see Chap. 46) [23,25]. A key point is that receptor affinity as measured by ligand binding does not change markedly with aging.

Age-related changes in synaptic chemistry and physiology are robust phenomena in a few neural systems, in which the scheme from gene expression to synaptic functions is partly mapped for aging changes [23–26]. Hippocampus (HC), striatum (ST) and cerebral cortex (CTX) of aging rodents show different features of cholinergic aging, in conjunction with changes in anatomy and other neurotransmitters, particularly DA (Table 30-4).

The ST has some of the most consistent neurochemical aging changes in mammals. Progressive declines of D2R are shown by ligand binding in mice, rats, rabbits and human brain and by positron emission tomographic (PET) imaging (see Chap. 54) in humans [25,26]. These declines can be detected during midlife, when they are not confounded by age-related pathology, and appear to be progressive, reaching net decreases of 20 to 40% by the life span. DA loss is smaller and more irregular in rodents than in humans but far less in any case during aging than in PD [2,23]. The loss of D2R is paralleled by a decrease of D2R mRNA in aging rodents [15]. These changes are attributed to two causes: a 20% loss of intrinsic ST cholinergic neurons, a major location of the D2R, and a slowed synthesis of the D2R. Despite their 10 to 50% decrease, D2R show no age-related dysfunctions in the sensitivity of DA release to haloperidol in perfused slices. Impairments in DA-activated adenylyl cyclase (see Chap. 12) are reported consistently, but there is no consensus on age changes in the D1R.

Cholinergic controls over transmitter release show marked but selective impairments of DA and acetylcholine (ACh) release in ST and of ACh release in HC and CTX of aging rats. The details of cholinergic receptor types are discussed in Chapter 11. Most reports agree on sizable age-related decreases in nicotinic and muscarinic M_2-binding sites in HC, CTX and ST [23,24,27]. Although no age changes are found in mRNAs for some M_1, M_3 and M_4 receptors in ST or in other brain regions, the mRNA for the M_2R has not been resolved for possible effects of age. Major impairments were identified with the M_2 control of DA release. Muscarinic control of ACh release, presumably via M_2 autoreceptors,

TABLE 30-4. **AGE-RELATED CHANGES IN MAMMALIAN BRAIN NEUROTRANSMITTERS, RE-CEPTORS AND RESPONSES**[a]

Region	Species/strain	Finding
	Acetylcholine	
Cortex, striatum, hippocampus/membrane	F344 and Wistar rats	No change in strain differences in ChAT, AChE and QNB binding
Neostriatal slices	F344 rats	↓Oxo-m-inhibited ACh release
Slices	F344 rats	↓KCl-stimulated ACh release
Striata (microdialysis)	F344 rats	↓KCl-stimulated ACh release
Cortical synaptosomes	Mice	↓KCl-stimulated ACh release
Striatal slices	Wistar rats	↓Muscarinic enhancement of KCl-evoked DA release
Cortex, striatum, ventral forebrain sections	Wistar rats	[3H]QNB-binding sites
Cortex, striatum, hippocampus/synaptosomes	C57/BL mice, F344 rats	↓[3H]QNB-binding sites and high-affinity form of receptor
Cortex	Sprague-Dawley rats	↓High-affinity nicotinic sites
Cortex, striatum	Human (PET)	↓[11C]methylbenzotropine sites
Neocortex/membranes	Rhesus monkeys	↓High-affinity form of M_1 receptor
Striatal slices	Wistar rats	↓Muscarinic enhancement of KCl-evoked DA release, M_1 and M_2 binding sites
Cortex, thalamus/synaptosomes	Human	↓M_1/M_2 in cortex and thalamus, same pattern for nicotinic receptors
Cortex, hippocampus/slices	F344 rats	↓IP_4 by carbachol
Striatal membranes	Wistar rats	↓Carbachol stimulation of low K_m GTPase
Cortical neurons	NMRI mice, dissociated cells	↑IP production by carbachol
Caudate/putamen accumbens	F344 rats	↓QNB binding
Cortex/synaptosomes	Wistar rats	↓Carbachol-stimulated arachidonic acid uptake
Cortex, striatum, hippocampus/slices	F344 rats	↓Carbachol-stimulated IP production
Hippocampus/temporal cortex slices	Long-Evans rats	↑Aged/impaired had carbachol-stimulated IP
	Dopamine	
Caudate, putamen	Human (PET)	No differences for [18F]fluorodopa uptake
Striatum	Wistar rats	Decreased DA, increased DOPAC:HVA ratio
Striatum	F344 rats	Decreased [3H]mazindol and [3H]DA binding
Caudate, putamen	Human postmortem tissue	Decreased DA and HVA:DA ratio
Substantia nigra	Human postmortem tissue	Decreased mRNA for DA transporter
Striatum	Human (PET)	Decreased [18F]fluorodopa uptake
Striatum	Wistar rats	Decreased turnover of DA
Striatum (microdialysis)	F344 rats	Decreased amphetamine-stimulated DA release
Striatum	Wistar rats	Decreased D2R and DA neurons
Striatum	Wistar rats	Decreased D2R-binding sites
Striatum	Wistar rats	Decreased D2R mRNA
Substantia nigra	Human postmortem tissue	No change in D1R or D2R-binding sites
Striatum, cortex, hippocampus	F344 rats	Decreased D1R stimulation of IP production
Striatum, substantia nigra, nucleus accumbens	Sprague-Dawley rats	Decreased receptor turnover
Striatum, hippocampus	Sprague-Dawley rats	Decreased D2R mRNA and D2L:D_2S ratio
Striatum	Human (PET)	Decreased D2R-binding sites
Striatum, frontal cortex	Human (PET)	Decreased D2R-binding sites
Striatum, substantia nigra	Wistar Kyoto rats	Decreased D2R mRNA in striatum

continued

Region	Species/strain	Finding
Caudate/putamen, cortex	Wistar rats	Decreased D1R-binding sites in nucleus accumbens, caudate, putamen; increased D1R-binding sites in parietal cortex
Striatum	Human (PET study)	Decreased D2R-binding sites
	GABA	
Inferior collicus	Sprague-Dawley/F344 rats	Decreased $GABA_A$ receptor-binding sites and GAD mRNA
Hippocampus membranes	F344 and Wistar rats	Increased high-affinity benzodiazepine-binding sites
Cortex	Wistar rats	Decreased $GABA_A$ receptor-binding sites, no change in benzodiazepine sites
	Glutamate	
Cortex, septum, hippocampus/synaptosomes	Wistar Kyoto and Brown Norway rats	No change in glutamate uptake with or without stress
Cortex, striatum, nucleus basalis, amygdala, thalamus/synaptosomes	Wistar rats	Decreased aspartate uptake between 4 and 12 months, no additional decrease after 12 months
Cortex	F344/Brown Norway rats	No change in aspartate uptake or KCl-evoked glutamate release
Telencephalon	Mice	Decreased immunoreactive AMPA-binding sites
Hippocampus	Wistar rats	Decreased mRNA for AMPA, Glu1, Glu2
Hippocampus, cortex slices	Long-Evans rats	Increased ACPD-stimulated IP_3 and DAG
Hippocampus	Human (postmortem)	No change in NMDA-, AMPA- or kainate-binding sites
Hippocampus	Rhesus and cynomolgus monkeys	Decreased NMDA-binding sites using monoclonal antibody for NMDA R1
	Serotonin	
Cortical slices	F344 rats	Decreased KCl-stimulated 5-HT release, PKC activity and PMA-stimulated translocation of PKC
Striatum, hippocampus, cortex	Han Wistar rats	Decreased 5-HT and 5-HIAA
Striatum	Human (PET)	Decreased S2-binding sites
Cortex	Human (postmortem)	Decreased $5-HT_{1D}$- and $5-HT_2$-binding sites
Cortex, nucleus accumbens	F344 rats	Decrease $5-HT_{2A}$-binding sites
Cortex/synaptosomes	Wistar rats	Decreased 5-HT-stimulated arachidonic acid uptake
Cortex	Human (PET)	Decreased S2-binding sites
	Norepinephrine	
Cortex	NMRI mice	Increased NE
Olfactory bulb	F344 rats	Increased NE, decreased MHPG
Cortex	Wistar rats	Decreased α_1-adrenergic receptors, increased NE stimulation of IP
Striatum	Wistar rats	Decreased NE-stimulated low K_m GTPase
Cortex	Human (postmortem)	Decreased α_2-adrenergic receptors
Cortex and hypothalamus	Human (postmortem)	Decreased high-affinity form of α_2-adrenergic receptors and G_i

[a] ChAT, choline acetyltransferase; AChE, acetylcholinesterase; ACh, acetylcholine; QNB, quinuclidinyl benzilate; DA, dopamine; IP, inositol phosphate; PET, positron emission tomography; DOPAC, 3,4-dihydroxyphenylacetic acid; HVA, homovanillic acid; GABA, γ-aminobutyric acid; GAD, glutamic acid decarboxylase; DAG, diacylglycerol; NMDA, N-methyl-D-aspartate; 5-HT, 5-hydroxytryptamine; PKC, protein kinase C; PMA, phorbol myristate acetate; 5-HIAA, 5-hydroxyindoleacetic acid; NE, norepinephrine; MHPG, 3-methoxylyhydroxyphenylglycol; Oxo-m, oxotremorine; AMPA, α-amino-3-hydroxy-5-methyl-4-isoxazole-4-proprionic acid; ACPD, aminocyclopentyl dicarboxylic acid. Table adapted from [25], which provides full references.

had a different pattern, with no age change in ST but marked impairments in HC and neocortex [25] (Fig. 30-2). These regional differences imply that the M_2 sites lost with aging in ST are not on local cholinergic neurons.

Postsynaptic receptor defects are implicated in several aging changes in HC, CTX and ST [25]. Unit recordings show a repeatable decrease in sensitivity of HC neurons to ACh *in vivo* and *in vitro*. The low-affinity GTPase activity stimulated by carbachol or oxotremorine was impaired by ≥30% in HC and ST. Of the many G proteins (described in Chap. 20), only the GTP-binding subunits $G_{\alpha i}$ and $G_{\alpha o}$ have been assayed; these showed no age change in ST or HC. In ST, in contrast to the reduced sensitivity to muscarinic agonists, the calcium ionophore A23087 and the signal transducer inositol 1,4,5-trisphosphate (IP_3) (Chap. 21) showed no age impairment in enhancing K^+-stimulated DA release. Reports of age changes in ACh-stimulated phosphoinositide metabolism (see Chap. 21) are not consistent. An impairment of Ca^{2+} regulation is implied at the ligand–muscarinic receptor interface.

Moreover, there are age-related changes of intraneuronal Ca^{2+} metabolism in HC and elsewhere. For example, Ca^{2+}-dependent, K^+-mediated afterhyperpolarization increases by 50% with age, as measured in HC slices [7,18]. Changes in corticosteroids and other hormones may contribute to disturbances in local or even systemic Ca^{2+} and inorganic phosphate (P_i) homeostasis during normal aging and AD [7,28]. Renal lesions and elevations of parathyroid and calcitonin hormones are common in aging rats [1] and may interact with brain aging. Normal intracellular Ca^{2+} regulation is detailed in Chapter 23.

Nerve growth factor (NGF) treatment partially reversed the perikaryal atrophy in cholinergic projections to the HC in aging rats and improved learning performance [2,29]. ChAT in the rat ST retains responsiveness to NGF throughout the life span and may even become more sensitive [2]. In view of the lack of change in NGF mRNA in aging rats or in AD, aging in these systems may not be attributed to deficits of NGF. There is some evidence of age-related diminution of the norepinephrine, serotonin, glutamate and GABA systems; as found for DA and cholinergic systems, these changes show regional differences [25,26].

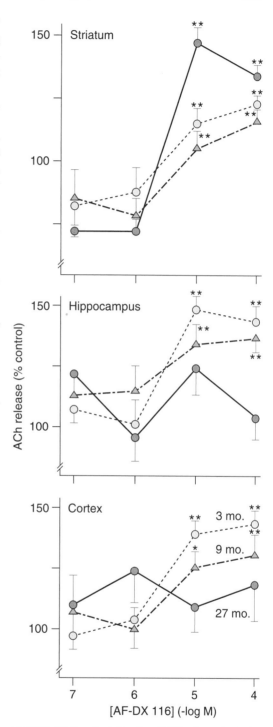

FIGURE 30-2. Acetylcholine *(ACh)* release by brain slices at increasing concentrations of the muscarinic agonist AF-DX 116 relative to controls (100%). Slices were taken from the indicated brain regions of male rats at the indicated ages. In cortex and hippocampus, slices from 27-month-old rats showed no enhancement of ACh release by AF-DX 116, whereas the striatum became more sensitive. (Redrawn from Araujo et al. [27] with permission.)

AGING PIGMENTS AND MEMBRANES

Intracellular pigments, such as lipofuscins and neuromelanins, show cell-type specificity and little relation to neuronal death

The accumulation of aging pigments or lipofuscin was historically one of the first brain aging changes to be established. These heterogeneous intracellular deposits include complex lipids, lysosome-type hydrolases and other proteins. They slowly accumulate in the myocardium and neurons throughout the body at rates that are cell-specific [1,2,30]. Aging pigments have a notable autofluorescence at 430 to 470 nm and may be iminopropenes. Despite the limited biochemistry, most distinguish the *lipofuscin* aging pigments from the *neuromelanins*. Neuromelanin granules accumulate from birth onward in the substantia nigra and certain other neurons of humans; in contrast, laboratory rodents do not have neuromelanins. Despite their accumulation, aging pigments show little toxicity. In the human inferior olivary nucleus, aging pigment depots grow large enough at late ages to displace the cell nucleus, yet the inferior olive shows no neuronal loss [2].

The accumulation rate of aging pigment may be related to cell activity. For example, in a 71-year-old woman who lost one eye at age 16, the alternate layers of the lateral geniculate differed in aging pigment, corresponding to the separation of optic fibers from each eye [1]. The protease inhibitor leupeptin rapidly causes pigment accumulation in brain and retina [30], which implicates inefficient protein-degradative pathways. This fits with DeDuve's lysosomal hypothesis about the origin of aging pigments. Conversely, aging pigment accumulation is inhibited in rodents by diet restriction, vitamin E and ergots [1].

Brain membrane compositional changes may influence membrane fluidity

Membranes in many cell types show trends for complex changes in composition and biophysical properties [31,32]. Of potential importance are the "lipid substitution groups" defined by G. Rouser [32a], for example, cerebrosides and sphingomyelin increase at the expense of phosphatidylcholine in human brain during aging. Oligodendroglia may be a source of increased myelin since the myelin around the pyramidal tracts continues to thicken long after maturation. A potentially important change is decreased brain membrane fluidity, which may influence receptor functions [31,32].

Vascular membrane changes may alter microperfusion and may contribute to brain age changes

Cerebrovascular atherosclerosis is ubiquitous to some degree in humans but is not recognized as a dysfunctional lesion in aging rodents. However, the microvasculature shows a general trend for increased hyalinization and histochemical staining with the periodic acid Schiff (PAS) reagent in normal human and rodent brain [2]. These histochemical changes imply alterations in basement membrane carbohydrates, which might alter local microperfusion without much change in regional blood flow (see Chap. 2).

ENERGY METABOLISM

Humans are the best characterized for resting brain metabolism during aging [33]. In neurologically normal individuals, basal cerebral glucose and oxygen consumption show modest declines of 10 to 30% over the life span (see Chaps. 31 and 54). These decreases are in the range of decreases in cerebral blood flow and of parenchymal atrophy. Overall, age contributes much less to the total variance than do intersubject variations. However, correlations in metabolism between cortical regions may be stronger in young adults than in the elderly, which implies decreased integration of cortical functions and would be consistent with the subtle age-related alterations in cognitive functions. These changes of normal aging are clearly distinct from the larger decreases of AD, which are associated with major atrophy and loss of neurons [31,33].

INSTABILITY IN THE NUCLEAR AND MITOCHONDRIAL GENOMES

Age-related changes show cell-type specificity

Two types of DNA damage have been found in the aging brain: I-spots, or chemically modified DNA bases [34], and mitochondrial DNA (mtDNA) deletions [35]. Neither type of lesion is detected in fetal brain, and both appear to accumulate slowly during adult life. I-spots in DNA from the cell nucleus result from treatment with chemical carcinogens in tissues with dividing cells. mtDNA deletions cause some degenerative diseases of muscle, such as Kearne-Sayers disease, through inhibiting oxidative phosphorylation (see Chap. 42). Age-related accumulation of mtDNA deletions is >100-fold more common in the DA-rich basal ganglia than in the cerebral CTX or cerebellum [ref. in 35], which is consistent with the suspected production of free radical damage by DA (see Chap. 45). However, remarkably low levels of mtDNA deletions are found during aging in the free radical-rich environment of the human retina [35]. The distribution of mtDNA deletions and DNA adducts among types of brain cell is unknown.

The Brattleboro rat strain has well-known deficiencies of vasopressin, which result from a frameshift mutation that prevents intracellular processing through the translated but abnormal C-terminal glycoprotein. However, from birth onward, the Brattleboro hypothalamus shows an increased number of solitary neurons with normal vasopressin and C-terminal glycoprotein [36]; these cells are hemizygous for the mutant and revertant protein (Fig. 30-3). cDNA cloned by polymerase chain reaction from older Brattleboro rats showed that reversions arose from further deletions. These remarkable findings were extended to normal proteins that acquire frameshifts during aging in the human hypothalamus [36] and Alzheimer brain [36a]. The mechanisms are not known, but appear to be post-transcriptional and sporadic at the cellular level [36a,37].

Demethylation of the rare nuclear DNA dinucleotide ^{Me}CpG during aging may be important in changes in gene expression. Loss of

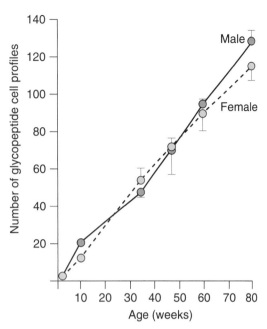

FIGURE 30-3.   Age-related increase of vasopressin-immunopositive hypothalamic neurons of Brattleboro rats which have a frameshift mutation in the vasopressin gene. Immunopositive neurons are represented by an increase of glycopeptide. All profiles on the ordinate axis. (From van Leewen et al. [53] with permission.)

^{Me}C in many vertebrate cells during differentiation often is correlated with increased gene expression. Several reports show age-related loss of methylation from nuclear DNA [1]. A comparison of brain DNA demethylation in two species showed a progressive loss of ^{Me}C that was faster in laboratory mice, which live half as long, than in *Peromyscus leucopus,* white-footed mice. Age-related loss of ^{Me}C could alter transcription by changing interactions of ^{Me}C-containing sequences with DNA-binding proteins.

GENE EXPRESSION

mRNA levels also show cell-type selectivity during aging

Evidence is now very strong that most age changes in transcription differ between cell types and are highly selective. The contrary belief was challenged by assaying the sequence complexity of brain polysomal poly(A)RNA populations.

Assay by saturation hybridization of mRNA to single-copy DNA estimates the number of different mRNA types, termed *complexity*. During development, brain and other organs show major shifts in mRNA subsets. However, there is no change in whole-brain mRNA mass or sequence inventory, termed *kinetic complexity*, during the life span as analyzed in two rat strains [4]. Brain cells still look like brain cells, even at the most advanced ages or in cases of AD. This implies the persistent expression of genes that specify cell-type mRNAs. Individual genes, however, show a range of changes, as shown in the following three examples.

Pro-opiomelanocortin (POMC) is a steroid-regulated neuropeptide precursor (detailed in Chap. 18) that decreases with aging in mice and rats and that shows age changes in post-translational processing, with increased levels of antagonist and *N*-acetylated forms that could be factors in the age-related impairment of gonadotropins [37a,38]. Moreover, hypothalamic POMC mRNA responsiveness to estrogen is lost at middle age (Fig. 30-4), when hypothala-

mic controls on the pituitary–ovary axis also are impaired [37a]. Because estrogen influences POMC transcription and because of decreased ovarian estrogen production during aging, it is necessary to control for changes in hormonal status. These data also show the importance of including intermediate ages to resolve whether the age change was progressive and related to maturation or to old age.

Cell-specific changes in different isoforms are shown by changes of mRNAs encoding Na,K-ATPase isoforms in aging rat cerebellum [39]. In young rats, $\alpha 1$ mRNA was prominent in the granular layer (GL) and less in molecular (ML) and Purkinje cell layers (PCL) and white matter (WM); during aging, $\alpha 1$ mRNA declined in GL, increased in WM but did not change in ML or PCL. With aging, $\alpha 3$ mRNA decreased by >80% in ML, PCL, Purkinje cells and GL but increased in WM (see Chap. 5). Such selective alterations may be due to signal-transduction processes that mediate motor control.

GFAP mRNA increases with age in hippocampus and other brain regions in association

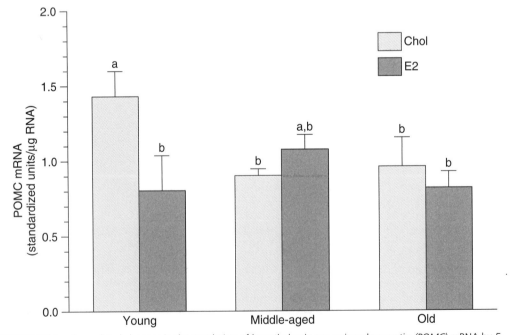

FIGURE 30-4. Age-related changes in the regulation of hypothalamic pro-opiomelanocortin *(POMC)* mRNA by E_2 (estradiol). Ovariectomized C57BL/6J mice of three ages (young, 4 months; middle-aged, 13 months; old, 25 months) were given 3 days of implants with *CHOL* (cholesterol) or E_2 (physiological concentrations). The middle-aged and old mice had lower levels of POMC mRNA that did not decrease further with E_2. (From Karelus and Nelson [37a].)

with the astrocytic hyperactivity of aging [4,5]. *In situ* hybridization for GFAP introns suggests that GFAP transcription is increased during aging [5]. This evidence for increased GFAP transcription during aging in the brain contrasts with the declining expression of many other genes in liver and other non-neural tissues [4,5]. Oxidative stress may be a factor because the increase of GFAP expression is delayed by food restriction (see below).

Age-related changes in gene expression may be mediated by steroid receptors

Age changes in gene expression may involve alteration in sex steroid receptors and other nuclear proteins which bind to specific DNA sequences as *trans*-acting regulators of transcription (see Chap. 49). Nuclear estrogen receptors (E_2R-α) consistently decrease in number in the hypothalamus of aging female rodents [37a,40,41]. A 35% loss of neurons containing β-endorphin suggests that neuronal loss could be a factor since these neurons also contain E_2R. Moreover, the nuclear retention of E_2 is shorter by middle age in female mice, which suggests the hypothesis that altered nuclear receptor dynamics cause the failure of E_2 to induce POMC (Fig. 30-4). In turn, dysregulation of POMC could impair the luteinizing hormone surge at middle age. The presence of multiple E_2Rs in the nucleus and membranes of cells in the brain and elsewhere (see Chap. 49) is expected to bear significance in aging research.

The two receptors for adrenal steroids are being studied during aging: mineralocorticoid and glucocorticoid receptors. Both receptor types show fairly consistent 35% decreases in hippocampus of aging male rats [8,41]. The loss of receptors may be greatest in the pyramidal layers, which also show neuronal loss. In the male rat hypothalamus, glucocorticoid receptors are also lost. Major open questions in transcriptional regulation in the brain during aging are the contributions of neuronal loss to receptor decreases and whether there are age changes in the interactions of receptors and DNA response elements.

PROTEINS

Altered proteins may increase through oxidative damage

Oxidation of proteins is prominent in the aging of many types of animal. In mammals, flies and nematodes, a portion of cellular enzymes becomes oxidized and inactive, although immunologically detectable [1,4,5,42,43]. Free radical-mediated oxidation may inactivate enzymes in brain and other tissues. Moreover, α-phenyl-*N*-tert-butylnitrone (PBN), a free radical quencher, reversed protein oxidation and improved learning in brains of middle-aged gerbils [42]. The causes of oxidation and other post-translational modifications during aging are unknown but may include the results of cumulative exposure to endogenous blood glucose, which tends to increase slowly during aging and to cause glycoxidation of proteins [44].

Slowing of protein synthesis could be a factor in slowed axoplasmic flow

Many studies conclude from the incorporation of amino acids that protein synthesis is slowed with age in brain and other organs of rodents by 20 to 50% [1,2,4]. The slowed axoplasmic transport in the sciatic nerve [45] is also generally consistent with slowed protein synthesis (see Chap. 28). However, because few brain mRNAs or enzymes show decreases with age, the rates of degradation must also be slowed to maintain steady state. Another outcome of slowed turnover might be the accumulation of intraneuronal proteins, such as neurofibrillary tangle (NFT) proteins in AD. In general, long-lived proteins are at risk for the accumulation of oxidative damage, as shown in detail for extracellular collagen. Glycoxidation occurs in senile plaques and NFT [44].

EXPERIMENTAL MANIPULATIONS OF BRAIN AGING

Diet restriction and hypophysectomy delay aging in many organs of rodents

Diet has major influences on aging in rodents, as represented by slowed aging in many peripheral tissues from diet restriction, in which rats are allowed 10 to 40% less than *ad libitum* intake but without deficiencies of micronutrients. Diet-restricted rats have impaired reproduction but are otherwise extremely healthy and, in parallel with the delay of age-related pathology, have increased life spans [1,4]. In the brain, diet restriction slowed the age-related loss of the D2R [5], as well the increased transcription of GFAP in the aging rat hippocampus [5]. Moreover, diet restriction also retards the normal age-related increases in protein carbonyl content of various mouse brain regions, especially the striatum [46]. These results are consistent with the retardation of striatal D2R loss and the protection against possible DA oxidation-related toxicity toward striatal neurons [47,48] discussed above. Diet restriction retarded the age-associated decline in mouse sensorimotor coordination while improving avoidance learning, also consistent with maintenance of motor function in rats [23,48]. Diet-restricted mice also have less 8-OH-guanosine, a product of DNA oxidation in various tissues including brain [47], and less of the oxidative age pigment lipofuscin [48]. Diet-restricted rats show less age-related production of reactive oxygen species in cortical synaptosomal membranes [32]. Both diet restriction and hypophysectomy also slow a demyelinating disease of spinal roots in aging rats, radiculoneuropathy, that may cause hindlimb paralysis [44]. The mechanisms are unclear but could arise from common effects of hypophysectomy and diet restriction on glucose metabolism.

Some hypothalamic and hippocampal aging changes are linked to steroid exposure

Two steroids are implicated in region-specific physiological and anatomical changes during aging in rodents: estradiol and corticosterone. In the hypothalamus of female mice and rats, chronic exposure to endogenous ovarian steroids, presumably estrogens, impairs the preovulatory gonadotropin surge in association with loss of the estrous cycle at midlife [40,41]. Ovariectomy of young rodents slows many hypothalamic and pituitary age changes, most of

which can be induced prematurely by chronic exposure of young rodents to exogenous estradiol [41]. We do not know the cell type(s) that mediates these effects of estradiol and the role of neuronal death vs. synaptic remodeling. There is no clear analog of estrogen-dependent hypothalamic aging in women since a preovulatory-like surge can be induced in postmenopausal women.

Certain features of hippocampal aging show adrenocorticosteroid-dependent aging with similar bidirectional responses to experimental manipulations. Pyramidal neuronal damage and astrocytosis during aging in male rats is slowed by adrenalectomy and, conversely, accelerated by exposure to stress or glucocorticoids [1,7,8]. As in the effects of estradiol in the hypothalamus, we do not know which hippocampal cells mediate these effects of stress or corticosterone. However, adrenalectomy partly reduced the Ca^{2+}-dependent afterhyperpolarization in pyramidal neurons [7]. This and other findings suggest that corticosteroids could interact with the cytotoxic effects of calcium [7,8]. The role of life-long exposure to endogenous corticosteroids is shown further by the improved cognitive performance and smaller neuronal loss during aging in rats which were handled neonatally and had lower basal blood corticosterone (see Chap. 49).

NEUROENDOCRINOLOGY AND SLEEP DURING AGING

The diurnal cycle has an important impact on age changes in central nervous system function, particularly for hormonal secretions. Elderly people exhibit an earlier onset of sleep, as well as an earlier morning awakening and a more shallow and fragmented sleep pattern overall [49], with reduced circadian amplitude of cortisol secretion in aged (67 to 84 years) compared to young (20 to 27 years) subjects. However, mean levels are normal. In addition, both waking and sleeping plasma thyroid-stimulating hormone (TSH) and growth hormone (GH) levels are decreased greatly in the older group, whereas prolactin and melatonin concentrations are reduced only during sleep [41]. Elderly individuals show earlier increases in cortisol, TSH and melatonin. Taken together, these observations suggest that aging affects important neuroendocrine mechanisms which regulate both awake/sleep cycles and hormonal secretion. Such fluctuation must be considered in interpreting studies on this subject.

MAMMALS ARE NOT THE ONLY ANIMAL MODELS FOR AGING

Mammals are not the only animals to show defined aging changes. Domestic fowl show aging in neuroendocrine functions, in which hypothalamic changes are implicated [1]; genotypic influences on reproductive decline and altered monamine metabolism are topics of interest for comparison with mammals. There are also major opportunities for studies on invertebrates which show evidence for aging in the nervous system: fruit flies *(Drosophila)* with a life span of 2 months, soil nematodes *(Caenorhabditis)* with a life span of 1 month, molluscs *(Aplysia californica)* with a life span 9 to 12 months and pond snails *(Lymnaea stagnalis)* with a life span of 24 to 30 months. Much is known about neural changes with aging in mollusks. *Aplysia* shows major behavioral age changes, which can be manipulated by sensory stimulation with increased acetylcholinesterase [50]. *Lymnaea* also has aging changes in neuroendocrine functions [1]. Although little is known about neural aging in *Drosophila* or *Caenorhabditis,* both models are being used to analyze functions of β-amyloid precursor-like proteins. Both flies and nematodes show marked changes in locomotion at later ages, which could be targets for genetic manipulation. Moreover, transgenic worms expressing Aβ under the control of a muscle-specific promoter developed deposits of aggregated Aβ (thioflavin-stained) in muscle cells [51].

In choosing a mammalian model, one must keep in mind that rodents and primates represent different evolutionary selections for reproductive schedules, as well as the 30 to 40 million years since the divergence of mice from rats or of rhesus from humans. The neuropathology of aging differs among mammals (Table 30-2). Although rodents are well justified as short-lived models by practicality, the genetic differences between rodents and humans could cause many species differences in responses to interventions.

Many argue for inbred strains of mice or rats to minimize the risk that the young and old individuals represent slightly different genotypes. Moreover, inbred strains favor replication of results between laboratories. Few brain age changes have been verified by different labs using the same rodent genotype. There is reason to extend findings from inbreds to hybrids and outbreds, to avoid bias by one genotype. The National Institute on Aging provides investigators with several different common strains and F1 hybrids from mice and rats; adult ages across the life span are provided at a subsidized cost.

The largest variety of genotypes is available in mice, which will continue to be the favored mammalian model for genetic approaches. The life span of most "normal" strains is 24 to 36 months; any with a life span less than 20 months suffer early-onset specific pathology, not accelerated aging. The differences between genotypes mostly influence the type or rate of progression of pathological lesions, such as benign tumors, kidney diseases, ectopic calcification, organ amyloid deposits and others [1]. No mutant genotype shows a uniform acceleration of all aging processes. The progerias in humans represent genetic disorders with segmental or mosaic features of aging. Similarly, senescence-accelerated mice develop systemic amyloid deposits in the liver with no relation to the amyloid of AD, PAS-staining deposits in the hippocampus and behavioral changes during the 1-year life span; they have a mutant serum lipoprotein [52]. The lineages of mouse strains commonly used for studies on aging are shown in Figure 30-5.

The growing interface between research on the immune and nervous systems impacts on the neurobiology of aging, such as in the recognition that complement and other inflammatory mediators are present in lesions of AD [6] and that the major histocompatibility complex (MHC) influences age changes in reproduction and immune functions [1]. Use of inbred mice developed for immunogenetics could help in analyzing inflammatory features of normal and pathological aging and the many interactions of glycoproteins encoded in the MHC.

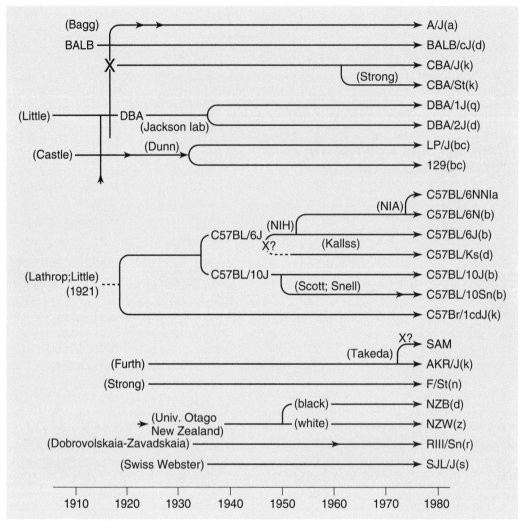

FIGURE 30-5. Origins of mouse strains commonly used for studies of aging. The histocompatibility allele set (H-2 haplotype) is given in parentheses on the right. (Reproduced from Finch [1] with permission.)

PROSPECTS

The neurochemistry of aging now offers many well-defined animal models and experimental paradigms for approaching the mechanisms of brain aging. We all want to know why the accumulation of amyloids is such a common outcome of aging in long-lived mammals. The burgeoning inventory of transgenic models will have a major impact on what is learned about the neurochemistry of aging. We also may anticipate a major impact from the genome-sequencing projects. The approaching avalanche of information on genes expressed in nervous tissues will give plenty to analyze in the study of the mechanisms of aging. These molecular approaches are expected to reveal the gene-regulation circuits that determine for a given genotype which cells are destined to degenerate, as well as the physiological circuits that maintain brain functions throughout the life span.

ACKNOWLEDGMENTS

Cited studies by C. E. Finch were partially supported by NIA grant 13499.

REFERENCES

1. Finch, C. E. *Longevity, Senescence, and the Genome.* Chicago: University of Chicago Press, 1990.
2. Finch, C. E. Neuron atrophy during aging: Programmed or sporadic? *Trends Neurosci.* 16:104–110, 1993.
3. West, M. J. Regionally specific loss of neurons in the aging human hippocampus. *Neurobiol. Aging* 14:287–293, 1993.
3a. Rasmussen, T., Schliemann, T., Sorenson, J. C., Zimmer, J., and West, M. J. Memory impaired aged rats: No loss of principal hippocampal and subicular neurons. *Neurobiol. Aging* 17:143–147, 1996.
4. Johnson, S. J., and Finch, C. E. Changes in gene expression during brain aging: A survey. In E. L. Schneider and J. W. Rowe (eds.), *Handbook of the Biology of Aging*, 3rd ed., San Diego: Academic Press, 1996, pp. 300–327.
5. Morgan, T. E., Rozovsky, I., Goldsmith, S. K., Stone, D. J., Yoshida, T., and Finch, C. E. Increased transcription of the astrocyte gene GFAP during middle-age is attenuated by food restriction: Implications for the role of oxidative stress. *Free Radic. Biol. Metab.* 23:524–528, 1997.
6. O'Banion, M. K., and Finch, C. E. (eds.). Inflammatory mechanisms and anti-inflammatory therapy in Alzheimer's disease. *Neurobiol. Aging* Special issue 17, (5), 1996.
7. Kerr, D. S., Campbell, L. W., Hao, S.-Y., and Landfield, P. W. Corticosteroid modulation of hippocampal potentials: Increased effect with aging. *Science* 245:1505–1509, 1989.
8. Sapolsky, R. M. *Stress, the Aging Brain, and the Mechanisms of Neuron Death.* Cambridge, MA: MIT Press, 1992.
9. Hsiao, K. K., Borchelt, D.R., Olson, K., et al. Age-related CNS disorder and early death in transgenic FVB/N mice overexpressing Alzheimer amyloid precursor proteins. *Neuron* 15(5): 1203–1218, 1995.
9a. Cole, G., Chapman, P., Nilsen, S., et al. Correlative memory deficits, Aβ-elevation and amyloid plaques in transgenic mice. *Science* 274:99–102, 1996.
10. Higgins, L. S., Rodems, J. M., Catalano, R., Quon, D., and Cordell, B. Early Alzheimer disease-like histopathology increases in frequency with age in mice transgenic for β-APP751. *Proc. Natl. Acad. Sci. USA* 92:4402–4406, 1995.
11. Citron, M., Westaway, D., Xia, W., et al. Mutant presenilins of Alzheimer disease increase production of 42-residue amyloid β-protein in both transfected cells and transgenic mice. *Nat. Med.* 3:67–72, 1997.
12. Yao, J., Kitt, C., and Reeves, R. H. Chronic elevation of S100 beta protein does not alter APP mRNA expression or promote β-amyloid deposition in the brains of aging transgenic mice. *Brain Res.* 702:32–36, 1995.
13. Farlie, P. G., Dringen, R., Rees, S. M., Kannourakis, G., and Bernard, O. Bcl-2 transgenic expression can protect neurons against developmental and induced cell death. *Proc. Natl. Acad. Sci. USA* 92:4397–4401, 1995.
14. Zhang, L., Kokkonen, G., and Roth, G. S. Identification of neuronal programmed cell death *in situ* in the striatum of normal adult rat brain and its relationship to neuronal death during aging. *Brain Res.* 677:177–179, 1995.
15. Shinkai, T., Zhang, L., Mathais, S. A., and Roth, G. S. Dopamine induces apoptosis in cultured rat striatal neurons; possible mechanism of D_2-dopamine receptor neuron loss during aging. *J. Neurosci. Res.* 47:393–399, 1997.
16. Bonnes-Taourel, D., Guerin, M. C., Torreilles, J., Ceballos-Picot, I., and de Paulet, A. C. 4-Hydroxynonenal content lower in brains of 25 month old transgenic mice carrying the human CuZn superoxide dismutase gene than in brains of their nontransgenic littermates. *J. Lipid Metab.* 8:111–120, 1993.
17. Cadet, J. L., Kujirai, K., Carlson, E., and Epstein, C. J. Autoradiographic distribution of [^{3}H] neurotensin receptors in the brain of superoxide dismutase transgenic mice. *Synapse* 14:24–33, 1993.
18. Barnes, C. A. Normal aging: Regionally specific changes in hippocampal synaptic transmission. *Trends Neurosci.* 17:13–18, 1994.
18a. Cotman, C. W., and Anderson, K. J. Synaptic plasticity and functional stabilization in the hippocampal formation: Possible role in Alzheimer's disease. *Adv. Neurol.* 47:313–335, 1988.
19. Schauwecker, P. E., Cheng, H. W., Serquinia, R. M. P., Morei, N., and McNeill, T. H. Lesion induced sprouting of commissural/associational axons and induction of GAP-43 mRNA in hilar and CA3 pyramidal neurons in the hippocampus are diminished in aged rats. *J. Neurosci.* 15:2642–2650, 1995.
20. Adler, J. E., and Black, I. B. Plasticity of substance P in mature and aged sympathetic neurons in culture. *Science* 225:1499–1500, 1984.
21. Morse, K., DeKosky, S. T., and Scheff, S. W. Neurotrophic effects of steroids on lesion-induced growth in the hippocampus. II, Hormone replacement. *Exp. Neurol.* 118:47–52, 1992.
22. Goudsmit, E., Fliers, E., and Swaab, R. Testosterone supplementation restores vasopressin in-

nervation in the senescent rat brain. *Brain Res.* 473:306–313, 1988.

23. Joseph, J. A., Roth, G. S., and Strong, R. The striatum, a microcosm for the examination of age-related alterations in the CNS: A selected review. *Rev. Biol. Res. Aging* 4:181–199, 1990.

24. Decker, M. W. The effects of aging on hippocampal and cortical projections of the forebrain cholinergic system. *Brain Res. Rev.* 12:423–438, 1987.

25. Kelly, J. F., and Roth, G. S. Changes in neurotransmitter signal transduction pathways in the aging brain. In M. P. Mattson and J. W. Geddes (eds.), *The Aging Brain: Advances in Gerontology.* Greenwich CT: JAI Press, 1997, pp. 243–278.

26. Morgan, D. G., and May, P. C. Age-related changes in synaptic neurochemistry. In E. L. Schneider and J. W. Rowe (eds.), *Handbook of the Biology of Aging,* 3rd ed. San Diego: Academic Press, pp. 219–254, 1990.

27. Araujo, D. M., Lapchak, P. A., Meany, M. J., Collier, B., and Quirion, R. Effects of aging on nicotinic and muscarinic autoreceptor function in the rat brain: Relationship to presynaptic cholinergic markers and binding sites. *J. Neurosci.* 10:3069–3078, 1990.

28. Landfield, P. W., Applegate, M. D., Schmitzer-Osborne, S. E., and Naylor, C. E. Phosphate/calcium alterations in the first stages of Alzheimer's disease: Implications for etiology and pathogenesis. *J. Neurol. Sci.* 106:221–229, 1991.

29. Fisher, W., Bjorklund, A., Chen, K., and Gage, F. H. NGF improves spatial memory in aged rodents as a function of age. *J. Neurosci.* 11:1889–1906, 1991.

30. Ivy, G. O., Schottler, F., Wenzel, J., Baudry, M., and Lynch, G. Inhibitors of lysosomal enzymes: Accumulation of lipofuscin-like dense bodies in the brain. *Science* 226:985–987, 1984.

31. Pettegrew, J. W., McClure, R. J., Kanfer, J. N., Mason, P. R. P., Panchalingam, K., and Klunk, W. E. The role of membranes and energetics in Alzheimer disease. In R. D. Terry, R. Katzman, and K. L. Bick (eds.), *Alzheimer Disease.* New York: Raven Press, pp. 369–386, 1994.

32. Choi, J. H., and Yu, B. P. Brain synaptosomal aging: Free radicals and membrane fluidity. *Free Radic. Biol. Med.* 18:133–139, 1995.

32a.Rauser, G. Kritchevsky G., Yamamoto, A., and Baxter, C. Lipids in the nervous system of different species as a function of age. Brain, spinal cord, peripheral nerve, purified whole cell preparations, and subcellular particulates: Regulatory mechanisms and membrane structures. In R. Paoletti and D. Kritchevsky (eds.), *Advances in Lipid Research,* New York, Academic Press, 1972, pp. 261–360.

33. Foster, N. L. PET imaging. In R. D. Terry, R. Katzman, and K. L. Bick (eds.), *Alzheimer Disease.* New York: Raven Press, 1994, pp. 87–103.

34. Randerath, K., Randerath, E., and Filburn, C. Genomic and mitochondrial DNA alterations with aging. In E. L. Schneider and J. W. Rowe (eds.), *Handbook of the Biology of Aging,* 4th ed. San Diego: Academic Press, 1995, pp. 198–214.

35. Soong, N. W., Dang, M. H., Hinton, D. R., and Arnheim, N. Mitochondrial DNA deletions are rare in the free radical-rich retinal environment. *Neurobiol. Aging* 17:827–831, 1996.

36. Evans, D. A. P., Burbach, J. P. H., et al. Mutant vasopressin precursors in the human hypothalamus: Evidence for neuronal somatic mutations in man. *Neuroscience* 71:1025–1030, 1996.

36a.van Leuwen, F. W., deKleijn, D. P. V., van den Hurk, H. H., et al. Frameshift mutants of β amyloid precursor protein and ubiquitin-B in Alzheimer's and Down patients. *Science* 279:242–247, 1998.

37. Finch, C. E., and Goodman, M. F. Relevance of 'adaptive' mutations arising in non-dividing cells of microorganisms to age-related changes in mutant phenotypes of neuron. *TINS* 20:501–507, 1997.

37a.Karelus, K., and Nelson, J. F. Aging impairs estrogenic suppression of hypothalamic propiomelanocortin mRNA in the mouse. *Neuroendocrinology* 55:627–633, 1992.

38. Joshi, D., Bennett, H. P. J., James, S., Tousignant, P., and Miller, M. M. Hypothalamic processing of β-endorphin in female C57B1/6J mice is altered at middle age. *J. Neuroendocrinol.* 144:405–415, 1995.

39. Chauhan, N., and Siegel, G. Differential expression of Na,K-ATPase α-isoform mRNAs in aging rat cerebellum. *J. Neurosci. Res.* 47:287–299, 1997.

40. Wise, P. M., Krajnak, K. M., and Kashon, M. L. Menopause: The aging of multiple pacemakers. *Science* 273:67–70, 1996.

41. Mobbs, C. V. Neuroendocrinology of aging. In E. L. Schneider and J. W. Rowe (eds.), *Handbook of the Biology of Aging,* 4th ed. San Diego: Academic Press, pp. 234–282, 1995.

42. Floyd, R. A. Oxidative damage to behavior during aging. *Science* 254:1597, 1991.

43. Martin, G. M., Austad, S., and Johnson, T. E. Genetic analysis of aging and the role of oxidative damage and environmental stresses. *Nat. Genet.* 13:25–34, 1996.

44. Finch, C. E., and Cohen, D. M. Aging, metabolism, and Alzheimer disease: Review and hypotheses. *Exp. Neurol.* 143:82–102, 1997.

45. McQuarrie, I. G., Brady, S. T., and Lasek, R. J. Retardation in the slow axonal transport of cytoskeletal elements during maturation and aging. *Neurobiol. Aging* 10:359–365, 1989.

46. Dubey, A., Forster, M. J., Lal, H., and Sohal, R. S. Effect of age and caloric intake on protein oxidation in different brain regions and on behavioral functions of the mouse. *Arch. Biochem. Biophys.* 333:189–197, 1996.

47. Sohal, R. S., Agarwal, S., Candas, M., Forster, M. J., and Lal, H. Effect of age and caloric restriction on DNA oxidative damage in different tissues of C57BL/6 mice. *Mech. Ageing Dev.* 76:215–224, 1994.

48. Moore, W. A., Davey, V. A., Weindruch, R., Walford, R., and Ivy, G. O. The effect of caloric restriction on lipofuscin accumulation in mouse brain with age. *Gerontology* 41(Suppl. 2):173–185, 1995.

49. Van Cauter, E., Leproult, R., and Kupfer, D. J. Effects of gender and age on the levels and circadian rhythmicity of plasma cortisol. *J. Clin. Endocrinol. Metab.* 81:2468–2473, 1996.

50. Peretz, B., and Srivastava, M. Chronic stimulation increases acetylcholinesterase in old *Aplysia. Behav. Brain Res.* 80:203–210, 1996.

51. Link, C. D. Expression of human β-amyloid peptide in transgenic *Caenorhabditis elegans. Proc. Natl. Acad. Sci. USA* 92:9368–9372, 1995.

52. Takeda, T. (ed.) The SAM model of senescence. *Excerpta Medica Int. Congress Ser. 1062.* Amsterdam: Elsevier Science V, 1994.

53. van Leeuwan, F., van der Beck, E., Seger, M., Burbach, P., and Ivel, R. Age-related development of a heterozygous phenotype in solitary neurons of the homozygous Brattleboro rat. *Proc. Natl. Acad. Sci. USA* 86: 6417–6420, 1989.

Metabolism

31

Circulation and Energy Metabolism of the Brain

Donald D. Clarke and Louis Sokoloff

Basic Neurochemistry: Molecular, Cellular and Medical Aspects, 6th Ed., edited by G. J. Siegel et al. Published by Lippincott–Raven Publishers, Philadelphia, 1999. Correspondence to Donald D. Clarke, Chemistry Department, Fordham University, Bronx, New York 10458.

The biochemical pathways of energy metabolism in the brain are in most respects like those of other tissues, but special conditions peculiar to the central nervous system *in vivo* limit full expression of its biochemical potentialities. In no tissue are the discrepancies between *in vivo* and *in vitro* properties greater or the extrapolations from *in vitro* data to conclusions about *in vivo* metabolic functions more hazardous. Valid identification of normally used substrates and products of cerebral energy metabolism, as well as reliable estimations of their rates of utilization and production, can be obtained only in the intact animal; *in vitro* studies identify pathways of intermediary metabolism, mechanisms and potential rather than actual performance.

Although the brain is said to be unique among tissues in its high rate of oxidative metabolism, the overall cerebral metabolic rate for O_2 ($CMRO_2$) is of the same order as the unstressed heart and renal cortex [1]. Regional fluxes in the brain may greatly exceed $CMRO_2$, however, and these are closely coupled to changes in metabolic demand.

INTERMEDIARY METABOLISM

ATP production in brain is highly regulated

Oxidative steps of carbohydrate metabolism normally contribute 36 of the 38 high-energy phosphate bonds ($\sim$P) generated during aerobic metabolism of a single glucose molecule. About 15% of brain glucose is converted to lactate and does not enter the Krebs cycle, also termed the citric acid cycle. However, this might be matched by a corresponding uptake of ketone bodies. The total net gain of $\sim$P is 33 equivalents per mole of glucose utilized. The steady-state concentration of ATP is high and represents the sum of very rapid synthesis and utilization. On average, half of the terminal phosphate groups turn over in about 3 sec; this is probably much faster in certain regions [2]. The level of $\sim$P is kept constant by regulation of ADP phosphorylation in relation to ATP hydrolysis. The active adenylyl kinase reaction, which forms equivalent amounts of ATP and AMP from ADP, prevents any great accumulation of ADP. Only a small amount of AMP is present under steady-state conditions; thus, a relatively small decrease in ATP may lead to a relatively large increase in AMP, which is a positive modulator of many reactions that lead to increased ATP synthesis. Such an amplification factor provides a sensitive control for maintenance of ATP levels [3]. Between 37 and 42°C, the brain metabolic rate increases about 5% per degree.

The concentration of creatine phosphate (CRP) in brain is even higher than that of ATP, and creatine phosphokinase (CPK) is extremely active. The CRP level is exquisitely sensitive to changes in oxygenation, providing $\sim$P for ADP phosphorylation and, thus, maintaining ATP levels. The CPK system also may function in regulating mitochondrial activity. In neurons with a very heterogeneous mitochondrial distribution, the CRP shuttle may play a critical role in energy transport [4]. The BB isoenzyme of CPK is characteristic of, but not confined to, brain. Thus, its presence in body fluids does not necessarily indicate disruption of neural tissue.

Glycogen is a dynamic but limited energy store in brain

Although present in relatively low concentration in brain (3.3 mmol/kg brain in rat), glycogen is a unique energy reserve that requires no energy (ATP) for initiation of its metabolism. As with glucose, glycogen levels in brain appear to vary with plasma glucose concentrations. Biopsies have shown that human brain contains much more glycogen than rodent brain, but the effects of anesthesia and pathological changes in the biopsied tissue may have contributed. Glycogen granules are seen in electron micrographs of glia and neurons of immature animals but only in astrocytes of adults. Barbiturates decrease brain metabolism and increase the number of granules seen, particularly in astrocytes of synaptic regions; however, biochemical studies show that neurons do contain glycogen and that enzymes for its synthesis and metabolism are present in synaptosomes. Astrocyte glycogen may form a store of carbohydrate made available to neurons by still undefined mechanisms. Associated with the granules are enzymes involved in glycogen synthesis and, perhaps, degradation. The increased glycogen found in areas of brain injury may be due to glial changes or to decreased utilization during tissue preparation.

The accepted role of glycogen is that of a carbohydrate reserve utilized when glucose falls below need. However, rapid, continual breakdown and synthesis of glycogen occur at a rate of 19 μmol/kg/min. This is about 2% of the normal glycolytic flux in brain and is subject to elaborate control mechanisms. This suggests that, even under steady-state conditions, local carbohydrate reserves are important for brain function. However, if glycogen were the sole supply, normal glycolytic flux in brain would be maintained for less than 5 min.

The enzymes which synthesize and catabolize glycogen in other tissues are found in brain also, but their kinetic and regulatory properties do differ [5]. Glycogen metabolism in brain, unlike in other tissues, is controlled locally. It is isolated from the tumult of systemic activity, evidently by the blood–brain barrier (BBB). Although glucocorticoid hormones that penetrate the BBB increase glycogen turnover, circulating protein hormones and biogenic amines have no effect. Beyond the BBB, cells are sensitive to local amine concentrations; drugs that cross the BBB and modify local amine concentrations or membrane receptors thus cause metabolic changes (see Chap. 32).

Separate systems for the synthesis and degradation of glycogen provide a greater degree of control than if glycogen were degraded by simply reversing its synthesis (Fig. 31-1). The amount of glucose-6-phosphate (G6P), the initial synthetic substrate, usually varies inversely with the rate of brain glycolysis because of greater facilitation of the phosphofructokinase step relative to transport and phosphorylation of glucose. Thus, a decline in G6P during energy need slows glycogen formation.

The glucosyl group of uridine diphosphoglucose (UDP-glucose) is transferred to the terminal glucose of the nonreducing end of an amylose chain in an α-1,4-glycosidic linkage (Fig. 31-1). This reaction, catalyzed by glycogen synthetase (GS), is rate-controlling for glycogen synthesis [5]. In brain, as in other tissues, GS occurs in both a phosphorylated (D) form, which depends on G6P as a positive modulator, and a dephosphorylated, independent (I) form sensitive to, but not dependent on, the modulator. Although in brain the I form of GS requires no stimulator, it has a relatively low affinity for UDP-glucose. At times of increased energy demand, not only is there a change from the D to the I form but also an I form with even lower affinity for substrate develops. Inhibition of glycogen synthesis is enhanced, and this increases the availability of G6P for energy needs. Goldberg and O'Toole [5] hypothesize that the I form in brain is associated with inhibition of glycogen synthesis under conditions of energy demand, whereas the D form causes a relatively

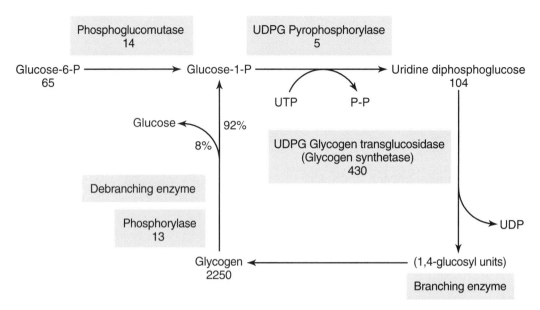

FIGURE 31-1. Glycogen metabolism in brain. Enzyme data from mouse brain homogenates. Numerals below each enzyme represent maximal velocity (V_{max}) at 38°C in millimoles per kilogram wet weight per minute; metabolite concentrations from quick-frozen adult mouse brain are in micromoles per kilogram wet weight. *P-P*, pyrophosphate. (Metabolic data from [41]; enzyme data from [42]).

small regulated synthesis under resting conditions. Regulation of the D form may reduce glycogen formation in brain to approximately 5% of its potential rate. In liver, where large amounts of glycogen are synthesized and degraded, the I form of GS is associated with glycogen formation. At present, it appears that the two tissues use the same biochemical apparatus in different ways to bring about their different overall metabolic patterns.

Under steady-state conditions, it is probable that less than 10% of phosphorylase in brain (Fig. 31-1) is in the unphosphorylated *b* form (requiring AMP), which is inactive at the very low AMP concentrations present normally. When a steady state is disturbed, there may be an extremely rapid conversion of enzyme to the *a* form, which is active at low AMP. Brain phosphorylase *b* kinase is activated indirectly by cAMP and by the molar concentrations of Ca^{2+} released during neuronal excitation (see Chap. 22). The endoplasmic reticulum of brain, like muscle, is capable of taking up Ca^{2+} to terminate its stimulatory effect. These reactions provide energy from glycogen during excitation and when cAMP-forming systems are activated. It has not been possible to confirm directly that the conversion from phosphorylase *b* to *a* is a control point of glycogenolysis *in vivo*. Norepinephrine and, probably, dopamine activate glycogenolysis through cAMP; but epinephrine, vasopressin and angiotensin II do so by another mechanism, possibly involving Ca^{2+} or a Ca^{2+}-mediated proteolysis of phosphorylase kinase.

Hydrolysis of the α-1,4-glycoside linkages leaves a limit dextrin that turns over at only half the rate of the outer chains (see also Chap. 42). The debrancher enzyme that hydrolyzes the α-1,6-glycoside linkages may be rate-limiting if the entire glycogen granule is utilized. Because one product of this enzyme is free glucose, approximately one glucose molecule for every 11 of G6P is released if an entire glycogen molecule is degraded (Fig. 31-1). α-Glucosidase, also termed acid maltase, is a lysosomal enzyme whose precise function in glycogen metabolism is not known. In Pompe's disease, which is the hereditary absence of α-glucosidase, glycogen accumulates in brain as well as elsewhere (see Chap. 42). The steady-state concentration of glycogen is regulated precisely by the coordination of synthetic and degradative processes through enzymatic regulation at several metabolic steps [6].

Brain glycolysis is regulated mainly by hexokinase and phosphofructokinase

Aerobic and anaerobic glycolysis have been defined historically as the amount of lactate produced under conditions of "adequate" oxygen and no oxygen, respectively. More recently, glycolysis refers to the Embden-Meyerhoff glycolytic sequence from glucose, or glycogen glucosyl, to pyruvate. Glycolytic flux is defined indirectly: it is the rate at which glucose must be utilized to produce the observed rate of ADP phosphorylation.

Figure 31-2 outlines the flow of glycolytic substrates in brain. Glycolysis first involves phosphorylation by hexokinase. The reaction is essentially irreversible and is a key point in the regulation of carbohydrate metabolism in brain. The electrophoretically slow-moving (type I) isoenzyme of hexokinase is characteristic of brain. In most tissues, hexokinase may be soluble and may exist in the cytosol or be attached firmly to mitochondria. Under conditions in which no special effort is made to stop metabolism while isolating mitochondria, 80 to 90% of brain hexokinase is bound. In the live steady state, however, when availability of substrate keeps up with metabolic demand and end products are removed, an equilibrium exists be-

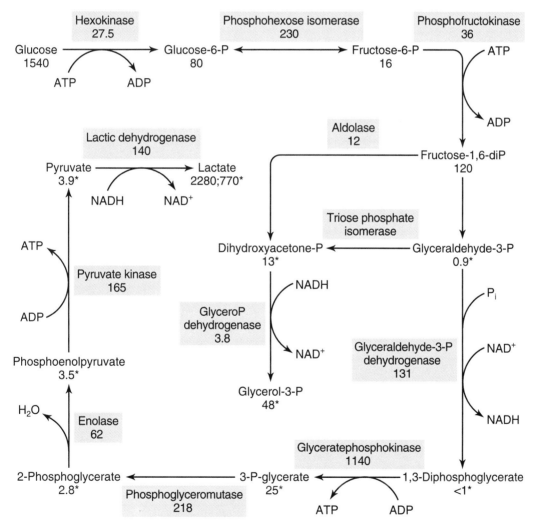

FIGURE 31-2.   Glycolysis in brain. Enzyme and metabolic data expressed as in Figure 31-1. *Ten-day-old mouse brain [43]. (Data from [44].)

tween the soluble and the bound enzyme. Binding changes the kinetic properties of hexokinase and its inhibition by G6P so that the bound enzyme on mitochondria is more active. The extent of binding is inversely related to the ATP: ADP ratio, so conditions in which energy utilization exceeds supply shift the solubilization equilibrium to the bound form and produce a greater potential capacity for initiating glycolysis to meet the energy demand. This mechanism allows ATP to function both as the substrate of the enzyme and, at another site, as a regulator to decrease ATP production through its influence on enzyme binding. It also confers preference on glucose in the competition for the $MgATP^{2-}$ generated by mitochondrial oxidative phosphorylation. Thus, a process that will sustain ATP production continues at the expense of other uses of energy. Because energy reserves are exhausted rapidly postmortem, it is not surprising that brain hexokinase is bound almost entirely.

The significance of reversible binding of other enzymes to mitochondria is not clear. The measured glycolytic flux, when compared with the maximal velocity of hexokinase, indicates that in the steady state the hexokinase reaction is inhibited 97%. Brain hexokinase is inhibited by its product G6P, to a lesser extent by ADP and allosterically by 3-phosphoglycerate and several nucleoside phosphates, including cAMP and free ATP^{4-}. The ratio of ATP to Mg^{2+} also may have a regulatory action. In addition to acting on enzyme kinetics, G6P solubilizes hexokinase, thus reducing the efficiency of the enzyme when the reaction product accumulates. The sum total of these mechanisms is a fine tuning of the activity of the initial enzyme in glycolysis in response to changes in the cellular environment. Glucokinase, also termed low-affinity hexokinase, a major component of liver hexokinase, has not been found in brain.

G6P represents a branch point in metabolism because it is a common substrate for enzymes involved in glycolytic, pentose phosphate shunt and glycogen-forming pathways. There is also slight but detectable G6Pase activity in brain, the significance of which is not clear. The liver requires this enzyme to convert glycogen to glucose. The differences between the hexokinases and the modes of glycogen metabolism

of liver and brain can be related to the function of liver as a carbohydrate storehouse for the body, whereas brain metabolism is adapted for rapid carbohydrate utilization for energy needs. In glycolysis, G6P is the substrate of phosphohexose isomerase. This is a reversible reaction, with a small free energy change and a 5:1 equilibrium ratio in brain that favors G6P.

Fructose-6-phosphate is the substrate of phosphofructokinase, a key regulatory enzyme controlling glycolysis [3]. The other substrate is $MgATP^{2-}$. Like other regulatory reactions, it is essentially irreversible. It is modulated by a large number of metabolites and cofactors, whose concentrations under different metabolic conditions have a great effect on glycolytic flux. Prominent among these are availability of ~P and citrate concentrations. Brain phosphofructokinase is inhibited by ATP, Mg^{2+} and citrate and stimulated by NH_4^+, K^+, PO_4^{2-}, 5'-AMP, 3',5',-cAMP, ADP and fructose-1,6-bisphosphate.

When oxygen is admitted to cells metabolizing anaerobically, utilization of O_2 increases, whereas utilization of glucose and production of lactate drop; this is known as the Pasteur effect. Modulation of the phosphofructokinase reaction can account directly for the Pasteur effect. In the steady state, ATP and citrate concentrations in brain apparently are sufficient to keep phosphofructokinase relatively inhibited as long as the concentration of positive modulators, or disinhibitors, is low. When the steady state is disturbed, activation of this enzyme produces an increase in glycolytic flux, which takes place almost as fast as events changing the internal milieu.

Fructose-1,6-bisphosphate is split by brain aldolase to glyceraldehyde-3-phosphate and dihydroxyacetone phosphate. Dihydroxyacetone phosphate is the common substrate for both glycerophosphate dehydrogenase, an enzyme active in reduced nicotinamide adenine dinucleotide (NADH) oxidation and lipid pathways (see Chap. 3), and triose phosphate isomerase, which maintains an equilibrium between dihydroxyacetone phosphate and glyceraldehyde-3-phosphate; the equilibrium strongly favors accumulation of dihydroxyacetone phosphate.

After the reaction with glyceraldehyde-3-phosphate dehydrogenase, glycolysis in brain proceeds through the usual steps. Brain enolase, also termed D-2-phosphoglycerate hydrolyase, which catalyzes dehydration of 2-phosphoglycerate to phosphoenolpyruvate, is present as two related dimers, one of which (γ) is associated specifically with neurons and the other (α) with glia. The neuronal subunit is identical to the neuron-specific protein 14-3-2. Immunocytochemical determination of the enolases makes them useful in determining neuron:glia ratios in tissue samples, but neuron-specific enolase is not confined to neural tissue. Brain phosphoenolpyruvate kinase controls an essentially irreversible reaction that requires not only Mg^{2+}, as do several other glycolytic enzymes, but also K^+ or Na^+. This step also may be regulatory.

Brain tissue, even when at rest and well oxygenated, produces a small amount of lactate, which is removed in the venous blood, accounting for 13% of the pyruvate produced by glycolysis. The measured lactate concentration in brain depends on success in rapidly arresting brain metabolism prior to tissue processing. Five lactate dehydrogenase isoenzymes are present in adult brain; the one that electrophoretically moves most rapidly toward the anode, termed band 1, predominates. This isoenzyme is generally higher in tissues that are more dependent on aerobic processes for energy; the slower moving isoenzymes are relatively higher in tissues such as white skeletal muscle, which is better adapted to function at suboptimal oxygen levels. The distribution of lactate dehydrogenase isoenzymes in various brain regions, layers of the retina, brain neoplasms and brain tissue cultures and during development indicates that their synthesis might be controlled by tissue oxygen concentrations. Lactate dehydrogenase functions in the cytoplasm to oxidize NADH, which accumulates as a result of the activity of glyceraldehyde-3-phosphate dehydrogenase in glycolysis. This permits glycolytic ATP production to continue under anaerobic conditions. Lactate dehydrogenase also functions under aerobic conditions because NADH cannot easily penetrate mitochondrial membranes. Oxidation of NADH in the cytoplasm depends on this reaction and on the activity of shuttle mechanisms that transfer reducing equivalents to mitochondria.

Glycerol phosphate dehydrogenase is another enzyme indirectly associated with glycolysis that participates in cytoplasmic oxidation of NADH. This enzyme reduces dihydroxyacetone phosphate to glycerol-3-phosphate, oxidizing NADH in the process. Under hypoxic conditions, α-glycerophosphate and lactate increase initially at comparable rates, although the amount of lactate produced greatly exceeds that of α-glycerophosphate. The relative concentrations of the oxidized and reduced substrates of these reactions indicate much higher local concentrations of NADH in brain than are found by gross measurements. In fact, the relative proportions of oxidized and reduced substrates of the reactions that are linked to the pyridine nucleotides may be a better indicator of local redox states (NAD^+/NADH) in brain than the direct measurement of pyridine nucleotides themselves [3,7].

An aspect of glucose metabolism that has led to much confusion is the observation that labeled glucose appears in carbon dioxide much more slowly than might be suggested from an examination of the glycolytic pathway plus the citric acid cycle [8]. Glucose flux is 0.5 to 1.0 μmol/min/g wet weight of brain in a variety of species. The concentration of glycolytic plus Krebs cycle intermediates is 2 μmol/g. Hence, the intermediates might turn over every 2 to 4 min and $^{14}CO_2$ production might reach a steady state in 5 to 10 min. This is not seen experimentally. Also, large amounts of radioactivity are trapped in amino acids related to the Krebs cycle (70 to 80%) from 10 to 30 min after a glucose injection. This is due to high transaminase activity in comparison with flux through the Krebs cycle, and amino acids made by transamination of cycle intermediates behave as if they are part of the cycle. When pools of these amino acids (~20 μmol/g) are added to the Krebs cycle components plus glycolytic intermediates, the calculated time for $^{14}CO_2$ evolution is increased by a factor of 10, in agreement with experimental results.

In contrast, in liver, amino acids related to the Krebs cycle are present at much lower steady-state values, and approximately 20% of the radioactivity from administered glucose is trapped in these amino acids shortly after injection. Thus, ignoring the radioactivity trapped in amino acids has a relatively small effect on estimates of glycolytic fluxes in liver but makes an enormous difference in brain. Immature brain resembles liver more nearly in this respect. The relationship of the Krebs cycle to glycolysis undergoes a sharp change during development, coincident with the metabolic compartmentation of amino acid metabolism characteristic of adult brain.

The pyruvate dehydrogenase complex plays a key role in regulating oxidation

Pyruvate dehydrogenase has an activity of 14 nmol/min/mg protein in rat brain and controls the rate of pyruvate entry into the Krebs cycle as acetyl coenzyme A (acetyl-CoA). Pyruvate dehydrogenase, or decarboxylase, is part of a mitochondrial multienzyme complex that also includes the enzymes lipoate acetyltransferase and lipoamide dehydrogenase; the coenzymes thiamine pyrophosphate, lipoic acid, CoA and flavine; and nicotinamide adenine dinucleotides. It is inactivated by being phosphorylated at the decarboxylase moiety by a tightly bound Mg^{2+}/ATP^{2-}-dependent protein kinase and activated by being dephosphorylated by a loosely bound Mg^{2+}- and Ca^{2+}-dependent phosphatase. About half the brain enzyme is usually active. Pyruvate protects the complex against inactivation by inhibiting the kinase. ADP is a competitive inhibitor of Mg^{2+} for the inactivating kinase. Under conditions of greater metabolic demand, increases in pyruvate and ADP and decreases in acetyl-CoA and ATP make the complex more active. Pyruvate dehydrogenase is inhibited by NADH, decreasing formation of acetyl-CoA during hypoxia and allowing more pyruvate to be reduced by lactate dehydrogenase, thus forming the NAD^+ necessary to sustain glycolysis. Pyruvate dehydrogenase defects do occur in several mitochondrial enzyme-deficiency states (see below and Morgan-Hughes [9], also Chap. 42).

Although acetylcholine synthesis normally is controlled by the rate of choline uptake and choline acetyltransferase activity (see Chap. 11), the supply of acetyl-CoA can be limiting under adverse conditions. Choline uptake is, however, independent of acetyl-CoA concentration. The mitochondrial membrane is not permeable to the acetyl-CoA produced within it, but there is efflux of its condensation product, citrate. Acetyl-CoA can then be formed from citrate in the cytosol by ATP citrate lyase. The acetyl moiety of acetylcholine is formed in a compartment, presumably the synaptosome, with rapid glucose turnover. The cytosol of cholinergic endings is rich in citrate lyase, and it is possible that citrate shuttles the acetyl-CoA from the mitochondrial compartment to the cytosol. During hypoxia or hypoglycemia, acetylcholine synthesis can be inhibited by failure of the acetyl-CoA supply.

Energy output and oxygen consumption are associated with high rates of enzyme activity in the Krebs cycle

The actual flux through the Krebs cycle depends on glycolysis and acetyl-CoA production, which can "push" the cycle, the possible control at several enzymatic steps of the cycle and the local ADP concentration, which is a prime activator of the mitochondrial respiration to which the Krebs cycle is linked. The steady-state concentration of citrate in brain is about one-fifth that of glucose. This is relatively high compared with glycolytic intermediates or isocitrate.

As in other tissues, there are two isocitrate dehydrogenases in brain. One is active primarily in the cytoplasm and requires nicotinamide adenine dinucleotide phosphate ($NADP^+$) as cofactor; the other, bound to mitochondria and requiring NAD^+, is the enzyme that participates in the citric acid cycle. The NAD^+-linked enzyme catalyzes an essentially irreversible reaction, has allosteric properties, is inhibited by ATP and NADH and may be stimulated by ADP. The function of cytoplasmic $NADP^+$ isocitrate dehydrogenase is uncertain, but it has been postulated that it supplies the NADPH necessary for many reductive synthetic reactions. The relatively high activity of this enzyme in immature brain and white matter is consistent with such a role. α-Ketoglutarate (α-KG) dehydrogenase, which oxidatively decarboxylates α-KG, requires the same cofactors as does the pyruvate decarboxylation step.

Succinate dehydrogenase, the enzyme that catalyzes the oxidation of succinate to fumarate, is bound tightly to the mitochondrial membrane. In brain, succinate dehydrogenase also may have a regulatory role when the steady state is disturbed. Isocitrate and succinate concentrations in brain are affected little by changes in the flux of the citric acid cycle as long as an adequate glucose supply is available. The highly unfavorable free energy change of the malate dehydrogenase reaction is overcome by the rapid removal of oxaloacetate, which is maintained at low concentrations under steady-state conditions by the condensation reaction with acetyl-CoA [6].

Malic dehydrogenase is one of several enzymes in the citric acid cycle present in both the cytoplasm and mitochondria. The function of the cytoplasmic components of these enzyme activities is not known, but they may assist in the transfer of hydrogen equivalents from the cytoplasm into mitochondria.

The Krebs cycle functions as an oxidative process for energy production and as a source of various amino acids, for example, glutamate, glutamine, γ-aminobutyrate (GABA), aspartate and asparagine. To export net amounts of α-KG or oxaloacetate from the Krebs cycle, the supply of dicarboxylic acids must be replenished. The major route for this seems to be the fixation of CO_2 to pyruvate or other substrates at the three-carbon level. Thus, the CO_2 fixation rate sets an upper limit at which biosynthetic reactions can occur. In studies of acute ammonia toxicity in cats, this has been estimated as 0.15 μmol/g wet weight brain/min, or approximately 10% of the flux through the citric acid cycle (see below). Liver seems to have ten times the capacity of brain for CO_2 fixation, as is appropriate for an organ geared to making large quantities of protein for export [10]. In brain, pyruvate carboxylase, which catalyzes CO_2 fixation, appears to be largely an astrocytic enzyme. Pyruvate dehydrogenase seems to be the rate-limiting step for the entry of pyruvate into the Krebs cycle from glycolysis.

The pentose shunt, also termed the hexose monophosphate pathway, is active in brain

Under basal conditions 5 to 8% of brain glucose is likely to be metabolized via the pentose shunt in the adult monkey and 2.3% in the rat [8]. Both shunt enzymes and metabolic flux have been found in isolated nerve endings. The pentose pathway has relatively high activity in developing brain, reaching a peak during myelination. Its main contribution is probably to produce the NADPH needed for reductive reactions necessary for lipid synthesis (see Chap. 3). Shunt enzymes and metabolic flux are found in synaptosomes. Although the capacity of the pathway, as determined using nonphysiological electron acceptors, remains constant throughout the rat life span, activity with physiological acceptors could not be detected in middle-aged (18 months) and older animals. It seems that the shunt serves as a reserve pathway for use under such stresses as the need for increased lipid synthesis or repair or reduction of oxidative toxins. The shunt pathway also provides pentose for nucleotide synthesis; however, only a small fraction of the activity of this pathway would be required. As with glycogen synthesis, turnover in the pentose phosphate pathway decreases under conditions of increased energy need, for example, during and after high rates of stimulation. Pentose phosphate flux apparently is regulated by the concentrations of G6P, $NADP^+$, glyceraldehyde-3-phosphate and fructose-6-phosphate. Since transketolase, an enzyme in this pathway, requires thiamine pyrophosphate as a cofactor, poor myelin maintenance in thiamine deficiency may reflect failure of this pathway to provide sufficient NADPH for lipid synthesis [6].

Glutamate in brain is compartmented into separate pools

The pools that subserve different metabolic pathways for glutamate equilibrate with each other only slowly. This compartmentation is a vital factor in the separate regulation of special functions of glutamate (see Chap. 15) and GABA (see Chap. 16), such as neurotransmission, and of general functions, such as protein biosynthesis. Glutamate metabolism in brain shows at least two distinct pools; in addition, the Krebs cycle intermediates associated with these pools are distinctly compartmented. Mathematical models to fit data from radiotracer experiments that require separate Krebs cycles to satisfy the hypotheses of compartmentation have been developed. A key assumption of current models is that GABA is metabolized at a site different from its synthesis. The best fit of kinetic data is obtained when glutamate from a small pool actively converted to glutamine flows back to a larger pool (8 μmol/g), which is converted to GABA. Of possible relevance to this is the finding that glutamate decarboxylase (GAD) is localized at or near nerve terminals, whereas GABA transaminase, the major degradative enzyme, is mitochondrial.

Evidence points to an inferred small pool of glutamate (2 μmol/g) as probably glial. Glutamate released from nerve endings appears to be taken up by glia or neurons, converted to glutamine and recycled to glutamate and GABA (see Chaps. 5 and 15). Various estimates of the proportion of glucose carbon that flows through the GABA shunt have been made, but the most definitive experiments show this to be about 10% of the total glycolytic flux. While this may seem small, that portion of the Krebs cycle flux used for energy production, including ATP synthesis and maintenance of ionic gradients, does not require CO_2 fixation, while the portion used for biosynthesis of amino acids does. Recycling the carbon skeleton of some of the glutamate released in neurotransmission through glutamine and GABA to succinate diminishes the need for dicarboxylic acids to replenish intermediates of the Krebs cycle when export of α-KG to make amino acids takes place.

It is difficult to get good estimates of the extent of CO_2 fixation in brain; the maximum capability measured during ammonia stress, when glutamine increases rapidly, suggests that CO_2 fixation occurs at 0.15 μmol/g/min in cat and 0.33 μmol/g/min in rat; this is about the same rate as for the GABA shunt.

For comparison, only about 2% of the glucose flux in whole brain goes toward lipid synthesis and approximately 0.3% is used for protein synthesis. Thus, turnover of neurotransmitter amino acids is a major biosynthetic activity in brain.

Metabolic compartmentation of glutamate usually is observed when labeled ketogenic substrates are administered to animals. It is interesting that acetoacetate and β-hydroxybutyrate do not show this effect, apparently because ketone bodies are a normal substrate for brain and are taken up in all kinds of cells. Acetate and similar substrates, which are not taken up into brain efficiently, appear to be more readily taken up or activated, or both, in glia. This is believed to lead to the observed abnormal glutamine/glutamate ratio. Similarly, metabolic inhibitors, like fluoroacetate, appear to act selectively in glia and to produce their neurotoxic action without marked inhibition of the overall Krebs cycle flux in brain. This difference in behavior has led to suggestions that acetate and fluoroacetate may be useful markers for the study of glial metabolism by autoradiography [11].

A nonuniform distribution of metabolites in living systems is a widespread occurrence. Steady-state concentrations of GABA vary from 2 to 10 mM in discrete brain regions, and it has been estimated that GABA may be as high as 50 mM in nerve terminals. Observations in brain indicate the existence of pools of metabolites with half-lives of many hours for mixing, which is most unusual. The discovery of subcellular, morphological compartmentation, that is, different populations of mitochondria in cerebral cortex that have distinctive enzyme complements, may provide a somewhat better perspective by which to visualize such a separation of metabolic function [12].

In addition to the phasic release of both excitatory and inhibitory transmitters, there may be a continuous tonic release of GABA, dependent only on the activity of the enzyme responsible for its synthesis and independent of the depolarization of the presynaptic membrane. Such inhibitory neurons could act tonically by constantly maintaining an elevated threshold in the excitatory neurons so that the latter would start firing when a decrease occurred in the continuous release of GABA acting on them. This is consistent with a known correlation between the inhibition of GAD and the appearance of convulsions after certain drug treatments. GABA is depleted by some convulsant drugs and elevated by others.

DIFFERENCES BETWEEN *IN VITRO* AND *IN VIVO* BRAIN METABOLISM

In addition to the usual differences between *in vitro* and *in vivo* studies that pertain to all tissues, there are two unique conditions that pertain only to the central nervous system.

In contrast to cells of other tissues, individual nerve cells do not function autonomously

They are generally so incorporated into a complex neural network that their functional activity is integrated with that of various other parts of the central nervous system and with somatic tissues. In addition, neurons and adjacent glia are linked in their metabolism. Any procedure that interrupts the structural and functional integrity of the network inevitably would alter quantitatively and, perhaps, qualitatively its normal metabolic behavior.

The blood–brain barrier selectively limits the rates of transfer of soluble substances between blood and brain

This barrier discriminates among various potential substrates for cerebral metabolism (see Chap. 32). The substrate function is confined to those compounds in the blood that are not only suitable substrates for cerebral enzymes but also can penetrate from blood to brain at rates adequate to support the considerable energy demands of brain. Substances that can be readily oxidized by brain slices, minces or homogenates *in vitro* and that are utilized effectively *in vivo* when formed endogenously within the brain often are incapable of supporting cerebral energy metabolism and function when present in the blood because of restricted passage through the BBB. The *in vitro* techniques establish only the existence and potential capacity of the enzyme systems required for the use of a given substrate; they do not define the extent to which such a pathway actually is used *in vivo*. This can be done only in intact animals, and it is this aspect of cerebral metabolism with which this part of the chapter is concerned.

CEREBRAL ENERGY METABOLISM *IN VIVO*

Numerous methods have been used to study the metabolism of the brain *in vivo;* these vary in complexity and in the degree to which they yield quantitative results. Some require such minimal operative procedures on the laboratory animal that no anesthesia is required, and there is no interference with the tissue except for the effects of the particular experimental condition being studied. Some of these techniques are applicable to normal, conscious human subjects, and consecutive and comparative studies can be made repeatedly in the same subject. Other methods are more traumatic and either require the animal to be killed or involve such extensive surgical intervention and tissue damage that the experiments approach an *in vitro* experiment carried out *in situ*. All, however, are capable of providing specific and useful information.

Behavioral and central nervous system physiology are correlated with blood and cerebrospinal fluid chemical changes

The simplest way to study the metabolism of the central nervous system *in vivo* is to correlate spontaneous or experimentally produced alterations in the chemical composition of the blood, spinal fluid or both with changes in cerebral physiological functions or gross central nervous system-mediated behavior. The level of consciousness, the reflex behavior or the electroencephalogram (EEG) generally is used to monitor the effects of chemical changes on functional and metabolic activities of brain. Such methods first demonstrated the need for glucose as a substrate for cerebral energy metabolism; hypoglycemia produced by insulin or other means altered various parameters of cerebral function that could not be restored to normal by administering substances other than glucose.

The chief virtue of these methods is their simplicity, but they are gross and nonspecific and do not distinguish between direct effects of the agent on cerebral metabolism and those secondary to changes produced initially in somatic tissues. Also, negative results are often inconclusive, for there always remain questions of insufficient dosage, inadequate cerebral circulation and delivery to the tissues or impermeability of the BBB.

Brain samples are removed for biochemical analyses

The availability of analytical chemical techniques makes it possible to measure specific metabolites and enzyme activities in brain tissue at selected times during or after exposure of the animal to an experimental condition. This approach has been very useful in studies of the intermediary metabolism of brain. It has permitted estimation of the rates of flux through the various steps of established metabolic pathways and the identification of control points in the pathways where regulation may be exerted. Such studies have helped to define more precisely changes in energy metabolism associated with altered cerebral functions, for example, those produced by anesthesia, convulsions or hypoglycemia. While such methods require killing animals and analyzing tissues, in effect, they are *in vivo* methods since they attempt to describe the state of the tissue while it is still in the animal at the moment of killing. They have encountered their most serious problems with regard to this point. Postmortem changes in brain are extremely rapid and not always retarded completely even by the most rapid freezing techniques available. These methods have proved to be very valuable, nevertheless, particularly in the area of energy metabolism.

Radioisotope incorporation can identify and measure routes of metabolism

The technique of administering radioactive precursors followed by the chemical separation and assay of products in the tissue has added greatly to the armamentarium for studying cerebral metabolism *in vivo*. Labeled precursors are administered by any of a variety of routes; at selected later times the brain is removed, the precursor and the various products of interest are isolated and the radioactivity and quantity of the compounds in question are assayed. Such techniques facilitate identification of metabolic routes and rates of flux through various steps of a pathway. In some cases, comparison of specific activities of the products and precursors has led to the surprising finding of higher specific activities in products than in precursors. This is conclusive evidence of the presence of compartmentation. These methods have been used effectively in studies of amine and neurotransmitter synthesis and metabolism, lipid metabolism, protein synthesis, amino acid metabolism and the distribution of glucose carbon through the various biochemical pathways present in brain.

Radioisotope incorporation methods are particularly valuable for studies of intermediary metabolism, which generally are not feasible by most other *in vivo* techniques. They are without equal for the qualitative identification of the pathways and routes of metabolism. They suffer, however, from a disadvantage: only one set of measurements per animal is possible because the animal must be killed. Quantitative interpretations often are confounded by the problems of compartmentation. Also, all too frequently, they are misused; unfortunately, quantitative conclusions are drawn incorrectly based on radioactivity data without appropriate consideration of the specific activities of precursor pools.

Oxygen utilization in the cortex is measured by polarographic techniques

The O_2 electrode has been used for measuring the amount of O_2 consumed locally in the cerebral cortex *in vivo* [13]. The electrode is applied to the surface of the exposed cortex, and the local partial pressure for O_2 (PO_2) is measured continuously before and during occlusion of the blood flow to the local area. During occlusion, PO_2 falls linearly as O_2 is consumed by tissue metabolism, and the rate of fall is a measure of the rate of O_2 consumption locally in the cortex. Repeated measurements can be made successively in the animal, and the technique has been used to demonstrate the increased O_2 consumption of the cerebral cortex and the relation between changes in the EEG and the metabolic rate during convulsions [13]. The technique is limited to measurements in the cortex and, of course, to O_2 utilization.

Arteriovenous differences identify substances consumed or produced by brain

The primary functions of the circulation are to replenish the nutrients consumed by the tissues and to remove the products of their metabolism.

These functions are reflected in the composition of the blood traversing the tissue. Substances taken up by a tissue from the blood are higher in concentration in the arterial inflow than in the venous outflow, and the converse is true for substances released by the tissue. The convention is to subtract the venous concentration from the arterial concentration so that a positive arteriovenous difference represents net uptake and a negative difference, net release. In nonsteady states, as after a perturbation, there may be transient arteriovenous differences that reflect changes in tissue concentrations and re-equilibration of the tissue with the blood. In steady states, in which it is presumed that the tissue concentration remains constant, positive and negative arteriovenous differences mean net consumption or production of the substance by the tissue, respectively. Zero arteriovenous differences indicate neither consumption nor production.

This method is useful for all substances in blood that can be assayed with enough accuracy, precision and sensitivity to enable the detection of arteriovenous differences. The method is useful only for tissues from which mixed representative venous blood can be sampled. Arterial blood has essentially the same composition throughout and can be sampled from any artery. In contrast, venous blood is specific for each tissue, and to establish valid arteriovenous differences the venous blood must represent the total outflow or the flow-weighted average of all of the venous outflows from the tissue under study, uncontaminated by blood from any other tissue. It is not possible to fulfill this condition for many tissues.

The method is fully applicable to the brain, particularly in humans, in whom the anatomy of venous drainage is favorable for such studies. Representative cerebral venous blood, with no more than approximately 3% contamination with extracerebral blood, is readily obtained from the superior bulb of the internal jugular vein in humans. The venipuncture can be made percutaneously under local anesthesia; therefore, measurements can be made during conscious states undistorted by the effects of general anesthesia. Using this method with monkeys is similar, although the vein must be exposed surgically before

puncture. Other common laboratory animals are less suitable because extensive communication between cerebral and extracerebral venous beds is present and uncontaminated representative venous blood is difficult to obtain from the cerebrum without major surgical intervention. In these cases, one can sample blood from the confluence of the sinuses, also termed the torcular herophili, even though it does not contain fully representative blood from the brainstem and some of the lower portions of the brain.

The chief advantages of these methods are their simplicity and applicability to unanesthetized humans. They permit the qualitative identification of the ultimate substrates and products of cerebral metabolism. They have no applicability, however, to those intermediates that are formed and consumed entirely within brain without being exchanged with blood or to those substances that are exchanged between brain and blood with no net flux in either direction. Furthermore, they provide no quantification of the rates of utilization or production because arteriovenous differences depend not only on the rates of consumption or production by the tissue but also on blood flow (see below). Blood flow affects all of the arteriovenous differences proportionately, however, and comparison of the arteriovenous differences of various substances obtained from the same samples of blood reflects their relative rates of utilization or production.

Combining cerebral blood flow and arteriovenous differences permits measurement of rates of consumption or production of substances by brain

In a steady state, the tissue concentration of any substance utilized or produced by brain is presumed to remain constant. When a substance is exchanged between brain and blood, the difference in its steady state of delivery to brain in the arterial blood and removal in the venous blood must be equal to the net rate of its utilization or production by brain. This relation can be expressed as follows:

$$CMR = CBF(A - V)$$

where $(A - V)$ is the difference in concentration in arterial and cerebral venous blood, *CBF* is the rate of cerebral blood flow in volume of blood per unit time and cerebral metabolic rate *(CMR)* is the steady-state rate of utilization or production of the substance by brain.

If both the rate of cerebral blood flow and the arteriovenous difference are known, then the net rate of utilization or production of the substance by brain can be calculated. This has been the basis of most quantitative studies of cerebral metabolism *in vivo*.

The most reliable method for determining cerebral blood flow is the inert gas method of Kety and Schmidt [14]. Originally, it was designed for use in studies of conscious, unanesthetized humans, and it has been employed most widely for this purpose; but it also has been adapted for use in animals. The method is based on the Fick principle, which is an equivalent of the law of conservation of matter; and it utilizes low concentrations of a freely diffusible, chemically inert gas as a tracer substance. The original gas was nitrous oxide, but subsequent modifications have substituted other gases, such as ^{85}Kr, ^{79}Kr or hydrogen, which can be measured more conveniently in blood. During a period of inhalation of 15% N_2O in air, for example, timed arterial and cerebral venous blood samples are withdrawn and analyzed for their N_2O contents. The cerebral blood flow in milliliters per 100 g of brain tissue per minute can be calculated from the following equation:

$$CBF = 100 \, \lambda \, V(T)/\int_0^T [A(t) - V(t)] \, dt$$

where $A(t)$ and $V(t)$ are the arterial and cerebral venous blood concentrations of N_2O, respectively, at any time t; $V(T)$ is concentration of N_2O in venous blood at the end of the period of inhalation, that is, time T; λ is the partition coefficient for N_2O between brain tissue and blood; t is variable time in minutes; T is total period of inhalation of N_2O, usually 10 min or more; and $\int_0^T [A(t) - V(t)] \, dt$ is the integrated arteriovenous difference in N_2O concentrations over the total period of inhalation.

The partition coefficient for N_2O is approximately 1 when equilibrium has been achieved between blood and brain tissue; at least 10 min

of inhalation is required to approach equilibrium. At the end of this interval, the N_2O concentration in brain tissue is about equal to the cerebral venous blood concentration. Because the method requires sampling of both arterial and cerebral venous blood, it lends itself readily to the simultaneous measurement of arteriovenous differences of substances involved in cerebral metabolism. This method and its modifications have provided most of our knowledge of the rates of substrate utilization or product formation by brain *in vivo*.

REGULATION OF CEREBRAL METABOLIC RATE

The brain consumes about one-fifth of total body oxygen utilization

The brain is metabolically one of the most active of all organs in the body. This consumption of O_2 provides the energy required for its intense physicochemical activity. The most reliable data on cerebral metabolic rate have been obtained in humans. Cerebral O_2 consumption in normal, conscious, young men is approximately 3.5 ml/100 g brain/min (Table 31-1); the rate is similar in young women. The rate of O_2 consumption by an entire brain of average weight (1,400 g) is then about 49 ml O_2/min. The magnitude of this rate can be appreciated more fully when it is compared with the metabolic rate of the whole body. An average man weighs 70 kg and con-

TABLE 31-1.	**CEREBRAL BLOOD FLOW AND METABOLIC RATE IN A NORMAL YOUNG ADULT MAN**[a]	
Function	Per 100 g of brain tissue	Per whole brain (1,400 g)
Cerebral blood flow (ml/min)	57	798
Cerebral O_2 consumption (ml/min)	3.5	49
Cerebral glucose utilization (mg/min)	5.5	77

[a] Based on data derived from the literature, in Sokoloff [16].

sumes about 250 ml O_2/min in the basal state. Therefore, the brain, which represents only about 2% of total body weight, accounts for 20% of the resting total body O_2 consumption. In children, the brain takes up an even larger fraction, as much as 50% in the middle of the first decade of life [15].

O_2 is utilized in the brain almost entirely for the oxidation of carbohydrate [16]. The energy equivalent of the total cerebral metabolic rate is, therefore, approximately 20 W, or 0.25 kcal/min. If it is assumed that this energy is utilized mainly for the synthesis of high-energy phosphate bonds, that the efficiency of the energy conservation is approximately 20% and that the free energy of hydrolysis of the terminal phosphate of ATP is approximately 7 kcal/mol, then this energy expenditure can be estimated to support the steady turnover of close to 7 mmol, or approximately 4×10^{21} molecules, of ATP per minute in the entire human brain. The brain normally has no respite from this enormous energy demand. Cerebral O_2 consumption continues unabated day and night. Even during sleep there is only a relatively small decrease in cerebral metabolic rate; indeed, it may even be increased in rapid eye movement (REM) sleep (see below).

The main energy-demanding functions of the brain are those of ion flux related to excitation and conduction

The brain does not do mechanical work, like that of cardiac and skeletal muscle, or osmotic work, as the kidney does in concentrating urine. It does not have the complex energy-consuming metabolic functions of the liver nor, despite the synthesis of some hormones and neurotransmitters, is it noted for its biosynthetic activities. Considerable emphasis has been placed on the extent of macromolecular synthesis in the central nervous system, an interest stimulated by the recognition that there are some proteins with short half-lives in brain. However, these represent relatively small numbers of molecules, and in fact, the average protein turnover and the rate of protein synthesis in mature brain are slower than in most other tissues, except perhaps muscle. Clearly, the functions of nervous tissues are

mainly excitation and conduction, and these are reflected in the unceasing electrical activity of the brain. The electrical energy ultimately is derived from chemical processes, and it is likely that most of the energy consumption of the brain is used for active transport of ions to sustain and restore the membrane potentials discharged during the processes of excitation and conduction (see Chaps. 5 and 6).

Not all of the O_2 consumption of the brain is used for energy metabolism. The brain contains a variety of oxidases and hydroxylases that function in the synthesis and metabolism of a number of neurotransmitters. For example, tyrosine hydroxylase is a mixed-function oxidase that hydroxylates tyrosine to 3,4-dihydroxyphenylalanine (DOPA), and dopamine β-hydroxylase hydroxylates dopamine to form norepinephrine. Similarly, tryptophan hydroxylase hydroxylates tryptophan to form 5-hydroxytryptophan in the pathway of serotonin synthesis. The enzymes are oxygenases, which utilize molecular O_2 and incorporate it into the hydroxyl group of the hydroxylated products. O_2 also is consumed in the metabolism of these monoamine neurotransmitters, which are deaminated oxidatively to their respective aldehydes by monoamine oxidases. All of these enzymes are present in brain, and the reactions catalyzed by them use O_2. However, the total turnover rates of these neurotransmitters and the sum total of the maximal velocities of all oxidases involved in their synthesis and degradation can account for only a very small, possibly immeasurable, fraction of the total O_2 consumption of brain.

Continuous cerebral circulation is absolutely required to provide sufficient oxygen

Not only does the brain utilize O_2 at a very rapid rate, but it is absolutely dependent on uninterrupted oxidative metabolism for maintenance of its functional and structural integrity. There is a large Pasteur effect in brain tissue, but even at its maximal rate anaerobic glycolysis is unable to provide sufficient energy. Since the O_2 stored in brain is extremely small compared with its rate of utilization, the brain requires continuous replenishment of its O_2 by the circulation. If cerebral blood flow is interrupted completely, consciousness is lost within less than 10 sec, or the amount of time required to consume the O_2 contained within the brain and its blood content. Loss of consciousness as a result of anoxemia, caused by anoxia or asphyxia, takes only a little longer because of the additional O_2 present in the lungs and the still-circulating blood. The average critical level of O_2 tension in brain tissues, below which consciousness and the normal EEG pattern are invariably lost, lies between 15 and 20 mm Hg. This seems to be so whether the tissue anoxia is achieved by lowering the cerebral blood flow or the arterial oxygen content. Cessation of cerebral blood flow is followed within a few minutes by irreversible pathological changes within the brain, readily demonstrated by microscopic anatomical techniques. In medical crises, such as cardiac arrest, damage to the brain occurs earliest and is most decisive in determining the degree of recovery.

Cerebral blood flow must be able to maintain the avaricious appetite of the brain for O_2. The average rate of blood flow in the human brain as a whole is approximately 57 ml/100 g tissue/min (see Table 31-1). For a whole brain this amounts to almost 800 ml/min, or approximately 15% of the total basal cardiac output. This must be maintained within relatively narrow limits, for the brain cannot tolerate any major drop in its perfusion. A fall in cerebral blood flow to half its normal rate is sufficient to cause loss of consciousness in normal, healthy, young men. There are, fortunately, numerous reflexes and other physiological mechanisms to sustain adequate levels of arterial blood pressure at the head level, such as the baroreceptor reflexes, and to maintain cerebral blood flow, even when arterial pressure falls in times of stress for example, autoregulation. There are also mechanisms to adjust cerebral blood flow to changes in cerebral metabolic demand.

Regulation of cerebral blood flow is achieved mainly by control of the tone or the degree of constriction, or dilation, of the cerebral vessels. This in turn is controlled mainly by local chemical factors, such as $PaCO_2$, PaO_2, pH and others still unrecognized. High $PaCO_2$, low PaO_2

and low pH, which are products of metabolic activity, tend to dilate the blood vessels and increase cerebral blood flow; changes in the opposite direction constrict the vessels and decrease blood flow [17]. Cerebral blood flow is regulated through such mechanisms to maintain homeostasis of these chemical factors in the local tissue. The rates of production of these chemical factors depend on the rates of energy metabolism; therefore, cerebral blood flow is adjusted to the cerebral metabolic rate [17].

Local rates of cerebral blood flow and metabolism can be measured by autoradiography and are coupled to local brain function

The rates of blood flow and metabolism presented in Table 31-1 and discussed above represent the average values in the brain as a whole. The brain is not homogeneous, however; it is composed of a variety of tissues and discrete structures that often function independently or even inversely with respect to one another. There is little reason to expect that their perfusion and metabolic rates would be similar. Indeed, experiments clearly indicate that they are not. Local cerebral blood flow in laboratory animals has been determined from the local tissue concentrations, measured by a quantitative autoradiographic technique, and from the total history of the arterial concentration of a freely diffusible, chemically inert, radioactive tracer introduced into the circulation [18]. The results reveal that blood-flow rates vary widely throughout the brain, with average values in gray matter approximately four to five times those in white matter [18].

A method has been devised to measure glucose consumption in discrete functional and structural components of the brain in intact, conscious laboratory animals [19]. This method also employs quantitative autoradiography to measure local tissue concentrations but utilizes 2-deoxy-D-[^{14}C]glucose as the tracer. The local tissue accumulation of [^{14}C]deoxyglucose as [^{14}C]deoxy-G6P in a given interval of time is related to the amount of glucose that has been phosphorylated by

A

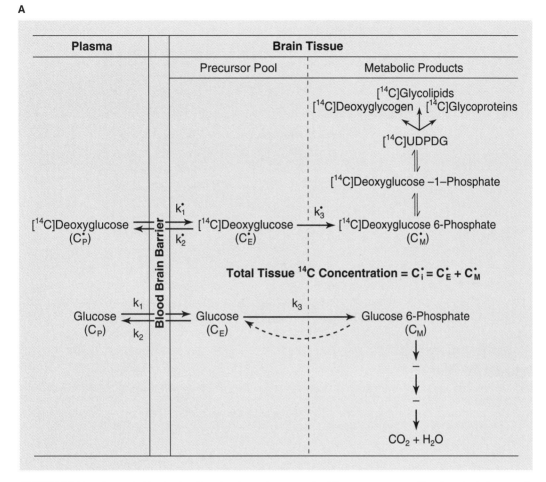

FIGURE 31-3. Theoretical basis of radioactive deoxyglucose method for measurement of local cerebral glucose utilization. **A:** Theoretical model. C_i^* represents the total ^{14}C concentration in a single homogeneous tissue of the brain. C_p^* and C_p represent the concentrations of $[^{14}C]$deoxyglucose and glucose in the arterial plasma, respectively; C_E^* and C_E represent their respective concentrations in the tissue pools that serve as substrates for hexokinase. C_M^* represents the concentration of $[^{14}C]$deoxyglucose-6-phosphate in the tissue. k_1^*, k_2^* and k_3^* represent the rate constants for carrier-mediated transport of $[^{14}C]$deoxyglucose from plasma to tissue, for carrier-mediated transport back from tissue to plasma and for phosphorylation by hexokinase, respectively. k_1, k_2 and k_3 are the equivalent rate constants for glucose. $[^{14}C]$Deoxyglucose and glucose share and compete for the carrier that transports them both between plasma and tissue and for hexokinase, which phosphorylates them to their respective hexose-6-phosphates. *Dashed arrow* represents the possibility of glucose-6-phosphate hydrolysis by glucose-6-phosphatase activity, if any. *UDPDG,* UDP-deoxyglucose. (*Figure continues on next page.*)

hexokinase over the same interval, and the rate of glucose consumption can be determined from the $[^{14}C]$deoxy-G6P concentration by appropriate consideration of (i) the relative concentrations of $[^{14}C]$deoxyglucose and glucose in the plasma, (ii) their rate constants for transport between plasma and brain tissue and (iii) the kinetic constants of hexokinase for de-

oxyglucose and glucose. The method is based on a kinetic model of the biochemical behavior of 2-deoxyglucose and glucose in brain. The model (diagrammed in Fig. 31-3) has been analyzed mathematically to derive an operational equation that presents the variables to be measured and the procedure to be followed to determine local cerebral glucose utilization.

B

General equation for measurement of reaction rates with tracers:

$$\text{Rate of reaction} = \frac{\text{Labeled Product Formed in Interval of Time, 0 to T}}{\left[\begin{array}{c}\text{Isotope effect}\\\text{correction factor}\end{array}\right]\left[\begin{array}{c}\text{Integrated specific activity}\\\text{of precursor}\end{array}\right]}$$

Operational equation of [^{14}C]deoxyglucose method:

Labeled Product Formed in Interval of Time, 0 to T

$$R_i = \frac{\overbrace{C_i^*(T)}^{\substack{\text{Total }^{14}\text{C in tissue}\\\text{at time T}}} - \overbrace{k_1^* \, e^{-(k_2^* + k_3^*)T} \int_0^T C_p^* \, e^{(k_2^* + k_3^*)t} \, dt}^{\substack{^{14}\text{C in precursor}\\\text{remaining in tissue at time T}}}}{\underbrace{\left[\dfrac{\lambda \cdot V_m^* \cdot K_m}{\Phi \cdot V_m \cdot K_m^*}\right]}_{\substack{\text{Isotope effect}\\\text{correction}\\\text{factor}}} \underbrace{\left[\int_0^T \left(\dfrac{C_p^*}{C_p}\right) dt - e^{-(k_2^* + k_3^*)T} \int_0^T \left(\dfrac{C_p^*}{C_p}\right) e^{(k_2^* + k_3^*)t} \, dt\right]}_{\substack{\text{Integrated plasma}\quad\quad\text{Correction for lag in tissue}\\\text{specific activity}\quad\quad\text{equilibration with plasma}}}}$$

FIGURE 31-3. *(Continued.)* **B:** Functional anatomy of the operational equation of the radioactive deoxyglucose method. *T* represents the time at the termination of the experimental period; λ equals the ratio of the distribution space of deoxyglucose in the tissue to that of glucose; Φ equals the fraction of glucose that, once phosphorylated, continues down the glycolytic pathway; K_m^*, V_m^* and K_m, V_m represent the familiar Michaelis-Menten kinetic constants of hexokinase for deoxyglucose and glucose, respectively. Other symbols are the same as those defined in **A.** (From [19].)

To measure local glucose utilization, a pulse of [^{14}C]deoxyglucose is administered intravenously at time zero and timed arterial blood samples are drawn for determination of the plasma [^{14}C]deoxyglucose and glucose concentrations. At the end of the experimental period, usually about 45 min, the animal is decapitated, the brain is removed and frozen and 20-μm-thick brain sections are autoradiographed on X-ray film along with calibrated [^{14}C]methyl-methacrylate standards. Local tissue concentrations of ^{14}C are determined by quantitative densitometric analysis of the autoradiographs. From the time courses of the arterial plasma [^{14}C]deoxyglucose and glucose concentrations and the final tissue ^{14}C concentrations, determined by quantitative autoradiography, local glucose utilization can be calculated by means of the operational equation for all components of the brain identifiable in the autoradiographs. The procedure is designed so that the autoradiographs reflect mainly the relative local concentrations of [^{14}C]deoxy-G6P. The autoradiographs, therefore, are pictorial representations of the relative rates of glucose utilization in all of the structural components of the brain.

Autoradiographs of the striate cortex in monkey in various functional states are illustrated in Figure 31-4. This method has demonstrated that local cerebral consumption of glucose varies as widely as blood flow throughout the brain (Table 31-2). Indeed, in normal animals, there is remarkably close correlation between local cerebral blood flow and glucose consumption [20]. Changes in functional activity produced by physiological stimulation, anesthesia or deafferentation result in corresponding changes in blood flow and glucose consumption [21] in the structures involved in the functional change. The [^{14}C]deoxyglucose method for the measurement of local glucose utilization has been used to map the functional visual pathways and to identify the locus of the visual cortical

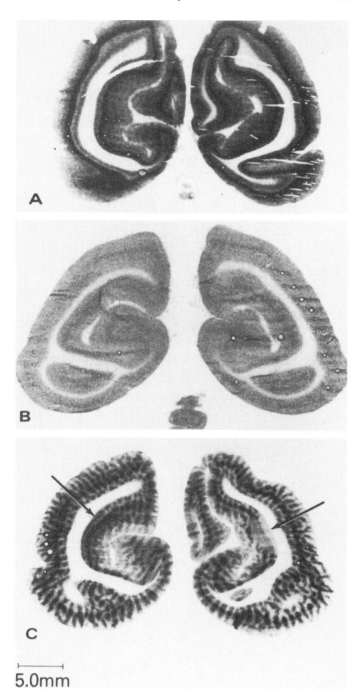

5.0mm

FIGURE 31-4. Autoradiograms of coronal brain sections from rhesus monkeys at the level of the striate cortex. **A:** Animal with normal binocular vision. Note the laminar distribution of the density; the *dark band* corresponds to layer IV. **B:** Animal with bilateral visual deprivation. Note the almost uniform and reduced relative density, especially the virtual disappearance of the dark band corresponding to layer IV. **C:** Animal with right eye occluded. The half-brain on the **left** represents the left hemisphere contralateral to the occluded eye. Note the alternate dark and light striations, each approximately 0.3 to 0.4 mm in width, representing the ocular dominance columns. These columns are most apparent in the dark lamina corresponding to layer IV but extend through the entire thickness of the cortex. *Arrows* point to regions of bilateral asymmetry, where the ocular dominance columns are absent. These are presumably areas that normally have only monocular input. The one on the **left,** contralateral to the occluded eye, has a continuous dark lamina corresponding to layer IV that is completely absent on the side ipsilateral to the occluded eye. These regions are believed to be the loci of the cortical representations of the blind spots. (From [21].)

TABLE 31-2.	REPRESENTATIVE VALUES[a] FOR LOCAL CEREBRAL GLUCOSE UTILIZATION IN THE NORMAL CONSCIOUS ALBINO RAT AND MONKEY (μmol/100g/min)		

Structure	Albino rat[b]	Monkey[c]
Gray matter		
Visual cortex	107 ± 6	59 ± 2
Auditory cortex	162 ± 5	79 ± 4
Parietal cortex	112 ± 5	47 ± 4
Sensorimotor cortex	120 ± 5	44 ± 3
Thalamus: lateral nucleus	116 ± 5	54 ± 2
Thalamus: ventral nucleus	109 ± 5	43 ± 2
Medial geniculate body	131 ± 5	65 ± 3
Lateral geniculate body	96 ± 5	39 ± 1
Hypothalamus	54 ± 2	25 ± 1
Mammillary body	121 ± 5	57 ± 3
Hippocampus	79 ± 3	39 ± 2
Amygdala	52 ± 2	25 ± 2
Caudate putamen	110 ± 4	52 ± 3
Nucleus accumbens	82 ± 3	36 ± 2
Globus pallidus	58 ± 2	26 ± 2
Substantia nigra	58 ± 3	29 ± 2
Vestibular nucleus	128 ± 5	66 ± 3
Cochlear nucleus	113 ± 7	51 ± 3
Superior olivary nucleus	133 ± 7	63 ± 4
Inferior colliculus	197 ± 10	103 ± 6
Superior colliculus	95 ± 5	55 ± 4
Pontine gray matter	62 ± 3	28 ± 1
Cerebellar cortex	57 ± 2	31 ± 2
Cerebellar nuclei	100 ± 4	45 ± 2
White matter		
Corpus callosum	40 ± 2	11 ± 1
Internal capsule	33 ± 2	13 ± 1
Cerebellar white matter	37 ± 2	12 ± 1
Weighted average for whole brain		
	68 ± 3	36 ± 1

[a] Values are the means plus or minus standard errors from measurements made in ten rats or seven monkeys.
[b] From Sokoloff and co-workers [19].
[c] From Kennedy and co-workers [22].

representation of the retinal "blind spot" in the brain of rhesus monkey [21] (Fig. 31-4). These results establish that local energy metabolism in the brain is coupled to local functional activity and confirm the long-held belief that local cerebral blood flow is adjusted to metabolic demand in local tissue. The method has been applied to humans by use of 2-[^{18}F]-fluoro-2-deoxy-D-glucose and positron emission tomography (PET), with similar results (see Chap. 54).

SUBSTRATES OF CEREBRAL METABOLISM

Normally, the substrates are glucose and oxygen and the products are carbon dioxide and water

In contrast to most other tissues, which exhibit considerable flexibility with respect to the nature of the foodstuffs extracted and consumed from the blood, the normal brain is restricted almost exclusively to glucose as the substrate for its energy metabolism. Despite long and intensive efforts, the only incontrovertible and consistently positive arteriovenous differences demonstrated for the human brain under normal conditions have been for glucose and oxygen [16]. Negative arteriovenous differences, significantly different from zero, have been found consistently only for CO_2, although water, which has never been measured, also is produced. Pyruvate and lactate production have been observed occasionally, certainly in aged subjects with cerebral vascular insufficiency but also irregularly in subjects with normal oxygenation of the brain.

In the normal *in vivo* state, glucose is the only significant substrate for energy metabolism in the brain. Under normal circumstances, no other potential energy-yielding substance has been found to be extracted from the blood in more than trivial amounts. The stoichiometry of glucose utilization and O_2 consumption is summarized in Table 31-3. The normal, conscious human brain consumes oxygen at a rate of 156 μmol/100 g tissue/min. CO_2 production is the same, leading to a respiratory quotient (RQ) of 1.0, further evidence that carbohydrate is the ultimate substrate for oxidative metabolism. O_2 consumption and CO_2 production are equivalent to a rate of glucose utilization of 26 μmol/100 g tissue/min, assuming 6 μmol of O_2 consumed and of CO_2 produced for each micromole of glucose completely oxidized to CO_2 and H_2O. The actual glucose utilization measured is, however, 31 μmol/100 g/min, which indicates that glucose consumption not only is sufficient to account for total O_2 consumption but is in excess by 5 μmol/100 g/min. For complete oxidation of glucose, the theoretical ratio of O_2: glucose utilization is 6.0; the excess glucose utilization is re-

Function	Value[a]
O_2 consumption (μmol/100 g brain tissue/min)	156
Glucose utilization (μmol/100 g brain tissue/min)	31
O_2:glucose ratio (mol/mol)	5
Glucose equivalent of O_2 consumption (μmol glucose/100 g brain tissue/min)	26[b]
CO_2 production (μmol/100 g brain tissue/min)	156
Cerebral respiratory quotient (RQ)	0.97

TABLE 31-3. RELATIONSHIP BETWEEN CEREBRAL OXYGEN CONSUMPTION AND GLUCOSE UTILIZATION IN A NORMAL YOUNG ADULT MAN

From Sokoloff [16].
[a] Values are the median of values reported in the literature.
[b] Calculated on the basis of 6 mol of O_2 required for complete oxidation of 1 mol of glucose.

sponsible for a measured ratio of only 5.5 μmol O_2/μmol glucose. The fate of the excess glucose is unknown, but it probably is distributed in part in lactate, pyruvate and other intermediates of carbohydrate metabolism, each released from the brain into the blood in insufficient amounts to be detectable as significant arteriovenous differences. Some of the glucose must be utilized not for the production of energy but for synthesis of the chemical constituents of brain.

Some oxygen is used for oxidation of substances not derived from glucose, for example, in the synthesis and metabolic degradation of monoamine neurotransmitters, as mentioned above. The amount of O_2 used for these processes is, however, extremely small and is undetectable in the presence of the enormous O_2 consumption used for carbohydrate oxidation.

The combination of a cerebral RQ of unity, an almost stoichiometric relationship between O_2 uptake and glucose consumption and the absence of any significant arteriovenous difference for any other energy-rich substrate is strong evidence that the brain normally derives its energy from the oxidation of glucose. Thus, cerebral metabolism is unique because no other tissue, except for testis [23], relies only on carbohydrate for energy.

This does not imply that the pathways of glucose metabolism in the brain lead, like combustion, directly and exclusively to production of CO_2 and H_2O. Various chemical and energy transformations occur between uptake of the primary substrates glucose and O_2 and liberation of the end products CO_2 and H_2O. Compounds derived from glucose or produced through the energy made available from glucose catabolism are intermediates in the process. Glucose carbon is incorporated, for example, into amino acids, protein, lipids and glycogen. These are turned over and act as intermediates in the overall pathway from glucose to CO_2 and H_2O. There is clear evidence from studies with [^{14}C]glucose that not all of the glucose is oxidized directly and that at any given moment some of the CO_2 being produced is derived from sources other than glucose that enter the brain at the same moment or just prior to that moment. That O_2 and glucose consumption and CO_2 production are essentially in stoichiometric balance and that no other energy-laden substrate is taken from the blood means, however, that the net energy made available to the brain ultimately must be derived from the oxidation of glucose. It should be noted that this is the situation in the normal state; as discussed later, other substrates may be used in special circumstances or in abnormal states.

In brain, glucose utilization is obligatory

The brain normally derives almost all of its energy from the aerobic oxidation of glucose, but this does not distinguish between preferential and obligatory utilization of glucose. Most tissues are largely facultative in their choice of substrates and can use them interchangeably more or less in proportion to their availability. This does not appear to be so in the brain. Except in some unusual and very special circumstances, only the aerobic utilization of glucose is capable of providing the brain with sufficient energy to maintain normal function and structure. The brain appears to have almost no flexibility in its choice of substrates *in vivo*. This conclusion is derived from the following evidence.

Glucose deprivation is followed rapidly by aberrations of cerebral function. Hypoglycemia, produced by excessive insulin or occurring spontaneously in hepatic insufficiency, is associated with changes in mental state ranging from mild, subjective sensory disturbances to coma, the severity depending on both the degree and the duration of the hypoglycemia. The behavioral effects are paralleled by abnormalities in EEG patterns and cerebral metabolic rate. The EEG pattern exhibits increased prominence of slow, high-voltage δ rhythms, and the rate of cerebral oxygen consumption falls. In studies of the effects of insulin hypoglycemia in humans [24], it was observed that when arterial glucose fell from a normal concentration of 70 to 100 mg/100 ml to an average of 19 mg/100 ml, subjects became confused and cerebral oxygen consumption fell to 2.6 ml/100 g/min, or 79% of normal. When arterial glucose fell to 8 mg/100 ml, a deep coma ensued and cerebral O_2 consumption decreased even further to 1.9 ml/100 g/min (Table 31-4).

These changes are not caused by insufficient cerebral blood flow, which actually increases slightly during coma. In the depths of coma, when the blood glucose content is very low, there is almost no measurable cerebral uptake of glucose from the blood. Cerebral O_2 consumption, although reduced, is still far from negligible; and there is no longer any stoichiometric relationship between glucose and O_2 uptakes by the brain, evidence that the O_2 is utilized for the oxidation of other substances. The cerebral RQ remains approximately 1, however, indicating that these other substrates are still car-

bohydrate, presumably derived from the endogenous carbohydrate stores of the brain. The effects are clearly the result of hypoglycemia and not of insulin in the brain. In all cases, the behavioral, functional and cerebral metabolic abnormalities associated with insulin hypoglycemia are reversed rapidly and completely by the administration of glucose. The severity of the effects is correlated with the degree of hypoglycemia and not the insulin dosage, and the effects of insulin can be prevented completely by the simultaneous administration of glucose with the insulin.

Similar effects are observed in hypoglycemia produced by other means, such as hepatectomy. Inhibition of glucose utilization at the phosphohexose isomerase step with pharmacological doses of 2-deoxyglucose also produces all of the cerebral effects of hypoglycemia despite an associated elevation in blood glucose content.

In hypoglycemia, substrates other than glucose may be utilized. The hypoglycemic state provides convenient test conditions to determine whether a substance is capable of substituting for glucose as a substrate of cerebral energy metabolism. If it can, its administration during hypoglycemic shock should restore consciousness and normal cerebral electrical activity without raising the blood glucose concentration. Numerous potential substrates have been tested in humans and animals. Very few can restore normal cerebral function in hypoglycemia, and of

TABLE 31-4.	EFFECTS OF INSULIN HYPOGLYCEMIA ON CEREBRAL CIRCULATION AND METABOLISM IN HUMANS[a]		
	Control	Insulin-induced hypoglycemia without coma	Insulin-induced hypoglycemic coma
Arterial blood			
Glucose concentration (mg%)	74	19	8
O_2 content (vol%)	17.4	17.9	16.6
Mean blood pressure (mm Hg)	94	86	93
Cerebral circulation			
Blood flow (ml/100 g/min)	58	61	63
O_2 consumption (ml/100 g/min)	3.4	2.6	1.9
Glucose consumption (mg/100 g/min)	4.4	2.3	0.8
Respiratory quotient	0.95	1.10	0.92

[a]From Kety et al. [24].

these all but one appear to operate through a variety of mechanisms to raise the blood glucose concentration rather than by serving directly as a substrate (Table 31-5).

Mannose appears to be the only substance that can be utilized by the brain directly and rapidly enough to restore or maintain normal function in the absence of glucose [25]. It traverses the BBB and is converted to mannose-6-phosphate. This reaction is catalyzed by hexokinase as effectively as the phosphorylation of glucose. The mannose-6-phosphate is then converted to fructose-6-phosphate by phosphomannose isomerase, which is active in brain tissue. Through these reactions mannose can enter directly into the glycolytic pathway and replace glucose.

Maltose also is effective occasionally in restoring normal behavior and EEG activity in hypoglycemia but only by raising the blood glucose concentration through its conversion to glucose by maltase activity in blood and other tissues [16]. Epinephrine is effective at producing arousal from insulin coma, but this is achieved through its well-known stimulation of glycogenolysis and the elevation of blood glucose concentration. Glutamate, arginine, glycine, GABA and succinate also act through adrenergic effects that raise glucose concentrations of the blood [16].

It should be noted, however, that failure to restore normal cerebral function in hypoglycemia is not synonymous with an inability of the brain to utilize the substance. Many of the substances that have been tested and found ineffective are compounds normally formed and utilized within the brain and are normal intermediates in its intermediary metabolism. Lactate; pyruvate; fructose-1,6-bisphosphate; acetate; β-hydroxybutyrate; and acetoacetate can be utilized by brain slices, homogenates or cell-free fractions; and the enzymes for their metabolism are present in brain. Enzymes for the metabolism of glycerol or ethanol, for example, may not be present in sufficient amounts. For other substrates, for example, D-β-hydroxybutyrate and acetoacetate, the enzymes are adequate but the substrate is not available to the brain because of inadequate blood levels or restricted transport through the BBB.

TABLE 31-5. EFFECTIVENESS OF VARIOUS SUBSTANCES IN PREVENTING OR REVERSING THE EFFECTS OF HYPOGLYCEMIA OR GLUCOSE DEPRIVATION ON CEREBRAL FUNCTION AND METABOLISM[a]

Effectiveness	Substance	Comments
Effective	Epinephrine	Raises blood glucose concentration
	Maltose	Converted to glucose and raises blood glucose concentration
	Mannose	Directly metabolized and enters glycolytic pathway
Partially or occasionally effective	Glutamate	Occasionally effective by raising blood glucose concentration
	Arginine	
	Glycine	
	ρ-Aminobenzoate	
	Succinate	
Ineffective	Glycerol	Some of these substances can be metabolized to various extents by brain tissue and conceivably could be effective if it were not for the blood–brain barrier
	Ethanol	
	Lactate	
	Glyceraldehyde	
	Hexose diphosphates	
	Fumarate	
	Acetate	
	β-Hydroxybutyrate	
	Galactose	
	Lactose	
	Insulin	

[a]Summarized from the literature, in Sokoloff [16].

Nevertheless, nervous system function in the intact animal depends on substrates supplied by the blood, and no satisfactory, normal, endogenous substitute for glucose has been found. Glucose, therefore, must be considered essential for normal physiological behavior of the central nervous system.

The brain utilizes ketones in states of ketosis

In special circumstances, the brain may fulfill its nutritional needs partly, although not completely, with substrates other than glucose. Normally, there are no significant cerebral arteriovenous differences for D-β-hydroxybutyrate and acetoacetate, which are "ketone bodies" formed in the course of the catabolism of fatty acids by liver. Owen and coworkers [26] observed, however, that when human patients were treated for severe obesity by complete fasting for several weeks, there was considerable uptake of both substances by the brain. If one assumed that the substances were oxidized completely, their rates of utilization would have accounted for more than 50% of the total cerebral oxygen consumption, more than that accounted for by the glucose uptake. D-β-hydroxybutyrate uptake was several times greater than that of acetoacetate, a reflection of its higher concentration in the blood. The enzymes responsible for their metabolism, D-β-hydroxybutyrate dehydrogenase, acetoacetate-succinyl-CoA transferase and acetoacetyl-CoA-thiolase, are present in brain tissue in sufficient amounts to convert them into acyl-CoA and to feed them into the tricarboxylic acid cycle at a sufficient rate to satisfy the metabolic demands of the brain [27].

Under normal circumstances, that is, ample glucose and few ketone bodies in the blood, the brain apparently does not oxidize ketones in any significant amounts. In prolonged starvation, the carbohydrate stores of the body are exhausted and the rate of gluconeogenesis is insufficient to provide glucose fast enough to meet the requirements of the brain; blood ketone concentrations rise as a result of the rapid fat catabolism. The brain then apparently turns to the ketone bodies as the source of its energy supply.

Cerebral utilization of ketone bodies appears to follow passively their concentrations in arterial blood [27]. In normal adults, ketone concentrations are very low in blood and cerebral utilization of ketones is negligible. In ketotic states resulting from starvation; fat-feeding or ketogenic diets; diabetes; or any other condition that accelerates the mobilization and catabolism of fat, cerebral utilization of ketones is increased more or less in direct proportion to the degree of ketosis [27]. Significant utilization of ketone bodies by the brain is, however, normal in the neonatal period. The newborn infant tends to be hypoglycemic but becomes ketotic when it begins to nurse because of the high fat content of the mother's milk. When weaned onto the normal, relatively high-carbohydrate diet, the ketosis and cerebral ketone utilization disappear. Studies have been carried out mainly in the infant rat, but there is evidence that the situation is similar in the human infant.

The first two enzymes in the pathway of ketone utilization are D-β-hydroxybutyrate dehydrogenase and acetoacetyl-succinyl-CoA transferase. These exhibit a postnatal pattern of development that is well adapted to the nutritional demands of the brain. At birth, the activity of these enzymes in the brain is low; activity rises rapidly with the ketosis that develops with the onset of suckling, reaches its peak just before weaning and then gradually declines after weaning to normal adult rates of approximately one-third to one-fourth the maximal rates attained [27,28].

It should be noted that D-β-hydroxybutyrate is incapable of maintaining or restoring normal cerebral function in the absence of glucose in the blood. This suggests that, although it can partially replace glucose, it cannot fully satisfy the cerebral energy needs in the absence of some glucose consumption. One explanation may be that the first product of D-β-hydroxybutyrate oxidation, acetoacetate, is metabolized further by its displacement of the succinyl moiety of succinyl-CoA to form acetoacetyl-CoA. A certain rate of glucose utilization may be essential to drive the tricarboxylic cycle, to provide enough succinyl-CoA to permit the further oxidation of acetoacetate and, hence, to pull along the oxidation of D-β-hydroxybutyrate.

AGE AND DEVELOPMENT INFLUENCE CEREBRAL ENERGY METABOLISM

Metabolic rate increases during early development

The energy metabolism of the brain and the blood flow that sustains it vary considerably from birth to old age. Data on the cerebral metabolic rate obtained directly *in vivo* are lacking for the early postnatal period, but the results of *in vitro* measurements in animal brain preparations and inferences drawn from cerebral blood flow measurements in intact animals [29] suggest that cerebral oxygen consumption is low at birth, rises rapidly during the period of cerebral growth and development and reaches a maximal level at about the time maturation is completed. This rise is consistent with the progressive increase in the levels of a number of enzymes of oxidative metabolism in the brain. The rate of blood flow in different structures of the brain reaches peak levels at different times, depending on the maturation rate of the particular structure. In structures that consist predominantly of white matter, the peaks coincide roughly with maximal rates of myelination. From these peaks, blood flow and, probably, cerebral metabolic rate decline to the levels characteristic of adulthood.

Metabolic rate declines and plateaus after maturation

Reliable quantitative data on the changes in cerebral circulation and metabolism in humans from the middle of the first decade of life to old age are summarized in Table 31-6. By 6 years of age, cerebral blood flow and oxygen consumption already have attained high rates, and they decline thereafter to the rates of normal young adulthood [15]. Cerebral oxygen consumption of 5.2 ml/100 g brain tissue/min in a 5- to 6-year-old child corresponds to total oxygen consumption by the brain of approximately 60 ml/min, or more than 50% of the total body basal oxygen consumption, a proportion markedly greater than that occurring in adulthood. The reasons for the extraordinarily high cerebral metabolic rates in children are unknown, but presumably they reflect the extra energy requirements for the biosynthetic processes associated with growth and development.

Tissue pathology, but not aging, produces secondary changes in metabolic rate

Whole-brain cerebral blood flow and oxygen consumption normally remain essentially unchanged between young adulthood and old age. In a population of normal elderly men in their eighth decade of life, who were selected carefully for good health and freedom from all disease including vascular disease, both blood flow and oxygen consumption were not significantly different from rates of normal young men 50 years younger (see Table 31-6) [30]. In a comparable group of elderly subjects, who differed only by the presence of objective evidence of minimal arteriosclerosis, cerebral blood flow was signifi-

TABLE 31-6.   CEREBRAL BLOOD FLOW AND OXYGEN CONSUMPTION IN HUMAN FROM CHILDHOOD TO OLD AGE AND SENILITY[a]

Life period and condition	Age (years)	Cerebral blood flow (ml/100 g/min)	Cerebral O_2 consumption (ml/100 g/min)	Cerebral venous O_2 tension (mm Hg)
Childhood	6[b]	106[b]	5.2[b]	—
Normal young adulthood	21	62	3.5	38
Aged				
Normal elderly	71[b]	58	3.3	36
Elderly with minimal arteriosclerosis	73[b]	48[b]	3.2	33[b,c]
Elderly with senile psychosis	72[b]	48[b,c]	2.7[b,c]	33[b,c]

[a]From Kennedy and Sokoloff [15] and Sokoloff [30].
[b]Statistically significant difference from normal young adult (p < 0.05).
[c]Statistically significant difference from normal elderly subjects (p < 0.05).

cantly lower. It had reached a point at which the oxygen tension of the cerebral venous blood declined, an indication of relative cerebral hypoxia. However, normal cerebral oxygen consumption was maintained through extraction of larger than normal proportions of the arterial blood oxygen. In senile, psychotic patients with arteriosclerosis, cerebral blood flow was no lower but cerebral oxygen consumption had declined. These data suggest that aging per se need not lower cerebral oxygen consumption and blood flow but that, when blood flow is reduced, it is probably secondary to vascular disease, which produces cerebral vascular insufficiency and chronic relative hypoxia in the brain, or to another tissue pathology that decreases function, such as dementia (see Chap. 46). Because arteriosclerosis and Alzheimer's disease are so prevalent in the aged population, most individuals probably follow the latter pattern. However, age-related changes in local regulation are possible and are the subject of research (see Chap. 30).

CEREBRAL METABOLIC RATE IN VARIOUS PHYSIOLOGICAL STATES

Cerebral metabolic rate is determined locally by functional activity in discrete regions

In organs such as heart or skeletal muscle that perform mechanical work, increased functional activity clearly is associated with increased metabolic rate. In nervous tissues outside the central nervous system, electrical activity is an almost quantitative indicator of the degree of functional activity; and in structures such as sympathetic ganglia and postganglionic axons, increased electrical activity produced by electrical stimulation definitely is associated with increased utilization of oxygen. Within the central nervous system, local energy metabolism also is correlated closely with the level of local functional activity. Studies using the [14C]deoxyglucose method have demonstrated pronounced changes in glucose utilization associated with altered functional activity in discrete regions of the central nervous system specifically related to that

function [21]. For example, diminished visual or auditory input depresses glucose utilization in all components of the central visual or auditory pathways, respectively (Fig. 31-4). Focal seizures increase glucose utilization in discrete components of the motor pathways, such as the motor cortex and the basal ganglia (Fig. 31-5).

Convulsive activity, induced or spontaneous, often has been employed as a method of increasing electrical activity of the brain (see Chap. 37). Davies and Remond [13] used the oxygen electrode technique in the cerebral cortex of cat and found increases in oxygen consumption during electrically induced or drug-induced convulsions. Because the increased oxygen consumption either coincided with or followed the onset of convulsions, it was concluded that the elevation in metabolic rate was the consequence of the increased functional activity produced by the convulsive state (see Chaps. 37 and 54).

Metabolic rate and nerve conduction are related directly

The [14C]deoxyglucose method has defined the nature and mechanisms of the relationship between energy metabolism and functional activity in nervous tissues. Studies in the superior cervical ganglion of the rat have shown almost a direct relationship between glucose utilization in the ganglion and spike frequency in the afferent fibers from the cervical sympathetic trunk [31]. A spike results from the passage of a finite current of Na^+ into the cell and of K^+ out of the cell, ion currents that degrade the ionic gradients responsible for the resting membrane potential. Such degradation can be expected to stimulate Na,K-ATPase activity to restore the ionic gradients to normal, and such ATPase activity in turn would stimulate energy metabolism. Indeed, Mata et al. [32] have found that, in the posterior pituitary *in vitro*, stimulation of glucose utilization due to either electrical stimulation or opening of Na^+ channels in the excitable membrane by veratridine is blocked by ouabain, a specific inhibitor of Na,K-ATPase activity (see Chap. 5). Most, if not all, of the stimulated energy metabolism associated with increased functional activity is confined to the axonal terminals

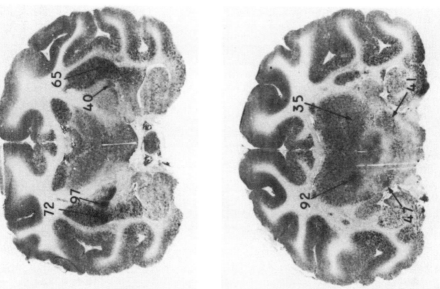
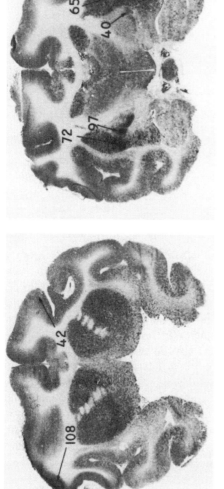

FIGURE 31-5. Local glucose utilization during penicillin-induced focal seizures. Penicillin was applied to the hand and face area of the left motor cortex of a rhesus monkey. The left side of the brain is on the **left** in each of the autoradiograms in the figure. Numbers are rates of local cerebral glucose utilization in micromoles per 100 g tissue per minute. Note the following: **upper left,** motor cortex in region of penicillin application and corresponding region of contralateral motor cortex; **lower left,** ipsilateral and contralateral motor cortical regions remote from area of penicillin applications; **upper right,** ipsilateral and contralateral putamen and globus pallidus; **lower right,** ipsilateral and contralateral thalamic nuclei and substantia nigra. (From [21].)

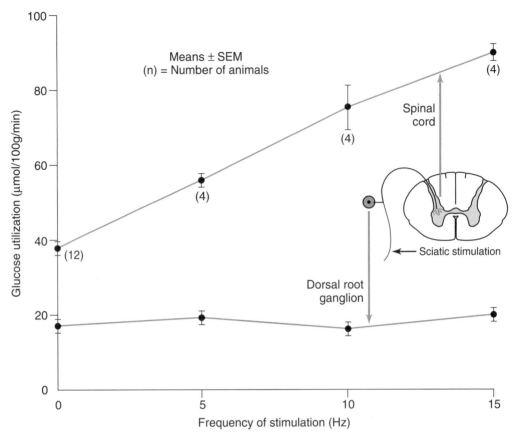

FIGURE 31-6. Effects of electrical stimulation of sciatic nerve on glucose utilization in the terminal zones in the dorsal horn of the spinal cord and in the cell bodies in the dorsal root ganglion. (From [33].)

rather than to the cell bodies in a functionally activated pathway (Fig. 31-6) [33]. Astrocytes also contribute to the increased metabolism [34].

It is difficult to define metabolic equivalents of consciousness, mental work and sleep

Mental work. Convincing correlations between cerebral metabolic rate and mental activity have been obtained in humans in a variety of pathological states of altered consciousness [35]. Regardless of the cause of the disorder, graded reductions in cerebral oxygen consumption are accompanied by parallel graded reductions in the degree of mental alertness, all the way to profound coma (Table 31-7). It is difficult to define or even to conceive of the physical equivalent of mental work. A common view equates concentrated mental effort with mental work, and it is

fashionable to attribute a high demand for mental effort to the process of problem solving in mathematics. Nevertheless, there appears to be no increased energy utilization by the brain during such processes. From resting levels, total cerebral blood flow and oxygen consumption remain unchanged during the exertion of the mental effort required to solve complex arithmetical problems [35]. It may be that the assumptions that relate mathematical reasoning to mental work are erroneous, but it seems more likely that the areas that participate in the processes of such reasoning represent too small a fraction of the brain for changes in their functional and metabolic activities to be reflected in the energy metabolism of the brain as a whole.

Sleep. Physiological sleep is a naturally occurring, periodic, reversible state of unconsciousness; and the EEG pattern in deep, slow-wave

TABLE 31-7.	RELATIONSHIP BETWEEN LEVEL OF CONSCIOUSNESS AND CEREBRAL METABOLIC RATE[a]	
Level of consciousness	Cerebral blood flow (ml/100 g/min)	Cerebral O_2 consumption (ml/100 g/min)
Mentally alert Normal young men	54	3.3
Mentally confused Brain tumor Diabetic acidosis Insulin hypoglycemia Cerebral arteriosclerosis	48	2.8
Comatose Brain tumor Diabetic coma Insulin coma Anesthesia	57	2.0

[a] From Sokoloff [35].

sleep is characterized by high-voltage, slow rhythms very similar to those often seen in pathological comatose states. As found in the pathological comatose states, cerebral glucose metabolism is depressed more or less uniformly throughout the brain of rhesus monkeys in stages 2 to 4 of normal sleep studied by the [^{14}C]deoxyglucose method [36]. There are no comparable data available for the state of paradoxical sleep, also termed REM sleep, or for normal sleep in humans. During the stages of sleep as studied by PET scanning in humans, regional blood flow measurements suggest selective deactivation in certain regions of association cortex during slow-wave sleep and selective activation in other regions during REM sleep [37]. Regional metabolic measurements show activation in the same regions in association with rapid eye movements during REM sleep as with saccadic eye movements during wakefulness [38].

CEREBRAL ENERGY METABOLISM IN PATHOLOGICAL STATES

The cerebral metabolic rate of the brain as a whole is normally fairly stable and varies over a relatively narrow range under physiological conditions. There are, however, a number of pathological states of the nervous system and other organs that affect the functions of the brain either directly or indirectly, and some of these have profound effects on cerebral metabolism.

Psychiatric disorders may produce effects related to anxiety

In general, disorders that alter the quality of mentation but not the level of consciousness (described in Chaps. 51 and 52), such as the functional neuroses, psychoses and psychotomimetic states, have no apparent effect on the average blood flow and oxygen consumption of the brain as a whole. Thus, no gross changes in either function are observed in schizophrenia [35] or LSD intoxication (Table 31-8) [35]. There is still uncertainty about the effects of anxiety, mainly because of the difficulties in evaluating quantitatively the intensity. It is generally believed that ordinary degrees of anxiety, or "nervousness," do not affect the cerebral metabolic rate but that severe anxiety, or "panic," may increase cerebral oxygen consumption [35]. This may be related to the level of epinephrine circulating in the blood. Small doses of epinephrine that raise heart rate and cause some anxiety do not alter cerebral blood flow and metabolism, but large doses that are sufficient to raise the arterial blood pressure cause significant increases in both.

TABLE 31-8.	CEREBRAL BLOOD FLOW AND METABOLIC RATE IN SCHIZOPHRENIA AND IN NORMAL YOUNG MEN DURING LSD-INDUCED PSYCHOTOMIMETIC STATE[a]	
Condition	Cerebral blood blow (ml/100 g/min)	Cerebral O_2 consumption (ml/100 g/min)
Normal	67	3.9
LSD intoxication	68	3.9
Schizophrenia	72	4.0

[a] From Sokoloff [35].

Coma and systemic metabolic diseases depress brain metabolism

Coma is correlated with depression of cerebral oxygen consumption; progressive reductions in the level of consciousness are paralleled by corresponding graded decreases in cerebral metabolic rate (Table 31-7). There are almost innumerable derangements that can lead to depression of consciousness. Table 31-9 includes only a few typical examples that have been studied by the same methods and by the same or related groups of investigators. Metabolic encephalopathy is discussed in detail in Chapter 38.

Inadequate cerebral nutrient supply leads to decreases in the level of consciousness, ranging from confusional states to coma. The nutrition of the brain can be limited by lowering the oxygen or glucose concentrations of arterial blood, as in anoxia or hypoglycemia, or by impairment of their distribution to the brain through lowering cerebral blood flow, as in brain tumors. Consciousness is then depressed, presumably because of inadequate supplies of substrate to support the energy metabolism necessary to sustain function of brain.

In a number of conditions, the causes of depression of both consciousness and the cerebral metabolic rate are unknown and must, by exclusion, be attributed to intracellular defects in the brain. Anesthesia is one example. Cerebral oxygen consumption always is reduced in the anesthetized state regardless of the anesthetic agent used, whereas blood flow may or may not be decreased and may even be increased. This reduction is the result of decreased energy demand and not insufficient nutrient supply or a block of intracellular energy metabolism. There is evidence that general anesthetics interfere with the balance of excitatory and inhibitory synaptic transmission, particularly by an agonist action at GABA-ergic inhibitory synapses, thus reducing neuronal interaction, functional activity and, consequently, metabolic demands (see Chap. 16).

Several metabolic diseases with broad systemic manifestations also are associated with disturbances of cerebral function. Diabetes mellitus, when allowed to progress to states of acidosis and ketosis, leads to mental confusion and, ultimately, deep coma, with parallel proportionate decreases in cerebral oxygen consumption (see Table 31-9) [39]. The abnormalities usually are reversed com-

TABLE 31-9. CEREBRAL BLOOD FLOW AND METABOLIC RATE IN HUMANS WITH VARIOUS DISORDERS AFFECTING MENTAL STATE[a]

Condition	Mental state	Cerebral blood flow (ml/100 g/min)	Cerebral O_2 consumption (ml/100 g/min)
Normal	Alert	54	3.3
Increased intracranial pressure (brain tumor)	Coma	34[b]	2.5[b]
Insulin hypoglycemia			
Arterial glucose level			
74 mg/100 ml	Alert	58	3.4
19 mg/100 ml	Confused	61	2.6[b]
8 mg/100 ml	Coma	63	1.9[b]
Thiopental anesthesia	Coma	60[b]	2.1[b]
Convulsive state			
Before convulsion	Alert	58	3.7
After convulsion	Confused	37[b]	3.1[b]
Diabetes			
Acidosis	Confused	45[b]	2.7[b]
Coma	Coma	65[b]	1.7[b]
Hepatic insufficiency	Coma	33[b]	1.7[b]

[a] All studies listed were carried out by Kety and/or his associates, employing the same methods. For references, see Kennedy and Sokoloff [15] and Sokoloff [35].
[b] Denotes statistically significant difference from normal level ($p < 0.05$).

pletely by adequate insulin therapy. The cause of the coma or depressed cerebral metabolic rate is not known. Deficiency of cerebral nutrition cannot be implicated because the blood glucose concentration is elevated and cerebral blood flow and oxygen supply are more than adequate. Neither is insulin deficiency, presumably the basis of the systemic manifestations of the disease, a likely cause of the cerebral abnormalities since no absolute requirement of insulin for cerebral glucose utilization or metabolism has been demonstrated. Ketosis may be severe in this disease, and there is evidence that a rise in the blood concentration of at least one of the ketone bodies, acetoacetate, can cause coma in animals. In studies of human diabetic acidosis and coma, a significant correlation between the depression of cerebral metabolic rate and the degree of ketosis has been observed, but there is an equally good correlation with the degree of acidosis [39]. Hyperosmolarity itself may cause coma. Ketosis, acidosis, hyperosmolarity or a combination may be responsible for the disturbances in cerebral function and metabolism.

Coma occasionally is associated with severe impairment of liver function, or hepatic insufficiency (see Chap. 38). In human patients in hepatic coma, cerebral metabolic rate is depressed markedly (see Table 31-9). Cerebral blood flow also is depressed moderately but not sufficiently to lead to limiting supplies of glucose and oxygen. Blood ammonia usually is elevated in hepatic coma, and significant cerebral uptake of ammonia from the blood is observed. Ammonia toxicity, therefore, has been suspected as the basis for cerebral dysfunction in hepatic coma. Because ammonia can, through glutamic dehydrogenase activity, convert α-KG to glutamate by reductive amination, it has been suggested that ammonia might thereby deplete α-KG and, thus, slow the Krebs cycle (see Chaps. 15 and 38). The correlation between the degree of coma and blood ammonia is far from convincing, however, and coma has been observed in the absence of an increase in blood ammonia concentration. Although ammonia may be involved in the mechanism of hepatic coma, the mechanism remains unclear, and other causal factors probably are involved.

Depression of mental functions and of the cerebral metabolic rate has been observed in association with kidney failure and uremic coma

(see Chap. 38). The chemical basis of the functional and metabolic disturbances in the brain in this condition also remains undetermined.

In the comatose states associated with these systemic metabolic diseases, there is depression of both conscious mental activity and cerebral energy metabolism. From the available evidence, it is impossible to distinguish which, if either, is the primary change. It is more likely that the depressions of both functions, although well correlated with each other, are independent reflections of a more general impairment of neuronal processes by some unknown factors incident to the disease.

Measurement of local cerebral energy metabolism in humans

Most of the *in vivo* measurements of cerebral energy metabolism described above, and all of those in humans, were made in the brain as a whole and represent the mass-weighted average of the metabolic activities in all of the component structures of the brain. The average, however, often obscures transient and local events in the individual components, and it is not surprising that many of the studies of altered cerebral function, both normal and abnormal, have failed to demonstrate corresponding changes in energy metabolism (see Table 31-8). The [^{14}C]deoxyglucose method [19] has made it possible to measure glucose utilization simultaneously in all of the components of the central nervous system, and it has been used to identify regions with altered functional and metabolic activities in a variety of physiological, pharmacological and pathological states [21]. As originally designed, the method utilized autoradiography of brain sections for localization, which precluded its use in humans. However, later developments with PET [40] made it possible to adapt it for human use, which is described fully in Chapter 54.

REFERENCES

1. Maker, H. S., and Nicklas, W. Biochemical responses of body organs to hypoxia and ischemia. In E. D. Robin (ed.), *Extrapulmonary Manifestations of Respiratory Disease.* New York: Dekker, 1978, pp. 107–150.

2. Gatfield, P. D., Lowry, O. H., Schulz, D. W., and Passoneau, J. V. Regional energy reserves in mouse brain and changes with ischaemia and anaesthesia. *J. Neurochem.* 13:185–195, 1966.

3. Lowry, O. H., and Passoneau, J. V. The relationships between substrates and enzymes of glycolysis in brain. *J. Biol. Chem.* 239:31–32, 1964.

4. Meyer, R. A., and Sweeney, H. L. A simple analysis of the "phosphocreatine shuttle." *Am. J. Physiol.* 246:365–377, 1984.

5. Goldberg, N. D., and O'Toole, A. G. The properties of glycogen synthetase and regulation of glycogen biosynthesis in rat brain. *J. Biol. Chem.* 244:3053–3061, 1969.

6. Matthews, C. K., and van Holde, K. E., *Biochemistry,* 2nd. ed. Redwood City, California: Benjamin, Cummings, 1996, pp. 474–477.

7. Stewart, M. A., and Moonsammy, G. I. Substrate changes in peripheral nerve recovering from anoxia. *J. Neurochem.* 13:1433–1439, 1966.

8. Gaitonde, M. K., Evison, E., and Evans, G. M. The rate of utilization of glucose via hexosemonophosphate shunt in brain. *J. Neurochem.* 41:1253–1260, 1983.

9. Morgan-Hughes, J. A. Mitochondrial disease. *Trends Neurosci.* 9:15–19, 1986.

10. Waelsch, H., Berl, S., Rossi, C. A., Clarke, D. D., and Purpura, D. P. Quantitative aspects of CO_2 fixation in mammalian brain *in vivo. J. Neurochem.* 11:717–728, 1964.

11. Clarke, D. D. Fluoroacetate and fluorocitrate: Mechanism of action. *Neurochem. Res.* 16:1055–1058, 1991.

12. Leong, S. F., Lai, J. C. K., Lim, L., and Clark, J. B. The activities of some energy metabolizing enzymes in non synaptic (free) and synaptic mitochondria derived from selected brain regions. *J. Neurochem.* 42:1308–1312, 1984.

13. Davies, P. W., and Remond, A. Oxygen consumption of the cerebral cortex of the cat during metrazole convulsions. *Res. Publ. Assoc. Nerv. Ment. Dis.* 26:205–217, 1946.

14. Kety, S. S., and Schmidt, C. F. The nitrous oxide method for the quantitative determination of cerebral blood flow in man: Theory, procedure, and normal values. *J. Clin. Invest.* 27:476–483, 1948.

15. Kennedy, C., and Sokoloff, L. An adaptation of the nitrous oxide method to the study of the cerebral circulation in children; normal values for cerebral blood flow and cerebral metabolic rate in childhood. *J. Clin. Invest.* 36:1130–1137, 1957.

16. Sokoloff, L. The metabolism of the central nervous system *in vivo.* In J. Field, H. W. Magoun, and V. E. Hall (eds.), *Handbook of Physiology–Neurophysiology.* Washington, D.C.: American Physiological Society, 1960, Vol. 3, pp. 1843–1864.

17. Sokoloff, L., and Kety, S. S. Regulation of cerebral circulation. *Physiol. Rev.* 40(Suppl. 4):38–44, 1960.

18. Freygang, W. H., and Sokoloff, L. Quantitative measurements of regional circulation in the central nervous system by the use of radioactive inert gas. *Adv. Biol. Med. Phys.* 6:263–279, 1958.

19. Sokoloff, L., Reivich, M., Kennedy, C., et al. The [^{14}C]deoxyglucose method for the measurement of local cerebral glucose utilization: Theory, procedure, and normal values in the conscious and anesthetized albino rat. *J. Neurochem.* 28:897–916, 1977.

20. Sokoloff, L. Local cerebral energy metabolism: Its relationships to local functional activity and blood flow. In M. J. Purves and L. Elliott (eds.), *Cerebral Vascular Smooth Muscle and Its Control* (Ciba Foundation Symposium 56). Amsterdam: Elsevier/Excerpta Medica/North Holland, 1978, pp. 171–197.

21. Sokoloff, L. Relation between physiological function and energy metabolism in the central nervous system. *J. Neurochem.* 29:13–26, 1977.

22. Kennedy, C., Sakurada, O., Shinohara, M., Jehle, J., and Sokoloff, L. Local cerebral glucose utilization in the normal conscious Macaque monkey. *Ann. Neurol.* 4:293–301, 1978.

23. Himwich, H. E., and Nahum, L. H. The respiratory quotient of testicle. *Am. J. Physiol.* 88:680–685, 1929.

24. Kety, S. S., Woodford, R. B., Harmel, M. H., Freyhan, F. A., Appel, K. E., and Schmidt, C. F. Cerebral flow and metabolism in schizophrenia. The effects of barbiturate seminarcosis, insulin coma, and electroshock. *Am. J. Psychiatry* 104:765–770, 1948.

25. Sloviter, H. A., and Kamimoto, T. The isolated, perfused rat brain preparation metabolizes mannose but not maltose. *J. Neurochem.* 17:1109–1111, 1970.

26. Owen, O. E., Morgan, A. P., Kemp, H. G., Sullivan, J. M., Herrera, M. G., and Cahill, G. F., Jr. Brain metabolism during fasting. *J. Clin. Invest.* 46:1589–1595, 1967.

27. Krebs, H. A., Williamson, D. H., Bates, M. W., Page, M. A., and Hawkins, R. A. The role of ketone bodies in caloric homeostatis. *Adv. Enzyme Regul.* 9:387–409, 1971.

28. Klee, C. B., and Sokoloff, L. Changes in D(−)-β-hydroxybutyric dehydrogenase activity during brain maturation in the rat. *J. Biol. Chem.* 242:3880–3883, 1967.

29. Kennedy, C., Grave, G. D., Jehle, J. W., and Sokoloff, L. Changes in blood flow in the component structures of the dog brain during postnatal maturation. *J. Neurochem.* 19:2423–2433, 1972.

30. Sokoloff, L. Cerebral circulatory and metabolic changes associated with aging. *Res. Publ. Assoc. Nerv. Ment. Dis.* 41:237–254, 1966.

31. Yarowsky, P., Kadekaro, M., and Sokoloff, L. Frequency-dependent activation of glucose utilization in the superior cervical ganglion by electrical stimulation of cervical sympathetic trunk. *Proc. Natl. Acad. Sci. USA* 80:4179–4183, 1983.

32. Mata, M., Fink, D. J., Gainer, H., et al. Activity-dependent energy metabolism in rat posterior pituitary primarily reflects sodium pump activity. *J. Neurochem.* 34:213–215, 1980.

33. Kadekaro, M., Crane, A. M., and Sokoloff, L. Differential effects of electrical stimulation of sciatic nerve on metabolic activity in spinal cord and dorsal root ganglion in the rat. *Proc. Natl. Acad. Sci. USA* 82:6010–6013, 1985.

34. Takahashi, S., Driscoll, B. F., Law, M. J., and Sokoloff, L. Role of sodium and potassium ions in regulation of glucose metabolism in cultured astroglia. *Proc. Natl. Acad. Sci. USA* 92:4616–4620, 1995.

35. Sokoloff, L. Cerebral circulation and behavior in man: Strategy and findings. In A. J. Mandell and M. P. Mandell (eds.), *Psychochemical Research in Man.* New York: Academic, 1969, pp. 237–252.

36. Kennedy, C., Gillin, J. C., Mendelson, W., et al. Local cerebral glucose utilization in non-rapid eye movement sleep. *Nature* 297:325–327, 1982.

37. Braun, A. R., Balkin, T. J., Wesenten, N. J., et al. Regional cerebral blood flow through the sleep–wake cycle. An $H_2[^{15}O]$ PET study. *Brain* 120:1173–1197, 1997.

38. Hong, C. C., Gillin, J. C., Dow, B. M., Wu, J., and Buchsbaum, M. S. Localized and lateralized cerebral glucose metabolism associated with eye movements during REM sleep and wakefulness: A positron emission tomography (PET) study. *Sleep* 18:570–580, 1995.

39. Kety, S. S., Polis, B. D., Nadler, C. S., and Schmidt, C. F. Blood flow and oxygen consumption of the human brain in diabetic acidosis and coma. *J. Clin. Invest.* 27:500–510, 1948.

40. Reivich, M., Kuhl, D., Wolf, A., et al. The $[^{18}F]$fluorodeoxyglucose method for the measurement of local cerebral glucose utilization in man. *Circ. Res.* 44:127–137, 1979.

41. Passoneau, J. V., Lowry, O. H., Schulz, D. W. and Brown, J. G. Glucose-1,6-diphosphate formation by phosphoglucomutase in mammalian tissues. *J. Biol. Chem.* 244:902–909, 1969.

42. Breckenridge, B. M. and Crawford E. T. The quantitative histochemistry of the brain. *J. Neurochem.* 7:234–240, 1961.

43. Matchinsky, F. M. Energy metabolism of the microscopic structures of the cochlea, the retina, and the cerebellum in biochemistry of simple neuronal models. E. Costa and E. Giacobini (eds.). *Adv. Biochem. Psychopharm.* 2:217–243, 1970.

44. McIlwain, H. *Biochemistry and the Central Nervous System,* 3rd ed. Boston: Little, Brown, 1966, pp. 1–26.

32

Blood–Brain–Cerebrospinal Fluid Barriers

John Laterra, Richard Keep, A. Lorris Betz and Gary W. Goldstein

Basic Neurochemistry: Molecular, Cellular and Medical Aspects, 6th Ed., edited by G. J. Siegel et al. Published by Lippincott–Raven Publishers, Philadelphia, 1999. Correspondence to A. Lorris Betz, Departments of Pediatrics, Surgery and Neurology, University of Michigan, D3227 Medical Professional Building, Ann Arbor, Michigan 48109-0718.

CONSTANCY OF THE INTERNAL ENVIRONMENT OF THE BRAIN

In no other organ is constancy of the internal environment more important than in the brain. Elsewhere in the body, the extracellular concentrations of hormones, amino acids and potassium undergo frequent fluctuations, particularly after meals and exercise or during times of stress. In the central nervous system, a similar change in the composition of the interstitial fluid could lead to uncontrolled brain activity because catecholamines and certain amino acids are centrally acting neurotransmitters and potassium influences the threshold for activation of synapses. Consequently, the cerebrospinal fluid (CSF) concentrations of many solutes are maintained lower than concentrations in plasma (Table 32-1). The blood–brain–CSF barriers isolate brain cells from the normal variations in body fluid composition and regulate the composition of the extracellular fluid in the brain to provide a stable environment for nerve cell interactions.

The concept of the blood–brain–CSF barriers was developed in the late nineteenth century when Ehrlich observed that vital dyes administered intravenously stained all organs except the brain. He concluded that the dyes had a lower affinity for binding to brain than to other tissues. In 1913, however, Goldmann disproved the binding hypothesis by administering trypan blue dye directly into the CSF. By this route, the dye readily stained the entire brain substance but was restricted to the brain and spinal cord and did not enter the bloodstream to reach other organs. The studies with vital dyes agreed well with the parallel work of Biedl and Kraus in 1898 on bile acids and of Lewandowsky in 1900 on ferrocyanide. These compounds were not neurotoxic when administered by vein but caused seizures and coma when injected directly into the brain. These experiments established that the central nervous system is separated from the bloodstream by blood–brain and blood–CSF barriers. The cellular basis for these barriers was not established until 50 years later, when the development of electron microscopy permitted examination of the ultrastructure of the brain microvasculature and choroid plexus.

MEMBRANE TRANSPORT PROCESSES

Contemporary research has focused on how selected molecules are able to enter and leave the brain and how CSF is formed. This work has led to an appreciation of the important role played by membrane transport processes in the function of the blood–brain–CSF barriers [1,2]. Monographs about the blood–brain and blood–CSF barriers are available for readers interested in a more complete review [3,4].

Physical and biological processes determine molecular movement across membranes of the blood–brain–cerebrospinal fluid barriers

The processes that determine molecular movement across membranes are diffusion, pinocytosis, carrier-mediated transport and transcellular transport [5]. The types of carrier-mediated transport are described in Chapter 5.

Diffusion is the process by which molecules in solution move from an area of higher to lower concentration. With this type of transport, the net rate of solute flux is directly proportional to the difference in concentration between the two areas. In biological systems, this process is an important mechanism for the movement of molecules within a fluid compartment; however, diffusion across a lipid membrane, such as the cell membranes of the blood–brain barrier, is possible only when the solute is lipid-soluble or when the membrane contains specialized channels. Diffusion is the primary mechanism for blood–brain exchange of respiratory gases and other highly lipid-soluble compounds.

Pinocytosis is a process by which extracellular fluid is engulfed by invaginating cell membranes, forming a vesicle that then separates from the membrane. This vesicle may move through the cell cytoplasm and release its contents on the other side of the cell layer by means of exocytosis. Under normal conditions, pinocytosis is thought to contribute little to the transport of solutes across the blood–brain barrier. Instead, the few vesicles that are observed within

TABLE 32-1. TYPICAL CEREBROSPINAL FLUID (CSF) AND PLASMA CONCENTRATIONS OF VARIOUS SUBSTANCES[a]

Substance	CSF	Plasma	CSF/ plasma ratio
Electrolytes (mEq/l)			
Na^+	138	138	1.0
K^+	2.8	4.5	0.6
Cl^-	119	102	1.2
HCO_3^-	22	24	0.9
Ca^{2+}	2.1	4.8	0.4
Mg^{2+}	2.3	1.7	1.4
PO_4^{3-}	0.5	1.8	0.3
Metabolites (mM)			
Glucose	3.3	5.0	0.7
Lactate	1.6	1.0	1.6
Pyruvate	0.08	0.11	0.7
Urea	4.7	5.4	0.9
Creatinine	0.09	0.14	0.7
Amino acids (μM)			
Alanine	26.0	350	0.1
Arginine	22.4	80.9	0.3
Aspartic acid	0.2	2.0	0.1
Asparagine	13.5	112	0.1
Glutamic acid	26.1	61.3	0.4
Glutamine	552	641	0.9
Glycine	5.9	283	0.02
Histidine	12.3	79.8	0.2
Isoleucine	6.2	76.7	0.1
Leucine	14.8	155	0.1
Lysine	20.8	171	0.1
Methionine	2.5	27.7	0.1
Ornithine	3.8	73.5	0.1
Phenylalanine	9.9	64.0	0.2
Phosphoethanolamine	5.4	5.1	1.0
Phosphoserine	4.2	8.3	0.6
Serine	29.5	140	0.2
Taurine	7.6	77.2	0.1
Threonine	35.5	166	0.2
Tyrosine	9.5	73.0	0.1
Valine	19.9	309	0.1
Proteins (mg/l)			
Total protein	350	70,000	0.005
Albumin	155	36,600	0.004
Transferrin	14.4	2,040	0.007
IgG	12.3	9,870	0.001
IgA	1.3	1,750	0.001
IgM	0.6	700	0.001

[a] Values are from Fishman [18].

brain capillary endothelial cells are probably destined to fuse with lysosomes. Nevertheless, some proteins may traverse the brain endothelial cell through a process that has been called absorptive-mediated transcytosis [6].

Transcellular transport across a layer of cells requires the presence of carrier or channel molecules on the luminal and antiluminal sides of the cells. Facilitated and active transport are defined in Chapter 5. In transcellular facilitated diffusion, the carriers on opposite sides of the cell are usually similar and solutes are not moved against concentration gradients. Active transport across a cell layer, however, requires a special arrangement of transport proteins within the plasma membranes. The active transport system is found on only one side of the cell and usually is associated with a nonactive transport system on the other side of the cell. With this arrangement, a solute accumulates within the cell by active transport through one membrane and subsequently leaves the cell by a channel or facilitated transport process through the opposite membrane. When plasma membranes of two surfaces of a cell have different properties, that cell is said to be polar. Cellular polarity underlies active transcellular transport and secretion of fluid by epithelial cells in the choroid plexus.

When fluid is secreted at one site and absorbed at another, there is bulk flow of fluid. This means that solutes of various sizes move together with the solvent as a bulk liquid. This process is important in the circulation and absorption of CSF, which is secreted by the choroid plexus, circulated through the ventricular and subarachnoid spaces and absorbed through arachnoid villi into the bloodstream.

Transport processes combine to provide stability for constituents of cerebrospinal fluid and brain extracellular fluid

Bradbury and Stulcova [7] defined stability of the blood–CSF systems as follows. If a substance is present in CSF at concentration C_{CSF} and in plasma at concentration C_{pl}, stability occurs when, as a result of a change in plasma concentration, a new steady state is reached so that

$$\Delta C_{CSF} < \Delta C_{pl}$$

At steady state, the flux of this substance from plasma to CSF, J_{in}, must equal its flux out, J_{out}, so that for any change in plasma concentration, ΔC_{pl} stability of CSF will occur when

$$\Delta J_{in}/\Delta C_{pl} < \Delta J_{out}/\Delta C_{CSF}$$

where J_{in} and J_{out} represent transport processes

that need not be identical. For instance, one process might be passive and the other active. If the carrier involved in J_{in} is saturated at the usual plasma concentration, then the ratio $\Delta J_{in}/\Delta C_{pl}$ will approach zero. Such carrier-mediated transport is probably the most common mechanism controlling the flow of water-soluble substances from the capillary lumen to the brain, but carrier systems also have been found to operate for outward flux. Here, the greatest stability is achieved when the carrier system operates well below saturation so that the ratio $\Delta J_{out}/\Delta C_{CSF}$ is a positive number. Such asymmetrical carrier mechanisms have been implicated in the maintenance of a stable K^+ concentration in CSF and may exist for some amino acids and organic acids.

BLOOD–BRAIN BARRIER

Endothelial cells in brain capillaries are the site of the blood–brain barrier

Studies of Reese and Karnovsky and Brightman and Reese demonstrated that brain endothelial cells differ from endothelial cells in capillaries of other organs in two important ways [8]. First, continuous tight junctions are present between the endothelial cells, which prevent transcapillary movement of polar molecules varying in size from proteins to ions. Second, there are no detectable transendothelial pathways. Thus, there is an absence of transcellular channels and fenestrations as well as a paucity of plasmalemmal and intracellular vesicles. As a result of these special anatomical features, the endothelial cells in brain provide a continuous cellular barrier between the blood and the interstitial fluid (Fig. 32-1). Not all areas of the brain contain capillaries that produce a barrier. In these nonbarrier regions, the morphological features of the capillaries are similar to those of systemic microvascular beds. Thus, the tight junctions are discontinuous, there are more plasmalemmal vesicles and some endothelial cells even exhibit fenestrations. Table 32-2 lists the brain regions that contain capillaries of this type. The absence of a blood–brain barrier in many of these regions may relate to their feedback role in the regulation of peptide hormone release.

Surrounding the capillary endothelial cell is

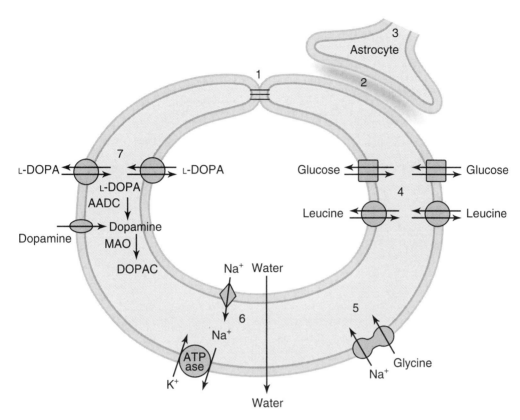

FIGURE 32-1. Schematic diagram of brain capillary. The continuous tight junctions (1) that join endothelial cells in brain capillaries limit the diffusion of large and small solutes across the blood–brain barrier. The basement membrane (2) provides structural support for the capillary and, along with the astrocytic foot processes (3) that encircle the capillary, may influence endothelial cell function. Transport carriers (4) for glucose and essential amino acids facilitate the movement of these solutes into brain, while secondary transport systems (5) appear to cause the efflux of small, nonessential amino acids from brain to blood. Sodium ion transporters on the luminal membrane and Na,K-ATPase on the antiluminal membrane (6) account for the movement of sodium from blood to brain, and this may provide an osmotic driving force for the secretion of interstitial fluid by the brain capillary. The enzymatic blood–brain barrier (7) consists of the uptake of neurotransmitter precursors such as L-DOPA into the endothelial cells via the large neutral amino acid carrier and their subsequent metabolism to 3,4-dihydroxyphenylacetic acid (DOPAC) by the aromatic amino acid decarboxylase (AADC) and monoamine oxidase (MAO) present within the endothelial cell. Neurotransmitters in the interstitial fluid also may be accumulated and metabolized by the brain capillary.

a collagen-containing extracellular matrix. Embedded within this basement membrane are contractile pericytes. These cells may regulate endothelial cell proliferation and, under certain pathological conditions, take on phagocytic functions. Almost the entire outer surface of the basement membrane is covered with foot processes from astrocytes. This close association suggests an interaction between astrocytes and endothelial cells that is important for the function of the blood–brain barrier. Support for this hypothesis is found in brain tumors and non-barrier regions of the brain, where the absence of intimate astrocyte–endothelial cell contact is associated with the absence of a blood–brain barrier. More direct evidence comes from cell culture studies in which astrocytes or their secreted cell products induce endothelial cells to differentiate morphogenically into vascular structures [9] and to increase their interendothelial tight junctional complexes [10].

Substances with a high lipid solubility may move across the blood–brain barrier by simple diffusion

Diffusion is the major entry mechanism for most psychoactive drugs. As shown in Figure 32-2, the

TABLE 32-2.	AREAS OF BRAIN WITHOUT A BLOOD–BRAIN BARRIER

Pituitary gland
Median eminence
Area postrema
Preoptic recess
Paraphysis
Pineal gland
Endothelium of the choroid plexus

rate of entry of compounds that diffuse into the brain depends on their lipid solubility, as estimated by oil/water partition coefficients. For example, the permeability of very lipid-soluble compounds, such as ethanol, nicotine, iodoantipyrine and diazepam, is so high that they are extracted completely from the blood during a single passage through the brain. Hence, their uptake by the brain is limited only by blood flow, and this provides the basis for use of iodoantipyrine to measure cerebral blood flow rate. In contrast, polar molecules, such as glycine and catecholamines, enter the brain only slowly, thereby isolating the brain from neurotransmitters in the plasma. Uptake in the brain of some compounds, such as phenobarbital and phenytoin, is lower than predicted from their lipid solubility as a result of binding to plasma proteins.

Water readily enters the brain by diffusion. Using intravenously administered deuterium oxide as a tracer, the measured half-time of exchange of brain water varies between 12 and 25 sec, depending on the vascularity of the region studied. Although this rate of exchange is rapid compared with the rate of exchange of most solutes, it is limited both by the permeability of the capillary endothelium and by the rate of cerebral blood flow. In fact, the calculated permeability constant of the cerebral capillary wall to the diffusion of water is about the same as that estimated for its diffusion across lipid membranes (Fig. 32-2).

As a consequence of its high permeability, water moves freely into or out of the brain as the osmolality of the plasma changes. This phenomenon is clinically useful since the intravenous administration of poorly permeable compounds such as mannitol (Fig. 32-2) will osmotically dehydrate the brain and reduce intracranial pressure. For example, when plasma osmolality is raised from 310 to 344 mOsm, a 10% shrinkage of the brain will result, with half of the shrinkage taking place in 12 min.

Gases, such as CO_2, O_2, N_2O and Xe, and volatile anesthetics diffuse rapidly into the brain. As a consequence, the rate at which their concentration in the brain comes into equilibrium with the plasma is limited primarily by the cerebral blood flow rate. Hence, the inert gases, such as N_2O and Xe, can be used to measure cerebral blood flow. An interesting contrast is found between CO_2 and H^+ with regard to their effects on brain pH. Since the blood–brain barrier permeability of CO_2 greatly exceeds that of H^+, the pH of the brain interstitial fluid will reflect blood pCO_2 rather than blood pH. Consequently, in a patient with a metabolic acidosis and a compensatory respiratory alkalosis, the brain is alkalotic.

Carrier-mediated transport enables molecules with low lipid solubility to traverse the blood–brain barrier

Although D-glucose and L-glucose are stereoisomers, extraction of D-glucose in the brain is more than 100-fold greater than that of L-glucose (Fig. 32-2). This apparently anomalous relationship also is observed for other metabolically essential compounds (Table 32-3). The high permeability of these polar compounds is mediated by specific transport proteins (see Chap. 5) in the plasma membranes of the endothelial cells (Fig. 32-1).

Glucose is the primary energy substrate of the brain, and its metabolism accounts for nearly all of the oxygen consumption in the brain (see Chap. 31). Since entry of glucose into the brain is critical, mechanisms for glucose transport across the blood–brain barrier have been studied particularly well [11]. Stereospecific, but insulin-independent, GLUT-1 glucose transporters are highly enriched in brain capillary endothelial cells (Fig. 32-3) and mediate the facilitated diffusion of this polar substrate through the blood–brain barrier [12]. The activ-

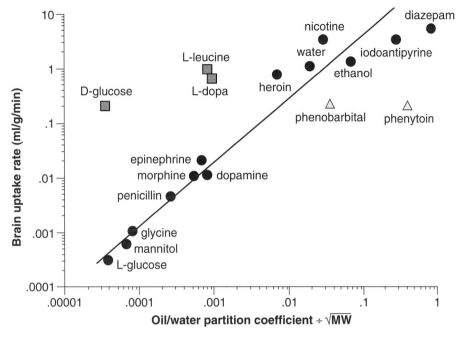

FIGURE 32-2. Relationship between lipid solubility and brain uptake of selected compounds. The distribution into octanol relative to water for each test substance serves as a measure of its lipid solubility. This value is adjusted for differences in molecular weight *(MW)* and plotted on the x-axis. The brain uptake rate for radiolabeled solutes (•), measured as the product of the blood–brain barrier permeability and surface area (PS product), is plotted on the y-axis. In general, the higher the oil–water partition coefficient, the greater the brain uptake. Uptake of the two anticonvulsants phenobarbital and phenytoin (△) is lower than predicted from their lipid solubility partly because of their binding to plasma proteins. Uptake of D-glucose, L-leucine and L-DOPA (■) is greater than predicted by their lipid solubility because specific carriers facilitate their transport across the brain capillary. Data are estimates based on several sources [14,32,36–39].

ity of these transporters is sufficient to transport two to three times more glucose than normally is metabolized by the brain.

Diminished blood–brain barrier GLUT-1 expression that is substantial enough to compromise energy substrate delivery to the brain has been found in a series of children with seizures, mental retardation, compromised brain development and low CSF glucose concentrations. GLUT-1 protein concentrations in red blood cells obtained from these patients is approximately 50% of normal, consistent with a heterozygous GLUT-1 genomic mutation. Interestingly, the seizures in these patients are particularly responsive to therapy with a ketogenic diet that replaces glucose with ketone bodies as the principal energy substrate for the brain. This is the first recognized example of disease attributed to a blood–brain barrier transport defect.

The stereospecificity of the glucose-transport system permits D-glucose, but not L-glucose, to enter the brain. Hexoses, such as mannose and maltose, also are transported rapidly into the brain; the uptake of galactose is intermediate, whereas fructose is taken up very slowly. 2-Deoxyglucose is taken up quickly and will competitively inhibit the transport of glucose. Once within neurons and glia, 2-deoxyglucose is phosphorylated but not metabolized further. If 2-deoxyglucose is used in tracer quantities, the amount of the phosphorylated tracer in the brain reflects the rate of glucose metabolism (see Chap. 31).

Monocarboxylic acids, including L-lactate, acetate, pyruvate and ketone bodies, are transported by a separate stereospecific system [13]. The rate of entry of these substances is significantly lower than that of glucose; however,

TABLE 32-3. TRANSPORT SYSTEMS THAT OPERATE FROM BLOOD TO BRAIN

Transport system	Typical substrate	Transport rate
Metabolic substrates		
Hexose	Glucose	700
Monocarboxylic acid	Lactate	60
Large neutral amino acid	Phenylalanine	12
Basic amino acid	Lysine	3
Acidic amino acid	Glutamate	0.2
β-amino acid	Taurine	0.4
Amine	Choline	0.2
Purine	Adenine	0.006
Nucleoside	Adenosine	0.004
Saturated fatty acid	Octanoate	
Vitamins and cofactors		
Thiamine	Thiamine	
Pantothenic acid	Pantothenic acid	
Biotin	Biotin	
Vitamin B_6	Pyridoxal	
Riboflavin	Riboflavin	
Niacinamide	Niacinamide	
Carnitine	Carnitine	
Inositol	*myo*-Inositol	
Electrolytes		
Sodium	Sodium	200
Potassium	Potassium	12
Chloride	Chloride	140
Hormones		
Thyroid hormone	T_3	
Vasopressin	Arginine vasopressin	
Insulin	Insulin	
Other peptides		
Transferrin	Transferrin	
Enkephalins	Leu-enkephalin	

[a]Transport rates (nmol/g/min) are estimated from experimentally determined uptake rates [14,13,18] and the normal plasma concentrations of the typical substrate.

they are important metabolic substrates in neonates and during starvation. The rate and capacity of monocarboxylic acid transport are elevated substantially in suckling neonates, consistent with the unique metabolic requirements of the developing brain and the elevated concentrations of monocarboxylic acids in breast milk.

Neutral L-amino acids have various rates of movement into the brain [13,14]. Phenylalanine, leucine, tyrosine, isoleucine, valine, tryptophan, methionine, histidine and L-dihydroxy-

phenylalanine (L-DOPA) may enter as rapidly as glucose. These essential amino acids cannot be synthesized by the brain and, therefore, must be supplied from protein breakdown and diet (see Chap. 33). Several are precursors for neurotransmitters synthesized in the brain (see Chaps. 12–14). Transport of these large neutral amino acids into the brain is inhibited by the synthetic amino acid 2-aminonorbornane-2-carboxylic acid (BCH) but not by 2-(methyl-amino)-isobutyric acid (MeAIB); hence, the transport system in the blood–brain barrier is similar to the leucine-preferring (L) transport

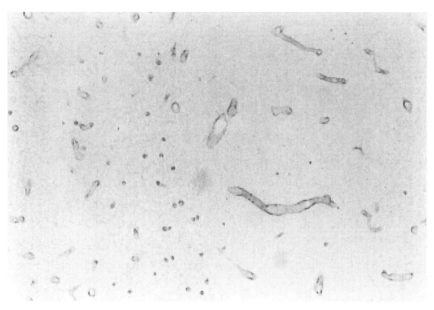

FIGURE 32-3. Expression of glucose transporter (GLUT-1) in microvessels of rat brain. Using a rabbit polyclonal antibody generated against the C terminus of the rat brain/human erythrocyte GLUT-1 protein, 5-μm-thick sections of rat cerebral cortex embedded in paraffin blocks were stained for expression of the transporter. Biotinylated goat anti-rabbit immunoglobulin was used to demonstrate the distribution of the primary antibody. The selective staining of brain microvessels is consistent with their role in the passage of glucose through the blood–brain barrier. (GLUT-1 antibody obtained from Dr. L. R. Drewes.)

system defined by Christensen (see [5]). Since a single type of transport carrier mediates the transcapillary movement of structurally related amino acids, these compounds compete with each other for entry into the brain. Therefore, an elevation in the plasma concentration of one will inhibit uptake of the others (Fig. 32-4). This may be important in certain metabolic diseases, such as phenylketonuria (PKU), where high concentrations of phenylalanine in plasma reduce brain uptake of other essential amino acids (see Chap. 44).

Small neutral amino acids, such as alanine, glycine, proline and γ-aminobutyric acid (GABA), are markedly restricted in their entry into the brain (for example, glycine in Fig. 32-2). These amino acids are synthesized by the brain, and several are putative neurotransmitters (see Chaps. 16 and 18). This restriction is consistent with the inability of MeAIB to inhibit brain uptake of amino acids and suggests that the alanine-preferring (A) transport system [5] is not present on the luminal surface of the blood–brain barrier. In contrast, these small neutral amino acids appear to be transported out of the brain across the blood–brain barrier, suggesting that the A-system carrier is present on the antiluminal surface of the brain capillary [15]. This may explain why the CSF: plasma concentration ratios are particularly low for these amino acids (Table 32-1). Thus, essential amino acids that serve as precursors for catecholamine and indoleamine synthesis are readily transported into the brain (L system), whereas amino acids synthesized by the brain, including those amino acids that act as neurotransmitters, not only are limited in their entry but also are transported actively out of the brain (A system).

In addition, there are distinct transport systems that facilitate the brain uptake of basic, acidic and β-amino acids (Table 32-3). Lysine and arginine are essential amino acids and, therefore, must be provided from the blood. The acidic amino acids glutamate and aspartate are both important metabolic intermediates as well as neurotransmitters (see Chap. 15). While the

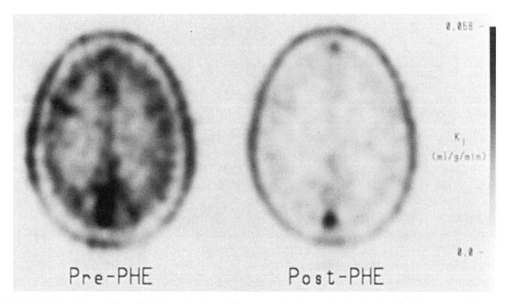

FIGURE 32-4. Competitive inhibition of amino acid transport in human brain. Regional brain uptake of the neutral amino acid analog ^{11}C-aminocyclohexane carboxylic acid (ACHC) was determined in a normal volunteer using positron emission tomography (see Chap. 54) before *(Pre-PHE)* and after *(Post-PHE)* oral ingestion of phenylalanine. Higher values for the influx rate constant (K_i) are noted by darker shading. Note the marked reduction of ACHC uptake rate in brain following ingestion of phenylalanine. In contrast, there is little or no effect on ACHC entry into the scalp or on the ACHC present in cerebral veins (dark spots at top and bottom of image). The reduced uptake of ACHC after ingestion of phenylalanine indicates that phenylalanine competes with ACHC for transport into the brain. For more details on methodology, see Koeppe et al. [40].

brain content of these amino acids is maintained primarily by *de novo* synthesis, they also can be transported into the brain at a slow rate across the blood–brain barrier. The β-amino acid taurine is present at high concentrations in the brain and is involved in volume regulation.

Choline enters the central nervous system through a carrier-mediated transport process that can be inhibited by molecules such as dimethyl aminoethanol, hemicholinium and tetraethyl ammonium chloride. Since choline cannot be synthesized by the brain, it has been proposed that blood–brain barrier transport may regulate the formation of acetylcholine in the central nervous system [16].

Vitamins are, by definition, substances that cannot be synthesized by mammalian organisms but are required in small amounts to support normal metabolism. Since vitamins cannot be synthesized by the brain, they must be obtained from the blood. Thus, specific transport systems are present in the blood–brain barrier for most

vitamins (Table 32-3) [17]. These transport systems generally have a low capacity since the brain requires only small amounts of the vitamins and efficient homeostatic mechanisms preserve brain vitamin content without the need for a rapid influx from the blood. Nevertheless, dietary deficiency of some vitamins can produce neurological disease (see Chaps. 33 and 44).

Metal ions are exchanged between plasma and brain very slowly compared with other tissues

Intravenously administered $^{42}K^+$, for example, exchanges with muscle K^+ in 1 hr, but K^+ exchange in brain is only half completed in 24 to 36 hr. Na^+ exchange is somewhat faster, with half-exchange into brain occurring in 3 to 8 hr. Despite its relatively slow entry into the brain, Na^+ exchange across the blood–brain barrier appears to occur by mediated transport [18]. This occurs, in part, through brain capillary Na,K-ATPase (see Chap. 5), which is located primarily on the antiluminal membrane of the endothelial cell (Fig. 32-1). Na,K-ATPase in the brain capillary also may mediate removal of interstitial fluid K$^+$ from the brain and thereby may maintain a constant brain K$^+$ concentration in the face of fluctuating plasma concentrations. In addition, the antiluminal location of Na,K-ATPase may underlie the proposed role of the brain capillary in secretion of interstitial fluid, an extrachoroidal source of CSF.

Some proteins cross the blood–brain barrier by binding to receptors or by absorption on the endothelial cell membrane

Receptor-mediated transcytosis. Most proteins in the plasma are not able to cross the blood–brain barrier because of their size and hydrophilicity. Consequently, concentrations of plasma proteins in the brain are very low (Table 32-1). However, concentrations of certain proteins, such as insulin and transferrin, vary as the plasma concentrations change, and uptake of these peptides in the brain is greater than expected based on their size and lipid solubility. Furthermore, the brain uptake of some proteins is saturable. These properties suggest the presence of a specific transport process. It is now believed that proteins such as insulin, transferrin, insulin-like growth factors and vasopressin cross the blood–brain barrier by a process called receptor-mediated transcytosis [6]. The brain capillary endothelial cell is highly enriched in receptors for these proteins, and following binding of protein to the receptor, a portion of the membrane containing the protein–receptor complex is endocytosed into the endothelial cell to form a vesicle. Although the subsequent route of passage of the protein through the endothelial cell is not known, there is eventual release of intact protein on the other side of the endothelial cell.

Absorptive-mediated transcytosis. Polycationic proteins and lectins cross the blood–brain barrier by a similar but nonspecific process called absorptive-mediated transcytosis [5]. Rather than binding to specific receptors in the membrane, these proteins absorb to the endothelial cell membrane based on charge or affinity for sugar moieties of membrane glycoproteins. The subsequent transcytotic events are probably similar to receptor-mediated transcytosis; however, the overall capacity of absorptive-mediated transcytosis is greater because it is not limited by the number of receptors present in the membrane. Thus, cationization may provide a mechanism for enhancing brain uptake of almost any protein.

Metabolic processes within the brain capillary endothelial cells are important to blood–brain barrier function

Most neurotransmitters present in the blood do not enter the brain because of their low lipid solubility and lack of specific transport carriers in the luminal membrane of the capillary endothelial cell. This is illustrated for dopamine in Figure 32-2. In contrast, L-DOPA, the precursor for dopamine, has affinity for the large neutral amino acid-transport system and more easily enters the brain from the blood than would be predicted by its lipid solubility (Figs. 32-1 and 32-2). This is why patients with Parkinson's disease are treated with L-DOPA rather than with dopamine (see Chap. 45); however, the penetration of L-DOPA into the brain is limited by the presence of the enzymes L-DOPA decarboxylase and monoamine oxidase within the capillary endothelial cell [19]. This "enzymatic blood–brain barrier" limits transendothelial passage of L-DOPA into the brain and explains the need for large doses of L-DOPA in the treatment of Parkinson's disease. Therapy is enhanced by concurrent treatment with an inhibitor of peripheral L-DOPA decarboxylase.

Intracapillary monoamine oxidase also may play a role in the inactivation of neurotransmitters released by neuronal activity since monoamines are accumulated actively and metabolized by brain capillaries [19]. The fact that monoamines show very little uptake when presented from the luminal side suggests that the uptake systems are present only on the antiluminal membrane of the brain capillary endothelial cell (Fig. 32-1).

The brain capillary contains a variety of other neurotransmitter-metabolizing enzymes, such as cholinesterases, GABA transaminase, aminopeptidases and endopeptidases. In addition, several drug- and toxin-metabolizing enzymes typically found in the liver are also found in brain capillaries [20]. Thus, the "enzymatic blood–brain barrier" protects the brain not only from circulating neurotransmitters but also from many toxins.

Carrier-mediated blood–brain barrier transport protects the brain from blood-borne neurotoxins and drugs

P-glycoproteins are transmembranous, ATP-dependent pumps originally discovered for their ability to confer *multidrug resistance* to neoplastic cells. P-glycoproteins typically are expressed by epithelial barriers and blood–brain barrier endothelial cells. Humans have only one drug-transporting P-glycoprotein, which is the product of the *MDR1* gene. Mice express two drug-transporting P-glycoproteins, mdr1a and mdr1b, the former of which is expressed by the blood–brain barrier. Blood–brain barrier P-glycoprotein is absent in *mdr1a* $(-/-)$ transgenic mice, which also display substantially enhanced entry into the brain of systemically administered P-glycoprotein substrates, such as ivernectin, vinblastine, cyclosporine A, domperidone and digoxin [21]. Thus, P-glycoprotein can efficiently limit the blood–brain barrier permeability of hydrophobic P-glycoprotein substrates by pumping them from barrier endothelial cells back to the blood.

The blood–brain barrier undergoes development

The development of the cerebral microvasculature and the morphological changes attributed to its expression of the blood–brain barrier have been described in detail by Bar and Wolff and Stewart and colleagues [22]. The brain blood vessels that are destined to express the blood–brain barrier are derived from endothelial cells that originate from a plexus of nonbarrier vessels on the surface of the developing brain. The endothelial cells of these primitive vessels are fenestrated and surrounded by a poorly organized extracellular matrix and rela-

tively undifferentiated mesenchymal cells. As these primitive vessels migrate into the brain, their morphology and function take on blood–brain barrier properties. This includes the ensheathment of endothelial cells by astroglial foot processes, their association with pericytes, the formation of a well-defined periendothelial basement membrane, the rapid loss of fenestrations and the more gradual maturation of interendothelial tight junctional complexes. This process involves the loss of large interendothelial junctional clefts that provide a paracellular diffusion pathway in immature cerebral vessels. In the rat, the loss of junctional clefts best coincides with the 30-fold diminution of paracellular diffusion as vessels achieve their most mature level of differentiation.

Developmental changes also occur in the endothelial cell carrier transport systems that selectively deliver nutrients from blood to the developing brain. Brain uptake of substrates such as β-hydroxybutyrate, tryptophan, adenine and choline is substantially higher in neonates relative to adults. The converse is true for glucose. These changes reflect the relative requirements of the developing and adult brain for specific energy and macromolecular substrates.

These developmental observations taken together with *in vivo* and *in vitro* experimental findings support the hypothesis that signals derived from brain parenchyma, more specifically perivascular astrocytes, induce endothelial cell expression of the blood–brain barrier phenotype. Transplantation studies indicate that endothelial cell expression of the blood–brain barrier is not intrinsic to brain endothelial cells since systemic endothelial cells can be induced to express barrier properties by transplanted brain tissue. A requirement for astroglial–endothelial cell interactions is supported by observations that brain endothelial cells continue to express blood–brain barrier proteins when surrounded by tumor cells of astroglial origin in the absence of neurons and stop expressing barrier proteins if surrounded by tumor cells of epithelial origin, such as in carcinoma cells that have metastasized to brain. Furthermore, more reductionist experiments *in vitro* show that brain endothelial cells lose all barrier properties when isolated from the brain and cultured under routine conditions but express certain barrier properties if cultured in the presence of astrocytes or their conditioned medium.

BLOOD–CEREBROSPINAL FLUID BARRIER

The choroid plexus epithelial cells and the arachnoid membrane form the blood–cerebrospinal fluid barrier

The choroid plexus is a vascular tissue found in all cerebral ventricles (Fig. 32-5). The functional unit of the choroid plexus, composed of a capillary enveloped by a layer of differentiated ependymal epithelium, is shown in Figure 32-6. Unlike the capillaries that form the blood–brain barrier, choroid plexus capillaries are fenestrated and have no tight junctions. The endothelium, therefore, does not form a barrier to the movement of small molecules. Instead, the blood–CSF barrier at the choroid plexus is formed by the epithelial cells and the tight junctions that link them. The other part of the blood–CSF barrier is the arachnoid membrane, which envelops the brain. The cells of this membrane also are linked by tight junctions.

Cerebrospinal fluid is secreted primarily by the choroid plexus

The major site of CSF formation is the choroid plexus, and from a morphological viewpoint, the epithelial cells of this tissue are similar to other secretory cells. There is also some extrachoroidal secretion, which may result from ion transport by brain capillaries, as discussed above. In humans, the rate of CSF secretion is 0.3 to 0.4 ml/min, about one-third the rate at which urine is formed. The total volume of CSF is estimated to be 100 to 150 ml in normal adults, such that CSF is replaced totally three or four times each day. Several constituents are maintained at concentrations different in CSF from those in plasma (Table 32-1), indicating that CSF is not

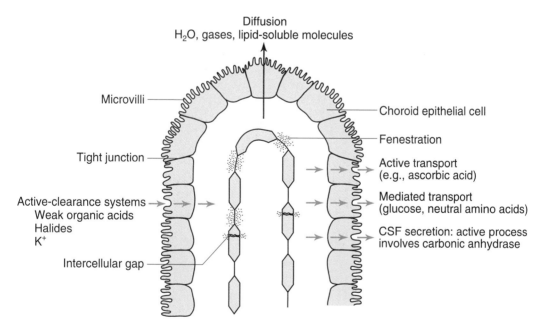

FIGURE 32-5. Blood–CSF barrier. The capillaries in the choroid plexus differ from those of the brain in that there is free movement of molecules across the endothelial cell through fenestrations and intercellular gaps. The blood–CSF barrier is at the choroid plexus epithelial cells, which are joined together by tight junctions. Microvilli are present on the CSF-facing surface. These greatly increase the surface area of the apical membrane and may aid in fluid secretion. Diffusion, facilitated diffusion and active transport into CSF, as well as active transport of metabolites from CSF to blood, have been demonstrated in the choroid plexus.

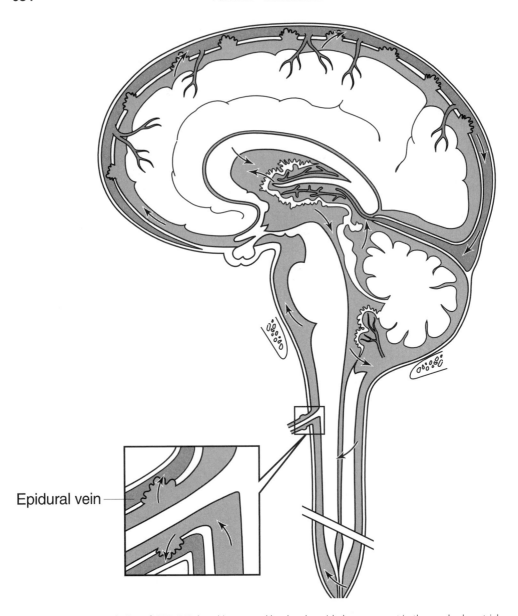

Epidural vein

FIGURE 32-6. Circulation of CSF. CSF *(gray)* is secreted by the choroid plexus present in the cerebral ventricles and by extrachoroidal sources. It subsequently circulates through the ventricular cavities and into the subarachnoid space. Absorption into the venous blood *(dark orange)* occurs through the arachnoid villi in the superior sagittal sinus and along the optic, olfactory and spinal nerve sheaths *(inset)*. (From Fishman [18], with permission.)

simply a protein-free ultrafiltrate of plasma. Instead, CSF production by the choroid plexus is driven by active ion transport that results in a net secretion of Na^+ and Cl^-, the main ionic constituents of CSF. The exact mechanisms involved have yet to be determined fully, but Figure 32-7 represents one model.

In contrast to most epithelia, Na,K-ATPase is found on the apical, or CSF-facing, microvilli of the choroid plexus [23]. Ouabain, an inhibitor of Na,K-ATPase, reduces CSF secretion. Na,K-ATPase is probably the main transporter of Na^+ from the epithelium to the CSF. It also provides the electrochemical gradient for basolateral, or blood-facing, Na^+ entry into the epithelium, which probably occurs via a Na^+/H^+ antiport system (see Chap. 5).

Cl^- influx into the epithelium is via a Cl^-/HCO_3^- exchanger on the basolateral membrane [24]. This exchanger can be inhibited directly with stilbenes or indirectly using acetazolamide, an inhibitor of carbonic anhydrase which reduces the intracellular production of HCO_3^-. Cl^- efflux from the epithelium to the CSF is primarily via a cotransporter, which is either of the K^+/Cl^- or $Na^+/K^+/Cl^-$ type [25]. This cotransporter can be inhibited by furosemide and bumetanide. Therapeutically, acetazolamide and furosemide are used to decrease the rate of CSF formation in hydrocephalus. Acetazolamide is generally a more effective agent at decreasing CSF production. This may reflect the involvement of a cotransporter in moving ions from CSF to the epithelium (Fig. 32-7).

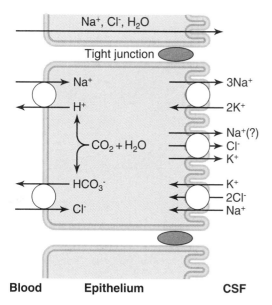

FIGURE 32-7. Model of ion transport at the choroid plexus epithelium. Net transport of Na^+ and Cl^- across the epithelium results in the secretion of CSF. Cl^- efflux from the epithelium to CSF is mediated by a cotransporter. It is uncertain whether that transporter is of the $Na^+/K^+/2Cl^-$ or K^+/Cl^- form. The generation of H^+ and HCO_3^- by carbonic anhydrase is important in the secretion of CSF.

The choroid plexus receives a number of different forms of innervation, most notably a sympathetic input from the superior cervical ganglia. It also has many hormone receptors [26]. For example, the choroid plexus epithelium has a tenfold greater density of 5-hydroxytryptamine (5-HT)$_{2C}$ receptors than any other brain tissue, although it does not appear to receive direct serotonergic innervation. A number of these neuroendocrine mechanisms modify choroid plexus blood flow or solute transport by the epithelium, indicating their potential role in controlling CSF secretion rate or composition.

Cerebrospinal fluid circulates through the ventricles, over the surface of the brain, and is absorbed at the arachnoid villi and at the cranial and spinal nerve root sheaths

The CSF circulation is from the lateral ventricles through the foramina of Monro into the third ventricle, the aqueduct of Sylvius, and then into the fourth ventricle. The fluid passes from the fourth ventricle through the foramina of Luschka and Magendie to the cisterna magna and then circulates into the cerebral and spinal subarachnoid spaces (Fig. 32-5).

There is evidence that absorption of CSF by the arachnoid villi occurs by a valve-like process, permitting the one-way flow of CSF from the subarachnoid spaces into the venous sinuses. CSF absorption does not occur until CSF pressure exceeds the pressure within the sinuses. Once this threshold is reached, the rate of absorption is proportional to the difference between CSF and sinus pressures. A normal human can absorb CSF at a rate up to six times the normal rate of CSF formation with only a moderate increase in intracranial pressure.

If obstructions occur at the foramina between the ventricles, the ventricle upstream from the obstruction will enlarge, producing obstructive hydrocephalus. Occasionally, disease processes affect CSF removal. For example, obliteration of the subarachnoid space by inflammation or thrombosis of the sinuses will prevent clearance of fluid. When this occurs, CSF pressure increases and hydrocephalus develops without obstruction of the ventricular foramina. This is called communicating hydrocephalus.

The choroid plexus is the major route of blood–brain barrier exchange for some compounds

The movement of substances from the blood into the CSF is, in many ways, analogous to that from the blood into the brain, with many of the same transporters present in both tissues. Quantitatively, however, there are major differences between transport by the choroid plexus and by the blood–brain barrier. Thus, in terms of O_2, CO_2, glucose and amino acid entry into the brain, the blood–brain barrier predominates. For some other compounds, however, the choroid plexus is the major site of entry. This is the case for Ca^{2+}, where the CSF influx rate constant is tenfold greater than the blood–brain barrier value. This reflects the role of the choroid plexus in not only CSF but also brain Ca^{2+} homeostasis. The choroid plexus also may be involved in the transport of hormones into the CSF or may be a source of those hormones. For example, the choroid plexus may secrete insulin-like growth factor-II into the CSF; it also produces and secretes transthyretin, a carrier of thyroxine and retinol, into the CSF [26].

Other active transport systems in the choroid plexus are linked to the efflux of specific solutes [27]. For example, iodide and thiocyanate are transported from the CSF by saturable carrier mechanisms that can be competitively inhibited by perchlorate. This system must be active because transport can be carried out against unfavorable electrochemical gradients. Another important transport system removes weak organic acids from the CSF. Among the molecules cleared by this mechanism are penicillin and neurotransmitter metabolites, such as homovanillic acid and 5-hydroxyindoleacetic acid. This clearance system, which transports against an unfavorable CSF to blood gradient, is saturable and inhibited by probenecid. Clearance of organic acids by a probenecid-sensitive transport mechanism also may occur across the blood–brain barrier in brain capillaries.

The composition of the CSF when it enters the subarachnoid space may be modified by the arachnoid membrane. This tissue is part of the blood–CSF barrier and, like the choroid plexus and the cerebral capillaries, may not be a purely passive barrier but capable of actively modifying CSF composition.

Cerebrospinal fluid has a number of functions

A number of functions have been ascribed to the CSF [28]. The fluid-filled system around the brain has a buoyancy effect that may protect the brain from injury. Also, the rigidity of the skull means that increases in brain volume, such as those that occur from vasodilation or parenchymal cell swelling, could cause marked rises in intracranial pressure. The fluid in the CSF system, which can be displaced, limits such changes in pressure. Similarly, if the brain is dehydrated, the CSF acts as a source of fluid to rehydrate it.

As described above, the CSF system is the major source of entry of a number of substances into the brain. Why certain substances should enter via the blood–CSF barrier while others enter at the blood–brain barrier is uncertain. It might reflect the difference in the passive permeability of the two barriers since the tight junctions of the blood–CSF barrier are quantitatively leakier than those of the blood–brain barrier. Alternately, it may reflect the requirements of regions adjacent to the ventricular system.

The combination of bulk absorption of solute and solvent by the arachnoid villi and the selective removal of molecules by the choroid plexus means that there can be a concentration gradient for molecules reaching the interstitial fluid of the brain to diffuse into the CSF. Those molecules are then cleared by bulk flow or active transport. This function of the CSF, known as its sink action, helps to maintain the low concentration of many substances in both brain and CSF compared with plasma concentrations.

The CSF system also may play a role in signal transduction. It may provide a route for hormones to move within the brain, but it also may be a route of communication from the brain to the rest of the body. The bulk flow of CSF along the optic and olfactory nerves drains through lymphatic tissue, and antigenic material in the CSF may produce a systemic immune reaction.

CEREBROSPINAL FLUID–BRAIN INTERFACE

The absence of tight junctions between some ependymal and pial cells permits the free diffusion of small hydrophilic molecules from the CSF into the interstitium of the brain and *vice versa.* Large molecules, such as proteins, also penetrate but more slowly. Quantitative studies of the movement of substances between CSF and brain suggest that the concentration of ions in extracellular fluid in the brain should be the same as that in the CSF. This relationship has been demonstrated directly for K^+ using ion-specific electrodes placed in the interstitial space of the brain. Brain interstitial K^+ concentration is approximately 3 mM, similar to that of CSF and independent of the plasma K^+ concentration [29].

BYPASSING THE BARRIERS WITH DRUGS

A number of agents of potential therapeutic importance do not readily enter the brain because they have low lipid solubility and are not transported by the specific carriers present in the blood–brain barrier or choroid plexus. To overcome this limitation, schemes to enhance drug entry into the central nervous system have been developed.

The most obvious method of circumventing the barriers is to inject the agents directly into the CSF. Although ventricular or cisternal access sites may be used, intrathecal administration of antineoplastic agents usually is accomplished by intralumbar injection. Because of limited drug penetration into brain substance, these routes are used most often in patients who have a disease process such as chronic meningitis or neoplastic cells in the CSF.

Enhanced delivery of drug into the brain can be accomplished by raising its concentration in the blood, but this approach often is limited by the occurrence of systemic side effects. It is possible to achieve similar high concentrations of drug in the brain vasculature by infusing the drug directly into the carotid artery. In this way, the same total systemic dose produces a much higher concentration gradient across the blood–brain barrier and leads to a greater uptake by the brain.

Another way to enhance delivery is to increase the permeability of the blood–brain barrier. The disease itself may produce this effect, and this is why the rate of penicillin passage into the brain is highest early in the course of meningitis; however, when the capillaries are intact, some intervention is necessary to open the barrier. Infusion of hyperosmolar solutions into the carotid circulation alters blood–brain barrier permeability in laboratory animals [30] and is used in the treatment of patients with brain tumors. The change in permeability appears to be caused by the osmotic reduction in endothelial cell volume which separates the tight junctions that normally seal together the endothelial cells in brain capillaries. The permeability of brain microvessels associated with pathophysiological processes can be enhanced selectively by certain vasoactive compounds, such as bradykinin, leukotrienes and histamine, which do not alter the permeability of normal brain vessels. This observation has led to the development of pharmacological agents that selectively enhance the delivery of chemotherapeutic drugs to brain tumors [31]. One such agent, RMP-7, a bradykinin derivative, enhances the therapeutic response of experimental gliomas to systemically administered chemotherapy and is presently undergoing clinical trials in humans.

The design of drugs with high blood–brain barrier permeability is a more selective way to improve delivery into the brain. In fact, most neuroactive drugs are effective because they dissolve in lipid and easily enter the brain. A good example of the importance of structure and lipid solubility is provided by comparison of the brain uptake of heroin and morphine [32]. These compounds are very similar in structure except for two acetyl groups that make heroin more lipid-soluble. The greater lipid solubility of heroin explains its more rapid onset of action. Once within the brain, the acetyl groups on heroin are removed enzymatically to produce morphine, which leaves the brain only slowly. By analogy, it would seem ideal to develop new therapeutic drugs that readily enter and then are trapped within the central nervous system.

A similar strategy for enhancing brain uptake of drugs involves producing prodrugs that have affinity for one of the blood–brain barrier transport systems. For example, the large neutral amino acid system appears to tolerate a considerable range of side-chain structures [14]. The attachment of drugs to proteins to form chimeric peptides that enter the brain by receptor- or absorption-mediated endocytosis also may prove to be a useful and flexible approach [6]. This strategy has been used in experimental models to increase the blood–brain barrier permeability and brain response to proteins covalently conjugated to antitransferrin receptor antibodies. Conjugate proteins administered intravenously or by intracarotid perfusion bind to blood–brain barrier endothelial cell transferrin receptors and enter the brain via transferrin receptor-mediated endocytosis [33]. Clearly, an understanding of transport processes will be crucial to developing the next generation of drugs useful in treating various brain diseases.

The advent of gene-transfer techniques has opened the possibility of genetic approaches to bypassing the blood–brain barrier for therapeutic purposes [34,35]. Replication-defective viruses, such as herpes simplex virus and adenovirus, can be used to deliver therapeutic transgenes to brain parenchymal cells, which then synthesize therapeutic transgenic proteins at relatively high levels directly within the brain. Virus-based gene transfer to the brain has been used successfully to treat experimental brain tumors and to correct metabolic brain defects in experimental models of metabolic brain diseases. Adenovirus and herpes virus-based gene therapy of brain neoplasms is presently in clinical trial. Alternatively, cells engineered *in vitro* to express therapeutic transgenes can be implanted in the brain or spinal cord, where they then secrete biologically active transgenic proteins. Fibroblasts, myoblasts, brain endothelial cells and neural progenitor cells have been used successfully in experimental systems. Neural progenitor cells differentiate and integrate into the brain in what appears to be a functionally appropriate manner. Similarly, implanted immortalized brain endothelial cell lines integrate with the host brain vasculature and secrete transgenic

proteins at concentrations adequate to inhibit brain tumor growth or to protect brain from injury. The development of host immune responses to viral vector proteins or implanted cells and the transient expression of therapeutic transgenes due to promoter inefficiencies remain obstacles to the practical application of these molecular therapies.

ACKNOWLEDGMENTS

This work was supported by Grants NS32148, NS23870, HL18575, NS34709 and NS33728 from the National Institutes of Health.

REFERENCES

1. Fishman, R. A. *Cerebrospinal Fluid in Diseases of the Nervous System.* Philadelphia: W. B. Saunders, 1980.
2. Goldstein, G. W., and Betz, A. L. The blood–brain barrier. *Sci. Am.* 254:74–83, 1986.
3. Spector, R., and Johanson, C. E. The mammalian choroid plexus. *Sci. Am.* 261:68–74, 1989.
4. Bradbury, M. *The Concept of a Blood–Brain Barrier.* Chichester: Wiley, 1979.
5. Kotyk, A., and Janacek, K. *Cell Membrane Transport.* New York: Plenum, 1975.
6. Pardridge, W. M. *Peptide Drug Delivery to the Brain.* New York: Raven, 1991.
7. Bradbury, M. W. B., and Stulcova, B. Efflux mechanism contributing to the stability of the potassium concentration in cerebrospinal fluid. *J. Physiol. (Lond.)* 208:415–430, 1970.
8. Brightman, M. Morphology of blood–brain interfaces. *Exp. Eye Res.* 25:1–25, 1977.
9. Laterra, J., Indurti, R. R., and Goldstein, G. W. Regulation of *in vitro* glia-induced microvessel morphogenesis by urokinase. *J. Cell Physiol.* 158:317–324, 1994.
10. Rubin, L. L., Hall, D. E., Porter, S. B., et al. A cell culture model of the blood–brain barrier. *J. Cell Biol.* 115:1725–1735, 1991.
11. Lund-Anderson, H. Transport of glucose from blood to brain. *Physiol. Rev.* 59:305–352, 1979.
12. Kalaria, R. N., Gravina, S. A., Schmidley, J. W., Perry, G., and Harik, S. I. The glucose transporter of the human brain and blood–brain barrier. *Ann. Neurol.* 24:757–764, 1988.
13. Pardridge, W. M. Brain metabolism: A perspec-

tive from the blood–brain barrier. *Physiol. Rev.* 63:1481–1535, 1983.

14. Smith, Q. R., Momma, S., Aoyagi, M., and Rapoport, S. I. Kinetics of neutral amino acid transport across the blood–brain barrier. *J. Neurochem.* 49:1651–1658, 1987.

15. Betz, A. L., and Goldstein, G. W. Polarity of the blood–brain barrier: Neutral amino acid transport into isolated brain capillaries. *Science* 202:225–227, 1978.

16. Cohen, E., and Wurtman, R. J. Brain acetylcoline synthesis: Control by dietary choline. *Science* 191:561–562, 1976.

17. Spector, R. Micronutrient homeostasis in mammalian brain and cerebrospinal fluid. *J. Neurochem.* 53:1667–1674, 1989.

18. Schielke, G. P., and Betz, A. L. Electrolyte transport. In: M. W. B. Bradbury (ed.), *Physiology and Pharmacology of the Blood–Brain Barrier.* Heidelberg: Springer-Verlag, 1992, pp. 221–243.

19. Hardebo, J. E., and Owman, C. Barrier mechanisms for neurotransmitter monoamines and their precursors at the blood–brain barrier. *Ann. Neurol.* 8:1–31, 1979.

20. Minn, A., Ghersi-Egea, J. F., Perrin, R., Leininger, B., and Siest, G. Drug metabolizing enzymes in the brain and cerebral microvessels. *Brain Res.* 16:65–82, 1991.

21. Schinkel, A. H., Smit, J. J. M., Vantellingen, O., et al. Disruption of the mouse mdr1a P-glycoprotein gene leads to a deficiency in the blood–brain barrier and to increased sensitivity to drugs. *Cell* 77:491–502, 1994.

22. Laterra, J., Stewart, P., and Goldstein, G. Development of the blood–brain barrier. In R. A. Polin and W. W. Fox (eds.), *Neonatal and Fetal Medicine—Physiology and Pathophysiology.* Philadelphia: W.B. Saunders, 1991, pp. 1525–1531.

23. Ernst, S. A., Palacios, J. R., and Siegel, G. J. Immunocytochemical localization of Na^+, K^+-ATPase catalytic polypeptide in mouse choroid plexus. *J. Histochem. Cytochem.* 34:189–195, 1986.

24. Lindsey, A. E., Schneider, K., Simmons, D. M., Baron, R., Lee, B. S., and Kopito, R. R. Functional expression and subcellular localization of an anion exchanger cloned from choroid plexus. *Proc. Natl. Acad. Sci. USA* 87:5278–5282, 1990.

25. Zeuthen, T. Secondary active transport of water across ventricular cell membrane of choroid plexus epithelium of necturus maculosus. *J. Physiol. (Lond.)* 444:153–173, 1991.

26. Nilsson, C., Lindvall-Axelsson, M., and Owman, C. Neuroendocrine regulatory mechanisms in the choroid plexus–cerebrospinal fluid system. *Brain Res. Rev.* 17:109–138, 1992.

27. Lorenzo, A. V. Factors governing the composition of the cerebrospinal fluid. *Exp. Eye Res.* 25:205–228, 1977.

28. Johanson, C. E. Ventricles and cerebrospinal fluid. In P. Conn (ed.), *Neuroscience in Medicine.* Philadelphia: J. B. Lippincott, 1995, pp. 171–196.

29. Jones, H. C., and Keep, R. C. The control of potassium concentration in the cerebrospinal fluid and brain interstitial fluid of developing rats. *J. Physiol.* 383:441–453, 1987.

30. Rapoport, S. I., Fredericks, W. R., Ohno, K., and Pettigrew, K. D. Quantitative aspects of reversible osmotic opening of the blood–brain barrier. *Am. J. Physiol.* 238:R421–R431, 1980.

31. Elliott, P. J., Hayward, N. J., Huff, M. R., Nagle, T. L., Black, K. L., and Bartus, R. T. Unlocking the blood–brain barrier: A role for RMP-7 in brain tumor therapy. *Exp. Neurol.* 141:214–224, 1996.

32. Oldendorf, W. H. The blood–brain barrier. *Exp. Eye Res.* 25:177–190, 1977.

33. Granholm, A. C., Backman, C., Bloom, F., et al. NGF and anti-transferrin receptor antibody conjugates: Short- and long-term effects on survival of cholinergic neurons in intraocular septal transplants. *J. Pharmacol. Exp. Ther.* 268:448–459, 1994.

34. Bloomer, U., Naldini, L., Verma, J. M., Trono, D., and Gage, F. H. Applications of gene therapy to the CNS. *Hum. Mol. Genet.* 5:1397–1404, 1996.

35. Xiao, X., Li, J., McCown, T. J., and Samulski, R. J. Gene transfer by adeno-associated virus vectors in the CNS. *Exp. Neurol.* 144:113–124, 1997.

36. Oldendorf, W. H. Clearance of radiolabeled substances by brain after arterial injection using a diffusible internal standard. In N. Marks and R. Rodnight (eds.), *Research Methods in Neurochemistry.* New York: Plenum, 1981, pp. 91–112.

37. Fenstermacher, J. D. Drug transfer across the blood–brain barrier. In D. D. P. Breimer (ed.), *Topics in Pharmaceutical Sciences 1983.* Amsterdam: Elsevier Science, 1983, pp. 143–154.

38. Cornford, E. M., Braun, L. D., Oldendorf, W. H., and Hill, M. A. Comparison of lipid mediated blood–brain barrier penetrability in neonates and adults. *Am. J. Physiol.* 243:C161–C168, 1982.

39. Hironaka, T., Fuchino, K. F., and Fujii, T. Absorption of diazepam and its transfer through the blood–brain barrier after intraperitoneal administration in the rat. *J. Pharmacol. Exp. Ther.* 299:809–815, 1984.

40. Koeppe, R. A., Mangner, T., Betz, A. L., et al. Use of ^{11}C aminocyclohexanecarboxylate for the measurement of amino acid uptake and distribution volume in human brain. *J. Cereb. Blood Flow Metab.* 10:727–739, 1990.

33

Nutrition and Brain Function

Gary E. Gibson and John P. Blass

Basic Neurochemistry: Molecular, Cellular and Medical Aspects, 6th Ed., edited by G. J. Siegel et al. Published by Lippincott–Raven Publishers, Philadelphia, 1999. Correspondence to Gary E. Gibson, Cornell University Medical College, Burke Medical Research Institute, 785 Mamaroneck Avenue, White Plains, New York 10605.

Nutrition affects brain chemistry in humans and other animals. Everyone experiences the fact that food and nutrition alter mood and behavior. Indeed, food can be a strong conditioning stimulus. One exposure to an adverse stimulus coupled with a particular food can cause a lifetime aversion to that food (see Chap. 50). The neurochemical mechanisms of how diet alters brain function are beginning to be known. Alterations of diet and nutrition based on sound neurochemical and other scientifically valid observations allow the use of diet as a rational and "natural" way to deal with disabilities related to the nervous system, including certain diseases.

The brain is sensitive to changes in diet. It depends on a continuous supply of nutrients from the blood, some of which are synthesized in other organs of the body, such as choline. Others, which cannot be synthesized in mammalian systems at all, are "essential" components that must be furnished by the diet. These essential nutrients include vitamins, amino acids and fatty acids. Studies of deficiencies of vitamins and other nutrients and elements, such as iodine, provide important insights into understanding brain metabolism.

Nutrition can alter brain function in short time frames, for example, by altering neurotransmitters and neuronal firing, and in the long-term, such as by altering membrane structure. The importance of proper nutrition during brain development has been appreciated for several decades. That the nutritional requirements of the brain of mature and aged individuals may differ from those of the young was established more recently. Genetics also affects dietary needs. Although classic vitamin and other nutritional "deficiencies" are major public health concerns in underdeveloped countries, they also occur in industrialized societies. Vitamin insufficiencies can occur secondary to alcohol or drug abuse or other psychiatric disorders, as a result of genetic variation or because particular age groups have special requirements. Nutritional therapy of neurodegenerative disorders in children has been successful in the past and may eventually provide a productive approach to the treatment of common adult neurodegenerative disorders, such as Alzheimer's and Parkinson's diseases, that encompass complex interactions of genetics and the environment. In this chapter, the effects of diet on normal brain function are discussed and the implications for brain disease are presented.

NUTRITION AND FUNCTIONAL NEUROCHEMISTRY

The availability of some nutrients can have immediate effects on behavior, especially on the ability to respond to stimulation. Several studies suggest that brain function, including cognitive processing, responds to changes in nutrients.

Nutrition can influence neurotransmitter concentrations and associated behaviors

Important neurotransmitters are synthesized from compounds which are essential dietary constituents. For instance, norepinephrine (NE) and serotonin are formed from the essential amino acids tyrosine and tryptophan, respectively. However, elevation of a precursor in the blood does not necessarily elevate its concentration in the brain. For example, increasing the blood concentration of large neutral amino acids such as phenylalanine, as occurs in phenylketonuria (see Chap. 44), reduces tryptophan uptake into the brain because these two compounds share a common carrier across the blood–brain barrier (see Chap. 32). Furthermore, the response to an increased concentration of precursor often depends on the demand, such as firing frequency of the neurons. En-

TABLE 33-1.	DIETARY MANIPULATION OF NEUROTRANSMITTERS: INCREASES IN PRECURSOR AVAILABILITY INCREASE THE ABILITY OF MANY NEUROTRANSMITTERS TO RESPOND TO INCREASED DEMAND		
Nutrient (precursor)	**Neurotransmitter**	**Process known to be changed**	**Disease where manipulation may be important**
Choline →	Acetylcholine	Memory	Alzheimer's disease, tardive dyskinesia,
Glucose →			Down's syndrome
Tryptophan →	Serotonin	Sleep	Depression, sleeplessness, hyperactive behaviors
Tyrosine →	Norepinephrine	Blood pressure	Hypertension, maze performance
→	Epinephrine	Learning	

hanced precursor availability may matter only when physiological demand is increased.

Choline for acetylcholine (ACh) synthesis can be obtained from either brain choline, the phosphatidylcholine in the membranes or serum choline (Table 33-1). It is taken up by a high-affinity choline-uptake system at the synapse (see Chap. 11). Although choline can be made in the body, its synthesis can be limited by the availability of "single-carbon" units in the diet. Ingestion of choline together with phosphatidylcholine can increase brain choline and ACh concentrations and enhance the ability of ACh synthesis to increase upon demand. For example, increased dietary choline permits the brain to make excess ACh following stimulation with atropine. Dietary phosphatidylcholine simultaneously increases memory and the ACh content of the brains of "demented" mice, which normally have reduced brain ACh concentrations [1]. Increasing choline prenatally and postnatally improves the working and reference memory of young rats.

Glucose normally provides the acetyl moiety of ACh. Extensive evidence indicates that relatively modest increases in circulating glucose concentrations can also increase ACh release and has been claimed to enhance learning and memory. The relative safety of glucose administration has permitted tests of its effects on cognitive functions in humans. Glucose enhances learning and memory in healthy aged humans and improves several other cognitive functions in subjects with severe cognitive pathologies, including individuals with Alzheimer's disease and Down's syndrome. Thus, moderate increases in circulating glucose concentrations may have robust and broad influences on brain functions that span many neural and behavioral measures and cross readily from rodents to humans. Considerable evidence suggests that these effects are mediated via ACh. Increasing glucose availability can increase the amount of ACh released during conditions of increased demand [2] (Fig. 33-1) (see also Chaps. 11 and 31).

Tryptophan, like tyrosine, crosses the blood–brain barrier predominantly by the carrier system for long-chain neutral amino acids. As a result, a protein-rich meal can actually increase blood tryptophan but reduce the passage of tryptophan into the brain by elevating at the same time the concentrations of other amino acids, such as phenylalanine, that compete for that carrier. Serotonin (5-hydroxytryptamine, 5-HT) synthesis depends on brain tryptophan, which in turn depends on blood tryptophan concentrations, which can be manipulated by varying the diet (Table 33-1). Elevating tryptophan in the brain produces physiologically important changes in the serotonergic system (see Chap. 13). Animals that are poor in brain tryptophan have a heightened sensitivity to painful stimuli that can be reversed with tryptophan ingestion, which rapidly elevates brain serotonin. Therapeutically, tryptophan has been reported to be useful in treating subgroups of patients with depression, sleeplessness or hyperactive behaviors.

Tyrosine is the precursor of NE and epinephrine (Table 33-1). Increasing tyrosine reduces blood pressure in both normotensive and hypertensive animals. The action of tyrosine on blood pressure occurs via CNS mechanisms since co-ad-

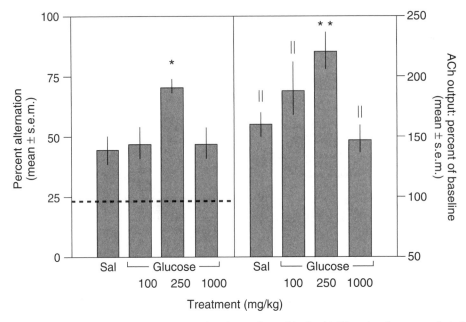

FIGURE 33-1. The relation of glucose levels to the release of acetylcholine (ACh) and performance of a behavioral task. Increasing glucose availability by intraperitoneal injection can increase the release of ACh during conditions of increased demand. A glucose-stimulated increase in hippocampal ACh is associated with improved performance on a memory task involving spontaneous attenuation in a maze. *, p<0.05 vs. saline; ‖, p<0.01 vs. baseline level; **, p<0.02 vs. saline. (From [2], with permission.)

ministering other large neutral amino acids that reduce the uptake of tyrosine into the brain blocks the effect. The antihypertensive action of tyrosine appears to be mediated by an acceleration in NE or epinephrine release within the CNS; injection of tyrosine produces a concurrent increase in brain concentrations of 3-methoxy-4-hydroxyphenylethylglycol sulfate, a catecholamine metabolite [3]. Tyrosine induces increased NE and alters NE and α and β receptor densities in hippocampus, providing further evidence of its physiological role. Furthermore, dietary restriction to 40% of normal food intake diminishes maze performance, and this effect can be reversed by administration of tyrosine.

Nutrition can influence brain energy reserve

Brain energy is more resistant to changes in fasting or overfeeding than that in liver or muscle. For example, severe fasting decreases liver ATP concentrations and ATP: phosphocreatine ratios, while brain energy metabolism is preserved. However, brain energy metabolism can be manipulated by diet. A high-fat (90% of caloric value), carbohy-drate-free ketogenic diet low in protein (10%) does not significantly alter regional brain glucose utilization or cerebral concentrations of glucose, glycogen, lactate or citrate. However, a high-carbohydrate diet (78%) low in fat (12%) and low in protein (10%) markedly decreases brain glucose utilization and increases cerebral concentrations of glucose 6-phosphate. These findings indicate that long-term, moderate ketonemia does not significantly alter brain glucose phosphorylation. However, even marginal protein dietary deficiency when coupled with a carbohydrate-rich diet depresses cerebral glucose utilization to a degree often seen in metabolic encephalopathies (see Chap. 38) [4].

Carnitine participates in mitochondrial reactions. Like choline, it can be synthesized by mammals if dietary sources of one-carbon groups are adequate. It participates in the transfer of acyl groups across mitochondrial membranes (Chap. 42). These include acetyl groups for ACh synthesis. Both carnitine and acetylcarnitine cross the blood–brain barrier (BBB), but the more lipid-soluble acetyl-L-carnitine has been described as having a variety of effects on the nervous system in experimental animals not seen with carnitine.

Hereditary deficits in the ability to transport carnitine or to synthesize its acyl derivatives have been associated with diseases of skeletal and cardiac muscle and, to a variable extent, with metabolic encephalopathy (see Chap. 34). Secondary deficiency of carnitine has been described in a number of disorders of mitochondrial oxidation, due in part to the detoxification and urinary excretion of potentially damaging short-chain acids as the carnitine derivatives [5]. The anticonvulsant valproic acid can increase carnitine requirements in susceptible individuals [6]. Treatment with acetylcarnitine has been reported to slow the progression of Alzheimer's disease [7].

Vitamins can regulate normal neuronal activity

Many vitamins function as cofactors in fundamental pathways, such as glycolysis, the Krebs cycle, the respiratory chain and amino acid metabolism. Although all tissues have these vitamin-dependent pathways, they take on increased importance in the brain because of its high metabolic rate and dependence on continuous metabolism. In fact, the discovery of vitamins was closely linked to the sensitivity of the brain to deficiency, specifically that of thiamine [8]. Furthermore, in the brain these pathways are linked to neurotransmitter synthesis.

Vitamin B$_1$ (thiamine) is critical to normal brain function. Thiamine pyrophosphate (TPP) functions as a cofactor of key enzymes of the Krebs cycle: the pyruvate and α-ketoglutarate dehydrogenase complexes (PDHC and KGDHC, respectively), the branched-chain dehydrogenase complex (BCDHC) and the pentose shunt enzyme transketolase (TK) (Table 33-2). These dehydrogenase complexes share a common enzyme component, lipoamide dehydrogenase. TK rearranges sugars (see Chap. 31). A kinase can convert a membrane-bound form of TPP to thiamine triphosphate (TTP), and a specific phosphatase hydrolyzes TTP to the diphosphate. TTP appears to play a role in nerve membrane function, notably in Na$^+$ gating. The cDNAs for a number of TPP-requiring enzymes have been obtained, and a TPP-binding motif has been proposed that is partially conserved in yeast, rat and human.

Thiamine deficiency is a classical and well-studied example of the interaction of nutrition with brain function. Research on thiamine deficiency continues to attract considerable interest. In developed countries, clinically significant thiamine deficiency is rare except as a complication of severe alcoholism or other conditions that impair nutrition [9]. It is more common in developing countries in which polished rice is the staple grain. It can be detected by measuring the "TPP effect," the percentage increase in red cell TK activity upon addition of exogenous TPP *in vitro,* and has been widely used in laboratory as well as in epidemiological studies of thiamine deficiency.

After 5 to 6 days of a diet deficient in thiamine, healthy young men developed a nonspecific syndrome of lassitude, irritability, muscle cramps and electrocardiographic changes, which were reversed by dietary thiamine.

Prolonged thiamine deficiency frequently leads to damage to peripheral nerves (see Chap. 36). This neuropathy tends to be worse distally than proximally, involves myelin more than ax-

Vitamin	Functional form	Examples of reactions	Influenced neuronal system
Thiamine	Thiamine pyrophosphate	Pyruvate dehydrogenase, α-ketoglutarate dehydrogenase, transketolase	Acetylcholine
Pyridoxine	Pyridoxal phosphate	Decarboxylation	GABA, serotonin, dopamine
Niacin	NAD$^+$, NADP$^+$	Oxidative reactions	Coupling to acetylcholine synthesis
Vitamin E	Tocopherol	Free radical quenching	Neurodegeneration
Vitamin C	Ascorbate	Free radical quencing	Neurodegeneration

TABLE 33-2.   ROLE OF VITAMINS IN BRAIN FUNCTION: THESE VITAMINS ARE CRITICAL FOR NORMAL BRAIN FUNCTION AND ARE REQUIRED IN THE DIET

ons and is often painful. The neuropathy may be linked to deficiencies in multiple water-soluble vitamins known for historical reasons as the vitamin B complex.

Wernicke-Korsakoff syndrome consists of an acute (Wernicke) phase and a chronic (Korsakoff) phase [9]. The acute syndrome consists of staggering gait, paralysis of eye movements and confusion, associated with small hemorrhages along the third and fourth ventricles and with reduced cerebral metabolic rate as measured by cerebral blood flow. Injections of thiamine can be lifesaving, with clinical improvement often evident within minutes. It is believed that prompt treatment with thiamine can prevent the onset of the chronic Korsakoff phase. In Korsakoff's syndrome, a striking loss of working memory accompanies relatively little loss of reference memory (see Chap. 50). Affected patients characteristically make up stories, or confabulate, in response to leading questions. In this phase, patients do not respond to thiamine treatment. The neuropathological lesions responsible for Korsakoff's syndrome have been debated; severe damage to the cholinergic neurons of the nucleus basalis complex has been reported.

Thiamine requirements can be altered genetically or environmentally. Among genetic disorders, thiamine-dependent maple syrup urine disease is due to a reduced affinity of BCDHC for TPP (see Chap. 44). A rare form of lactate acidosis is due to reduced affinity of PDHC for TPP. Both disorders respond to treatment with large doses of thiamine. Wernicke-Korsakoff syndrome is associated with a variant form of TK having a decreased affinity for TPP [9]. This variation, which may be more common in chronic alcoholics, puts patients at risk when on a diet marginal or deficient in thiamine. Subacute necrotizing encephalomyelopathy (SNE) of Leigh is an uncommon, autosomal recessive disorder in which the neuropathology resembles Wernicke-Korsakoff syndrome. Patients with SNE in whom a defect in PDHC has been documented at the cDNA level have been described. The role of thiamine in this disorder is controversial.

Environmentally, a number of dietary constituents are known to impair the absorption of thiamine, including ethanol. Severe illness or in-

jury also has been reported to increase thiamine requirements. Rarely, patients have been found who are intolerant to very large doses of thiamine. Thiamine-dependent enzymes are reduced in the brains of patients with a variety of neurodegenerative diseases, including Alzheimer's, Huntington's and Parkinson's diseases.

Thiamine-deficient animals model many aspects of human thiamine deficiency [10]. Experimentally, thiamine deficiency is frequently induced by the combination of a thiamine-deficient diet and a thiamine antagonist, either pyrithiamine or oxythiamine. However, pyrithiamine can directly inhibit action potentials and oxythiamine does not enter the brain efficiently. In the pyrithiamine model in mice, abnormal neuropsychological responses develop within 5 to 7 days, gross neurological abnormalities in 8 to 9 days and death usually by 10 to 11 days. Strain significantly modifies the response to experimental thiamine deficiency in mice (Fig. 33-2). In rats, abnormalities of motor performance occur by day 3, additional neurological symptoms by day 12 and death within 2 weeks. Thiamine deficiency leads to a selective cell death that is accompanied by accumulation of amyloid precursor protein in surrounding neurons. It causes severe memory disruption and loss of cholinergic function. The activities of thiamine-dependent enzymes decline in early stages of thiamine deficiency, but surprisingly, selective cell death is not related to the cellular or regional distribution of thiamine-dependent enzymes or to their response to thiamine deficiency. Instead, the general reduction in thiamine-dependent enzymes predisposes particular brain regions to other insults. The earliest known change that reflects selective vulnerability is an alteration in the BBB that is accompanied by oxidative stress, which causes increased ferritin and iron deposition, and induction of nitric oxide synthase. The results suggest that cerebrovascular endothelial cells of these brain regions may be particularly vulnerable to thiamine deficiency [10].

Vitamin B$_3$ (niacin) deficiency in humans leads to pellagra, which is characterized by dementia, dermatitis, diarrhea and eventually death. The deficiency was recognized in the eighteenth cen-

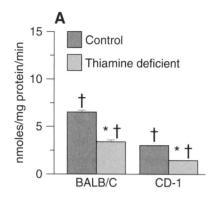
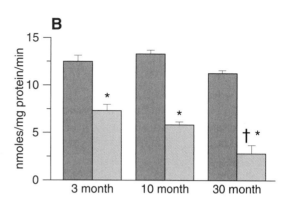

* Denotes a significant effect of thiamin deficiency.
† Denotes a significant effect between strains.

* Denotes a significant effect of thiamin deficiency.
† Denotes a significant effect of aging.

FIGURE 33-2. Strain and age differences in response to thiamine deficiency in mice. **A:** Transketolase activity in the brains of thiamine-deficient and pair-fed control Balb/C and CD-1 mice. **B:** β-Ketoglutarate dehydrogenase complex activity in the brains of thiamine-deficient and pair-fed control Balb/C mice of different ages. (Data derived from [34], with permission.)

tury, shortly after the introduction of American corn (maize) into Europe [8].

Niacin and niacinamide refer to nicotinic acid and its amide, respectively. Although these pyrimidine derivatives can be synthesized from tryptophan in mammals, perhaps at least in part by intestinal bacteria, 60 mg of dietary tryptophan are required to synthesize 1 mg of the vitamin. Niacin is considered to be a vitamin because most human diets do not contain enough tryptophan to fulfill the normal human requirement for the vitamin of 10 to 30 mg/day.

Hartnup's syndrome is a hereditary disorder in which tryptophan transport is impaired and requirements for dietary niacin increase. Phenylketonuria and hyperphenylalaninemia can increase niacin requirements by increasing the concentrations of amino acids that compete with tryptophan for transport systems (see also Chap. 44). A high-corn diet predisposes to niacin deficiency since the major storage protein of American corn (zein) has relatively little tryptophan relative to other amino acids that compete for the same carrier. Addition of purified niacin to the diet has largely abolished pellagra, which was once a common disease in areas where corn was a dietary staple.

Niacin is incorporated into the coenzymes NAD^+ and $NADP^+$ and their reduced

forms. These cofactors are involved in numerous oxidation/reduction reactions, including the coupling of the Krebs cycle to the respiratory chain. Antimetabolites, particularly 6-aminonicotinamide and 3-acetylpyridine, have been particularly useful in determining the role of niacin deficiency in the brain in experimental animals. Newborn mice that received a single intraperitoneal injection of 6-aminonicotinamide consistently developed lesions in the CNS, the skin and the intestinal tract. Anterior horn cells in the spinal cord as well as motor neurons in the brain exhibit the ultrastructural features of neuronal chromatolysis, while glial and ependymal cells show edematous changes. 3-Acetylpyridine administration leads to selective neuropathological lesions in the brainstem. Although the pathological features of antimetabolite-treated mice are not identical to those of human pellagra, possible contributory mechanisms in the development of pellagra lesions, including dementia and selective cell loss, may be elucidated with this experimental model [11].

Vitamin B₆ (pyridoxine) is necessary for the biosynthesis of several neurotransmitters. It is a pyridine derivative that can exist as an alcohol, amine or aldehyde. The concentration in brain is normally about 100-fold higher than that in the blood. The active coenzyme is the phosphorylated derivative pyridoxal phosphate, which readily forms Schiff bases. This coenzyme participates in decarboxylation reactions, including those that form GABA from glutamate, 5-HT from 5-hydroxytryptophan and probably DOPA from dihydroxyphenylalanine. It is also involved in transaminations, including that converting α-ketoglutarate to glutamate. The conversion of tryptophan to nicotinamide requires pyridoxyl phosphate as a cofactor, and the excretion of xanthurenic acid after a tryptophan load is widely used to test the adequacy of pyridoxine nutriture. In vitamin B_6 deficiency in rats, biochemical and morphological abnormalities, including decreased dendritic arborization and reduced numbers of myelinated axons and synapses, are associated with behavioral changes, such as epileptiform seizures and movement disorders. Reduced seizure threshold and delayed neuronal recovery are related to the significantly reduced brain regional GABA and elevated glutamate concentrations in pyridoxine-deficient rats [12]. In addition, vitamin B_6 deficiency during gestation and lactation alters the function of N-methyl-D-aspartate (NMDA) receptors.

Pyridoxine deficiency has occurred in human infants fed a formula from which vitamin B_6 had been inadvertantly omitted. The prominent finding was intractable seizures which responded promptly to injections of the vitamin. Deficiency of pyridoxine can contribute to the polyneuropathy of B-complex deficiency. However, very large doses of pure pyridoxine can lead to a persistant sensory neuropathy [13] (Chap. 36).

Like those of other nutrients, requirements for pyridoxine can be altered by genetic or environmental factors and are increased in a number of disorders of the nervous system [8,14,15]. Treatment of "pyridoxine-deficient" infants may require doses of pyridoxine several hundredfold the normal daily requirement. Maintenance with doses at least tenfold the normal requirement typically permits normal development if irreversible brain damage has not yet occurred. It has been suggested that mild forms of pyridoxine dependence may be a relatively common cause of intractable seizures and mental retardation, but neurochemical studies of these patients are limited. In homocystinuria and cystothioninuria, two disorders of amino

acid metabolism, some patients respond to large doses of pyridoxine. In these patients, the mutations appear to reduce the affinity of the relevant enzymes for pyridoxal phosphate (see Chap. 44).

Environmentally, hydrazides and oximes can increase pyridoxine requirements. Large doses of pyridoxine are routinely given with the antituberculous medication isonicotinic hydrazide, to prevent drug-induced neuropathy.

Vitamin B_{12} (cobalamin) deficiency is commonly associated with neurological syndromes. The cobalamins are a series of porphyrin-like compounds [16]. The active forms contain a cobalt ion linked to one of the methylene groups. The cobalamins are synthesized by many microorganisms but not by higher plants or animals. A rich dietary source is meat, particularly liver. Effective absorption requires a series of transport proteins, including a glycoprotein intrinsic factor secreted by gastric parietal cells. Conversion to the active coenzymes adenosylcobalamin and methylcobalamin requires at least two reductase reactions and an adenosyltransferase step. The reductases are flavoproteins that require NAD^+ as a cofactor. Thus, B_{12} metabolism involves at least three vitamins: B_{12} itself, niacin and riboflavin. Body stores of cobalamins are normally large enough to maintain health for over 2 years without a dietary source of the vitamin.

Cobalamins have two well-established biochemical functions. Adenosylcobalamin is the cofactor for the mutase that converts methylmalonyl CoA to succinyl CoA. This reaction is part of the pathway of metabolism of propionic acid, which itself derives from the metabolism of odd-chain fatty acids and from certain amino acids. Methylcobalamin is the cofactor for the methyltransferase that converts homocysteine to the amino acid methionine. This reaction is important in folate metabolism as well. Its impairment appears to foster folate deficiency by an accumulation of N^5-methyltetrahydrofolate in a "folate trap." Deficiency of cobalamins or of folate or of both can restrict the supply of metabolically available one-carbon groups for metabolic pathways, including those of nucleic acid synthesis.

Cobalamin deficiencies are relatively common clinically [16]. Pure dietary deficiency responding promptly to treatment with oral cobalamins has been described in a few children of strict vegan mothers. A more common syndrome is caused by failure of absorption due to an inadequate supply of the glycoprotein intrinsic factor, usually on an autoimmune basis. The most characteristic abnormality is pernicious anemia, characterized by enlarged erythrocytes, called megaloblasts, and abnormal leukocytes. Neurological symptoms occur in many of these patients and can precede the hematological changes [17].

Combined system disease is the most common B_{12}-mediated neurological syndrome. Affected patients develop unpleasant tingling sensations (paresthesias), followed by loss of vibratory sensation, particularly in the legs, and spastic weakness. The characteristic neuropathology is a spongy demyelination in the long tracts of the spinal cord, particularly prominent in the posterior columns as well as corticospinal tracts. Combined system disease responds poorly to treatment with cobalamins.

Cobalamin deficiency is characteristically associated with malaise that does respond dramatically to treatment, even before the hematological response is evident. Relatively low serum concentrations of B_{12} have been reported in subgroups of psychiatric patients, including patients with Alzheimer's disease, but responses to treatment with the vitamin have, in general, not been dramatic. Recent studies indicate that elevated concentrations of serum or cerebrospinal fluid methylmalonate can identify patients whose neuropsychiatric manifestations benefit from B_{12} treatment, even though the amounts of vitamin in serum are not in the deficient range [17].

Whether the damage to the nervous system relates to decreased activity of the methylmalonyl mutase or of the methyltransferase or of both remains unsettled. Increased excretion of methylmalonate has been reported to be a marker for patients whose neuropsychiatric manifestations will improve with B_{12} treatment, but clinically normal children with a mutase deficiency are known. Children with homocystinuria and related disorders do not develop the clinical or pathological stigmata of combined system disease (see Chap. 44). An infant with an apparent reduction in methyltransferase activity was clinically normal when reported at age 1 year. Patients with severe inherited deficiencies in the activities of both enzymes secondary to a defect in the metabolism of the cobalamins do develop profound disease of the nervous system, with some characteristics of combined system disease.

As with other nutrients, requirements for cobalamin can be modified by genetic and environmental influences. Genetic factors apparently predispose to intrinsic factor deficiencies with resultant cobalamin deficiency. Furthermore, at least six different inherited methylmalonic acidurias have been described [16]: absence of the mutase, decreased affinity of the mutase for adenosylcobalamin, deficiency of mitochondrial cobalamin reductase, deficiency of a mitochondrial cobalamin adenyltransferase and two distinguishable defects associated with abnormal cytosolic metabolism of cobalamin (see Chap. 44). Other conditions leading to increased cobalamin requirements include surgical removal of the stomach, excessive destruction of cobalamins in the gut by bacteria in a blind loop or destruction by certain kinds of intestinal tapeworm.

Folic acid contains a pterin moiety linked to para-aminobenzoic acid, which is linked to one or more glutamate residues [18]. It plays a key role in the transfer of one-carbon (active methylene) groups, including the conversion of serine to glycine and the cobalamin-dependent transfer from homocysteine to methionine. Dietary deficiency of folate with normal cobalamin leads to anemia without significant neurological signs. However, both genetic and environmental disorders of folate metabolism have been associated with disease of the nervous system. Genetic defects in the relevant enzyme reactions are discussed further in Chapter 44.

Genetic disorders of folate absorption, intraconversion and utilization are rare [18]. They have occasionally been associated with phenocopies of well-known psychiatric syndromes. A boy with apparent deficiency of hepatic dihydrofolate reductase was treated with folate and developed a sociopathic personality in his teens. A folate-responsive form of mental retardation with catatonia has been described in an adolescent girl with N^5,10-methylenetetrahydrofolic acid reductase deficiency. Her younger sister was mentally impaired with "psychosis"; an unrelated boy with a defect of the same enzyme had seizures and proximal muscle weakness without notable psychiatric problems. Most patients with glutamate formiminotransferase deficiency have had a syndrome of psychomotor retardation in infancy, but a few have been entirely normal clinically.

Environmentally, a number of common medications, including phenytoin and certain antitumor agents, increase requirements for dietary folate. Treatment with folate can mask the hematological signs of cobalamin deficiency without affecting the progressive damage to the nervous system.

Pantothenic acid is a substituted hydroxybutyric acid that is a constituent of CoA [19]. Experimental induction of pantothenic acid deficiency leads to signs of peripheral nerve damage, for example, demyelination in laboratory animals and paresthesias in humans. Late signs of CNS damage in animals may relate as well to the adrenal failure that is a prominent part of the syndrome.

The brain depends on select vitamins and closely related compounds as antioxidants to control potentially damaging free radicals

The main antioxidants in brain are vitamin E (tocopherol), vitamin C (ascorbic acid) and glutathione (Table 33-2). The first two can be easily manipulated by diet, whereas the latter is more difficult to control. Dietary α-lipoate appears to be a useful compound to regenerate the antioxidant capacity of these other compounds (see below). Dietary manipulation of antioxidants has practical implications for brain function. Aging has been associated with free radical damage in the brain (see Chap. 34). In aged patients tested over a 22-year period, free recall, recognition and vocabulary correlated positively with ascorbic acid and β-carotene in blood, even after controlling for possible confounding variables, such as age, education and gender. These results indicate the important role played by antioxidants in brain aging and may have implications for prevention of progressive cognitive impairments [20].

Vitamin E (α-tocopherol) deficiency produces a characteristic neurological syndrome. It presumably results from increased oxidative stress arising from a reduction in antioxidant capacity. Vitamin E deficiency in neural tissues increases endogenous lipid peroxidation, as evidenced in brain tissues by the appearance of thiobarbituric acid-reactive substances such as malondialdehyde. The brain is more susceptible to the deficiency than muscle. Within the brain, the cortex, striatum and cerebellum are the most sensitive regions. Isolated fractions from myelinated nerve tracts show that the axoplasmic membranes and organelles are particularly vulnerable to oxidative stress [21]. Vitamin E deficiency reduces tyrosine hydroxylase-immunopositive neurons in the substantia nigra but not in the adjacent ventral tegmental area. The enhanced sensitivity of the nigrostriatal pathway to oxidative stress could have important implications for the pathogenesis of Parkinson's disease (see Chap. 45). A diet deficient in vitamin E increases glutamate and GABA and decreases tryptophan concentrations in the substantia nigra. The increase of nigral glutamate suggests possible links to degenerative processes through glutamatergic excitotoxicity. These results suggest that vitamin E may play a significant role in the degeneration of the substantia nigra and that this tissue may be particularly sensitive to oxidative stress. Furthermore, these findings support the widely held view that oxidative stress in the substantia nigra is important in the pathophysiology of Parkinson's disease.

Vitamin C (ascorbate) deficiency leads to extensive oxidative damage of proteins and protein loss in the microsomes, as evidenced by accumulation of carbonyl groups on proteins as well as tryptophan loss. This oxidative damage is reversed by ascorbate therapy. Ascorbate deficiency also leads to lipid peroxidation in microsomes, as evidenced by accumulation of conjugated dienes, malondialdehyde and fluorescent pigment. Lipid peroxides disappear after ascorbate therapy but not after treatment with vitamin E. These results indicate that vitamin C may exert a powerful protection against degenerative changes in the brain associated with oxidative damage [22].

Oxidation of vitamin E and C is maintained by glutathione, the predominant thiol antioxidant in the brain. Glutathione cannot be directly manipulated by diet, whereas the metabolic antioxidant α-lipoate can be absorbed from the diet and cross the BBB to reduce oxidized glutathione and vitamins A and C (Fig. 33-3). α-Lipoate is taken up and reduced in cells and tissues to dihydrolipoate, which is also exported to the extracellular space; hence, protection is afforded to both intracellular and extracellular environments. Both α-lipoate and dihydrolipoate are potent antioxidants that regenerate other antioxidants, like vitamins C and E, and raise intracellular glutathione concentrations. Protective effects by antioxidants have been reported in cerebral ischemia–reperfusion, excitotoxic amino acid brain injury, mitochondrial dysfunction, diabetes and diabetic neuropathy, inborn errors of metabolism and other causes of acute

or chronic damage to the brain or neural tissue. Thus, α-lipoate administration may prove to be an effective treatment in numerous neurodegenerative disorders [20].

Trace nutrients in the diet have a vital role in maintaining normal brain function

Zinc (Zn^{2+}) influences numerous cellular functions, including immune mechanisms, actions of several hormones and enzyme activities. More than 200 enzymes are known to be Zn^{2+}-dependent, including mRNA-editing enzymes, superoxide dismutase, metalloproteins and a "Zn^{2+}-finger" family of sequence-specific DNA-binding proteins that regulate transcription. Metallothionein binds excess Zn^{2+}, thus maintaining its steady-state concentration and preventing inhibition of an extensive number of sulfhydryl-containing enzymes and receptor sites; hence, it protects against metal-related neurotoxicity. Metallothionein donates Zn^{2+} to an extensive number of Zn^{2+}-activated, pyridoxal phosphate-mediated biochemical reac-

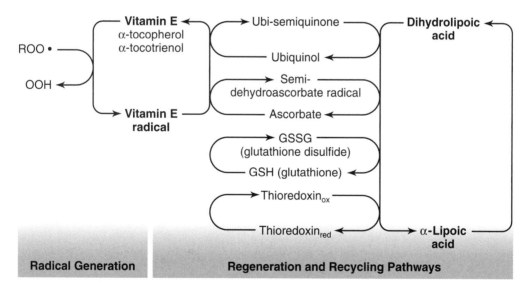

FIGURE 33-3. Interaction of various aspects of the oxidative status of the brain that depend on diet. The elaborate mechanisms of the brain to minimize free radical formation depend on many dietary constituents, including vitamin C, vitamin E, α-lipoate, the selenium-dependent enzyme glutathione peroxidase and the niacin that is part of the NADPH necessary for regeneration of glutathione. The figure shows the pathways by which dihydrolipoate recycles vitamin E and other antioxidants. (From [20] with permission.)

tions. The complex nature of the interactions of Zn^{2+} with multiple enzymes is exemplified by the observation that epileptic seizures that are blocked by GABA can be blocked by either deficiency or excess of either Zn^{2+} or pyridoxal phosphate. A proposed explanation of these observations is that at physiological concentrations Zn^{2+} stimulates the activity of hippocampal pyridoxal kinase, enhancing the formation of pyridoxal phosphate and of GABA via glutamate decarboxylase formation, whereas at higher doses Zn^{2+} inhibits the activity of glutamate decarboxylase by preventing the binding of pyridoxal phosphate [23]. Severe Zn^{2+} deficiency during the period of rapid brain growth has effects similar to that seen with protein-calorie malnourishment, including altered regulation of emotions; food motivation; lethargy (reduced activity and responsiveness), and deficits in learning, attention and memory. In addition to the many deficits produced by Zn^{2+} deficiency in the brain, the severe effect of Zn^{2+} deficiency on other tissues leads to additional peripheral mechanisms that alter brain function [24]. Although Zn^{2+} is essential at low concentrations, higher concentrations are toxic. For example, high Zn^{2+} concentrations enhance and prolong the firing rate of neurons, significantly depress paired-pulse potentiation, block the action of NMDA on cortical neurons, enhance quisqualate receptor-mediated injury and inhibit the Ca^{2+}-dependent release of transmitter by inhibiting the entry of Ca^{2+} into nerve terminals.

Copper is an integral component of multiple cellular enzymes, including the cytochromes and superoxide dismutase. Copper deficiency produces clinical signs analogous to those of Parkinson's disease and results in low dopamine concentration in the corpus striatum. Neuropathology in experimental animals occurs in only part of the copper-deficient population and is dam- and litter-related, suggesting the presence of a genetic component that alters the response to copper deficiency. Insight into the role of copper in brain function is provided by two genetic diseases.

Wilson's disease is an inherited disorder that leads to copper accumulation, causing damage primarily to the liver and the brain (see Box 45-1). Psychiatric and behavioral abnormalities occur in 30 to 100% of Wilson's disease patients and are often the initial symptoms. The most common of the psychiatric and behavioral manifestations include personality changes, such as irritability and low anger threshold; depression, sometimes leading to suicidal ideation and attempts; and deteriorating academic and work performance, which is present in almost all neurologically affected patients [25].

Menke's disease is caused by a genetic deficiency of serum copper and of copper-dependent enzymes and is characterized by neurological degeneration and mental retardation, connective tissue and vascular defects, brittle and depigmented hair and death in early childhood (see Box 45-1). Despite excessive accumulation of the metal in various tissues, a functional copper deficiency is evident, caused by a defective intracellular copper-transport protein. A large amount of copper accumulates in the organelle-free cytoplasm, whereas mitochondria are in a state of copper deficiency, indicating that the Menke's mutation probably affects copper transport from the cytosol to the intracellular organelles [26]. *Brindled* is a murine mutation that produces similar copper-transport deficits, and studies of this animal model show that the copper deficit in organelles causes reductions in critical copper-dependent enzymes, such as cytochrome oxidase. It has been hypothesized that the Wilson's disease gene is a copper-transporting ATPase with homology to the Menke's disease gene. Dietary copper deficiency can affect brain development [27] (see below).

Selenium is vital in maintaining the antioxidant capacity of the brain. Glutathione peroxidase is a selenium-dependent enzyme that is important for maintaining the antioxidant capacity of brain glutathione (Fig. 33-2) and is reduced in selenium-deficient animals. Selenium supplementation significantly elevates Na,K-ATPase activity and significantly decreases lipid peroxide formation. Since Na,K-ATPase activity is known to be inhibited by oxygen free radicals, selenium supplementation appears to exert its beneficial effect on the Na,K-ATPase activity by preventing free radical-induced damage. Selenium significantly reduces the production of thiobarbituric acid-reactive substances, a measure of lipid peroxidation, in response to an oxidative challenge in blood and different regions of the brain [28]. Selenium deficiency increases dopamine turnover in the substantia nigra but not in the striatum. These results suggest that dietary selenium protects the brain, particularly the substantia nigra, against oxidative damage.

Trace compounds are also important in brain function. *Chromium*-deficient patients develop severe diabetic symptoms, including glucose intolerance, weight loss, impaired energy utilization and nerve and brain disorders. Low dietary *boron* is reported to cause significantly poorer performance on various cognitive and psychomotor tasks. Additional research is likely to reveal additional trace components of the diet that may be critical to normal brain function.

NUTRITION AND STRUCTURAL ASPECTS OF THE BRAIN

Dietary manipulation of membrane content and fluidity can have profound effects on brain function and has implications for changes seen in aging and disease. The nervous system has the second greatest tissue concentration of lipids (after adipose tissue), and brain lipids are remarkably sensitive to diet (Table 33-3). These lipids participate directly in membrane functioning and affect the activities of enzymes and receptors. It is necessary to ensure that nerve cells receive an adequate supply of essential lipids during their differentiation and multiplication and in adulthood.

The essential polyunsaturated fatty acids belong to two families, ω6 and ω3, that are characterized by the indicated number of carbons of the first double bond from the methyl terminal

Neither of these is synthesized in humans or animals (Chap. 3). The principal dietary source of the ω6 polyunsaturated fatty acids is linoleic acid (18:2ω6). The ω3 polyunsaturated fatty acids are derived mainly from α-linolenic acid (18:3ω3). Other polyunsaturated acids with similarly positioned unsaturated bonds are synthesized from these compounds. For example, linoleic acid is the basis for synthesis of eicosatrienoic (20:3ω6) and arachidonic (20:4ω6) acids. Docosahexaenoic acid (DHA) (22:6ω3) is derived from α-linolenic acid (18:3ω3).

The effects of α-linolenic acid (18:3ω3) deficiency on brain composition have been studied extensively. Feeding rats diets low in α-linolenic

| TABLE 33-3. | DIETARY FATTY ACIDS AND BRAIN FUNCTION: SINCE THE BRAIN CANNOT MAKE CERTAIN FATTY ACIDS, A REDUCTION IN THEIR CONCENTRATIONS IN THE DIET DIMINISHES THEIR BRAIN CONCENTRATIONS; CHANGES IN BRAIN FATTY ACIDS PRODUCE NEUROCHEMICAL AND BEHAVIORAL EFFECTS | | |

Diet	Brain	Neurochemical effect	Behavioral effect
Low α-linolenic acid (18:3ω3)	Reduced 22:6ω3 Increased 22:5ω6	Reduced Na,K-ATPase, reduced 5′ nucleotidase, altered membrane fluidity	Impaired learning and memory, resistance to toxins, reduction in synaptic vesicles
High linoleic acid (18:2ω6)	Increased 22:5(ω6) Increased 22:4(ω6) Decreased 22:6(ω3)	Altered esterase transition temperature, decreased membrane fluidity	
High saturated fatty acids	Polyunsaturated: saturated ratio decreased	Decreased membrane fluidity, lower β-adrenergic receptor binding,	
Decreased cholesterol	Decreased cholesterol	Increased membrane fluidity	Increased activity, improved memory

acid content results in reduced amounts of DHA in all brain cells and organelles and in various other organs. The reduction is compensated for by an increase in 22:5ω6, thus maintaining the total content of polyunsaturated fatty acids approximately constant. Restoration to normal brain composition from such conditions is extremely slow for brain cells, organelles and microvessels, in contrast to other organs. During cerebral development, there is a linear relation between ω3 fatty acid content in the brain and the ω3 fatty acids in the diet, and the shift in ω3 content can alter the properties of enzymes and membranes. A decrease in the ω3 series of fatty acids in the membranes produces a 40% reduction in the Na,K-ATPase of nerve terminals, a 20% reduction in 5′-nucleotidase and altered membrane fluidity in rats. A diet low in ω3 fatty acids has little effect on motor function and activity, but learning is reportedly markedly impaired. The inferior learning performance in the ω3 fatty acid-deficient group is associated with a nearly 30% reduction in the average densities of synaptic vesicles in the terminals of the hippocampal CA1 region. The diet-induced morphological changes in synapses in the hippocampus of rats are thus associated with differential learning performance. The presence of ω3 fatty acids in the diet also confers resistance to certain neurotoxic agents, such as triethyl-lead [29].

A diet high in 18:2ω6 (linoleic acid) and in the 18:2(ω6):18:3(ω3) ratio does not change synaptosomal cholesterol, total lipid phosphorus or phospholipid class composition. However, synaptosomal fatty acid composition is influenced by this diet. The proportion of 22:6ω3 is decreased, while 22:4ω6 and 22:5ω6 are increased. The monoene content, especially 18:1, is also reduced in synaptosomes. Although the activity of synaptosomal acetylcholinesterase is unaffected by this diet, higher transition temperatures for this enzyme are seen, indicating decreased membrane fluidity. The data suggest that a diet high in 18:2ω6 and/or a high 18:2ω6/18:3ω3 ratio compromises normal fatty acid accretion and physical properties of brain synaptosomal membranes.

The fatty acid composition of individual phospholipids in the brain can also be manipulated by diet. Feeding a derived ω3 fatty acid concentrate containing eicosapentaenoic acid (20:5ω3, EPA) and DHA to growing rats alters brain fatty acids. EPA becomes significantly enriched in all phospholipid fractions in the brain, including phosphatidylcholine, phosphatidylethanolamine, phosphatidylserine and phosphatidylinositol. Corresponding changes also occur in the 22:5ω3 contents, with little or no elevation in DHA. In contrast, the percentages by weight of the ω6 fatty acids, including 18:2ω6, 20:4ω6 (arachidonic acid), 22:4ω6 and 22:5ω6, are generally lower in the various phospholipids. These results indicate that dietary ω3 fatty acids can greatly affect the fatty acid composition of the various membrane phospholipids in nervous tissues. These alterations may be important for functional changes, including altered membrane fluidity, cellular responses, ion transport and the biosynthesis of prostaglandins and leukotrienes (Chap. 35).

Feeding isoenergetic diets rich in saturated fatty acids alters the response of neurotransmitter receptors

Binding affinities of the β-adrenergic receptor in the hypothalamus and cortex are significantly lower in the saturated fatty acid group, while those of the α receptor do not differ between the two groups. The polyunsaturated-to-saturated fatty acid ratio and the fluidity of plasma membranes in the hypothalamus and cortex are lower in saturated fatty acids. These results suggest that a diet rich in saturated fatty acids decreases membrane fluidity by altering the fatty acid composition of plasma membranes [30].

Dietary manipulation of cholesterol also alters brain neurochemistry. Feeding 3-month-old rats a diet that lowered the cholesterol in the hippocampus and cortex increased membrane fluidity. The animals also had a higher activity and better learning performance compared to animals on a normal diet.

NUTRITION AND BRAIN DEVELOPMENT

This area of active research has received extensive attention for several decades. Nutrition is one of the most important environmental influences on the fetus and the neonate. Many of the effects of early diet on the brain are permanent. Malnutrition produces a variety of minimal brain dysfunction-type syndromes, including attentional processes and learning disabilities. Malnutrition often produces a distributed, nonfocal brain pathology.

Iodine deficiency constitutes one of the most common preventable causes of mental deficiency in the world. Iodine deficiency causes cretinism, deaf mutism and cerebral palsy by altering neuronal and dendritic growth [31].

Copper deficiency during development leads to smaller, shorter and narrower cell nuclei in the infrapyramidal and suprapyramidal arms of the dentate gyrus and smaller cell nuclei in region CA3 of the hippocampus. All alterations in the groups fed low-copper diets are consistent with slowed cell nuclear maturation. The findings indicate that copper is required for maturation of the dentate gyrus and hippocampus.

Arachidonic acid (20:4ω6) and DHA (22:6ω3) are deposited in large amounts in the nonmyelin membranes of the developing CNS. Inadequate supplies of ω6 and ω3 fatty acids during CNS development are of concern because of possible long-term changes in learning ability and reduced visual function. Current evidence suggests that the newborn is able to synthesize 20:4ω6 and 22:6ω3 from linoleic acid (18:2ω6) and α-linolenic acid (18:3ω3), respectively [32].

Prenatal protein malnutrition produces differential morphological changes on CA3 pyramidal cells. Significant decreases occur in the somal size, length of apical dendrites, apical and basal dendritic branching and spine density. Thus, prenatal protein malnutrition affects normal development and produces long-term effects on CA3 pyramidal cells [33].

NUTRITION AND AGING OF THE NERVOUS SYSTEM

Nutritional requirements vary with age, and the aged brain is particularly sensitive to nutritional deficiencies. For example, while the activity of the enzyme α-ketoglutarate dehydrogenase does not change with age, thiamin deficiency induces a much larger change in the activity of α-ketoglutarate dehydrogenase in aged than in young animals [34] (Fig. 33-2). This sensitivity to other insults might be one of the factors that predisposes the aged brain to the development of neurodegenerative disorders.

Antioxidants may provide an important way to delay aging of the brain

Oxidative stress with overproduction of reactive oxygen species has been implicated in a variety of neurodegenerative disorders and in the aging process itself. Vitamin E deficiency of young adult animals causes changes in brain intracellular ionic content, synaptic contact areas and synaptic and perykaryal mitochondria similar to that seen in "normal," old animals. As described previously, antioxidant concentrations in the brain can be manipulated effectively with diet.

Restricting intake of a balanced diet is an effective means of extending life span and of reducing several measures of oxidative stress in the brain under laboratory conditions in rodents and primates

Dietary restriction suppresses the amount of reactive oxygen species produced by synaptosomal membranes from both young and old animals. Age-related decreases in membrane fluidity are diminished by dietary restriction in rats. Age-related increases in the cholesterol-to-phospholipid ratio occur in both normal and diet-restricted groups, so the improvement in fluidity may be influenced by factors other than cholesterol, such as decreased lipid peroxidation. Dietary restriction lowers lipofuscin deposition in the neurons of hippocampus and frontal cortex. Protein carbonyl concentrations, a measure of protein oxidation, increase with age in most regions of the mouse brain, with the most notable accumulations occurring in the striatum and hippocampus, regions strongly implicated in age-associated functional loss. Dietary restriction reverses age-associated regional trends in protein carbonyl concentrations, the largest improvements occurring within the striatum. Dietary restriction also lowers age-related increases in concentrations of 8-hydroxydeoxyguanosine, a product of DNA oxidation in skeletal muscle, brain and heart, tissues which are composed primarily of long-lived, postmitotic cells, to levels comparable to those seen in young mice. Dopamine receptor concentrations in striata of aged rats that had been on a restricted diet since weaning are 50% higher than those of control animals of the same age and comparable to those seen in young control rats. These findings suggest that the beneficial effects of dietary restriction on brain function and life span may depend on a reduction in steady-state levels of oxidative stress [35]. In parallel with these neurochemical improvements, dietary restriction diminishes age-associated reductions of sensorimotor coordination and improves performance of aged mice in an avoidance learning task. Diet-restricted mice also learn faster and perform better on the radial maze task than do control rats.

Other treatments can also diminish age-related increases in oxidative stress

Chronic treatment with the spin-trapping compound N-tert-butyl-α-phenylnitrone (PBN) reverses increases in oxidized protein, as assessed by carbonyl residues, as well as the decreases in glutamine synthetase that accompany aging in gerbils. Old gerbils make more errors than young animals and, when treated with PBN, fewer errors in a radial arm maze test for temporal and spatial memory than untreated, aged controls. Thus, a variety of results support the hypothesis that oxidative damage may be important during aging and that these changes can be manipulated in part by diet, including caloric restriction and/or ingestion of antioxidants (Chap. 34).

NUTRITION AND THE TREATMENT OF NEURODEGENERATIVE DISEASE

An understanding of the interaction of brain and nutrition permits the use of diet to treat neuro-

logical disorders. One of the best-known examples is phenylketonuria. This disease results from the near absence of phenylalanine hydroxylase, an enzyme which converts phenylalanine to tyrosine. This deficit results in excessive phenylalanine in the blood and severe mental retardation. Dietary control of phenylalanine largely protects the brain from this otherwise devastating condition (see Chap. 44). Diet can also be used to bypass inborn errors in oxidative metabolism (see Chap. 44). The neurological status of patients with diminished pyruvate dehydrogenase activity can be improved with a diet that is high in ketones, which bypasses the pyruvate dehydrogenase step in brain metabolism. A diet enriched in antioxidants may be particularly useful in treating neurodegenerative disorders. Treatment with vitamin E of patients with moderately severe impairment from Alzheimer's disease has been reported to slow the progression of disease [36]. Nutritional approaches to ameliorate age-related changes in the brain are discussed above.

The concentration of Zn^{2+} is altered in many disorders of the CNS. For example, chronic alcoholism is associated with low serum Zn^{2+}. Low brain Zn^{2+} may enhance NMDA excitotoxicity and ethanol-withdrawal seizure susceptibility. Also, Zn^{2+} deficiency can produce neuronal damage through increased free radical formation. Zn^{2+} replacement therapy may be a rational approach to the treatment of alcohol-withdrawal seizures and alcohol-related brain dysfunction. Other diseases said to be associated with low serum Zn^{2+} include Alzheimer-type dementia, amyotrophic lateral sclerosis, Down's syndrome, epilepsy, Friedreich's ataxia, Guillain-Barré syndrome, hepatic encephalopathy, multiple sclerosis, Parkinson's disease, Pick's disease, retinitis pigmentosa, retinal dystrophy, schizophrenia and Wernicke-Korsakoff syndrome. The status of metallothionein isoforms and other low-molecular-weight, Zn^{2+}-binding proteins in these conditions is unknown. Several of these disorders are associated with oxidative stress: since metallothioneins are able to prevent the formation of free radicals, induction of metallothioneins may provide long-lasting protection against oxidative damage [37].

NUTRITION AND GENETICS

Genetic factors may determine susceptibility to chronic disease as well as the response to diet

The response to thiamine deficiency provides a striking example of this predisposition. In rodents, large, strain-dependent differences occur in the concentrations of thiamine-dependent enzymes [34] (Fig. 33-2). Among humans, Asians and Europeans respond to thiamine deficiency differently: Asians tend to develop a wet beri-beri characterized by heart problems, whereas Europeans tend to develop a dry beri-beri accompanied by severe neurological problems, including extensive memory deficits. Wernicke-Korsakoff syndrome, a thiamine-deficiency syndrome associated with alcoholism and severe memory problems, does not develop in all alcoholics. It has been proposed that individuals who develop Wernicke-Korsakoff syndrome have TK with a high K_m for TPP so that they require more thiamine. Such individuals thus have a genetic predisposition for developing a neurodegenerative disease related to nutrition. There are other instances where the interaction is not quite so direct. For example, individuals with the E4 alleles of the APOE gene (ApoE4) have higher cholesterol levels and bear a higher risk for cardiovascular disease and for Alzheimer's disease than individuals with ApoE3. ApoE genetic variations thus can influence the response to diet. For example, men with ApoE4/E3 phenotype show the greatest improvement in their low-density to high-density lipoprotein ratios when there is a high polyunsaturated to saturated fatty acid ratio in the diet.

Nutrients are involved in gene transcription, mRNA processing, mRNA stability and mRNA translation

Dietary constituents modulate the nuclear events governing gene transcription and transcript processing. For example, transcription of the fatty acid synthase gene is inhibited by specific polyunsaturated fatty acids, the pyruvate kinase gene contains a specific carbohydrate response element and editing of ApoB-100 to ApoB-48 lipoproteins is enhanced by dietary carbohydrate. Nutrients such as iron and glucose control mRNA stability and translational rates of selected transcripts by regulating the interaction of cytosolic proteins with specific nucleotide sequences [38]. Diet strongly influences glucose transport into tissues by altering both the expression of the glucose transporter genes (GLUT-1 and GLUT-4) and the functional activity of the gene products. Dietary regulation of GLUT-1 and GLUT-4 is tissue-specific. In the starved state, there is a profound downregulation of glucose transporter gene expression in adipose cells, while expression of the same transporter genes is somewhat increased in skeletal muscle. Studies of brain RNA of animals on diets with varying protein contents show that brain insulin-like growth factor-II mRNA is decreased by 57% with a low-protein diet.

Chronic acetyl-L-carnitine administration abolishes the age-associated reduction of p75 nerve growth factor (NGF) receptor mRNA concentrations in the basal forebrain and cerebellum of old rats. The results suggest a neuroprotective effect for acetylcarnitine on central cholinergic neurons exerted at the level of receptor transcription. The restoration of p75NGF receptor concentrations could increase trophic support by NGF of these CNS cholinergic neurons, which are implicated in degenerative events associated with aging [39]. Long-term treatment with acetylcarnitine completely prevents the loss of choline acetyltransferase activity in the CNS of aged rats.

Clearly, much remains to be learned about the regulation by diet of gene expression in the brain.

NEURONAL CONTROL OF FOOD INTAKE

The control of food intake by the brain is an integral part of nutrition. An explosion of interest in this area has accompanied the identification of the so-called "obesity genes" that produce the OB protein, also termed leptin. Leptin is secreted by adipose cells and acts as a negative feedback on the brain centers that control food intake and energy balance. Leptin is deficient in some obese animals, while other obese strains are leptin receptor-deficient or leptin-unresponsive. Injection of leptin into brain reduces food intake. Leptin receptors are colocalized in the ventromedial hypothalamus with neuropeptide Y neurons. Leptin administration reduces neuropeptide Y production, while neuropeptide Y stimulates food intake. Thus, the interaction of neuropeptide Y with leptin forms an important axis in the regulation of food intake [40].

SUMMARY

Adequate and deficient nutrition have important consequences for brain function. Nutrition of the developing brain is important for optimal brain capacity over the lifetime of an animal or person. Proper nutrition of the aged brain may be important not only for normal function but also for minimizing some of the consequences of aging and of neurodegenerative diseases.

REFERENCES

1. Chung, S. Y., Moriyama, T., Uezu, E., et al. Administration of phosphatidylcholine increases brain acetylcholine concentration and improves memory in mice with dementia. *J. Nutr.* 125:1484–1489, 1995.

2. Ragozzino, M. E., Unick, K. E., and Gold, P. E. Hippocampal acetylcholine release during memory testing in rats: Augmentation by glucose. *Proc. Natl. Acad. Sci. USA* 93:4693–4698, 1996.

3. Avraham, Y., Bonne, O., and Berry, E. M. Behavioral and neurochemical alterations caused by diet restriction—the effect of tyrosine administration in mice. *Brain Res.* 732:133–144, 1996.

4. al-Mudallal, A. S., Levin, B. E., Lust, W. D., and Harik, S. I. Effects of unbalanced diets on cerebral glucose metabolism in the adult rat. *Neurology* 45:2261–2265, 1995.

5. Stumpf, D. A., Parker, W. D., and Angelini, C. Carnitine deficiency, organic acidemias, and Reyes syndrome. *Neurology* 35:1014–1045, 1985.

6. Triggs, W. J., Bohan, T. P., Lin, S. N., and Willmore, L. J. Valproate-induced coma with ketosis

and carnitine insufficiency. *Arch. Neurol.* 47:1131–1133, 1990.

7. Spagnoli, A., Lucca, U., Menasce, G., et al. Long-term acetylcarnitine treatment in Alzheimer's disease. *Neurology* 41:1726–1732, 1991.

8. McIlwain, H., and Bachelard, H. S. Nutritional factors and the central nervous system. In *Biochemistry and the Central Nervous System*, 5th ed. London: Churchill Livingstone, 1985, pp. 244–281.

9. Blass, J. P., and Gibson, G. E. Deleterious aberrations of a thiamine-requiring enzyme in four patients with Wernicke-Korsakoff syndrome. *N. Engl. J. Med.* 297:1367–1370, 1977.

10. Calingasan, N., Baker, H., Sheu, K. F. R., Gandy, S. E., and Gibson, G. E. Thiamine deficiency as a model of selective neurodegeneration with chronic oxidative deficits. In G. Fiskum (ed.), *Neurodegenerative Diseases.* New York: Plenum Press, 1995, pp. 193–201.

11. Gibson, G. E., and Blass, J. P. Oxidative metabolism and acetylcholine synthesis during acetylpyridine treatment. *Neurochem. Res.* 10:453–467, 1985.

12. Sharma, S. K., Bolster, B., and Dakshinamurti, K. Picrotoxin and pentylene tetrazole induced seizure activity in pyridoxine-deficient rats. *J. Neurol. Sci.* 121:1–9, 1994.

13. Bendich, A., and Cohen, M. Vitamin B_6 safety issues. *Ann. N.Y. Acad. Sci.* 585:321–330, 1990.

14. Lott, I. B., Coulombe, T., DiPaolo, R. V., Richardson, E. P., and Levy, H. L. Vitamin B_6-dependent seizures: Pathology and chemical findings in brain. *Neurology* 28:47–54, 1978.

15. Sokoloff, L., Lassen, N. A., McKhann, G. M., Tower, D. B., and Albers, W. Effects of pyridoxine withdrawal on cerebral circulation and metabolism in a pyridoxine-dependent child. *Nature* 173:751–753, 1959.

16. Rosenberg, L. E. Disorders of propionate and methylmalonate metabolism. In J. B. Stanbury, J. B. Wyngaarden, D. S. Fredrickson, J. L. Goldstein, and M. S. Brown (eds.), *The Metabolic Basis of Inherited Diseases,* 5th ed. New York: McGraw-Hill, 1976, pp. 474–497.

17. Lindenbaum, J., Healton, E. B., Savage, D. G., et al. Neuropsychiatric disorders caused by cobalamin deficiency in the absence of anemia or macrocytosis. *N. Engl. J. Med.* 318:1720–1728, 1988.

18. Erbe, R. W. Inborn errors of folate metabolism. *N. Engl. J. Med.* 293:807–812, 1975.

19. Bean, W. B., and Hodges, R. E. Pantothenic acid deficiency induced in human subjects. *Proc. Soc. Exp. Biol. Med.* 86:693–698, 1954.

20. Packer, L., Tritschler, H. J., and Wessel, K. Neuroprotection by the metabolic antioxidant α-lipoic acid. *Free Radic. Biol. Med.* 22:359–378, 1997.

21. MacEvilly, C. J., and Muller, D. P. Lipid peroxidation in neural tissues and fractions from vitamin E-deficient rats. *Free Radic. Biol. Med.* 20:639–648, 1996.

22. Ghosh, M. K., Chattopadhyay, D. J., and Chatterjee, I. B. Vitamin C prevents oxidative damage. *Free Radic. Res.* 25:173–179, 1996.

23. Ebadi, M., Murrin, L. C., and Pfeiffer, R. F. Hippocampal zinc thionein and pyridoxal phosphate modulate synaptic functions. *Ann. N.Y. Acad. Sci.* 585:189–201, 1990.

24. Golub, M. S., Keen, C. L., Gershwin, M. E., and Hendrick, A. G. Developmental zinc deficiency and behavior. *J. Nutr.* 125(Suppl. 8): 2263S–2271S, 1995.

25. Akil, M., and Brewer, G. J. Psychiatric and behavioral abnormalities in Wilson's disease. *Adv. Neurol.* 65:171–178, 1995.

26. Horn, N., Tonnesen, T., and Tumer, Z. Menkes disease: An X-linked neurological disorder of copper metabolism. *Brain Pathol.* 2:351–362, 1992.

27. Olivares, M., and Mauy, R. Copper as an essential nutrient. *Am. J. Clin. Nutr.* 63:791S–796S, 1996.

28. al-Deeb, S., al-Moutaery, K., Bruyn, G. W., and Tariq, M. Neuroprotective effect of selenium on iminodipropionitrile-induced toxicity. *J. Psychiatry Neurosci.* 20:189–192, 1995.

29. Bourre, J. M., Bonneil, M., Clement, M., et al. Function of dietary polyunsaturated fatty acids in the nervous system. *Prostaglandins Leuko. Essent. Fatty Acids* 48:5–15, 1993.

30. Matsuo, T., and Suzuki, M. Brain β-adrenergic receptor binding in rats with obesity induced by a beef tallow diet. *Metab. Clin. Exp.* 46:18–22, 1997.

31. Pharoah, P. O., and Connolly, K. J. Iodine and brain development. *Dev. Med. Child Neurol.* 37:744–748, 1995.

32. Innis, S. M. The 1993 Borden Award Lecture. Fatty acid requirements of the newborn. *Can. J. Physiol. Pharmacol.* 72:1483–1492, 1994.

33. Diaz-Cintra, S., Garcia-Ruiz, M., Corkidi, G., and Cintra, L. Effects of prenatal malnutrition and postnatal nutritional rehabilitation on CA3 hippocampal pyramidal cells in rats of four ages. *Brain Res.* 662:117–126, 1994.

34. Freeman, G. B., Nielsen, P. N., and Gibson, G. E. Effect of age on behavioral and enzymatic changes during thiamin deficiency. *Neurobiol. Aging* 8:429–434, 1987.

35. Dubey, A., Forster, M. J., Lal, H., and Sohal, R. S. Effect of age and caloric intake on protein oxidation in different brain regions and on behavioral functions of the mouse. *Arch. Biochem. Biophys.* 333:189–197, 1996.

36. Sano, M., Ernesto, C., Thomas, R. G., et al. A controlled trial of selegiline, α-tocopherol, or both as treatment for Alzheimer's disease. The Alzheimer's Disease Cooperative Study. *N. Engl. J. Med.* 336:1216–1222, 1997.

37. Ebadi, M., Iversen, P. L., Hao, R., et al. Expression and regulation of brain metallothionein. *Neurochem. Int.* 27:1–22, 1995.

38. Clarke, S. D., and Abraham, S. Gene expression: Nutrient control of pre- and posttranscriptional events. *FASEB J.* 6:3146–3152, 1992.

39. Foreman, P. J., Perez-Polo, J. R., Angelucci, L., Ramacci, M. T., and Taglialatela, G. Effects of acetyl-L-carnitine treatment and stress exposure on the nerve growth factor receptor (p75NGFR) mRNA level in the central nervous system of aged rats. *Prog. Neuropsychopharmacol. Biol. Psychiatry* 19:117–133, 1995.

40. Wang, Q., Bing, C., Al-Barazanji, K., et al. Interactions between leptin and hypothalamic neuropeptide Y neurons in the control of food intake and energy homeostasis in the rat. *Diabetes* 46:335–341, 1997.

34

Hypoxic-Ischemic Brain Injury and Oxidative Stress

Laura L. Dugan and Dennis W. Choi

Basic Neurochemistry: Molecular, Cellular and Medical Aspects, 6th Ed., edited by G. J. Siegel et al. Published by Lippincott–Raven Publishers, Philadelphia, 1999. Correspondence to Laura L. Dugan, Washington University, Department of Neurology, 660 South Euclid Avenue, St. Louis, Missouri 63110.

HYPOXIA-ISCHEMIA AND BRAIN INFARCTION

Hypoxic-ischemic brain injury continues to be the third leading cause of death in the United States, affecting over half a million new victims each year. Of these, nearly one-third will die and another third will be left with severe and permanent disability. Unlike ischemic injury to many other tissues, the severity of disability is not predicted well by the amount of brain tissue lost. For example, damage to a small area in the medial temporal lobe may lead to severe disability, such as loss of speech, while damage to a greater volume elsewhere has little effect on function. The degree of disability does not simply reflect the severity or distribution of impaired blood supply. Populations of cells lying side by side in the brain can display dramatically different vulnerabilities to equivalent degrees of ischemia. Although a great deal has been learned about how nervous system anatomy, physiology and biochemistry interact to modify hypoxic-ischemic brain injury, much remains to be learned about what features contribute to the special vulnerability of the brain to stroke and of specific cell populations to hypoxic-ischemic injury during stroke.

Energy failure, an early consequence of hypoxia-ischemia, causes disruption of ionic homeostasis and accumulation of extracellular neurotransmitters

As discussed in Chapter 31, normal energy metabolism in the brain has several unusual features, including a high metabolic rate, limited intrinsic energy stores and critical dependence on aerobic metabolism of glucose. Reflecting this special metabolic status, as well as the existence of several unique injury mechanisms discussed below, the brain exhibits higher vulnerability to ischemic injury than most other tissues. Ischemic brain injury occurs in several clinical settings. The most common is *stroke,* focal disruption of blood supply to a part of the brain. Other settings include transient impairment of blood flow to the entire brain, *global ischemia,* as occurs during cardiac arrest.

When brain hypoxia or ischemia occurs, tissue energy demands cannot be met, so ATP levels fall. Loss of ATP results in decreased function of active ion pumps, such as the Na,K-ATPase, the most important transporter for maintaining high intracellular concentrations of K^+ ($\sim$155 mM) and low intracellular concentrations of Na^+ ($\sim$12 mM) (see Chap. 5). Loss of ion pump function allows rundown of transmembrane ion gradients (Fig. 34-1), leading to membrane depolarization, the opening of voltage-sensitive ion channels and a cascade of subsequent events, which, if sustained, lead ultimately to cell death. Depending on the circumstances, this death may be restricted to selectively vulnerable neuronal populations or may involve all cells, termed tissue infarction.

Within seconds of an ischemic insult, normal brain electrical activity ceases due to the activation of membrane K^+ channels and widespread neuronal hyperpolarization [1]. The hyperpolarization may be due to opening of K^+ channels responding to acute changes in local concentrations of ATP, H^+ or Ca^{2+}, or it may reflect altered nonheme metalloprotein association with and regulation of specific K^+ channels [2]. This response, presumably protective, however fails to preserve high-energy phosphate levels in tissue as concentrations of phosphocreatine (PCr) and ATP fall within minutes after ischemia onset [3]. The fall in pO_2 during ischemia leads to enhanced lactic acid production

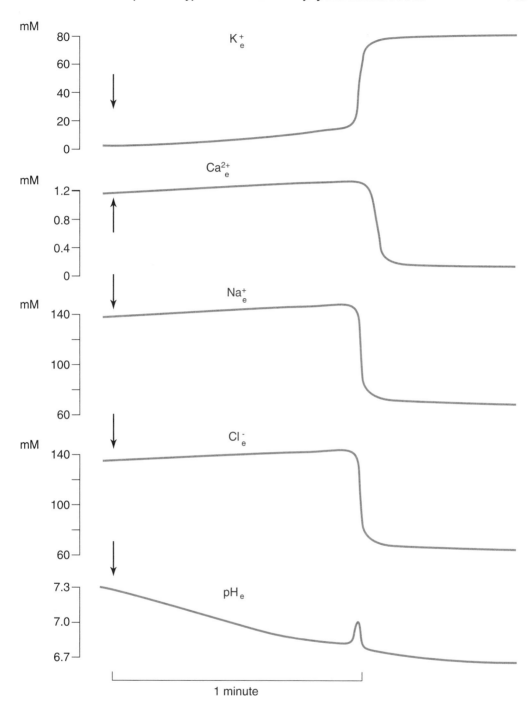

FIGURE 34-1.   Changes in extracellular ion concentrations following ischemia. Extracellular pH begins to decrease immediately after the onset of ischemia. This change is accompanied by slight increases in the extracellular concentrations of K^+, Cl^- and Na^+. After about 1 min of ischemia, a dramatic shift of ions occurs, with K^+ leaving cells and Ca^{2+}, Cl^- and Na^+ leaving the extracellular space. (From [1], with permission.)

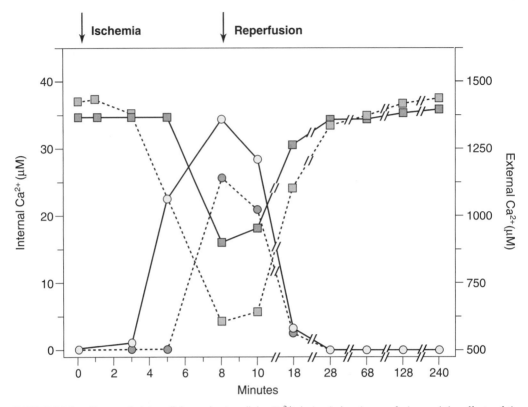

FIGURE 34-2. Changes in intracellular and extracellular Ca^{2+} during ischemia-reperfusion and the effects of the *N*-methyl-D-aspartate receptor antagonist MK-801. Intracellular Ca^{2+}, *circles;* extracellular Ca^{2+}, *squares;* with MK-801, *dark orange;* without MK-801, *light orange or gray.* (From Silver and Erecinska, in [3].)

as cells undergo a Pasteur shift from a dependence on aerobic metabolism to a dependence on glycolysis. The resulting lactic acidosis decreases the pH of the ischemic tissue from the normal 7.3 to intra-ischemic values ranging from 6.8 to 6.2, depending, in part, on the preischemic quantities of glucose available for conversion to lactic acid. In addition, efflux of K^+ from depolarizing neurons results in prolonged elevations in extracellular $[K^+]$ (Fig. 34-1) and massive cellular depolarization, a state known as *spreading depression,* which can propagate in brain tissue. Rapid inactivation of O_2-sensitive K^+ channels by decreased pO_2 may represent one mechanism whereby neurons put a brake on this ongoing K^+ efflux [2]. Other cellular ion gradients are also lost; thus, intracellular Na^+ and Ca^{2+} rise (Fig. 34-2) and intracellular Mg^{2+} falls.

Extracellular concentrations of many neurotransmitters are increased during hypoxia-ischemia. Depolarization-induced entry of Ca^{2+} via voltage-sensitive Ca^{2+} channels stimulates release of vesicular neurotransmitter pools, including the excitatory amino acid neurotransmitter glutamate. At the same time, Na^+-dependent uptake of certain neurotransmitters, including glutamate, is impaired (Chap. 5). High-capacity uptake of glutamate by the glutamate transporter couples the uptake of one glutamate and two Na^+ with the export of one K^+ and one HCO_3^- (or OH^-) (see Fig. 15-7). When the cellular ion gradients are discharged, the driving force for glutamate uptake is lost. In addition, glutamate uptake by the widely expressed astrocyte high-affinity glutamate transporter GLT-1, or excitatory amino acid transporter-2 (EAAT2), and the neuronal transporter, or EAAT3, can be downregulated by free radical-mediated oxidation of a redox site on the transporter [4]. Furthermore, since the transporter is electrogenic, that is, normally transferring a positive charge inward, membrane depolarization can lead to reversal of the transporter, producing glutamate efflux [5]. Thus, both impaired glutamate uptake and enhanced glutamate release contribute to sustained elevations of extracellular glutamate in the ischemic brain. Microdialysis of ischemic rat brain has detected an increase from the resting extracellular glutamate concentrations of 1 to 2 μM up to concentrations in the high micromolar or even low millimolar range.

Focal and global ischemia produce different distributions of injury

Ischemic injury to the brain can result from several different processes. Focal ischemia, which accounts for a majority of strokes, occurs when an artery supplying a region of the brain is occluded, either by an embolus, which is generally material broken off from a plaque in a large artery or a thrombus in the heart, or by a thrombus or platelet plug which forms directly in the affected artery (Fig. 34-3A–C). While focal ischemic insults generally reflect the distribution of vascular supply to a region, the area of infarction is typically less than the entire distribution of the occluded artery due to the presence of collateral circulation at the borders of the region supplied by the occluded vessel. The ultimate area of infarction will depend on the duration and degree of vascular occlusion and the availability of collateral blood supply [6]. The region of the brain supplied uniquely by the occluded artery develops the most severe injury, termed the *ischemic core,* while the rim of tissue surrounding the core, termed the *penumbra,* which has the benefit of some maintained blood flow supplied by collateral circulation, sustains less severe injury. Focal ischemia may also accompany other acute brain insults, such as intracerebral hemorrhage or trauma.

Reversible global ischemia, such as occurs during cardiac arrest and resuscitation, reflects a transient loss of blood flow to the entire brain and generally results in the death of certain selectively vulnerable neuronal populations. Hypoxia accompanies ischemic insults but may also occur without loss of blood flow, for example, during near drowning or carbon monoxide poisoning.

Hypoglycemia produces brain injury that has several features in common with ischemic injury. Neurons are more susceptible than glial cells to ischemia, hypoxia or hypoglycemia; and the phylogenetically newer regions of the brain, including the cortex and cerebellum, are affected to a greater extent than the brainstem [6].

"Selective vulnerability" of certain neurons is not explained by vascular distribution

As recognized by Vogt and Vogt (see in [6]), the juxtaposition of relatively vulnerable and relatively resistant neuronal populations within a single vascular distribution suggests that intrinsic tissue factors contribute heavily to ischemic neuronal vulnerability. For example, pyramidal neurons in the CA1 subfield of the hippocampus die after 5 to 10 min of global ischemia, while neurons in the nearby CA3 region are preserved. Populations of neurons that are selectively vulnerable to ischemia include cortical pyramidal neurons, cerebellar Purkinje cells, hippocampal CA1 pyramidal neurons and subpopulations in the amygdala, striatum, thalamus and brainstem nuclei (Fig. 34-4). Some of the mechanisms that may contribute to selective vulnerability of certain cell populations to ischemic injury are discussed further below.

MICROVASCULAR INJURY IN HYPOXIA-ISCHEMIA

Hypoxia-ischemia disrupts the blood–brain barrier and damages endothelial cells

Damage to the blood–brain barrier (BBB), which occurs gradually following ischemia-reperfusion, reflects the vulnerability of the cellular components of the BBB to damage, both directly by the ischemic insult itself and indirectly as a consequence of brain parenchymal responses. Damage to microvascular endothelial cells can lead to vasospasm and promote adhesion of platelets and leukocytes, leading to vessel plugging. Maneuvers which limit the postischemic recruitment of inflammatory cells to the

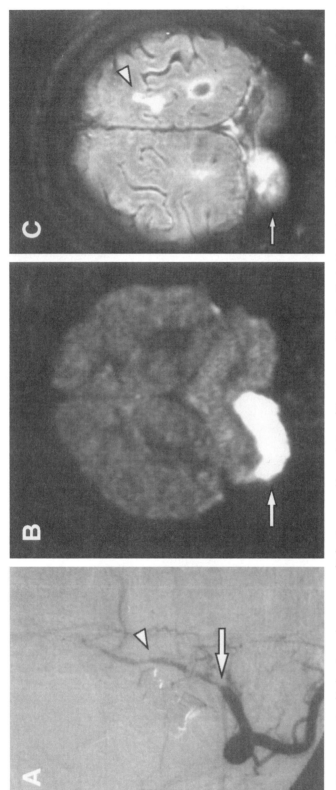

FIGURE 34-3. Focal ischemia produces a core of infarction caused by occlusion of the vessel supplying the affected brain tissue. A 53-year-old man presented with imbalance, various cranial neuropathies and hiccups. **A:** Angiography revealed high-grade stenosis and clot in his right vertebral artery *(arrow)* and nonfilling *(arrowhead)* of his posterior inferior cerebellar artery *(PICA).* **B:** Diffusion-weighted magnetic resonance *(MR)* study demonstrates infarction and edema in the right inferior cerebellum *(arrow),* in the distribution of the occluded PICA. **C:** Fluid-attenuated inversion recovery *(FLAIR)* MR image: in addition to the cerebellar infarct *(arrow),* a small infarct in the left occipital lobe *(arrowhead)* was found, likely resulting from an embolus into the left posterior cerebral artery from plaques in the vertebral artery. (Images kindly provided by Dr. DeWitte Cross, Mallinckrodt Institute of Radiology, Washington University School of Medicine.)

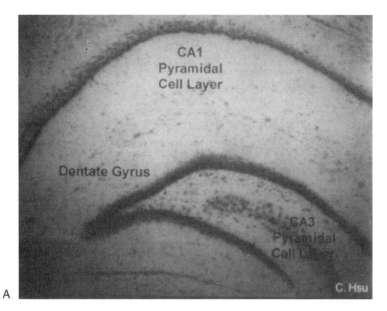

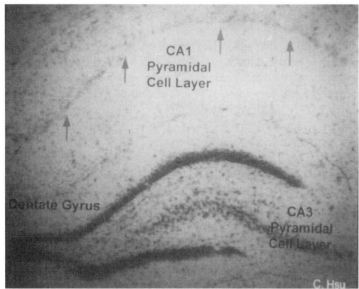

FIGURE 34-4.   Rat hippocampus showing neuronal populations that are selectively vulnerable to ischemic damage. **A:** control; **B:** ischemia. A brief period of global ischemia causes nearly complete loss of neurons in the CA1 region *(arrows)* of the hippocampus, while neurons in the nearby CA3 region are almost completely spared. (Images kindly provided by Dr. Chung Y. Hsu, Washington University School of Medicine.)

ischemic zone and the subsequent inflammatory response can protect the integrity of the BBB and improve postischemic cerebral blood flow [3]. Transgenic mice which do not express intercellular adhesion molecule-1 (ICAM-1), a protein which is important in promoting adhesion of leukocytes to endothelial cells (see Chap. 7), are less vulnerable to ischemic injury than littermate controls and have improved cerebral blood flow. Besides increased ischemia, another consequence of damage to the endothelial cells or astrocytes that comprise the BBB may be the entry of components of the vascular compartment, such as cytokines and inflammatory cells, to the brain parenchyma. Agents which protect endothelial cells, such as antioxidants, can help preserve BBB integrity following ischemia-reperfusion [7].

The response of nonvascular or parenchymal cells to the ischemic insult also affects BBB function. For example, *N*-methyl-D-aspartate (NMDA) receptor antagonists, which reduce neuronal death and tissue infarction after focal ischemia (see below), decrease BBB disruption, possibly by blocking neuronal production of reactive oxygen species (ROS) triggered by NMDA receptor activation, thus reducing their deleterious effects on endothelial or astrocyte cell function. The function of the BBB and the role of inflammation in BBB breakdown are discussed further in Chapters 32 and 35, respectively.

Edema may lead to secondary ischemia, which can produce further brain damage

Due to the breakdown of the BBB after ischemia, the tissue content of water in the affected area of the brain may increase, leading to swelling or edema of the ischemic region. Some of the increased tissue water is intracellular, reflecting impaired cellular ion homeostasis due to energy failure, as well as the action of glutamate, which triggers excess cation influx in neurons and glia (Chap. 15). Some of the increased tissue water is extracellular due to breakdown of the BBB, followed by leakage of solute and water from the intravascular space. Tissue swelling in the rigid intracranial cavity can restrict blood flow, thus causing secondary ischemia. If edema is substan-

tial, uncal or central brain herniation may result, leading to respiratory arrest and death.

EXCITOTOXIC INJURY IN HYPOXIA-ISCHEMIA

NMDA and AMPA/kainate receptors contribute to excitotoxic neuronal degeneration

Excitotoxicity (toxic glutamate receptor activation) is a key mediator of central neuronal loss consequent to hypoxic-ischemic insults [8]. While brain gray matter contains glutamate concentrations in the average range of 10 mM, much of which is stored in synaptic vesicles for release as a neurotransmitter, the extracellular concentration of glutamate is normally maintained in the range of ~1 μM by Na$^+$ flux-coupled transport (see Chap. 5). During hypoxia-ischemia, as cellular energy reserves and Na$^+$ gradients fall, increased release and impaired uptake of glutamate mediate a toxic buildup of extracellular glutamate, leading to overstimulation of glutamate receptors and consequent neuronal cell death. Excitotoxicity can be exacerbated by decreased cellular energy stores.

In vitro studies on excitotoxicity suggest that while both NMDA and α-amino-3-hydroxy-5-methyl-4-isoxazole propionic acid (AMPA)/kainate (KA) receptors can mediate excitotoxicity (see Chap. 15), these classes of glutamate receptors do not do so equally. Experiments with cortical or hippocampal cell cultures suggest that much of the neuronal death associated with brief, intense glutamate exposure is mediated by NMDA receptor activation, probably because this can induce lethal amounts of Ca^{2+} influx more rapidly than can AMPA/KA receptor stimulation. However, overactivation of AMPA or KA receptors can also lead to intracellular Ca^{2+} overload and neurodegeneration. This may be especially true under conditions where NMDA-receptor activity is reduced by extracellular acidity or a buildup of extracellular Zn^{2+} [9]. It is also true with respect to specific neuronal subpopulations that express AMPA-sensitive Ca^{2+} channels (see Chap. 15). G protein-linked metabotropic glutamate receptors (mGluRs) appear not to mediate excitotoxicity directly but, rather, to modify excitotoxicity either upward or downward.

Excitotoxicity leads to increased Ca^{2+} influx, which can activate cytotoxic intracellular pathways

The prolonged availability of extracellular glutamate during hypoxia-ischemia is transduced by neuronal membrane receptors into potentially lethal intracellular ionic derangements, in particular, intracellular Na^+ and Ca^{2+} overload. Excitotoxic neuronal cell death, which tends to occur by necrosis, correlates well with measures of total Ca^{2+} influx, and removal of extracellular Ca^{2+} attenuates glutamate-induced neuronal death.

Sustained elevations in intracellular Ca^{2+} can initiate "toxic cascades," which are capable of ultimately killing the cell (Fig. 34-5). These

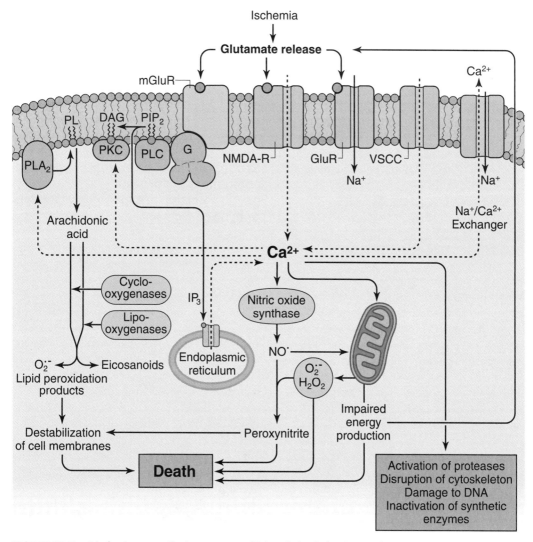

FIGURE 34-5. Mechanisms contributing to neuronal injury during ischemia-reperfusion. Simplified diagram showing several pathways believed to contribute to excitotoxic neuronal injury in ischemia. *mGluR*, metabotropic glutamate receptor; *NMDA-R*, N-methyl-D-aspartate receptor; *GluR*, AMPA/Kainate type of glutamate receptors; *PL*, phospholipids; *PLA₂*, phospholipase A₂; *DAG*, diacylglycerol; *PLC*, phospholipase C; *PKC*, protein kinase C; *G*, G protein; *PIP₂*, phosphatidylinositol 4,5-bisphosphate; *IP₃*, inositol 1,4,5-trisphosphate; *NO•*, nitric oxide; $O_2^{•-}$, superoxide radical; *H₂O₂*, hydrogen peroxide; *VSCC*, voltage-sensitive Ca^{2+} channel.

cascades include activation of catabolic enzymes, such as proteases, phospholipases and endonucleases [10]. Elevated concentrations of intracellular Ca^{2+} can further lead to initiation of protein-kinase (Chap. 24) and lipid-kinase (Chap. 21) cascades, impairment of metabolism and generation of ROS. While many of these events occur early and can result in rapid cell death, others, such as energy compromise and ROS formation, may initiate more delayed death processes, discussed in more detail in the next section. In addition, most of these Ca^{2+}-dependent events may be common to both NMDA and AMPA/KA receptor-mediated excitotoxicity.

Ca^{2+}-dependent activation of the cysteine protease calpain occurs early in ischemia and may lead to disruption of the cytoskeleton in ischemia-reperfusion [3]. Endonuclease activation can be triggered by influx of large amounts of Ca^{2+}, which may lead to DNA breakdown during hypoxia-ischemia [11]. Increased intracellular Ca^{2+} also activates a variety of protein kinases. In particular, Ca^{2+}/calmodulin kinase (CaMK) and the classical Ca^{2+}-dependent isoforms of protein kinase C (PKC) can modify the function of many ion channels, including NMDA and AMPA/KA receptor-gated channels and voltage-gated Ca^{2+} channels [12].

An especially important deleterious consequence of Ca^{2+} overload following excitotoxic glutamate receptor activation is formation of ROS. Free radical production is linked to elevated $[Ca^{2+}]_i$ in several ways: (i) Ca^{2+}-dependent activation of phospholipase A_2, with liberation of arachidonic acid and further metabolism, leading to "by-product" free radical production and lipid peroxidation (Chaps. 3 and 35); (ii) stimulation of NMDA receptors, leading to activation of nitric oxide synthase (NOS) and the release of nitric oxide (NO), which can then interact with ROS from other sources to generate highly reactive peroxynitrite [13]; and (iii) uncoupling of mitochondrial electron transport, enhancing mitochondrial production of free radicals [14].

Activation of NMDA receptors triggers Ca^{2+}-dependent production of ROS from the mitochondrial electron-transport chain. In cell cultures, ROS production is stimulated by concentrations of NMDA which are not neurotoxic,

and in awake rats, NMDA receptors are responsible for a low baseline production of ROS, suggesting that even "physiological" NMDA receptor activity may trigger production of ROS. However, cell culture studies suggest that substantially greater amounts of mitochondrial ROS are generated when NMDA receptors are overstimulated sufficiently to produce excitotoxicity. Since AMPA/KA receptor activation, possibly in conjunction with the group 1 metabotropic glutamate receptors (see Chap. 15), may also elicit enhanced mitochondrial ROS production, it is likely that excitotoxicity may be an important trigger for mitochondrial free radical production in ischemia-reperfusion injury. Supporting the idea that free radicals are important downstream mediators of excitotoxicity, treatment with free radical scavengers can attenuate NMDA or AMPA receptor-mediated neuronal death.

Excitatory amino acid-receptor antagonists can provide neuroprotection in experimental models of hypoxia-ischemia

Supporting the glutamate hypothesis of hypoxic-ischemic brain damage, substantial evidence indicates that antagonists of ion channel-linked glutamate receptors can reduce infarct volume in animal models of focal brain ischemia. This is true both for NMDA antagonists and for AMPA/KA antagonists [8]. The magnitude of infarct reduction is model-dependent but is typically on the order of 25 to 30%, and the reduction can exceed 50%.

An additional injury mechanism, ischemic apoptosis (discussed below), may evolve in parallel with excitotoxic necrosis, but apoptosis has little chance to be manifested under circumstances in which fulminant excitotoxicity predominates. Evidence favoring the concurrence of apoptosis and necrosis can be found in the observation that the application of an NMDA antagonist drug together with a drug designed to inhibit apoptosis leads to greater neuroprotection than does either drug treatment alone. Each agent alone, administered at optimal doses systemically just after the ischemic insult, reduces infarction by about half, but combination therapy reduces infarct volume by ~80%.

Zn²⁺ AND HYPOXIA-ISCHEMIA

New evidence suggests that the ubiquitous metal ion Zn^{2+} may contribute to neuronal injury during cerebral ischemia-hypoxia. Zn^{2+} is necessary for the proper function of many metalloenzymes and transcription factors (see Chaps. 26 and 33). In the nervous system, Zn^{2+} appears to serve an additional function as a mediator of central neural signaling [9]. Low concentrations of Zn^{2+} can modify the function of Na^+, K^+ and Ca^{2+} channels as well as certain subtypes of $GABA_A$ receptors, and Zn^{2+} strongly attenuates activation of the NMDA subclass of glutamate receptors. Free Zn^{2+} is present in synaptic vesicles within excitatory boutons throughout the brain, and the neuropil of the hippocampus and neocortex is especially rich in releasable pools of Zn^{2+}. Neuronal firing causes a Ca^{2+}-dependent release of Zn^{2+}; with intense neuronal activity, it has been estimated that Zn^{2+} concentrations of several hundred micromolar could be achieved in synaptic clefts.

A pathogenic role for Zn^{2+} in ischemic brain damage has been suggested, based on the following observations: presynaptic Zn^{2+} translocates into selectively vulnerable hippocampal hilar neurons, which degenerate after transient forebrain ischemia, and into limbic or cortical neurons, which degenerate after seizures induced by KA or perforant path stimulation; and chelation of extracellular Zn^{2+} by Ca^{2+}-EDTA reduces selective neuronal death in multiple regions of rat brain in an experimental model of transient global ischemia [15].

ISCHEMIC APOPTOSIS

Hypoxia-ischemia may initiate apoptosis in parallel with necrosis

In 1972, Wyllie and co-worker (see [15a]) described two distinct patterns of cell death. One form, apoptosis, progressed through a set of morphological changes characterized by condensation and margination of large nuclear chromatin aggregates and extrusion of membrane-bound cytoplasmic and nuclear material, termed apoptotic bodies, with progressive loss of cell volume. Since these features were prominent in cells dying by programmed cell death during normal development, the concept emerged that apoptosis reflects the execution of a death "program," in many cases requiring new protein synthesis. The mechanisms underlying apoptosis [16] are outlined in more detail in Chapters 23 and 27.

As discussed above, growing evidence has implicated not only excitotoxicity, but also apoptosis as important processes leading to brain cell death after hypoxic-ischemic insults. Inhibitors of macromolecular synthesis and of caspase activity can limit apoptotic death of neurons exposed to hypoxia-ischemia [17]. In addition, transgenic mice overexpressing the antiapoptotic gene *bcl-2* have smaller infarcts than their littermates after hypoxia-ischemia.

Triggers of ischemic apoptosis may include decreased supply of or reduced sensitivity to neurotrophins, development of oxidative stress and exposure to inflammatory cytokines

One factor that may promote apoptosis after ischemic insults is deprivation of growth factor support. Deprivation may result from damage to neuronal or glial targets responsible for providing growth factor support. However, tissue concentrations of several growth factors increase in the brain following hypoxic-ischemic insults, suggesting that there may be either decreased sensitivity of neurons to neurotrophins after ischemia or increased concentrations of neurotrophins are required to counter proapoptotic stimuli, such as free-radical exposure. Addition of exogenous growth factors, such as nerve growth factor (NGF) or basic fibroblast growth factor (bFGF) (see Chap. 19) [18], can reduce hypoxic-ischemic damage. However, while neurotrophins may attenuate ischemic apoptosis, they may, in contrast, have deleterious effects by enhancing the excitotoxic necrosis induced by ischemia.

In addition, oxidative stress may trigger apoptosis following hypoxia-ischemia. Exposure of neurons to a free radical stress, either by application of H_2O_2, exposure to UV irradiation or depletion of antioxidant defenses, such as glutathione or superoxide dismutase (SOD; see below), may trigger apoptosis. Free radicals not only may serve as inducers of apoptotic cell death, they may also be a signal in the apoptotic cascade; neurons deprived of growth factors demonstrate an early increase in oxygen free radical formation and can be rescued from growth factor deprivation-induced apoptosis by application of antioxidants [19]. Thus, free radicals may serve as triggers, signals or effectors of neuronal apoptosis.

Persistent impairment of cellular energy metabolism after an ischemic insult may also play a role in triggering apoptotic neuronal degeneration. Studies in cell culture and animal models of stroke suggest that inhibition of mitochondrial function by mitochondrial toxins such as 3-nitropropionic acid or rotenone not only worsens excitotoxic injury but also can trigger apoptotic neuronal death. Prolonged deficits in mitochondrial function and energy metabolism have been observed after ischemia-reperfusion and may represent a trigger for apoptotic neurodegeneration after ischemia.

Increased expression and enhanced concentrations of inflammatory cytokines, such as interleukin-1β (IL-1β), tumor necrosis factor α (TNFα) and transforming growth factor β (TGFβ) (Chap. 35), are observed in brain following ischemia and may derive from inflammatory cells, such as macrophages or microglia, as well as neurons and glia. Because cytokines are capable of triggering apoptosis in many cell types, including neurons [20], increased concentrations of these molecules might be expected to trigger apoptotic cell death in vulnerable cells. Thus, ischemic apoptosis may be induced by free radicals, cytokines, metabolic insults and changes in growth factor sensitivity, which may result from excitotoxic damage to intracellular systems such as the cytoskeleton and axonal transport.

FREE RADICALS IN HYPOXIA-ISCHEMIA

The brain has a number of characteristics which make it especially susceptible to free radical-mediated injury. Brain lipids are highly enriched in polyunsaturated fatty acids (PUFA), and many regions of the brain, for example, the substantia nigra and the striatum, have high concentrations of iron. Both of these factors increase the susceptibility of brain cell membranes to lipid peroxidation (see also Chap. 45). Because the brain is critically dependent on aerobic metabolism, mitochondrial respiratory activity is higher than in many other tissues, increasing the risk of free radical "leak" from mitochondria; conversely, free radical damage to mitochondria in brain may be tolerated relatively poorly because of this dependence on aerobic metabolism.

Oxygen free radicals are required intermediates in many biological reactions but may damage macromolecules during oxidative stress

Free radicals are molecules which posses an outer electron orbital with a solitary unpaired electron; these include the hydrogen atom ($H^\bullet$); the diatomic oxygen molecule O_2, which possesses two unpaired electrons with the same spin in two separate orbitals; $NO^\bullet$; superoxide ($O_2^{\bullet-}$); hydroxyl radical ($^\bullet OH$); and transition metals, such as copper and iron. While O_2 qualifies as a radical by having two unpaired electrons, its reactivity with nonradical compounds is limited because the unpaired electrons in O_2 have the same spin state. The two electrons in a covalent bond have opposite spins, so in order for O_2 to react with a nonradical, one of the electrons must undergo "spin inversion" so that both are anti-spin to the electrons on O_2, an extremely slow process. O_2 does react readily with radicals, accepting one electron at a time to form the very reactive superoxide radical $O_2^{\bullet-}$, which has one unpaired electron [21].

Although some radical species may persist for prolonged periods, most are generally unstable and will attempt to donate their unpaired electron to a nearby molecule or to remove or "abstract" a second electron, usually in the form of a hydrogen atom, from a neighboring molecule to pair with their free electron. Free-radical reactions are intrinsic to a majority of the metabolic and synthetic reactions carried out by eukaryotic cells and, as such, are required for life. ATP production by the mitochondrial electron chain, for example, uses a controlled set of oxygen radical reactions to couple the reduction of free-radical electrons with the movement of protons across the mitochondrial membrane. Cytochrome oxidase, complex IV of the mitochondrial electron transport chain (Chap. 42), catalyzes transfer of these free electrons to molecular oxygen as the final acceptor with water as the end product.

The addition of oxygen to macromolecules, such as in the metabolism of arachidonic acid to the eicosanoids or the oxidation of small molecules by P450 enzymes, requires "activation" of molecular O_2 to permit transfer of atomic oxygen ($O^\bullet$) from O_2 to the biological compound. Most enzymes which catalyze biological radical reactions bind a metal ion (Fe, Cu, Co or the group VI element Se), which destabilizes the O_2 molecule. These reactions also involve cofactors such as flavin adenine dinucleotide (FAD) or flavin mononucleotide (FMN) to help stabilize the resulting oxygen atoms until the reaction is complete.

Although such reactions are generally very efficient, there is often some small amount of leak of ROS encompassing radicals such as $O_2^{\bullet-}$, its acid HO_2, hydroxyl radical ($^\bullet OH$) and $NO^\bullet$, as well as nonradicals such as hydrogen peroxide (H_2O_2), singlet oxygen ($^1O\Delta g$) and hypochlorous acid (HOCl). While H_2O_2 is not a free radical, it can be rapidly decomposed via the *Fenton reaction:*

$$Fe^{2+} + H_2O_2 \rightarrow Fe^{3+} + {}^\bullet OH + OH^-$$

In addition, superoxide, hydrogen peroxide and hydroxyl radicals can be interconverted via the so-called *Haber-Weiss reaction:*

$$\begin{array}{c} Fe^{3+} + O_2^{\bullet-} \leftrightarrow Fe^{2+} + O_2 \\ \underline{Fe^{2+} + H_2O_2 \rightarrow Fe^{3+} + {}^\bullet OH + OH^-} \\ O_2^{\bullet-} + H_2O_2 \rightarrow {}^\bullet OH + OH^- + O_2 \end{array}$$

Cuprous and cupric ions may substitute for ferrous and ferric ions in the Haber-Weiss reaction [21]. Peroxynitrite can be formed from the reaction of NO with superoxide:

$$NO^\bullet + O_2^{\bullet-} \rightarrow ONOO^- \rightarrow NO_2^{\bullet-} + {}^\bullet OH$$

Oxidative stress generally describes a condition in which cellular antioxidant defenses are inadequate to completely detoxify the free radicals being generated, due to excessive production of ROS, loss of antioxidant defenses or, typically, both [22]. This condition may occur locally, as antioxidant defenses may become overwhelmed at certain subcellular locations while remaining intact overall, and selectively with regard to radical species, as antioxidant defenses are radical-specific, for example, SOD for superoxide and catalase or glutathione peroxidase for H_2O_2.

A major consequence of oxidative stress is damage to cellular macromolecules. Addition of the free "radical" electron to a fatty acid causes fragmentation of the lipid or alteration of its chemical structure (Fig. 34-6). For example, the unconjugated *cis* double bonds in unsaturated fatty acids may be shifted to produce a conjugated *trans* double bond system (see Chap. 2). Peroxyl or hydroxyl groups may be added to the unsaturated fatty acid, or the fatty acid carbon chain may be cleaved during reaction with the free electron to generate a fatty aldehyde, both processes termed *lipid peroxidation*. Fatty aldehydes such as 4-hydroxynonenal can then react with free thiol groups such as cysteines on proteins to produce thioesters, which may affect protein function and stability [21]. Free-radical damage to proteins may cause cross-linking, carbonyl formation and protein denaturation. DNA bases may be modified by oxidation, resulting in single- and double-strand breaks or mispairing of purine and pyrimidine during DNA replication.

Reactive oxygen species generated during ischemia-reperfusion contribute to the injury

Evidence for free radical production and oxidative stress during ischemia-reperfusion comes from a variety of studies. While free radicals may be generated to a small extent during ischemia, far greater production of reactive oxygen intermediates occurs after reintroduction of oxygen during reperfusion. Early studies with animal models of ischemia-reperfusion injury showed decreased brain concentrations of antioxidants such as ascorbic acid, vitamin E and glutathione,

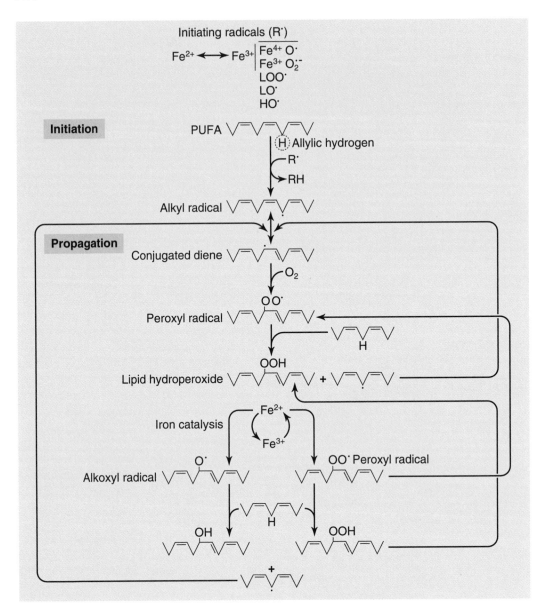

FIGURE 34-6. Lipid peroxidation leads to fragmentation or oxidation of polyunsaturated fatty acids (PUFA). *LOO•*, lipid peroxyl radical; *LO•*, lipid alkoxylradical; *HO•*, hydroxyl radical; *O₂•⁻*, superoxide radical; *O•*, atomic oxygen radical. (From Hall in [3].)

as well as production of aldehydic lipid peroxidation products, detected as thiobarbituric acid-reactive substances. Additional evidence for ROS generation has been obtained with intra-ischemic microdialysis with solutions containing salicylic acid or spin-trapping agents, which react with ROS to form relatively stable products that can be detected in the microdialysis solu-

tion. Oxidative damage to macromolecules has provided another index of ROS-mediated injury in ischemia-reperfusion. Lipid- and protein-oxidation products as well as DNA-oxidation products have been detected in brain tissue after ischemia-reperfusion.

Treatment with antioxidants, such as vitamin E; 21-aminosteroids; and spin-trapping agents, such as phenyl tert-butyl *N*-nitrone (PBN), can reduce ischemic brain infarction. In addition, transgenic mice which overexpress the cytosolic antioxidant enzyme CuZn-SOD (SOD1) (see below) [23] or the extracellular SOD3 [24] are resistant to ischemic brain injury compared to wild-type controls. Conversely, reduction of cellular antioxidant defenses can potentiate ischemic injury. Transgenic mice that are *sod1−/−* exhibit enhanced susceptibility to ischemic brain injury, even though they have a grossly normal CNS phenotype under unstressed conditions, for example, in the absence of ischemia or nerve transection. This suggests that other antioxidant defenses are adequate to handle physiological concentrations of cytosolic superoxide anion. In contrast, mice lacking the mitochondrial antioxidant enzyme Mn^{2+}-SOD (SOD2) die soon after birth [3]. This suggests that extracellular SOD3 or other antioxidant systems may be able to compensate partially for loss of cytosolic, but not mitochondrial, SOD activity.

Mitochondria, nitric oxide synthase and arachidonic acid metabolism are sources of reactive oxygen species during ischemia-reperfusion injury

ROS generation during ischemia-reperfusion may come from several sources, including NOS activity, mitochondrial electron transport, multiple steps in the metabolism of arachidonic acid and, in some species, xanthine oxidase, which is produced by hydrolysis of xanthine dehydrogenase. In addition, the decreased intracellular pH accompanying ischemia may alter the binding of transition metals such as iron, increasing their participation in the Haber-Weiss reaction [21]. P450 enzymes and NAD(P)H oxidase are two additional potential sources of oxygen radicals whose contribution to enhanced radical production during CNS ischemia has not been systematically explored.

Mitochondria were among the earliest sites of cellular ROS production to be identified. Studies on isolated mitochondria have suggested that as much as 3% of oxygen utilization by resting mitochondria may be lost as leak of ROS, although this estimate may be high. Mitochondrial production of ROS can be enhanced by increased electron-transport activity, as well as by disturbances in electron transfer down the transport chain [25]. The lipid electron-transport molecule ubiquinone (Q_9, Q_{10}) is the major site of free radical leak from mitochondria via the ubiquinone cycle. Ubiquinone undergoes a two-electron reduction, first to a semiquinone and then to a diol, at mitochondrial complex I (NADH dehydrogenase, NADH:ubiquinone oxidoreductase) or complex II (succinate dehydrogenase) and subsequently delivers the two electrons to the iron–sulfur center of complex III (cytochrome bc_1 in mammalian mitochondria). Inhibition of either complex I or complex III will impair the efficiency of electron transfer and may allow a free semiquinone to be produced. The semiquinone can then interact with O_2 to generate $O_2^{\bullet-}$ (Fig. 34-7). Elevated intracellular Ca^{2+}, exposure to fatty acids or other molecules which alter the physical properties of the mitochondrial membrane and inhibition of mitochondrial respiratory components may enhance this leak of ROS from mitochondria.

Mitochondria appear to be an important and, perhaps, even dominant source of free radicals in brain tissue subjected to ischemia-reperfusion. Microdialysis studies using salicylate to detect ROS release from ischemic brain cortex show that mitochondrial inhibitors such as rotenone eliminate ROS production during ischemia-reperfusion. Elevated concentrations of intracellular Ca^{2+} and Na^+, a consequence of energy failure and excitotoxic glutamate receptor stimulation, can be expected to inhibit complex I as well as overproduction of superoxide anion. The resultant oxidative stress may lead to further inhibition of mitochondrial respiratory components, promoting further free radical production in a vicious, feed-forward cycle.

Nitric oxide and peroxynitrite contribute to oxidative damage

NOS has been identified as another source of ROS with special relevance to pathological conditions. NOS is homologous to P450 cytochrome *c* reductase; cofactors in the reaction are FMN, FAD, tetrahydrobiopterin and NAD(P)H (Fig. 34-7). NOS normally converts arginine and molecular oxygen to citrulline and

Sources of Oxygen Radicals

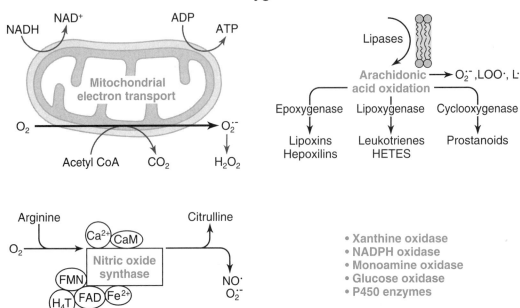

FIGURE 34-7. Sources of free radical formation which may contribute to injury during ischemia-reperfusion. Nitric oxide synthase, the mitochondrial electron-transport chain and metabolism of arachidonic acid are among the likely contributors, *LOO•*, lipid peroxyl radical; *L•*, lipid alkoxyl radical; *HETES*, hydroxyeicosatetraenoic acids; *H_4T*, tetrahydrobiopterin; *$O_2^{•-}$*, superoxide radical; *CaM*, calcium/calmodulin; *NO•*, nitric oxide; *FAD*, flavin adenine dinucleotide; *FMN*, flavin mononucleotide.

NO•, a free radical gas; this process is itself leaky and associated with free radical generation [13]. NO•, originally identified as endothelial-derived relaxing factor (EDRF), is a potent vasodilator. NO• also binds to guanylyl cyclase to increase GTP production and can nitrosylate the small G protein Ras on a specific cysteine to cause constitutive activation. Three family members have been identified: Ca^{2+}/calmodulin-activated brain NOS (nNOS), endothelial NOS (eNOS) and inducible NOS (iNOS). High concentrations of nNOS are found in a subpopulation of neurons previously identified as NAD(P)H-diaphorase cells.

NO•, which has limited radical reactivity, can combine readily with $O_2^{•-}$ and possibly H_2O_2 to produce a highly oxidizing, nonradical compound, peroxynitrite [13]. When protonated, peroxynitrite has reactivity similar to that of •OH. Cell culture studies suggest that while NO• itself is relatively nontoxic, peroxynitrite is quite neurotoxic. Peroxynitrite reacts with pro-

tein tyrosine residues to produce nitrotyrosine. Potential targets of tyrosine nitrosylation include many important cellular proteins, including Cu,Zn-SOD, aconitase, Mn-SOD and cytochrome oxidase (mitochondrial complex IV), all of which are inactivated by nitrosylation. Peroxynitrite may cause lipid peroxidation but may also generate nitrosolipids, which decrease lipid peroxidation by acting as peroxidation "chain-breakers." In addition, peroxynitrite targets DNA, leading to chain breaks and DNA base oxidation. Involvement of nNOS as a mediator of ischemic injury is suggested by the ability of nNOS inhibitors to reduce ischemic injury and by the neuroprotective effect of nNOS gene deletion in knockout mice.

Peroxynitrite-mediated DNA damage can activate poly(ADP-ribose) polymerase (PARP or PARS), an enzyme involved in DNA repair. It has been suggested that activation of PARP, which catalyzes extensive hydrolysis of ATP to produce polyADP ribosylation of damaged

DNA, contributes to ischemic injury by hastening energy depletion. Pharmacological studies *in vitro* and experiments with PARP knockout mice have suggested that inhibition of PARP provides substantial neuroprotection against ischemic neuronal injury.

Production of eicosanoids from polyunsaturated fatty acids such as arachidonic acid may generate reactive oxygen species

Arachidonic acid metabolism may also be a source of ROS production [26,27]. As discussed in Chapters 3 and 35, arachidonic acid undergoes an extensive array of reactions to biologically active lipids, the eicosanoids. These reactions may be accompanied by free-radical production. In particular, cyclooxygenase isoforms and 5-lipoxygenase contain heme iron and may generate a low concentration of superoxide anion constitutively. 12-Lipoxygenases, which possess nonheme iron, may not release superoxide anion but may induce lipid peroxidation after translocation to membranes.

The role of xanthine oxidase in human stroke is unclear

In rodent models of ischemia, xanthine oxidase inhibitors, such as allopurinol or oxypurinol, decrease ROS formation; but since these drugs also can serve as hydroxyl radical scavengers, it has been difficult to determine which of these effects is responsible for neuroprotection. Analyses of human tissues have shown high concentrations of xanthine dehydrogenase in liver and intestine but neither xanthine dehydrogenase nor xanthine oxidase in brain parenchyma and little in cerebral endothelial cells.

Brain antioxidant defenses modify ischemia-reperfusion injury

The high metabolic rate of brain cells implies a high baseline ROS production, and brain cells possess high concentrations of both enzymatic and small molecule antioxidant defenses. SOD1 may represent as much as 1% of total protein in brain; it converts $O_2^{\bullet-}$ to H_2O_2, which is then further metabolized to water and oxygen by catalase and glutathione peroxidase. The *SOD1* gene is located on chromosome 21 and codes for a 16- to 18-kDa subunit, which binds one Cu^{2+} and one Zn^{2+}; the active enzyme is a homodimer. SOD2 is a homotetramer and the gene is on chromosome 6. An extracellular, glycosylated form, SOD3, has been shown in rodents to overlap in activity with SOD1. Several other enzymes unrelated to CuZn-SOD, for example, the *atx1-HAH* gene product, are also capable of acting as SODs. It remains to be determined to what extent SOD3 and these alternative dismutases complement SOD1 and SOD2 as antioxidant systems in humans.

Catalase and glutathione peroxidase provide two important cellular systems for eliminating H_2O_2. Catalase, a 56-kDa cytosolic hemeprotein homotetramer that can act without a cofactor, although it may bind NAD(P)H, functions as a peroxidase to convert H_2O_2 to water. It can be irreversibly inactivated by oxidation and demonstrates decreased activity after ischemia-reperfusion. Catalase is more abundant in astrocytes than in neurons and in white matter than in gray matter, but it can be induced in neurons by neurotrophins. There is substantially less catalase activity in brain than in other tissues, such as liver.

The human genes have been identified for four members of the glutathione peroxidase family of selenoproteins. Classical glutathione peroxidase (GPx1) is a complex of four 23-kDa subunits. Plasma GPx (GPx3), GPx2 and a fourth enzyme, phospholipid hydroperoxide glutathione peroxidase (PHGPx), are monomers with extensive homology to classical GPx1. All four enzymes contain one selenium atom per subunit in the form of a selenocysteine and all use glutathione (GSH) as a cofactor to convert H_2O_2 to water. PHGPx is unique in its ability to detoxify not only H_2O_2 but fatty acid and cholesterol lipid hydroperoxides directly. In addition, it has a cytosolic isoform and an isoform with a mitochondrial targeting sequence. Both GPx1 and PHGPx proteins are present in the brain. The components of the glutathione peroxidase system, GPx, GSH, glutathione reductase and NAD(P)H, are present in the mitochondria as well as the cytoplasm. Several other proteins, including glutathione *S*-transferase, may contribute minor peroxidase activity.

Small-molecule antioxidants include glutathione, ascorbic acid (vitamin C), vitamin E and a number of dietary flavenoids. Because humans, in contrast to most other animals, are unable to synthesize vitamin C, this important antioxidant must be supplied entirely from dietary intake (see Chap. 33). Other proteins, such as thioredoxin and metallothionine, may also contribute to some extent to the cellular antioxidant pool.

Reactive oxygen species may modify both the excitotoxic and the apoptotic components of ischemic brain damage

In addition to direct effects of oxidative injury during ischemia-reperfusion, ROS may modify ischemic excitotoxicity by downregulating current through NMDA receptors. However, exposure to oxidative stress can be expected to enhance NMDA receptor-mediated neurotoxicity by depleting intracellular antioxidant defenses. Free radicals also contribute to apoptosis at several points in the apoptotic cascade, serving as initiators, early signals and possibly late effectors of apoptotic neuronal death. It may be this interaction of injury mechanisms, including excitotoxicity, ischemic apoptosis, oxidative injury, inflammation and impaired metabolism, which, in part, makes the brain so vulnerable to ischemic damage.

REFERENCES

1. Kristian, T., and Siesjo, B. K. Changes in ionic fluxes during cerebral ischaemia. *Int. Rev. Neurobiol.* 40:27–45, 1997.
2. Haddad, G. G., and Jiang, C. O_2-sensing mechanisms in excitable cells: Role of plasma membrane K^+ channels. *Annu. Rev. Physiol.* 59:23–43, 1997.
3. Welch, K. M. A., Caplan, L. R., Reis, D. J., Siesjo, B. K., and Weir, B. (eds.), *Primer on Cerebrovascular Diseases.* San Diego: Academic Press, 1997.
4. Trotti, D., Rizzini, B. L., Rossi, D., et al. Neuronal and glial glutamate transporters possess an SH-based redox regulatory mechanism. *Eur. J. Neurosci.* 9:1236–1243, 1997.
5. Nicholls, D., and Attwell, D. The release and uptake of excitatory amino acids. *Trends Pharmacol. Sci.* 11:462–468, 1990.
6. Graham, D. I., and Brierly, J. B. Vascular disorders of the central nervous system. In J. H. Adams, J. A. N. Corsellis and L. W. Duchen. (eds.), *Greenfield's Neuropathology.* New York: John Wiley & Sons, 1984, pp. 157–207.
7. Hall, E. D., Andrus, P. K., Smith, S. L., et al. Neuroprotective efficacy of microvascularly-localized versus brain-penetrating antioxidants. *Acta Neurochir. Suppl. (Wien)* 66:107–113, 1996.
8. Choi, D. W., and Rothman, S.M. The role of glutamate neurotoxicity in hypoxic-ischemic neuronal death. *Annu. Rev. Neurosci.* 13:171–182, 1990.
9. Frederickson, C. J. Neurobiology of zinc and zinc-containing neurons. *Int. Rev. Neurobiol.* 131:145–238, 1989.
10. Choi, D. W. Calcium: Still center-stage in hypoxic-ischemic neuronal death. *Trends Neurosci.* 18:58–60, 1995.
11. Chopp, M., Chan, P. H., Hsu, C. Y., Cheung, M. E., and Jacobs, T. P. DNA damage and repair in central nervous system injury: National Institute of Neurological Disorders and Stroke Workshop Summary. *Stroke* 27:363–369, 1996.
12. Smart, T. G. Regulation of excitatory and inhibitory neurotransmitter-gated ion channels by protein phosphorylation. *Curr. Opin. Neurobiol.* 7:358–367, 1997.
13. Beckman, J. S., and Koppenol, W. H. Nitric oxide, superoxide, and peroxynitrite: The good, the bad, and ugly. *Am. J. Physiol.* 71:C1424–C1437, 1996.
14. Dykens, J. A. Isolated cerebral and cerebellar mitochondria produce free radicals when exposed to elevated Ca^{2+} and Na^+: Implications for neurodegeneration. *J. Neurochem.* 63:584–591, 1994.
15. Koh, J. Y., Suh, S. W., Gwag, B. J., He, Y. Y., Hsu, C. Y., and Choi, D. W. The role of zinc in selective neuronal death after transient global cerebral ischemia. *Science* 272:1013–1016, 1996.
15a. Wyllie, A. H., Kerr, J. F., and Currie, A. R. Cell death: The significance of apoptosis. *Int. Rev. Cytol.* 68:251–306, 1980.
16. Fraser, A., McCarthy, N., and Evan, G. I. Biochemistry of cell death. *Curr. Opin. Neurobiol.* 6:71–80, 1996.
17. Hara, H., Friedlander, R. M., Gagliardini, V., et al. Inhibition of interleukin 1 beta converting enzyme family proteases reduces ischemic and excitotoxic neuronal damage. *Proc. Natl. Acad. Sci. USA* 94:2007–2012, 1997.
18. Koketsu, N., Berlove, D. J., Moskowitz, M. A., Kowall, N. W., Caday, C. G., and Finklestein, S. P. Pretreatment with intraventricular basic fibroblast growth factor decreases infarct size following focal cerebral ischemia in rats. *Ann. Neurol.* 35:451–457, 1994.

19. Greenlund, L. J., Deckwerth, T. L., and Johnson, E. M., Jr. Superoxide dismutase delays neuronal apoptosis: A role for reactive oxygen species in programmed neuronal death. *Neuron* 14:303–315, 1995.

20. Licinio, J. Central nervous system cytokines and their relevance for neurotoxicity and apoptosis. *J. Neural Transm. Suppl.* 49:169–175, 1997.

21. Halliwell, B. Reactive oxygen species and the central nervous system. *J. Neurochem.* 59:1609–1623, 1992.

22. Davies, K. J. Oxidative stress: The paradox of aerobic life. *Biochem. Soc. Symp.* 61:1–31, 1995.

23. Chan, P. H. Role of oxidants in ischemic brain damage. *Stroke* 27:1124–1129, 1996.

24. Sheng, S., Bart, R. D., Oury, T. D., Pearlstein, R. D., Crapo, J. D., and Warner, D. S. Mice overexpressing extracellular superoxide dismutase have increased resistance to focal cerebral ischemia. *J. Neurosci.* (in press), 1998.

25. Beal, M. F., Howell, N., and Bodis-Wollner, I. (eds.), *Mitochondria and Free Radicals in Neurodegenerative Diseases.* New York: John Wiley & Sons, 1997.

26. Schreiber, J., Eling, T. E., and Mason, R. P. The oxidation of arachidonic acid by the cyclooxygenase activity of purified prostaglandin H synthase: Spin trapping of a carbon-centered free radical intermediate. *Arch. Biochem. Biophys.* 249:126–136, 1986.

27. Kontos, H. A. Oxygen radicals from arachidonate metabolism in abnormal vascular responses. *Am. Rev. Respir. Dis.* 136:474–477, 1987.

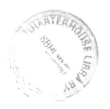

35

Eicosanoids, Platelet-Activating Factor and Inflammation

Nicolas G. Bazan

SOURCES OF BIOACTIVE LIPIDS

Excitable membranes maintain and rapidly modulate substantial transmembrane ion gradients in response to stimuli. This function requires the presence of ion pumps and channels, neurotransmitter receptors and other associated membrane proteins. Excitable membranes have a phospholipid composition that differs from other membranes, a property assumed to be related to their highly specialized functions. Several molecular species of phospholipids of

Basic Neurochemistry: Molecular, Cellular and Medical Aspects, 6th Ed., edited by G. J. Siegel et al. Published by Lippincott–Raven Publishers, Philadelphia, 1999. Correspondence to Nicolas G. Bazan, Neuroscience Center of Excellence, Louisiana State University Medical Center, School of Medicine, 2020 Gravier Street, Suite D, New Orleans, Louisiana 70112-2272.

excitable membranes are reservoirs of bioactive lipids that act as messengers (see Chap. 3). Signals, such as those resulting from receptor occupancy, trigger the release of phospholipid moieties via the activation of phospholipases. Some of the breakdown products are bioactive, such as inositol 1,4,5-trisphosphate (IP_3), diacylglycerol (DAG) and arachidonic acid (AA, 20:4n-3). Another product, lyso-platelet-activating factor (lyso-PAF), upon further metabolism, gives rise to the bioactive lipid, PAF (1-0-alkyl-2-acetyl-*sn*-3-glycerol-3-phosphocholine). Eicosanoids are derived from enzyme-mediated oxygenation of AA. Synaptic membranes are enriched in phospholipids esterified with the polyunsaturated fatty acids, AA and docosahexaenoic acid (DHA, 22:6 n-6), which form a significant proportion of the free fatty acids (FFA) rapidly released during ischemia, seizure activity and other types of brain traumas. AA and its metabolites function as intra- and intercellular messengers. In contrast, the roles of DHA remain an enigma. DHA-containing phospholipids may provide a specific milieu in which the membrane proteins of excitable membranes function. For example, the high concentrations of DHA phospholipids of outer segments of retinal rod photoreceptors provide a highly specialized membrane environment for rhodopsin (Chap. 47).

Mammalian phospholipids generally contain polyunsaturated fatty acyl chains almost exclusively esterified to the second carbon of glycerol (Chap. 3). The activity of phospholipase A_2 (PLA_2) contributes significantly to the release of the corresponding FFA. Nonetheless, FFA may also be released by the actions of various lipases secondary to the actions of other classes of phospholipases. There are a number of potential fates for the phospholipase products. They may be reincorporated into lipids or, in the case of AA, further metabolized to biologically active derivatives. The remaining lysophospholipid can be either re-esterified and reincorporated into a membrane phospholipid or further metabolized.

This chapter surveys the neurochemistry of bioactive lipids that are messengers, as well as the mechanisms by which bioactive lipids accumulate upon stimulation in response to injury, cerebral ischemia, seizures, neurotrauma or neurodegenerative diseases, and, thus, contribute to pathophysiology. Emphasis is placed on two groups of bioactive lipids: AA and its metabolites, known collectively as eicosanoids, and PAF, a highly potent ether phospholipid. Both have initially been studied in terms of their roles in classical inflammatory responses, such as increased vascular permeability and the activation of and infiltration by inflammatory cells. It is now becoming apparent, however, that these bioactive lipids have significant neurobiological roles in ion channel functions, receptors, neurotransmitter release, synaptic plasticity and neuronal gene expression. Moreover, bioactive lipids may be considered dual messengers: they modulate cell functions as messengers, and they become part of the response of the nervous tissue to injury, broadly referred to as the inflammatory response. This response occurs in ischemia-reperfusion damage associated with stroke, various forms of neurotrauma, infectious diseases and neurodegenerative diseases such as Alzheimer's disease. Inflammation in the nervous system differs from that in other tissues. If the blood–brain barrier is broken, blood-borne inflammatory cells invade the intercellular space and glial cells are activated, particularly microglia, which play a prominent role in the inflammatory response, and as a consequence, may lead to neuronal death [1]. In addition, ischemia, seizures and other forms of injury upregulate signaling in neurons, mainly through *N*-methyl-D-aspartate (NMDA)-type glutamate receptors (see Chap. 34). As a consequence, PLA_2 is activated, arachidonic acid is released, eicosanoids and PAF are synthesized and COX-2 is induced in neurons. Other neuronal correlates of the inflammatory response include signaling by cytokines, nitric oxide and various growth factors.

Identification of lipids with biological activity has progressed remarkably over the last several years. While the inositol phosphates have been known for some time to play fundamental roles in cell biology, others, such as lysophosphatidic acids, previously considered only as intermediates in phospholipid metabolism, have recently been found to possess important functions, and a lysophosphatidic acid receptor has recently been cloned [2–4]. Although the specific roles of many of these bioactive lipids and lipid derivatives in neuroscience remain sparsely explored, this review should give the reader a broad appreciation of the diversity of bioactive lipids, particularly eicosanoids and PAF, which are produced in brain under injury, seizures and inflammatory conditions.

PHOSPHOLIPASES A$_2$

PLA_2 catalyzes the cleavage of the fatty acyl chain from the second carbon of the glycerol backbone of phospholipids. There are a wide variety of PLA_2 types [5], and current investigations aim at defining those affected by ischemia and other pathological conditions. For example, in addition to the role(s) of intracellular PLA_2 in lipid messenger formation, it has recently been suggested that a low-molecular-weight secretory PLA_2 ($sPLA_2$) synergizes glutamate-induced neuronal damage [6]. Whereas pathways leading to PLA_2 activation are part of normal neuronal function, ischemia-reperfusion enhances these events, overproducing PLA_2-derived lipid messengers, such as (i) enzymatically produced AA oxygenation metabolites and (ii) nonenzymatically generated lipid peroxidation products and other reactive oxygen species (ROS), all of which may be involved in neuronal damage (see Chap. 34). Among the consequences of PLA_2 activation by ischemia are alterations in mitochondrial function by the rapid increase in the brain FFA pool size, for example, the uncoupling of oxidative phosphorylation from electron transport in the mitochondrial respiratory chain and the generation of ROS (see Chap. 34). Intracellular PLA_2 types are located either in the cytosol or in noncovalent association with membranes and are comprised of Ca^{2+}-dependent types ($cPLA_2$), which require micromolar concentrations of Ca^{2+}, and Ca^{2+}-independent types ($iPLA_2$).

Calcium ion-dependent phospholipases A$_2$ with a preference for arachidonoyl chains are involved in bioactive lipid formation

$cPLA_2$ is regulated by transcription, post-translational modulation of enzyme activity and

membrane translocation. Membrane translocation of $cPLA_2$ to endoplasmic reticulum and nuclear membranes is mediated via a specific Ca^{2+}-dependent domain similar to those seen in protein kinase C, phospholipase C and GTPase-activating protein [7,8]. This site is consistent with that of other enzymes of AA metabolism, such as prostaglandin G/H synthases (PGS), also termed cyclooxygenases (COX-1 or -2) [9], as well as 5-lipoxygenase and its activator protein [10].

The intrinsic catalytic activities of $cPLA_2$ are stimulated by phosphorylation catalyzed by the mitogen-activated protein kinase (MAPK) at Ser_{505}. This modification stimulates enzyme activity only, indicating that translocation and phosphorylation are independent mechanisms of $cPLA_2$ regulation [8].

Synaptic stimulation, ischemia or seizures activate phospholipases A$_2$ and release arachidonic acid

Ischemia or seizures trigger accumulation of free AA, as well as of other FFA in the brain. This reflects PLA_2 activation in excitable membranes [11]. While little is known about the mechanisms that control its activity, the importance of $cPLA_2$ in ischemic brain injury is strongly supported by the recent finding that $cPLA_2$ knockout mice have substantially reduced infarcts and neurological deficits in a model of stroke [12].

Shifts in intracellular pH may be another mechanism by which intracellular PLA_2 activity can be regulated. Glutamate-induced AA release in mouse cortical neuronal cultures is mediated in part by a membrane-associated PLA_2 activity, which is upregulated in alkaline pH and, thus, is sensitive to the shifts in pH induced by excitatory neurotransmission.

There are also mechanisms in the brain for the downregulation of intracellular PLA_2 activity by lipocortins, a family of Ca^{2+} and phospholipid-binding proteins that act as endogenous inhibitors of PLA_2. The steroid-inducible lipocortin-1 is present in neuronal and glial cells, especially in the hippocampus, where it may act as an endogenous neuroprotective agent [13]. Exogenous lipocortin-1 administered intracerebroventricularly to rats significantly reduces the infarct size and edema induced by cerebral ischemia and attenuates excitotoxic damage mediated by NMDA receptors. Glucocorticoid hormones inhibit lipocortin synthesis.

Secretory phospholipases A₂ require millimolar Ca²⁺ concentrations, as found in the extracellular milieu, for catalytic activity

These are of relatively low molecular weight, 13,000–18,000, and have a high number of disulfide bridges, making them resistant to denaturation. The sPLA₂ types have classically been described in terms of their roles in digestion and snake and bee venom toxicity but are now known to have even more diverse roles. The mammalian sPLA₂ types can be subdivided on the basis of amino acid sequence into pancreatic, or group I sPLA₂, the members of which function in pancreatic secretions, smooth muscle contraction, cell proliferation and fertilization, and synovial, or group II PLA₂, the members of which function in inflammatory responses.

There are high-affinity receptors that bind sPLA₂ [11,14]. The muscle (M-type) and neuronal (N-type) receptors are structurally and pharmacologically distinct. The M-type consists of a single ~180-kDa subunit and binds both OS_1 and OS_2 sPLA₂ (purified from the venom of the Australian taipan snake *Oxyuranus scutellatus scutellatus*). The N-type is composed of three major polypeptides of 34, 48 and 82 kDa and binds OS_2 and bee venom sPLA₂ but not OS_1. Expression of the M- and N-type receptors is not limited to their nominal sites. In fact, both types are widely distributed in different cells and tissues. The M-type receptor has been cloned from rabbit and human tissues and, independently, from mouse and bovine tissues; it mediates group I sPLA₂ cellular actions. The receptor consists of a single 180- to 200-kDa glycoprotein subunit that bears significant sequence homology to the macrophage mannose receptor and to other members of the C-type lectin superfamily. The recombinant receptor binds both mammalian group I and group II sPLA₂ with high affinity. Studies using enzymatically inactive mutants of group I sPLA₂ to stimulate prostaglandin E₂ (PGE₂) synthesis in rat mesan-

gial cells suggest that at least some of the effects mediated through the receptor are independent of sPLA₂ enzymatic activity. Potential ligands for the N-type receptor may be the group II sPLA₂ induced in rat brain during ischemia.

EICOSANOIDS

AA is converted to a variety of biologically active metabolites by COXs and lipoxygenases (Fig. 35-1). These metabolites, referred to collectively as eicosanoids, are potent messengers that modulate neural cell function and that are also involved in pathophysiological processes. COXs are inhibited by nonsteroidal anti-inflammatory drugs (NSAIDs), such as aspirin or ibuprofen. Mainly as a consequence of studies on NSAIDs, the significance of prostaglandins as critical modulators of immune responses, pain, fever, inflammation, mitogenesis and apoptosis have been established.

Prostaglandins are very rapidly released from neurons and glial cells

Synaptic activation and certain forms of injury, such as ischemia-reperfusion or seizures, trigger prostaglandin synthesis and rapid efflux into the intercellular media [15]. These lipid mediators, in turn, elicit their signaling actions through autocrine and paracrine routes. Several prostaglandin receptors have been cloned. Figure 35-2 depicts the selective PGE₂ receptor, also called the EP receptor, that in turn generates cAMP by activating adenylyl cyclase. The PGE₂ receptor belongs to the seven-transmembrane-domain receptor family and is coupled via G proteins to the cAMP-signaling route (see Chap. 22). This depends on the activity of protein kinase A (PKA), a heteromeric enzyme that, upon binding cAMP to its regulatory subunit, releases the catalytic subunit. The catalytic subunit, in turn, activates gene transcription by phosphorylation of a DNA-binding protein, namely, the cAMP-response element–binding (CREB) protein (Chap. 26). Several genes contain consensus sequences for CREB. Expression of these genes in turn is modulated by this lipid signaling pathway, as well as by other means. CREB has been

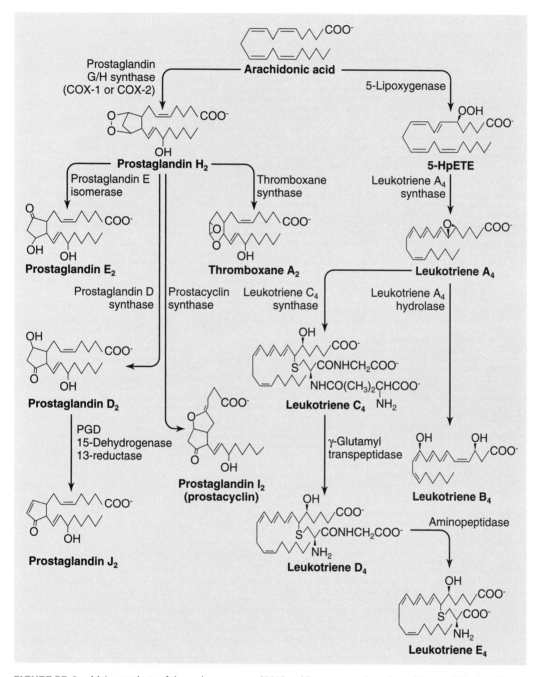

FIGURE 35-1.   Major products of the cyclooxygenase *(COX)* and lipoxygenase branches of the arachidonic acid cascade. PGD, prostaglandin D; $5H_pETE$, hydroxyperoxyeicosatrienoic acid.

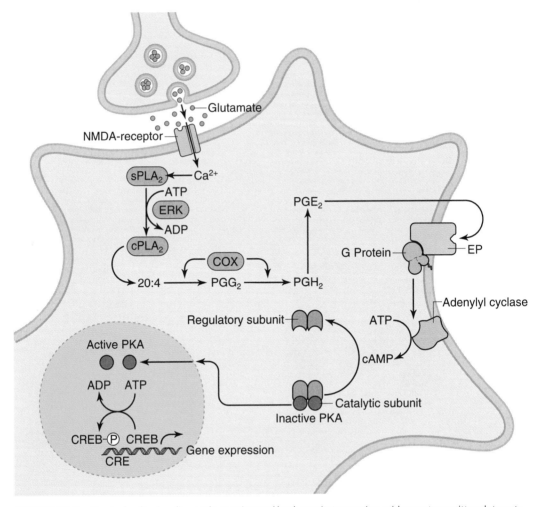

FIGURE 35-2.   Prostaglandin signaling pathway triggered by the excitatory amino acid neurotransmitter glutamate. *cPLA₂*, calcium-dependent phospholipases A_2; *sPLA₂*, secretory phospholipase A_2; *ERK,* extracellular signal-regulated kinase; *COX,* cyclooxygenase; *PGG₂* and *PGH₂* are short-lived intermediates in the synthesis of prostaglandin E_2 (PGE₂); *CREB,* cAMP-response element–binding protein; CRE, cAMP response element; *EP receptor,* prostaglandin E_2 receptor; *PKA,* protein kinase A; NMDA, *N*-methyl-D-aspartate.

implicated in plasticity changes of synaptic circuits as well as in behavior (see Chap. 50). The cloning of a second COX isoenzyme in 1991 was a major step in the effort to obtain a better understanding of the physiological significance and pathological role of prostaglandins.

AA is also the substrate for lipoxygenase and, as in the case of COX, molecular oxygen is required. The exact mechanisms controlling the channeling of AA through COXs or lipoxygenases are not clearly understood. However, there is growing evidence that subcellular compartmentalization is a major factor in the channeling of AA through either pathway.

PLATELET-ACTIVATING FACTOR

Neural membrane phospholipids are important participants in synaptic signaling as well as targets for cerebral ischemia and seizures. Phospholipid molecules of membranes from neurons and glial cells store a wide variety of lipid messengers. Receptor-mediated events and changes in $[Ca^{2+}]_i$, such as occur during excitatory neurotransmission and activity-dependent synaptic plasticity, activate phospholipases that catalyze the release of bioactive moieties from phospholipids, which then participate in intra- and/or intercellular signaling pathways.

Cerebral ischemia (Chap. 34) or seizures (Chap. 37) disrupt the tightly regulated events that control the production and accumulation of lipid messengers, such as free AA, DAG and PAF, under physiological conditions (Fig. 35-3). Rapid activation of phospholipases, particularly of PLA$_2$, occurs at the onset of cerebral ischemia or seizures and is involved during these pathophysiological conditions [11].

PAF is a very potent and short-lived lipid messenger. It is known to have a wide range of actions: as a mediator of inflammatory and immune responses, as a second messenger and as a potent inducer of gene expression in neural systems. Thus, in addition to its acute roles, PAF can potentially mediate longer-term effects on cellular physiology and brain functions.

PAF enhances glutamate release in synaptically paired rat hippocampal neurons in culture [14]. The PAF analog, methylcarbamoyl (mc-PAF), but not the biologically inactive compound lyso-PAF, increases excitatory synaptic responses. Action of the inhibitory neurotransmitter GABA is unaffected by mc-PAF under these conditions. The presynaptic PAF receptor antagonist BN 52021 blocks the mc-PAF-enhanced glutamate release. In addition, mc-PAF increases presynaptic glutamate release since it does not augment the effects of exogenously added glutamate, and it evokes spontaneous synaptic responses characteristic of enhanced neurotransmitter release. Therefore, as a modulator of glutamate release, PAF participates in long-term potentiation [17,18], synaptic plasticity and memory formation [19,20].

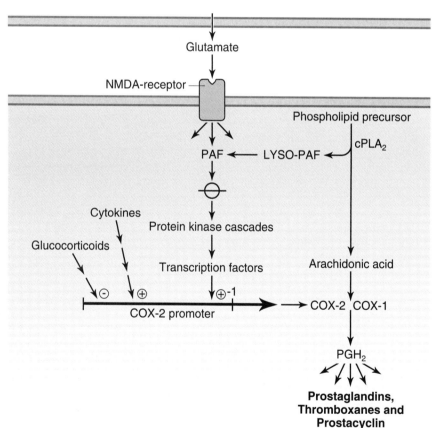

FIGURE 35-3. Seizures or ischemia-triggered signaling events linking synapse activation and cyclooxygenase-2 *(COX-2)* gene expression in neurons. *N*-methyl-ᴅ-aspartate (NMDA) receptor activation by glutamate leads to phospholipase A$_2$ (PLA$_2$) activation and the generation of platelet-activating factor *(PAF)* and of arachidonic acid. PAF is synthesized through other metabolic routes as well [16]. PAF activates COX-2 gene expression through protein kinase cascades and transcription factors. The COX-2 promoter is also a target for cytokines (activation) and glucocorticoids (inhibition). COX-2 protein then catalyzes the conversion of arachidonic acid into prostaglandin H$_2$ (PGH$_2$), the precursor of eicosanoids. Constitutive activity of COX-1 also catalyzes this metabolic step.

Ischemia and seizures increase PAF content in the brain [21]. Furthermore, the brain is endowed with a variety of degradative enzymes that rapidly convert PAF to biologically inactive lyso-PAF [22]. Presynaptic membranes display PAF binding that can be displaced by BN 52021, a terpenoid extracted from the leaf of the *Ginkgo biloba* tree. It is likely that this PAF-binding site is identical to a seven-transmembrane PAF receptor. BN 52021 inhibits both PAF-induced glutamate release [14] and long-term potentiation [17]. Moreover, this antagonist is neuroprotective in ischemia-reperfusion damage in the gerbil brain [23]. These findings together indicate that PAF, when overproduced at the synapse during ischemia, will promote enhanced glutamate release, which in turn, will contribute to excitotoxicity through the activation of postsynaptic receptors.

CYCLOOXYGENASES

COX-1 is a constitutive enzyme that converts AA to prostaglandin H_2. In 1991, a COX isoenzyme was found [9]. This enzyme, PGS-2, also known as COX-2 and tetradecanoylphorbol-13-acetate (TIS-10), is inducible by several cytokines, glutamate, growth factors, PAF and other mediators and is inhibited by glucocorticoids. COX-2 is encoded by an early-response gene, and its mRNA has a short half life (Table 35-1). In the human neocortex, the half-life is about 3 hr, as compared to 12 hr for COX-1 mRNA. In most tissues, stimulation, injury, inflammatory stimuli and other forms of cellular stress trigger expression of the COX-2 gene. However, brain, macula densa of kidney, testes and the female reproductive system also display constitutive levels of COX-2. In brain, the relatively high constitutive COX-2 expression appears to be almost exclusively neuronal. Dendrites and the perinuclear region are enriched in COX-2. Moreover, COX-2 expression seems to be regulated by synaptic activity [24].

COX-2 and COX-1 thus catalyze the same first committed step of the AA cascade. COX-2, however, is expressed in response to mitogenic and inflammatory stimuli and encoded by an early-response gene. In contrast, COX-1 expression is not subject to short-term regulation. Neurons in the hippocampus, as well as in a few other brain regions, are unlike other cells in that they display basal COX-2 expression [24]. This expression is modulated by synaptic activity, such as long-term potentiation, and involves the NMDA class of glutamate receptors [24,25] (Chap. 50).

PAF is a transcriptional activator of COX-2 as PAF induces mouse COX-2 promoter-driven luciferase activity transfected in neuroblastoma cells, such as NG108-15 or SH-SY5Y, and in NIH 3T3 cells. The intracellular PAF antagonist BN 50730 inhibits PAF activation of this construct [26].

The abundance in brain of several early-response gene transcripts shows rapid and transient increases during cerebral ischemia and after seizures. Several early-response genes encode tran-

TABLE 35-1.	CHARACTERISTICS OF CYCLOOXYGENASES (COX) OR PROSTAGLANDIN SYNTHETASES (IUPAC:IUB EC 1.14.99.1)	
	COX-1	**COX-2**
	Constitutive	Inducible in neurons, macula densa of kidney; testes and female reproductive system also contain constitutive COX-2.
Chromosome localization		1q25 10 exons, 7.5 kb
mRNA	~5.2 kb ~2.8 kb	~4.3–4.6 kb ~2.8 kb
Half-life	≥12 hr	≤3 hr (human neocortex) ~1–2 hr (IMR-90 cells) ~1–3 hr (IM9, HUVEC)
Function	Primarily cellular homeostasis	Inflammation and mitogenesis, neuronal Constitutive COX-2 is involved in synaptic plasticity. Plays a role in neurodegenerative disease, epilepsy and stroke.

scription factors, which in turn modulate the expression of other genes, whereas others encode inducible enzymes. The glutamate analog, kainic acid, promotes extensive neuronal damage, particularly in the hippocampus, and induces early-response genes such as the transcription factor *zif*-268. COX-2 is also induced under these conditions, but there are striking differences in the magnitude and duration of the induction of COX-2 as compared with *zif*-268. COX-2 mRNA, 2 hr after kainic acid injection, showed a 35-fold increase in hippocampus, as compared to only a 5.5-fold increase for *zif*-268 [27]. Also, a peak in COX-2 mRNA abundance was evident at 3 hr, a 71-fold increase, as compared with 1 hr for *zif*-268, a 10-fold increase. The *zif*-268 mRNA time course of changes in the hippocampus corresponds to the expected profile of early-response genes, that is, a rapid decrease in abundance after the peak. COX-2, however, displayed sustained upregulation for several hours after kainic acid injection, a 5.2-fold increase remaining at 12 hr [27].

LIPID SIGNALING PATHWAYS AND NEUROINFLAMMATION

A platelet-activating factor–stimulated signal-transduction pathway is a major component of the kainic acid–induced cyclooxygenase-2 expression in hippocampus

Both PAF [28] and COX-2 are potent mediators of the injury/inflammatory response (Fig. 35-4).

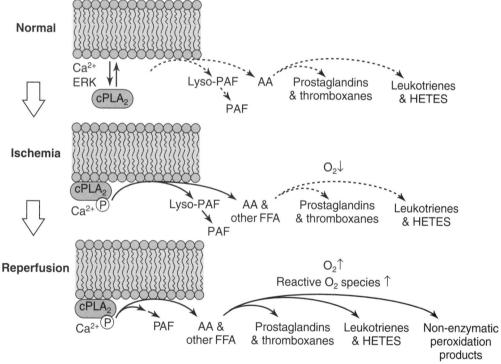

FIGURE 35-4. Calcium-dependent phospholipases A_2 *(cPLA$_2$)* and the generation of bioactive lipids during ischemia and reperfusion. During the ischemic phase, phospholipase overactivation and the down regulation of oxidative and energy metabolism, and hence reincorporation of cPLA$_2$ metabolites, promote the accumulation of arachidonic acid *(AA)* and lysophospholipids such as lyso-platelet-activating factor *(lyso-PAF)*. The reperfusion state permits the completion of PAF and eicosanoid synthesis but at the expense of the accumulation of pathophysiologically high amounts of these mediators. Reactive oxygen species are generated at rates that can overload the antioxidant and free radical scavenger systems of the brain, thus allowing free radical damage to a range of molecules, including peroxidation of polyunsaturated fatty acids. ERK, extracellular signal-regulated kinase; FFA, free fatty acids; HETES, hydroxyeicosatrienoic acid.

PAF and COX-2 are also interrelated in neuronal plasticity. The PAF transcriptional activation of COX-2 may provide clues about novel neuronal cell death pathways. In fact, the delayed induction of COX-2 by kainic acid precedes selective neuronal apoptosis by this agonist in the hippocampus [27,29].

In cerebrovascular diseases, the phospholipase A$_2$-related signaling triggered by ischemia-reperfusion may be part of a delicate balance between neuroprotection and neuronal cell death

Events that would tilt the balance toward the neuroprotection are of interest as possible therapeutic targets. It is interesting to note that PAF, being short-lived and rapidly degraded by PAF acetylhydrolase [30], is a long-term signal with consequences to neurons [31], through COX-2 sustained expression. Overexpression of hippocampal COX-2 during cerebral ischemia [32] and seizures may in turn lead to the formation of neurotoxic metabolites, such as ROS (see Chap. 34). The regulatory subunit of PAF-acetylhydrolase (intracellular) is the *Lis-1* gene, mutated in Miller-Diecker syndrome, a neuronal disease characterized by the absence of gyri and sulci in the cerebral cortex (lissencephaly). A defect in neuronal migration during brain development may underlie the smooth cerebrum of people afflicted with the syndrome, and PAF and PAF-acetylhydrolase may be involved in neuronal migration [33]. Current investigations aim at determining whether other messengers, such as nitric oxide, cooperate to enhance neuronal damage and to what extent astrocytes and microglial cells are involved. Further understanding of these potentially neurotoxic events involving lipid messengers and COX-2 will contribute to the identification of new therapeutic strategies for the management of cerebrovascular diseases, neurodegenerative diseases and other pathological conditions involving neuroinflammation (see Fig. 35-4).

REFERENCES

1. Giulian, D. Microglia and diseases of the nervous system. *Curr. Neurol.* 12:23–27, 1992.

2. Hecht, J. H., Weiner, J. A., Post, S. R., and Chun, J. Ventricular zone gene-1 (vzg-1) encodes a lysophosphatidic acid receptor expressed in neurogenic regions of the developing cerebral cortex. *J. Cell Biol.* 135:1071–1083, 1996.

3. Guo, Z., Liliom, K., Fischer, D. J., et al. Molecular cloning of a high-affinity receptor for the growth factor-like mediator lysophosphatidic acid from *Xenopus* oocytes. *Proc. Natl. Acad. Sci. USA* 93:14367–14372, 1996.

4. An, S., Dickens, M. A., Bleu, T., Hallmark, O. G., and Goetzl, E. J. Molecular cloning of the human EDG2 protein and its identification as a functional cellular receptor for lysophosphatidic acid. *Biochem. Biophys. Res. Commun.* 231:619–622, 1997.

5. Dennis, E. A. Diversity of group types, regulation and function of phospholipase A$_2$. *J. Biol. Chem.* 304:417–422, 1994.

6. Kolko, M., DeCoster, M. A., Rodriguez de Turco, E. B., and Bazan, N. G. Synergy by secretory phospholipase A$_2$ and glutamate on inducing cell death and sustained arachidonic acid metabolic changes in primary cortical neuronal cultures. *J. Biol. Chem.* 271:32722–32728, 1996.

7. Tay, A., Maxwell, P., Li, Z. G., Goldberg, H., and Skorecki, K. Cytosolic phospholipse A$_2$ gene expression in rat mesangial cells is regulated posttranscriptionally. *Biochem. J.* 304:417–422, 1994.

8. Clark, J. D., Lin, L.-L., Kriz, R. W., et al. A novel arachidonic acid-selective cytosolic PLA$_2$ contains a Ca^{2+}-dependent translocation domain with homology to PKC and GAP. *Cell* 65:1043–1051, 1991.

9. Herschman, H. R. Prostaglandin synthase 2. *Biochim. Biophys. Acta* 1299:125–140, 1996.

10. Brock, T. G., McGish, R. W., and Peters-Golden, M. Translocation and leukotriene synthetic capacity of nuclear 5-lipoxygenase in rat basophilic leukemia cells and alveolar macrophages. *J. Biol. Chem.* 270:21652–21658, 1995.

11. Bazan, N. G., Rodriguez de Turco, E. B., and Allan, G. Mediators of injury in neurotrauma: Intracellular signal transduction and gene expression. *J. Neurotrauma* 12:789–911, 1995.

12. Bonventre, J. V., Huang, Z., Taheri, M. R., et al. Reduced fertility and postischaemic brain injury in mice deficient in cytosolic phospholipase A$_2$. *Nature* 390:622–625, 1997.

13. Flower, R. J., and Rothwell, N. J. Lipocortin-1: Cellular mechanisms and clinical relevance. *Trends Pharmacol. Sci.* 15:71–76, 1994.

14. Clark, G. D., Happel, L. T., Zorumski, C. F., and Bazan, N. G. Enhancement of hippocampal exci-

tatory synaptic transmission by platelet-activating factor. *Neuron* 9:1211–1216, 1992.

15. Birkle, D. L., and Bazan, N. G. Effect of biculculine-induced status epilepticus on prostaglandins and hydroxyeicosatetraenoic acids in rat brain subcellular fractions. *J. Neurochem.* 48: 1768–1778, 1987.

16. Bazan, N. G. Inflammation: A signal terminator. *Nature* 374:501–502, 1995.

17. Kato, K., Clark, G. D., Bazan, N. G., and Zorumski, C. F. Platelet activating factor as a potential retrograde messenger in CA1 hippocampal long-term potentiation. *Nature* 367:175–179, 1994.

18. Wieraszko, A., Li, G., Kornecki, E., Hogan, M. V., and Ehrlich, Y. H. Long-term potentiation in the hippocampus induced by platelet-activating factor. *Neuron* 10:553–557, 1993.

19. Izquierdo, I., Fin, C., Schmitz, P. K., et al. Memory enhancement by intrahippocampal, intraamygdala, or intraentorhinal infusion of platelet-activating factor measured in an inhibitory avoidance task. *Proc. Natl. Acad. Sci. USA* 92:5047–5051, 1995.

20. Packard, M. G., Teather, L., Bazan, N. G. Effects of intrastriatal injections of platelet-activating factor and the PAF antagonist BN 52021 on memory. *Neurobiol. Learn. Mem.* 66:177–182, 1996.

21. Kumar, R., Harvary, S., Kester, M., Hanahan, D., and Olsen, M. Production and effects of platelet-activating factor in the rat brain. *Biochim. Biophys. Acta* 963:375–390, 1988.

22. Bito, H., Nakamura, M., Honda, Z., et al. Platelet-activating factor (PAF) receptor in rat brain: PAF mobilizes intracellular Ca^{2+} in hippocampal neurons. *Neuron* 9:285–294, 1992.

23. Panetta, T., Marcheselli, V. L., Braquet, P., Spinnewyn, B., Bazan, N. G. Effects of a platelet-activating factor antagonist (BN52021) on free fatty acids, diacylglycerols, polyphosphoinositides and blood flow in the gerbil brain: Inhibition of ischemia-reperfusion induced cerebral injury. *Biochem. Biophys. Res. Comm.* 149:580–587, 1987.

24. Kaufmann, W. E., Worley, P. F., Pegg, J., Bremer, M., and Isakson, P. COX-2, a synaptically induced enzyme, is expressed by excitatory neurons at postsynaptic sites in rat cerebral cortex. *Proc. Natl. Acad. Sci. USA* 93:2317–2321, 1996.

25. Yamagata, K., Andreasson, K. I., Kaufmann, W. E., Barnes, C. A., and Worley, P. F. Expression of a mitogen-inducible cyclooxygenase in brain neurons: Regulation by synaptic activity and glucocorticoids. *Neuron* 11:371–386, 1993.

26. Bazan, N. G., Fletcher, B. S., Herschman, H. R., and Mukherjee, P. K. Platelet-activating factor and retinoic acid synergistically activate the inducible prostaglandin synthase gene. *Proc. Natl. Acad. Sci. USA* 91:5252–5256, 1994.

27. Marcheselli, V. L., and Bazan, N. G. Sustained induction of prostaglandin endoperoxide synthase-2 by seizures in hippocampus. Inhibition by a platelet-activating factor antagonist. *J. Biol. Chem.* 271:24794–24799, 1996.

28. Prescott, S. M., Zimmerman, G. A., and McIntyre, T. M. Platelet-activating factor antagonist. *J. Biol. Chem.* 265:17381–17384, 1990.

29. Chen, J., Marsh, T., Zhang, J. S., and Graham, S. H. Expression of cyclooxygenase 2 in rat brain following kainate treatment. *Neuroreport* 6: 245–248, 1995.

30. Stafforini, D. M., McIntyre, T. M., Zimmerman, G. A., and Prescott, S. M. Platelet-activating factor acetylhydrolases. *J. Biol. Chem.* 272: 17895–17898, 1997.

31. Bazan, N. G., and Allan, G. Platelet-activating factor and other bioactive lipids. In M. D. Ginsberg, J. Bogousslavsky (eds). *Cerebrovascular Disease, Pathophysiology, Diagnosis and Management.* Blackwell Science Publishers, Malden, MA, 1998, pp. 532–555.

32. Nogawa, S., Zhang, F., Ross, M. E., and Iadecola, C. Cyclooxygenase-2 gene expression in neurons contributes to ischemic brain damage. *J. Neurosci.* 17:2746–2755, 1997.

33. Hattori, M., Adachi, H., Tsujimoto, M., Arai, H., and Inoue, K. Miller-Dieker lissencephaly gene encodes a subunit of brain platelet-activating factor acetylhydrolase. *Nature* 370:216–218, 1994.

36

Neuropathy

David E. Pleasure

Basic Neurochemistry: Molecular, Cellular and Medical Aspects, 6th Ed., edited by G. J. Siegel et al. Published by
Lippincott–Raven Publishers, Philadelphia, 1999. Correspondence to David E. Pleasure, The Children's Hospital of Philadelphia, Room 516A Abramson Research Building, 3517 Civic Center Boulevard, Philadelphia, Pennsylvania 19104.

REGENERATION IN THE CENTRAL AND PERIPHERAL NERVOUS SYSTEMS

The peripheral and central nervous systems have many anatomical and molecular features in common

Somatic motor and sensory neurons that give rise to peripheral nervous system (PNS) axons maintain large fractions of their total protoplasmic bulk within the central nervous system (CNS). Extracellular matrix components involved in the guidance of CNS development are employed for the same purpose in the PNS. PNS microglia-like cells, as microglia in the CNS, are bone marrow-derived and have a similar repertoire of responses to activation. Both oligodendroglia and Schwann cells speed axonal action potential propagation by assembling and maintaining myelin. Capillary endothelial cells linked by tight junctions serve to restrict entry of polar molecules into the PNS, as into the CNS.

One substantial difference between the PNS and CNS is that PNS regeneration is robust, a difference attributable in part to the contrasting inhibitory effect of oligodendroglia and the stimulatory effect of Schwann cells on axonal elongation. We provide here a short description of common patterns of PNS degeneration and regeneration.

Despite the resemblances between the PNS and CNS, there are many PNS-specific diseases. Some of the reasons for PNS disease selectivity are listed in Table 36-1. We briefly discuss a few of these PNS-selective diseases (Table 36-2) and some disorders affecting the CNS as well as the PNS (Table 36-3). The chapter concludes with a short consideration of the enteric nervous system (ENS), a clinically important but relatively neglected region of the nervous system.

Cellular and molecular properties of the peripheral nervous system are important in disease susceptibility and regenerative capacity

Whereas in the CNS, oligodendroglia invest large axons in myelin and astroglia regulate ion and metabolite concentrations in the neuropil, these functions are the combined responsibility of Schwann cells in the PNS. There are two major Schwann cell phenotypes: myelinating Schwann cells, which ensheath single axons greater than 1 μm in diameter for hundreds of microns and synthesize myelin-specific molecules, such as P_0 [1], and nonmyelinating Schwann cells, which invest multiple small axons and do not synthesize myelin (see Chaps. 1 and 4). The choice between myelin-forming and nonmyelinating Schwann cell specializations is determined by the caliber of the axons with which the Schwann cells are in contact [2]. Reciprocally, Schwann cells regulate the cytoskeletal organization and axonal caliber of the axons they invest [3].

Myelin, a paracrystalline array of lipid-rich glial or Schwann cell plasma membranes, supports saltatory, rapid conduction of nerve impulses by providing a high-resistance, low-ca-

TABLE 36-1. **MECHANISMS OF PNS-SPECIFIC DISEASE PATHOGENESIS**

Mutations affecting genes expressed exclusively in PNS
Autoimmune disorders targeting PNS-specific constituents
Penetration of blood–nerve barrier by toxins or antibodies
Lack of redundancy of the endoneurial arterial supply
Great length of some PNS axons
Vulnerability of the PNS to trauma

TABLE 36-2.	EXAMPLES OF DISEASES AFFECTING EXCLUSIVELY OR PRINCIPALLY THE PNS

Acute motor axonal neuropathy

Botulism

Charcot-Marie-Tooth disease types 1A, 1B and 1X

Cisplatin neuropathy

Diabetic neuropathy

Diphtheritic neuropathy

Familial amyloid neuropathy

Guillain-Barré syndrome

Lambert-Eaton syndrome

Leprosy

Neuropathy with IgM_1 anti-myelin-associated glycoprotein

Pyridoxine neuropathy

Refsum's disease

pacitance sheath around large axons. Unlike oligodendroglia, Schwann cells form myelin around no more than one axon. Both PNS and CNS myelin contain various isoforms of P_1 myelin basic protein [4]; multiple isoforms of myelin-associated glycoprotein (MAG), which is involved in glia–axon adhesion [5]; abundant cholesterol and phospholipids; and the galactosphingolipids galactocerebroside and sulfatide. While proteolipid protein (PLP) is the most abundant protein in CNS myelin [6] and is made by Schwann cells as well [7], it is only a minor PNS myelin constituent. Myelin proteins present in PNS myelin but not in CNS myelin of most higher vertebrates include P_0 and P_2 (see Chap. 4).

PNS sensory and motor axons may exceed 1 m in length. Since PNS axons lack ribosomes, the supply of essential structural proteins and enzymes to distal regions derived from the neuronal perikaryon must be transported through the axons for great distances (see Chap. 28). The proteins that polymerize to form neurofilaments and microtubules as well as many enzymes move centrifugally at 1 to 10 mm/day. Organelles such as neurotransmitter vesicles and mitochondria are transported through the axoplasm at velocities of greater than 100 mm/day by a process involving interactions between kinesin and microtubules [8]. Conversely, proteins internalized by the nerve terminal are translocated toward the neuronal perikaryon at approximately 100 mm/day, employing a mechanism in which dynein and microtubules play roles [9]. PNS neurons with long axons are particularly vulnerable to disorders that compromise either perikaryal synthesis of axonal proteins or the local axonal machinery responsible for axoplasmic transport. Long axons are also more likely to sustain localized damage owing to trauma, ischemia or other noxious influences.

Wallerian degeneration. When Schwann cell–axon contact is lost, as occurs in the distal stump of nerves undergoing Wallerian degeneration, mononuclear cells from the bloodstream enter the trauma zone and assist resident Schwann cells and microglia-like cells in catabolizing fragmented myelin. These cells secrete cytokines (for example, interleukin-1 and platelet-derived growth factor), which stimulate Schwann cell proliferation. These cycling Schwann cells downregulate expression of myelin components and form tubular cellular aggregates ("bands of Büngner"), which facilitate axonal regeneration. In the nerves of young animals undergoing Wallerian degeneration, some of these excess Schwann cells generated during Wallerian degeneration undergo apoptosis [10]. Myelin-forming and nonmyelinating Schwann cell phenotypes are restored as axonal regeneration through the distal stump occurs.

TABLE 36-3.	EXAMPLES OF DISEASES AFFECTING BOTH PNS AND CNS

Acute intermittent porphyria

Adrenoleukodystrophy

AIDS

Amyotrophic lateral sclerosis

Friedreich's ataxia

Lyme disease

Metachromatic leukodystrophy

Neurofibromatosis types 1 and 2

Syphilis

Thiamine deficiency

Segmental demyelination. Schwann cells injured by immune-mediated mechanisms or subjected to trauma may lose axonal contact, proliferate and participate in the catabolism of myelin fragments. If several successive internodes along an axon are demyelinated, nerve action potential conduction through the demyelinated segment is blocked, resulting in clinically detectable neurological dysfunction. Since thousands of Schwann cells are required to myelinate long PNS axons, the likelihood is high that a pathological process that randomly compromises the capacity of Schwann cells to maintain myelin will interfere with saltatory conduction along such a fiber. Thin, regenerating myelin sheaths permit nerve action potential propagation but at markedly diminished velocity. Excess Schwann cells generated during the phase of Schwann-cell proliferation that are not successful in re-establishing contact with an axon are pruned from the nerve, perhaps by apoptosis. Repeated cycles of demyelination and remyelination, which may occur in various inherited and acquired demyelinative neuropathies, lead to the deposition of layers of redundant Schwann cells, which encircle demyelinated or partially remyelinated axons, forming "onion bulbs" [11]. Under these circumstances, full regeneration of normal PNS anatomy may become impossible.

Clinical features of polyneuropathies reflect vulnerability of the longest axons to degeneration and segmental demyelination

Typically, patients manifest symmetrical distal sensory disturbances, usually first in the feet. Distal muscles are weakened more than proximal muscles, and distal tendon reflexes are lost prior to proximal tendon reflexes. This pattern of clinical deficit is referred to as *symmetrical distal polyneuropathy*. In some instances, symmetrical distal polyneuropathy causes selective impairment of transmission of motor function, such as acute motor axonal neuropathy [12], or of sensory and autonomic function, such as familial amyloid neuropathy [13]. Signs of autonomic neuropathy include defective regulation of blood pressure, heart rate, pupillary responses and bowel motility. Other clinical patterns of

PNS disease include mononeuropathy, which is the dysfunction of a single peripheral nerve, and mononeuropathy multiplex, which involves several to many, but not all, peripheral nerves. Mononeuropathy multiplex is caused most commonly by diseases affecting PNS blood flow, including periarteritis nodosa and diabetes mellitus [14].

Extracellular matrix. Flattened, basal lamina-lined perineurial cells [15] delineate nerve fascicles, providing a barrier to movement of ionic compounds and macromolecules between non-neural tissues and the endoneurium (see also Chap. 32). Fibroblasts constitute roughly 10% of total cells within the endoneurium and are far more uncommon in the CNS. The collagens are a family of extracellular structural proteins characterized by a triple α-helical configuration and a high content of hydroxyproline, hydroxylysine and glycine. Collagens comprise 30% or more of total PNS protein and are present in the endoneurium both in the form of interstitial collagen fibrils and as a component of the basal lamina surrounding the processes of Schwann cells and perineurial cells, in addition to lining the outer aspect of endoneurial capillaries. The bulk of interstitial collagen fibrils are synthesized by fibroblasts, although Schwann cells and perineurial mesothelial cells secrete the more heavily glycosylated basal lamina forms of collagen. Fibroblasts augment production of interstitial collagen both in a traumatized nerve segment and distal to it. This increases the tensile strength of the damaged nerve and provides the collagenous framework required for axonal ensheathment by Schwann cells. The extracellular accumulation of collagen in the injured PNS [16] contrasts sharply with the astrogliosis and increased intracellular glial fibrillary acidic protein (GFAP) elicited by trauma in the CNS. As regeneration proceeds, axonal growth cones penetrate the scar and extend into the tubular Schwann cell aggregates.

Compression injury. Movements of the limbs subject nerves to repeated stretch. Although collagen fibrils afford tensile strength, there is some waviness in the course of axons that permits a degree of nerve elongation without axonal ripping. However, stretch that is too great causes axonal disruption. Nerves in exposed regions, for example, the median nerve at the wrist, the ulnar nerve at the elbow and the common peroneal nerve at the knee, are vulnerable to compression that can cause either demyelination or axonal transection if it is sufficiently severe. Such compression also can interrupt blood flow, causing nerve infarction. In addition to these mechanical injuries, superficial nerves experience considerable thermal fluctuations that can kill cells directly or predispose nerves to damage by precipitation of cold-insoluble proteins or other mechanisms (see discussion of leprosy, for example, below).

Blood–nerve barrier. Both the CNS and PNS demonstrate local regions of incompetence of their respective blood–tissue barrier systems, and in both tissues these regions have specific physiological functions. In the CNS, for example, the function of medullary chemosensory nuclei requires free passage of polar molecules from the blood. In the PNS, trophic proteins secreted by target organs gain access to axon terminals that are not invested in a perineurial sheath. Lectins and other proteins useful as anatomical tracers also gain access to the PNS at nerve terminals, and some viruses are able to penetrate at this site [9]. Another region of relative incompetence of the blood–nerve barrier is at the level of the dorsal root ganglia. Neurotoxic molecules may gain entry to the PNS at this point, producing degeneration of sensory neurons [17,18].

EXAMPLES OF PERIPHERAL NERVOUS SYSTEM-SPECIFIC DISEASES

Examples of disorders exclusively or predominantly of the PNS are listed in Table 36-2. Some are quite common, for example, lepromatous neuropathy, diabetic neuropathy [14], Guillain-Barré syndrome and acute motor axonal neuropathy [12]. Others are rare, for example, botulism [19], Lambert-Eaton syndrome [20], acute intermittent porphyria [21] and familial amyloid neuropathy [13], but merit mention because they illustrate pathogenetic mechanisms.

The lepromatous form of leprosy is characterized by loss of cutaneous sensibility

Neuropathy is a consequence of damage caused by the growth of Hansen's bacilli in Schwann cells around affected cutaneous nerves. Hansen's bacilli, fastidious organisms that proliferate only at temperatures below that maintained by most mammals, grow in subcutaneous Schwann cells because these nerves are in an environment that is often cooler than the CNS and other deeper tissues.

Diphtheria causes a demyelinative neuropathy

Corynebacterium diphtheriae, a bacterium that colonizes the pharynx, secretes a protein exotoxin that gains access to endoneurial fluid, binds to a Schwann cell plasma membrane receptor and catalyzes ADP-ribosylation and inactivation of an elongation factor required for Schwann cell protein synthesis.

Excess vitamin B_6 causes a progressive, purely sensory axonal polyneuropathy

This is usually the result of inappropriate self-medication and affects predominantly the largest fibers emanating from the dorsal root ganglion neurons. A similar purely sensory axonal polyneuropathy with dorsal root ganglion neuropathy is seen in patients given cisplatin as a chemotherapeutic agent for the treatment of gynecologic or bladder carcinoma. In both instances, the toxin is able to penetrate the blood–nerve barrier, particularly at the level of the dorsal root ganglia. Neurotropin-3 treatment is effective in protecting dorsal root ganglion neurons against these sensory neuronal toxins [17,18]. Deficiency of vitamin B_6 is discussed in Chapter 33.

Botulinus exotoxin impedes release of neurotransmitter vesicles from cholinergic terminals at neuromuscular junctions

This toxin is ingested with food or, in infants, synthesized *in situ* by anaerobic bacteria that colonize the gut [19]. A characteristic electrophysiological feature of botulinus paralysis is that strength increases when motor nerve electrical stimulation is repeated at low frequency, a phenomenon attributable to the recruitment of additional cholinergic vesicles with repetitive depolarization of the neuromuscular presynaptic terminals (see also Chap. 43).

Immune-mediated neuropathies may be related to various sources of antigens

Lambert-Eaton syndrome. This disorder, which sometimes is seen in patients with small cell lung carcinoma, is characterized clinically by weakness of the limbs and trunk and hyporeflexia and is caused by autoantibodies against motor nerve terminal Ca^{2+} channels (Chap. 43). The antibodies inhibit cholinergic vesicle release [20]. The electrophysiological phenomena are very similar to those in botulism.

Experimental allergic neuritis (EAN). This disorder can be elicited in various experimental animals, including Lewis rats and monkeys, by sensitization to myelin P_2 epitopes [22], and rabbits, by immunization with the myelin glycolipid galactocerebroside (galC) [23] (see Chap. 39). Although both types of EAN are primarily demyelinative, P_2-EAN is mediated primarily by sensitized T lymphocytes and galC-EAN primarily by galC antibodies. The reasons for PNS selectivity of the two EANs are also distinct. Although T lymphocytes can penetrate the CNS as well as PNS, myelin P_2 basic protein is restricted to the PNS, and P_2-sensitized T lymphocytes are, therefore, more likely to set up an inflammatory reaction in the PNS than the CNS. GalC, on the other hand, is a constituent of the plasma membranes of oligodendroglia as well as Schwann cells and of CNS myelin as well as PNS myelin. PNS selectivity of galC-EAN presumably reflects the more ready ingress of complement-fixing galC antibodies to the PNS than the CNS.

Acute idiopathic demyelinative polyneuritis. This disease, also called Guillain-Barré syndrome, often occurs 1 or 2 weeks after a viral infection. Typically, no virus can be isolated from the PNS. Most patients recover completely, particularly if treated early in the course by plasmapheresis or immunoglobulin infusion. Guillain-Barré syndrome resembles P_2-EAN (see Chap. 39) both clinically and pathologically, being characterized by segmental demyelination and infiltration of the endoneurium by lymphocytes and macrophages. Although most likely due to an autoimmune mechanism, the responsible neural antigen has not yet been identified. *Acute motor axonal neuropathy* resembles acute idiopathic demyelinative polyneuritis in its favorable long-term prognosis but affects primarily axons rather than myelin sheaths. This neuropathy often follows an antecedent *Campylobacter jejuni* infection and is a consequence of injury to the plasma membrane of motor axons caused by attack by antiganglioside antibodies and complement [12].

IgM$_k$ paraproteinemia. Elderly men with a plasma cell-proliferative disorder occasionally develop a slowly progressive polyneuropathy characterized pathologically by focally abnormal compaction of PNS myelin lamellae. In some cases, the paraproteinemic immunoglobulin has been observed to bind to intact myelin and to MAG (see Chap. 4). The PNS specificity of this syndrome, despite the greater abundance of MAG in myelin of the CNS than the PNS, may be due to greater penetration of the paraprotein into the PNS than the CNS. Alternatively, the higher incidence in the PNS may be due to glycolipids in PNS myelin that share epitopes with MAG.

Amyloid neuropathy. Amyloid is the generic term applied to acquired and inherited disorders characterized by abnormal deposition of protease-resistant protein aggregates in tissue (see also Chap. 46). Acquired amyloid neuropathy fits within the group of immune-mediated neuropathies in that insoluble aggregates of immunoglobulin light chains accumulate in the nerves of patients with multiple myeloma or other plasma cell dyscrasias. This leads both to compressive neuropathies and to selective dysfunction of autonomic and nonmyelinated sensory fibers. Patients with dominantly inherited amyloid neuropathies, caused by mutations that diminish the solubility of transthyretin or gelsolin, present with autonomic dysfunction together with a progressive distal sensory neuropathy that particularly affects pain and temperature perception. Transthyretin is synthesized in the liver, and liver transplantation has shown promise in preventing progression of amyloid neuropathy caused by transthyretin mutations [13].

Demyelinative polyneuropathies may be genetic in origin

Refsum's disease. Refsum's disease is inherited as an autosomal recessive trait and is characterized clinically by polyneuropathy that is hypertrophic and demyelinative, retinitis pigmentosa, ichthyosis and deafness. Biochemically, it is characterized by elevation in plasma levels of phytanic acid, a long-chain, branched fatty acid derived from the diet. Refsum's disease is caused by deficient peroxisomal activity of phytanic acid α-hydroxylase [24] and is treated by diminution in dietary intake of phytanic acid and by plasmapheresis to remove circulating phytanic acid (see Chap. 41).

Hereditary motor and sensory neuropathy. This disease, also known as Charcot-Marie-Tooth (CMT) syndrome, is a diverse group of polyneuropathies with varying patterns of inheritance, including dominant, recessive and X-linked patterns. Demyelinative forms of CMT are characterized by reduced velocity of nerve action potentials, prominent segmental demyelination and Schwann cell proliferation, sometimes with onion-bulb formation; axonal forms manifest distal Wallerian degeneration. A 1.5-megabase duplication in chromosome 17p11.2-12 is the cause of dominantly inherited CMT1A. This duplicated segment contains the gene encoding the PNS myelin protein PMP22; thus, patients with CMT1A have three copies of this gene. A reciprocal deletion of this region of chromosome 17 causes *hereditary neuropathy with predisposition to pressure palsies* (HNPP). Patients with this dominantly inherited disorder, who have only one copy of the PMP22 gene, develop repeated focal demyelinative mononeuropathies, and many also have a mild demyelinative polyneuropathy. Histological examination of nerves demonstrates segmental demyelination and scattered sausage-shaped myelin sheath swellings, hence, the alternative name for HNPP, *tomaculous neuropathy* [25]. Point mutation of the PMP22 gene is responsible for recessively inherited demyelinative polyneuropathy in the *trembler* mouse [26]. CMT1B is caused by a variety of mutations in the major P_0 glycoprotein of PNS myelin, presumably impairing its capacity to stabilize the major dense or intraperiod lines. The *X-linked form of CMT* (CMT1X) is a demyelinative polyneuropathy caused by mutations of a gene encoding the gap-junction protein connexin32 [27]. Gap junctions containing connexin32 are expressed in Schmidt-Lantermann incisures, in paranodal myelin by myelinating Schwann cells and by oligodendroglia in the CNS; but their functions are not as yet clear.

Diabetes mellitus is the most common cause of peripheral neuropathy in the United States

The usual clinical pattern of diabetic neuropathy is a slowly progressive, mixed sensorimotor and autonomic polyneuropathy. More acute, asymmetrical motor neuropathies are also seen, typically affecting the lumbosacral plexus, particularly in older persons with non-insulin-dependent diabetes mellitus [14]. Patients with diabetes mellitus are also prone to develop isolated palsies of cranial nerve III or VII, and there is a very high incidence of asymptomatic focal demyelination in the distal median nerve.

Among the pathogenetic mechanisms that have been proposed for diabetic neuropathy are excess glycation of neural proteins, alteration in nerve polyol metabolism induced by hyperglycemia and nerve ischemia, as well as, in some cases, an immune mechanism. In hyperglycemic rats, endoneurial blood flow is diminished by what may be an endothelin-dependent mechanism [28,29]. The presence of small vessel disease in human diabetic nerves suggests that diminished endoneurial blood flow plays a role in human diabetic neuropathy, particularly with respect to the scattered infarctions of the proximal regions of peripheral nerves seen at autopsy in some patients with diabetic neuropathy [14,30]. Antibodies found in the serum of some diabetic patients with neuropathy are potentially neurotoxic [31].

DISEASES AFFECTING BOTH THE PERIPHERAL AND CENTRAL NERVOUS SYSTEMS

Because of the similarities between the PNS and CNS, it is not surprising that many diseases affect both (Table 36-3). It should be noted, however, that the clinical expression of such diseases is variable and sometimes restricted to the PNS. For example, patients with thiamine deficiency often display symmetrical distal sensorimotor polyneuropathy without accompanying brainstem or thalamic degeneration. Infection with human immunodeficiency virus (HIV) may cause early chronic demyelinative polyneuropathy, with dementia appearing months later. The spirochetal diseases, syphilis and Lyme disease, may involve the PNS or the CNS or both together [32]. Sulfatidase deficiency, also termed *metachromatic leukodystrophy* [33], may cause polyneuropathy initially, with CNS dysfunction becoming clinically apparent only years thereafter. In some instances, this apparent PNS specificity is simply an ascertainment artifact; that is, although both the CNS and PNS are involved, only the PNS component is detectable in the early stages. In other cases, subtle host factors or as yet unappreciated etiologic variables dictate PNS selectivity. We briefly discuss a few of the inherited, combined PNS/CNS diseases which are genetically determined (see also Chap. 40).

Neurofibromatosis type 1, von Recklinghausen's disease, is the most frequent dominantly inherited disorder affecting the nervous system

Neurofibromatosis type 1 (NF1) has an incidence of about 1 in 2,000 persons. Among its diagnostic features are benign Schwann cell tumors arising from small cutaneous nerves, termed *subcutaneous neurofibromas,* or within larger nerves, *plexiform neurofibromas;* cuta-

neous accumulations of melanocytes, termed *café-au-lait spots;* focal accumulations of pigmentary cells in the iris, termed *Lisch nodules;* and a variety of orthopaedic deformities, including absence of a segment of the sphenoid bone, tibial nonunion and others. While all of these features can be attributed to abnormalities of neural crest- or placode-derived tissues, patients with NF1 may also manifest various CNS abnormalities, including mental retardation and gliomas, particularly of the optic nerves or chiasm. Patients with NF1 are prone to develop both Schwann cell malignancies, termed *neurofibrosarcomas,* and other forms of cancer. NF1 is caused by a variety of mutations in the neurofibromin gene, situated on chromosome 17, which encodes a large tumor-suppressor protein with a GTPase-activating domain and many other domains of unknown function. Most neurobiological attention has been devoted to a search for intrinsic abnormalities in Schwann cell behavior in NF1, and it has been demonstrated that NF1-deficient Schwann cells do contain elevated levels of Ras-GTP [34] (see Chap. 20). There are also data to suggest that other cellular components of neurofibromas contribute to tumor growth in NF1. Neurofibromin-deficient embryonic sensory neurons have an enhanced capacity to survive in the absence of exogenous neurotrophins [35], and neurofibromin-deficient fibroblasts have an impaired capacity to form perineurium [36].

Neurofibromatosis type 2 is a much rarer dominantly inherited disease

NF2 is caused by various mutations affecting a chromosome 22q tumor-suppressor gene, which encodes a protein named merlin or schwannomin. The functions of this protein are unknown. Clinical features of NF2 include bilateral acoustic nerve Schwann cell tumors, lenticular opacities and CNS glial tumors [37].

Acute intermittent porphyria is a dominantly inherited partial deficiency of porphobilinogen deaminase

This enzyme is involved in heme biosynthesis [21]. Patients with acute intermittent porphyria

(AIP) may present with acute abdominal pain, rapidly progressive sensorimotor axonal polyneuropathy or psychosis and have elevated concentrations of the heme precursor δ-aminolevulinic acid in the urine. Symptoms may be precipitated by treatment with barbiturates or other drugs and are suppressed by treatment with hematin.

Adrenoleukodystrophy is an X-linked disorder caused by mutations of a gene encoding a peroxisomal protein

These mutations result in impaired β-oxidation of very long-chain fatty acids [38] (see Chap. 41). Affected men may present with symmetrical distal axonal polyneuropathy, adrenocortical insufficiency or CNS demyelination, while occasional heterozygous women demonstrate deficits suggestive of multiple sclerosis. Manipulation of dietary fatty acid intake has had some minimal therapeutic effect, while bone marrow transplantation has diminished deficits in a few patients.

Friedreich's ataxia is an autosomal recessive disorder

This disease is caused by an unstable, expanded GAA repeat in an intron in the frataxin gene on chromosome 9q13. Children with this disease show a symmetrical distal axonal polyneuropathy, corticospinal tract deficits, ataxia and nystagmus [39] (see Chap. 40).

Inherited motor neuron diseases may entail death of motor neurons in the spinal cord and brainstem, resulting in motor axonal degeneration in the peripheral nervous system

Two inherited human motor neuron diseases have been defined. One, *X-linked bulbospinal muscular atrophy,* also termed *Kennedy's syndrome,* like Friedreich's ataxia, is caused by an unstable expanded repeat. The repeat, however, is a CAG, situated in the first exon of the androgen receptor gene. Affected men demonstrate progressive proximal limb and bulbar weakness together with gynecomastia. As in Friedreich's

ataxia and other neurological disorders associated with unstable triplet expansions (see Chap. 40), there is a tendency toward earlier onset and greater severity of symptoms with each succeeding generation in a family, which correlates with increasing repeat number [40]. The second form of human motor neuron disease that has been characterized is a dominantly inherited disorder that is due to gain-of-function mutations of the Cu,Zn superoxide dismutase gene [41].

DISEASES OF THE ENTERIC NERVOUS SYSTEM

The enteric nervous system (ENS) is derived from the neural crest. Neurons in enteric ganglia resemble various classes of CNS neurons in neurotransmitter specificity and growth factor requirements. Enteric neuroglia resemble astroglia in expressing GFAP and glutamine synthetase. Many diseases that affect the PNS also involve the ENS. Among these are infections such as Chagas' disease and herpes simplex and metabolic disorders such as diabetes mellitus, AIP and amyloidosis. Some disorders selectively involve the ENS. Among these is Hirschsprung's disease, which presents typically in infancy with massive segmental dilatation of the colon. The dilatation is the result of segmental absence of colonic enteric ganglia, among the causes of which are mutations of the RET receptor tyrosine kinase and of the endothelin B receptor [42] (tyrosine kinases are discussed in Chap. 25). The observation that most patients with Parkinson's syndrome have a deficiency of dopaminergic ENS neurons [43] may explain the constipation commonly observed and suggests that it may be profitable to investigate the ENS in Alzheimer's disease, Huntington's disease and other chronic neuronal degenerative disorders. These observations draw attention to the ENS as a potential neuronal graft donor site [44].

REFERENCES

1. Shapiro, L., Doyle, J. P., Hensley, P., Colman, D. R., and Hendrickson, W. A. Crystal structure of the extracellular domain from P_0, the major

structural protein of peripheral nerve myelin. *Neuron* 17:435–449, 1996.

2. Voyvodic, J. T. Target size regulates calibre and myelination of sympathetic axons. *Nature* 346:430–433, 1989.

3. de Weegh, S. M., Lee, V. M., and Brady, S. T. Local modulation of neurofilament phosphorylation, axonal caliber, and slow axonal transport by myelinating Schwann cells. *Cell* 68:451–463, 1992.

4. Beniac, D. R., Luckevich, M. D., Czarnota, G. J., et al. Three-dimensional structure of myelin basic protein. I. Reconstruction via angular reconstitution of randomly oriented single particles. *J. Biol. Chem.* 272:4261–4268, 1997.

5. Yang, L. J., Zeller, C. B., Shaper, N. L., et al. Gangliosides are neuronal ligands for myelin-associated glycoprotein. *Proc. Natl. Acad. Sci. USA* 93:814–818, 1996.

6. Shapiro, L., Doyle, J. P., Hensley, P., Colman, D. R., and Hendrickson, W. A. Crystal structure of the extracellular domain from P_0, the major structural protein of peripheral nerve myelin. *Neuron* 17:435–449, 1996.

7. Kamholz, J., Sessa, M., Behrman, T., et al. Structure and expression of proteolipid protein in the peripheral nervous system. *J. Neurosci. Res.* 31:231–244, 1992.

8. Okada, Y., Yamazaki, H., Sekine-Aizawa, Y., and Hirokawa, N. The neuron-specific kinesin superfamily protein K1F1A is a unique monomeric motor for anterograde axonal transport of synaptic vesicle precursors. *Cell* 81:769–780, 1995.

9. Topp, K. S., Meade, L. B., and LaVail, J. H. Microtubule polarity in the peripheral processes of trigeminal ganglion cells: Relevance for the retrograde transport of herpes simplex virus. *J. Neurosci.* 14:318–325, 1994.

10. Grinspan, J. B., Marchionni, M. A., Reeves, M., Coulaloglou, M., and Scherer, S. S. Axonal interactions regulate Schwann cell apoptosis in developing peripheral nerve: Neuregulin receptors and the role of neuregulins. *J. Neurosci.* 16:6107–6118, 1996.

11. Sereda, M., Griffiths, I., Puhlhofer, A., et al. A transgenic rat model of Charcot-Marie-Tooth disease. *Neuron* 16:1049–1060, 1996.

12. Hafer-Macko, C., Hsieh, S. T., Li, C. Y., et al. Acute motor axonal neuropathy: An antibody-mediated attack on axolemma. *Ann. Neurol.* 40:635–644, 1996.

13. Coelho, T. Familial amyloid polyneuropathy: New developments in genetics and treatment. *Curr. Opin. Neurol.* 9:355–359, 1996.

14. Said, G., Goulon-Goeau, C., Lacroix, C., and Moulonguet, A. Nerve biopsy findings in different patterns of proximal diabetic neuropathy. *Ann. Neurol.* 35:559–569, 1994.

15. Bunge, M. B., Wood, P. M., Tynan, L. B., Bates, M. L., and Sanes, J. R. Perineurium originates from fibroblasts: Demonstration *in vitro* with a retroviral marker. *Science* 213:229–231, 1989.

16. Eather, T. F., Pollock, M., and Myers, D. B. Proximal and distal changes in collagen content of peripheral nerve that follow transection and crush lesions. *Exp. Neurol.* 92:299–310, 1986.

17. Gao, W. Q., Dybdal, N., Shinsky, N., et al. Neurotrophin-3 reverses experimental cisplatin-induced peripheral sensory neuropathy. *Ann. Neurol.* 38:30–37, 1995.

18. Helgren, M. E., Cliffer, K. D., Torrento, K., et al. Neurotrophin-3 administration attenuates deficits of pyridoxine-induced large-fiber sensory neuropathy. *J. Neurosci.* 17:372–382, 1997.

19. Montecucco, C., and Schiavo, G. Mechanism of action of tetanus and botulinum neurotoxins. *Mol. Microbiol.* 13:1–8, 1994.

20. Lennon, V. A., Kryzer, T. J., Griesmann, G. E., et al. Calcium-channel antibodies in the Lambert-Eaton syndrome and other paraneoplastic syndromes. *N. Engl. J. Med.* 332:1467–1474, 1995.

21. Lindberg, R. L., Porcher, C., Grandchamp, B., et al. Porphobilinogen deaminase deficiency in mice causes a neuropathy resembling that of human hepatic porphyria. *Nat. Genet.* 12:195–199, 1996.

22. Weishaupt, A., Gold, R., Gaupp, S., Giegerich, G., Hartung, H. P., and Toyka, K. V. Antigen therapy eliminates T cell inflammation by apoptosis: Effective treatment of experimental autoimmune neuritis with recombinant myelin protein P_2. *Proc. Natl. Acad. Sci. USA* 94:1338–1343, 1997.

23. Saida, T., Saida, K., Dorfman, S. H., et al. Experimental allergic neuritis induced by sensitization with galactocerebroside. *Science* 204:1103–1106, 1979.

24. Pahan, K., Khan, M., and Singh, I. Phytanic acid oxidation: Normal activation and transport yet defective alpha-hydroxylation of phytanic acid in peroxisomes from Refsum disease and rhizomelic chondrodysplasia punctata. *J. Lipid Res.* 37:1137–1143, 1996.

25. Chance, P. F., Abbas, N., Lensch, M. W., et al. Two autosomal dominant neuropathies result from reciprocal DNA duplication/deletion of a region on chromosome 17. *Hum. Mol. Genet.* 3:223–228, 1994.

26. Suter, U., Moskow, J. J., Welcher, A. A., et al. A leucine-to-proline mutation in the putative first

transmembrane domain of the 22-kDa peripheral myelin protein in the trembler-J mouse. *Proc. Natl. Acad. Sci. USA* 89:4382–4386, 1992.

27. Bergoffen, J., Scherer, S. S., Wang, S., et al. Connexin mutations in X-linked Charcot-Marie-Tooth disease. *Science* 262:2039–2042, 1993.

28. Cameron, N. E., and Cotter, M. A. Effects of a nonpeptide endothelin-1 ETA antagonist on neurovascular function in diabetic rats: Interaction with the renin-angiotensin system. *J. Pharmacol. Exp. Ther.* 278:1262–1268, 1996.

29. Zochodne, D. W., Cheng, C., and Sun, H. Diabetes increases sciatic nerve susceptibility to endothelin-induced ischemia. *Diabetes* 45:627–632, 1996.

30. Giannini, C., and Dyck, P. J. Ultrastructural morphometric abnormalities of sural nerve endoneurial microvessels in diabetes mellitus. *Ann. Neurol.* 36:408–415, 1994.

31. Pittenger, G. C., Lise, D., and Vinick, A. I. The apoptotic death of neuroblastoma cells caused by serum from patients with insulin-dependent diabetes and neuropathy may be Fas-mediated. *J. Neuroimmunol.* 76:153–160, 1997.

32. Roberts, E. D., Bohm, R. P., Jr., Cogswell, F. B., et al. Chronic lyme disease in the rhesus monkey. *Lab. Invest.* 72:146–160, 1995.

33. Hess, B., Saftig, P., Hartmann, D., et al. Phenotype of arylsulfatase A-deficient mice: Relationship to human metachromatic leukodystrophy. *Proc. Natl. Acad. Sci. USA* 93:14821–14826, 1996.

34. Kim, H. A., Rosenbaum, T., Marchionni, M. A., Ratner, N., and DeClue, J. E. Schwann cells from neurofibromin deficient mice exhibit activation of p21ras, inhibition of cell proliferation and morphological changes. *Oncogene* 11:325–335, 1995.

35. Vogel, K. S., Brannan, C. I., Jenkins, N. A., Copeland, N. G., and Parada, L. F. Loss of neurofibromin results in neurotrophin-independent survival of embryonic sensory and sympathetic neurons. *Cell* 82:733–742, 1995.

36. Rosenbaum, T., Boissy, Y. L., Kombrinck, K., et al. Neurofibromin-deficient fibroblasts fail to form perineurium *in vitro*. *Development* 121:3583–3592, 1995.

37. Lutchman, M., and Rouleau, G. A. Neurofibromatosis type 2: A new mechanism of tumor suppression. *Trends Neurosci.* 19:373–377, 1996.

38. Watkins, P. A., Gould, S. J., Smith, M. A., et al. Altered expression of ALDP in X-linked adrenoleukodystrophy. *Am. J. Hum. Genet.* 57:292–301, 1995.

39. Campuzano, V., Montermini, L., Molto, M. D., et al. Friedreich's ataxia: Autosomal recessive disease caused by an intronic GAA triplet repeat expansion. *Science* 271:1423–1427, 1996.

40. La Spada, A. R., Roling, D. B., Harding, A. E., et al. Meiotic stability and genotype–phenotype correlation of the trinucleotide repeat in X-linked spinal and bulbar muscular atrophy. *Nat. Genet.* 2:301–304, 1992.

41. Yim, M. B., Kang, J. H., Yim, H. S., Kwak, H. S., Chock, P. B., and Stadtman, E. R. A gain-of-function of an amyotrophic lateral sclerosis-associated Cu,Zn-superoxide dismutase mutant: An enhancement of free radical formation due to a decrease in K_m for hydrogen peroxide. *Proc. Natl. Acad. Sci. USA* 93:5709–5714, 1996.

42. Goyal, R. K., and Hirano, I. The enteric nervous system. *N. Engl. J. Med.* 334:1106–1115, 1996.

43. Singaram, C., Ashraf, W., Gaumnitz, E. A., et al. Dopaminergic defect of enteric nervous system in Parkinson's disease patients with chronic constipation. *Lancet* 346:861–864, 1995.

44. Tew, E. M., Anderson, P. N., Saffrey, M. J., and Burnstock, G. Transplantation of the postnatal rat myenteric plexus into the adult rat corpus striatum: An electron microscopy study. *Exp. Neurol.* 129:120–129, 1994.

37

Epileptic Seizures and Epilepsy

Brian Meldrum and Astrid Chapman

Basic Neurochemistry: Molecular, Cellular and Medical Aspects, 6th Ed. edited by G. J. Siegel et al. Published by Lippincott–Raven Publishers, Philadelphia, 1999. Correspondence to Brian Meldrum, Department of Clinical Neurosciences, Institute of Psychiatry, De Crespigny Park, Denmark Hill, London SE5 8AF, United Kingdom.

EPILEPSIES ARE DISORDERS CHARACTERIZED BY SPONTANEOUS, RECURRENT SEIZURES

"Epilepsy" refers to an etiologically and clinically diverse group of neurological disorders characterized by spontaneous, recurrent, paroxysmal cerebral discharges, called seizures. The latter may have varied subjective, behavioral or motor manifestations; but the common factor has been assumed for the last 100 years to be the paroxysmal, excessive and synchronous discharge of a group of neurons. Only limited progress has been made in understanding the molecular and cellular basis of either the proneness to epileptic seizures or their acute manifestations (for detailed reviews, see [1,2]).

EPILEPTOGENESIS

Epilepsy sometimes has a genetic basis

Some forms of epilepsy in humans appear to have an autosomal dominant inheritance. These include *benign familial neonatal convulsions*, 2- to 3-Hz spike and wave absence attacks and juvenile myoclonic epilepsy [3]. Many inborn errors of metabolism are associated with seizures (see below and Chaps. 42 and 44). Genetic factors also contribute to seizures that are secondary to some other ac-

quired pathology, such as a head injury or a space-occupying lesion.

Inbred strains of chickens, rodents and primates can show specific types of reflex or sensory epilepsy. Many specific mutations leading to neurological syndromes with seizures are known in mice.

The approximate chromosomal localization for the genes determining epilepsy is now known for many of the human and murine epileptic syndromes. Mutant genes responsible for three recessive syndromes in mice that show brief spike and wave discharges (SWD) resembling those associated with absence attacks in children have been identified (Table 37-1). In a rare familial syndrome with focal seizures occurring during sleep, termed *autosomal dominant nocturnal frontal lobe epilepsy*, a mutation has been found affecting the α_4 subunit of the nicotinic cholinergic receptor (see Chap. 11). *Benign familial neonatal convulsions* commonly show autosomal dominant inheritance with linkage to chromosome 20q or 8q. On chromosome 20, five different mutations involving a voltage-gated K^+ channel (KCNQ$_2$) have been identified [4,5]. A mutation involving a related K^+ channel gene (KCNQ$_3$) has been found on chromosome 8. The responsible mutation has also been identified in several genetic defects that produce either developmental abnormality (see below) or degenerative changes, as in *progressive myoclonic epilepsy* (Table 37-1). The epilepsy is here secondary to the malformation or degeneration.

TABLE 37-1. EPILEPTIC SYNDROMES IN MICE AND HUMANS WITH SINGLE GENE DEFECTS

Syndrome	Mutation	Phenotype pathology/seizures
Mice		
Lethargic (lh/lh)	VS Ca^{2+} channel β4 subunit	6 to 8 Hz S & W, XS GABA$_B$ receptors
Tottering (tg/tg)	VS Ca^{2+} channel α1A subunit	6 to 8 Hz S & W XS noradrenergic innervation, XS α$_2$, β$_1$, GABA$_A$ subunits
Slow-wave epilepsy	Na$^+$/H$^+$ exchanger	2 to 3 Hz S & W
Humans		
Autosomal dominant nocturnal frontal lobe epilepsy (ADNFLE)	α4 subunit of nAChR serine at 248 in TM2 replaced by phenylalanine	Brief focal seizures during sleep
Benign familial neonatal convulsions (BFNC)	Voltage-gated K$^+$ channel (KCNQ$_2$, KCNQ$_3$)	Generalized seizures from age 3 days to 3 months
Progressive myoclonus epilepsy (EPM1), Unverricht-Lundborg type	Cystatin B (protease inhibitor)	Degeneration in cerebellum and thalamus
Tuberous sclerosis	Tuberin	Neuronal migration defects

VS, voltage sensitive; nAChR, nicotinic acetylcholine receptor; S & W, spike and wave; XS, excess.

Some developmental disorders are associated with epilepsy

The major developmental disorders giving rise to epilepsy are those of neuronal migration [6]. These may have genetic or intrauterine causes. Abnormal patterns of neuronal migration through the cortex give rise to various forms of agyria or pachygyria. In type I lissencephaly, there is a highly abnormal cortex of four layers and a very high incidence of focal or generalized seizures beginning early in childhood. Lesser degrees of failure of neuronal migration represented by neuronal heterotopia in the subcortical white matter may favor the development of primary generalized or focal epilepsies at later stages in life. Tuberous sclerosis is a developmental disorder with an autosomal dominant mutation in the gene for tuberin. This defect leads to focally disordered neuronal migration and, frequently, epilepsy.

Traumatic injury and focal lesions can be epileptogenic

Epilepsy is commonly a delayed consequence of head injury. It has shown a consistent incidence after penetrating head injuries in the major wars of this century. It occurs with a lower incidence after closed head injury. An epileptogenic action of blood or iron may be involved, as may the hyperexcitability that follows cortical deafferentation. The long latent interval between the injury and the onset of epilepsy indicates that slow processes, possibly of degeneration and regeneration, are involved. Other forms of focal injury, including those produced by benign or malignant tumors, by abscesses and by parasitoses such as cerebral malaria and cysticercosis, also can lead to focal epilepsy [6].

Metabolic disorders may trigger seizures

Circumstances impairing energy metabolism may produce cerebral seizures of various types when cerebral functions are partially impaired or may induce tonic spasms or other forms of brainstem seizures when cortical activity has essentially ceased but some brainstem electrical activity persists. These phenomena are seen in hypoglycemia and cerebral hypoxia and when oxidative metabolism is poisoned, as by cyanide or fluorocitrate (see also Chaps. 34 and 38). When seizures are caused by a transient, nonrecurrent metabolic disturbance, the disorder is not referred to as epilepsy.

Certain mitochondrial disorders are characterized by myopathy and myoclonus or seizures, such as myoclonus epilepsy with ragged red fibers in the skeletal muscle (MERRF). The mitochondrial disorders may show maternal transmission. They are biochemically and genetically heterogeneous, but the myopathy and the myoclonus, or epilepsy, are thought to be directly related to defects in the electron-transport chain (see Chap. 42).

A very wide range of other metabolic disorders may show seizures as a secondary feature, ranging from pyridoxine dependence, where a defective synthesis of GABA contributes to the seizures (Chap. 33), to phenylketonuria, where the primary defect is in phenylalanine 4-hydroxylase in the liver (see Chap. 44).

Hyperthermia often lowers the seizure threshold or triggers seizures in human children aged 6 months to 5 years and in young kittens or rodents. The mechanism involved is not known.

EPILEPSY MODELS

Maximal electroshock triggers seizures

A brief electrical pulse delivered via corneal electrodes triggers seizures with tonic hindlimb extension in rodents. Historically, this has been a major test system for screening potential antiepileptic drugs that are active against generalized tonic–clonic seizures in humans.

Convulsions can be induced by drugs

Drugs may act on ion channels or on inhibitory or excitatory neurotransmission (Table 37-2). Potassium channel blockers such as 4-aminopyridine are potent convulsant agents. Convulsions can also be induced by cholinergic agents, most notably by muscarinic agonists, such as pilocarpine, and by cholinesterase inhibitors, such as physostigmine and diisopropylfluorophosphonate (see Chap. 11).

TABLE 37-2.   BIOCHEMICAL ACTIONS OF CONVULSANT DRUGS

Drug	Effect
Drugs that affect ion transport or ionic conductance	
Ouabain	Na,K-ATPase inhibitor
4-Aminopyridine	K^+ channel blocker
Drugs that block energy metabolism	
Fluoroacetate	Inhibits Krebs cycle
Fluorocitrate	Inhibits Krebs cycle
Drugs that block inhibitory transmission	
Strychnine, brucine	Antagonists at glycine receptor in spinal cord
Bicuculline, penicillin	Antagonists at GABA receptor
Convulsant barbiturates (CHEB, DMBB)	Antagonists at GABA complex
Convulsant β-carbolines (DMCM)	Inverse agonists at benzodiazepine site
Allylglycine, 3-mercaptopropionic acid, pyridoxal phosphate antagonists	Block GABA synthesis by inhibiting glutamic acid decarboxylase activity
Tetanus toxin	Blocks GABA release
Drugs that enhance cholinergic excitatory transmission	
Physostigmine, DFP	Anticholinesterases that enhance synaptic acetylcholine concentration
Pilocarpine	Agonist at muscarinic receptor
Drugs that enhance glutamatergic excitatory transmission	
Kainate, domoate	Agonists at kainate receptor
Quisqualate, AMPA	Agonists at AMPA receptor
NMDA, ibotenate, quinolinate	Agonists at NMDA receptor
3,5-Dihydroxyphenylglycine	Agonist at metabotropic receptor

CHEB, 5-(2-cyclohexylidene ethyl)-5-ethyl barbituric acid; DMBB, 5-(1,3-dimethylbutyl)-5 ethyl barbituric acid; DMCM, methyl-6,7-dimethoxy-4-ethyl-β-carboline-3-carboxylate; DFP, diisopropylfluorophosphonate.

Many chemical convulsants impair inhibition mediated by GABA (see Chap. 16). Some do this by blocking its synthesis; 3-mercaptopropionic acid, a competitive inhibitor of glutamic acid decarboxylase (GAD), induces seizures with a short latency, consistent with the very rapid turnover of GABA. Compounds that interfere with the synthesis or coenzymatic function of pyridoxal phosphate induce seizures by impairing GABA synthesis. Compounds such as bicuculline and benzylpenicillin that compete with GABA for binding at the $GABA_A$-recognition sites are powerful convulsants. Convulsions are also produced by certain compounds, termed inverse agonists, that act at the benzodiazepine site. Methyl-6,7-dimethoxy-4-ethyl-β-carboline-3-carboxylate (DMCM) is an example. Yet other convulsants, such as picrotoxin, ethylbicyclophosphate and tetramethylene-disulfotetramine, act at the $GABA_A$ receptor complex to block the chloride ion channel [7].

Agonist compounds acting at glutamate receptors (GluR) are convulsant following intracerebral or systemic injection. Antibodies to $GluR_3$, as found in sera of children with Rasmussen's encephalitis, enhance neuronal excitability and are associated with seizures (Chap. 15). Kainate and domoate, which are synthesized by marine plants, induce limbic seizures, apparently by acting at high-affinity kainate receptors in the CA3 subfield of the hippocampus. Presynaptically, they inhibit GABA release; postsynaptically, they are depolarizing. Eating mussels containing domoate has induced limbic seizures acutely in humans with, in some cases, secondary hippocampal pathology and enduring anterograde amnesia. Seizures can also be induced by agonists acting on the other subtypes of ionotropic receptor, that is, N-methyl-D-aspartate (NMDA) and quinolinate acting on NMDA receptors and quisqualate or α-amino-3-hydroxy-5-methyl-4-isoxazole propionic acid (AMPA) acting on AMPA receptors (see Chap. 15). Type I glutamate metabotropic receptor agonists, such as 3,5-dihydroxyphenylglycine, are convulsant. They are depolarizing and potentiate NMDA receptor responses.

Compounds that act as $GABA_B$ receptor agonists, such as baclofen, facilitate cortical SWDs of the sort associated with absence attacks. This is seen particularly in the model of absence attacks provided by certain Wistar rats.

Seizure-susceptible inbred strains of rodents exhibit spontaneous or evoked seizures

In addition to the incidence of naturally occurring epilepsy in domestic or wild animals, there are strains of rodents that have been selected and bred for seizure susceptibility. Some of the strains exhibit spontaneous seizures, while the majority have seizures in response to a specific stimulus, such as sound or vestibular stimulation, for example, DBA/2 mice, EL mice and genetically epilepsy prone rats. The underlying gene defects responsible for the seizure susceptibility are unknown in these syndromes.

Absence seizures in rodents resemble absence epilepsy in humans

A number of rodent strains exhibit a syndrome with many of the clinical features of human absence epilepsy: similar EEG abnormalities, such as synchronous SWDs accompanied by behavioral arrest; similar corticothalamic distribution of SWD; suppression of SWD by clinical anti-absence drugs, such as ethosuximide and valproate; and in contrast to most clonic–tonic seizures in rodents and humans, aggravation of the syndrome by agonists acting at the $GABA_A$ and $GABA_B$ receptors. However, $GABA_B$ antagonists, including some saclofen derivatives, suppress SWD.

Single-gene mutations in voltage-sensitive calcium ion channels form the basis of spontaneous absence seizures in two of the mouse strains (lh/lh and tg/tg) as shown in Table 37-1.

After an initial episode of severe status epilepticus, rats develop recurrent, spontaneous seizures

Recurrent, spontaneous limbic seizures in rats after an earlier episode of prolonged status epilepticus (SE), which is typically induced by a convulsant dose of the cholinergic drug pilocarpine or by the glutamatergic agonist kainic acid, resemble complex partial epilepsy developing after prolonged febrile convulsions in childhood. There is a similar delayed development of seizures, a similar pathology including mossy fiber sprouting and a similar antiepileptic pharmacology [8]. The spontaneous seizures in this model are accompanied by enhanced glutamate release measured by *in vivo* microdialysis (see below).

Kindling, which is recurrent, subconvulsant stimulation, provides an experimental model of epileptogenesis

A brief burst of electrical stimulation sufficient to induce a local after discharge but not sufficient to trigger a seizure will eventually trigger a seizure if repeated frequently. This phenomenon is referred to as "kindling" [9]. It can be most readily induced by stimulating the structures that comprise the limbic system. The changes responsible for the lowered seizure threshold occur diffusely in the brain and are permanent. They appear to involve voltage-sensitive ion channels and several neurotransmitter systems, including GABA, acetylcholine and glutamate. Enhanced sensitivity of NMDA and metabotropic glutamate receptors (see Chap. 15) is particularly important in facilitating epileptiform discharges [10]. Some of the changes related to synaptic function in the kindled brain are listed in Table 37-3.

The kindling process is a model for epileptogenesis and, like long-term potentiation (LTP) (see Chap. 50), it is dependent on activation of NMDA receptors. It can be retarded or pre-

vented by the administration of NMDA receptor antagonists prior to the episodes of kindling stimulation [11].

Spontaneous seizures are observed in transgenic mice with a wide range of gene deletions or overexpressions

Mice with deletion of the β_3 subunit of the $GABA_A$ receptor are behaviorally abnormal and show seizures [12], as do mice with K^+-channel deletions, such as MKv1.1 and inward rectifying K^+ channel 2 (GIRK2). Limbic seizures are observed in mice with a deletion of Ca^{2+}/calmodulin-dependent kinase II [13]. These observations help to identify candidate genes or gene classes that may be mutated in human genetic syndromes (reviewed in [14]). Thus, the Angelman syndrome, which is a neurodevelopmental disorder with mental retardation and epilepsy, has a deletion on chromosome 15q that includes the $GABA_A$ β_3 subunit. Data from knockout mice suggest that this loss contributes to the onset of seizures.

BASIC ELECTROPHYSIOLOGY

Macroelectrodes show spikes, while intracellular microelectrodes show paroxysmal depolarizing shifts

Macroelectrodes on the scalp, on the cerebral surface or in the depths of the brain record the net resultant electrical potential of many cells around the electrode. These records show high-voltage spikes as the most characteristic feature of epilepsy. These spikes may occur in isolation, in continuous or rhythmic bursts or in association with intervening slow waves. Intracellular records show that, corresponding to the macrorecordings of spikes, episodes that look like giant excitatory synaptic potentials occur synchronously in many single cells. These are referred to as "paroxysmal depolarizing shifts." Intracellular records show a large, sustained depolarization of the membrane associated with a burst of action potentials, which are largely Na^+-dependent at the begin-

---

TABLE 37-3.   **SYNAPTIC FUNCTIONAL CHANGES IN KINDLED RATS**

Enhancement of
  Voltage-sensitive Ca^{2+} conductance
  Glutamate metabotropic polyphosphoinositide hydrolysis
  Glutamate release in hippocampus (CA3)
  GABA release in hippocampus (CA1)
  Sensitivity of NMDA receptors in hippocampus (dentate granule cells, CA3 pyramidal cells)
  Protein kinase C activity
Decrease in
  Calbindin immunoreactivity in hippocampus
  Type II Ca^{2+}/calmodulin kinase activity

ning of the burst and Ca^{2+}-dependent at the end (see also Chap. 10).

Ionic movements occur in brain during seizures

Measurements with ion-specific electrodes in brain slices or *in vivo* show that there is a drop in the extracellular concentration of calcium ion, $[Ca^{2+}]_e$, that begins at the same time the seizure discharge is recorded. The fall is significant in more or less all types of epilepsy and in some cases can be so marked as to probably prevent presynaptic release of neurotransmitters [15]. Extracellular $[K^+]$ rises, often with a slight delay compared to $[Ca^{2+}]_e$, and reaches a plateau around 10 to 12 mM (Table 37-4). There is also a moderate fall in $[Na^+]_e$ and a smaller rise in $[Cl^-]_e$ (see Chaps. 5 and 6).

Inhibition and excitation have roles in the synaptic synchronization that spreads through anatomical networks

Multiple recordings in hippocampus or cortex show that during a seizure many neurons fire synchronously, as a result of synchronous excitatory inputs. This pattern of activity may spread locally by progressive recruitment in the cortex or by spread from the CA3 to the CA1 subfield in the hippocampus. Spread also occurs by distal recruitment of subcortical or limbic structures. *In vitro* studies with hippocampal or cortical slices have shown that the initiation and spread of synchronous discharges can be facilitated by ionic changes, such as high $[K^+]_e$ or low $[Mg^{2+}]_e$; by factors decreasing GABA-mediated inhibition; or by factors enhancing excitation, such as the enhanced sensitivity of the NMDA

TABLE 37-4. TYPICAL METABOLIC RESPONSE TO ONSET OF SEIZURES

Extracellular ion concentrations *(immediate onset)*

Calcium influx	Decrease from 1.3 to 0.6–0.8 mM
Potassium efflux	Increase from 3 to 8–12 mM

Metabolic rate parameters *(immediate onset, sustained at elevated rates for duration of seizure activity)*

Cerebral blood flow	2- to 3-fold increase, initially higher
Oxygen consumption	2- to 3-fold increase
Glucose consumption	2- to 3-fold increase, initially higher

Metabolite tissue concentrations *(immediate onset, usually transient with partial recovery)*

Phosphocreatine	Decrease (30 to 50%)
ATP	Decrease (10%)
Glucose, glycogen	Decrease (30 to 70%), sustained
Lactate	Increase (3- to 10-fold), sustained
Free fatty acids (18:0, 20:4)	Increase (2- to 4-fold)
Prostaglandins (PGF$_2\alpha$, PGE$_2$, PGD$_2$)	Increase (20- to 100-fold)
cAMP, cGMP	Increase (3- to 5-fold)
Adenosine, inosine, hypoxanthine	Increase (10- to 300-fold)

Amino acid tissue concentrations *(gradual onset 1 to 30 min, varied response according to model)*

Glutamate, aspartate	Usually decrease
Glutamine	Usually increase
GABA	Often increase

Transmitter release (extracellular concentrations measured by microdialysis; *immediate onset, transient change, more pronounced in chronic seizure models; conflicting results in acute seizure models*)

Glutamate, aspartate	Usually increase
GABA	Usually increase
Noradrenaline	Usually increase
Dopamine	Usually increase

Gene expression *(gradual onset 10 to 60 min)*

Induction of immediate early genes (*c-fos, c-jun, junB*), heat shock protein, neurotrophins (neurotrophin 3, nerve growth factor), dynorphin, GAP-43, ornithine decarboxylase, proteases, lipases, protein kinases, calcium-binding proteins, nitric oxide synthase

Generalized seizures, global changes; focal seizures, changes restricted to brain regions involved in seizure progression.

receptor induced by low $[Mg^{2+}]_e$ (see Chaps. 15 and 16).

CHANGES IN NEUROTRANSMITTER SYSTEMS UNDERLYING EPILEPSY

GABA and benzodiazepine receptors decrease in some conditions

A decrease in the relative proportion of GABAergic terminals has been observed in cortical epileptic foci induced in monkeys with alumina cream. However, there do not appear to be any similar, consistent decreases in the temporal lobes of humans with complex partial epilepsy, the principal form of focal epilepsy in humans [16]. It is proposed that GABAergic interneurons in the hippocampus become "dormant" through failure of their excitatory input [17].

Decreases in ligand binding to benzodiazepine receptors in the midbrain have been shown by autoradiography in certain rodent species with genetic epilepsy. Patients with complex partial seizures show decreases in benzodiazepine receptor density in the temporal lobe as measured by flumazenil binding in positron emission tomography (PET) studies [18] (see Chap. 54).

Glutamate sensitivity at *N*-methyl-D-aspartate receptors may increase

An increased sensitivity to the action of glutamate at NMDA receptors is seen in hippocampal slices from kindled rats and in cortical slices from, or adjacent to, cortical foci in human epilepsy [19]. This leads to an enhanced entry of Ca^{2+} into neurons during synaptic activity [20] (see Chap. 15).

Noradrenergic innervation may increase or decrease in rodent models

In various genetically determined rodent models of epilepsy, either excesses or deficiencies of noradrenergic innervation may be found. In the *tottering mouse*, an absence-like syndrome consisting of intermittent episodes of behavioral arrest associated with 6- to 7-Hz cortical spike-wave EEG discharges is linked to a noradrenergic hyperinnervation of the forebrain. Selective destruction of the ascending noradrenergic system at birth prevents the onset of the syndrome in the adolescent mouse, implying a causal role for the noradrenergic abnormality, although the genetic defect involves a voltage-sensitive Ca^{2+} channel.

Opioid peptides have both convulsant and anticonvulsant actions

In experimental studies, opioids and opioid peptides have both convulsant and anticonvulsant actions. Peptides with a μ agonist action given intraventricularly induce hippocampal or limbic seizures, perhaps by inhibiting interneurons. In patients with complex partial seizures, μ receptor density is increased in the temporal cortex, as shown by [11C]-carfentanil binding in PET studies [21]. Opioid peptides and their receptors are discussed further in Chapter 18.

ANTICONVULSANT DRUG MECHANISMS

About 16 drugs are in clinical use as antiepileptic medications (Table 37-5). Some are effective predominantly in complex partial seizures and generalized tonic–clonic seizures; these include phenytoin, barbiturates, carbamazepine and vigabatrin. Those used in SE include the benzodiazepines; those used predominantly in absence seizures include ethosuximide and trimethadione; and those broadly active include valproate and lamotrigine. These drugs are largely derived from animal screening tests employing acutely induced electrical or chemical seizures [22]. Their mechanisms of action are only partially understood (Table 37-5). Some act predominantly on ion channels in the neuronal membrane; others act on synaptic transmission [23]. Phenytoin, carbamazepine and lamotrigine suppress rapid repetitive firing in cultured neurons by prolonging the inactivation time of Na^+ channels (see Chap. 6). Ethosuximide and related drugs that suppress absence seizures decrease activity in voltage-sensitive Ca^{2+} channels

TABLE 37-5. **ANTICONVULSANT DRUGS: MECHANISMS OF ACTION**

Drug	Na$^+$ channel[a]	Ca^{2+} channel[b] T	Ca^{2+} channel[b] N, P/Q	GABA[c]	Glutamate[d]
Phenytoin	++				
Carbamazepine	++				
Lamotrigine	++		+		
Valproate	++				
Ethosuximide		++			
Phenobarbitone	+			+	+
Diazepam	+			++	
Vigabatrin				(++)	
Tiagabine				(++)	
Topiramate	+			+	+

[a] Prolonged inactivation of the voltage-dependent Na$^+$ channel.
[b] Blockade of the T calcium current or of the N, P/Q calcium currents.
[c] Enhancement of GABA-mediated inhibition, by inhibition of GABA-transaminase with vigabatrin and of GABA uptake with tiagabine.
[d] Antagonist action at the AMPA receptor.
++, Strong action at clinically relevant concentration; +, action of possible significance.

of the T type [24]. Benzodiazepines and barbiturates enhance inhibition mediated via GABA/benzodiazepine receptors. Antagonists of excitatory amino acid neurotransmission, acting on glutamate receptors of the NMDA or non-NMDA type, are also anticonvulsant in animal models of epilepsy, but their clinical usefulness is not yet identified. Acetazolamide has a modest anticonvulsant action in absence seizures, apparently due to inhibition of carbonic anhydrase activity and the resultant in changes in pH.

METABOLIC CONSEQUENCES OF SEIZURES

Energy metabolism in the discharge pathway is massively increased during seizures

During seizure activity, there is a greater increase in cerebral metabolic rate (CMR) than under any other circumstance (see Chaps. 31 and 54). This is seen in measurements of oxygen consumption (CMRO$_2$) and glucose uptake and metabolism (reviewed in [25]). It is also reflected in a marked increase in cerebral blood flow (CBF). The metabolic activation is confined to the brain regions involved in the seizure propagation; for example, during limbic seizures, such as those in-

duced by kainic acid, the increases in CBF and CMRO$_2$ and the metabolic changes described in Table 37-4 are confined to the limbic system. In contrast, generalized, global seizures cause metabolic activation to a varying degree in all brain regions. During seizures, there is commonly both an increase in arterial blood pressure and a marked local vasodilation, the latter partly due to local formation of nitric oxide and adenosine. The increase in CBF often exceeds the increase in CMRO$_2$ so that the oxygen content of the venous blood is increased. Provided that arterial blood pressure, arterial oxygenation and blood glucose concentration are maintained, this enhanced metabolism can also be maintained in excess of an hour of seizure activity.

Energy metabolites decrease rapidly

Despite the sharp increase in oxygen and glucose supply to the brain, the massive increase in energy demand associated with the onset of seizure activity causes a rapid fall in brain energy metabolites. Tissue stores of glycogen and glucose are rapidly depleted, and concentrations of phosphocreatine and, to a lesser extent, ATP fall rapidly and transiently. Associated with the fall in nucleotide is a concomitant sharp rise in nucleosides, including adenosine and free bases, for example, hypoxanthine.

Concentrations of lactate and certain amino acids change rapidly

Seizure activity is associated with a doubling or more of brain lactate, ammonia and alanine contents within 1 min [25]. There is a modest fall in the intracellular pH at the same time. The lactate increase occurs in the absence of hypoxia and reflects the relatively greater increase in the glycolytic rate than in $CMRO_2$, the maximally activated pyruvic acid dehydrogenase being the rate-limiting step. Glutamate, aspartate and GABA concentrations initially remain constant, but if seizure activity is prolonged, glutamate and aspartate usually fall and glutamine and GABA rise [26].

Second messengers change rapidly

There are dramatic changes in all of the second messengers that reflect increased release of neurotransmitters acting on metabotropic receptors within the first minute of seizure activity (see Chaps. 10, 15 and 20–22). Increases in cAMP are partly due to activation of α-adrenergic receptors (see Chap. 12). Increases in cGMP are partly due to formation of nitric oxide, following ionotropic glutamate receptor (NMDA) activation. Activation of glutamate, α_1-adrenergic or muscarinic metabotropic receptors causes phospholipase C (PLC) activation and phosphoinositide breakdown (see Chaps. 21 and 35). The lipase activity results in the formation of diacylglycerol, which activates protein kinase C, and of inositolphosphate, which causes release of Ca^{2+} from nonmitochondrial stores (see Chap. 23). There is also a marked increase in intracellular Ca^{2+} concentration, $[Ca^{2+}]_i$, due to enhanced Ca^{2+} entry, through receptor and voltage-operated calcium ion channels (see Chap. 23).

The effects of these changes are to phosphorylate many enzymes, ion channels and cell membrane receptors and to directly activate calcium-dependent enzymes (see Chap. 24). Among the latter is phospholipase A_2, leading to the formation of free fatty acids, in particular arachidonic acid (see below and Chap. 35).

Free fatty acids and prostaglandins increase

Primarily due to activation of phospholipases, free fatty acids are liberated during seizure activity. The greatest increase during seizures induced by electroshock or bicuculline is in the unsaturated fatty acid arachidonic acid, 20:4, which acts as a precursor for various prostaglandins (Table 37-4) (see Chaps. 34 and 35).

Release of neurotransmitter amino acids is rapidly increased at the beginning of a seizure

The synaptic release of amino acid neurotransmitters was studied by *in vivo* microdialysis. In patients with epileptic foci in the temporal lobe, the extracellular hippocampal concentrations of glutamate and aspartate increase directly prior to or at the moment of seizure onset; the extracellular concentration of GABA rises with a slight delay in both the epileptic focus and the contralateral temporal lobe [27]. A similar enhanced release of aspartate, glutamate and GABA is seen associated with the onset of seizures in chronically seizure-prone rodents, kindled rats or rats with spontaneous, recurrent seizures. It is more difficult to demonstrate an enhanced release of excitatory amino acids or GABA at the onset of acute, evoked seizures in rats, perhaps due to an optimally functioning amino acid-transporter system during these conditions.

Seizures produce changes in gene expression and protein synthesis

Seizure activity has a dramatic effect on gene transcription. This has been studied in rats by *in situ* hybridization with mRNA probes (see Chap. 26). There are increases in expression of the immediate early genes c-*fos,* c-*jun, junB* and tissue plasminogen activator (tPA) in many structures involved in seizure activity, notably in the granule cells of the dentate gyrus (Table 37-4). Immunocytochemistry with specific antisera reveals that synthesis of the proteins en-

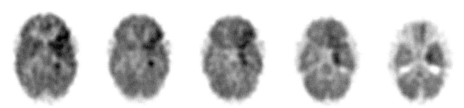

FIGURE 37-1. Ictal PET scan images with [^{18}F]2-fluoro-2-deoxy-D-glucose. The scan, performed during continuous partial seizures originating in the left frontal and temporal cortices, shows asymmetrical hypermetabolism of the left frontal motor cortex, orbitofrontal cortex and hippocampus (right side of images). There are secondary activations of the ipsilateral basal ganglia and the contralateral cerebellum. Biopsy showed Rasmussen's encephalitis. (Courtesy of Dr. K. A. Frey.)

coded by the immediate early genes is also enhanced [28].

There are also selective increases in the mRNAs for various trophic factors, such as nerve growth factor and neurotrophin 3. These factors are detailed in Chapter 19. These changes have a longer latency of approximately 1 hr and a longer duration than the changes in the immediate early genes. With a longer latency still, there are increases in the expression of the genes encoding various peptide neurotransmitters and their precursors (Table 37-4) (see also Chap. 18).

Although the synthesis of some proteins, such as those mentioned above and the enzyme ornithine decarboxylase, is increased by seizures, the synthesis of most proteins is impaired during or after prolonged seizures in rats or newborn marmosets. When studied with labeled amino acid precursors and autoradiography, protein synthesis is impaired in those regions showing the greatest metabolic activa-

tion. The rate of protein synthesis depends on the cellular GDP:GTP ratio, with GDP increases being inhibitory.

Positron emission tomography studies show ictal hypermetabolism and interictal hypometabolism

PET (see Chap. 54) can be used to study the regional metabolism of the human brain during seizures and in the interictal period (Figs. 37-1 and 37-2). Regional glucose uptake can be studied with [^{18}F]fluorodeoxyglucose and oxygen extraction with [^{15}O]oxygen (see Chap. 31). In partial epilepsy, enhanced metabolism is usually seen in the zone of seizure initiation during a seizure. Interictal studies in partial epilepsy commonly show a large zone of hypometabolism, which may be more extensive than the presumed focal zone. Children with absence attacks show a marked diffuse increase in cerebral metabolism during

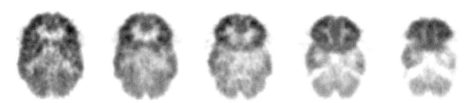

FIGURE 37-2. Interictal PET scan images with [^{18}F]2-fluoro-2-deoxy-D-glucose. The images depict typical reduction in metabolic rate in both the mesial and lateral temporal cortex on the side of the seizure focus (right side of images). Note also the bilateral reduction in cerebellar metabolic rate, which is seen in approximately one third of patients with epilepsy refractory to anticonvulsant medication. Surgical specimen showed hippocampal sclerosis. (Courtesy of Dr. K. A. Frey.)

the attack and normal interictal metabolism [2].

PATHOLOGICAL CHANGES SECONDARY TO SEIZURES OR RELATED TO EPILEPTOGENESIS

Status epilepticus causes damage in vulnerable neurons

It has long been known that a very prolonged severe seizure can induce nerve cell death in selectively vulnerable neurons [29]. These include pyramidal neurons in hippocampus CA1; neurons in amygdala; small pyramidal neurons in cortical laminae III, V and VI; cerebellar Purkinje cells; and some thalamic nuclei [4]. Such damage is commonly seen in children or adults experiencing SE lasting more than 2 hr especially if the body temperature is elevated.

Brain injury of a similar nature can be reproduced in rats or baboons by inducing seizures lasting over 1.5 hr with chemical convulsants such as bicuculline, allylglycine, kainate or pilocarpine. The early cellular changes are characteristic of excitotoxic damage (see Chap. 34), that is, postsynaptic changes involving focal dendritic swelling, mitochondrial dilation and Ca^{2+} accumulation. Such changes are seen 1 to 4 hr after SE in most of the selectively vulnerable neurons, for example, the CA1 and CA3 subfields of the hippocampus. Subsequently, proliferation of astrocytes and microglia may be seen.

Many experimental studies have shown that selective neuronal death in the hippocampus is related to the local excessive neuronal discharge and not to systemic or local vascular factors. Excessive entry of Ca^{2+} and failure of intracellular calcium buffering and of ATP-dependent Ca^{2+} extrusion (see Chap. 23) are thought to be key events [29]. Activation by Ca^{2+} of proteases, such as calpain, protein kinases and phospholipases, is thought to play a role in determining cell death (see Chaps. 23 and 34). NMDA receptor antagonists (see Chap. 15) can prevent most of the epileptic damage even when kainate is used to induce seizures, and their overall duration is not decreased by the NMDA antagonist [29], indicating that the burst pattern of firing and the activation of NMDA receptors play crucial roles in causing the damage.

Febrile convulsions in early childhood are normally benign. If they are repeated within 24 hr or prolonged for more than 30 min, especially if unilateral, they may be associated with a higher incidence in later childhood and adolescence of either primary, generalized tonic–clonic seizures or complex, partial temporal lobe seizures. Experimental studies support the concept that prolonged or closely repeated febrile convulsions give rise to cell loss in the CA1 and hilar regions of the hippocampus and that this lesion may subsequently be a cause of focal limbic seizures.

Epileptogenesis is associated with regenerative sprouting in the hippocampus

A regenerative phenomenon referred to as "sprouting" is seen in the kindling model of epilepsy after focal hippocampal damage following kainate seizures and in the hippocampus of patients with temporal lobe epilepsy [6]. This particularly concerns the mossy fiber system, which contains the axons that derive from the dentate granule cells and that stain for zinc with Timm's stain and for dynorphin by immunocytochemistry. This sprouting becomes prominent in the inner molecular layer of the dentate gyrus and in the dendritic fields of CA1. This axonal sprouting may be in response to enhanced release of growth factors triggered by seizure activity or it may be a response to local degeneration of terminals (see also Chaps. 19 and 29). The new terminals are excitatory but may be ending on inhibitory interneurons. A loss of certain types of hilar interneurons, which contain somatostatin and neuropeptide Y, may be functionally important as these normally provide an excitatory feedback to inhibitory interneurons.

The changes that follow injury and contribute to epileptogenesis are very complex. Multiple changes in ion channels, receptors and neuronal morphology have been identified, but the significance of these changes cannot yet be specified.

REFERENCES

1. Delgado-Escueta, A. V., Wilson, W. A., Olsen, R. W., and Porter, R. (eds.) *Basic Mechanisms of the Epilepsies.* New York: Lippincott-Raven, 1998.

2. Engel, J. *Seizures and Epilepsy.* Philadelphia: F. A. Davis, 1989.

3. Noebels, J. L. Molecular genetics and epilepsy. In T. A. Pedley and B. S. Meldrum (eds.), *Recent Advances in Epilepsy*, Vol. 5. Edinburgh: Churchill-Livingstone, 1992, pp. 1–13.

4. Singh, N. A., Charlier, C., Stauffer, D., et al. A novel potassium channel gene *KCNQ2* is mutated in an inherited epilepsy of newborns. *Nature Gen.* 18:25–29, 1998.

5. Bievert, C., Schroeder, B. C., Kubisch, C. et al. A potassium channel mutation in neonatal human epilepsy. *Science* 279:403-406, 1998.

6. Honavar, M., and Meldrum, B. S. Epilepsy. In D. I. Graham and P. L. Lantos (eds.), *Greenfield's Neuropathology*, 6th ed. London: Edward Arnold, 1997, pp. 931–971.

7. Meldrum, B. Epilepsy. In A. N. Davison and H. S. Thompson (eds.), *The Molecular Basis of Neuropathology.* London: Edward Arnold, 1981, pp. 265–301.

8. Cavalheiro, E. A., Leite, J. P., Bortolotto, Z. A., Turski, W. A., Ikonomidou, C., and Turski, L. Long-term effects of pilocarpine in rats: Structural damage of the brain triggers kindling and spontaneous recurrent seizures. *Epilepsia* 32:778–782, 1991.

9. Wada, J. *Kindling 3.* New York: Raven Press, 1985.

10. Akiyama, K., Daigen, A., Yamada, N., et al. Long-lasting enhancement of metabotropic excitatory amino acid receptor-mediated polyphosphoinositide hydrolysis in the amygdala/pyriform cortex of deep prepyriform cortical kindled rats. *Brain Res.* 569:71–77, 1992.

11. Holmes, K. H., Bilkey, D. K., Laverty, R., and Goddard, G. V. The *N*-methyl-D-aspartate antagonists aminophosphonovalerate and carboxypiperazinephosphate retard the development and expression of kindled seizures. *Brain Res.* 506:227–235, 1990.

12. Homanics, G. E., DeLorey, T. M., Firestone, L. L., et al. Mice devoid of gamma-aminobutyrate type A receptor B3 subunit have epilepsy, cleft palate, and hypersensitive behavior. *Proc. Natl. Acad. Sci. USA* 94:4143–4148, 1997.

13. Butler, L. S., Silva, A. J., Abeliovich, A., Watanabe, Y., Tonegawa, S., and McNamara, J. O. Limbic epilepsy in transgenic mice carrying a Ca^{2+}/calmodulin-dependent kinase II alpha subunit mutation. *Proc. Natl. Acad. Sci. USA* 92:6852–6855, 1995.

14. Noebels, J. L. Targeting epilepsy genes. *Neuron* 16:241–244, 1996.

15. Heinemann, U. Changes in the neuronal microenvironment and epileptiform activity. In H. G. Wieser, E. J. Speckmann, and J. Engel (eds.), *The Epileptic Focus.* London: John Libbey, 1987, pp. 27–44.

16. Babb, T. L. Research on the anatomy and pathology of epileptic tissue. In H. Luders (ed.), *Neurosurgery of Epilepsy.* New York: Raven Press, 1991, p. 719.

17. Sloviter, R. S. Permanently altered hippocampal structure, excitability, and inhibition after experimental status epilepticus in the rat: The "dormant basket cell" hypothesis and its possible relevance to temporal lobe epilepsy. *Hippocampus* 1:41–66, 1991.

18. Savic, I., Widen, L., Thorell, J. O., Blomqvist, G., Ericson, K., and Roland, P. Cortical benzodiazepine receptor binding in patients with generalized and partial epilepsy. *Epilepsia* 31:724–730, 1990.

19. Hwa, G. G., and Avoli, M. Excitatory synaptic transmission mediated by NMDA and non-NMDA receptors in the superficial/middle layers of the epileptogenic human neocortex maintained *in vitro. Neurosci. Lett.* 143:83–86, 1992.

20. Louvel, J., and Pumain, R. *N*-Methyl-D-aspartate-mediated responses in epileptic cortex in man: An *in vitro* study. In S. Avanzini, J. Engel, J., R. Forello, and U. Heinemann (eds.), *Neurotransmitters in Epilepsy.* Amsterdam: Elsevier, 1992, pp. 361–367.

21. Mayberg, H. S., Sadzot, B., Meltzer, C. C., et al. Quantification of mu and non-mu opiate receptors in temporal lobe epilepsy using positron emission tomography. *Ann. Neurol.* 30:3–11, 1991.

22. Meldrum, B. S. Identification and preclinical testing of novel antiepileptic compounds. In *4th International Merritt-Putnam Symposium: The Development of Antiepileptic Drugs. Current Status and Future Directions (Epilepsia* Supplement). Philadelphia: Lippincott-Raven, 1997, pp. S7–S15.

23. Macdonald, R. L., and Meldrum, B. S. General principles. Principles of antiepileptic drug action. In R. Levy, R. Mattson, and B. Meldrum (eds.), *Antiepileptic Drugs*, 4th ed. New York: Raven Press, 1995, pp. 61–77.

24. Coulter, D. A., Huguenard, J. R., and Prince, D. A. Differential effects of petit mal anticonvulsants and convulsants on thalamic neurones: Calcium current reduction. *Br. J. Pharmacol.* 100:800–806, 1990.

25. Chapman, A. G. Cerebral energy metabolism and seizures. In T. A. Pedley, and B. S. Meldrum (eds.), *Recent Advances in Epilepsy.* Edinburgh: Churchill-Livingstone, 1985, pp. 19–63.

26. Chapman, A. G., Meldrum, B. S., and Siesjo, B. K. Cerebral metabolic changes during prolonged epileptic seizures in rats. *J. Neurochem.* 28:1025–1035, 1977.

27. During, M. J., and Spencer, D. D. Extracellular hippocampal glutamate and spontaneous seizure in the conscious human brain. *Lancet* 341:1607–1610, 1993.

28. Kiessling, M., and Gass, P. Immediate early gene expression in experimental epilepsy. *Brain Pathol.* 3:381–393, 1993.

29. Meldrum, B. S. Epileptic brain damage: A consequence and a cause of seizures. The first Alfred Meyer Memorial Lecture. *Neuropathol. Appl. Neurobiol.* 23:185–202, 1997.

38

Metabolic Encephalopathies

Roger F. Butterworth

Basic Neurochemistry: Molecular, Cellular and Medical Aspects, 6th Ed., edited by G. J. Siegel et al. Published by Lippincott–Raven Publishers, Philadelphia, 1999. Correspondence to Roger F. Butterworth, Clinical Research Center, University of Montreal, Campus Saint-Luc, 1058 Rue Saint Denis, Montreal, Quebec H2X 3J4, Canada.

The metabolic encephalopathies comprise a series of neurological disorders not caused by primary structural abnormalities; rather, they result from systemic illness, such as diabetes, liver disease, renal failure and heart failure (Table 38-1). Metabolic encephalopathies usually develop acutely or subacutely and are reversible if the systemic disorder is treated. If left untreated, however, metabolic encephalopathies may result in secondary structural damage to the brain.

There are two major types of metabolic encephalopathies, namely those due to lack of glucose, oxygen or metabolic cofactors (which are usually vitamin-derived) and those due to peripheral organ dysfunction (Table 38-1).

Abnormalities of brain chemistry sufficient to cause encephalopathy and coma are numerous and represent a wide array of disorders. Vitamin deficiencies (Chap. 33), inherited disease, (Chaps. 40, 41 and 44) and some neuroendocrine disorders (Chap. 49) may at some stage disrupt brain metabolic processes and result in encephalopathy. Exposure to various heavy metals and organic solvents also may cause a toxic encephalopathy. Of particular significance is ethanol because it is widely used and, in excessive amounts, can produce permanent brain damage, particularly in association with avitaminoses and malnutrition (see Chap. 33). Clinically, hepatic encephalopathy secondary to alcoholic cirrhosis is not infrequently associated with brain damage resulting from previous acute alcoholic episodes.

Clinical signs and symptoms of metabolic encephalopathies consist of a generalized depression of cerebral function, including consciousness. The effects on consciousness may be a consequence of decreased integrative capacity of the neocortex [1]. Arousal of the neocortex and other forebrain structures involved in cognition is mediated by specific brainstem nuclei and their projecting fiber tracts, which together constitute the ascending reticular activating system (ARAS). Activating pathways ascend from the ARAS via thalamic synaptic relays to the neocortex. Metabolic encephalopathies result from alterations of brain chemistry at both neocortical and brainstem ARAS centers. Respiration may be diminished and pupils appear small but reactive. As encephalopathy progresses, asterixis, also termed "flapping tremor," is encountered, particularly in hepatic disease, uremia and sedative intoxication. Asterixis results from the loss of postural tone in voluntary muscles of the limbs, trunk, head or tongue. More advanced stages of metabolic encephalopathy may be characterized by seizures, for example, in hypoglycemia, acute liver failure and, ultimately, Cheyne-Stokes pattern of respiration resulting from loss of brainstem respiratory control. In addition, many metabolic encephalopathies, including those caused by vitamin deficiencies and ingestion of toxic substances, are characterized by focal metabolic changes in basal ganglia and cerebellar structures, resulting in disorders of movement control and coordination. Vitamin deficiencies and their effects on CNS function are discussed in Chapter 33.

BRAIN ENERGY METABOLISM

The brain has an absolute dependence on the blood for its immediate supply of oxygen and energy substrates. Interruption of oxygen or substrate supply by compromise of pulmonary or cardiovascular function or metabolic factors results in encephalopathy and, ultimately, cell death. The brain utilizes approximately 20% of the total oxygen supply of the body. While glucose remains the primary energy substrate for the brain, alternative substrates may be used, under certain circumstances. For example, in the developmental period as well as during fast-

TABLE 38-1.	CLASSIFICATION OF THE MAJOR METABOLIC ENCEPHALOPATHIES

Due to lack of glucose, oxygen or metabolic cofactors
　Hypoglycemia
　Ischemia
　Hypoxia
　Hypercapnia
　Vitamin deficiencies
Due to peripheral organ dysfunction
　Hepatic encephalopathy
　Uremic and dialysis encephalopathies

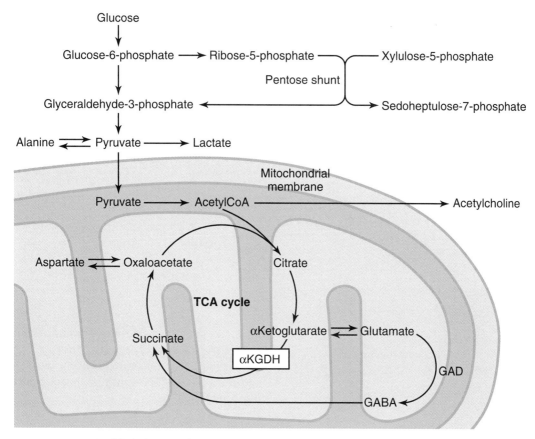

FIGURE 38-1. Simplified schematic diagram of the major metabolic pathways linking glycolysis and tricarboxylic acid (*TCA*) cycle flux to the synthesis of neurotransmitters: acetylcholine, GABA, glutamate and aspartate. *αKGDH,* α-ketoglutarate dehydrogenase; *GAD,* glutamic acid decarboxylase.

ing in the adult, ketone bodies are generated and blood concentrations may become sufficiently high to afford an alternative energy substrate. The appropriate enzymes required for ketone body utilization are maintained in both developing and adult brain in readiness for an emergency such as prolonged fasting or starvation. In conditions such as hypoglycemia, alternative energy substrates, such as glycogen and amino acids, may be used, but the limited pool size and compartmentation of these substrates limits their ability to support cerebral energy requirements (Chap. 31).

Given the high dependency of cerebral energy production and neurotransmitter synthesis on glucose and oxygen (Fig. 38-1), any limitations in the supply of these substrates can result in metabolic encephalopathy.

HYPOGLYCEMIC ENCEPHALOPATHY

Hypoglycemia usually results from insulin overdose, hepatic disease resulting in decreased hepatic gluconeogenesis or renal disease

Hypoglycemia is sometimes encountered in other medical conditions, such as malignancies and chronic alcoholism. Early clinical signs in hypoglycemia reflect the appearance of physiological protective mechanisms initiated by hypothalamic sensory nuclei [1]. Such symptoms include sweating, also termed diaphoresis, tachycardia, anxiety and hunger. If unheeded, these symptoms give way to a more serious CNS disorder progressing through confusion,

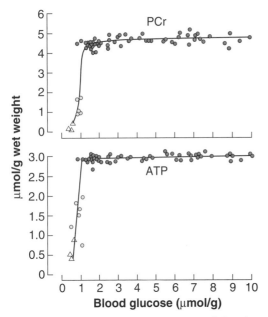

FIGURE 38-2. Neocortical concentrations of phosphocreatine *(PCr)* and ATP in rats subjected to graded hypoglycemia. Samples of frozen neocortex were used for these measurements. ●, EEG non-isoelectric; ◐, EEG isoelectric for 3 min prior to freezing brain; △, EEG isoelectric for 6 to 28 min prior to freezing brain. (From [2], © 1978 by John Wiley & Sons, Inc., with permission.)

lethargy and delirium followed by seizures and coma. Prolonged hypoglycemia may lead to irreversible brain damage.

During the progression of hypoglycemic encephalopathy, as blood glucose falls below 2.5 mM, a stage at which confusion and delirium occur, the cerebral metabolic rate for glucose (CMR_{glc}) falls more rapidly than does the cerebral metabolic rate for oxygen ($CMRO_2$), a finding which signifies the utilization of substrates other than glucose by the brain. Such substrates include tricarboxylic acid cycle (TCA) intermediates as well as amino acids, particularly glutamine and glutamate. However, these substrates are quickly used up and support cerebral energy requirements for only a few minutes in the absence of glucose. As blood glucose concentrations fall below 2 mM, the electroencephalogram (EEG) initially shows increased amplitude and decreased frequency, followed by decreased amplitude and frequency as blood glucose concentrations approach 1 mM. Below 1 mM blood glucose concentrations, brain ATP levels be-

come depleted [2] (Fig. 38-2), the EEG becomes isoelectric and coma develops. Similar conclusions have been drawn from ^{31}P nuclear magnetic resonance spectroscopic experiments with brain slices, in which perfusion of guinea pig slices in buffered medium containing various concentrations of glucose revealed that lowering of glucose concentrations from 10 to 0.2 mM was necessary before the ATP and phosphocreatine (PCr) contents of the slices were significantly reduced [3].

Clinically, hypoglycemia results in depression of CNS function, with rostral brain regions being affected before more caudally situated regions. For example, in severe hypoglycemia associated with isoelectric EEG tracings, cerebral cortical activity is absent but medullary function persists, as indicated by the maintenance of effective respiratory and cardiovascular activity.

Reduced synthesis of neurotransmitters rather than a global cerebral energy deficit explains the neurological symptoms and EEG changes in moderate hypoglycemia

Regional susceptibility to hypoglycemic insult is not reflected in selective regional changes in glucose, glycolytic or TCA cycle intermediates, pyruvate, lactate or ATP. However, glucose oxidation by the brain not only provides energy in the form of the anhydride bonds of ATP but also provides precursors for the synthesis of some neurotransmitters, including acetylcholine (ACh), γ-amino-butyric acid (GABA) and glutamate (Fig. 38-1). Most evidence now suggests that the neurological symptoms characteristic of hypoglycemic encephalopathy prior to isoelectric EEG stages result from "neurotransmission failure" involving one or more of these neurotransmitter systems.

Pyruvate derived from glucose is the major precursor of the acetyl group of ACh (Fig. 38-1). Inhibition of pyruvate oxidation results in reduced ACh synthesis both *in vitro* and *in vivo*. Incorporation of [^{14}C]choline into ACh in brain *in vivo* is decreased in rats with insulin-induced hypoglycemia [4]. That hypoglycemia results in decreased synthesis of the neurotransmitter pool of ACh is supported by the observation that administration of the CNS cholinesterase inhibitor physostigmine to hypoglycemic animals delays the onset of seizures and coma.

Similar findings of an adverse effect of hypoglycemia on the synthesis of the amino acid neurotransmitters GABA and glutamate have also been reported. Utilization of amino acids such as glutamate and glutamine as alternative energy substrates in moderate to severe hypoglycemia results in accumulation of aspartate and ammonia in the brain [5]. Hypoglycemia also produces a transient but substantial increase in extracellular concentrations of glutamate, GABA and dopamine, as measured using *in vivo* cerebral microdialysis [6]. Alterations of neurotransmission mediated by ACh, glutamate, GABA and/or dopamine (DA) could therefore contribute to the neurological signs and symptoms that characterize moderate hypoglycemia.

As hypoglycemia progresses below 1mM, the EEG becomes isoelectric and neuronal cell death ensues. As is the case in some other metabolic encephalopathies, cell death is not global in distribution; rather, certain brain structures, in particular hippocampal and cortical structures, are selectively vulnerable to hypoglycemic insult. Pathophysiological mechanisms responsible for neuronal cell death in hypoglycemia include the involvement of glutamate excitotoxicity. Severe and prolonged hypoglycemia results in increased release of glutamate in the brain, leading to membrane depolarization. This is followed by cerebral energy failure and neuronal cell death, particularly in the hippocampus. Glutamate neurotoxicity is thus implicated in the pathogenesis of hypoglycemia-induced neuronal death, and Ca^{2+} calmodulin-dependent protein kinase II appears to be one of the intracellular targets for glutamate neurotoxicity in hypoglycemia [7]. Glutamate excitotoxicity is discussed in Chapter 34.

HYPOXIC ENCEPHALOPATHY

An uninterrupted supply of oxygen is vital for cerebral function

Although it is possible to metabolize glucose to lactate and supply some energy needs as ATP, this represents only a small fraction of that resulting from oxidative metabolism, as can be seen by comparing the following reactions:

$$\text{glucose} + 6O_2 \rightarrow 6CO_2 + 6H_2O + 32ATP \text{ (aerobic)}$$

$$\text{glucose} \xrightarrow{\text{absence of } O_2} 2 \text{ lactate} + 2 \text{ ATP (anaerobic)}$$

Thus, anaerobic glycolysis cannot sustain the energy requirements of adult brain for more than a few minutes (see Chap. 31). Normal human brain consumes 3.3 ml of oxygen per 100 g of brain per minute ($CMRO_2$), a value which remains relatively stable during periods of wakefulness and sleep and represents ~20% of total body resting oxygen consumption despite the fact that the brain represents only ~2% of body weight. With impaired cerebral function, $CMRO_2$ declines in parallel with the severity of cerebral depression.

Experimental studies demonstrate that cerebral energy metabolism remains normal when mild to moderate hypoxia (PaO_2 = 25-40 mm Hg) results in severe cognitive dysfunction in human volunteers [1,2,8]. In mild hypoxia, cerebral blood flow (CBF) increases in order to maintain oxygen delivery to the brain. However, CBF can increase only about twofold; beyond this, $CMRO_2$ starts to fall and symptoms of hypoxia occur. In normal individuals exposed acutely to high altitudes (Table 38-2), difficulties with complex learning tasks and short-term memory appear at altitudes of around 10,000 feet as PaO_2 falls below 45 mm Hg, and above 20,000 feet, where PaO_2 = 30 mm Hg, cognitive disturbances and problems with motor coordination start to appear. Acute hypoxia of less than PaO_2 = 20 mm Hg generally results in coma. Graded hypoxia in experimental animals reveals that brain ATP levels remain normal at PaO_2 = 20 to 25 mm Hg (Fig. 38-3) despite EEG slowing and attenuated sensory evoked responses.

Glycolysis is stimulated to maintain brain ATP levels in moderate hypoxia

Studies on experimental animals reveal that at PaO_2 = 50 mm Hg an oxygen tension well in excess of that necessary to cause impaired ATP

TABLE 38-2. **HYPOXIC THRESHOLDS FOR CNS DYSFUNCTION**[a]

Simulated altitude (ft)	F_iO_2 (%)	PaO_2 (mm Hg)	Neurological status
Sea level	21	90	Normal
5,000	17	80	Impaired dark vision
8,000–10,000	15–14	55–45	Impaired short-term memory, difficulty learning complex tasks
15,000–20,000	11–9	40–30	Loss of judgment, euphoria, obtundation
>20,000	<9	<25	Coma

[a] Values derived from young volunteers subjected to acute (minutes) decompression hypoxia. F_iO_2, fractional percentage of ambient oxygen.

synthesis (Fig. 38-3), an increase in the [lactate]/[pyruvate] ratio and a decrease in brain tissue pH are observed. Increased lactate production is accompanied by a rise in CMR_{glc} [8], indicating accelerated glycolysis. The cytosolic redox potential measured by the $NADH:NAD^+$ ratio is shifted toward a more reduced state at PaO_2 below 45 mm Hg. PCr concentrations start to decline (Fig. 38-3), falling precipitously below a PaO_2 of 20 mm Hg. This steep fall in PCr coincides with a decrease in ATP and reflects failure of mitochondrial respiration and oxidative phosphorylation.

All forms of hypoxia result in alterations of neurotransmitter synthesis and release

Hypoxic hypoxia is a condition in which insufficient oxygen reaches the blood; this may result from either low oxygen tension in the environment, as encountered at high altitudes (Table 38-2), or the inability of oxygen to reach and cross the alveolar capillary membrane, as encountered in pulmonary disease.

Decreasing the oxygen content in the inspired air of anesthetized rats from 30 to 10% reduces the PaO_2 from 120 to 42 mm Hg; arteriovenous differences for oxygen decrease by 25%, but this is offset by an increase in CBF so that the $CMRO_2$ is unchanged. However, below 15% oxygen, glycolysis in brain is stimulated, leading to increased cerebral glucose utilization [8] and increased brain lactate. Neurotransmitter synthesis in brain is exquisitely sensitive to hypoxia. When rats are made to breathe 10% oxygen, ACh synthesis is decreased by 68%. This means

that ACh synthesis in the brain is decreased during hypoxia when $CMRO_2$ is maintained at normal values [9]. Hypoxia of a similar magnitude also results in altered synthesis and release of other neurotransmitters, including those derived from glucose. Arterial oxygen tension of below 50 mm Hg results in reductions in synthesis of glutamate and GABA in brain [10]. Synthesis of the biogenic amines may also be susceptible to hypoxia since tyrosine hydroxylase and tryptophan hydroxylase, the rate-limiting enzymes in monoamine neurotransmitter synthesis, require molecular oxygen, for which the K_m (O_2) is 12 μM, equivalent to 7 mm Hg [10].

Anemic hypoxia results when sufficient oxygen reaches the blood but the quantity of hemoglobin needed to bind and transport it is

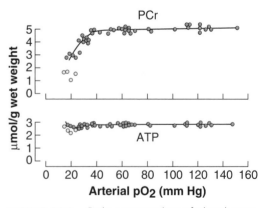

FIGURE 38-3. Brain concentrations of phosphocreatine *(PCr)* and ATP in rats anesthetized with 70% N_2O and subjected to graded hypoxia for periods of 15 to 30 min. ●, Animals with ≤120 mm Hg mean arterial pressure; ◐, animals with >80 mm Hg mean arterial pressure. (From [2], with permission.)

decreased. Either low hemoglobin due to anemia or chemical modifications of hemoglobin, for example, in carbon monoxide poisoning, may result in anemic hypoxia. Anemic hypoxia resulting from treatment of rats with sodium nitrite decreases synthesis of ACh, glutamate, GABA and the biogenic amines. Decreased neurotransmitter synthesis occurs at degrees of hypoxia which do not result in decreases in brain concentrations of ATP or adenylate energy charge [4,10].

Histotoxic hypoxia occurs when the ability of the tissue to utilize oxygen is impaired due to, for example, cyanide poisoning, which interferes with oxidative phosphorylation. Treatment of rats with potassium cyanide leads to reductions in synthesis of ACh and of glucose-derived amino acids in the brain [10].

In addition to decreased synthesis of neurotransmitters, hypoxia results in alterations in their release. In striatal slices, hypoxia increases the evoked release of glutamate, DA and, to a lesser extent, ACh. The effects of hypoxia on neurotransmitter release are mediated by cytosolic free Ca^{2+} or on neurotransmitter release (see Chap. 5).

HEPATIC ENCEPHALOPATHY

Hepatic encephalopathy is a neuropsychiatric disorder occurring in both acute and chronic liver diseases

Depending upon the duration and severity of liver dysfunction, hepatic encephalopathy (HE) may present as one of two major types [11]. Portal-systemic encephalopathy (PSE) results from portal-systemic shunting of venous blood. This shunting of blood may arise spontaneously due to increased pressure in the portal vein, resulting in the formation of collaterals, or it may be induced surgically in order to relieve portal hypertension arising from liver disease. Neurologically, PSE evolves slowly. Early symptoms include altered sleep patterns and personality changes, followed by shortened attention span and asterixis progressing through stupor to coma as the severity of liver disease progresses.

PSE is commonly precipitated by a gastrointestinal hemorrhage or use of a sedative. HE in acute liver failure, in contrast to PSE, progresses rapidly through altered mental status to stupor and coma within hours or days. Seizures are occasionally encountered and mortality rates are high. Death most frequently results from brainstem herniation caused by increased intracranial pressure as a consequence of brain edema.

Edema is rarely encountered in PSE; rather, the latter is characterized neuropathologically by astrocytic changes known as Alzheimer type II astrocytosis. The Alzheimer type II astrocyte has a characteristic swollen shape with a large, pale nucleus, prominent nucleolus and margination of chromatin [12]. In addition to these morphological changes, astrocytes in PSE manifest many neurochemical alterations, including reduced expression of key astrocytic proteins, such as glial fibrillary acidic protein (GFAP); of astrocytic enzymes, including glutamine synthetase; and of monoamine oxidase type B (MAO-B), as well as increased expression of astrocytic, "peripheral-type" benzodiazepine receptors (PTBRs)[13]. These changes suggest that normal key astrocytic functions, such as ammonia metabolism and the uptake and metabolism of monoamine and amino acid neurotransmitters, are impaired; and it has been proposed that PSE results from a disorder of "neuron–astrocyte trafficking" of these key substrates [11].

Liver failure, whether acute or chronic, leads to the accumulation in brain of neurotoxic substances

These are normally eliminated by hepatic or biliary routes. Two such substances have been identified, ammonia and manganese. Magnetic resonance imaging (MRI) reveals increased signal intensity in pallidum of T_1-weighted images in the majority of patients with chronic liver disease, suggesting the presence of a paramagnetic substance in this region of the brain. Evidence to date suggests that this substance is manganese, a metal which is normally excreted in the bile. Blood manganese concentrations are increased in cirrhotic patients, and a positive correlation has been found between blood manganese content and the magnitude of pallidal signal hyperintensity on MRI in these cases [14]. Manganese deposition in the basal ganglia could explain the extrapyramidal symptoms frequently encountered in cirrhotic patients, such as tremor and rigidity (see Chap. 45).

Both ammonia and manganese may be responsible for the astrocytic morphological changes observed in HE. Exposure of cultured astrocytes to ammonia results in decreased expression of GFAP, decreased capacity of cells to take up glutamate and increased expression of PTBRs [12,15], phenomena which are consistently observed *in situ* in the brains of humans or experimental animals with HE. Similar changes in glutamate uptake capacity and PTBRs are observed following exposure of cultured astrocytes to manganese, and both ammonia and manganese have been reported to cause Alzheimer type II astrocytosis, the cardinal neuropathological feature of PSE.

Ammonia concentrations in arterial blood of patients with liver failure rise to 0.5 to 1 mM, in contrast to the normal range of 0.01 to 0.02 mM. Using positron emission tomography (PET) (see Chap. 54) and $^{13}NH_3$, increases of the cerebral metabolic rate for ammonia (CMRA), that is, the rate at which ammonia is taken up and metabolized by the brain, have been reported (Fig. 38-4) [16]. Furthermore, increased CMRA was accompanied by increases in the permeability/surface area product (PS), a measure of blood–brain barrier permeability to ammonia. The apparent ease with which ammonia is taken up into the brain offers a possible explanation for the hypersensitivity of patients with chronic liver disease to ammoniagenic conditions such as a dietary protein load or gastrointestinal bleeding and for the sometimes imperfect correlation between the degree of neurological impairment and blood ammonia concentrations in these patients.

Ammonia has deleterious effects on cerebral function by both direct and indirect mechanisms

Concentrations of ammonia in the 1 to 2 mM range, equivalent to those reported in the brain in experimental liver failure, impair postsynaptic

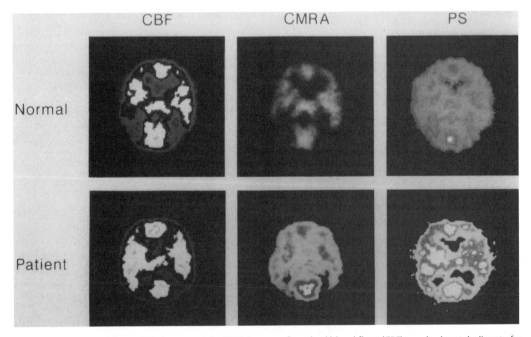

FIGURE 38-4. Positron emission tomography (PET) images of cerebral blood flow *(CBF)*, cerebral metabolic rate for ammonia *(CMRA)* and permeability/surface area product *(PS,* a measure of blood–brain barrier permeability) of a normal subject with an arterial ammonia concentration of 26 μM compared to a patient with liver disease, subclinical encephalopathy and a 66 μM arterial ammonia concentration. (From [16], with permission.) See text.

inhibition in cerebral cortex and brainstem by a direct effect on Cl^- extrusion from the post-synaptic neuron, rendering the inhibitory neuro-transmitter ineffective [17]. Millimolar concentrations of ammonia also inhibit excitatory neurotransmission. Synaptic transmission from Schaffer collaterals to CA1 hippocampal neurons is reversibly depressed by 1 mM ammonia, and the firing of CA1 neurons by iontophoretic application of glutamate is inhibited by 2 mM ammonia, suggesting a direct inhibitory action of ammonia on excitatory synaptic transmission [18].

Since brain is devoid of an effective urea cycle, ammonia removal depends almost entirely on glutamine formation via glutamine synthetase, an enzyme with a predominantly astrocytic localization. Glutamine concentrations are increased five- to ten-fold in cerebrospinal fluid (CSF) and brain of experimental animals and humans with liver failure. While glutamine is not neurotoxic, its rapid accumulation in astrocytes has been linked to the pathogenesis of brain edema in acute liver failure and to the increased uptake of aromatic amino acids into the brain in acute and chronic liver diseases (see below).

If sufficiently elevated, ammonia may depress metabolic energy reserves

In patients with HE, $CMRO_2$ and CBF decline in parallel with the decline in neurological function. In portacaval shunted rats, with chronic low-grade hyperammonemia, the addition of an ammonia load tolerated by sham-operated controls results in EEG abnormalities, stupor, coma and reductions in $CMRO_2$ and CBF. Addition of millimolar concentrations of ammonia to brain preparations results in inhibition of α-ketoglutarate dehydrogenase (αKGDH) in rat brain preparations [19]. αKGDH is a rate-limiting enzyme of the TCA cycle, and, consistent with decreased oxidation of pyruvate and α-ketoglutarate, both acute and chronic liver failure result in increased brain lactate concentrations (Fig. 38-1). In hyperammonemic rats, increases in the cerebral lactate:pyruvate ratio are accompanied by increases in the cytoplasmic $NADH:NAD^+$ ratio. Since mitochondria are impervious to cytoplasmically generated NADH, electrons must cross the inner mitochondrial membrane via the malate-aspartate shuttle (MAS) (Fig. 38-5). Ammonia-induced changes in lactate:pyruvate and $NADH:NAD^+$ ratios suggest an action on the MAS, an impairment which could further compromise cerebral energy metabolism [20]. Thus, brain concentrations of ammonia in both acute and chronic liver failure are sufficiently elevated to cause impaired cerebral energy metabolism via two independent routes: inhibition of αKGDH and of the MAS. Ammonia-precipitated coma in portacaval-shunted rats results in decreased brain ATP, but these changes are not apparent until late, preterminal stages associated with prolonged coma [20]. ^{31}P-Nuclear magnetic resonance studies should have the potential to resolve the issue of cerebral energy metabolism in HE in patients with acute or chronic liver failure, but to date, data from such studies have been inconsistent.

Hepatic encephalopathy is a disorder of multiple neurotransmitter systems

As discussed above, in common with hypoglycemic and hypoxic encephalopathies, HE does not result, at least at early stages, from a cerebral energy deficit; rather, it is associated with alterations of multiple neurotransmitter systems in the brain. In most cases, these changes appear to be directly or indirectly the consequence of ammonia or of manganese toxicity.

Ammonia metabolism is linked to the synthesis and turnover of a number of amino acids, two of which, glutamate and aspartate, are major excitatory neurotransmitters (see Chap. 15). The essential steps in the synthesis of glutamate and its relationship to cerebral ammonia metabolism are shown in a simplified schematic form in Figure 38-6. Regulation at the glutamate synapse requires a functional interaction between the presynaptic nerve terminal and the neighboring astrocyte, a phenomenon frequently referred to as "neuron–astrocyte trafficking" or the "glutamate–glutamine cycle." Glutamate released by the nerve terminal interacts with receptors on the postsynaptic or astrocytic membranes and is then inactivated by high-affinity transport systems mainly into astrocytes, where it is converted into glutamine by the action of glutamine

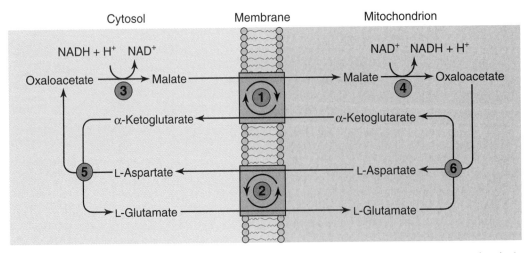

FIGURE 38-5. The malate–aspartate shuttle for the transport of reducing equivalents between cytosol and mitochondria: *1,* α-ketoglutarate–malate carrier; *2,* glutamate–aspartate carrier; *3,* cytosolic malate dehydrogenase; *4,* mitochondrial malate dehydrogenase; *5,* cytosolic aspartate aminotransferase; *6,* mitochondrial aspartate aminotransferase. The enzymatic steps are reversible, but a directionality is imposed via the energy-requiring, one-way passage of aspartate from mitochondria to the cytosol. Glutamate and aspartate are consistently lowered in the brain of hyperammonemic animals. These changes may slow both the glutamate–aspartate exchange and flux through the transaminases. The mitochondrial enzyme may be particularly susceptible to changes in glutamate since its apparent K_m for glutamate is approximately 20 mM. (From [30], copyright 1985 by John Wiley & Sons, Inc., with permission.)

synthetase. The glutamine formed is then available for reuse by the presynaptic nerve terminal as the preferred, immediate precursor of releasable glutamate (see Chaps. 10 and 15).

Several lines of evidence suggest that this neuron–astrocyte trafficking of substrates is impaired due to excessive amounts of ammonia or manganese and that this impairment results in glutamatergic synaptic dysregulation, a phenomenon which could contribute to the pathogenesis of HE [11]. Glutamate uptake into cultured astrocytes is reduced by exposure to submillimolar concentrations of manganese and by millimolar concentrations of ammonia [14]. Furthermore, consistent with diminished clearance of glutamate from the synaptic cleft in HE, microdialysis studies in animals with experimental acute liver failure reveal increased extracellular concentrations of glutamate as a function of the degree of neurological impairment [21], and reduction of expression of the astrocytic glutamate transporter (GLT-1) has been reported in experimental acute liver failure [11]. Studies of glutamate-binding sites in the brain demonstrate a significant loss of the α-amino-3-hydroxy-5-methyl-4-isoxazole propionic acid (AMPA)/kainate sites in animals with acute liver failure.

Increased synthesis of glutamine in the brain, resulting from increased ammonia concentrations in liver failure, leads to increased brain uptake of the aromatic amino acids tyrosine, phenylalanine and tryptophan [22]. Since tryptophan is the amino acid precursor of serotonin and its hydroxylation, the rate-limiting step in serotonin synthesis, is not saturated at usual brain concentrations of tryptophan, increases in its availability could lead to increased brain serotonin synthesis in liver failure. Many of the neuropsychiatric symptoms in early PSE, such as altered sleep patterns, are signs that have classically been attributed to modifications of serotonergic neurotransmission. Serotonin turnover, as indicated by the ratio of the concentrations of the serotonin metabolite 5-hydroxyindoleacetic acid to serotonin, is increased in brain in both human and experimental PSE [11]. Other tryptophan metabolites, including quinolinic acid and the neuroactive trace amine tryptamine, have also been found to be elevated in brain in PSE.

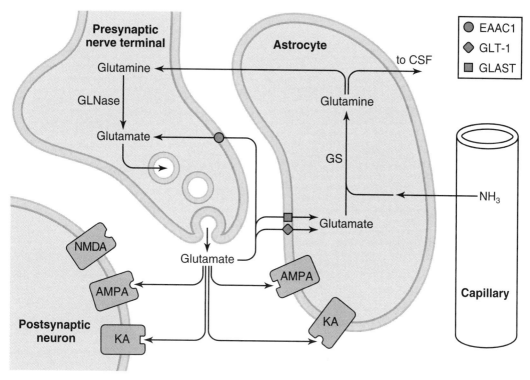

FIGURE 38-6. Major steps in glutamatergic neurotransmission. Glutamate released from the presynaptic neuron is taken up into the perineuronal astrocyte via the glutamate transporter-1 (*GLT-1*) and the glutamate–aspartate transporter (*GLAST*) or the neuronal excitatory amino acid carrier-1 (*EAAC1*). Glutamate receptors are expressed on neurons (*NMDA, AMPA*, kainate [*KA*] subtypes) and astrocytes (*AMPA, KA* subtypes). Ammonia (NH_3) removal by glutamine synthetase (*GS*) occurs only in the astrocyte. In acute liver failure, decreased expression of GLT-1 and concomitant increases of extracellular glutamate may signify impaired neuron–astrocyte trafficking. *GLNase*, glutaminase; *CSF*, cerebrospinal fluid.

A widely publicized theory has suggested that HE results from increased central "GABAergic tone" [23]. While electrophysiological similarities are seen in metabolic encephalopathy and from GABA receptor modulators, such as the benzodiazepines, the precise nature and origins of the GABAergic changes in encephalopathy remain unclear (see Chap. 16). Original reports of alterations of GABA-related enzymes, blood–brain uptake of GABA or changes in GABA/benzodiazepine receptors in either human or experimental HE have not been confirmed. However, increases in CSF and brain concentrations of substances which bind to the GABA-related benzodiazepine receptor in human HE have been verified [24,25]. Concentrations of benzodiazepine receptor ligands were considered sufficient to have contributed to HE in some of these patients, and subsequent clinical trials with the benzodiazepine receptor antagonist flumazenil revealed a beneficial effect in some patients with HE. The origin of these endogenous, benzodiazepine-like compounds in liver failure is unclear. In some cases, they may simply be active pharmaceutical benzodiazepine metabolites left over from earlier treatment of liver disease patients with benzodiazepine medication; in other cases, they may have been synthesized *in situ*. Further studies will be required to resolve this issue.

The PTBR is expressed in higher amounts in hepatic encephalopathy. It is a hetero-oligomeric protein complex located on the outer mitochondrial membrane. In the CNS, PTBRs are localized mainly on the mitochondrial membranes of astrocytes. Therefore, they are not allosterically coupled to the GABA$_A$ receptor. Increases of expression and maximal binding site densities of PTBRs have consistently been described in brain and peripheral tissues of animals following portacaval anastomosis [13] and in human HE brain. Increased PTBR expression also occurs in cultured astrocytes exposed to ammonia or manganese. Precisely how the increased expression of PTBRs in brain is related to the neuropsychiatric symptoms in HE is unclear, but it has been demonstrated that activation of PTBRs may lead to the production of neurosteroids, such as 3-α-hydroxy-5α-pregnan-20-one, a compound which has a high affinity for the GABA$_A$ receptor, and for which it is a positive allosteric modulator. Concentrations of an endogenous PTBR agonist, also termed the diazepam-binding inhibitor (DBI), are increased in the CSF of HE patients, and a positive correlation is reported between CSF DBI concentrations and severity of encephalopathy [26]. These findings suggest that PTBR activation could contribute to the phenomenon of "increased GABAergic tone" in HE via the production of neurosteroids.

Finally, there is an emerging body of evidence to suggest that the endogenous opioid system of the brain may be involved in the mediation of some of the effects of chronic liver disease on cerebral function. Patients with chronic liver disease are hypersensitive to the effects of morphine, and rats with portacaval shunts show increased pain sensitivity, phenomena which are related to the endogenous opioid system. Increased plasma concentrations of the endogenous opioid peptide met-enkephalin have been described in patients with primary biliary cirrhosis, and β-endorphin concentrations are increased in the brains of rats following portacaval shunting together with alterations of μ and δ opioid-binding sites [27].

HYPERCAPNIC ENCEPHALOPATHY

Respiratory acidosis leads to decreased brain pH

Patients with chronic pulmonary disorders may exhibit lethargy, confusion, memory loss and stupor. The combined insults of hypoxia and hypercapnia, which result in CO_2 retention, con-

tribute to the encephalopathy, but neurological symptoms correlate best with the degree of CO_2 retention. Acute moderate hypercapnia, 5 to 10% CO_2 in the expired air, leads to arousal and excitability, whereas higher CO_2 concentrations, >35% in the expired air, are anesthetic.

Although CO_2 is a normal metabolite, it is toxic at elevated levels. CO_2 exists in equilibrium with carbonic acid (H_2CO_3) and with bicarbonate (HCO_3^-), a major H^+ buffer. Renal conservation of HCO_3^- is generally sufficient to buffer hypercapnia; however, an added insult, such as an infection, fatigue or ingestion of a sedative, may further compromise pulmonary function, resulting in further CO_2 retention and disruption of the normal buffering mechanisms. The respiratory acidosis associated with CO_2 retention in blood leads to a proportional increase in brain tissue $[H^+]$.

The combination of hypoxia and hypercapnia in pulmonary insufficiency results in cerebral vasodilation and increased CBF and may lead to increased intracranial pressure. Arteriovenous differences for oxygen across the brain generally decrease as a function of increased CBF, leaving CMRO$_2$ unchanged [28].

Acute hypercapnic acidosis leads to an increase in concentrations of glycolytic intermediates above the phosphofructokinase step, and a decrease below this step is likely due to inhibition of phosphofructokinase by $[H^+]$. Brain ATP concentrations are unchanged in hypercapnia, and it is generally believed that decreased CMR$_{glc}$ is the result of decreased neuronal activity and, hence, reduced fuel, that is, glucose requirements. Neurotransmitter-related mechanisms which could contribute to hypercapnic encephalopathy include decreased neurotransmitter glutamate pools and decreased synthesis of acetylcholine.

UREMIC AND DIALYSIS ENCEPHALOPATHIES

Patients with renal failure continue to manifest neuropsychiatric symptoms despite significant advances in therapeutics and management. Patients with renal failure who are not yet on dialysis develop an array of symptoms, including clouding of consciousness, disturbed sleep patterns, tremor, asterixis and even coma and death.

Uremia is characterized by retention in the blood of urea, phosphates, proteins, amines and a number of poorly defined low-molecular-weight compounds. Despite acidemia, the pH of brain, muscle and CSF are normal in humans with renal failure. Whereas brain water, K^+ and Mg^{2+} content are normal, Al^{3+} and Ca^{2+} concentrations are significantly increased [29].

Uremia leads to alterations in the characteristics of the blood–brain barrier

Uremia results in increased permeability of the blood–brain barrier to sucrose and inulin; K^+ transport is enhanced, whereas Na^+ transport is impaired. There is an increase in brain osmolarity in acute renal failure due to the increase in urea concentrations. However, in contrast to acute renal failure, the increase in osmolarity in chronic renal failure results from the presence of idiogenic osmoles in addition to urea. CBF is increased in uremic patients, but $CMRO_2$ and CMR_{glc} are decreased. In the brains of rats with acute renal failure, ATP, PCr and glucose are increased, whereas AMP, ADP and lactate are decreased most likely as a result of decreased energy demands.

Parathyroid hormone may be implicated in the pathogenesis of uremic encephalopathy

Parathyroid hormone (PTH) produces CNS effects in normal subjects, and neuropsychiatric symptoms are frequently encountered in patients with primary hyperparathyroidism, where EEG changes resemble those described in acute renal failure. Circulating PTH is not removed by hemodialysis. In uremic patients, both EEG changes and neuropsychiatric symptoms are improved by either parathyroidectomy or medical suppression of PTH. The mechanism whereby PTH causes disturbances of CNS function is not well understood, but it has been suggested that increased PTH might facilitate the entry of Ca^{2+} into the cell, resulting in cell death.

Aluminum toxicity may play a role in the pathogenesis of dialysis encephalopathy

This condition, also termed "dialysis dementia," is a progressive, frequently fatal neurological disorder which occurs in patients treated with chronic hemodialysis. Symptoms progress through personality changes, psychosis, seizures and dementia. Many cases of dialysis dementia may result from aluminum accumulation in brain. Aluminum content of cerebral gray matter from patients with dialysis dementia is 11 times higher than normal and three times higher than that observed in patients on chronic hemodialysis but without dialysis dementia. Aluminum is normally excreted by the kidney.

Epidemiological studies have shown a strong association between aluminum content of the water used to prepare dialysates and the incidence of dialysis dementia. Reducing water aluminum content below 20 µg/l appears to prevent the onset of the disease in patients who have just started dialysis.

REFERENCES

1. Pulsinelli, W. A., and Cooper, A. J. L. Metabolic encephalopathies and coma. In G. J. Siegel, B. W. Agranoff, R. W. Albers and P. B. Molinoff (eds.), *Basic Neurochemistry: Molecular, Cellular and Medical Aspects*, 5th ed. New York: Raven Press, 1994, pp. 841–857.
2. Siesjo, B. K. (eds.) *Brain Energy Metabolism.* New York: John Wiley & Sons, 1978, pp. 380–446.
3. Cox, D. W. G., Morris, P. G., Feeney, J., and Bachelard, H. S. ^{31}P-NMR studies on cerebral energy metabolism under conditions of hypoglycaemia and hypoxia *in vitro*. *Biochem. J.* 212:365–370, 1983.
4. Gibson, G. E., and Blass, J. P. Impaired synthesis of acetylcholine in brain accompanying hypoglycemia and mild hypoxia. *J. Neurochem.* 27:37–42, 1976.
5. Butterworth, R. F. Metabolism of glutamate and related amino acids in insulin hypoglycaemia. In L. Hertz, E. Kvamme, E. G. McGeer, and A. Schousboe (eds.), *Glutamine, Glutamate and GABA in the Central Nervous System.* New York: Alan R. Liss, 1983, pp. 595–608.
6. Butcher, S. P., Sandberg, M., Hagberg, H., and Hamberger, A. Cellular origin of endogenous

amino acids released into the extracellular fluid of the rat striatum during severe insulin-induced hypoglycemia. *J. Neurochem.* 48:722–728, 1987.

7. Hu, B. R., Kurihara, J., and Wieloch, T. Persistent translocation and inhibition of Ca^{2+}/calmodulin-dependent protein kinase II in the crude synaptosomal fraction of the vulnerable hippocampus following hypoglycemia. *J. Neurochem.* 64:1361–1369, 1995.

8. Pulsinelli, W. A., and Duffy, T. E. Local cerebral glucose metabolism during controlled hypoxemia in rats. *Science* 204:626–629, 1979.

9. Gibson, G. E., Pulsinelli, W., Blass, J. P., and Duffy, T. E. Brain dysfunction in mild to moderate hypoxia. *Am. J. Med.* 70:1247–1254, 1981.

10. Gibson, G. E., and Huang, H. M. Animal models of brain hypoxia. In A. Boulton, G. Baker, and R. F. Butterworth (eds.), *Neuromethod 22: Animal Models of Neurological Disease II.* Clifton, NJ: Humana Press, 1992, pp. 51–91.

11. Butterworth, R. F. The neurobiology of hepatic encephalopathy. *Semin. Liver Dis.* 16:235–244, 1996.

12. Norenberg, M. D. The role of astrocytes in hepatic encephalopathy. *Neurochem. Pathol.* 6:13–33, 1987.

13. Giguère, J. F., Hamel, E., and Butterworth, R. F. Increased densities of binding sites for the "peripheral-type" benzodiazepine receptor ligand [³H]PK11195 in rat brain following portacaval anastomosis. *Brain Res.* 594:150–154, 1992.

14. Spahr, L., Butterworth, R. F., Fontaine, S., et al. Increased blood manganese in cirrhotic patients: Relationship to pallidal magnetic resonance signal hyperintensity and neurological symptoms. *Hepatology* 24:1116–1120, 1996.

15. Bender, A. S., and Norenberg, M. D. Effects of ammonia on L-glutamate uptake in cultured astrocytes. *Neurochem. Res.* 21:567–573, 1996.

16. Lockwood, A. H., Yap, E. W. H., and Wong, W. H. Cerebral ammonia metabolism in patients with severe liver disease and minimal hepatic encephalopathy. *J. Cereb. Blood Flow Metab.* 11:337–341, 1991.

17. Raabe, W. Synaptic transmission in ammonia intoxication. *Neurochem. Pathol.* 6:145–166, 1987.

18. Szerb, J. C., and Butterworth, R. F. Effect of ammonium ions on synaptic transmission in the mammalian central nervous system. *Prog. Neurobiol.* 39:135–153, 1992.

19. Lai, J. C. K., and Cooper, A. J. L. Brain α-ketoglutarate dehydrogenase: Kinetic properties, regional distribution and effects of inhibitors. *J. Neurochem.* 47:1376–1386, 1986.

20. Hindfelt, B., Plum, F., and Duffy, T. E. Effect of acute ammonia intoxication on cerebral metabolism in rats with portacaval shunts. *J. Clin. Invest.* 59:386–396, 1977.

21. Michalak, A., Rose, C., Butterworth, J., and Butterworth, R. F. Neuroactive amino acids and glutamate (NMDA) receptors in frontal cortex of rats with experimental acute liver failure. *Hepatology* 24:908–913, 1996.

22. Jonung, T., Rigotti, P., James, J. H., Bradett, K., and Fischer, J. E. Methionine sulfoximine reduces the brain uptake index and the brain concentrations of neutral amino acids after portacaval anastomosis. *Surg. Forum* 34:38–40, 1980.

23. Schafer, D. F., and Jones, E. A. Hepatic encephalopathy and the γ-aminobutyric acid system. *Lancet* 1:18–20, 1982.

24. Basile, A. S., Hughes, R. D., Harrison, P. M., et al. Elevated brain concentrations of 1,4-benzodiazepines in fulminant hepatic failure. *N. Engl. J. Med.* 325:473–478, 1991.

25. Olasmaa, M., Rothstein, J. D., Guidotti, A., et al. Endogenous benzodiazepine receptor ligands in human and animal hepatic encephalopathy. *J. Neurochem.* 55:2015–2023, 1990.

26. Rothstein, J. D., McKhann, G., Guarneri, P., Barbaccia, M. L., Guidotti, A., and Costa, E. Cerebrospinal fluid content of diazepam binding inhibitor in chronic hepatic encephalopathy. *Ann. Neurol.* 26:57–62, 1989.

27. De Waele, J. P., Audet, R. M., Leong, D. K., and Butterworth, R. F. Portacaval anastomosis induces region-selective alterations of the endogenous opioid system in the rat brain. *Hepatology* 24:895–901, 1996.

28. Miller, A. L. Carbon dioxide narcosis. In D. W. McCandless (ed.), *Cerebral Energy Metabolism and Metabolic Encephalopathy.* New York: Plenum Press, 1985, pp. 143–162.

29. Fraser, C. L. Neurologic manifestations of the uremic state. In A. I. Arieff, and R. C. Griggs, (eds.), *Metabolic Brain Dysfunction in Systemic Disorders.* Boston: Little Brown, 1992, pp. 139–166.

39

Diseases Involving Myelin

Richard H. Quarles, Pierre Morell and Henry F. McFarland

GENERAL CLASSIFICATION 784

A deficiency of myelin can result either from failure to produce the normal amount of myelin during development or from myelin breakdown after it is formed **784**

Many of the biochemical changes associated with central nervous system demyelination are similar regardless of etiology **784**

ACQUIRED DISORDERS OF MYELIN 785

Damage in many acquired allergic and infectious demyelinating diseases is directed specifically against myelin or myelin-forming cells **785**

Experimental allergic encephalomyelitis is an animal model of autoimmune demyelination **785**

A number of animal diseases caused by viruses involve primary demyelination and often are associated with inflammation **786**

Multiple sclerosis is the most common demyelinating disease of the central nervous system in humans **786**

Some human peripheral neuropathies involving demyelination are thought to be immune-mediated **791**

Other acquired disorders affecting myelin in humans may be secondary to viral infections, neoplasias or immunosuppressive therapy **793**

GENETIC DISORDERS OF MYELIN 793

Spontaneous mutations in experimental animals provide insights about the structure and assembly of myelin **793**

The human leukodystrophies are inherited disorders affecting central nervous system white matter **795**

Deficiencies of peripheral nerve myelin in several inherited neuropathies are caused by genetic mutations in sheath proteins **797**

TOXIC AND NUTRITIONAL DISORDERS OF MYELIN 798

Biological toxins can produce myelin loss **798**

Many chemical toxins can impair myelin formation or cause its breakdown **798**

General undernourishment or dietary deficiencies of specific substances can lead to a preferential reduction in myelin formation **798**

Basic Neurochemistry: Molecular, Cellular and Medical Aspects, 6th Ed., edited by G. J. Siegel et al. Published by Lippincott–Raven Publishers, Philadelphia, 1999. Correspondence to Richard H. Quarles, Laboratory of Molecular and Cellular Neurobiology, National Institute of Neurological Disorders and Stroke, National Institutes of Health, Bethesda, Maryland 20892.

The integrity of myelin sheaths is dependent on the normal functioning of myelin-forming oligodendrocytes in the CNS and Schwann cells in the PNS, as well as on the viability of the axons that they ensheath. Neuronal death inevitably leads to subsequent degeneration of both axons and the myelin surrounding them. The title of this chapter was chosen to emphasize that myelin cannot be considered an isolated entity in disease processes. Deficiencies of myelin can result from a multitude of causes, including viral infections, autoimmunity, inherited disorders, toxic agents, malnutrition and mechanical trauma that affects myelin, myelin-forming cells or myelinated neurons.

GENERAL CLASSIFICATION

A deficiency of myelin can result either from failure to produce the normal amount of myelin during development or from myelin breakdown after it is formed

An impediment of normal myelin formation is referred to as *hypomyelination* or, in some cases, as *dysmyelination*. According to the definition of Poser, dysmyelination is a genetically determined disorder of myelinogenesis in which "myelin initially formed was abnormally constituted, thus inherently unstable, vulnerable, and liable to degeneration" (see [1]). Diseases involving loss of normal myelin after it is formed, which is termed *demyelination*, can be subdivided into primary and secondary categories on the basis of morphological observations. *Primary demyelination* involves the early destruction of myelin with relative sparing of axons; subsequently, other structures may be affected. *Secondary demyelination* includes disorders in which myelin is involved after damage to neurons and axons. The classification used in this chapter is based on etiology as well as comparative neuropathology. Disorders causing hypomyelination and demyelination are included in four categories: (i) acquired allergic and infectious diseases, (ii) genetically determined disorders, (iii) toxic and nutritional disorders and (iv) disorders primarily affecting neurons with secondary involvement of myelin.

Many of the biochemical changes associated with central nervous system demyelination are similar regardless of etiology

The most pronounced changes occur in white matter, where there is a marked increase in water content, a decrease of myelin proteins and lipids and, in many demyelinating diseases, the appearance of cholesterol esters and/or glial fibrillary acidic protein (GFAP) (Chap. 8) [1]. Particularly noteworthy with regard to lipids are dramatic decreases in galactocerebroside, ethanolamine plasmalogens and cholesterol, all of which are enriched in myelin membranes (see Chap. 4). The major structural proteins of CNS myelin, myelin basic protein (MBP) and proteolipid protein (PLP), also are invariably decreased. These changes can be explained by the breakdown and gradual loss of myelin, which is relatively rich in solids, and its replacement by extracellular fluid, astrocytes and inflammatory cells, which are more hydrated, relatively lipid-poor and free of myelin-specific constituents. The frequent appearance of cholesterol esters in demyelinating diseases apparently is related to the fact that cholesterol is not readily degraded and is esterified by phagocytes, often remaining at the site of the lesion for some time. Since cholesterol esters are essentially absent from normal mature brain, their presence in myelin disorders is indicative of inflammation and recent demyelination. Such compounds are also responsible for the neutral fat staining, or sudanophilia, demonstrated histochemically in many demyelinating diseases. In the CNS, GFAP is specific to astrocytes, and an increase of this protein during demyelination is due to reactive astrocytes associated with the pathology (see Chap. 1). The magnitude of the changes mentioned above varies considerably from disease to disease and from specimen to specimen in the same disease, depending on the severity, location, duration and activity of the pathological processes.

ACQUIRED DISORDERS OF MYELIN

Damage in many acquired allergic and infectious demyelinating diseases is directed specifically against myelin or myelin-forming cells

In most of these disorders, the lesions are disseminated and characterized by perivenular demyelination and inflammation, macrophage activity, sudanophilic deposits consisting of myelin degradation products and relative sparing of axons. The extent to which these criteria are fulfilled depends on the particular type and phase of disease. Furthermore, it is not always clear whether the immunological activity is autoimmune in nature or whether it is related primarily to an antecedent viral infection, nor is the amount of damage directly caused by the virus always clear. Most of the diseases discussed here are reviewed in more detail elsewhere [1–3].

Experimental allergic encephalomyelitis is an animal model of autoimmune demyelination

The animal model thought to most clearly resemble multiple sclerosis (MS) is experimental allergic encephalomyelitis (EAE). EAE is an acute or chronic demyelinating disease of the CNS, which is induced by immunization of susceptible animals with either myelin or various components of myelin that are encephalitogenic, meaning that they can induce EAE. The EAE model

initially was identified through efforts to understand the cause of cases of encephalomyelitis developing after inoculation of patients with the Pasteur rabies vaccine. Since the vaccine was made from virally infected neural tissue, animals were inoculated with either the vaccine or, for controls, uninfected neural tissue; some animals receiving uninfected neural tissue developed an encephalomyelitis. Since that time, the EAE model has been studied extensively. A detailed examination of the EAE model and the extensive immunological data that have been obtained using it is beyond the scope of this chapter, but readers are referred to recent reviews [2,3]. In brief, EAE can be induced by immunization with several encephalitogenic proteins from myelin, most notably MBP and PLP. The disease is mediated by CD4+ major histocompatability complex (MHC) class II-restricted T cells and can be transferred from an immunized animal to a naive animal using CD4+ T cells. There is considerable variation in susceptibility of various animals, and this variation is largely due to the genetic background, especially MHC genes. It is now understood that elements of the three components of antigen recognition, the T-cell receptor (TCR), antigen and the MHC molecule that presents antigen, together known as the trimolecular complex, are central to disease induction. For example, in the SJL mouse, which is $H2^s$, the principal encephalitogenic portion of MBP is the middle of the molecule spanning amino acids 88 to 102. In contrast, in the PL/J mouse, which is $H2^u$, the immunodominant region is the N-terminal portion of the molecule. Also, in some animals, encephalitogenic T cells use the same TCR, a condition known as restricted TCR usage. The exquisite specificity seen for the trimolecular complex of encephalitogenic T cells has resulted in the development of numerous therapies that target the trimolecular complex and can modify disease. These include generating an immune response to the TCR or administration of a peptide that binds to MHC but does not activate T cells.

The most characteristic component of the EAE lesion is perivascular inflammation; the extent of demyelination will vary between species. Evidence from studying EAE in the rat or mouse indicates that activated T cells, regardless of specificity, can cross the blood–brain barrier (BBB) and enter the nervous system. If the T cell encounters its antigen, the cell will be further activated and begin production of proinflammatory cytokines, such as γ interferon and tumor necrosis factor (TNF) α, which in turn activate the endothelial cells, with upregulation of cell adhesion molecules promoting an inflammatory response. The outcome of this process, at least in some animals, is myelin damage. The actual effector mechanism for myelin damage is uncertain. Possibilities include a direct toxic effect of TNFα or nitric oxide (NO) on oligodendrocytes or damage mediated by macrophages and microglial cells. The latter possibility could be enhanced by the presence of antibodies which may bind to myelin and provide a ligand for activated monocytes. Indeed, demyelination associated with EAE in several animals, including the rat, mouse and marmoset, a non-human primate, can be increased by the presence of antibodies to surface components of myelin, such as galactocerebroside or myelin oligodendrocyte glycoprotein (MOG). In fact, immunization of rodents with MOG alone induces a relapsing-remitting demyelinating disease with both cellular and humoral immunity to this glycoprotein [4].

A number of animal diseases caused by viruses involve primary demyelination and often are associated with inflammation

These diseases are studied as animal models, which may provide clues about how a viral infection could lead to immune-mediated demyelination in humans [1,2,5]. *Canine distemper* virus causes a demyelinating disease, and the lesions in dog brain show a strong inflammatory response with some similarities to acute disseminated encephalomyelitis in humans [1]. *Visna* is a slowly progressive demyelinating disease caused by a retrovirus of sheep [1,2]. *Border disease* is another disorder of myelin in sheep and results from prenatal infection with a pestivirus [1,6]. However, in contrast to the other viral diseases described here, which cause demyelination, this is a condition in which the virus interferes with myelinogenesis during development, resulting in a hypomyelination similar to that in the genetic mutants discussed later.

Two neurotropic viruses of mice are of particular interest with regard to how immune-me-

diated demyelination of the CNS can be induced by a viral infection. *JHM virus* is a neurotropic strain of mouse hepatitis virus in the coronavirus family that infects oligodendrocytes and produces acute and chronic inflammatory demyelination in rodents [1,2,5]. The acute phase is probably a direct cytopathic effect from the infection of oligodendrocytes, but the chronic phase appears to involve immune mechanisms directed against myelin. Rats infected with JHM virus develop T-cell sensitization to both viral antigens and MBP, and lymphocytes from these animals produce typical EAE when transferred to normal recipients. *Theiler's virus* encephalomyelitis is a chronic, picornavirus-induced disease of the CNS in which many cell types are infected [2,5]. Although there are inflammatory demyelinating lesions in this disease, the immune response does not appear to be directed against myelin itself but rather against viral antigens, some of which may be expressed on the surfaces of infected oligodendrocytes. It has been postulated that the demyelination is caused by a "bystander" effect in which humoral and/or cell-mediated immunity to the virus damages myelin or oligodendrocytes.

Multiple sclerosis is the most common demyelinating disease of the central nervous system in humans

MS appears to be due to a combination of immunological, genetic and environmental factors. It is a chronic demyelinating disease affecting the CNS [1–3]. The disease primarily affects young adults and is characterized by a highly variable course. Most often, the disease begins in the third or fourth decade of life, and the initial course is characterized by acute episodes of neurological dysfunction, such as decreased vision, followed by subsequent recovery. This course is known as relapsing-remitting MS. Over time, the improvement after attacks may be incomplete and the relapsing-remitting course may evolve into one of increasing progression of disability, termed secondary progressive MS. A small number of patients develop a form of disease that begins as a slowly progressive process, without acute episodes of worsening followed by improvement, which has been termed primary progressive MS. A few patients have a very aggressive course, which can lead to death over a short period.

The diagnosis of MS is dependent on clinical evidence of CNS involvement separated in both time and space. Thus, evidence that two areas of the CNS are involved and a history that this involvement occurred at two different times and without any other identifiable cause is necessary to establish a diagnosis of clinically definite MS. While there is no diagnostic test specific for MS, alterations in cerebrospinal fluid (CSF), as well as abnormalities in electrophysiological tests and imaging, particularly magnetic resonance imaging (MRI), can help to identify subclinical lesions and to establish the diagnosis. Of all of these tests, the use of MRI probably has resulted in the greatest change in our understanding of MS. The use of T2-weighted MRI is extremely effective in identifying MS lesions. The areas of increased signal seen on T2-weighted images reflect increased water and, thus, are neither specific for MS nor able to distinguish new from old lesions since both inflammation as well as tissue loss associated with demyelination or gliosis will result in increased signal. A second

technique, T1-weighted imaging done after the administration of a gadolinium salt, which normally does not cross the BBB, can identify new lesions. Serial studies of patients with early relapsing-remitting MS have shown that the first event in the development of a new MS lesion is disruption of the BBB seen on a T2-weighted, gadolinium-enhanced MRI. Thus, post-contrast MRI provides a very sensitive technique for following at least one aspect of disease activity. Using this approach, several groups of investigators have shown that MS is an active and progressive disease even in the early relapsing-remitting phase and during periods of clinical stability in many patients. Newer imaging techniques now hold promise for providing greater specificity for the various stages of lesion development.

MS lesions, or plaques, can be identified grossly at autopsy (Fig. 39-1) and are sharply demarcated from the surrounding tissue. Plaques occur throughout the white matter, but areas of predilection, such as the periventricular white matter, are well known. Microscopic examina-

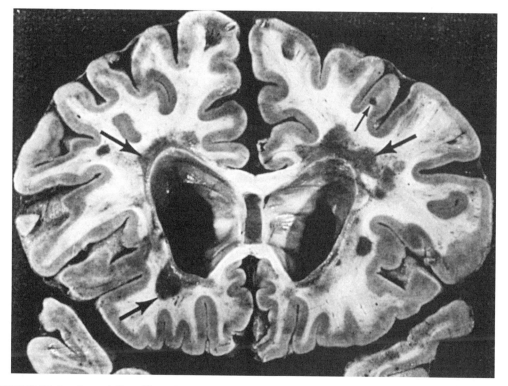

FIGURE 39-1. Coronal slice of brain from a patient who died with multiple sclerosis. Demyelinated plaques are clearly visible in white matter *(large arrows)*. Small plaques are also observed at the boundaries between gray and white matter *(small arrows)*. (From [29], with permission.)

tion characteristically shows loss of myelin with preservation of axons, reflecting primary demyelination. Plaques develop around venules, and "early" lesions contain many lymphocytes, plasma cells and macrophages. The greatest cellularity is found at the margins of acute lesions and is believed to be the location at which some of the earliest changes associated with myelin loss occur. For many years, there has been discussion about whether the primary pathological effect in this disease is directed at oligodendrocytes or myelin sheaths. Detailed examination of MS lesions has indicated that some exhibit demyelination with the preservation of oligodendrocytes, others show demyelination with concomitant destruction of oligodendrocytes and still others exhibit primary oligodendrocyte destruction with secondary demyelination [7]. These findings were interpreted to indicate that the demyelinated plaque may be a common end point resulting from a variety of different immunological and pathological mechanisms. Older chronic lesions are sharply defined and contain bare, nonmyelinated axons and many fibrous astrocytes. Although the most prominent pathology in MS is primary demyelination, there have been indications over the years that there is also some axonal pathology. A recent investigation using techniques of immunocytochemistry and confocal microscopy has clearly demonstrated that transected axons are common in MS lesions [7a]. These findings suggest that axonal loss may account for much of the irreversible neurological impairment in MS and raise the possibility that therapeutic strategies designed to protect axons from injury could be beneficial.

The biochemistry of demyelination in MS has been reviewed in detail [8]. Affected areas of MS white matter exhibit the expected decrease of myelin constituents and a buildup of cholesterol esters. For example, polyacrylamide gel electrophoresis of homogenates of macroscopically normal appearing white matter, outer periplaque, inner periplaque and plaque shows the expected decline of MBP and PLP in going from the normal appearing white matter to the center of the plaque in both chronic and acute lesions (Fig. 39-2). There is a virtual absence of these myelin proteins in the center of the chronic plaque and an accumulation of GFAP indicative

of astrogliosis (Fig. 39-2B). A plaque center from a more acute lesion is not demyelinated completely, as indicated by the presence of some MBP and PLP, and there is no accumulation of GFAP (Fig. 39-2C). The more acute plaque contains albumin due to breakdown of the BBB. Immunocytochemical and quantitative biochemical analyses of myelin proteins have revealed that myelin-associated glycoprotein (MAG) often is decreased more than other myelin proteins at the periphery of plaques, and this may be indicative of early pathological events in the distal periaxonal regions of oligodendroglial processes, where MAG is selectively localized [9]. A number of biochemical studies have indicated that myelin constituents are reduced significantly even in some areas of macroscopically normal appearing white matter of MS brain in comparison to control white matter [8], and this most likely is explained by the presence of microlesions throughout the affected brain. Although the yield of myelin from MS tissue is reduced, most studies indicate that there is no compositional difference between isolated MS and control myelin, suggesting that the etiology of MS is unlikely to be due to an underlying defect in myelin composition. This conclusion may have to be re-evaluated in light of recent findings of a relative increase in MS tissue of an isoform of MBP with a relatively low positive charge because of the conversion of arginine residues to citrulline [10]. This citrulline-rich isoform of MBP is characteristic of immature myelin and may render the myelin less stable. However, it is not yet entirely clear whether this modification of MBP composition in MS reflects an inborn abnormality of myelin structure or whether somehow it is brought on by the disease process.

The cause of MS is not known, but most evidence points to an immunologically mediated disease with important genetic and environmental risk factors [1–3]. The evidence for an autoimmune process is largely circumstantial, based in part on animal models of autoimmune demyelinating diseases such as EAE. In addition to providing insights into the natural history of the disease and a tool that can be used to monitor new treatments, MRI provides insights into the nature of the MS lesion. As indicated previously, BBB disruption seems to be the initial event in lesions,

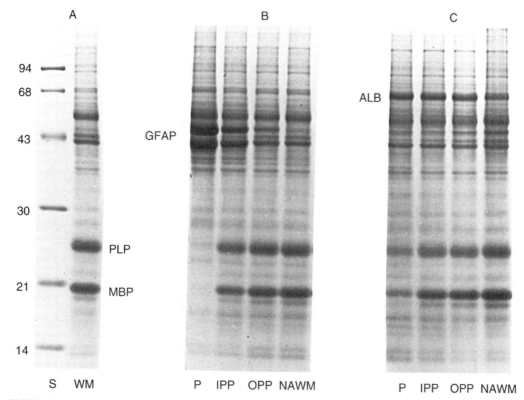

FIGURE 39-2. Polyacrylamide gel electrophoresis of proteins in control and multiple sclerosis (MS) tissue. Total proteins of the tissue samples were solubilized with a detergent (sodium dodecyl sulfate) and electrophoresed on a polyacrylamide gel system that separates proteins according to size. After electrophoresis, proteins were stained with Coomassie brilliant blue dye. **A:** Molecular weight standards *(S)* labeled according to molecular mass in kilodaltons and the proteins of control white matter *(WM)*. **B:** Samples from a region of a chronic MS plaque. **C:** Samples from a region of an acute MS plaque. Tissue samples: *P,* plaque center; *IPP,* inner periplaque; *OPP,* outer periplaque; *NAWM,* macroscopically normal appearing white matter near the plaque. Proteins: *PLP,* proteolipid protein; *MBP,* myelin basic protein; *GFAP,* glial fibrillary acidic protein; *ALB,* serum albumin. (From [30].)

and pathological studies suggest that enhancement on MRI is often reflective of acute inflammation. Based on findings derived from studies of EAE, it is likely that migration of activated T cells represents the initial step in lesion development. What is not clear is the specificity of the T cells. Numerous studies of T-cell reactivity to myelin antigens, such as MBP, PLP and MOG, all of which are encephalitogenic in animals, have been done. To date, the evidence taken as a whole has failed to demonstrate a substantially increased response to these antigens in most patients with MS compared to healthy controls. It may be that several myelin antigens play a role in MS and that the relative importance of different antigens varies among individuals depending on the immunogenetic background and environmental factors.

Further, studies of TCR usage generally have failed to provide evidence for a restricted or limited TCR usage in myelin antigen-specific T cells. What has emerged from studies of the T-cell response to antigens such as MBP is that some regions of the molecule are immunodominant and these can be encephalitogenic in some animal models. Also, the human lymphocyte antigen (HLA) types that most readily present MBP to MBP-specific T cells are those that are over-represented in patients with MS, such as Drw15 (DR2), DR4 and DR6. Thus, it can be postulated that the T-cell response to myelin antigens could represent one component of lesion development but one that, alone, is not sufficient for disease. Other factors could include those which influence the integrity of the BBB and regulation of cytokines.

Once a T cell enters the CNS and encounters antigen, it is postulated that a proinflammatory cytokine cascade is initiated, which produces further disruption of the BBB and amplifies the inflammatory response, eventually resulting in demyelination. The cause of myelin damage is not known. Possibilities include direct toxic effects of some cytokines, such as TNF or NO, on oligodendrocytes or macrophage-mediated damage either through production of proteases or through ligand-mediated interaction with the myelin membrane. Electron microscopy of active MS lesions indicates that one mechanism for myelin destruction is the direct removal of myelin lamellae from the surface of intact sheaths by macrophages. This involves the attachment of superficial lamellae to coated pits at the macrophage surface, implying the presence of receptors that bind to a ligand on the myelin. The Fc receptors on the macrophages may bind to immunoglobulins attached to the myelin, and as mentioned previously, studies of EAE have shown that antibodies to surface molecules of myelin, such as galactocerebroside or MOG, can augment demyelination.

There is much evidence indicating that proteases and other catabolic enzymes are involved in the myelin loss in MS [8]. MBP is highly susceptible to proteases even when present in myelin membranes. A neutral protease released by stimulated macrophages catalyzes the conversion of plasminogen to plasmin, which rapidly degrades MBP. Acid proteinase and other degradative enzymes, presumably lysosomal and of macrophage origin, are elevated in affected MS tissue and are likely to be involved in breakdown of myelin proteins and lipids. In addition, protease activities intrinsic to myelin sheaths, such as Ca^{2+}-activated neutral protease, may facilitate myelin destruction. Immunologically reactive, proteolytic fragments of MBP appear in the CSF and urine of MS patients during exacerbations of the disease and presumably reflect myelin breakdown. However, the presence of this material is not specific for MS since it occurs in other conditions with myelin damage, such as stroke and encephalitis.

Three therapies that are thought to modify immunopathogenic aspects of the disease have been approved for use in treating patients with relapsing-remitting MS: interferon β1a, interferon β1b and copolymer-1 (COP-1) [11]. The mechanism of action of the β interferons is not known. Nevertheless, it is postulated that the interferons modify antigen presentation by reducing the expression of HLA class II molecules. It is also possible that the interferons may modify events responsible for BBB disruption, such as expression of cell adhesion molecules. The mechanism of COP-1 is also not well understood. It is postulated that COP-1, which is a random polymer composed of the amino acids L-alanine, L-glutamic acid, L-lysine and L-tyrosine, may result in peptides that selectively bind to HLA class II molecules and block antigen presentation. Generation of regulatory T cells also has been suggested. In addition to these approved therapies, a number of therapies targeting different steps thought to be involved in development of the MS lesion are under investigation [11]. Among the more interesting are therapies designed to modify T-cell reactivity, decrease the influx of inflammatory cells into the CNS and modify the action of proinflammatory cytokines. MRI provides a powerful tool for monitoring the initial testing of experimental therapies such as those mentioned above.

In addition to immunological elements, it is likely that both genetic and environmental factors contribute to disease susceptibility [1–3]. Two types of studies have provided data which favor a genetic component in MS. First, the prevalence of MS varies substantially among ethnic groups, with Caucasian populations showing a higher frequency than some other groups. For example, MS occurs at low frequency both in Japan and in Japanese Americans living in high-prevalence regions of the United States. Second, there is increased risk among first-degree relatives of individuals with the disease, especially in monozygotic twins, where the rate of concordance for the disease is 20 to 30% and even higher with careful examination by techniques such as MRI. Several possible genetic loci have been examined in MS, and, as mentioned above, a fairly consistent association, although weak, with HLA makeup has been found in most studies. Three studies have examined the entire genome in patients with MS. While some areas of possible significance have been found, it is certain that the effect of any single genetic locus is relatively small. It is almost certain that multiple genes are involved, each with a small influence on susceptibility.

Several types of evidence point to an environmental influence in MS. These include unequal geographic distribution of the disease, effect of migration between low and high risk areas on susceptibility and evidence for epidemics or clusters. Each of these sets of observations is open to variable interpretation, and in many cases, the genetic influence is difficult to separate from that of the environment. However, the bulk of evidence suggests that the environment contributes to risk. The nature of the environmental influence is not known, but a viral infection has long been suspected [1–3]. In animals, there are a number of naturally occurring and experimental disorders caused by viruses that have long incubation periods and involve primary demyelination with sparing of axons (see above). A possible viral etiology for MS has stimulated an extensive amount of research, leading to many reports of viruses associated with MS, and there is currently a substantial amount of interest in a possible involvement of human herpes viruses. However, at this time, a definite causative infectious agent has not been established. Nevertheless, a viral infection occurring before puberty and possibly modifying immune function, rather than resulting in a persistent infection, seems likely. Thus, although it is widely thought that MS is an autoimmune disease associated with an infectious agent, the putative antigen(s) and virus(es) remain elusive.

Some human peripheral neuropathies involving demyelination are thought to be immune-mediated

These include Guillain-Barré Syndrome (GBS), chronic inflammatory demyelinating polyneuropathy (CIDP), multifocal motor neuropathy (MMN) and neuropathy associated with IgM gammopathy. GBS is an acute inflammatory demyelinating polyneuropathy that is monophasic and self-limiting and frequently occurs following a bacterial or viral infection [2,12]. Generally, it is characterized by primary demyelination, although variants with severe axonal

involvement also exist. CIDP is similar but is progressive or relapsing-remitting, with a duration of many months or years [2,12]. With regard to potential target antigens for autoimmune diseases of the PNS, it should be kept in mind that although PNS and CNS myelin structures are morphologically similar, they differ significantly in chemical composition, especially in protein constituents (see Chap. 4). Cumulative evidence suggests that nerve injury in GBS and CIDP is mediated by immunological mechanisms, but, as in MS, the role of the patient's cell-mediated and humoral responses in causing the demyelination has not been fully defined. A role of humoral immunity in the diseases is suggested by findings that sera from GBS patients cause demyelination in appropriate test systems and that plasmapheresis and intravenous administration of immunoglobulin are effective therapies in many of these patients.

Although experimental allergic neuritis (EAN) often is considered to be a good animal model for GBS and the P2 myelin protein is implicated as an important antigen in this model (see Chap. 36), neither cellular nor humoral immunity to P2 or other myelin proteins has been detected consistently in GBS. Similarly, although antibodies to galactocerebroside have been shown to cause peripheral demyelination in experimental animals, evidence for significant concentrations of antibodies to this glycolipid in GBS is lacking. However, antibodies to more complex glycolipids, such as gangliosides, have been detected in some patients with GBS and other forms of demyelinating neuropathy [12,13]. For example, antibodies to GM1 ganglioside are particularly associated with a subset of GBS that occurs following *Campylobacter jejuni* infection. This type of GBS is particularly severe, has a high degree of axonal degeneration and presents with predominantly motor symptoms. Although these correlations have not been observed in all cases, this form of GBS appears to be a good example in which molecular mimicry between an immunogen of an infectious agent and a neural antigen causes an autoimmune disease (Fig. 39-3) because a carbohydrate configuration identical to that in GM1 ganglioside occurs in the lipopolysaccharide (LPS) of strains of *C. jejuni* that are associated with this subset of

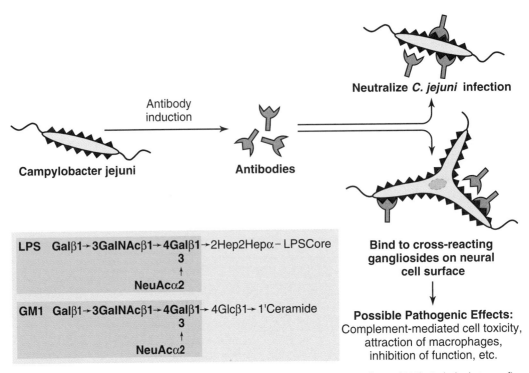

FIGURE 39-3. Molecular mimicry in subsets of patients with Guillain-Barré syndrome (GBS). Carbohydrate configurations *(black triangles)* in the lipopolysaccharide *(LPS)* of some strains of *Campylobacter jejuni* are the same as in GM1 ganglioside on neural membranes. The chemical structures of LPS and GM1 are shown in the **inset**, with the shared terminal tetrasaccharide in boldface. Antibodies produced in response to LPS during a *C. jejuni* infection are intended to fight the infection but may cross-react with GM1 on neural cells, causing pathogenic effects in GBS by mechanisms such as those listed in the **lower right** of the figure. Similarly, the LPS in other strains of *C. jejuni* have carbohydrate structures similar to those in GQ1b ganglioside, and these strains are associated with the Miller-Fisher variant of GBS, with prominent cranial nerve involvement, ataxia and areflexia. Antibodies to GQ1b are found in essentially all patients with this variant.

GBS. Antibodies to GM1 ganglioside are also found frequently in a distinct chronic progressive neuropathy defined by multifocal motor conduction blocks. This condition, known as multifocal motor neuropathy (MMN), is characterized by weakness, muscle atrophy and motor nerve demyelination, while sensory function is normal or only slightly affected. Generally, there appears to be a strong correlation between antibodies to GM1 ganglioside and motor nerve disorders that include GBS, MMN and the neuropathies in association with monoclonal gammopathy described below. Furthermore, there is evidence from *in vitro* and *in vivo* animal models that the anti-GM1 antibodies cause the motor nerve pathology in these patients [13].

Neuropathies also occur in association with monoclonal gammopathy, also termed parapro-

teinemia, in which there is expansion of a clone of plasma cells, leading to large amounts of a monoclonal antibody in the patient's serum. It is thought that the neuropathies in these patients may be caused by binding of the monoclonal antibodies to neural antigens [13]. One of the best known examples of this is a demyelinating sensory or mixed sensorimotor neuropathy in which a monoclonal IgM antibody binds to a carbohydrate epitope in MAG. It is noteworthy that the reactive carbohydrate epitope in MAG is shared with some glycolipids and other glycoproteins present in the PNS but generally absent from the CNS. The principal antigenic glycolipid is sulfate-3-glucuronyl paragloboside (SGPG), and P_0 glycoprotein and peripheral myelin protein-22 (PMP-22) of compact PNS myelin also express the reactive epitope. The specificity of these human antibodies is very similar to that of the HNK-1 antibody, which reacts with a number of adhesion proteins in the nervous system (see Chap. 4). Several animal models involving administration of the human anti-MAG/SGPG antibodies or immunization with SGPG strongly suggest that this disease is caused by the antibodies, but the relative importance of the potential glycolipid and glycoprotein target antigens in contributing to the pathology remains to be established. About half of patients with neuropathy in association with IgM gammopathy have antibodies of this specificity, and monoclonal IgM antibodies in other patients with neuropathy that are MAG/SGPG-negative frequently react with ganglioside antigens [13]. For example, some of these patients have monoclonal IgM anti-GM1 antibodies in association with motor neuropathy (see above). The relatively high frequency with which antibodies that react with acidic glycolipid antigens, such as gangliosides or SGPG, occur in patients with neuropathy may be significant with regard to pathogenic mechanisms. Furthermore, there is a growing body of experimental evidence indicating that these antibodies contribute to the neuropathies in many cases, although the precise molecular and cellular mechanisms causing the pathogenesis remain to be established.

Other acquired disorders affecting myelin in humans may be secondary to viral infections, neoplasias or immunosuppressive therapy

Acute disseminated encephalomyelitis, also called postinfectious or postimmunization encephalitis, represents a group of disorders of usually mixed viral–immunological etiology. The condition is most commonly related to a spontaneous viral infection, such as measles, smallpox or chickenpox [1,2]. The demyelination occurring in these conditions is likely to be mediated at least in part by immune mechanisms since T cells sensitized to MBP are detected in many of these patients.

The nervous system is affected in a high proportion of patients with acquired immunodeficiency syndrome (AIDS) [14]. Abnormalities related to myelin include a generalized myelin pallor observed histologically, vacuolar myelopathy and

focal demyelination. Although it was originally thought that the widespread myelin pallor could be indicative of substantial demyelination, it now appears that the reduced staining is related to accumulation of fluid because of breakdown of the BBB and not to extensive myelin loss. It is generally accepted that human immunodeficiency virus (HIV) infection in the nervous system *in vivo* is largely restricted to macrophages and microglia, and the myelin and oligodendrocyte damage associated with HIV may be mediated by cytokines released by infected macrophages (see section on toxins below). Nevertheless, there continues to be interest in the observations that galactocerebroside and sulfatide can bind the GP120 surface protein of HIV, suggesting that they could act as alternate receptors to CD4, thereby allowing some virus into oligodendrocytes [15].

Progressive multifocal leukoencephalopathy (PML) is a rare demyelinating disease that usually is associated with disorders of the reticuloendothelial system, neoplasias and immunosuppressive therapy [1]. However, it has become more important in clinical medicine because it is frequently seen as one of the opportunistic secondary infections associated with immunocompromised persons with AIDS. PML is characterized by noninflammatory focal lesions that are caused by infection of oligodendrocytes with the JC papovavirus.

GENETIC DISORDERS OF MYELIN

Spontaneous mutations in experimental animals provide insights about the structure and assembly of myelin

These mutants often have names relating to their characteristic tremor due to the myelin deficit, such as *shiverer*, *jimpy*, *quaking* and *trembler* mice. Although some of the mutants have been studied for many years [1], it is only recently that recombinant DNA techniques have led to identification of the primary genetic defects in many of them. Some of them are good models for inherited human diseases affecting myelin, as described below. Furthermore, the naturally occurring mouse mutants, which may express abnormal myelin proteins, sometimes have phenotypes that differ from null mutants produced experimentally by homologous recombination (see Chap. 4) and are thereby instructive with regard to the mechanisms of myelin formation and loss. Analyses of whole homogenates of CNS or PNS tissue from the mutants generally reveal a deficiency of all characteristic myelin lipids, such as galactocerebroside and phosphatidylethanolamine, and proteins, even when the genetic defect directly affects only one of the myelin proteins [16]. This implies that there is a coordinated expression of myelin lipids and proteins which is interrupted when one component is abnormal. The magnitude of the deficiency varies with the severity of the hypomyelination. Generally, the deficiencies of proteins of compact myelin, MBP, PLP and P_0 glycoprotein are greater than those of cyclic nucleotide phosphohydrolase (CNPase) and MAG, presumably because the mutants exhibit a greater deficiency of compact myelin than of associated oligodendroglial or Schwann cell membranes in which the latter components are localized (see Chap. 4).

Mutation of either of the major structural proteins of CNS myelin, MBP and PLP, can lead to a severe hypomyelination. MBP is mutated in *shiverer* and myelin-deficient (mld) mice [17], and PLP is mutated in *jimpy* mice and several other animal mutants [18,19]. Ultrastructural abnormalities in the small amount of myelin that is formed by these mutants have been informative with regard to the structural roles of these proteins in compact CNS myelin. Thus, the cytoplasmic surfaces of the spiraled oligodendrocyte membranes do not compact to form a major dense line in the absence of MBP in *shiverer* mutants, and the intraperiod line is abnormal in *jimpy* mice, which express very little PLP (see Chap. 4). The ultrastructure of PNS myelin is normal in both of these mutants since PLP is not in peripheral myelin, and P_0 appears to be capable of stabilizing both the intraperiod and major dense lines of myelin of the PNS in the absence of MBP.

The *shiverer* phenotype can be corrected by introducing normal MBP into transgenic mutant mice, resulting in almost complete correction of the shivering, early death and failure of CNS myelin compaction. The gene for PLP is on the X-chromosome, so all of the mutants in which PLP is altered exhibit sex-linked inheritance; however, the severity of the myelin deficiency varies from mutant to mutant. In addition to the severe deficiency and abnormal structure of CNS myelin, *jimpy* mice exhibit a profound loss of oligodendrocytes. Furthermore, attempts to correct the *jimpy* phenotype by introducing the normal gene have not been successful. This is because the small amount of abnormal PLP produced in this mutant is toxic, causing failure of oligodendrocyte differentiation and producing cell death with morphological features of apoptosis. This failure of oligodendrocyte development, rather than the absence of PLP in the myelin, appears to be the primary cause of the severe hypomyelination in *jimpy* mice. Thus, mutation of the PLP gene in another position in *rumpshaker* mice does not cause oligodendrocyte death and produces a much milder phenotype. Furthermore, experimentally produced null-mutants for PLP have relatively normal myelination with regard to the number and thickness of CNS sheaths, although they exhibit abnormal compaction of the intraperiod line similar to that of *jimpy* mice (see Chap. 4). The PLP mutants provide a good illustration of the fact that a null allele can produce a milder phenotype than other abnormal alleles because simple loss of function may not be as harmful as the effects of an abnormal protein.

The *trembler* mutation is autosomal dominant and specific for the PNS [20]. Two allelic forms of this mutant are caused by different point mutations in transmembrane domains of PMP-22. The *trembler* phenotypes are characterized by hypomyelination, continued Schwann cell proliferation and partial paralysis of the limbs. These mutants are animal models for some of the inherited human neuropathies caused by abnormalities of the PMP-22 gene (see below). However, because the function of PMP-22 is unknown (see Chap. 4), the mechanism by which the point mutations in PMP-22 cause the *trembler* phenotype is not known.

A number of spontaneous animal mutants have been described that are not due to lesions in one of the proteins of compact myelin but appear to be caused by a defect in some cellular process needed for myelin assembly or maintenance. One example is the autosomal recessive *quaking* mutation in mice, resulting in hypomyelination of both the CNS and PNS [1]. Unlike the *shiverer* and *jimpy* mice, which form almost no myelin and die early, *quaking* mice generate more myelin and live to adulthood. However, the myelin sheaths are thin and poorly compacted, especially in the CNS, which is affected more severely than the PNS. The myelin isolated from the CNS of this mutant has all of the known myelin proteins, but its overall composition resembles that of very immature 7- to 10-day-old normal mice. Although the *quaking* mouse was one of the first dysmyelinating mutants to be described and has been studied extensively, the genetic lesion has only recently been identified by positional cloning [21]. The mutated protein appears to be one that links signal transduction of extracellular information to some aspect of RNA metabolism, possibly alternative splicing of mRNAs. In this regard, it is of interest that several of the myelin proteins occur in developmentally regulated isoforms due to alternative splicing of mRNA (see Chap. 4), and this regulation is abnormal in *quaking* mice.

A mutation that affects myelination in the CNS occurs in the "taiep" rat [22]. Taiep is an acronym for the progression of symptoms with development: trembling, ataxia, immobility, epilepsy and paralysis. These mutants exhibit an impaired accumulation of myelin for up to 2 months, followed by a period of demyelination so that adults have only 10 to 25% of the normal amount of myelin. The primary genetic lesion has not been identified, but mutant oligodendrocytes exhibit an abnormal accumulation of microtubules during development, suggesting that a microtubule-associated protein might be involved. Biochemical evidence suggests that the accumulation of microtubules could interfere with the transport of myelin proteins or their mRNAs, eventually leading to a failure of myelin maintenance.

The human leukodystrophies are inherited disorders affecting central nervous system white matter

These disorders are characterized by a diffuse deficiency of myelin caused by a variety of genetic lesions, and often begin prior to 10 years of age (Table 39-1). Some are caused by a variety of different mutations in the PLP gene and resemble the PLP animal mutants described above [18,19]. As with the animal models, depending on the site of the mutation, they vary from a severe form in connatal Pelizaeus-Merzbacher disease (PMD) to an intermediate phenotype in classical PMD to a mild phenotype in spastic paraplegia.

Other leukodystrophies are associated with lysosomal and peroxisomal disorders in which specific lipids or other substances accumulate due to a deficiency in a catabolic enzyme, as in Krabbe's disease, metachromatic leukodystrophy (MLD) and adrenoleukodystrophy (ALD) (see Chap. 41) [23]. Similarly, disorders of amino acid metabolism, such as phenylketonuria and Canavan's disease, lead to hypomyelination (see Chap. 44) [23]. The composition of myelin in genetically determined disorders may be normal or have a specific alteration reflecting the genetic lesion. In some, myelin may show a nonspecific pathological composition, which is found in many myelin disorders. The composition of the small amount of myelin isolated from Krabbe's disease is normal, and the hypomyelination is believed to be caused by the accumulation of galactosylsphingosine, which has a cytotoxic effect on myelin-forming cells. By contrast, myelin isolated from postmortem MLD brain is enriched in sulfatide (Table 39-2). It is not known whether the myelin formed in MLD is unstable and, therefore, degenerates because of the excess sulfatide or whether the excess sulfatide is due to sulfatide-enriched micelles that are coisolated during myelin purification.

In some genetic disorders, such as ALD and Canavan's disease, as well as in a wide variety of disorders involving secondary demyelination, myelin preparations have similar, abnormal chemical compositions. This is shown in Table 39-2 for Canavan's disease and subacute sclerosing panencephalomyelitis (SSPE). Certain experimental disorders induced in animals by toxic agents show the same type of abnormal myelin. In each case, the isolated pathological myelin has a generally normal ultrastructural appearance but much more cholesterol, less cerebroside and less phosphatidalethanolamine than normal myelin. Myelin with this abnormal

TABLE 39-1. GENETICALLY DETERMINED DISORDERS AFFECTING MYELIN IN HUMANS

Disorder	Inheritance[a]	Genetic lesion	Comments	References
Adrenoleukodystrophy	X-linked	Peroxisomal membrane protein in the ABC transporter family	Decreased peroxidation of saturated, very long-chain fatty acids, causing their accumulation in brain, adrenals and other tissues; variable phenotypes with regard to hypomyelination; see text and Table 39-2	1, 23, 24 and Chap 41
Canavan's disease (spongy degeneration)	AR	Aspartoacylase	Widespread edema in white matter with diminished myelin; *N*-acetylaspartic aciduria; see text and Table 39-2	1, 23 and Chap 44
Charcot-Marie-Tooth disease and other inherited neuropathies	AD or X-linked	PMP-22, P_0 or connexin-32	Variable degrees of myelin deficiency specific for the PNS; see text	1, 19 and 20
Krabbe's leukodystrophy	AR	Galactocerebroside, β-galactosidase	Globoid cells contain galactocerebroside; see text	1, 23 and Chap 41
Metachromatic leukodystrophy	AR	Arylsulfatase A	Accumulation of sulfatide in brain; see text and Table 39-2	1, 23 and Chap 41
Pelizaeus-Merzbacher disease (classical and connatal forms) and spastic paraplegia	X-linked	PLP	Variable hypomyelination due to different mutations in the major structural protein of CNS myelin; similar to rodent mutants, such as the *jimpy* mouse	1, 18 and 19
Phenylketonuria	AR	Phenylalanine hydroxylase	White matter is up to 40% deficient in myelin, hypomyelination may be caused by inhibition of amino acid transport and/or protein synthesis by the high concentration of phenylalanine that accumulates	1, 23 and Chap 44
Refsum's disease	AR	Oxidation of branched-chain fatty acids	Increase of branched-chain phytanic acid, especially prominent in PNS myelin	1, 23 and Chap 41

[a]AR, autosomal recessive; AD, autosomal dominant.

composition is referred to as the "nonspecific pathological type" and probably represents a partially degraded form.

X-linked ALD has long been known to be a peroxisomal disease that involves a defect in the β oxidation of very long-chain fatty acids (VLCFAs), leading to their accumulation in complex lipids [24], and it was thought that the genetic defect would be in an enzyme such as VLCFA-CoA synthetase (Chap. 41). However, the positional cloning approach surprisingly showed that the defective gene is a 70-kDa peroxisomal membrane protein in the ATP-binding cassette transporter protein family (see Chap. 5). Members of this family are involved in transporting a variety of ligands, and it may be that the mutated protein is needed to import VLCFA-CoA synthetase into peroxisomes. An interesting aspect of ALD is that the phenotype can vary from a major neurological problem in

TABLE 39-2. **HUMAN MYELIN COMPOSITION IN THREE DISEASES COMPARED WITH CONTROLS**[a]

Lipids[b]	Control	Spongy degeneration	SSPE	MLD
Total lipid (% of dry weight)	70.0	63.8	73.7	63.2
Cholesterol	27.7	58.0	43.7	21.2
Cerebrosides	22.7	8.0	18.8	9.0
Sulfatides	3.8	2.0	2.8	28.4
Total phospholipids	43.1	33.4	36.6	36.1
Ethanolamine phosphatides	15.6	9.8	9.7	8.1
Plasmalogen[c]	12.3	—	9.1	5.3
Lecithin	11.2	11.3	10.4	10.7
Sphingomyelin	7.9	5.9	8.8	7.1
Serine phosphatides	4.8	5.5	4.6	3.8
Phosphatidylinositol	0.6	0.8	1.4	3.1

[a] SSPE, subacute sclerosing panencephalitis; MLD, metachromatic leukodystrophy; source of data is Tables I and II in [31].
[b] Individual lipids expressed as weight percentage of total lipid.
[c] Most of the plasmalogen is phosphatidalethanolamine and is included in the ethanolamine phosphatides column.

the childhood form with a severe deficiency of myelin in the brain to a milder form known as adrenomyeloneuropathy, which occurs in young men and affects primarily spinal cord and peripheral nerve, to less common phenotypes without neurological involvement. This clinical variability cannot be accounted for by the severity of the biochemical abnormality or the nature of the gene defect, and it is thought that the action of an autosomal modifier gene is the most likely explanation. The involvement of another parameter in causing the neurological pathology is also indicated by gene targeting research in several laboratories that produced mice not expressing the peroxisomal membrane protein that is mutated in human ALD (see [24a] for example). These knockout mice exhibit the same biochemical abnormalities with the accumulation of VLCFAs, but no neurological involvement was noted in developing or young adult mice. Unlike most other lipid-storage diseases, active ALD brain lesions are characterized by perivascular accumulation of lymphocytes, and it has been hypothesized that the severity of CNS pathology may relate to an autoimmune reaction which varies from patient to patient. Since ALD involves inflammation, it is not surprising that substantial amounts of cholesterol ester accumulate in the brain. In ALD and other disorders in which myelin debris is phagocytosed,

most of the cholesterol esters are in an abnormal floating fraction of lower density than the isolated myelin when tissue homogenates are fractionated on sucrose gradients.

Deficiencies of peripheral nerve myelin in several inherited neuropathies are caused by genetic mutations in sheath proteins

Remarkable progress in understanding the inherited neuropathies has been achieved in recent years [19,20] (see Chap. 36). The most common inherited neuropathies, Charcot-Marie-Tooth (CMT) disease type 1A and hereditary neuropathy with liability to pressure palsies (HNPP), are caused by dominant abnormalities of the PMP-22 gene. CMT1A, usually due to duplication of the PMP-22 gene with onset in the second or third decade of life, is characterized by segmental demyelination, remyelination and onion bulb formation. HNPP is a milder neuropathy, brought on by pressure or trauma to an affected nerve, caused by a heterozygous deletion of the PMP-22 gene. These human disorders caused by over- and underexpression of PMP-22, respectively, illustrate the importance of dosage of some myelin proteins for myelin stability (see Chaps. 4 and 36). CMT1B is caused by mutations in the major P_0 protein of myelin. There is also an X-linked form of CMT that is caused by mutations in the gap junction protein connexin 32 (CX32), localized in the paranodal membranes and incisures of peripheral myelin sheaths, which may be involved in maintenance of the sheaths.

TOXIC AND NUTRITIONAL DISORDERS OF MYELIN

Biological toxins can produce myelin loss

These toxins can be produced by exogenous infectious agents in diseases such as diphtheria or endogenously by lymphocytes and macrophages. Diphtheric neuropathy [1] is a possible complication of *Corynebacterium diphtheriae* infection and is characterized by vacuolation and fragmentation of myelin sheaths in the PNS. A similar disorder can be caused by injection of animals with the toxin, which may act by inhibiting protein synthesis in Schwann cells or by binding to myelin and producing channels in the membrane (Chap. 36).

Some cytokines released by lymphocytes and macrophages, such as TNF and lymphotoxin, are toxic to oligodendrocytes in culture [25]. Activated macrophages and microglia can release oxygen radicals and NO, which are also harmful to oligodendrocytes [25]. As a result, there is much ongoing research concerning the role of cytokines in demyelinating diseases, such as EAE and MS, that are associated with immune reactions [2,3,25]. These toxins could lead to myelin destruction independent of whether the immune reaction is targeted against myelin or an exogenous infectious agent. Damage to myelin by an immune reaction directed to an unrelated antigen is referred to as a "bystander effect."

Many chemical toxins can impair myelin formation or cause its breakdown

These include lead, cuprizone, lysolecithin, organotin, hexachlorophene and tellurium. Lead is a common environmental pollutant that causes hypomyelination and demyelination [1]. Cuprizone and lysolecithin are toxins that frequently have been used experimentally in the context of investigating remyelination [1,5] (see below). Systemically administered cuprizone has a direct toxic effect on oligodendrocytes, whereas lysolecithin causes lysis of myelin sheaths themselves when administered focally. Triethyltin and hexachlorophene cause an edematous demyelination with splitting at the intraperiod line but without apparent damage to myelin-forming cells [1]. Tellurium treatment of young rats causes a highly synchronous demyelination and remyelination in sciatic nerve that is associated with the inhibition of cholesterol synthesis by some metabolite of this element [26]. A detailed description of the effects of these and other chemical toxins on the biochemistry of myelin is beyond the scope of this chapter, but they have been covered in more detail in earlier editions of this book or in other sources [1].

General undernourishment or dietary deficiencies of specific substances can lead to a preferential reduction in myelin formation

Much of the CNS myelin in mammals is formed during a relatively restricted time period, corresponding to the final prenatal months and the first few years of postnatal life in humans and 15 to 30 days of postnatal life in rats. Just before this rapid deposition of myelin, there is a burst of oligodendroglial proliferation. During these restricted periods of time, large portions of the metabolic activity and synthetic capacity of the brain are involved in myelinogenesis. Any metabolic insult during this "vulnerable" period may lead to a preferential reduction in myelin formation [1]. The most vulnerable period appears to be the time of oligodendroglia proliferation since animals deprived of food in this period have an irreversible deficit of myelin-forming cells and hypomyelination. However, animals deprived at a later age often demonstrate significant recovery with regard to the amount of myelin when nutritional rehabilitation is instigated after a period of underfeeding. Failure to myelinate properly and demyelination also are associated with deficiencies of dietary protein, essential fatty acids and several vitamins, including thiamine, B_{12} and B_6 [1]

(see Chap. 33). Hypomyelination also is caused by copper deficiency in animals and in the sex-linked inherited disorder Menkes' kinky hair disease, in which there is a disorder of copper transport (see Chap. 5 and Box 45-1) [1].

DISORDERS PRIMARILY AFFECTING NEURONS WITH SECONDARY INVOLVEMENT OF MYELIN

Many insults to the nervous system initially cause damage to neurons but eventually result in regions of demyelination as a consequence of neuronal degeneration. These include mechanical trauma, infarcts, tumors, viral diseases such as SSPE, genetic disorders like Tay-Sachs disease and motor neuron disease.

The archetypical model for secondary demyelination is Wallerian degeneration

When a nerve in the PNS or a myelinated tract in the CNS is cut or crushed, the proximal segment often survives and regenerates [1]. In the distal segment, Wallerian degeneration occurs, with both axons and myelin disappearing (see Chap. 36). Debris is phagocytosed by neural cells and macrophages. From such experiments, it is clear that the integrity of the myelin sheath depends on continued contact with a viable axon. Any disease that causes injury to neurons may result in axonal degeneration and lead to the onset of myelin breakdown secondary to the neuronal damage. During Wallerian degeneration in the PNS, there is a rapid loss of myelin-specific lipids within a period of 1 to 2 weeks and even more rapid loss of myelin-specific proteins. There is also a concomitant increase in many lysosomal enzymes. Between the second and fourth week after nerve section, most of the myelin debris has been removed and remyelination of regenerating axons begins. Wallerian degeneration has been studied in the CNS by enucleating eyes in rats and examining the optic nerve at different times. Degeneration of myelin is a much slower process in the CNS than in the PNS and takes place within macrophages.

Secondary demyelination occurs in subacute sclerosing panencephalitis and other diseases of the central nervous system

The first human disease to be studied with respect to myelin composition during secondary demyelination was SSPE, a CNS disease caused by a defective measles virus infection [1]. It is probable that this disease involves destruction of both neurons and oligodendroglia. The isolated myelin has a grossly normal ultrastructural appearance and a normal lipid:protein ratio. However, it has the typical nonspecific changes, with more cholesterol, less cerebroside and less ethanolamine phosphatides than normal human myelin (Table 39-2). No cholesterol esters were found in the myelin, although they were abundant in the white matter. Abnormal myelin of this type also has been isolated from such sphingolipidoses as Tay-Sachs disease, generalized gangliosidosis and Niemann-Pick disease (see Chap. 41).

REMYELINATION

The capacity for remyelination is generally greater in the peripheral than in the central nervous system

Much of this chapter has considered biochemical mechanisms of myelin loss, but the capacity of nervous tissue to repair the damage by remyelination is also an important factor in the eventual clinical outcome of disorders affecting myelin. Following transection of the peripheral nerve, as described in the previous section, myelination of the regenerating axons occurs soon after the final clean up of myelin debris by Schwann cells [1]. The Schwann cells that form the new myelin are probably not the same ones that phagocytose the debris but appear to arise by cell division. The smaller capacity for remyelination in the CNS in comparison to the PNS may lie in the nature of the myelin-forming cells in that oligodendrocytes myelinate many axons, in contrast to the single segments of myelin formed by Schwann cells. Under some circumstances, such as in EAE and MS, Schwann cells will migrate into the spinal cord and remyelinate demyelinated CNS axons.

Remyelination in the central nervous system can be promoted by various treatments

Substantial remyelination can occur in the CNS depending on the nature of the pathogenic insult. For example, rapid remyelination by oligodendrocytes occurs following acute demyelination caused by toxins such as cuprizone and lysolecithin, although the myelin sheaths are thinner than normal [5]. The failure of significant remyelination in other circumstances may relate to the continuing effect of pathogenic processes. Thus, studies in experimental animals with autoimmune demyelination have shown that various immunosuppressive treatments promote remyelination in addition to combating demyelination [5]. Even in MS, careful observations of acute lesions have demonstrated the presence of healthy oligodendrocytes and regeneration of myelin in the presence of myelin breakdown [7]. Although the remyelination attempt eventually fails and oligodendrocytes are lost from lesions that progress to advanced demyelinated plaques, such observations raise the possibility that management of patients with demyelinating diseases of the CNS eventually may involve treatments that take advantage of the capacity of oligodendrocytes for remyelination.

Research on experimental animals indicates that remyelination can occur by proliferation and differentiation of host progenitor cells, which are quiescent in normal adult tissue. Several approaches are being used to attempt to enhance the natural capacity of oligodendrocytes or their progenitors to remyelinate. Because a large number of growth factors, such as epidermal growth factor, basic fibroblast growth factor, platelet-derived growth factor, ciliary neurotrophic factor and insulin-like growth factor, affect the survival, proliferation, migration and differentiation of oligodendrocyte progenitors, it is feasible that remyelination is promoted in patients by treatment with one or more of these factors [27]. For example, insulin-like growth factor-1 promotes remyelination and clinical improvement in the EAE model of autoimmune demyelination. Another somewhat surprising observation that may have relevance for enhancing remyelination is that various immunoglobu-

lin preparations containing antibodies that react with surface antigens of oligodendrocytes have the capacity to promote remyelination in experimental animals [5]. Finally, an approach actively being pursued at this time involves the capacity of transplants of myelin-forming glial cells to repair demyelinated lesions [28]. Much of this research involves the transplantation of Schwann cells, oligodendrocytes, oligodendrocyte progenitors or glial cell lines into hypomyelinated mutants or focally demyelinated lesions and has clearly demonstrated that transplanted cells have the capacity to remyelinate. It appears that oligodendrocyte progenitors may possess the best combination of properties for extensive remyelination with regard to survival, proliferation, migration and differentiation to the myelinating stage. Furthermore, it may be that a combination of treatments, such as glial transplants plus growth factors, will provide the best results. Further research is needed to evaluate the success of these approaches in the presence of astrocytic gliosis and inflammation. Nevertheless, it appears likely that treatment of myelin disorders in humans eventually may involve promotion of remyelination as well as prevention of myelin breakdown.

REFERENCES

1. Morell, P. *Myelin.* New York: Plenum Press, 1984.
2. McFarland, H., and McFarlin, D. Immunologically mediated demyelinating diseases of the central and peripheral nervous system. In M. Frank and M. Samter (eds.), *Immunologic Diseases.* Boston: Little Brown, 1995, pp. 1081–1101.
3. Martin, R., and McFarland, H. F. Immunological aspects of experimental allergic encephalomyelitis and multiple sclerosis. *Crit. Rev. Clin. Lab. Sci.* 32:121–182, 1995.
4. Bernard, C. C., Johns, T. G., Slavin, A., et al. Myelin oligodendrocyte glycoprotein: A novel candidate autoantigen in multiple sclerosis. *J. Mol. Med.* 75:77–88, 1997.
5. Miller, D. J., Asakura, K., and Rodriguez, M. Central nervous system remyelination: Clinical application of basic neuroscience principles. *Brain Pathol.* 6:331–344, 1996.

6. Moller, J. R., McLenigan, M., Potts, B. J., and Quarles, R. H. Effects of congenital infection of sheep with border disease virus on myelin proteins. *J. Neurochem.* 61:1808–1812, 1993.

7. Lucchinetti, C. F., Bruck, W., Rodriguez, M., and Lassmann, H. Distinct patterns of multiple sclerosis pathology indicate heterogeneity on pathogenesis. *Brain Pathol.* 6:259–274, 1996.

7a. Trapp, B. D., Peterson, J., Ransohoff, R. M., Rudick, R., Mork, S., Bo, L. Axonal transection in the lesions of multiple sclerosis. *N. Engl. J. Med.* 338:278–285, 1998.

8. Cuzner, M. L., and Norton, W. T. Biochemistry of demyelination. *Brain Pathol.* 6:231–242, 1996.

9. Quarles, R. Glycoproteins of myelin sheaths. *J. Mol. Neurosci.* 8:1–12, 1997.

10. Wood, D. D., Bilbao, J. M., O'Connors, P., and Moscarello, M. A. Acute multiple sclerosis (Marburg type) is associated with developmentally immature myelin basic protein. *Ann. Neurol.* 40:18–24, 1996.

11. Martin, R., Holfield, R., and McFarland, H. F. Multiple sclerosis. In T. Brant, L. Caplan, J. Dichgans, H. Diener, and C. Kennard (eds.), *Neurological Disorders: Course and Treatment.* San Diego: Academic Press, 1996, pp. 483–505.

12. van der Meche, F. V. D., and van Doorn, P. V. Guillain-Barre syndrome and chronic inflammatory demyelinating polyneuropathy: Immune mechanisms and update on current therapies. *Ann. Neurol.* 37S:S14–S31, 1995.

13. Quarles, R. H. The spectrum and pathogenesis of antibody mediated neuropathies. *Neuroscientist* 3:195–204, 1997.

14. Price, R. W. Understanding the AIDS dementia complex (ADC). The challenge of HIV and its effects on the central nervous system. *Res. Publ. Assoc. Res. Nerv. Ment. Dis.* 72:1–45, 1994.

15. Harouse, J. M., Collman, R. G., and Gonzales-Scarano, F. Human immunodeficiency virus type 1 infection of SK-N-MC cells: Domains of gp120 involved in entry into a CD4-negative, galactosyl ceramide/3′ sulfo-galactosyl ceramide-positive cell line. *J. Virol.* 69:7383–7390, 1995.

16. Quarles, R. H. The biochemistry of myelin in X-linked mutants. *Ann. N. Y. Acad. Sci.* 605:135–145, 1990.

17. Mikoshiba, K., Aruga, J., Ikenaka, K., and Okano, H. Shiverer and allelic mutant mld mice. In R. Martenson (ed.), *Myelin: Biology and Chemistry.* Boca Raton, FL: CRC Press, 1992, pp. 723–744.

18. Nave, K., and Boespflug-Tanguy, O. X-Linked developmental defects of myelination: From mouse mutants to human genetic diseases. *Neuroscientist* 2:33–43, 1996.

19. Scherer, S. S. Molecular genetics of demyelination: New wrinkles on an old membrane. *Neuron* 18:13–16, 1997.

20. Snipes, G. J., Suter, U., Welcher, A. A., and Shooter, E. M. The molecular basis of the neuropathies of mouse and human. *Prog. Brain Res.* 105:319–325, 1995.

21. Ebersole, T. A., Chen, Q., Justice, M. J., and Artzt, K. The quaking gene product necessary in embryogenesis and myelination combines features of RNA binding and signal transduction proteins. *Nat. Genet.* 12:260–265, 1996.

22. Möller, J., Durr, P., Quarles, R., and Duncan, I. Biochemical analysis of myelin proteins in a novel neurological mutant: The taiep rat. *J. Neurochem.* 69:773–779, 1997.

23. Scriver, C., Beaudet, A., Sly, W., and Vallee, D. *The Metabolic and Molecular Bases of Inherited Diseases.* New York: McGraw-Hill, 1995.

24. Moser, H. W. Adrenoleukodystrophy. *Curr. Opin. Neurol.* 8:221–226, 1995.

24a. Lu, J. F., Lawler, A. M., Watkins, P. A., et al. A mouse model for X-linked adrenoleukodystrophy. *Proc. Natl. Acad. Sci. U.S.A.* 94:9366–9371, 1997.

25. Merrill, J. E., and Benveniste, E. N. Cytokines in inflammatory brain lesions: Helpful and harmful. *Trends Neurosci.* 19:331–338, 1996.

26. Morell, P., Toews, A. D., Wagner, M., and Goodrum, J. F. Gene expression during tellurium-induced primary demyelination. *Neurotoxicology* 15:171–180, 1994.

27. McMorris, F. A., and McKinnon, R. D. Regulation of oligodendrocyte development and CNS myelination by growth factors: Prospects for therapy of demyelinating disease. *Brain Pathol.* 6:313–329, 1996.

28. Duncan, I. D. Glial cell transplantation and remyelination of the central nervous system. *Neuropathol. Appl. Neurobiol.* 22:87–100, 1996.

29. Raine, C. S. The neuropathology of myelin diseases. In: P. Morell (ed.) *Myelin.* New York: Plenum Press, 1984.

30. Johnson, D., Sato, S., Quarles, R. H., Inuzuka, T., Brady, R. O., and Tourtellotte, W. W. Quantitation of myelin-associated glycoprotein in human nervous tissue from controls and multiple sclerosis patients. *J. Neurochem.* 46:1086–1093, 1986.

31. Norton, W. T., and Cammer W. Isolation and characterization of myelin. In P. Morell (ed.) *Myelin.* New York: Plenum Press, 1984, pp. 147–195.

Inherited and Neurodegenerative Diseases

40

Genetics of Inherited Diseases

Kunihiko Suzuki

GENETIC NEUROLOGICAL DISORDERS

Traditional molecular biological approaches to genetic neurological disorders, in which the defective gene products responsible for the phenotypes are known, have been well devel-oped and are providing a powerful tool for our understanding and eventual therapy for these disorders. The traditional approach starts with the knowledge of the defective gene products, such as an enzyme deficiency, and reaches the gene and its characterization through purifi-cation of the gene products and cloning of the

Basic Neurochemistry: Molecular, Cellular and Medical Aspects, 6th Ed., edited by G. J. Siegel et al. Published by Lippincott–Raven Publishers, Philadelphia, 1999. Correspondence to Kunihiko Suzuki, Neuroscience Center, CB7250, Departments of Neurology and Psychiatry, University of North Carolina School of Medicine, Chapel Hill, North Carolina 27599.

gene. Examples of the approaches and recent advances in such genetic disorders are illustrated elsewhere in this book (see Chap. 41). However, the genetic disorders in this category constitute a relatively small proportion of the over 3,000 known human genetic disorders of Mendelian inheritance [1,2]. Methodological advances have allowed us to approach the genetic causes of the remaining disorders without knowledge as to which genes are responsible for the disease. Since the flow of logic in this approach is in the reverse direction of the traditional approach, it is often termed "reverse genetics" because one first tries to obtain the gene responsible for the disorder without knowing its function and then tries to understand its function and the pathophysiology of the disease. The cloning strategy is also termed "positional cloning" since the genes are cloned on the basis of position in the genome only [3]. The ongoing project of mapping and sequencing the entire human genome is expected to greatly facilitate the search for the genes responsible for all types of genetic disorders [4].

If the present revolutionary advances in our molecular genetic understanding of hereditary neurodegenerative disorders are to be of pragmatic value in the future, strategies to achieve the ultimate gene therapy are of utmost importance. Technological progress in this direction has also been noteworthy. A large number of prokaryotic and eukaryotic systems that allow expression of cloned genes have been developed. Gene-transfer technology is progressing rapidly, either vector-mediated or as transgenes in the whole animal. Furthermore, homologous recombination is being used to generate mouse mutant strains in which specific genes are artificially and intentionally rendered inactive, termed "gene targeting." This approach allows production of authentic murine models of human genetic disorders when naturally occurring mutants do not exist among the easily manipulated small laboratory animals. Many murine models that are genetic equivalents of known human genetic disorders have already been generated using this approach (See Chap. 41).

Reverse genetics involves linkage analysis, positional cloning and diagnosis using linked markers

Linkage analysis can localize a disease-causing gene to a region of a chromosome without knowledge of its function. When the abnormal gene product responsible for a given genetic disease is not known, one would like to know first the location of the responsible gene within the genome. The strategy of locating the gene to a single chromosome and then to as specific a region as possible within the chromosome is referred to as *linkage analysis*. The traditional approach for this analysis is based on two principles. First, the primary sequence of the human genome is not fixed but varies in different individuals; this phenomenon is known as polymorphism. Such polymorphisms are statistically more common within introns and other noncoding regions of the genome, which constitute most of the genomic sequences. In addition, there are regions of the human genome which are particularly polymorphic. Since such polymorphisms often either generate a new restriction site or abolish an existing site, they can be identified by digestion with appropriate restriction enzymes and observing the size of the generated fragments with a probe spanning the region, which is known as a restriction fragment length polymorphism (RFLP). Second, during meiosis, two corresponding pairs of chromosomes line up together and then are separated into two daughter cells that eventually generate the germ cells. Thus, two regions of the genome which are on the same chromosome tend to stay together, while those on different chromosomes distribute to the germ cells independently from each other. However, the two corresponding chromosomes do not always separate cleanly from each other after coming together in meiosis. A crossover can occur, and the two chromosomes exchange an equivalent portion, generating a new pair of chromosomes. Therefore, even two regions on the same chromosome can be separated onto two chromosomes if a crossover occurs between the two regions. It then follows that the closer the two regions are on the chromosome, the more likely they are to stay together. In the extreme case when the polymorphic marker site is within the gene responsible for the disease, the marker will always be together with the gene. The strategy is, therefore, to find a polymorphic marker which is closely "linked" to affected individuals within the family being analyzed and, thus, to the disease-causing gene. The physical map of the human genome is being developed rapidly, with locations of known DNA sequences marked [5]. Many of those sequences are polymorphic, such that they provide different RFLPs in different individuals and, thus, can be used as markers for linkage analyses.

A successful linkage analysis requires DNA materials from family members of affected patients, preferably from as many generations as possible. A set of known polymorphic markers are chosen as probes, and genomic DNA is prepared from individuals. The genomic DNA is then digested by appropriate restriction enzymes and the RFLP patterns examined for each of the markers. Any markers which do not segregate with or against the disease state are discarded. In X-linked diseases, the chromosomal localization is known and only the markers on the X-chromosome need to be selected for the study. As should be clear from this description, linkage analysis is essentially a statistical procedure requiring assistance of the computer. Software programs have been developed specifically for analyses of the results of complex linkage studies. The results are expressed as the *lod* score [6,7], which gives a statistical estimate, in decimal logarithm, of the relative closeness of the given polymorphic marker to the disease-causing gene. A *lod* score of at least 3, preferably greater, is considered to be an indication that the gene being searched for is "linked" to the marker.

Linkage analysis has been used to map the genes responsible for a number of genetic neurological disorders to specific chromosomes. The first spectacular success of linkage analysis was the localization of the gene responsible for Huntington's disease [8]. The study was successful partly because of the availability of an enormous pedigree in the Lake Maracaibo region of Venezuela. Since then, chromosomal localization of many genes responsible for neurodegen-

erative disorders have been identified, including familial retinoblastoma, neurofibromatosis I, Charcot-Marie-Tooth disease, myotonic dystrophy, three different forms of Batten disease and ataxia telangiectasia. The catalogue of such diseases continues to expand [9].

A few caveats must be kept in mind. Linkage analyses are effective for Mendelian disorders where single genes are responsible for the disease states. This is not because the principle of linkage analysis is not applicable for multigenic disorders but, rather, that the increase in the number of genes that must be taken into consideration logarithmically increases the complexity of the linkage analysis. Another potentially complicating factor is that genetically different diseases can manifest themselves with similar clinical phenotypes. For example, what had been classified as Sanfilippo's syndrome has turned out to consist of four distinct genetic diseases caused by genetic defects in four different genes (see Chap. 41). If families gathered for a linkage analysis of what is considered to be one genetic disease in fact represent more than one genetically distinct disorder, the results of the linkage analysis may obscure the location of the gene. It is essential, therefore, to ascertain that all individuals included in a linkage analysis be within a single genetic complementation group. The complementation test is based on the principle that if the genetic cause of two patients with a similar phenotype lies in the same gene, fusion of the cells from these patients will show the phenotype. Furthermore, the disease phenotype should disappear in the fused cells if defects in two different genes are the causes of the similar phenotype. Despite these theoretical constraints, linkage analysis is being applied to potentially highly complex genetic disorders, such as manic-depressive disorder and schizophrenia.

In some instances, cytologically identifiable deletions or other chromosomal abnormalities associated with the disease can provide the crucial clue as to the location of the responsible gene. Such abnormalities were used in the positional cloning of the dystrophin gene, which is responsible for Duchenne's and Becker's muscular dystrophy [10]. Association of the disease with another phenotype due to a known gene can provide a useful hint at the location of the disease-causing gene. For example, the frequent association of X-linked adrenoleukodystrophy with color blindness indicated the close proximity of the two genes. More recently, the chromosomal localization of the gene responsible for Niemann-Pick type C disease was determined by taking advantage of the fact that an equivalent disease exists in both humans and mice. In this approach, artificially constructed mouse microcells, each containing a single copy of a human chromosome, were used as the human chromosome donor. When fused with cells from affected mice, the biochemical phenotype of the disease could be corrected only when human chromosome 18 was introduced. The gene localization could be narrowed down further because those cells that lost a portion of chromosome 18 in subsequent subcloning reverted back to the Niemann-Pick type C phenotype. Finally, the gene responsible for the major complementation group of Niemann-Pick type C disease was cloned, several mutations were identified and the homology search suggests that it is related to known cholesterol homeostasis genes [11].

Positional cloning. Localizing the gene to a chromosome, even to a specific region of a chromosome, is obviously the first step for cloning and characterization of the gene responsible for the disorder. It is generally desirable to obtain more than one linked marker, particularly two markers that flank the target gene. While a variety of ways to reach the target gene have been devised, the basic principle is to extend the DNA sequence information from the identified linked marker region toward the gene, either contiguously or discontinuously. These procedures are often referred to as "chromosomal walking" and "jumping." Genomic DNA libraries in the λ phage, cosmids and, more recently, in the form of the yeast artificial chromosome (YAC) are commonly used to track down the target gene. Human chromosome-specific YAC clones that collectively give the complete contiguous chromosomal DNA sequence have been constructed. In the primitive "walking," a segment of genomic DNA containing the identified marker is sequenced from the marker region. A new primer is made from the newly sequenced region

and used for further sequencing, slowly extending along the stretch of DNA toward the target. For this strategy to be effective, the marker must be reasonably close to the target gene because the number of nucleotides that can be sequenced in one step is still limited. Another variation is "jumping," in which the genomic DNA containing the marker sequence is circularized with the marker region on one end and sequenced across the ligated region, thus obtaining the sequence information some distance away from the marker for the next "jumping."

These procedures are slow and tedious as attested to by the search for the Huntington's disease gene, which took 10 years to be cloned after it was localized to a chromosome [12]. The positional cloning approach has been successful in many disorders when no other approaches were feasible. Some notable examples of neuromuscular disorders for which the responsible gene has been cloned by this strategy include familial retinoblastoma, myotonic dystrophy, fragile X syndrome, neuronal ceroid-lipofuscinosis, Duchenne/Becker muscular dystrophy and neurofibromatosis-I, also known as von Recklinghausen's disorder. Although not a neurological disorder, the cloning of the gene responsible for cystic fibrosis also provides an excellent example of how the positional cloning strategy has been successfully employed [13].

The final step of the positional cloning strategy for genetic diseases is elucidation of the cloned gene function and mutational analysis in affected individuals. When the cloned gene is homologous to genes with known functions, elucidation of its function is aided enormously. Otherwise, the search for the function of the cloned gene can be as tedious as the cloning process itself. It is *a priori* evident that if the correct gene has been obtained, the gene structure and the function of its product should be abnormal in affected patients.

Diagnosis. When the marker is sufficiently close to the target gene, the polymorphism of the marker sequence itself can be used for diagnosis of affected individuals. This is true even when the gene responsible for the disease has not been identified because essentially no crossover occurs on the chromosome between the disease-causing gene and the marker. As in DNA diagnosis based on the disease-causing mutation within the responsible gene, knowledge of the nature of the polymorphism in the family is a prerequisite. Conceptually, the disease-causing mutation is merely a polymorphism within the gene. It is no different from a polymorphism in the marker sequence which is so close to the gene that no crossover occurs.

NATURE OF MUTATIONS IN GENETIC DISORDERS

Mutations are constantly occurring in the genome. Mammalian genes have evolved over billions of years, and thus, most random alterations to their structures are statistically likely to be detrimental to their functions. Polymorphisms in the general population are mutations that do not result in functional impairment. Since alterations in the nucleotide sequence within introns are generally less likely to affect gene functions than those occurring within exons, introns contain more polymorphisms than exons. Several categories of mutation and the respective underlying mechanisms are known, including single-base-pair substitutions, deletions, insertions, duplications, retrotranspositions and trinucleotide expansions, which are being recognized as particularly important in many neurodegenerative disorders [14–16].

Point mutations, or single-base substitutions, are the most common form of mutations

Any nucleotide in the genomic sequence may be substituted with another, either through transition between two purine or pyrimidine bases or transversion between a purine base and a pyrimidine base. Many point mutations are silent functionally. Those that occur within introns and other noncoding sequences may not have any functional effect. Since many amino acids are encoded by more than a single genetic code, many base substitutions within exons have no effect on the translation products. In some instances, mutations may not affect the function of the products even when they result in changes in the primary amino acid sequence. Statistically, however, a majority of point mutations that alter the primary amino acid sequence of the translation products result in impaired gene function at various stages. If a point mutation affects the function of a regulatory sequence, the gene may not be transcribed properly. If a mutation is at or near an intron–exon junction, processing of the primary transcript may be abnormal and an intron may remain or exons may be skipped in the processed mRNA. Sometimes a point mutation creates a consensus sequence for splicing which generates abnormally spliced mRNA. Loss of the polyadenylation signal also will result in abnormally processed mRNA. Within the coding sequence, if a mutation affects the initiation codon, no translation product can be generated. Single-base substitution can change the codon to another amino acid, termed a sense mutation, or generate a stop codon, termed a nonsense mutation. A sense mutation can alter the folding of the protein; affect sites important in post-translational modifications, such as the proteolytic cleavage, phosphorylation and glycosylation sites; or modify the translation products in other ways. Statistically, most of these will result in loss of the function of the translation product.

Many point mutations appear to occur randomly. Fidelity of DNA polymerase and slipped mispairing at the time of DNA duplication are often suggested as the main mechanisms for random point mutations [14]. However, there is one mechanism that appears to occur frequently. The sequence CpG is known as a mutation hot spot because spontaneous chemical methylation and deamination result in C-to-T and G-to-A transitions. Many disease-causing point mutations are known at the "CpG island."

Deletion, insertion and duplication also are frequent causes of many genetic disorders

Segments of the genomic sequence, ranging in size from a single nucleotide to regions of the chromosome large enough to be visible microscopically, can be either deleted, inserted or duplicated. Deletions or insertions that are not multiples of three and that occur within the protein coding sequence result in a frameshift in translation. The amino acid sequence downstream from the mutation is then abnormal and a stop codon is encountered 21 or 22 codons downstream, on the average. Larger deletions or insertions naturally will affect the structure and, consequently, the function of the gene more drastically. These larger deletions or insertions are often readily detectable by appropriate restriction digestion of genomic DNA and Southern analysis. The mechanisms for these mutations are multiple. Relatively small deletions or insertions can occur during DNA replication as the result of slippage mispairing or homologous and unequal recombination, particularly between repetitive sequences, such as the *Alu* element. Rare retrotransposition may also be responsible for some of the large insertions [14].

Gene duplication can be considered as a large-scale insertion. This mechanism appears to have played an important role in the genomic evolution of higher organisms. If both the original and the duplicated genes are functional, the organism will acquire a double dose of that gene. However, most of the time, the duplication is not complete and can be the cause of a genetic disorder. For example, the *mld* mutant mouse has a duplicated and partially inverted myelin basic protein gene in close proximity to the native gene. This results in a decreased level and an abnormal temporal schedule of myelin basic protein synthesis with a clinical phenotype milder than that of the allelic *shiverer* mutant [17].

Trinucleotide expansion is one of the most important categories of mutation underlying neurodegenerative disorders

The dynamically expanding trinucleotide repeat is an important class of abnormality that causes some genetic disorders [15,16]. It was first reported in fragile X syndrome in 1992. The expanding triplets can be CAG, CGG, GCC, CTG or GAA. As of this writing, there are at least a dozen genetic disorders which have triplet expansions as the underlying gene abnormality (Table 40-1). They are commonly classified into two groups, those with very long expansions that are not translated and those with moderate CAG expansions that result in a polyglutamine stretch in the translation products. The repeating sequence in the first group can be extremely long, from a few hundred to thousands. The repeating sequence in the second group is usually moderate, approximately 40 to 120 triplets. Most of the disorders in the second group are inherited as dominant traits. Thus, acquired toxic function is often postulated as the pathogenetic mechanism. The location may be within the coding sequence, on either side of the coding sequence but within exons, in the promoter region or within an intron. For unknown reasons, all of these disorders are neuromuscular in phenotype. In some disorders, such as myotonic dystrophy and spinocerebellar atrophy 1, a positive correlation is found between the length of the repeat and the clinical severity of the disease. The exact mechanism for the expansion is not known. The rule of the triplet repeat expansion has been extended to include a repeated stretch of 12 nucleotides in the cystatin B gene in progressive myoclonus epilepsy of the Unverricht type [18]. We can expect that more genetic disorders will be found in the near future that are due to dynamic expansions of repeated nucleotide sequences within the genome.

GENE TRANSFER AND EXPRESSION

Cloned genes can be expressed in many different ways on different levels

When reverse genetics, or positional cloning, is successful and the gene involved in a particular genetic disorder is identified, the next major step is elucidation of its function. Once segments of the gene are available, isolation of transcripts in the form of cDNA is a relatively straightforward procedure in principle with the standard recombinant DNA technology. Thus, we assume that both the genomic and cDNA sequences are characterized and available. This also means that the primary amino acid sequence of the gene product is known. Not infrequently, the sequence information itself may suggest the function of the product by its similarity to other proteins of known function. It may be homologous, that is, evolutionarily related, to other proteins or similar due to similar functions. The up-to-date data of

TABLE 40-1.   GENETIC NEUROMUSCULAR DISORDERS CAUSED BY DYNAMIC EXPANSION OF NUCLEOTIDE REPEATS

Disease	Inheritance	Repeat sequence	Gene	Repeat location
Polyglutamine disorders (expansions usually moderate)				
Spinobulbar muscular atrophy (Kennedy's disease)	X-linked recessive	CAG	Androgen receptor	Coding sequence
Huntington's disease	Autosomal recessive	CAG	Huntingtin	Coding sequence
Spinocerebellar atrophy (SCA) 1 and 2	Autosomal recessive	CAG	Ataxins 1 and 2	Coding sequence
SCA 6	Autosomal recessive	CAG	α1A Calcium channel	Coding sequence
Machado-Joseph disease (SCA 3)	Autosomal recessive	CAG	Ataxin 3	Coding sequence
Dentatorubro-pallidoluysian atrophy	Autosomal recessive	CAG	Atrophin	Coding sequence
Non-coding (expansions often enormous)				
Fragile X	X-linked dominant	CGG	FMR1	5'-UTR[a]
Fragile XE	X-linked recessive	CCG	FMR2	5'-UTR
Myoclonic dystrophy	Autosomal dominant	CTG	Serine/threonine kinase	3'-UTR
Friedreich's ataxia	Autosomal recessive	GAA	Frataxin	Intron
Progressive myoclonus epilepsy (Unverricht)	Autosomal recessive	Dodecamer	Cystatin B	5'-Promoter

[a]UTR, untranslated region.

recorded nucleotide sequences (NCBI-GenBank) and protein sequences (SWISS-PROT) can be readily accessed through the Internet as well as through self-standing software programs; these programs can be used to evaluate possible similarity of the gene and its product with those in the database. Beyond such arm-chair evaluation, many methodologies are available to transfer and express genes on different levels of organization.

Cell-free expression. For *in vitro* translation, the cDNA that includes the entire protein coding sequence can be subcloned into a suitable plasmid vector with flanking RNA polymerase promoters and then transcribed with a capping analog to a translatable mRNA. The protein coded by the cDNA can then be generated in any of the commercially available *in vitro* translation systems, such as those from rabbit reticulocytes or wheat germ lysate. The *in vitro* translation product is useful to test immunological reactivity but is often functionally inactive since no post-translational processing takes place. Proteolytic trimming, glycosylation, phosphorylation and other modifications are often essential for functional activity. The quantity of the gene product that can be generated by *in vitro* translation is very limited.

Expression in living cells. A large number of expression systems that use living cells, either in culture or in the form of frog oocyte, are available. Isolated genes, cDNAs or mRNAs generated from cDNAs can be expressed. They may be prokaryotic or eukaryotic, for transient or stable expression or integrated and regulated expression or overexpression systems. Each type has its own advantages and disadvantages and is used in accordance with the purpose of the experiment.

The frog oocyte system is a cellular equivalent of the *in vitro* translation system in that mRNA appropriately generated from cloned cDNA is injected directly into fertilized frog eggs. The frog produces unusually large eggs, which permit direct manual injection of a relatively large quantity of mRNA. The injected mRNA is translated by the intrinsic metabolic machinery within the egg and processed to form functional proteins. Thus, the function of the produced protein, if known or suspected, can be tested. This system allows only a brief, transient expression of the exogenously injected mRNA, and again, the quantity that can be generated is very small. Nevertheless, the system has been used widely in neurobiology because many expressed membrane proteins, such as receptors and channel proteins, are integrated into the oocyte membrane and their functions can be studied by sophisticated tools, such as patch clamping.

Perhaps one of the most commonly used mammalian cell types for transient expression is COS-1, transformed African green monkey kidney cells. When transfected by cDNAs subcloned into appropriate plasmid vectors that include a suitable transcriptional control element upstream of the cloned cDNA, COS-1 cells generate a gene product which can then be tested for its known or suspected function. Expression is transient, with peak activity between 1 and 4 days after transfection. Unless some mechanism is used to select the transfected cells, no more than 10 to 20% of the cells in the culture express the exogenous gene. Even for these limitations, this system is used widely for its simplicity and technical ease. For more stable expression of cloned genes, many hosts and suitable vectors have been devised which allow stable integration and expression of the exogenously introduced genes.

When a large quantity of the gene product is required, several overexpression systems can be utilized, some prokaryotic and others eukaryotic. For example, a prokaryotic system has been used successfully to produce milligram quantities of human GM2 activator protein. In this example, the gene product was generated by a recombinant plasmid, pHX17, in *Escherichia coli,* strain M15/pREP4. The gene product was expressed as a fusion protein attached to six histidine residues bridged to the mature activator protein sequence by a three-amino-acid sequence specific for the coagulation factor Xa. Characteristically for proteins generated by prokaryotes, the GM2 activator was not processed. However, the unprocessed fusion protein was fully functional in activating hydrolysis of GM2 ganglioside by β-hexosaminidase A. The fusion protein could be purified to near homogeneity by a single step of Nickel affinity chromatography. After renaturation, the GM2 activator protein identical in the primary amino acid sequence with the native mature, processed protein in the tissue could be obtained by digestion with Factor Xa.

While the prokaryotic overexpression system can produce preparative quantities of cloned gene products, the lack of post-translational processing limits its usefulness when the protein requires such modifications for functional activity. An extensively used system utilizes a unique property of an insect virus, baculovirus. This virus is pathogenic only to butterflies and moths and thus does not pose a hazard to human workers. It contains a gene coding for the polyhedrin protein, which is generated in an enormous quantity within infected insect tissues. When the cloned cDNA is inserted into the virus just downstream of the polyhedrin gene promoter, the infected insect cells produce large quantities of the protein coded by the cDNA. The protein is secreted into the culture medium. The quantity of the protein that can be produced by the baculovirus system varies widely from 1 to 100 mg per liter of culture medium. Recombinant baculovirus constructs, including the hexahistidine tail and either the Factor Xa or enterokinase cleavage sequence, have become commercially available, thus permitting the same one-step purification of the generated protein by Nickel affinity chromatography. Generally, proteins produced by the baculovirus system undergo post-translational processing similar to that for the native protein in mammalian tissues and are functionally active [19], although subtle differences, for example, in the glycosylation pattern, have been described. However, the large quantity of the generated protein tends to overload the intracellular processing machinery and only a small proportion actually undergoes normal processing. Most proteins expressed in this system are excreted without any processing or with only incomplete processing. One of the drawbacks of the baculovirus overexpression system is that the virus eventually kills the host insect cells. Thus, a large amount of desired protein can be obtained for a few days only. New infections need to be started with a new batch of cultured insect cells every time. To overcome this difficulty, continuous, stably transfected cell culture systems have been developed. While the production rate of introduced genes may not be as high as in baculovirus-infected cells, the system can be set up in such a way that the culture medium can be continuously or periodically removed for harvesting of the product and replaced by fresh medium. This type of "bioreactor" can generate more product over days and weeks than the transient systems, such as the baculovirus.

***In vivo* transfer and expression.** Various attempts have been made to introduce and express foreign genes directly in a living organism. A somewhat naive approach of direct injection of dystrophin cDNA into muscles proved to be effective in establishing reasonably stable local expression in tissue [20]. More usual are procedures that utilize various vectors, most commonly, viral vectors. Viruses have evolved to have an efficient machinery to introduce and replicate themselves into the host and to express their genetic materials. In principle, therefore, genes that are foreign to a virus can be inserted into the viral genome and expressed within infected hosts. Similarly, introduction and expression of foreign genes by transplantation of tissues or organs have been attempted extensively to treat genetic disorders and will be covered later.

Transgenic mice. The term transgenic mouse refers to mice genetically manipulated by a technology which permits stable integration and expression of exogenous DNA fragments into the genome of the entire organism [21,22]. The technology combines recombinant DNA and murine biology.

The principle of the conventional transgenic experiment involves construction of a suit-

able exogenous gene preparation with an appropriate promoter, which is injected into a fertilized mouse embryo at the stage of the zygote with a glass pipette. The injected zygote is then implanted back into the oviduct of a pseudopregnant host female mouse prepared by mating a virgin female mouse with a vasectomized male (Fig. 40-1). The injected DNA randomly integrates itself into the embryo genome with a certain statistical probability. The pseudopregnant mouse serves as the host to carry the embryo to term. Mice with the stably integrated exogenous gene will carry it in all cells of the body and should express its product. The efficiency of integration of the exogenous DNA into the mouse genome ranges from a few percent to over 10% of injected eggs. The transgene can be driven by its own native promoter or by an artificially introduced promoter according to the experimental design. When unregulated overexpression of the exogenous gene is desired, an unregulated strong promoter can be placed upstream of the injected gene. Attempts have been made to reg-

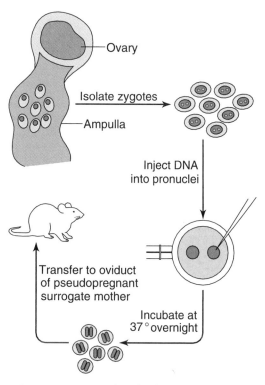

FIGURE 40-1. Procedure for the conventional transgenic experiment. (From [21], with permission.)

ulate gene expression in transgenic animals by using a developmentally regulated promoter, such as the native promoter for myelin protein genes, which should be turned on at the time of myelination and used only in actively myelinating cells. Similarly, inducible promoters, such as the metallothionein gene promoter, which can be regulated by exogenously provided heavy metals, have been employed. Traditional transgenic mice can express the introduced foreign gene as if it were a native gene in its genome. The source of the exogenous gene is not a factor in the conventional transgenic expression. In principle, genes from any eukaryotic sources can be expressed in mice. A major limitation of this technology is the randomness of the site of integration of the injected DNA. There is always a statistical probability that the exogenous DNA sequence is integrated in such a way that a native gene sequence is disrupted and, thus, rendered inactive. Such a transgene may be incompatible with life or may produce varying degrees of abnormality, depending on the function of the disrupted native gene. In fact, a whole group of transgenic mice with unintended insertional mutations of endogenous genes are known [23]. This unpredictable disruption of native genes must be kept in mind when the clinical and biochemical phenotypes of conventional transgenic mice are evaluated. Since the integration sites are random, a common phenotype among more than one founder mouse gives a reasonable assurance that it is the consequence of the transgenic expression rather than the result of inactivation of an endogenous gene.

Endogenous genes can be specifically targeted for inactivation or introduction of a mutation, allowing creation of murine models of genetic diseases

Unintended disruptions of endogenous genes can occur randomly and unpredictably in the conventional transgenic mouse. A recent development of homologous recombination technology and further manipulation of the mouse reproductive biology, however, have made it possible to target specific endogenous genes for disruption [22,24]. This technology, therefore, allows in principle the duplication of specific ge-

netic defects found in humans and mice. The aim of this manipulation is not to express exogenous genes but specifically to inactivate or otherwise to manipulate endogenous genes. The underlying mechanistic principle of this technology is homologous recombination. When an exogenous DNA sequence is integrated into the mouse genome, there is an extremely small but finite probability that it recombines itself at the site where the native sequence is similar to that of the exogenous sequence. For the homologous recombination to occur, the two sequences must be as close to identical as possible. Homologous genes from even closely related mammalian species may not be similar enough, particularly in the intron sequence. The probability of homologous recombination can be dramatically greater when the gene used to disrupt the endogenous gene is derived from the same strain of mouse as that of the recipient cells.

The principle of generating a murine model of a genetic disease involves the steps illustrated in Figure 40-2. Since the efficiency of

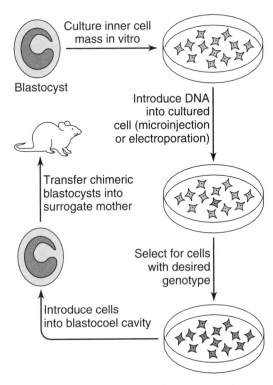

FIGURE 40-2.   Procedure for the gene-targeting experiment. (From [21], with permission.)

true homologous recombination is far below that of random integration, direct injection into individual zygotes is impractical. The critical additional component for this technology is the embryonic stem (ES) cells. These are undifferentiated multipotential cells from mouse blastocysts which can develop into any type of cell and organ in the body. Under certain specific culture conditions, they can be maintained with their multipotential intact. To increase the usefulness of recombinant ES cells, a mechanism for selection is usually constructed into the exogenously introduced DNA sequence. The selection mechanism may be either positive, such as resistance to antibiotics, or negative (tk). The exogenous DNA sequence is introduced into the ES cells most commonly by electroporation. Cells in which the introduced sequence is integrated into the homologous sequence in the host genome are selected and injected into the cavity of a mouse embryo at the blastocyst stage. The injected blastocyst is returned to a pseudopregnant host female mouse. Thus, the embryo consists of two types of cell, each with different genetic makeup: the native cells of the blastocyst and the injected ES cells. Since both are multipotential, the embryo develops to a whole animal which is chimeric, consisting of varying proportions of both cells. If, for example, strains of different fur colors are used for the host and the ES cells, the chimera will exhibit stripes and patches of two different fur colors, allowing for easy identification of the resultant chimeras.

Since the produced transgenic mice are genetically chimeric, an additional step is required to obtain a genetically homogeneous strain in which a specific gene is inactivated. It is necessary to select chimeras that produce recombinant germ cells. Unless the germ cells have the genotype of the ES cells, the resultant offspring will be of the host genotype. When the disrupted gene is located on the X chromosome, only male chimeras producing sperm of the recombinant genotype are needed. For autosomal genes, suitable males and females must be obtained. Since the statistical probability of both alleles being disrupted in an ES cell is infinitesimally small, these chimeras will be carriers of the disrupted gene. Crosses between chimeras thus produce

homozygous mice with both alleles inactivated. The strain then can be maintained as any other autosomal recessive mutant strain.

The number of artificially generated insertional mutations is increasing at an accelerated pace. Many known human genetic disorders have been replicated in the mouse (see Chap. 41). They provide invaluable tools for studies of pathogenesis and eventual gene therapy of these disorders. Many other "knockout" mice are being generated in order to gain insight into physiological function of the targeted gene. The technology further allows "double knockouts," in which more than one functionally related gene is simultaneously inactivated, a condition that is not known in humans because of the extremely low statistical probability of identifying such "double mutants." Furthermore, refinements of the technology allow modifications of the target gene that are less drastic than total inactivation, such as point mutations. We should keep a few important factors in mind when analyzing such models. For example, the hypoxanthine phosphoribosyltransferase (HPRT) gene was inactivated in the mouse for the purpose of producing a model of human Lesch-Nyhan disease (see Box 17-1). Despite the complete inactivation, "affected" mice were clinically normal. The most likely explanation is that the mouse has active uricase and, thus, can bypass the defective HPRT. Many murine lines in which supposedly important genes are inactivated have shown no or only very limited phenotypes. The concept of functional substitution of the lost gene product with another similar product, known as redundancy, is often invoked to explain the unexpected observations, unfortunately often without experimental data to support it.

Gene therapy provides ultimate hope and is steadily developing

In a broad sense, the term gene therapy should indicate any attempt at treating genetic diseases caused by defective genes by introduction and expression of normally functional genes [25–28]. Such attempts were made before the advent of molecular biological technologies in the form of organ and tissue transplantation and are still made to a limited extent. Organ transplantation has been employed to provide the body with normal gene products missing in patients. In some instances, transplantation was indicated for other medical reasons, such as kidney transplantation in Fabry's disease, in which kidney failure is common. Cultured fibroblasts were transplanted for their ready availability. The amniotic membrane was used because of its immunological inactivity. Generally, somatic organ implantations were of limited effectiveness. This is particularly true in genetic disorders that affect the central nervous system because the normal gene products produced by the implanted organs do not effectively reach the brain. However, promising results have been reported with normal bone marrow transplantation into patients with some genetic neurological disorders, most notably in mucopolysaccharidoses [29]. In the *twitcher* mouse mutant, which is a naturally occurring murine model of human globoid cell leukodystrophy, also known as Krabbe's disease or galactosylceramidase deficiency (see Chap. 41), allogenic bone marrow transplantation effectively alleviated the disease process and prolonged the life span of affected mice by a factor of 3 [30]. Bone marrow transplantation has also been attempted in other animal models.

The narrow definition of gene therapy is treatment of genetic diseases on the gene level utilizing recombinant DNA technologies. Organ and tissue transplantation therefore, is not within this narrow definition of the gene therapy. Direct injection of exogenous genes, such as the one described above for expression of dystrophin in muscle, appears to be of limited potential. Virus-mediated transfer and expression of normal genes currently are being actively pursued by many laboratories. Highly promising results have been obtained in tissue culture systems and in some animal models of human genetic diseases. One of the most commonly employed viral vectors is the retrovirus because of its efficient and relatively nondiscriminatory capacity to infect various cellular types. If a retrovirus is modified appropriately with an inserted exogenous gene, it can infect the target cells and produce the gene product lacking in the host cell. For stable expression of the viral genome, the retrovirus must be integrated into the host genome, and the inte-

gration requires mitosis of the host cells. This property seriously limits the usefulness of retroviruses as the vector for gene therapy of genetic diseases of the central nervous system because most neurons and glia in the mature brain are postmitotic. Replication-defective herpes simplex 1 overcomes this disadvantage of the retrovirus since it does not need to be integrated into the host cell genome for expression. Thus, the exogenous gene engineered into herpes simplex 1 virus can be expressed in postmitotic cells and actively replicating cells with similar efficiency. This ability to replicate and express its own genome independent of host cell replication provides a further advantage in that there is much less risk of inadvertently disrupting important host genes by random integration. Adenovirus is also capable of infecting postmitotic cells, such as the neurons and glial cells, and has been used for gene transfer into the central nervous system (CNS). However, applications of adenoviral vectors in gene therapy have been hampered by associated immunogenicity and cytopathogenicity. The adeno-associated virus (AAV) vector has been under intensive investigation as a potentially useful vehicle for transfer and expression of exogenous genes [31,32]. Its nonpathogenicity and wide host range make it a good candidate as a gene delivery system in the CNS. AAV is a small, nonenveloped parvovirus. The wild-type AAV-2 genome contains a single-strand DNA of 4,680 nucleotides. It consists of one structural gene (Cap) and one nonstructural gene (Rep) responsible for viral encapsulation and replication, respectively, as well as two inverted repeated sequences (ITRs) of 145 bases which are minimal essential *cis*-acting sequences required for viral replication, host integration and packaging. So far, no human disease has been reported to be associated with AAV. Coinfection by helper viruses, such as adenovirus or herpes simplex virus, is required for productive AAV infections. Without helper viruses, the genome integrates into the host chromosome DNA, preferentially into human chromosome 19.

Transfer and expression of normal genes as the means of treating genetic diseases, as described above, are applicable only to diseases in which the normal functions of the genes are lacking, also termed deficiency diseases. While some genetic diseases of autosomal dominant inheritance may well be caused by lack of sufficient quantity of the normal gene products, some others may be due to a detrimental effect of mutant gene products. In these disorders, providing normal genes and their products will not be an effective treatment. Similarly, gene therapy will not be effective in conditions in which a gene overdose might be the underlying mechanism, such as in Down's syndrome.

For obvious reasons, gene therapy along the experimental design of the transgenic mouse cannot be readily applied to human patients. However, transgenic technology has been shown to effectively "cure" the clinical, pathological and biochemical abnormalities in the murine model of β-glucuronidase deficiency (see Chap. 41) [33].

UNIQUE NATURE OF GENETIC DISORDERS AFFECTING THE BRAIN

Successful therapy of disorders involving the nervous system must overcome some unique features of the brain

We have considered molecular genetic approaches to genetic neurological disorders. While in principle there is no difference between neurological and non-neurological disorders, the biological uniqueness of the nervous system must always be taken into consideration. Delivery and expression of normal genes or their products are the first important considerations. Transplantation of normal bone marrow cells, transduced *ex vivo* by viral vector-mediated normal protective protein gene, was highly effective in alleviating systemic pathology but not neuropathology in the galactosialidosis knockout mouse [34]. The essentially postmitotic nature of most neurons and glial cells in the mature central nervous system and the consequent considerations for selection of suitable vectors for gene transfer have been discussed. There are other properties of the nervous system that differentiate it from other organs and tissues and, thus, limit the feasibility of gene therapy. First, the anatomical and cellular structure of the brain is much more complex

than that of other organs, consisting of specialized regions and cell types with unique functional roles, including neurons, astrocytes, oligodendroglia, microglia and other cell types. Expression of intrinsic genes is highly complex with respect to regions and cellular types, as well as during development. In fact, expression of certain genes is taken as a determinant or marker of the cell type, such as glial fibrillary acid protein in astrocytes or many myelin-specific proteins and UDP-galactose ceramide galactosyltransferase in the myelin-forming cells, the Schwann cells and oligodendrocytes. Some receptors may be specific for certain neurons in certain regions and perhaps only during a certain period in brain development. These factors surely render different regions and cellular components of the brain susceptible to different degrees to any genetic abnormalities in the various developmental stages. For example, in Huntington's disease, a dominantly expressed genetic disorder, an abnormality in only one of the pair of genes on chromosome 4, present in every single cell, causes a disease in which the nervous system develops and functions perfectly well until middle age, when a specific small group of neurons starts to degenerate while other brain constituents apparently continue to function normally. Thus, more than for any other organ, variables such as anatomical region, cell type and developmental stage are critical for the nervous system.

Equally critical is the question of plasticity of the developing brain, particularly when treatment of degenerative genetic disorders is contemplated. The brain repairs itself poorly compared to other organs. Even if an effective treatment is found for the disease, it would be of only academic interest if it could not be initiated before the brain sustained irreparable damage. Most genetic lysosomal disorders (see Chap. 41) affect the brain early and severely. Affected fetuses diagnosed and aborted at 20 weeks of gestation always show obvious neuropathology. Affected newborns, therefore, must have advanced damage to the brain. Even if a perfect cure is available, it may have to start *in utero* to be useful. These considerations point to the necessity of learning much more about the normal developmental processes of the brain and its plasticity than we know now.

REFERENCES

1. McKusick, V. A. *Mendelian Inheritance in Man*, 11th ed. Baltimore: Johns Hopkins University Press, 1994.
2. Beaudet, A. L., Scriver, C. R., Sly, W. S., and Valle, D. Genetics, biochemistry, and molecular basis of variant human phenotypes. In C. R. Scriver, A. L. Beaudet, W. S. Sly, and D. Valle (eds.), *The Metabolic and Molecular Basis of Inherited Disease*, 7th ed. New York: McGraw-Hill, 1995, pp. 53–118.
3. Lehrach, H., and Bates, G. Approaches to identifying disease gene. In J. Brosius, and R. T. Fremeau (eds.), *Molecular Genetic Approaches to Neuropsychiatric Diseases*. New York: Academic Press, 1991, pp. 3–17.
4. Green, E. D., Cox, D. R., and Myers, R. M. The human genome project and its impact on the study of human disease. In C. R. Scriver, A. L. Beaudet, W. S. Sly, and D. Valle (eds.), *The Metabolic and Molecular Basis of Inherited Disease*, 7th ed. New York: McGraw-Hill, 1995, pp. 401–436.
5. NIH/CEPH Collaborative Mapping Group. A comprehensive genetic linkage map of the human genome. *Science* 258:67–102, 1992.
6. Ott, J. Principle of human genetic linkage analysis. In J. Brosius and R. T. Fremeau (eds.), *Molecular Genetic Approaches to Neuropsychiatric Diseases*. New York: Academic Press, 1991, pp. 35–53.
7. Buckler, A., and Housman, D. *Methods of Genome Analysis. A Gene Hunter's Guide*. New York: W. H. Freeman, 1992.
8. Gusella, J. F., Wexler, N. S., Conneally, P. M., et al. A polymorphic DNA marker genetically linked to Huntington's disease. *Nature* 306:234–238, 1983.
9. Harding, A. E., and Rosenberg, R. N. A neurologic gene map. In R. N., Rosenberg, S. B. Prusiner, S. DiMauro, R. L. Barchi, and L. M. Kunkel (eds.), *The Molecular and Genetic Basis of Neurological Disease*. Boston: Butterworth-Heinemann, 1993, pp. 21–24.
10. Koening, M., Hoffman, E. P., Bertelson, C. J., Monaco, A. P., Feener, C., and Kunkel, L. M. Complete cloning of the Duchenne muscular dystrophy (DMD) cDNA and preliminary genomic organization of the DMD gene in normal and affected individuals. *Cell* 50:509–517, 1987.
11. Carstea, E. D., Morris, J. A., Coleman, K. G., et al. Niemann-Pick C1 disease gene: Homology to mediators of cholesterol homeostasis. *Science* 277:228–231, 1997.
12. Huntington's Disease Collaborative Research Group. A novel gene containing a trinucleotide repeat that is expanded and unstable on Huntington's disease chromosomes. *Cell* 72:971–983, 1993.
13. Tsui, L.-C., and Buchwald, M. Biochemical and molecular genetics of cystic fibrosis. *Adv. Hum. Genet.* 20:153–266, 1991.
14. Cooper, D. N., Krawczak, M., and Antonarakis, S. E. The nature and mechanisms of human gene mutation. In C. R. Scriver, A. L. Beaudet, W. S. Sly, and D. Valle (eds.), *The Metabolic and Molecular Basis of Inherited Disease*, 7th ed. New York: McGraw-Hill, 1995, pp. 259–291.
15. Gusella, J. F., and MacDonald, M. E. Trinucleotide instability: A repeating theme in human inherited disorders. *Annu. Rev. Med.* 47:201–209, 1996.
16. Paulson, H. L., and Fischbeck, K. H. Trinucleotide repeats in neurogenetic disorders. *Annu. Rev. Neurosci.* 19:79–107, 1996.
17. Popko, B., Puckett, C., Lai, E., et al. Myelin deficient mice: Expression of myelin basic protein and the generation of mice with varying levels of myelin. *Cell* 48:713–721, 1987.
18. Lalioti, M. D., Scott, H. S., Buresi, C., et al. Dodecamer repeat expansion in cystatin B gene in progressive myoclonus epilepsy. *Nature* 386:847–851, 1997.
19. Luckow, V. A., and Summers, M. D. Trends in the development of baculovirus expression vectors. *Biotechnology* 6:47–55, 1988.
20. Wolff, J. A., Malone, R. W., Williams, P., et al. Direct gene transfer into mouse muscle *in vivo*. *Science* 247:1465–1468, 1990.
21. Popko, B. Germ-line manipulation of the mouse in neuroscience. In J. Brosius and R. T. Fremeau (eds.), *Molecular Genetic Approaches to Neuropsychiatric Diseases*. New York: Academic Press, 1991, pp. 429–447.
22. Sedivy, J. M., and Joyner, A. L. *Gene Targeting*. New York: W. H. Freeman, 1992.
23. Meisler, M. H. Insertional mutation of "classical" and novel genes in transgenic mice. *Trends Genet.* 8:341–344, 1992.
24. Capecchi, M. R. Targeted gene replacement. *Sci. Am.* 270:52–58, 1994.
25. Verma, I. M. Gene therapy. *Sci. Am.* 262:68–84, 1990.
26. Wolff, J. A. Postnatal gene transfer into the central nervous system. *Curr. Opin. Neurobiol.* 3:743–748, 1993.
27. Suhr, S. T., and Gage, F. H. Gene therapy for neurological disease. *Arch. Neurol.* 50:1252–1268, 1993.

28. Friedmann, T. Gene therapy for neurological disorders. *Trends Genet.* 10:210–214, 1994.

29. Krivit, W., Shapiro, E. G., Lockman, L. A., et al. Bone marrow transplantation treatment for globoid cell leukodystrophy, metachromatic leukodystrophy, adrenoleukodystrophy and Hurler syndrome. In H. W. Moser (ed.), *Neurodystrophies and Neurolipidses.* Amsterdam: Elsevier, 1996, pp. 87–106.

30. Suzuki, K., and Suzuki, K. The twitcher mouse: A model for Krabbe disease and for experimental therapies. *Brain Pathol.* 5:249–258, 1995.

31. Kaplitt, M. G., Leone, P., Samulski, R. J., et al. Long-term gene expression and phenotypic correction using adeno-associated virus vectors in the mammalian brain. *Nat. Genet.* 8:148–154, 1994.

32. Du, B., Wu, P., Boldt-Houle, D. M., and Terwilliger, E. F. Efficient transduction of human neurons with an adeno-associated virus vector. *Gene Ther.* 3:254–261, 1996.

33. Kyle, J. W., Birkenmeier, E. H., Gwynn, B., et al. Correction of murine mucopolysaccharidosis VII by a human β-glucuronidase transgene. *Proc. Natl. Acad. Sci. USA* 87:3914–3918, 1990.

34. Zhou, X. Y., Morreau, H., Rottier, R., et al. Mouse model for the lysosomal disorder galactosialidosis and correction of the phenotype with overexpressing erythroid precursor cells. *Genes Dev.* 9:2623–2634, 1995.

41

Lysosomal and Peroxisomal Diseases

Kunihiko Suzuki and Marie T. Vanier

Many neurological disorders occur as the result of genetically determined abnormal metabolism of lipids, the carbohydrate moieties of glycoproteins or mucopolysaccharides. A majority of these differences have underlying metabolic abnormalities in the catabolic pathways catalyzed by a group of enzymes commonly referred to as lysosomal enzymes. A series of genetic defects of proteins normally involved in peroxisomal biogenesis or function have been attracting increasing attention in recent years. Details of the biochemical and molecular aspects of the individual lysosomal and peroxisomal disorders can be found in the standard reference volume [1].

Basic Neurochemistry: Molecular, Cellular and Medical Aspects, 6th Ed., edited by G. J. Siegel et al. Published by Lippincott–Raven Publishers, Philadelphia, 1999. Correspondence to Kunihiko Suzuki, Departments of Neurology and Psychiatry, Neuroscience Center, CB 7250, University of North Carolina School of Medicine, Chapel Hill, North Carolina 27599.

THE LYSOSOME

The concept of the lysosome as the subcellular organelle responsible for physiological turnover of cellular constituents was first proposed by de Duve. It contains catabolic enzymes that are generally glycoproteins themselves and have very low pH optima for their function. Defective catalytic activity of any of these enzymes results in a block in the digestive process of the cellular materials essential for normal function. In the mid-1960s, using glycogenosis type II, termed Pompe's disease, as the model, Hers defined a category of genetic diseases as "inborn lysosomal disorders," which satisfied two major criteria: (i) an acidic hydrolase normally localized in the lysosome is genetically defective and (ii) as a consequence, the substrate of the defective enzyme accumulates abnormally within pathologically altered secondary lysosomes [2]. Over the years, several important groups of genetic disorders have been identified as belonging to the inborn lysosomal diseases. Among them are the sphingolipidoses, mucopolysaccharidoses and oligosaccharidoses. These disorders are often referred to as storage diseases because the abnormal storage of the undigested substrate is often the most conspicuous clinical and pathological manifestation. The original concept of Hers has inevitably been expanded since its inception to include abnormalities in not only lysosomal enzymes but also in other noncatalytic lysosomal proteins, as well as abnormalities of more general lysosomal functions.

THE PEROXISOME

The peroxisome is another of the membrane-bound subcellular organelles. It had been known morphologically as microbodies before de Duve characterized it biochemically. Its physiological functions are more complex and diverse than those of the lysosome. Known functions of the peroxisome include metabolism of very long-chain fatty acids, pipecolic acid, dicarboxylic acids and phytanic acid and biosynthesis of plasmalogens and bile acids. By analogy to the lyso-

somal diseases, there is now recognized a group of inherited disorders caused by genetic defects in the peroxisomes themselves or the enzymes normally localized in the peroxisome. Many of these diseases manifest primarily as neurological disorders [3].

MOLECULAR GENETICS

The past decade has witnessed a dramatic transition in studies of lysosomal and peroxisomal disorders, from a focus on gene products to the genes themselves. For most of these genetic disorders, the normal cDNAs and the genes responsible for the respective disorders have been isolated and characterized, and in many instances, specific disease-causing mutations have been identified. As expected, information at the genetic level demonstrates the highly complex genetic heterogeneity of these diseases, even when they appear homogeneous in clinical manifestations, analytical biochemistry and enzymatic defects.

DIAGNOSIS AND TREATMENT

Earlier, diagnosis of this group of disorders was based primarily on clinicopathological findings and then on identification of abnormally stored materials by analytical biochemistry. Emphasis has shifted during the past two decades to enzymatic and other metabolic assays [4]. Enzymatic assays provide the means for relatively easy, noninvasive antemortem diagnosis because clinically available materials, such as serum, blood cells and cultured fibroblasts, can be used for this purpose. These procedures can generally be used for detection of heterozygous carriers with varying degrees of reliability. Identification of affected fetuses during pregnancy is generally possible with similar procedures. The most commonly used materials for prenatal diagnosis were cultured amniotic fluid cells. However, biopsied chorionic villi have gained popularity as the material of choice for prenatal diagnosis because diagnosis can be done immediately after the procedure at a much earlier stage of pregnancy. Unambiguous diagnosis of affected and carrier individuals is possible when specific mutations in the responsible genes are known. Unlike the enzymatic diagnosis, however, the DNA diagnosis will not replace earlier procedures because the DNA diagnosis is too specific. It requires prior information on the nature of the mutations in the family. Negative results for any number of known mutations do not exclude the possibility that the patient is affected due to as yet unidentified or untested mutations. Enzymatic and metabolic procedures have a theoretical advantage in that they test for functionality of a particular metabolic step irrespective of the nature of the underlying genetic abnormality.

Replacement of the defective enzyme with the normal enzyme has been attempted through various routes, including direct injection of purified enzyme or transplantation of various normal organs or bone marrow. Earlier trials have been at best partial successes. Long-term, pragmatic benefits to patients have been variable. A much more promising outcome has been reported with replacement of enzymes that have been modified to minimize undesirable uptake and removal from the circulation or to target the enzyme to the proper organs. The commercial availability of such modified enzyme preparations and consistent and long-lasting benefits to patients have made the large-scale enzyme replacement of non-neuronopathic forms of Gaucher's disease a real success story throughout the world. Long-term beneficial effects of bone marrow transplantation are also being reported with increasing frequency. Nevertheless, identification of affected fetuses and termination of pregnancy remain the best that can be offered for a large majority of families with these devastating genetic neurological disorders. The situation could change dramatically in the next decade or two if and when treatment at the genetic level becomes a reality. Extensive and intensive studies are under way in many laboratories focusing on the transfer and expression of genes involved in these disorders *in vitro* and, in some instances, in experimental animals (see Chap. 40).

ANIMAL MODELS

Many of the genetic lysosomal diseases in humans have equivalents among other mammalian species. Since most of the human diseases are rare and since there are serious ethical constraints in studying human patients, these animal models provide useful tools for studying all aspects of these disorders, including natural history of the disease processes, pathogenesis and therapeutic trials. These animal models, particularly those in smaller mammalian species, are expected to be used more extensively in the near future as vehicles for recombinant DNA experiments. It is now possible to generate artificial mouse mutant strains with specific gene deficiencies using homologous recombination and transgenic technology. Most of the genetic sphingolipidoses, some mucopolysaccharidoses and three peroxisomal disorders known in humans have been duplicated in mice with this approach; and in some instances, new genetic conditions, such as double mutants or gene defects not known in humans, have also been generated (Table 41-1) [5].

LYSOSOMAL DISEASE

Lysosomal diseases are traditionally classified according to the nature of the materials that accumulate abnormally. There is considerable overlap in substrate specificities of the enzymes, and consequently, the classification is merely for the purpose of convenience. For example, genetic β-galactosidase defects can result primarily in GM1-ganglioside accumulation (sphingolipidosis), or in bony abnormalities (mucopolysaccharidosis), depending on the nature of mutations. In both instances, degradation of carbohydrate chains of glycoproteins are also impaired (glycoprotein disorders).

Sphingolipidoses are caused by genetic defects in a series of lysosomal enzymes and other proteins essential for the catabolism of sphingolipids

These enzymes are involved in degradation of lipids that contain sphingosine as the basic

TABLE 41-1. ARTIFICIALLY GENERATED MURINE MODELS OF LYSOSOMAL AND PEROXISO-MAL DISEASE[a]

Inactivated gene	Equivalent human disease
Lysosomal disease	
Sphingomyelinase	Niemann-Pick, type A
Glucosylceramidase	Gaucher
α-Galactosidase A	Fabry
Arylsulfatase A (sulfatidase)	Metachromatic leukodystrophy (MLD)
β-Galactosidase	G_{M1}-gangliosidosis
β-Hexosaminidase α subunit	Tay-Sachs
β-Hexosaminidase β subunit	Sandhoff
β-Hexosaminidase α and β subunits	Unknown
G_{M2} activator	G_{M2}-gangliosidosis AB variant
Sphingolipid activator (prosaposin)	Total sphingolipid activator deficiency
β-Gal/sialidase protective protein	Galactosialidosis
Acid phosphatase	Unknown
N-Acetyl α-galactosaminidase	Schindler
Cation-dependent mannose 6-phosphate receptor	Unknown
Cation-independent mannose 6-phosphate receptor	Unknown
Mannose 6-phosphate receptors, double knockout	Unknown
α-Iduronidase	Hurler-Scheie (MPS I and V)
Arylsulfatase B	Maroteaux-Lamy (MPS VI)
Glycosylasparaginase	Aspartylglycosaminuria
Peroxisomal disease	
ALD protein	X-Linked adrenoleukodystrophy
PEX5	Zellweger
Fatty acid acyl-CoA oxidase	Pseudoneonatal adrenoleukodystrophy

[a] Two naturally occurring murine models of lysosomal disorders are known: twitcher (globoid cell leukodystrophy, Krabbe's disease) and β-glucuronidase deficiency (MPS VII). MPS, mucopolysaccharidosis.

building block (Fig. 41-1, Table 41-2) (Chap. 3). Since the nervous system is rich in these lipids, many disorders in this category manifest as neurological disorders. Sphingolipids are degraded by sequential removal of the terminal moieties of the hydrophilic chain: sulfate in the case of sulfatide, phosphorylcholine in the case of sphingomyelin and sialic acid or sugar moieties in others, to ceramide and then to sphingosine and fatty acid. Genetic disorders are known in humans affecting almost every step of the degradative pathway. The mode of inheritance is Mendelian autosomal recessive for all sphingolipidoses, except for Fabry's disease, which is an X-linked disorder (Fig. 41-1, Table 41-2).

Farber's disease, also termed ceramidosis, or Farber's lipogranulomatosis. Primary manifestations of this very rare disorder are painful, progressively deformed joints and subcutaneous granulomatous nodules in infants. Nervous system involvement is variable. The cutaneous nodules, lung and heart are the main sites of abnormal accumulation of ceramide. However, ceramide levels are also increased in the CNS. A mild and probably nonspecific accumulation of simpler gangliosides in the brain is commonly observed. Human ceramidase cDNA has been cloned and characterized.

Niemann-Pick disease. This disease was traditionally classified into types A, B, C and D, primarily according to clinical phenotypes. However, only types A and B are allelic and caused by primary genetic deficiency of lysosomal acid sphingomyelinase. The term Niemann-Pick should be used only for these two types. Patients with either type A or B disease exhibit hepatosplenomegaly and characteristic foamy cells in the bone marrow. Type A disease usually occurs in infants and is characterized by additional severe CNS involvement. Patients rarely survive beyond 5 years. On the other hand, type B patients are normal in intellect and free of neuro-

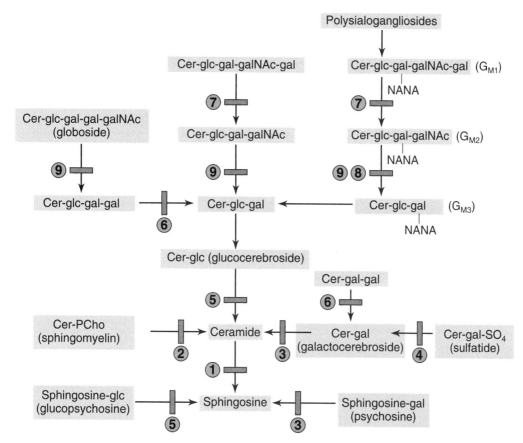

FIGURE 41-1. Chemical and metabolic relationships among the major sphingolipids. Normal catabolic pathways are indicated by *arrows* connecting adjacent compounds. Biosynthesis of these lipids occurs in the reverse direction. *Numbers* indicate locations of genetic metabolic blocks known in humans. *Numbers* correspond to those in Table 41-2.

logical manifestations. Onset may vary from birth to adulthood, with varying severity of organomegaly. In both types, there is an enormous accumulation of sphingomyelin in the liver and spleen. Up to a five-fold increase in sphingomyelin occurs in the CNS only in type A patients. The degree of the sphingomyelinase deficiency is similar in the two types when assayed *in vitro*. However, type A and type B can be differentiated from each other via the loading test, in which degradation of exogenously added sphingomyelin is assessed in living cultured fibroblasts: type B fibroblasts are capable of hydrolyzing a much higher percentage of the added sphingomyelin than type A fibroblasts. Mutation analyses have indicated close association of at least some mutations with clinical phenotypes [6].

Niemann-Pick type C. This disease was originally classified as a juvenile neurological subtype of Niemann-Pick disease because patients exhibit organomegaly, slowly progressive CNS signs and similar foam cells in bone marrow cells, with moderately increased amounts of sphingomyelin in liver and spleen. However, other lipids, in particular unesterified cholesterol and glucosylceramide, accumulate and sphingomyelinase activities, although partially decreased in cultured fibroblasts, are normal in leukocytes and solid tissues. Work during the past 10 years has convincingly shown that lysosomal sequestration of endocytosed low-density lipoprotein (LDL)-derived cholesterol and accompanying anomalies in intracellular sterol trafficking are the hallmark phenotypic features of the disease [6–8]. Impairment of cholesterol

TABLE 41-2. MAJOR SPHINGOLIPIDOSES*a*

Disease	Clinicopathological manifestations	Affected lipids	Enzymatic defects
1. Farber's disease (lipogranulomatosis)	Mostly infantile disease, tender swollen joints, multiple subcutaneous nodules, later flaccid paralysis and mental impairment	Ceramide	Acid ceramidase
2. Niemann-Pick disease (types A and B)	Neuropathic and non-neuropathic forms, hepatosplenomegaly, foamy cells in bone marrow, severe neurological signs in the neuropathic form (type A)	Sphingomyelin	Sphingomyelinase
3. Globoid cell leukodystrophy (Krabbe's disease)	Almost always infantile disease, white matter signs, peripheral neuropathy, high spinal fluid protein, loss of myelin, globoid cells in white matter	Galactosylceramide Galactosylsphingosine	Galactosylceramidase
4a. Metachromatic leukodystrophy	Late infantile, juvenile and adult forms; white matter signs; peripheral neuropathy; high spinal fluid protein; metachromatic granules in the brain, nerves, kidney and urine	Sulfatide	Arylsulfatase A ("sulfatidase")
4b. Multiple sulfatase deficiency	Similar to metachromatic leukodystrophy but additional gray matter signs, facial and skeletal abnormalities, organomegaly similar to mucopolysaccharidoses	Sulfatide, other sulfated compounds (see text)	Arylsulfatases A, B, C, (see text)
4c. Sulfatidase activator (*sap*-B) deficiency	Similar to later-onset forms of 4a	Sulfatide, globotriaosyl-ceramide	Sulfatidase activator (*sap*-B)
5a. Gaucher's disease	Neuropathic and non-neuropathic forms, hepatosplenomegaly, Gaucher cells in bone marrow, severe neurological signs in the neuropathic form, also an intermediate form (type III)	Glucosylceramide, glucosylsphingosine	Glucosylceramidase
5b. *sap*-C deficiency	Gaucher-like (type 3) clinical phenotype	Glucosylceramide	*sap*-C ("Gaucher's factor")
6. Fabry's disease	Primarily adult and non-neurological, angiokeratoma around buttocks, renal damage, X-linked	Trihexosylceramide (gal-gal-glc-cer) Digalactosylceramide	α-Galactosidase A (trihexosyceramidase)
7. G$_{M1}$-gangliosidosis	Slow growth, motor weakness, gray matter signs, infantile form with additional facial and skeletal abnormalities and organomegaly, swollen neurons	G$_{M1}$-ganglioside, galactose rich fragments of glycoproteins	G$_{M1}$-ganglioside β-galactosidase
8a. Tay-Sachs disease	Severe gray matter signs, slow growth, motor weakness, hyperacusis, cherry red spot, head enlargement, swollen neurons	G$_{M2}$-ganglioside	β-Hexosaminidase A
8b. B1 variant	Commonly later onset, slower progression but otherwise similar to Tay-Sachs disease, milder pathology	G$_{M2}$-ganglioside	β-Hexosaminidase A (normal against non-sulfated artificial substrates but deficient against G$_{M2}$-ganglioside and sulfated artificial substrate)
8c. AB variant	Similar to 8a	G$_{M2}$-ganglioside	G$_{M2}$ activator protein
9. Sandhoff's disease	Panethnic but otherwise indistinguishable from Tay-Sachs disease	G$_{M2}$-ganglioside, asialo-G$_{M2}$-ganglioside, globoside	β-Hexosaminidases A and B

*a*The numbers correspond to the steps of metabolic blocks in Figure 41-1.

egress from lysosomes appears as the key intracellular lesion, resulting in an array of cholesterol-processing errors, including delayed induction of homeostatic responses. Demonstration in cultured cells of a lysosomal accumulation of unesterified cholesterol by fluorescent staining with filipin and of impaired LDL-induced cholesterol esterification are the tests currently used for diagnosing patients.

The wide clinical spectrum of the disease has been discussed extensively [1,6] and is also illustrated by the various names under which patients have been described in the literature, including "juvenile dystonic lipidosis," "giant-cell hepatitis," "neurovisceral storage disease with vertical supranuclear ophthalmoplegia," "lipidosis with vertical gaze palsy," "lactosylceramidosis, maladie de Neville," "down-gaze paresis, ataxia, foam cells (DAF) syndrome" and "adult neurovisceral lipidosis." Cardinal neurological symptoms in the most common juvenile presentation include ataxia, dysarthria, cataplexia, learning difficulties and almost constantly, vertical supranuclear gaze palsy. Linkage and complementation analyses have shown that genetic defects in two separate genes, *NPC1*, which is mapped to 18q11, 90% of patients, and *NPC2,* induce similar clinical and biochemical phenotypes [9]. The so-called Niemann-Pick type D appears to be only one particular variant, the Nova-Scotian form, within group 1. These new findings clearly argue against the term Niemann-Pick for this disorder. Conceptually, there is no evidence that Neimann-Pick type C disease is a sphingolipidosis. The *NPC1* gene has been cloned and is homologous to known cholesterol homeostasis genes [10].

Globoid cell leukodystrophy (Krabbe's disease). This disorder and metachromatic leukodystrophy are two of the classical genetic myelin disorders simply because they involve abnormal degradation of two sphingolipids highly localized in the myelin sheath, galactosylceramide and sulfatide (Fig. 41-1) (see also Chap. 39). The disease is usually infantile, although rarer late-onset forms are also known. Clinicopathological manifestations are almost exclusively those of the white matter and the peripheral nerves. The unique globoid cells are hematogenous histiocytic cells that infiltrate the white matter in response to undigested

galactosylceramide. Unlike other storage diseases, the primary natural substrate of the defective enzyme, galactosylceramide (psychosine), not only does not accumulate abnormally but it is almost always much lower than normal because of a rapid and almost complete destruction of the oligodendroglia and the consequent early cessation of myelination. On the other hand, a toxic metabolite, galactosylsphingosine, does accumulate and appears to be responsible for the devastating pathology of the disease [11,12]. Effects of psychosine, including early cessation of myelination and possibly overlapping substrate specificities between the two lysosomal β-galactosidases, galactosylceramidase and GM1-ganglioside β-galactosidase, are important in understanding the pathogenesis of this disease [1]. The galactosylceramidase gene has been cloned, and over 60 disease-causing mutations have been identified, including the one underlying the classic Nordic infantile disease.

Metachromatic leukodystrophy. The enzymatic defect in metachromatic leukodystrophy is one step before that in Krabbe's disease (Fig. 41-1). While these two diseases share many common features, there are significant differences that suggest different pathogenetic mechanisms. Clinically, relatively large proportions of patients with metachromatic leukodystrophy are of juvenile or adult form. Pathologically, the reduction in the number of oligodendrocytes is less severe. Remaining oligodendrocytes contain acid-phosphatase-positive lamellar inclusions, which exhibit metachromasia, or yellow–brown staining with cresyl violet at acidic pH at the light microscopic level. Unlike in globoid cell leukodystrophy, the affected substrate, sulfatide, is always abnormally increased. Both cDNA and the gene coding for human arylsulfatase A have been cloned, and several mutations causing the clinical disease of metachromatic leukodystrophy have been described [1]. A pseudodeficiency allele occurs relatively frequently. Bone marrow transplantation treatment has been tried in patients with late-onset forms of the disease with some degree of positive effects. A metachromatic leukodystrophy-like disorder, which is due to a deficiency in the sulfatidase activator protein has also been observed (see below).

Multiple sulfatase deficiency (MSD). Phenotypically, this disease combines features of metachromatic leukodystrophy and mucopolysaccharidoses. In addition to clinical manifestations of metachromatic leukodystrophy, patients present with craniofacial abnormalities, skeletal deformities and hepatosplenomegaly. There is abnormal urinary excretion of sulfatide, dermatan sulfate and heparan sulfate. Pathological findings are also combinations of the two conditions. Inheritance is mendelian autosomal recessive. Nevertheless, activities of a series of sulfatases are deficient, including arylsulfatases A, B and C; steroid sulfatases; and sulfatases related to mucopolysaccharide degradation (see below). Greater understanding of the underlying genetic defect has been achieved by the discovery of a novel co- or post-translational modification common to many sulfatases [13]. The mechanism involves modification of a cysteine residue to formyl glycine, also termed 2-amino-3-oxypropionic acid. This modification appears to be prerequisite for catalytic activity of the sulfatases. In two sulfatases known to be deficient in MSD, this conversion did not take place. The exact metabolic mechanism for the conversion is not yet known.

Gaucher's disease. Traditionally Gaucher's disease has been classified as one of three types: type I, non-neuropathic, with a widely varying age of onset, and by far the most common; type II, infantile, severely neuropathic; and type III, intermediate phenotype. Type I is highly prevalent in the Jewish population, while a large distinct group of type III patients exists in northern Sweden. All types are allelic and are caused by defective glucosylceramidase activity. Glucosylceramide is present in great excess in the enlarged liver and spleen in all types of the disease. The brain, in which glucosylceramide is normally almost nonexistent, accumulates only small amounts of this substrate in type II patients. By analogy to Niemann-Pick disease, non-neuropathic Gaucher patients are free of neurological involvement and survive for decades, while type II neuropathic patients die within a few years with severe CNS involvement. The difference in the pathogenetic mechanisms in these phenotypes is not known. As is the case for globoid cell leukodystrophy, the accumulation of a toxic metabolite, glucosylsphingosine, may play an important role in the pathogenesis of Gaucher's disease. The degree of CNS involvement parallels the concentrations of glucopsychosine in the brain. The gene for glucosylceramidase has been cloned and characterized, and many mutations responsible for the disease state have been identified [1]. Genotypic and phenotypic correlations have been studied in large populations of patients. The most common N370S mutation has never been found associated with a neuropathic phenotype, either alone or in association with another mutation. On the other hand, patients with another frequent mutation, L444P, initially thought typical of type III, may also present as type I or II. The most intensive enzyme replacement therapy has been tried in patients with the non-neuropathic form of Gaucher's disease. With the use of purified or recombinant enzyme modified at the carbohydrate moiety to increase efficiency of macrophage targeting, the positive outcome of enzyme therapy has been established and is widely used as the standard treatment for non-neuropathic forms of the disease. See below for details of a Gaucher-like disorder which is due to deficiency of an endogenous activator protein.

Fabry's disease. Unlike most other sphingolipidoses, Fabry's disease is an X-linked disorder, occurring mostly in adults. It is also primarily a systemic disease, and neurological manifestations, when present, are largely secondary. Cutaneous angiokeratoma is the most conspicuous early sign. The affected lipids, trihexosylceramide (gal-gal-glc-ceramide) and digalactosylceramide, are nearly absent in neural tissues from normal individuals. There are some accumulations of these lipids in the brain of patients, thought to be contributed primarily by those in the blood vessels. Cerebrovascular pathology commonly results in secondary neurological symptoms. Most patients succumb to renal failure and other vascular diseases. Consequently, transplantation of normal kidney has been attempted as a form of treatment. However, the results were not sufficiently encouraging to pursue further. The enzyme responsible for degradation of these sphingolipids with the terminal α-galactose residue is α-galactosidase A, a mutation of which causes the disease. A normal cDNA coding for α-galactosidase A has been cloned, and several mutations have been identified [1]. An enzyme replacement therapy analogous to that for Gaucher's disease is being initiated.

GM1-gangliosidosis. The infantile form of this disease shows, in addition to psychomotor retardation and other neurological manifestations, mucopolysaccharidosis-like clinical features. The late-onset form is relatively free of systemic signs. Morquio's disease type B is a unique adult phenotype of this disorder, also caused by genetic defects in GM1-ganglioside β-galactosidase, also termed acid β-galactosidase (see below). These pleomorphic phenotypes are consequences of the wide substrate specificity of the defective enzyme, GM1-ganglioside β-galactosidase, which hydrolyzes not only GM1-ganglioside, asialo-GM1-ganglioside and lactosylceramide but also terminal β-galactosyl residues of carbohydrate chains of various glycoproteins and intermediate degradation products of keratan sulfate. Distinct mutations in the gene could differentially inactivate catalytic activity toward different substrates. Large accumulations of GM1-ganglioside occur primarily in the brains of patients with the infantile and late-infantile forms of the disease. The major materials accumulated in the systemic organs are fragments of glycopeptides. It is not known whether GM1-ganglioside accumulates in the brain of patients with Morquio's B disease. The human acid β-galactosidase cDNA and the gene have been isolated and characterized, and many mutations have been identified [1]. Within the relatively limited number of patients examined so far, there appears to be an excellent correlation between the clinical phenotypes and underlying mutations.

Tay-Sachs disease. The classic Tay-Sachs disease prevalent among the Ashkenazi Jewish population is the prototype of human sphingolipidoses. It is caused by a mutation in the β-hexosaminidase α-subunit gene. Normally, the hexosaminidase α and β subunits form two catalytically active isozymes, β-hexosaminidase A (αβ) and B (ββ). A defect in the α subunit thus results in defective hexosaminidase A with normal hexosaminidase B. Hexosaminidase A can hydrolyze all known natural substrates with terminal β-*N*-acetylgalactosamine or β-*N*-acetyl-

glucosamine residues, while hexosaminidase B hydrolyzes all of these substrates except GM2-ganglioside. As a result, a relatively specific accumulation of GM2-ganglioside occurs in genetic hexosaminidase α-deficiency states.

A few genetic variants are known on the basis of clinical and enzymatic criteria. Patients with the adult form may not develop clinical symptoms until the second or third decade of life. The enzymologically unique B1 variant is characterized by essentially normal hexosaminidases A and B when assayed with the standard artificial substrates but completely defective hexosaminidase A against the natural substrate GM2-ganglioside and an artificial substrate, 4-methylumbelliferyl glcNAc-6-sulfate. These enzymatic variants are caused by genetic defects in the hexosaminidase α-subunit gene. In contrast, the AB variant, which is phenotypically indistinguishable from the infantile hexosaminidase α defect, is caused by an entirely different genetic mechanism, a mutation in a specific activator protein (GM2 activator protein) (see below).

While all of these phenotypic and enzymological differentiations have been useful, a molecular genetic understanding of these diseases is progressing. Normal cDNA and the gene for the hexosaminidase α chain have been cloned and characterized [14]. Patients with some forms of the disease lack enzyme activity and exhibit an immunologically reactive α subunit, while others lack enzyme activity but exhibit immunoreactivity for the α subunit. Availability of cDNA for the α subunit has shown that the presence or absence of cross-reactive material largely corresponds to the presence or absence of the relevant mRNA. Both the classic Tay-Sachs disease and a phenotypically indistinguishable disease occurring in the French-Canadian population are mRNA-negative, while the B1 variant and some other unusual forms are mRNA-positive. Contrary to earlier expectations of a single mutation, two mutations underlying the classic Jewish infantile form of the disease have been identified: a splicing defect and a four-base insertion, the latter accounting for two-thirds to three-fourths of the Jewish infantile alleles [1]. The French-Canadian form showed a major deletion in the 5′ end of the hexosaminidase α gene of approximately 7 kb, spanning from the putative promoter region to beyond the first exon into the first intron. The first point mutation in the hexosaminidase α gene was identified in a patient with the B1 variant form of the disease [15]. The normal arginine at residue 178 was substituted by histidine. Computer analysis suggested substantial changes in the secondary structure of the enzyme protein around the mutation, consistent with the unusual enzymological characteristic of this variant. The possible origin of this particular mutation has been traced to northern Portugal. Since the mid-1980s, over 60 mutations that cause Tay-Sachs disease or its variants have been identified within the β-hexosaminidase α gene. The expected complexity of abnormalities at the level of the gene is likely to render the traditional clinical and enzymatic classification of the disease obsolete.

Sandhoff's disease. When the hexosaminidase β gene is genetically defective, it results in inactivation of both hexosaminidases A (αβ) and B (ββ). While the typical infantile form of Sandhoff's disease cannot be readily distinguished clinically from infantile hexosaminidase α defect, histochemical and biochemical studies reveal accumulation of additional materials other than GM2-ganglioside in the brain. All sphingolipids with the terminal β-hexosamine residue are affected, including GM2-ganglioside, asialo-GM2-ganglioside and globoside (Fig. 41-1). Since globoside is primarily a systemic lipid, it also accumulates in systemic organs. The cDNA and the gene for the hexosaminidase β subunit have also been cloned and many mutations characterized [1]. It is of interest that, despite the localization on different chromosomes, α on chromosome 15 and β on chromosome 5, hexosaminidase α and β chains are homologous. These two subunit genes, located on different chromosomes, appear to have been separated from a single gene relatively recently in the evolutionary time scale.

Activator deficiencies. *In vivo* degradation of the highly hydrophobic lipids often requires, in addition to the specific hydrolases, a third component, commonly referred to as the activator protein. These generally are small glycoproteins localized within the lysosomes but are not enzymes themselves. When such an activator protein is essential for *in vivo* degradation of the substrates and when it is genetically defective, the end results are very similar to deficiency of the enzyme itself. GM2-gangliosidosis AB variant is caused by genetic absence of the activator required for *in vivo* degradation of GM2-ganglioside. The degradative enzyme β-hexosaminidase A is normal in these patients. Conceptually similar diseases have been described in patients showing metachromatic leukodystrophy-like and Gaucher-like clinical phenotypes and in whom activator proteins, rather than the hydrolases arylsulfatase A and glucosylceramidase, respectively, were genetically defective. Both of these activator proteins, sulfatide activator, also termed sap-B or saposin B, and the glucosylceramidase activator, also termed sap-C or saposin C, are homologous proteins coded by a single gene. A single transcript generates a large polypeptide, which is subsequently proteolytically processed into four small, homologous proteins, including the sulfatide activator and the glucosylceramidase activator. The fourth domain, saposin D (sap-D) has been shown to stimulate ceramide degradation in cultured fibroblasts. Evidence exists that suggests that the first domain, saposin A (sap-A) also has sphingolipid activator function. No human disease is known to be caused by mutations in the A or D domain. Several mutations in these activator proteins responsible for the clinical diseases have been characterized, including a point mutation in the initiation codon resulting in complete loss of all four activator proteins and, consequently, a highly complex clinical and biochemical phenotype [1]. A murine model in which all saposins have been eliminated by gene targeting displayed characteristics of the human disease [16].

Mucopolysaccharidoses are caused by genetic enzymatic defects in the degradation of carbohydrate chains of glycosaminoglycans

The carbohydrate chains of glycosaminoglycans are sequentially degraded by a series of lysosomal enzymes (Table 41-3). By analogy to sphingolipidoses, genetic enzymatic defects in these degradative steps cause the accumulation of undegradable metabolites, resulting in the various forms of mu-

TABLE 41-3. MUCOPOLYSACCHARIDOSES

Disease	Clinicopathological manifestations	Affected compounds	Enzymatic defects
Hurler's disease, Scheie's disease (MPS IH and IS)[a]	Craniofacial abnormalities, cloudy cornea, bone and other mesodermal tissue abnormalities, severe to mild psychomotor retardation, organomegaly, lysosomal storage in mesodermal organs, zebra bodies in neurons	Dermatan sulfate, heparan sulfate	α-L-Iduronidase
Hunter's syndrome (MPS II)	Generally similar to but milder than Hurler-Scheie but X-linked, corneal clouding rare	Dermatan sulfate, heparan sulfate	α-Iduronate sulfatase
Sanfilippo's disease (MPS III)	Four genetically distinct (nonallelic) types, similar clinicopathological manifestations, severe psychomotor retardation, difficult to manage aggressive behavioral problems, relatively mild bone and other systemic involvement, zebra bodies in neurons	Heparan sulfate	Type A, heparan *N*-sulfatase; type B, *N*-acetyl α-glucosaminidase; type C, *N*-acetyl-CoA: α-glucosaminide *N*-acetyltransferase; type D, *N*-acetyl α-glucosaminide 6-sulfatase
Morquio's disease (MPS IV)	Two nonallelic forms, primarily bone abnormalities, corneal clouding, nervous system involvement secondary to bone changes, type B allelic to G$_{M1}$-gangliosidosis	Keratan sulfate	Type A, *N*-acetyl-galactosamine 6-sulfatase; type B, β-galactosidase
Maroteaux-Lamy disease (MPS VI)	Severe to mild clinical types, bone and corneal changes, nervous system involvement, generally mild	Dermatan sulfate	Arylsulfatase B (*N*-acetyl-galactosamine 4-sulfatase)
β-Glucuronidase deficiency (MPS VII)	Fetal hydrops, organomegaly, bone abnormalities, mild to no psychomotor retardation, inclusions in leukocytes	Dermatan sulfate, heparan sulfate	β-Glucuronidase

[a] MPS, mucopolysaccharidosis.

copolysaccharidoses. These materials are also excreted into urine in massive amounts. The standard classification of mucopolysaccharidoses is based on clinical manifestations and the nature of the accumulated and excreted materials. The enzymatic classification does not necessarily correspond to the traditional classification; a single classic disease often consists of more than one nonallelic disorder, while two disorders classified earlier as different may be allelic. All mucopolysaccharidoses are inherited as autosomal recessive traits, except for the X-linked Hunter's disease [1].

Hurler's disease and Scheie's disease (mucopolysaccharidosis IH and IS). Hurler's syndrome is the prototype of the mucopolysaccha-

ridoses. It is caused by a genetic deficiency in α-iduronidase activity. Scheie's disease was once considered to be a separate disease and classified as mucopolysaccharidosis V; it is now known to be a milder allelic variant of Hurler's syndrome. Neurons in the brain are commonly distended and contain characteristic lamellar inclusions, known as zebra bodies. They are the site of abnormal ganglioside accumulation commonly found in this and other mucopolysaccharidoses. While the increase is nonspecific and is mainly in normally minor monosialogangliosides, the degree of the increase is often substantial, up to several fold above normal. Polysulfated mucopolysaccharides are inhibitory to some lysosomal enzymes *in vitro*. Similar inhibition *in vivo* might be responsible for the ganglioside increase. Whether the ganglioside accumulation and neuronal distention contribute to the neurological manifestations of the disease is not known.

Hunter's syndrome (mucopolysaccharidosis II). Other than being an X-linked disorder and generally milder and slower in the clinical features and course, patients with Hunter's syndrome resemble closely those with Hurler syndrome. The responsible enzyme, α-iduronate sulfatase, has been cloned.

Sanfilippo's disease (mucopolysaccharidosis III). This is an excellent example of a disease identified on the basis of clinicopathological criteria, which has turned out to be a mixture of more than one genetically distinct disease. Four enzymatically different and nonallelic diseases are included under the eponym, Sanfilippo's disease. All four defective enzymes are involved at different steps of heparan sulfate degradation. Thus, the end results are essentially identical. Differential diagnosis cannot be established without appropriate enzyme assays.

Morquio's disease (mucopolysaccharidosis IV). Unlike other mucopolysaccharidoses, Morquio's disease is primarily a skeletal disorder. Neurological involvement is almost always secondary to skeletal abnormalities. The most common neurological complications are traumatic lesions of the spinal cord at the cervical level due to vertebral deformity. There are two genetically distinct types: type A, which is an *N*-acetylgalactosamine 6-sulfatase deficiency, and type B, which is a β-galactosidase deficiency. Patients with type A disease are clinically more severely affected. Since the type B disease is allelic with GM1-gangliosidosis, mutations responsible for Morquio's B phenotype have been identified in the β-galactosidase gene. *N*-Acetylgalactosamine 6-sulfatase has been cloned, and a few mutations responsible for the type A disease have been described.

Maroteaux-Lamy disease (mucopolysaccharidosis VI). This disease is another of the Hurler-like syndromes but can be differentiated from Hurler's syndrome by relatively well-preserved intellectual capacity. Urinary excretion of mucopolysaccharides is predominantly dermatan sulfate. Clinical severity and duration varies among apparently allelic cases.

β-Glucuronidase deficiency (mucopolysaccharidosis VII). The first case of this disease was reported by Sly et al. in 1973 [17]. While the general clinical picture is that of a mucopolysaccharidosis, the degrees of severity in skeletal abnormalities, organomegaly and nervous system involvement appear widely variable. β-Glucuronidase was one of the first lysosomal enzymes cloned [18]. A complete "cure" of the disease with restoration of β-glucuronidase activity has been reported in mutant mice genetically deficient in glucuronidase activity, when the normal human β-glucuronidase gene was transgenically introduced [19].

Glycoprotein disorders result from defects in lysosomal hydrolases

Natural substrates of certain lysosomal glycosidases are primarily carbohydrate chains of glycoproteins. When such enzymes are genetically defective, the results are accumulation and urinary excretion of undigested sugar chains and small glycopeptides since the protein backbone is usually degradable by proteases, which are genetically normal in patients (Table 41-4).

Sialidosis (neuraminidase deficiency, mucolipidosis I). Apparently, two dissimilar phenotypes result from enzymatic defects in the same lysosomal α-neuraminidase, also termed sialidase. The infantile form had been known as mucolipidosis I because of the mucopolysaccharidosis-like appearance of patients. Neurological involvement is severe to moderate, including impaired intellectual capacity. The second type occurs in the juvenile age group. Three findings stand out: typical macular cherry red spots, intractable myoclonic seizures and intact intellect. The α-neuraminidase deficient in sialidosis cleaves both α-2,6 and α-2,3 sialyl linkages but is apparently distinct from neuraminidase(s), which hydrolyzes sialic acid from gangliosides. Thus, patients accumulate and excrete excess

TABLE 41-4. GLYCOPROTEIN STORAGE DISEASES AND MUCOLIPIDOSES

Disease	Clinicopathological manifestations	Affected compounds	Enzymatic defects
Sialidosis (mucolipidosis I)	Two distinct phenotypes, mucolipidosis I (mucopolysaccharidosis-like features, severe to moderate psychomotor retardation) and the cherry red spot myoclonus syndrome	Sialyloligosaccharides	α-Neuraminidase (sialidase)
I-Cell disease and pseudo-Hurler's polydystrophy (mucolipidoses II and III)	Mucopolysaccharidosis-like features, severe psychomotor retardation, characteristic inclusions in fibroblasts, ML-II is a milder allelic disease	Multiple (see text)	Primary defect in UDP-glcNAc: lysosomal enzyme glcNAc phospho-transferase, secondary abnormality in multiple lysosomal enzymes (see text)
α-Mannosidosis	Mucopolysaccharidosis-like features, severe to moderate psychomotor retardation	Oligosaccharides with terminal α-mannose	Acid α-mannosidase
β-Mannosidosis	Infantile and late-onset forms, psychomotor retardation, Sanfilippo-like general clinical features	β-Mannosyl-glcNAc, heparan sulfate?	β-Mannosidase, heparan sulfamidase
α-Fucosidosis	Mucopolysaccharidosis-like features, severe to moderate psychomotor retardation	Fucose-containing oligosaccharides and glycolipids	α-Fucosidase
Galactosialidosis	Similar to late-onset form of G_{M1}-gangliosidosis, also more severe infantile form	"Protective protein" (secondary defect in G_{M1}-ganglioside β-galactosidase and sialidase)	Primary defect in carboxypeptidase activity due to "protective protein"

sialic acid-containing materials derived from complex carbohydrate chains of glycoproteins, but there is no evidence for increased levels of gangliosides in the brain and elsewhere as the consequence of the genetic defect. The lysosomal acid sialidase has been cloned and a few disease-causing mutations identified [20,21] (see Galactosialidosis, below).

I-Cell disease (mucolipidosis II) and pseudo-Hurler's polydystrophy (mucolipidosis III).

Among the disorders primarily affecting glycoprotein metabolism, I-cell disease and pseudo-Hurler's polydystrophy are conceptually unique. These two disorders had been considered separate entities on the basis of phenotypic manifestations. However, they are now known to be allelic variants of the same disease. Activities of many, but not all, lysosomal hydrolases are deficient in cultured fibroblasts. Notable exceptions are glucosylceramidase and acid phos-

phatase. Activities of those that are deficient in fibroblasts are dramatically much higher than normal in serum and other extracellular fluids, including the culture media in which patients' fibroblasts are grown. The primary genetic cause of the disease is not in any of the individual lysosomal enzymes but in the UDP-glcNAc:lysosomal enzyme glcNAc phospho-transferase, which is localized in the Golgi apparatus and is essential for the normal processing and packaging of lysosomal enzymes. Without this enzyme, lysosomal enzymes cannot acquire the mannose 6-phosphate recognition marker which allows them to be properly routed to the lysosome. As the result, lysosomal enzymes are abnormally routed out of the cell. While lack of lysosomal enzyme activities must be primarily responsible for clinicopathological manifestations, this disease does not rigorously satisfy the two classic criteria of Hers [2] for inherited lysosomal disease.

α-Mannosidosis. α-Mannosidases, which participate in the processing of carbohydrate chains of glycoproteins, are localized in the Golgi apparatus and are genetically intact in α-mannosidosis. The lysosomal α-mannosidase deficient in this disease degrades the carbohydrate chains. Therefore, abnormal accumulations and urinary excretion of undegraded oligosaccharides with terminal α-mannose residues derived from normally synthesized and processed glycoproteins occur as a consequence of the genetic defect. A plant toxin, swainsonine, inhibits α-mannosidases, and its chronic ingestion creates an experimental condition that mimics many aspects of genetic α-mannosidosis. A limitation of this model, however, is that swainsonine inhibits both lysosomal and Golgi α-mannosidases.

β-Mannosidosis. This is the only disorder among those dealt with in this chapter that was discovered first in another mammalian species before an equivalent disease was found in humans. For several years, β-mannosidase deficiency was known in the goat. Affected goats show severe neurological signs almost from birth. The goat disease is rapidly fatal, and an almost complete lack of myelination is the unique feature of the neuropathology. A human patient with β-mannosidase deficiency has now been identified [22]. Unlike in the goat disease, the clinical picture was relatively mild, presenting with Sanfilippo-like features. There was urinary excretion of a disaccharide, β-mannose-glcNAc, and heparan sulfate. The same disaccharide is excreted in the goat disease. It is thought to derive from the innermost mannose in the glycoprotein carbohydrate chains. The parents of the patient possessed intermediate activities of the enzyme, consistent with the deficiency being the primary genetic defect. There was also a concomitant lack of heparan sulfamidase activity, which was normal in one parent and intermediate in the other. Human β-mannosidosis occurring in infants has also been described. The clinical features are more similar to those of the goat disease.

α-Fucosidosis. α-Fucoside residues are present in carbohydrate chains of both sphingoglycolipids and glycoproteins. Although fucosylated glycolipids are quantitatively minor, they are functionally important tissue constituents. Many blood-group antigens are fucosylated glycosphingolipids. In patients with genetic α-fucosidase deficiency, accumulations and urinary excretion of fucose-terminated oligosaccharides and fucosylated sphingolipids are observed.

Galactosialidosis (combined sialidase–β-galactosidase deficiency). The concept of the protective protein is relatively new. Lysosomal β-galactosidase and sialidase appear to exist as a complex with a third small protein within the lysosome. This protein protects these enzymes from being degraded by acid proteases also present in the lysosome, and when it is absent, both enzymes are degraded rapidly. Genetic abnormality of this protective protein results in deficient activities of both sialidase and β-galactosidase [23]. The protein also possesses carboxypeptidase activity. Thus, assays for carboxypeptidase activity can be used for diagnosis. The disease is generally a slowly progressive neurological disorder, resembling the later-onset form of GM1-gangliosidosis. The cDNA and the gene coding for the protective protein have been cloned and several mutations characterized [1].

There are other genetic disorders due to abnormalities in lysosomal function

Some of the major disorders are listed here and readers are referred to appropriate chapters in Scriver et al. [1]: α-glucosidase deficiency, also termed Pompe's disease; acid lipase deficiency, also termed Wolman's disease and cholesterol ester storage disease; *N*-acetyl α-galactosaminidase deficiency, also termed Schindler's disease; pycnodysostosis (cathepsin K defect); aspartylglycosaminuria; sialic acid storage disease, also termed Salla's disease and generalized sialic acid storage disorder; and cystinosis. The last two disorders are caused by genetic defects in transport of sialic acid and cysteine, respectively, across the lysosomal membrane.

PEROXISOMAL DISEASE

This group comprises neurological disorders that occur as the result of defects in biogenesis of peroxisomes or, directly or indirectly, in enzymes that are normally localized in peroxisomes. For an overview of this rapidly evolving field, readers are referred to review articles [1,3,24–27]. In the following, only representative disorders are described. Table 41-5 summarizes the main biochemical abnormalities and the known genetic defects in these diseases.

Disorders of function can result from genetic defects in factors that are critical for peroxisomal formation

These disorders form a clinically and genetically heterogeneous group of severe autosomal recessive diseases [26]. Consequently, peroxisomes are either absent or abnormal morphologically, and there is a general failure of all metabolic functions normally associated with the peroxisome.

Zellweger spectrum. The term Zellweger spectrum (ZS) has been given to a complex group of

disorders with overlapping clinical features and common biochemical abnormalities [28]. Three major categories, ZS, neonatal adrenoleukodystrophy (NALD) and infantile Refsum's disease (IRD), are described here. However, it should be emphasized that this classification is based on clinical phenotypes but not on genetic causes. The metabolic abnormalities common among these disorders include accumulation of very long-chain fatty acids (VLCFA) and of phytanic acid, elevated bile acid intermediates and deficiency of plasmalogen biosynthesis. Peroxisomes are virtually absent in hepatocytes and fibroblasts, although peroxisomal membrane ghosts can be found. In spite of this common biochemical phenotype, genetic complementation analysis using cell hybridization has revealed the existence of at least nine different complementation groups (CGs), with no correlation to any given clinical phenotype. This clearly indicates the complexity of peroxisome biogenesis and of the genetic disorders that can result from abnormalities in any of the steps.

TABLE 41-5.   PEROXISOMAL DISEASES[a]

Disease	Biochemistry	Genetics and defective gene
Peroxisomal biogenesis disorders		Autosomal recessive, at least 11 CGs
The Zellweger syndrome spectrum Zellweger syndrome Neonatal adrenoleukodystrophy Infantile Refsum's disease	Accumulation of VLCFA, phytanic acid and bile acid intermediates; deficiency of plasmalogen biosynthesis and of multiple peroxisomal enzymes	CG1, *PEX1*; CG2, *PEX5* (PTS1 receptor); CG3, *PEX12* (IMP); CG4, *PEX6*; CG10, *PEX2* (IMP, paF1)
Rhizomelic chondrodysplasia punctata	Deficiency of plasmalogen synthesis, high phytanic acid, normal VLCFA	CG11, *PEX7* (PTS2 receptor)
Disorders of peroxisomal β-oxidation		Autosomal recessive
Pseudoneonatal adrenoleukodystrophy	Elevated VLCFA	Acyl-CoA oxidase
Peroxisomal bifunctional enzyme deficiency	Elevated VLCFA and bile acid intermediates, bifunctional enzyme deficiency	Bifunctional protein?
Pseudo-Zellweger syndrome	Elevated VLCFA and bile acid intermediates, thiolase deficiency	Thiolase?
X-Linked adrenoleukodystrophy (ALD)		X-Linked recessive
Childhood cerebral ALD Adrenomyeloneuropathy Adult cerebral ALD Adrenal insufficiency	Elevated VLCFA, impaired VLCFA oxidation, in many (but not all) cases absent ALD protein	ALD gene
Adult Refsum's disease	Elevated phytanic acid, phytanate-oxidase deficiency	Autosomal recessive, phytanoyl CoA hydroxylase (*PAHX*)

[a] CG, complementation group; VLCFA, very long-chain fatty acids; PTS, peroxisomal targeting signal; IMP, integral membrane protein; *PEX* genes, see [29].

Zellweger syndrome. The prototype of the generalized peroxisomal disorder is ZS, or cerebro-hepato-renal syndrome, in which the seminal discovery of an apparent lack of peroxisomes in hepatocytes and renal tubules was made quite early. Patients show a combination of craniofacial dysmorphia; neurological abnormalities, including pronounced hypotonia, epileptic seizures and severe psychomotor retardation; ocular abnormalities; and liver involvement. They die before the end of the first year. The brain shows micropolygyria. The most characteristic neuropathological abnormality is an impaired neuronal migration and severe demyelination.

Neonatal adrenoleukodystrophy. The first described patient with this disorder showed central demyelination and adrenal atrophy, hence the denomination, together with abnormalities similar to those seen in ZS, although milder. Today, NALD is considered as a less severe form of ZS.

Infantile Refsum's disease. IRD patients show no distinct abnormalities in the neonatal period and only minor dysmorphia. The main clinical features are mental retardation, retinitis pigmentosa, neurosensory deafness and growth retardation. Several reported patients were still alive in their late teens.

Rhizomelic   chondrodysplasia   punctata (RCDP). The characteristic clinical features of this disorder are rhizomelia: severe symmetrical shortening of upper extremities, profound growth failure, flexion contractures, cataract, ichthyosis, some degree of craniofacial dysmorphism, variable neurological signs and widespread epiphyseal calcifications. Biochemical peroxisomal abnormalities consist of a severe deficiency of plasmalogens, with combined deficiency of dihydroxyacetone-phosphate acyltransferase (DHAP-AT) and alkyl-DHAP synthetase. Deficient α-oxidation of phytanic acid is also present [27]. In spite of a defective import of peroxisomal thiolase, peroxisomal β oxidation does not seem to be compromised, as evidenced by normal plasma VLCFA. Peroxisomes are present but abnormal. Classic RCDP patients have been shown to belong to a common comple-

mentation group, CG11.

In disorders of peroxisomal biogenesis, an apparent lack of abnormal appearance of peroxisomes and mislocalization of several peroxisomal matrix proteins suggest a problem of protein import as the primary lesion. Considerable progress has been achieved in this field. Peroxisomal targeting signals, either C-terminal (PTS1, for most proteins) or N-terminal (PTS2, for thiolase and other yet unknown proteins) have been discovered and proteins involved in peroxisomal import, biogenesis, proliferation and inheritance isolated. The concerted action of such peroxisomal assembly proteins, peroxins, has been shown to govern import of matrix proteins into peroxisomes, and many of the corresponding *PEX* genes have been cloned, at least in yeast [29]. To date, defects in at least five *PEX* genes have been shown to cause human peroxisomal disorders. Mutations in *PEX5*, which encodes the PTS1 receptor, *PEX2* and *PEX12*, which encode two zinc-binding integral membrane proteins; and *PEX6*, which encodes vesicle-associated cytosolic ATPase, cause a Zellweger spectrum phenotype, while mutated *PEX7*, which encodes the PTS2 receptor, is associated with a RCDP phenotype (Table 41-5).

Disorders of the peroxisomal β-oxidation pathway result in a loss of peroxisomal function

A number of patients with clinical features mimicking those of the Zellweger spectrum but showing only an accumulation of VLCFA and possibly some abnormalities of bile acid intermediates have also been reported under the descriptive names of "pseudo-neonatal adrenoleukodystrophy" or "pseudo-Zellweger syndrome" [26]. Detailed investigations of the peroxisomal β-oxidation pathway revealed a single loss of peroxisomal function in these patients, either an acyl-CoA oxidase deficiency (pseudo-NALD), bifunctional enzyme deficiency or thiolase deficiency (pseudo-ZS).

X-Linked adrenoleukodystrophy (ALD) and adrenomyeloneuropathy (AMN). The name adrenoleukodystrophy was coined based on the features of a progressive genetic demyelinating disease associated with adrenal insufficiency manifesting in boys aged 5 to 13 years. This X-linked recessive disease, with an estimated frequency of 1/20,000 men, presents in a variety of phenotypes [24]. Different phenotypes are commonly observed in the same family or the same kindred. In the most severe late infantile or juvenile cerebral form, which has a mean age of onset of about 7 years and constitutes 40 to 50% of the cases, neurological symptoms predominate. Initial behavioral and school problems are followed by gait disturbances, visual and hearing impairment, varying alterations of cognitive functions with progressive dementia and a devastating downhill course toward an apparent vegetative state in 3 to 5 years. Adrenal insufficiency can be demonstrated in 90% of cases. Most patients die in adolescence. Severe and confluent demyelinating lesions involving the parieto-occipital region are observed most characteristically, but magnetic resonance imaging (MRI) studies have shown other topographic localizations, especially at an early stage of the disease. Correlations between the initial localization of demyelinating lesions and progression of the disease have been reported. A rare adult-onset cerebral form has been described. The second most frequent clinical variant, AMN, which accounts for 30 to 40% of cases, occurs in older individuals, with a mean age of onset of about 27 years. This form involves predominantly the spinal cord and peripheral nerves with the main clinical symptoms of spastic paraplegia and adrenal insufficiency, and the disease progresses slowly over decades. Some degree of cerebral involvement may occur in one-third to one-half of patients, as judged by brain MRI and cognitive functions. Approximately 10% of patients present only with symptoms characteristic of Addison's disease for a long time. A significant proportion of female carriers show varying degrees of clinical signs of the disease.

The most prominent biochemical finding is increased concentrations of VLCFA ($>C_{22}$) in the brain, adrenal, plasma, red cells and cultured fibroblasts. These fatty acids are present mostly in the forms of cholesterol esters, cerebrosides, gangliosides and sphingomyelin. There are no indications of other peroxisomal dysfunctions. The biochemical pathogenesis that leads to the massive demyelination is unclear because, even though the relative increase is large, the net concentrations of VLCFA in the tissue remain very low. Accumulation of VLCFA appears to be due to impaired activation of VLCFA-CoA, a reaction catalyzed by the peroxisomal enzyme VLCFA-CoA synthase. The gene responsible for X-linked ALD has been cloned and shown to be an ABC transporter protein (Chap. 5) [30]. To date, the substrate transported by the ALD protein and the relationship between its transport function and VLCFA-CoA synthase activation are unknown. Elucidation of its precise physiological function should provide insight into the pathogenetic mechanism of this disorder. More than 150 disease-causing mutations have been described. Interestingly, many of them, including 60% of mis-sense mutations, lead to undetectable levels of ALD protein by either Western blot or immunofluorescence [24]. A murine model has been generated [31].

Adult Refsum's disease. The classic form of Refsum's disease occurs in adults of both sexes, with hypertrophic polyneuropathy as the most prominent manifestation [25]. There is an abnormal elevation of a methylated fatty acid, phytanic acid, which is exogenously derived from chlorophyll in the food. There is no indication of other peroxisomal dysfunction. Peroxisomes appear morphologically normal in size and number. Since phytanic acid is exclusively exogenous in origin, chlorophyll-free dietary treatment can be quite effective in alleviating the disease. As indicated above, the so-called infantile Refsum's disease is genetically distinct from the classic adult Refsum's disease.

UPDATE ADDED IN PROOF

Neuronal ceroid lipofuscinosis. Abnormalities in lysosome-localized proteins/enzymes have recently been demonstrated as the causes for three members of an important group of neurogenetic disorders, collectively known as *neuronal ceroid lipofuscinosis* [32,33]. Defective palmitoyl protein thioesterase, the product of the CLN1 gene and an enzyme that deacylates S-acylated protein [34] underlies the infantile form of the disease prevalent in the Finnish population. This enzyme is targeted to lysosomes [35]. Utilizing mannose 6-phosphate modification of lysosomal proteins as a marker, the protein absent in the most common late infantile form of the disease, encoded by CLN2, has been identified as a pepstatin-insensitive peptidase [36]. Furthermore, the product of the positionally cloned CLN3 gene responsible for the juvenile form [37] has recently been localized to lysosomes by confocal immunofluorescence studies with appropriate markers [38]. These developments suggest that the entire group of neuronal ceroid lipofuscinosis may be lysosomal disorders.

Peroxisomal disease. Abnormalities in the PEX1 gene have been shown to be the cause for the most common complementation group 1 (CG1) of the Zellweger syndrome spectrum among the peroxisomal disease (Table 41-5) [39,40].

REFERENCES

1. Scriver, C. R., Beaudet, A. L., Sly, W. S., and Valle, D. (eds.) *The Metabolic and Molecular Basis of Inherited Disease*, 7th ed. New York: McGraw-Hill, 1995.
2. Hers, H. G. Inborn lysosomal disease. *Gastroenterology* 48:625–633, 1966.
3. Moser, H. W. Peroxisomal diseases. *Adv. Hum. Genet.* 21:1–106, 1993.
4. Suzuki, K. Enzymatic diagnosis of sphingolipidoses. *Methods Enzymol.* 138:727–762, 1987.
5. Suzuki, K., and Vanier, M. T. Lysosomal disorders. In B. Popko (ed.), *Mouse Models of Human Genetic Neurological Disease.* New York: Plenum Press, 1998, in press.
6. Vanier, M. T., and Suzuki, K. Niemann-Pick diseases. In H. W. Moser (ed.), *Neurodystrophies and Neurolipidoses.* Amsterdam: Elsevier, 1996, pp. 133–162.
7. Pentchev, P. G., Vanier, M. T., and Suzuki, K. Niemann-Pick disease type C: A cellular cholesterol lipidosis. In C. R. Scriver, A. L. Beaudet, W. S. Sly, and D. Valle (eds.), *The Metabolic and Molecular Basis of Inherited Disease*, 7th ed. New York: McGraw-Hill, 1995, pp. 2625–2639.
8. Pentchev, P. G., Comly, M. E., Kruth, H. S., et al. A defect in cholesterol esterification in Niemann-Pick disease (type C) patients. *Proc. Natl. Acad. Sci. USA* 82:8247–8251, 1985.
9. Vanier, M. T., Duthel, S., Rodriguez-Lafrasse, C., Pentchev, P., and Carstea, E. D. Genetic heterogeneity in Niemann-Pick C disease: A study using somatic cell hybridization and linkage analysis. *Am. J. Hum. Genet.* 58:118–125, 1996.
10. Carstea, E. D., Morris, J. A., Coleman, K. G. et al. Niemann-Pick C1 disease gene: Homology to mediators of cholesterol homeostasis. *Science* 277:228–231, 1997.
11. Miyatake, T., and Suzuki, K. Globoid cell leukodystrophy: Additional deficiency of psychosine galactosidase. *Biochem. Biophys. Res. Commun.* 48:538–543, 1972.
12. Svennerholm, L., Vanier, M.-T., and Månsson, J.-E. Krabbe disease: A galactosylsphingosine (psychosine) lipidosis. *J. Lipid Res.* 21:53–64, 1980.
13. Schmidt, B., Selmer, T., Ingendoh, A., and von Figura, K. A novel amino acid modification in sulfatases that is defective in multiple sulfatase deficiency. *Cell* 82:271–278, 1995.
14. Myerowitz, R., Piekarz, R., Neufeld, E. F., Shows, T. B., and Suzuki, K. Human β-hexosaminidase α chain: Coding sequence and homology with the β chain. *Proc. Natl. Acad. Sci. USA* 82:7830–7834, 1985.
15. Ohno, K., and Suzuki, K. Mutation in GM2-gangliosidosis B1 variant. *J. Neurochem.* 50:316–318, 1988.
16. Fujita, N., Suzuki, K., Vanier, M. T., et al. Targeted disruption of the mouse sphingolipid activator protein gene: A complex phenotype, including severe leukodystrophy and wide-spread storage of multiple sphingolipids. *Hum. Mol. Genet.* 5:711–725, 1996.
17. Sly, W. S., Quinton, B. A., McAlster, W. H., and Rimoin, D. L. β-Glucuronidase deficiency: Report of clinical, radiologic, and biochemical features of a new mucopolysaccharidosis. *J. Pediatr.* 82:249–257, 1973.
18. Catterall, J. F., and Leary, S. L. Detection of early changes in androgen-induced mouse renal β-glucuronidase messenger ribonucleic acid using cloned complementary deoxyribonucleic acid. *Biochemistry* 22:6049–6053, 1983.
19. Krivit, W., Shapiro, E. G., Lockman, L. A., et al. Bone marrow transplantation treatment for globoid cell leukodystrophy, metachromatic leukodystrophy, adrenoleukodystrophy and Hurler syndrome. In H. W. Moser (ed.), *Neurodystrophies and Neurolipidoses.* Amsterdam: Elsevier, 1996, pp. 87–106.
20. Bonten, E., Van der Spoel, A., Fornerod, M., Grosveld, G., and d'Azzo, A. Characterization of human lysosomal neuraminidase defines the

molecular basis of the metabolic storage disorder sialidosis. *Genes Dev.* 10:3156–3169, 1996.

21. Pshezhetsky, A. V., Richard, C., Michaud, L., et al. Cloning, expression and chromosomal mapping of human lysosomal sialidase and characterization of mutations in sialidosis. *Nat. Genet.* 15:316–320, 1997.

22. Wenger, D. A., Sujansky, E., Fennessey, P. V., and Thompson, J. N. Human beta-mannosidase deficiency. *N. Engl. J. Med.* 315:1201–1205, 1986.

23. d'Azzo, A., Hoogeveen, A., Reuser, A. J. J., Robinson, D., and Galjaard, H. Molecular defect in combined beta-galactosidase and neuraminidase deficiency in man. *Proc. Natl. Acad. Sci. USA* 79:4535–4539, 1982.

24. Aubourg, P. X-Linked adrenoleukodystrophy. In H. W. Moser (ed.), *Neurodystrophies and Neurolipidoses.* Amsterdam: Elsevier, 1996, pp. 447–483.

25. Skjeldal, O. H. Heredopathia atactica polyneuritoformis (Refsum's disease). In H. W. Moser (ed.), *Neurodystrophies and Neurolipidoses.* Amsterdam: Elsevier, 1996, pp. 485–503.

26. Wanders, R. J. A., Heymans, H. S. A., Schutgens, R. B. H., and Barth, P. G. Generalized peroxisomal disorders and disorders of peroxisomal fatty acid oxidation. In H. W. Moser (ed.), *Neurodystrophies and Neurolipidoses.* Amsterdam: Elsevier, 1996, pp. 505–524.

27. Heymans, H. S. A., and Wanders, R. J. A. Rhizomelic chondrodysplasia punctata. In H. W. Moser (ed.), *Neurodystrophies and Neurolipidoses.* Amsterdam: Elsevier, 1996, pp. 525–533.

28. Braverman, N., Steel, G., Obie, C., et al. Human *PEX7* encodes the peroxisomal PTS2 receptor and is responsible for rhizomelic chondrodysplasia punctata. *Nat. Genet.* 15:369–376, 1997.

29. Subramani, S. PEX genes on the rise. *Nat. Genet.* 15:331–333, 1997.

30. Mosser, J., Douar, A.-M., Sarde, C.-O., et al. Putative X-linked adrenoleukodystrophy gene shares unexpected homology with ABC transporters. *Nature* 361:726–730, 1993.

31. Kobayashi, T., Shinnoh, N., Kondo, A., and Yamada, T. Adrenoleukodystrophy protein-deficient mice represent abnormality of very long chain fatty acid metabolism. *Biochem. Biophys. Res. Commun.* 232:631–636, 1997.

32. Goebel, H. H. and Sharp, J. D. The neuronal ceroid-lipofuscinosis. Recent advances. *Brain Pathology* 8:151–162, 1998.

33. Boustany, R. M. Batten disease or neuronal ceroid lipofuscinosis. In H. W. Moser, editor. Neurodystrophies and neurolipidses. Amsterdam: Elsevier, 1996, pp. 671–700.

34. Vesa, J., Hellsten, E., Verkruyse, L. A., et al. Mutations in the palmitoyl protein thioesterase gene causing infantile neuronal ceroid lipofuscinosis. *Nature* 376:584–587, 1995.

35. Hellsten, E., Vesa, J., Olkkonen, V. M., Jalanko, A., and Peltonen, L. Human palmitoyl protein thioesterase: Evidence for lysosomal targeting of the enzyme and disturbed cellular routing in infantile neuronal ceroid lipofuscinosis. *EMBO J.* 15:5240–5245, 1996.

36. Sleat, D. E., Donnelly, R. J., Lackland, H., et al. Association of mutations in a lysosomal protein with classical late-infantile neuronal ceroid lipofuscinosis. *Science* 277:1802–1805, 1997.

37. International Batten Disease Consortium. Isolation of a novel gene underlying Batten Disease, CLN3. *Cell* 82:949–957, 1995.

38. Jarvela, I. E., Sainio, M., Rantamäki, T., et al. Biosynthesis and subcellular localization of the CLN3 protein defective in Batten disease. *J. Am. Soc. Hum. Genet.* 61:A253, Abst. 1469, 1997.

39. Reuber, B. E., Germain-Lee, E., Collins, C. S., et al. Mutations in *PEX1* are the most common cause of peroxisome biogenesis disorders. *Nat. Genet.* 17:445–448, 1997.

40. Portsteffen, H., Beyer, A., Becker, E., Epplen, C., Pawlak, A., Kunau, W.-H., and Dodt, G. Human *PEX1* is mutated in complementation group 1 of the peroxisome biogenesis disorders. *Nat. Genet.* 17:449–452, 1997.

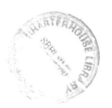

42

Diseases of Carbohydrate, Fatty Acid and Mitochondrial Metabolism

Salvatore diMauro and Darryl C. De Vivo

Basic Neurochemistry: Molecular, Cellular and Medical Aspects, 6th Ed., edited by G. J. Siegel et al. Published by Lippincott–Raven Publishers, Philadelphia, 1999. Correspondence to Salvatore diMauro, Department of Neurology, College of Physicians and Surgeons, Columbia University, New York, New York 10032.

Defects of energy metabolism cause profound disturbances in the function of muscle and brain. Such defects may present as a myopathy, encephalopathy or encephalomyopathy. Clinical features are best appreciated by understanding the preferred oxidizable substrates for brain and muscle.

Muscle in the resting state predominantly utilizes fatty acids. The immediate source of energy for muscle contraction is ATP, which is rapidly replenished at the expense of creatine phosphate by the phosphorylation of ADP by creatine kinase. During exercise of moderate intensity, the fuel choice depends on the duration of work. Initially, glycogen is the main fuel source; after 5 or 10 min, blood glucose becomes the more important fuel. As work continues, fatty acid utilization increases, and after approximately 4 hr, lipids are the primary source of energy. During high-intensity exercise, at near-maximal power, additional ATP is generated by the anaerobic breakdown of glycogen and by glycolysis. Intense exercise is performed in essentially anaerobic conditions, whereas mild or moderate exercise is accompanied by increased blood flow to exercising muscles, facilitating substrate delivery and favoring aerobic metabolism. This adaption is known as the "second-wind" phenomenon [1].

Brain utilizes glucose predominantly, with regional variations of the metabolic rate depending on the mental or motor task being performed [1]. As with muscle, the immediate intracellular energy source is ATP, buttressed by the creatine phosphate stores. Glycogen provides very little energy reserve because brain concentrations of glycogen are extremely low, approximately only one-tenth the amount found in muscle per gram wet weight. Therefore, brain is exquisitely sensitive to fluctuations in the blood glucose concentration. Movement of glucose across the blood–brain barrier is facilitated by a carrier protein, the glucose transporter (GLUT-1) [2]. The facilitated transport of glucose ensures adequate brain glucose concentrations to meet the needs of cerebral metabolism under normal conditions. During starvation, the brain uses little, if any, fatty acids. However, fatty acids of varying chain lengths may be taken up by brain, as the efficiency of transport across the blood–brain barrier is much greater for short- or medium-chain fatty acids than for long-chain fatty acids. Ketone bodies represent the preferred cerebral fuel source during starvation when glucose supply is limited [3] (see Chap. 31). Defective fatty acid oxidation, therefore, may affect muscle directly by blocking oxidation of this substrate and brain indirectly by limiting hepatic ketogenesis. Elevated circulating free fatty acids may also have a direct toxic effect on brain, but the precise mechanisms for this effect are poorly understood (see Chaps. 35 and 38).

Energy metabolism has been studied extensively in skeletal muscle, and several metabolic disorders have been documented [1,4]. Comparatively less is known about metabolic defects in cerebral energy metabolism. This may be because muscle tissue is more accessible for biochemical analysis and because certain cerebral enzyme defects are lethal.

DISEASES OF CARBOHYDRATE AND FATTY ACID METABOLISM IN MUSCLE

One class of glycogen or lipid metabolic disorders in muscle is manifest as acute, recurrent, reversible dysfunction

These disorders occur with exercise intolerance and myoglobinuria, with or without cramps. Among the glyogenoses, this is characteristic of deficiencies in phosphorylase, phosphofructokinase (PFK), aldolase, phosphoglycerate kinase (PGK), phosphoglycerate mutase (PGM) and lactate dehydrogenase (LDH). Among the disorders of lipid metabolism, this is characteristic of deficiencies in very-long-chain acyl-CoA dehydrogenase (VLCAD), trifunctional protein (TP), carnitine palmitoyltransferase II (CPT II) and short-chain 3-hydroxyacyl-CoA dehydrogenase (SCHAD). Figures 42-1 and 42-2 schematically illustrate the pathways of glycogen and fatty acid metabolism.

Phosphorylase deficiency (McArdle's disease, glycogenosis type V) is an autosomal recessive myopathy caused by a genetic defect of the mus-

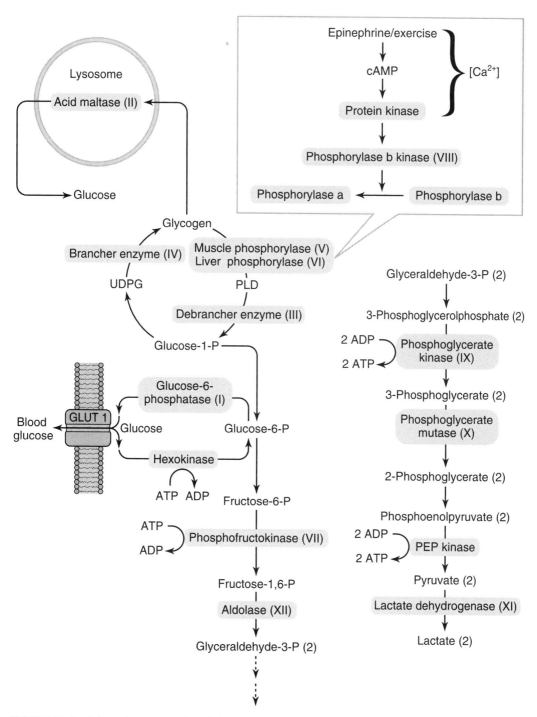

FIGURE 42-1. Schematic representation of glycogen metabolism and glycolysis. *Roman numerals* indicate the sites of identified enzyme defects: *I,* glucose-6-phosphatase; *II,* acid maltase; *III,* debrancher enzyme; *IV,* brancher enzyme; *V,* muscle phosphorylase; *VI,* liver phosphorylase; *VII,* phosphofructokinase; *VIII,* phosphorylase kinase; *IX,* phospho-glycerate kinase; *X,* phosphoglycerate mutase; *XI,* lactate dehydrogenase; *XII,* aldolase. *GLUT 1,* glucose transporter; *PLD,* phosphorylase-limit dextrin; *PEP,* phosphoenolpyruvate; *P,* phosphate; *UDPG,* uridine diphosphate glucose.

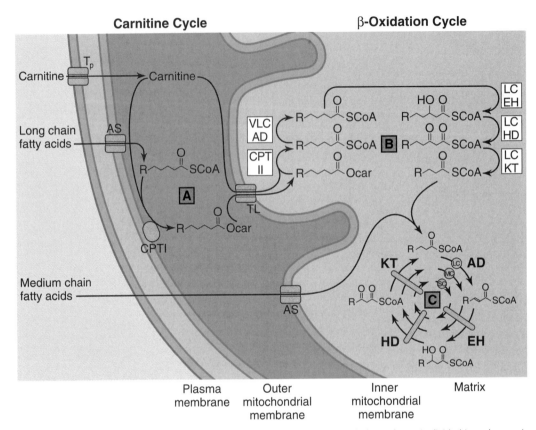

FIGURE 42-2. Schematic representation of fatty acid oxidation. This metabolic pathway is divided into the carnitine cycle [A], the inner mitochondrial membrane system [B], and the mitochondrial matrix system [C]. The carnitine cycle includes the plasma membrane transporter, carnitine palmitoyltransferase I (*CPT I*). The reactions shown in [B] occur in the inner mitochondrial membrane. The carnitine–acylcarnitine translocase system and carnitine palmitoyltransferase II (*CPT II*). The inner mitochondrial membrane system includes the very-long-chain acyl-CoA dehydrogenase (*VLCAD*) and the trifunctional protein with three catalytically active sites. Long-chain acylcarnitines enter the mitochondrial matrix by the action of CPT II to yield long-chain acyl-CoAs. These thioesters undergo one or more cycles of chain shortening catalyzed by the membrane-bound system. Chain-shortened acyl-CoAs are degraded further by the matrix β-oxidation system. Medium-chain fatty acids enter the mitochondrial matrix directly and are activated to the medium-chain acyl-CoAs before degradation by the matrix β-oxidation system. *Tp,* carnitine transporter; *TL,* carnitine-acylcarnitine translocase; *LC,* long chain; *EH,* 2-enoyl-CoA hydratase; *CoA,* coenzyme A; *VLC,* very long chain; *AD,* acyl-CoA dehydrogenase; *AS,* arginosuccinate; *HD,* 3-hydroxyacyl-CoA dehydrogenase; *CPT,* carnitine palmitoyltransferase; *KT,* 3-ketoacyl-CoA thiolase; *MC,* medium chain; *SC,* short chain; (From [6], with permission.)

cle isoenzyme of glycogen phosphorylase (Fig. 42-1). Intolerance of strenuous exercise is present from childhood, but usually onset is in adolescence, with cramps after exercise [1,5]. Myoglobinuria occurs in about one-half of patients. If they avoid intense exercise, most patients can live normal lives; however, about one-third of them develop some degree of fixed weakness, usually as a late-onset manifestation of the disease. In a few patients, weakness rather than exercise-related cramps and myoglobinuria characterizes the clinical picture.

In patients with myoglobinuria, renal insufficiency is a possible life-threatening complication. Physical examination between episodes of myoglobinuria may be completely normal or show some degree of weakness and, occasionally, wasting of some muscle groups.

Even between episodes, most patients have increased serum creatine kinase (CK); forearm ischemic exercise causes no rise of venous lactate concentration. This is a useful but nonspecific test in McArdle's disease. The electromyogram (EMG) at rest shows nonspecific myopathic features in about one-half of patients.

Muscle biopsy demonstrates subsarcolemmal blebs that contain periodic acid-Schiff (PAS)-positive material, a marker for glycogen. The histochemical stain for phosphorylase is negative, except in regenerating fibers. Biochemical documentation of the enzyme defect requires muscle biopsy because the defect is not expressed in more easily accessible tissues, such as leukocytes, erythrocytes and cultured fibroblasts. The gene encoding muscle phosphorylase has been assigned to chromosome 11, and a dozen distinct mutations have been identified in patients [5]. By far the most common among these is a nonsense mutation in codon 49 *(mut-49)*. This allows diagnosis of 90% of patients through molecular analysis of genomic DNA isolated from blood, thus making muscle biopsy unnecessary in most cases [5].

Phosphofructokinase deficiency (Tarui's disease, glycogenosis type VII) is an autosomal recessive myopathy caused by a genetic defect of the muscle (M) subunit of the rate-limiting enzyme of glycolysis, PFK (Fig. 42-1). Presenting symptoms are cramps after intense exercise, followed by myoglobinuria in some patients. A few patients may have mild jaundice, reflecting excessive hemolysis, or typical symptoms and signs of gout. In patients with typical presentation, fixed weakness appears to be less common than in phosphorylase deficiency. However, in PFK deficiency, as in phosphorylase deficiency, a few patients have only weakness, without cramps or myoglobinuria. In addition to renal insufficiency due to myoglobinuria, other possible complications include renal colic due to urate stones and gouty arthritis [1].

Physical examination may show slight jaundice. Neurological examination is normal. Serum CK is variably increased in most patients. Forearm ischemic exercise causes no rise of venous lactate concentration. Serum bilirubin is elevated in most patients, and the number of reticulocytes is increased. Serum uric acid is also increased in most patients. The EMG is usually normal. Muscle biopsy shows focal, mostly subsarcolemmal, accumulation of glycogen. In some patients, a small portion of the glycogen is

abnormal. By histochemical analysis, it is shown to be diastase-resistant; by electron microscopy, it appears finely granular and filamentous in structure. The enzyme defect can be demonstrated by a specific histochemical reaction for PFK. Although a partial defect of PFK activity is manifest in erythrocytes from patients, firm diagnosis usually requires biochemical studies of muscle. The gene encoding PFK-M is on chromosome 1, and several mutations have been identified in patients of different ethnic origins. Recognition of a specific mutation in genomic DNA from blood cells can eliminate the need for a muscle biopsy in suspected PFK-deficient patients [1].

The first patient with muscle aldolase deficiency was identified in 1996: this young boy suffered from a hemolytic trait but also complained of exercise intolerance and experienced several episodes of myoglobinuria during febrile illnesses [1].

Phosphoglycerate kinase deficiency is an X-linked recessive disease (type IX, Fig. 42-1). The most common clinical presentation includes hemolytic anemia with or without CNS involvement (see below). Thus far, only three patients have been described with a purely myopathic syndrome, characterized by exercise-induced cramps and myoglobinuria. Between episodes of myoglobinuria, physical and neurological examinations were normal. Forearm ischemic exercise caused contracture and no rise of venous lactate concentration.

Because the enzyme defect is expressed in all tissues except sperm, diagnosis can be made by biochemical studies of muscle, erythrocytes, leukocytes and cultured fibroblasts. Two distinct mutations have been identified in patients with myopathy [1].

Phosphoglycerate mutase deficiency is an autosomal recessive myopathy caused by a genetic defect of the muscle subunit of the enzyme PGM (type X, Fig. 42-1). Ten patients with this enzyme deficiency have been identified thus far.

The clinical picture includes cramps and recurrent myoglobinuria following intense exercise. Aside from episodes of myoglobinuria, none of the patients was weak. Forearm ischemic exercise caused a 1.5- to 2.0-fold increase in venous lactate concentration, an abnormally low but not absent response. Muscle biopsy showed normal or only moderately increased glycogen concentration. Because other accessible tissues, such as erythrocytes, leukocytes and cultured fibroblasts, express a different isoenzyme, the diagnosis of PGM-M subunit deficiency must be established by biochemical studies of muscle. Three different mutations have been identified in the PGM-M gene, which is located on chromosome 7 [1].

Lactate dehydrogenase deficiency is an autosomal recessive myopathy caused by a genetic defect of the muscle subunit, which is encoded by a gene on chromosome 11 (type XI, Fig. 42-1). Thus far, six Japanese families and three Caucasian patients with this disease have been described. The clinical picture is characterized by cramps and myoglobinuria after intense exercise.

Forearm ischemic exercise showed a subnormal rise of lactate concentration, contrasting with an increased rise of pyruvate. The diagnosis can be established by electrophoretic studies of LDH in serum, erythrocytes and leukocytes, showing lack of subunit M-containing isoenzymes. Nevertheless, it should be confirmed by biochemical studies of muscle or by molecular analysis of genomic DNA as five different mutations have been documented in patients [1].

Carnitine palmitoyltransferase deficiency is an autosomal recessive myopathy caused by a genetic defect of the mitochondrial enzyme CPT (Fig. 42-2). The disease is prevalent in men (male:female ratio, 5.5:1) and appears to be the most common cause of recurrent myoglobinuria in adults [4].

Clinical manifestations are limited to attacks of myoglobinuria, not preceded by contractures and usually precipitated by prolonged exercise, of several hours duration; prolonged fasting; or a combination of the two conditions. Less common precipitating factors include intercurrent infection, emotional stress and cold exposure, but some episodes of myoglobinuria occur without any apparent cause. Most patients have two or more attacks, probably because the lack of muscle cramps deprives them of a warning signal of impending myoglobinuria.

For unknown reasons, some women seem to have milder symptoms, such as myalgia, after prolonged exercise, without pigmenturia. This has been observed in sisters of men with recurrent myoglobinuria. The only serious complication is renal failure following myoglobinuria.

Physical and neurological examinations are completely normal. Prolonged fasting at rest, which should be conducted under close medical observation, causes a sharp rise of serum CK in about one-half of patients. Also, in about one-half of patients, ketone bodies fail to increase normally after prolonged fasting. Forearm ischemic exercise causes a normal increase of venous lactate concentration. Aside from episodes of myoglobinuria, the serum CK concentration and EMG are normal. A muscle biopsy specimen may appear completely normal or show variable, but usually moderate, accumulation of lipid droplets. Most patients with CPT deficiency benefit from a high-carbohydrate, low-fat diet, and the therapeutic response may serve as an indirect diagnostic clue. Because the enzyme defect appears to be generalized, tissues other than muscle, such as mixed leukocytes or isolated lymphocytes or platelets, can be used to demonstrate CPT deficiency; but the diagnosis should be confirmed in muscle.

The myopathic form of CPT deficiency is due to a defect of CPT II. The gene for CPT II has been localized to chromosome 1, and several mutations have been identified in patients [4]. As in the case of McArdle's disease (see above), one mutation, a serine-to-leucine substitution at codon 113, is far more common than the others and can be screened for in genomic DNA from blood cells, thus potentially avoiding muscle biopsy.

Very-long-chain acyl-CoA dehydrogenase and trifunctional protein are the two inner membrane-bound enzymes of fatty acid β-oxidation. Genetic defects of either can mimic the clinical presentation of CPT II deficiency by causing recurrent myoglobinuria in otherwise apparently healthy young adults. As in CPT II deficiency, precipitating factors include prolonged exercise, prolonged fasting, cold exposure, intercurrent illnesses or emotional stress [4].

Short-chain 3-hydroxyacyl-CoA dehydrogenase deficiency has been described in three patients. It is associated with additional defects of β-oxidation, which have been associated with limb weakness and attacks of myoglobinuria, and it is potentially fatal.

A second class of disorders of glucose and fatty acid metabolism causes progressive weakness

These disorders are associated with acid maltase, debrancher enzyme and brancher enzyme deficiencies among the glycogenoses. These are also associated with carnitine deficiency, some defects of β oxidation and other biochemically undefined lipid-storage myopathies among the disorders of lipid metabolism. Figures 42-1 and 42-2 schematically illustrate the pathways of glycogen and fatty acid metabolism.

Acid maltase deficiency (AMD) (glycogenosis type II) is an autosomal recessive disease caused by a genetic defect of the lysosomal enzyme acid maltase, an α-1,4- and α-1,6-glucosidase capable of digesting glycogen completely to glucose (Fig. 42-1). Two major clinical syndromes are caused by AMD. The first is Pompe's disease, which is a severe, generalized and invariably fatal disease of infancy; the second is a less severe neuromuscular disorder beginning in childhood or in adult life (see Chap. 41).

Infantile, generalized cardiomegalic AMD, or *Pompe's disease,* usually becomes manifest in the first weeks or months of life, with failure to thrive, poor suck, generalized hypotonia and weakness, also termed floppy infant syndrome. Macroglossia is common, as is hepatomegaly, which, however, is rarely severe. There is massive cardiomegaly, with congestive heart failure. Weak respiratory muscles make these infants susceptible to pulmonary infection; death usually occurs before the age of 1 year and invariably before the age of 2 years [1].

The *childhood- and adult-onset forms of AMD* cause signs and symptoms that are limited to the musculature, with progressive weakness of truncal muscles and of proximal, more than distal, limb muscles, usually sparing facial and extraocular muscles. In the childhood form, onset is in infancy or childhood and progression tends to be rapid. In the adult form, onset usually is in the third or fourth decade but occasionally even later and the course is slower [1].

The clinical picture in male children can closely resemble Duchenne-type muscular dystrophy; in adults, it mimics limb-girdle dystrophy or polymyositis. The early and severe involvement of respiratory muscles in most patients with AMD is a distinctive clinical clue. Respiratory failure and pulmonary infection are the most common causes of death.

Serum CK is consistently increased in all forms of AMD. Forearm ischemic exercise causes a normal rise of venous lactate concentration in patients with childhood or adult AMD. The electrocardiogram (ECG) is altered in Pompe's disease, with a short P-R interval, giant QRS complexes and left ventricular or biventricular hypertrophy, but is usually normal in the later-onset forms. The EMG shows myopathic features and fibrillation potentials, bizarre high-frequency discharges and myotonic discharges.

Muscle biopsy shows vacuolar myopathy of very severe degree affecting all fibers in Pompe's disease but of varying degree and distribution in childhood and adult AMD. In adult AMD, biopsy specimens from unaffected muscles may appear normal by light microscopy. The vacuoles contain PAS-positive material, a marker for glycogen. Electron microscopy shows abundant glycogen, both within membranous sacs, presumably lysosomes, and free in the cytoplasm.

The enzyme defect is expressed in all tissues, and the diagnosis can be made by biochemical analysis of urine, lymphocytes (mixed leukocytes do not give reliable results) or cultured skin fibroblasts. Fibroblasts cultured from amniotic fluid can be used for prenatal diagnosis of Pompe's disease. The gene encoding acid maltase is on chromosome 17, and numerous mutations have been identified in patients with both forms of AMD, confirming that infantile and late-onset AMD are allelic disorders. Predictably, more severe mutations are associated with Pompe's disease; however, many patients are compound heterozygotes, and there is no strict genotype/phenotype correlation [1].

Debrancher enzyme deficiency (glycogenosis type III, Cori's disease, Forbe's disease) is an autosomal recessive disease (Fig. 42-1). In its more common presentation, debrancher enzyme deficiency causes liver dysfunction in childhood, with hepatomegaly, growth retardation, fasting hypoglycemia and seizures [1]. Myopathy has been described in about 20 patients [1]. In most, onset of weakness was in the third or fourth decade. Wasting of distal leg muscles and intrinsic hand muscles is common, and the association of late-onset weakness and distal wasting often suggests the diagnosis of motor neuron disease or peripheral neuropathy. The course is slowly progressive. In a smaller number of patients, onset of weakness is in childhood, with diffuse weakness and wasting. The association of hepatomegaly and growth retardation facilitates the diagnosis.

There is no glycemic response to glucagon or epinephrine (Fig. 42-1), whereas a galactose load causes a normal glycemic response. Forearm ischemic exercise produces a blunted venous lactate rise or no response. Serum CK activity is variably, often markedly, increased. The ECG shows left ventricular or biventricular hypertrophy in most patients, and the EMG may show myopathic features alone or associated with fibrillations, positive sharp waves and myotonic discharges. This "mixed" EMG pattern in patients with weakness and distal wasting often reinforces the erroneous diagnosis of motoneuron disease. Motor nerve conduction velocities are moderately decreased in one-fourth of patients, suggesting a polyneuropathy.

Muscle biopsy shows severe vacuolar myopathy with glycogen storage. On electron microscopy, the vacuoles correspond to pools of glycogen free in the cytoplasm.

In most patients, the enzyme defect is generalized, and it has been demonstrated in erythrocytes, leukocytes and cultured fibroblasts. In patients with myopathy, the diagnosis is securely established by measurement of debrancher enzyme activity in muscle biopsy specimens or by studies of iodine adsorption spectra of glycogen isolated from muscle; there is a shift in the spectrum toward lower wavelengths, indicating that the polysaccharide has abnormally short peripheral branches. The gene for the debrancher enzyme has been assigned to chromosome 1, and the first mutations have been identified in patients [1].

Branching enzyme deficiency (glycogenosis type IV; Andersen's disease) is an autosomal recessive disease of infancy or early childhood, typically causing liver dysfunction with hepatosplenomegaly, progressive cirrhosis and chronic hepatic failure (Fig. 42-1). Death usually occurs in childhood. Although muscle wasting and hypotonia are mentioned in several reports, only three patients have had severe hypotonia, wasting, contractures and hyporeflexia, suggesting the diagnosis of spinal muscular atrophy [1].

There are no diagnostic laboratory tests. A muscle biopsy specimen may be normal or show focal accumulations of abnormal glycogen, which is intensely PAS-positive and partially resistant to diastase digestion. With the electron microscope, the abnormal glycogen is found to have a finely granular and filamentous structure. The gene that encodes the branching enzyme has recently been cloned and assigned to chromosome 3 [1].

Carnitine deficiency is a clinically useful term describing a diversity of biochemical disorders affecting fatty acid oxidation. Carnitine deficiency may be tissue-specific or generalized.

Tissue-specific carnitine deficiency has previously been termed myopathic carnitine deficiency because patients have generalized limb weakness, starting in childhood. Limb, trunk and facial musculature may be involved. The course is slowly progressive, but weakness may fluctuate in severity. Laboratory investigations show normal or near-normal serum carnitine concentrations and variably increased serum CK values. The EMG shows myopathic features with or without spontaneous activity at rest. Muscle biopsy reveals severe triglyceride storage, best seen with the oil red O stain in frozen sections. This condition is transmitted as an autosomal recessive trait. Originally, it was thought that the primary biochemical defect involved the active transport of carnitine from blood into muscle. However, no such defect has ever been documented [6]. Rather, an increasing number of patients have a tissue-specific defect involving the short-chain isoform of acyl-CoA dehydrogenase (SCAD). As such, the muscle carnitine deficiency is secondary to a primary enzyme defect.

Generalized carnitine deficiency, in its primary form and inherited as an autosomal recessive trait, is due to a defect of the specific high-affinity, low-concentration, carrier-mediated carnitine-uptake mechanism. The defect has been documented in cultured fibroblasts and muscle cultures, but the same uptake system is probably shared by heart and kidney, thus explaining the cardiomyopathy and the excessive "leakage" of carnitine into the urine. Oral L-carnitine supplementation results in dramatic improvement in cardiac function [4,6].

Systemic carnitine deficiency was first described in 1975 and is thought to represent a defect in the *de novo* biosynthesis of carnitine [4,6]. However, no such defect has been documented. Patients with systemic carnitine deficiency have a generalized decrease in the tissue and plasma concentrations of carnitine and an excessive urinary excretion of carnitine. Many of the patients originally reported to have systemic carnitine deficiency have been reinvestigated and found to have a primary enzyme defect, such as medium-chain acyl-CoA dehydrogenase deficiency (MCAD). This deficiency is the prototype of a defect in β oxidation that produces secondary carnitine deficiency. β-Oxidation defects also are associated with dicarboxylic aciduria. This finding is particularly prominent during a metabolic crisis and may be rather inconspicuous between attacks. The differential diagnosis of systemic carnitine deficiency and dicarboxylic aciduria includes other defects of β oxidation, such as deficiencies of the long-chain isoform of acyl-CoA dehydrogenase (LCAD), SCAD, electron transfer flavoprotein (ETF) and ETF oxidoreductase [4], the long- and short-chain isoforms of 3-hydroxyacyl CoA dehydrogenase (LCHAD, SCHAD), β-ketothiolase, and the newly described TP enzyme that includes the catalytic activities of enoyl hydratase, LCHAD and β-ketothiolase. Cardiac involvement is particularly prominent in conditions that involve the metabolism of long-chain fatty acids. Other genetically determined biochemical defects involving organic acid metabolism and respiratory chain function may produce secondary carnitine

deficiency. Carnitine deficiency also may result from acquired diseases, such as chronic renal failure treated by hemodialysis, renal Fanconi's syndrome, chronic hepatic disease with cirrhosis and cachexia, kwashiorkor and total parenteral nutrition in premature infants [6]. The mechanisms of carnitine depletion in these diverse conditions include excessive renal loss and excessive accumulation of acyl-CoA thioesters. These potentially toxic compounds are esterified to acylcarnitines and excreted in the urine, resulting in an excessive loss of carnitine.

The genetically determined defect of membrane carnitine transport is the only known condition that fulfills the criteria for primary carnitine deficiency [4,6,7]. This condition, like the other conditions involving the carnitine cycle, is not associated with dicarboxylic aciduria. It is transmitted as an autosomal recessive trait and produces a life-threatening cardiomyopathy in infancy or early childhood, which is effectively treated with carnitine supplementation. The untreated patient also manifests systemic features of hypotonia, failure to thrive and alterations of consciousness, including coma. Carnitine concentrations are extremely low in plasma and body tissues, and the excretion of carnitine in the urine is extremely high. The excessive urinary carnitine losses are caused by a defect in renal tubular uptake of filtered carnitine, resulting from the primary defect of the plasma membrane carnitine transporter. This condition can be documented by carnitine-uptake studies in cultured skin fibroblasts from patients. Uptake studies in parents give intermediate values, consistent with a heterozygous state.

A few patients have been described with a defect involving the carnitine–acylcarnitine translocase system, which facilitates the movement of long-chain acylcarnitine esters across the inner membrane of the mitochondrion (Fig. 42-2). These patients have extremely low carnitine concentrations and minimal dicarboxylic aciduria [4,6].

Carnitine concentrations are normal to high in patients with a primary defect of CPT I. Patients with CPT II have normal carnitine concentrations. Two clinical syndromes have emerged in relationship to CPT II. The more common syndrome, as discussed previously, involves recurrent myoglobinuria provoked by fasting or intercurrent infection and later is associated with fixed limb weakness. The less common syndrome involves infants and produces hypoketotic hypoglycemic coma with a Reye-like clinical signature. All cases thought to be recurrent Reye's syndrome should be investigated for defects involving fatty acid oxidation. Low serum carnitine concentrations and increased urinary dicarboxylic acids implicate a biochemical defect of β oxidation. Low serum carnitine concentrations and normal urinary dicarboxylic acids implicate a defect of the membrane carnitine transporter or the mitochondrial inner membrane carnitine–acylcarnitine translocase system. Normal to high serum carnitine concentrations and no dicarboxylic aciduria suggests a defect of CPT I or CPT II.

Oral administration of L-carnitine is lifesaving in patients with the genetically determined defect of the plasma membrane carnitine transporter [4,6,7]. It also is recommended as a supplement in all patients who have documented carnitine deficiency, even though clear evidence of benefit is lacking. Medium-chain triglyceride supplementation has proven beneficial in CPT I deficiency and should be beneficial also in the other defects of the carnitine cycle. Medium-chain fatty acids cross the plasma membrane and the mitochondrial membranes directly and are esterified to the thioesters in the mitochondrial matrix (Fig. 42-2). A ketonemic response to medium-chain triglycerides documents the biological integrity of β oxidation and implicates a biochemical defect of the carnitine cycle or of β oxidation involving the metabolism of the longer-chain fatty acids.

The impairment of energy production from carbohydrate, which is the common consequence of these defects, should result in similar, exercise-related signs and symptoms

Except for debrancher deficiency, this is the case [1]. Of the nine glycolytic enzyme defects described above, six affect glycogen breakdown or glycolysis: phosphorylase, debrancher, PFK, aldolase, PGK, PGM, LDH deficiencies. Patients with phosphorylase, PFK, aldolase, PGK, PGM,

or LDH deficiency have exercise intolerance manifested by premature fatigue, cramps and myoglobinuria. As predicted by the crucial role of glycogen as a fuel source, these patients are more prone to experience cramps and myoglobinuria when they engage in isometric exercise, such as lifting weights, or in intense dynamic exercise, such as walking uphill. Energy for these types of exercise derives mainly from anaerobic or aerobic glycolysis. The block of glycogen utilization leads to a shortage of pyruvate and, therefore, of acetyl CoA (Fig. 42-3), the pivotal substrate of the Krebs cycle, and to a decreased mitochondrial energy output. Moderate exercise typically causes premature fatigue and myalgia, but these symptoms usually resolve after brief rest or slowing of pace; thereafter, patients find that they can resume or continue exercise without problems. This second-wind phenomenon seems to be due to early mobilization of fatty acids and to increased blood flow to exercising muscles.

Conversely, patients with fatty-acid oxidation defects experience myalgia and myoglobinuria after prolonged, though not necessarily high-intensity, exercise. Fasting exacerbates these complaints. Thus, myoglobinuria occurs in CPT deficiency under metabolic conditions that favor oxidation of fatty acids in normal muscle [4,8]. This observation suggests that impaired cellular energetics are the common cause of myoglobinuria in diverse metabolic myopathies. However, biochemical proof of energy depletion is still necessary. No abnormal decrease of ATP concentration has yet been measured in muscle of patients with McArdle's disease during fatigue, which is defined as failure to maintain the required or expected force, or during ischemic exercise-induced contracture. It cannot be excluded, however, that contracture as well as necrosis may involve only a relatively small percentage of fibers. Measurements of ATP and phosphocreatine in whole muscle might fail to detect loss of high-energy phosphate compounds in selected fibers. Additionally, ATP deficiency may affect a specific subcellular compartment.

The cause of weakness is also poorly understood. Chronic impairment of energy provision is unlikely because two of the three glycogenoses causing weakness involve a glycogen-synthesiz-

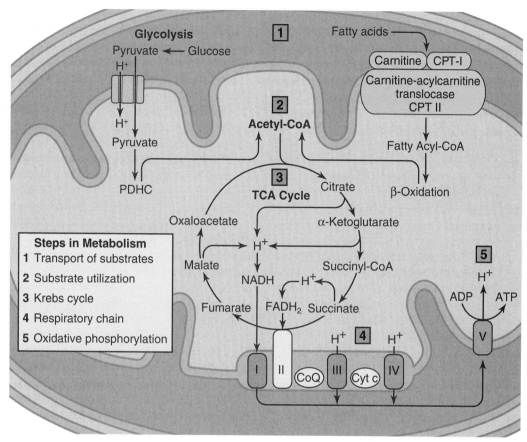

FIGURE 42-3. Schematic representation of mitochondrial metabolism. Respiratory chain complexes or components encoded exclusively by the nuclear genome are light orange. Complexes containing some subunits encoded by the nuclear genome and others encoded by mitochondrial DNA are dark orange. *CPT,* carnitine palmitoyltransferase; *PDHC,* pyruvate dehydrogenase complex; *CoA,* coenzyme A; *TCA,* tricarboxylic acid; *CoQ,* coenzyme Q; *Cyt c,* cytochrome c. (Modified from [12], with permission of McGraw-Hill, New York).

ing enzyme, branching enzyme deficiency, and a lysosomal glycogenolytic enzyme, acid maltase deficiency (Chap. 41), neither of which is directly involved in energy production [1].

A more likely explanation is that weakness may be due to a net loss of muscle fibers because regeneration cannot keep pace with the rate of degeneration. With fewer functioning fibers, the muscle cannot exert full force. EMG reinforces this interpretation: motor unit potentials are of smaller amplitude and briefer duration than normal due to loss of muscle fibers from a motor unit. Fibrillations are attributed to areas of focal necrosis of muscle fiber, isolating areas of the cell from the neuromuscular junction in a form of "microdenervation." Muscle fiber degeneration may be due to excessive storage of glycogen, as in

acid maltase and debrancher enzyme deficiencies, or lipid droplets, as in carnitine deficiency. In agreement with this hypothesis is the observation that in at least two of the glycogenoses causing weakness, infantile acid maltase deficiency and debrancher enzyme deficiency, glycogen storage is much more severe than in the glycogenoses causing cramps and myoglobinuria. Similarly, lipid storage is much more severe in carnitine deficiency than in CPT deficiency [4,6,7].

An additional cause of weakness may be involvement of the anterior horn cells of the spinal cord, which is very conspicuous in infantile acid maltase deficiency. All three glycogenoses causing weakness are in fact due to generalized enzyme defects, but histological signs of denervation are not evident.

DISEASES OF CARBOHYDRATE AND FATTY ACID METABOLISM IN BRAIN

The concentration of glycogen in brain is small: approximately 0.1 g per 100 g fresh tissue, compared with 1.0 g per 100 g in muscle and 6 to 10 g per 100 g in liver. The functional significance of glycogen in the brain is not completely understood, but it is generally assumed that it represents available energy to be tapped during glucose depletion; however, the limited glycogen reserve renders the brain vulnerable to injury within minutes of onset of hypoglycemia or hypoxia.

The role of fatty acids as oxidizable fuels for brain metabolism is negligible, but ketone bodies, derived from fatty acid oxidation, can be utilized, particularly in the neonatal period. Diseases of carbohydrate and fatty acid metabolism may affect the brain directly or indirectly [1,9].

Defective transport of glucose across the blood–brain barrier is caused by deficiency in the glucose transporter protein

Glucose crosses the blood–brain barrier by a mechanism of facilitated diffusion (Chaps. 5 and 32). This stereospecific system has a relatively high K_m for glucose, approximately 6 mM. Normally, transport of glucose across the blood–brain barrier is not rate-limiting for cerebral metabolism. Two patients were reported with a defect involving the GLUT-1 carrier protein [2]. The clinical presentation was infantile-onset seizures and developmental delay. One patient had deceleration of head growth with resulting microcephaly. The metabolic signature of this condition is a persistent hypoglycorrhachia with low-normal or low CSF lactate values. The patients responded to a ketogenic diet that was implemented to provide ketone bodies as an alternative fuel source for cerebral metabolism [2,3]. The GLUT-1 protein also is present in erythrocyte membranes. Decreased binding of cytochalasin B, a ligand that selectively binds to glucose transporters, was documented in both cases, and decreased uptake of 3-O-methylglucose by freshly isolated erythrocytes

was documented in one case. The molecular and genetic basis for this condition involves mutation in the GLUT-1 gene on chromosome 1 [9a]. These patients may be misdiagnosed as examples of cerebral palsy, suspected hypoglycemia or sudden infant death syndrome.

One class of carbohydrate and fatty acid metabolism disorders is caused by defects in enzymes that function in the brain

Acid maltase deficiency is characterized by large amounts of glycogen in the perikaryon of glial cells in both gray and white matter, whereas cortical neurons contain much smaller quantities of glycogen. In the spinal cord, the neurons of the anterior horn appear ballooned and contain glycogen, as shown by the abundant PAS-positive material that is digested by diastase. Schwann cells of both anterior and posterior spinal roots and of peripheral nerves also contain excessive glycogen. By electron microscopy, the most striking feature is the presence of glycogen granules within membrane-bound vacuoles. These glycogen-laden vacuoles are particularly abundant in anterior horn cells, in neurons of brainstem motor nuclei and in Schwann cells, whereas they are scarce in cortical neurons. Glycogen is increased in postmortem brain, and acid maltase activity is undetectable. The severe involvement of spinal and brainstem motor neurons and the massive accumulation of glycogen in muscle contribute to the profound hypotonia, weakness and hyporeflexia seen in Pompe's disease [1].

Debrancher enzyme deficiency appears to be generalized. Accordingly, although neither pathology nor debrancher enzyme activity has been reported, increased glycogen concentration has been observed in the brain of a patient. Thus, in debrancher enzyme deficiency, the nervous system seems to be involved biochemically, although clinical signs of brain dysfunction are limited to hypoglycemic seizures in childhood [1].

Branching enzyme deficiency has been described in multiple tissues, reflecting the fact that the enzyme is expressed as a single molecular form. Although signs and symptoms of brain dysfunction are not prominent in brancher enzyme deficiency, deposits of abnormal polysaccharide, in the form of PAS-positive spheroids, were seen in subpial and perivascular zones of the brainstem and spinal cord but never within neurons. Electron microscopy showed that the spheroids were composed of branched osmiophilic filaments, 600 nm in diameter, and located within distended astrocytic processes [1].

Phosphoglycerate kinase deficiency, as it is most commonly manifest, includes nonspherocytic hemolytic anemia and CNS dysfunction. Neurological problems vary in severity. All patients show some degree of mental retardation, with delayed language acquisition and behavioral abnormalities, and some have hemiplegia or seizures. The enzyme defect has been directly proven in the brain, and the severe brain involvement can be explained by impairment of the glycolytic pathway. The lack of symptoms of brain dysfunction in some patients with PGK deficiency, such as the two patients with recurrent myoglobinuria described above, are probably attributable to the presence of sufficient residual enzyme activity to prevent severe energy shortage.

Lafora and other polyglucosan-storage diseases manifest an accumulation of an abnormal glucose polymer resembling amylopectin, termed polyglucosan, in the CNS and PNS as well as in other tissues, but the biochemical defect(s) remains unknown [1].

Lafora's disease is transmitted as an autosomal recessive trait and is characterized by epilepsy, myoclonus and dementia. Other neurological manifestations include ataxia, dysarthria, spasticity and rigidity. Onset is in adolescence, and death occurs in most patients before 25 years of age.

The pathological hallmark of the disease is the presence in the brain of Lafora bodies: round, basophilic, PAS-positive intracellular inclusions varying in size from small, "dust-like" bodies less than 3 nm in diameter to large bodies up to 30 nm in diameter. Lafora bodies are typically seen in neuronal perikarya and processes, not in glial cells, and are more abundant in cerebral cortex, substantia nigra, thalamus, globus pallidus and dentate nucleus. Ultrastructural studies have shown that Lafora bodies consist of two components: amorphous electron-dense granules and irregular branched filaments.

Although the storage material is histochemically and biochemically similar to the polysaccharide that accumulates in branching enzyme deficiency, brancher enzyme activity was normal in brain and muscle from one patient. A different form of polyglucosan body disease was described in patients with a characteristic neurological syndrome consisting of progressive upper and lower motoneuron involvement, sensory loss, neurogenic bladder, and, in one-half of the patients, dementia without myoclonus or epilepsy. Onset is in the fifth or sixth decade, and the course varies between 3 and 30 years. Polyglucosan bodies are disseminated throughout the CNS and PNS in processes of neurons and astrocytes but not in perikarya. Other tissues are also affected, including liver, heart and skeletal and smooth muscle. In Ashkenazi Jewish patients with this disorder, but not in patients of different ethnic origins, branching enzyme activity is decreased in leukocytes, peripheral nerve and, presumably, brain but is normal in muscle [1]. The molecular basis for the differences in organs affected and clinical course between "typical" branching enzyme deficiency (see above) and polyglucosan body disease remains to be explained. The observation that branching deficiency in polyglucosan body disease is confined to Ashkenazi Jewish patients suggests that this disorder is biochemically heterogeneous.

Another class of carbohydrate and fatty acid metabolism disorders is caused by systemic metabolic defects that affect the brain

Glucose-6-phosphatase deficiency (glycogenosis type I, Von Gierke's disease) results in hypoglycemia and excessive intracellular accumulation of glucose-6-phosphate (Fig. 42-1). Hypoglycemia may produce lethargy, coma, seizures and brain damage in gluconeogenic and glycogen synthetase deficiencies [6]. As a result, there is formation of lactic acid, uric acid and lipids. A second form of the disease (type Ib) has been described. The defect in this form involves the glucose-6-phosphate translocation system that is important in facilitating the movement of the substrate into the microsomal compartment for enzymatic conversion to glucose by glucose-6-phosphatase. The clinical features of types Ia and Ib are similar, but normal enzyme activity is present in type Ib. Hepatomegaly, bleeding diathesis and neutropenia are present. The neurological signs result from the chronic hypoglycemia. Recent studies indicate that lactate may be used by the brain as an alternative cerebral metabolic fuel when hypoglycemia is associated with lactic acidosis. Nocturnal intragastric feeding and frequent daytime meals ameliorate most of the clinical and metabolic abnormalities of this condition.

Fructose-1,6-bisphosphatase deficiency, first described by Baker and Winegrad in 1970, has now been reported in approximately 30 cases. It is more common in women and is inherited as an autosomal recessive disorder. Initial manifestations are not strikingly dissimilar from those of glucose-6-phosphatase deficiency. Neonatal hypoglycemia is a common presenting feature, associated with profound metabolic acidosis, irritability or coma, apneic spells, dyspnea, tachycardia, hypotonia and moderate hepatomegaly. Lactate, alanine, uric acid and ketone bodies are elevated in the blood and urine [10]. The enzyme is deficient in liver, kidney, jejunum and leukocytes. Muscle fructose-1,6-bisphosphatase activity is normal.

Fructose-1,6-bisphosphatase is an important rate-limiting step in gluconeogenesis. This gluconeogenic step antagonizes the opposite reaction that forms fructose-1,6-bisphosphate from fructose-6-phosphate and ATP (see Chap. 31). A futile cycle exists between these two enzymes, one forming fructose-1,6-bisphosphate and the other disposing of this substrate. Small amounts of fructose-2,6-bisphosphate also are formed by the PFK reaction. This metabolite stimulates the PFK reaction and inhibits the fructose-1,6-bisphosphatase reaction. This finding nicely explains the subtle interplay between the key rate-limiting step in glycolysis, which is PFK-dependent, and the rate-limiting step in gluconeogenesis catalyzed by fructose-1,6-bisphosphatase.

Phosphoenolpyruvate carboxykinase (PEPCK) deficiency is a distinctly rare and even more devastating clinically than deficiencies of glucose-6-phosphatase or fructose-1,6-bisphosphatase. PEPCK activity is almost equally distributed between a cytosolic form and a mitochondrial form. These two forms have similar molecular weights but differ by their kinetic and immunochemical properties. The cytosolic activity is responsive to fasting and various hormonal stimuli. Hypoglycemia is severe and intractable in the absence of PEPCK [10]. A young child with cytosolic PEPCK deficiency had severe cerebral atrophy, optic atrophy and fatty infiltration of liver and kidney.

Pyruvate carboxylase deficiency has been documented in 36 cases [9,11]. This enzyme is mitochondrial in location and catalyzes the conversion of pyruvate to oxaloacetate in a biotin-dependent manner (Chaps. 35 and 39). The first report of pyruvate carboxylase deficiency involved an infant with subacute necrotizing encephalomyelopathy, or Leigh's syndrome. Subsequent reports have failed to confirm this causal relationship between pyruvate carboxylase deficiency and the neuropathological features of Leigh's syndrome. Leigh's syndrome has now been assigned to several other biochemical defects, including pyruvate dehydrogenase deficiency, cytochrome-oxidase deficiency, biotinidase deficiency and defects involving complex I and complex V of the respiratory chain.

Most patients with pyruvate-carboxylase deficiency present with failure to thrive, developmental delay, recurrent seizures and metabolic acidosis. Lactate, pyruvate, alanine, β-hydroxybutyrate and acetoacetate concentrations are elevated in blood and urine. Hypoglycemia is not a consistent finding despite the fact that pyruvate carboxylase is the first rate-limiting step in gluconeogenesis.

Sixteen patients had an associated hyperammonemia, citrullinemia and hyperlysinemia. This presentation is the most malignant, with death in early infancy. This French phenotype is commonly associated with the absence of any immunological cross-reacting material (CRM) corresponding to the pyruvate carboxylase apoenzyme protein.

The North American phenotype is associated with the presence of CRM. Possibly as a result, the clinical presentation is less devastating in early infancy, although the outcome is almost invariably fatal in later infancy or early childhood. These patients do not have the associated abnormalities of ammonia metabolism, and the serum aspartic acid concentrations are not as severely depleted. Only one patient has been described with the North American phenotype and a benign clinical syndrome. She has had recurrent episodes of metabolic acidosis requiring hospitalization. Otherwise, her growth and neurological development have been normal.

Prenatal and postnatal diagnoses can be made by enzyme assay of cultured amniocytes, fibroblasts or white blood cells. Treatment remains symptomatic. Sodium bicarbonate is necessary to correct the acidosis. Aspartic acid supplementation will improve the systemic condition but has no effect on the neurological disturbances. Biotin supplementation is of no value.

Biotin-dependent syndromes are manifest in infants, who may present with developmental delay and may demonstrate laboratory abnormalities resulting from deficiencies of the four biotin-dependent carboxylases (see Chap. 39). Three of the carboxylases, located in the mitochondria, are involved in organic acid metabolism. Multiple carboxylase deficiency, when present in the newborn period, is the result of a deficiency of holocarboxylase synthetase, the enzyme that catalyzes the binding of biotin to the apocarboxylase. These infants often die shortly after birth. Older infants gradually develop neurological signs, with developmental delay and seizures associated with alopecia, rash and immunodeficiency. There is a deficiency of biotinidase, the enzyme responsible for the breakdown of biocytin, the lysyl derivative of biotin, to free biotin. Biotinidase deficiency can be recognized at birth by measuring the serum activity. Biotinidase deficiency occurs in 1 in 41,000 live births, and it is eminently treatable by the oral administration of biotin.

Glycogen synthetase deficiency has been described in three families. It caused stunted growth and severe fasting hypoglycemia with ke-

tonuria. Mental retardation was reported in the three children who survived past infancy. The liver was virtually devoid of glycogen and showed fatty degeneration in all cases. In two patients, the brain showed diffuse, nonspecific changes in the white matter, seen as the presence of reactive astrocytes and increased microglia, which were considered secondary to prolonged hypoglycemia or anoxia. Biochemical studies showed that glycogen-synthetase activity was markedly decreased in liver but normal in muscle, erythrocytes and leukocytes, suggesting the existence of multiple tissue-specific isoenzymes under separate genetic control. It is not known whether brain glycogen synthetase is different from that in liver.

In *liver phosphorylase deficiency* (glycogenosis type VI, Hers' disease; Fig. 42-1) and in two genetic forms of *phosphorylase kinase deficiency*, one of which is X-linked recessive, the other of which is autosomal recessive, hypoglycemia is either absent or mild. Symptoms of brain dysfunction do not usually occur (type VIII, Fig. 42-1) [1].

Fatty acid oxidation defects often produce recurrent disturbances of brain function [4,6,9]. Drowsiness, stupor and coma occur during acute metabolic crises and mimic the Reye's syndrome phenotype. The neurological symptoms have been attributed to hypoglycemia, hypoketonemia and the deleterious effects of potentially toxic organic acids. Hypoglycemia is caused by a continuing demand for glucose by brain and other organs, resulting from the primary biochemical defect of fatty-acid oxidation (Fig. 42-2). Avoidance of catabolic circumstances that require the utilization of fatty acids is the basic principle of treatment. L-Carnitine supplementation is recommended for all conditions associated with generalized carnitine deficiency. Some patients may benefit from medium-chain triglyceride supplementation, as discussed previously. Certain forms of ETF-oxidoreductase deficiency respond to riboflavin supplementation. The riboflavin-responsive multiple acyl CoA dehydrogenase deficiency represents the milder form of glutaric aciduria type II.

DISEASES OF MITOCHONDRIAL METABOLISM

Mitochondrial dysfunction produces syndromes involving muscle and the central nervous system

Although some energy can be obtained quickly from glucose or glycogen through anaerobic glycolysis, most of the energy derives from oxidation of carbohydrates and fatty acids in the mitochondria. The common metabolic product of sugars and fats is acetyl-CoA, which enters the Krebs cycle. Oxidation of one molecule of acetyl-CoA results in the reduction of three molecules of NAD and one of FAD. These reducing equivalents flow down a chain of carriers (Fig. 42-3) through a series of oxidation-reduction events. The final hydrogen acceptor is molecular oxygen, and the product is water. The released energy "charges" the inner mitochondrial membrane, converting the mitochondrion into a veritable biological battery. This oxidation process is coupled to ATP synthesis from ADP and inorganic phosphate (P_i), catalyzed by mitochondrial ATPase [9,12,13]. Considering the enormous amount of information collected since 1960 on mitochondrial structure and function, it is surprising that diseases of terminal mitochondrial metabolism, that is, the Krebs cycle and respiratory chain, have attracted the attention of clinical investigators only recently [9,12–14].

Initial clues that some diseases might be due to mitochondrial dysfunction come from electron-microscopic studies of muscle biopsies showing fibers with increased numbers of structurally normal or abnormal mitochondria. These fibers have a "ragged red" appearance in the modified Gomori trichrome stain. Because the diagnosis was based on mitochondrial changes in muscle biopsies, these disorders were initially labeled mitochondrial myopathies. It soon became apparent, however, that many mitochondrial diseases with ragged red fibers were not confined to skeletal muscle but were multisystem disorders. In these patients, the clinical picture is often dominated by signs and symptoms of muscle and brain dysfunction, probably due to the great dependence of these tissues on oxidative metabolism. This group of disorders, often called mitochondrial encephalomyopathies, includes three more common syndromes (Table 42-1) [9,12,13].

The first, *Kearns-Sayre syndrome (KSS)*, is characterized by childhood onset of progressive external ophthalmoplegia and pigmentary degeneration of the retina. Heart block, cerebellar syndrome or high CSF protein may also appear. Almost all cases are sporadic. The second syndrome, *myoclonus epilepsy with ragged red fibers (MERRF)*, is characterized by myoclonus, ataxia, weakness and generalized seizures. The third syndrome, *mitochondrial myopathy, encephalopathy, lactic acidosis and stroke-like episodes (MELAS)*, affects young children, who show stunted growth, episodic vomiting and headaches, seizures and recurrent cerebral insults resembling strokes and causing hemipare-

TABLE 42-1. DISTINGUISHING FEATURES OF MITOCHONDRIAL ENCEPHALOMYOPATHIES

Clinical features	KSS	MERRF	MELAS
Ophthalmoplegia	+	−	−
Retinal degeneration	+	−	−
Heart block	+	−	−
CSF protein > 100 mg/dl	+	−	−
Myoclonus	−	+	−
Ataxia	+	+	+
Weakness	+	+	+
Episodic vomiting	−	−	+
Cerebral blindness	−	−	+
Hemiparesis, hemianopsia	−	−	+
Seizures	−	+	+
Dementia	+	+	+
Short stature	+	+	+
Sensorineural hearing loss	+	+	+
Lactic acidosis	+	+	+
Family history	−	+	+
Ragged red fibers	+	+	+
Spongy degeneration	+	+	+
mtDNA deletion	+	−	−
mtDNA point mutation	−	tRNA^{lys}	tRNA$^{leu(UUR)}$

KSS, Kearns-Sayre syndrome; MERRF, myoclonus epilepsy with ragged red fibers; MELAS, mitochondrial encephalomyopathy, lactic acidosis and stroke-like episodes; CSF, cerebrospinal fluid; boxes highlight differential features (see text).

sis, hemianopsia or cortical blindness. Unlike KSS, MERRF and MELAS are usually familial, and analysis of several pedigrees has documented non-Mendelian maternal inheritance [9,12,13].

Mitochondrial DNA is inherited maternally

What makes mitochondrial diseases particularly interesting from a genetic point of view is that the mitochondrion has its own DNA (mtDNA) and its own transcription and translation processes. The mtDNA encodes only 13 polypeptides; nuclear DNA (nDNA) controls the synthesis of 90 to 95% of all mitochondrial proteins. All known mitochondrially encoded polypeptides are located in the inner mitochondrial membrane as subunits of the respiratory chain complexes (Fig. 42-3), including seven subunits of complex I; the apoprotein of cytochrome b; the three larger subunits of cytochrome c oxidase, also termed complex IV; and two subunits of ATPase, also termed complex V.

In the formation of the zygote, almost all mitochondria are contributed by the ovum. Therefore, mtDNA is transmitted by maternal inheritance in a vertical, non-Mendelian fashion. Strictly maternal transmission of mtDNA has been documented in humans by studies of restriction fragment length polymorphisms (RFLPs) in DNA from platelets. In theory, diseases caused by mutations of mtDNA should also be transmitted by maternal inheritance: an affected mother ought to pass the disease to all of her children, were it not for the "threshold effect," which is described later, but only her daughters would transmit the trait to subsequent generations [9,12,13]. Characteristics that distinguish maternal from Mendelian inheritance include the following:

1. The number of affected individuals in subsequent generations should be higher than in autosomal dominant disease, again, were it not for the "threshold effect" (see below).
2. Inheritance is maternal, as in X-linked diseases, but children of both sexes are affected.
3. Because there are hundreds or thousands of copies of mtDNA in each cell, the phenotypic

expression of a mitochondrially encoded gene depends on the relative proportions of mutant and wild-type mtDNAs within a cell; this is termed the "threshold effect."
4. Because mitochondria replicate more often than do nuclei, the relative proportion of mutant and wild-type mtDNAs may change within a cell cycle.
5. At the time of cell division, the proportion of mutant and wild-type mtDNAs in the two daughter cells can shift, thus giving them different genotypes and, possibly, different phenotypes, a phenomenon called mitotic segregation.

Maternal inheritance has been documented in diseases due to point mutations of mtDNA, while most diseases due to mtDNA deletions or duplications are sporadic.

The genetic classification of mitochondrial diseases divides them into three groups

Defects of mtDNA include point mutations and deletions or duplications. From a biochemical point of view, these disorders will be associated with dysfunction of the respiratory chain because all 13 subunits encoded by mtDNA are subunits of respiratory chain complexes. Diseases due to point mutations are transmitted by maternal inheritance, and the number has rapidly increased during the past few years. The main syndromes include MERRF; MELAS (Table 42-1); Leber's hereditary optic neuropathy (LHON), a disorder causing blindness in young adult men; and neurogenic atrophy, ataxia and retinitis pigmentosa (NARP), which, depending on the relative proportion of mutant mitochondrial genomes in tissues, can cause a multisystem disorder in young adults or a devastating encephalomyopathy of childhood, termed Leigh's syndrome. Diseases due to deletions or duplications are usually sporadic, for reasons that are not completely clear. They include, besides KSS (Table 42-1), isolated progressive external ophthalmoplegia and Pearson's syndrome, a usually fatal infantile disorder dominated by sideroblastic anemia and exocrine pancreas dysfunction.

Defects of nuclear DNA also cause mitochondrial diseases. As mentioned above, the vast majority of mitochondrial proteins are encoded by nDNA, synthesized in the cytoplasm and "imported" into the mitochondria, through a complex series of steps. Defects of genes encoding the proteins themselves or controlling the importation machinery will cause mitochondrial diseases, which will be transmitted by Mendelian inheritance. From a biochemical point of view, all areas of mitochondrial metabolism can be affected (see below).

Defects of communication between nDNA and mtDNA can also cause mitochondrial diseases. The nDNA controls many functions of the mtDNA, including its replication. It is, therefore, conceivable that mutations of nuclear genes controlling these functions could cause alterations in the mtDNA. Two human diseases have been attributed to this mechanism [9,12,13]. The first is associated with multiple mtDNA deletions and is characterized clinically by ophthalmoplegia, weakness of limb and respiratory muscles and early death. Transmission is usually autosomal dominant, and it is assumed that a mutation in a nuclear gene makes the mtDNA prone to develop deletions. In fact, linkage analyses in a few large pedigrees have mapped the affected genes to two different loci, one on chromosome 3 and the other on chromosome 10, showing that these disorders are genetically heterogeneous [9,12,13]. The second disease is associated with mtDNA depletion in one or more tissues, more commonly in muscle. Depending on the tissue affected and the severity of the mtDNA decrease, the clinical picture can be a rapidly fatal congenital myopathy, a slightly more benign myopathy of childhood or a fatal hepatopathy. Transmission appears to be autosomal recessive or dominant, and it is postulated that an nDNA mutation may impair mtDNA replication. As expected, all subunits encoded by mtDNA are markedly decreased in the affected tissues.

The biochemical classification of mitochondrial DNA is based on the five major steps of mitochondrial metabolism

These steps are illustrated in Figure 42-3 and divide mitochondrial diseases into five groups: (i) defects of mitochondrial transport, (ii) defects of substrate utilization, (iii) defects of the Krebs cycle, (iv) defects of oxidation–phosphorylation coupling and (v) defects of the respiratory chain.

All disorders except those in group 5 are due to defects of nDNA and are transmitted by Mendelian inheritance. Disorders of the respiratory chain can be due to defects of nDNA, mtDNA or intergenomic communication. Usually, mutations of nDNA cause isolated, severe defects of individual respiratory complexes, whereas mutations in mtDNA or defects of intergenomic communication cause variably severe, multiple deficiencies of respiratory chain complexes. The description that follows is based on the biochemical classification.

Defects of mitochondrial transport interfere with the movement of molecules across the inner mitochondrial membrane, which is tightly regulated by specific translocation systems. The carnitine cycle is shown in Figure 42-2 and is responsible for the translocation of acyl-CoA thioesters from the cytosol into the mitochondrial matrix. The carnitine cycle involves four elements: the plasma membrane carnitine-transporter system, CPT I, the carnitine–acyl carnitine translocase system in the inner mitochondrial membrane and CPT II. Genetic defects have been described for each of these four steps, as discussed previously [4,6–8].

Defects of substrate utilization. Pyruvate dehydrogenase (PDH) deficiency can cause alterations of pyruvate metabolism, as can defects of pyruvate carboxylase, as discussed earlier. Over 200 patients have been described with a disturbance of the PDH complex (PDHC) [9]. The clinical picture includes several phenotypes ranging from a severe, devastating metabolic disease in the neonatal period to a benign, recurrent syndrome in older children. There is considerable overlap clinically and biochemically with other disorders (see below).

The PDHC catalyzes the irreversible conversion of pyruvate to acetyl-CoA (Fig. 42-3) and is dependent on thiamine and lipoic acid as cofactors (see Chap. 35). The complex has five enzymes: three subserving a catalytic function and two subserving a regulatory role. The catalytic components include PDH, E1; dihydrolipoyl transacetylase, E2; and dihydrolipoyl dehydrogenase, E3. The two regulatory enzymes include PDH-specific kinase and phospho-PDH-specific phosphatase. The multienzyme complex contains nine protein subunits, including protein X. Protein X anchors the E3 component to the E2 core of the complex. The E1 α subunit is encoded by a gene on the short arm of the X chromosome and a gene on chromosome 4. The E1 β subunit is encoded by a gene on chromosome 3, the E2 component is encoded by a gene on chromosome 11 and the E3 component is encoded by a gene on chromosome 7. Biochemical defects have been documented for the E1 α subunit, E2 (one case), E3 (six cases), protein X (two cases) and the phospho-PDH-specific phosphatase (four cases). The great majority of cases involve a mutation defect of the E1 α subunit. Both genders are equally represented despite the location of the E1 α-subunit gene on the X chromosome.

The most devastating phenotype of PDH deficiency presents in the newborn period. The majority of patients are male and critically ill with a severe metabolic acidosis. There is an elevated blood or CSF lactate concentration and associated elevations of pyruvate and alanine. These patients have seizures, failure to thrive, optic atrophy, microcephaly and dysmorphic features. Multiple brain abnormalities have been described, including dysmyelination of the cortex, cystic degeneration of the basal ganglia, ectopic olivary nuclei, hydrocephalus and partial or complete agenesis of the corpus callosum. A less devastating phenotype presents in early infancy. These patients demonstrate the histopathological features of Leigh's syndrome. Other patients affected in infancy survive with a chronic neurodegenerative syndrome manifested by mental retardation, microcephaly, recurrent seizures, spasticity, ataxia and dystonia.

Mutations involving the E1 α subunit behave clinically like an X-linked dominant condition. These mutations usually are lethal in boys during early infancy. The clinical spectrum in the heterozygous girl is more varied, ranging from a devastating condition in early infancy to a mild chronic encephalopathy with mental retardation. The least symptomatic woman may give birth to affected male and female progeny and pose a significant problem in clinical diagnosis and genetic counseling.

Treatment is largely symptomatic, and the prognosis ranges from dismal to guarded. Thiamine, lipoic acid, ketogenic diet and physostigmine have been tried in different concentrations and doses with equivocal results. Some patients with periodic ataxia resulting from PDHC deficiency may respond to acetazolamide.

Glutaric aciduria type II, which is a defect of β-oxidation, may affect muscle exclusively or in conjunction with other tissues. Glutaric aciduria type II, also termed multiple acyl-CoA dehydrogenase deficiency (Fig. 42-2), usually causes respiratory distress, hypoglycemia, hyperammonemia, systemic carnitine deficiency, nonketotic metabolic acidosis in the neonatal period and death within the first week. A few patients with onset in childhood or adult life showed lipid-storage myopathy, with weakness or premature fatigue [4,6]. *Short-chain acyl-CoA deficiency* (Fig. 42-2) was described in one woman with proximal limb weakness and exercise intolerance. Muscle biopsy showed marked accumulation of lipid droplets. Although no other tissues were studied, the defect appeared to be confined to skeletal muscle, suggesting the existence of tissue-specific isozymes [9,12,13].

Defects of the Krebs cycle. *Fumarase deficiency* was reported in three children with mitochondrial encephalomyopathy. Two of them had developmental delay since early infancy, microcephaly, hypotonia and cerebral atrophy; one died at 8 months of age. The third patient was a 3.5-year-old, mentally retarded girl. The laboratory hallmark of the disease is the excretion of large amounts of fumaric acid and, to a lesser extent, succinic acid in the urine. The enzyme defect has been found in muscle, liver and cultured skin fibroblasts [9,12,13].

Defects of oxidation–phosphorylation coupling. The best known example of such a defect is Luft's disease, or nonthyroidal hypermetabolism. Only two patients with this condition have been reported. Family history was noncontributory in both cases. Symptoms started in childhood or early adolescence with fever, heat intolerance, profuse perspiration, resting tachypnea and dyspnea, polydipsia, polyphagia and mild weakness. The basal metabolic rate was markedly increased in both patients, but all tests of thyroid function were normal. Muscle biopsies showed ragged red fibers and proliferation of capillaries. Other tissues were morphologically normal. Studies of oxidative phosphorylation in isolated muscle mitochondria from both patients showed maximal respiratory rate even in the absence of ADP, an indication that respiratory control was lost. Respiration proceeded at a high rate independently of phosphorylation, and energy was lost as heat, causing hypermetabolism and hyperthermia [13].

Abnormalities of the respiratory chain are usually identified based on polarographic studies showing differential impairment in the ability of isolated intact mitochondria to use different substrates. For example, defective respiration with NAD-dependent substrates, such as pyruvate and malate, but normal respiration with FAD-dependent substrates, such as succinate, suggests an isolated defect of complex I (Fig. 42-3). However, defective respiration with both types of substrates in the presence of activity of normal cytochrome c oxidase, also termed complex IV, localizes the lesions to complex III (Fig. 42-3).

Polarographic studies can be complemented by measurement of reduced-minus-oxidized spectra of cytochromes, showing decreased amounts of reducible cytochromes a and a3 in patients with complex IV deficiency and of reducible cytochrome b in many, but not all, patients with complex III deficiency (Fig. 42-3). Finally, electron transport through discrete portions of the respiratory chain can be measured directly. Thus, an isolated defect of NADH–cytochrome c reductase activity suggests a problem within complex I, while a simultaneous defect of NADH and succinate–cytochrome c reductase activities points to a biochemical error in complex III (Fig. 42-3). The function of complex III alone can be tested by measuring the activity of reduced coenzyme Q–cytochrome c reductase.

Abnormalities of the respiratory chain: defects of complex I. These have been described in about 25 patients and seem to cause two major clinical syndromes: pure myopathy, with exercise intolerance and myalgia presenting in childhood or adult life, and multisystem disorder. Patients with multisystem disorder were not clinically homogeneous: some had a fatal infantile form of the disease, causing severe congenital lactic acidosis, hypotonia, seizures, respiratory insufficiency and death before age 3 months; others had a less severe encephalomyopathy with onset in childhood or adult life and characterized by the association, in various proportions, of the following signs and symptoms: exercise intolerance, weakness, ophthalmoplegia, pigmentary retinopathy, optic atrophy, sensorineural hearing loss, dementia, cerebellar ataxia and pyramidal signs [12–14]. This clinical heterogeneity is hardly surprising when one considers the large number of proteins comprising complex I, but the molecular defect in most patients is not known (Fig. 42-3).

Abnormalities of the respiratory chain: defects of complex II. These have not been fully characterized in the few reported patients, and the diagnosis has often been based solely on a decrease of succinate–cytochrome c reductase activity (Fig. 42-3). The clinical picture is characterized by severe infantile myopathy, with lactic acidosis in two cases and encephalomyopathy in three cases [3,5,7,11]. However, partial complex II deficiency was documented in muscle and cultured fibroblasts from two sisters with clinical and neuroradiological evidence of Leigh's syndrome, and molecular genetic analysis showed that both patients were homozygous for a point mutation in the flavoprotein subunit of the complex [15]. This is the first documentation of a molecular defect in the nuclear genome associated with a respiratory chain disorder.

Abnormalities of the respiratory chain: coenzyme Q10 (CoQ10) deficiency. This disorder is characterized, based on four patients described thus far, by a triad of symptoms in muscle: (i) exercise intolerance and recurrent myoglobinuria; (ii) CNS dysfunction, with seizures or mental retardation; and (iii) ragged red fibers and markedly increased lipid droplets in the muscle biopsy. Biochemical analysis of muscle shows a partial block at the level of complex III. This syndrome is important to consider in the differential diagnosis of recurrent myoglobinurias because patients benefit considerably from CoQ10 administration [16,17].

Abnormalities of the respiratory chain: defects of complex III. These have a clinical picture that falls into one of two groups: (i) childhood- or adolescent-onset myopathy with or without involvement of extraocular muscles and (ii) encephalopathy with exercise intolerance, fixed weakness, pigmentary degeneration of the retina, sensorineural hearing loss, cerebellar ataxia, pyramidal signs and dementia [9,12–14].

Biochemically, some patients show lack of reducible cytochrome b, whereas others have normal cytochrome spectra. In patients with a normal amount of reducible cytochrome b, the defect may involve the nonheme iron sulfur protein, also termed Rieske protein or coenzyme Q (Fig. 42-3).

In a young woman with complex III deficiency myopathy, the bioenergetic capacity of muscle was studied by [^{31}P]-nuclear magnetic resonance (NMR). The ratio of phosphocreatine to inorganic phosphate concentration (PCr:P$_i$) was greatly reduced at rest, decreased further with mild exercise and returned to pre-exercise values very slowly. Treatment with menadione, vitamin K$_3$, and ascorbate, vitamin C, two compounds whose redox potentials permit them to function between coenzyme Q and cytochrome c (Fig. 42-3), was associated with marked improvement of exercise capacity. NMR showed increased PCr:P$_i$ ratios at rest and improved rates of recovery after exercise.

Abnormalities of the respiratory chain: defects of complex IV. These disorders, also termed cytochrome oxidase (COX) deficiency, have clinical phenotypes that fall into two main groups: one in which myopathy is the predominant or exclusive manifestation and another in which brain dysfunction predominates (Fig. 42-3). In the first group, the most common disorder is fatal infantile myopathy, causing generalized weakness, respiratory insufficiency and death before age 1 year. There is lactic acidosis and renal dysfunction, with glycosuria, phosphaturia

and aminoaciduria, also termed DeToni-Fanconi-Debre syndrome. The association of myopathy and cardiopathy in the same patient and myopathy and liver disease in the same family has also been described [12].

In patients with pure myopathy, COX deficiency is confined to skeletal muscle, sparing heart, liver and brain. The amount of immunologically reactive enzyme protein is markedly decreased in muscle by enzyme-linked immunosorbent assay (ELISA) and by immunocytochemistry of frozen sections. *Benign infantile mitochondrial myopathy,* in contrast, has been described in a few children with severe myopathy and lactic acidosis at birth, who then improve spontaneously and are virtually normal by age 2 years. This condition is due to a reversible COX deficiency. The enzyme activity is markedly decreased, <19% of normal, in muscle biopsies taken soon after birth but returns to normal in the first year of life. Immunocytochemistry and immunotitration show normal amounts of enzyme protein in all muscle biopsies. This finding differs from the virtual lack of CRM in patients with fatal infantile myopathy and may represent a useful prognostic test. The selective involvement of one or more tissues and the reversibility of the muscle defect in the benign form suggest the existence of tissue-specific and developmentally regulated COX isoenzymes in humans [12].

Subacute necrotizing encephalomyelopathy, also termed Leigh's syndrome, typifies the second group of disorders of complex IV, dominated by involvement of the CNS. Leigh's syndrome usually starts in infancy or childhood and is characterized by psychomotor retardation, brainstem abnormalities and apnea [12]. The pathological hallmark consists of focal, symmetrical necrotic lesions from thalamus to pons, involving the inferior olives and the posterior columns of the spinal cord. Microscopically, these spongy brain lesions show demyelination, vascular proliferation and astrocytosis. In these patients, COX deficiency is generalized, including cultured fibroblasts in most, but not all, cases. This may provide a useful tool for prenatal diagnosis in at least some families. Immunological studies show CRM in all tissues. Partial defects of COX have been reported in patients with progressive external ophthalmoplegia and proximal myopathy and in patients with encephalomyopathy. However, the precise pathogenic significance of COX deficiency in these disorders remains uncertain [12].

Abnormalities of the respiratory chain: defects of complex V, mitochondrial ATPase, have been reported in two patients. One was a young woman with congenital, slowly progressive myopathy; the other was a 17-year-old boy who, at age 10 years, was found to have muscle carnitine deficiency [13]. Later, he developed a multisystem disorder characterized by weakness, dementia, ataxia, retinopathy and peripheral neuropathy. In both patients, respiration of isolated mitochondria was decreased with all substrates but returned to normal after addition of the uncoupling agent 1,4-dinitrophenol. This finding suggested that the biochemical defect involved the phosphorylative pathway rather than the respiratory chain. ATPase activity was decreased and responded poorly to dinitrophenol stimulation.

ACKNOWLEDGMENTS

Some of the work discussed in this chapter was supported by USPHS grants NS11766 and NS176965 from the National Institute of Neurological and Communicative Disorders and Stroke, a grant from the Muscular Dystrophy Association and a laboratory grant from the Colleen Giblin Foundation for Pediatric Neurology Research. We are grateful to Ms. Alice H. Marti for typing the manuscript.

REFERENCES

1. DiMauro, S., Servidei, S., and Tsujino, S. Disorders of carbohydrate metabolism: Glycogen storage diseases. In R. L. Rosenberg, S. B. Prusiner, S. D. DiMauro, and R. L. Barchi (eds.), *The Molecular and Genetic Basis of Neurological Disease.* Boston: Butterworth-Heinemann, 1997, pp. 1067–1097.

2. De Vivo, D. C., Trifiletti, R. R., Jacobson, R. I., Ronen, G. M., Behmand, R. A., and Harik, S. I. Defective glucose transport across the blood–brain barrier as a cause of persistent hypoglycorrhachia, seizures, and developmental delay. *N. Engl. J. Med.* 325:703–709, 1991.

3. De Vivo, D. C. The effects of ketone bodies on glucose utilization. In J. V. Passonneau, R. A., Hawkins, W. D. Lust, and F. A. Welsh (eds.), *Cerebral Metabolism and Neural Function.* Baltimore: Williams & Wilkins, 1980, pp. 243–254.

4. DiDonato, S. Diseases associated with defects of beta-oxidation. In R. N. Rosenberg, S. B. Prusiner, S. DiMauro, and R. L. Barchi (eds.), *The Molecular and Genetic Basis of Neurological Disease.* Boston: Butterworth-Heinemann, 1997, pp. 939–956.

5. Tsujino, S., Shanske, S., and DiMauro, S. Molecular genetic heterogeneity of myophosphorylase deficiency (McArdle's disease). *N. Engl. J. Med.* 329:241–245, 1993.

6. Pons, R., and De Vivo, D. C. Primary and secondary carnitine deficiency syndromes. *J. Child. Neurol.* 10(Suppl. 2):S8-S24, 1995.

7. Treem, W. R., Stanley, C. A., Finegold, D. N., Hale, D. E., and Coates, P. W. Primary carnitine deficiency due to a failure of carnitine transport in kidney, muscle, and fibroblasts. *N. Engl. J. Med.* 319:1331–1336, 1988.

8. Tein, I., DiMauro, S., and De Vivo, D. C. Recurrent childhood myoglobinuria. In L. A. Barness, D. C. De Vivo, G. Morrow, F. Oski, and A. M. Rudolph (eds.), *Avances in Pediatrics,* vol. 37. Chicago: Mosby Year Book, 1990, pp. 77–119.

9. De Vivo, D. C., Hirano, M., and DiMauro, S. Mitochondrial disorders. In H. W. Moser (ed.), *Handbook of Clinical Neurology,* vol. 22. Amsterdam: Elsevier, 1996, pp. 389–446.

9a. Seidner, G., Alvarez, M. G., Yeh, J.–I., et al. GLUT-1 deficiency syndrome caused by haploinsufficiency of the blood–brain barrier hexose carrier. *Nat. Gen.* 18:188–191, 1998.

10. Haymond, M. W. Hypoglycemia. In A. M. Rudolph (ed.), *Pediatrics,* 20th ed. Norwalk, CT: Appleton & Lange, 1996, pp. 1828–1837.

11. Van Coster, R., Fernhoff, P. M., and De Vivo, D. C. Pyruvate carboxylase deficiency: A benign variant with normal development. *Pediatr. Res.* 30:1–4, 1991.

12. DiMauro, S., Hirano, M., Bonilla, E., and De Vivo, D. C. The mitochondrial disorders. In B. O. Berg (ed.), *Principles of Child Neurology.* New York: McGraw-Hill, 1996, pp. 1201–1232.

13. DiMauro, S., and Bonilla, E. Mitochondrial encephalomyopathies. In R. N. Rosenberg, S. B. Prusiner, S. DiMauro, and R. L. Barchi (eds.), *The*

Molecular and Genetic Basis of Neurological Disease. Boston: Butterworth-Heinemann, 1997, pp. 201–232.

14. Morgan-Hughes, J. A. Mitochondrial diseases. In A. G. Engel and C. Franzini-Armstrong (eds.), *Myology,* 2nd ed. New York: McGraw-Hill, 1994, pp. 1610–1660.

15. Bourgeron, T., Rustin, P., Chretien, D., et al. Mutation of a nuclear succinate dehydrogenase gene results in mitochondrial respiratory chain deficiency. *Nat. Genet.* 11:44–149, 1995.

16. Ogasahara, S., Engel, A. G., Frens, D., and Mack, D. Muscle coenzyme W10 deficiency in familial mitochondrial encephalomyopathy. *Proc. Natl. Acad. Sci. USA* 86:2379–2382, 1989.

17. Sobreita, C., Hirano, M., Shanske, S., et al. Mitochondrial encephalomyopathy with coenzyme Q10 deficiency. *Neurology* 48:1238–1243, 1997.

43

Disorders of Muscle Excitability

Robert L. Barchi

Basic Neurochemistry: Molecular, Cellular and Medical Aspects, 6th Ed., edited by G. J. Siegel et al. Published by Lippincott–Raven Publishers, Philadelphia, 1999. Correspondence to Robert L. Barchi, Institute of Neurological Sciences, University of Pennsylvania School of Medicine, 36th Street and Hamilton Walk, Philadelphia, Pennsylvania 19104.

Normal contraction of skeletal muscle requires that electrical signals originating in a motor nerve be transmitted across the neuromuscular junction, disseminated along the muscle surface membrane, propagated into the fiber interior along the T-tubular system and coupled to Ca²⁺ release from the sarcoplasmic reticulum, to ultimately cause actin–myosin interaction. Failure at any one of these steps will result in muscle weakness or paralysis even in the presence of a normal contractile apparatus. First, the molecular aspects of normal muscle contraction and of the membrane systems that link contraction to nerve excitation are briefly reviewed. Then, some of the pathobiological processes that can affect excitation in skeletal muscle are explored.

MUSCLE FIBERS ARE ORGANIZED IN REPEATING UNITS

Muscle contraction is due to relative sliding of two sets of filaments identified by light and electron microscopy

Light microscopists have long recognized that the physiological unit of muscle, the cell or fiber, contains repeating structures known as sarcomeres that are separated from each other by dark lines called Z disks. Within each sarcomere, the A and I bands are seen; the A band, lying between two I bands, occupies the center of each sarcomere and is highly birefringent. Within the A band is a central, lighter zone, the H band, and in the center of the H band is the darker M band. The Z disk is at the center of the I band (Fig. 43-1). The difference in birefringence between the A

and I bands produces the characteristic striated appearance of voluntary muscle when seen through the light microscope.

The repeating optical characteristics of the A and I bands in each sarcomere reflect the regular arrangement of two sets of filaments. The thin filaments have a diameter of ~180 Å, appear to be attached to the Z bands and are found in the I band and part of the A band. The thick filaments have a diameter of ~150 Å, occupy the A band and are connected crosswise by material in the M band. In cross section, the thick filaments are arranged in a hexagonal lattice and the thin filaments occupy the centers of the triangles formed by the thick filaments.

With the identification of two sets of discontinuous filaments in the sarcomere came the recognition that (i) the two kinds of filaments become cross-linked only on excitation and (ii) contraction of muscle does not depend on shortening the length of the filaments but rather on the relative motion of the two sets of filaments, termed the sliding-filament mechanism. Thus,

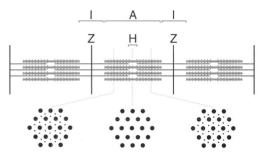

FIGURE 43-1. Schematic representation of the structure of striated muscle. Actin-containing thin filaments originate at Z lines. Note thick myosin-containing filaments that bear cross-bridges. The M disk lies in the center of the H band (see text). (From [46], with permission.)

the length of the muscle depends on the length of the sarcomeres and, in turn, variation in sarcomere length is based on variation in the degree of overlap between the thin and thick filaments. High-resolution electron micrographs have shown that cross-bridges emanate from the thick filaments; in active muscle, these structures are responsible both for the links with thin filaments [1] and for generation of the force that produces fiber translocation.

Actin and myosin form the chief components of the thin and thick filaments, respectively

In addition, other proteins are found in the two sets of filaments. Tropomyosin and a complex of three subunits collectively called troponin are present in the thin filaments and play an important role in the regulation of muscle contraction. Although the proteins constituting the M and the Z bands have not been fully characterized, they include α-actinin and desmin as well as the enzyme creatine kinase and a number of other proteins [2]. A continuous elastic network of proteins, such as connectin, surround the actin and myosin filaments, providing muscle with a parallel passive elastic element.

Actin forms the backbone of the thin filaments. The thin filaments of muscle are linear polymers of slightly elongated, bilobar actin subunits, each about 4 × 6 nm, arranged in a helical fashion, with the longer dimension roughly at right angles to the filament axis [1]. Each monomer has a molecular weight of about 42,000 and contains a single nucleotide-binding site. Hydrolysis of ATP to ADP takes place during actin polymerization but is not involved in muscle contraction.

A wide variety of proteins interact with actin in both muscle and nonmotile cells. They may affect the polymerization-depolymerization of actin and are involved in the attachment of actin to other cellular structures, including the Z disks in muscle as well as membranes in both muscle and nonmuscle cells. One protein interacting with actin in the Z disk, α-actinin, is also a component of the rod-like bodies found in nemaline myopathy.

Myosin, the chief constituent of thick filaments, is a multisubunit protein. It is a highly asymmetrical molecule of ~500 kDa with an overall length of ~150 nm (Fig. 43-2) [3]. Its width varies between about 2 and 10 nm. In contrast to actin, myosin consists of several peptide subunits. Each myosin molecule contains two heavy chains of ~200 kDa; these extend through the length of the molecule. Over most of their length, the two chains are intertwined to form a double α-helical rod; at one end they separate, each forming an elongated globular portion. The two globular portions contain the sites responsible for ATP hydrolysis and interaction with actin. In addition to the two heavy chains, each myosin molecule contains four light chains of ~20 kDa. These light chains modulate myosin activity. Some can be covalently modified by kinases in the muscle cell.

Myosin molecules form end-to-end aggregates involving the rod-like segments, which then grow into larger structures, that is, the thick filament [3]. The polarity of the myosin mole-

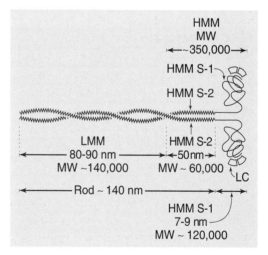

FIGURE 43-2. Schematic representation of the structure of the myosin molecule. The rod portion of the molecule has a coiled α-helical structure. Hinge regions postulated in the mechanism of contraction are at the junctions of heavy chain meromyosin (HMM) S-1 and HMM S-2 and of HMM S-2 and light chain meromyosin (LMM). It should be noted that HMM S-1 has one chief polypeptide chain, whereas other fragments have two. Note the light chains *(LC)* in the head region. The scheme suggests the presence of two different subunits in each HMM S-1. (From [47], with permission.)

cules is reversed on either side of the central portion of the filament. The globular ends of the molecules form projections, termed crossbridges, on the aggregates that interact with actin. Conformational changes within this region, driven by ATP hydrolysis, provide the force that propels the movement of actin fibrils with respect to the myosin filament.

The ATPase activity of myosin itself is stimulated by Ca^{2+} and is low in Mg^{2+}-containing media. The precise details of the conformational changes accompanying the hydrolysis of ATP and of the mechanism by which the free energy of ATP is converted into mechanical work are quite complicated [4] and will not be considered further here.

Tropomyosin and troponin regulate the interaction of actin and myosin

Tropomyosin and troponin are proteins located in the thin filaments, and together with Ca^{2+}, they regulate the interaction of actin and myosin [5] (Fig. 43-3). Tropomyosin is an α-helical protein consisting of two polypeptide chains; its structure is similar to that of the rod portion of myosin. Troponin is a complex of three proteins. If the tropomyosin–troponin complex is present, actin cannot stimulate the ATPase activity of myosin unless the concentration of free Ca^{2+} exceeds about 10^{-6} M, while a system consisting solely of purified actin and myosin does not show Ca^{2+} dependence. Thus, the actin–myosin interaction is controlled by Ca^{2+} in the presence of the regulatory troponin–tropomyosin complex.

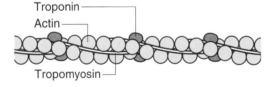

Troponin
Actin

Tropomyosin

FIGURE 43-3. Model of arrangements of actin, tropomyosin and troponin in the thin filament. Note that troponin itself is a complex of three proteins. Tropomyosin is close to the groove of the actin filaments in relaxed muscle. Note that, according to current views, the actin subunits are bilobar, with the long axis more or less perpendicular to the filament axis. The troponin complex also appears more elongated along the filament.

MEMBRANE SYSTEMS COUPLE NERVE EXCITATION TO MUSCLE CONTRACTION

The neuromuscular junction connects nerve to muscle

Synaptic transmission at the neuromuscular junction (NMJ) requires the integrated activity of complex macromolecular systems at both the presynaptic and the postsynaptic levels (Fig. 43-4). Defects in any of the elements can cause degradation in synaptic efficiency and block transmission of information. Synaptic failure at the NMJ produces muscle weakness, fatigability or paralysis. In many respects, synaptic transmission at the NMJ resembles that at other peripheral and central nerve synapses; molecular details of this process are provided in Chapter 10.

Terminal elements of motor nerves form specialized structures at the point of contact with muscle that constitute the NMJ. The distal arborizations of the motor neuron form enlarged presynaptic terminals containing large numbers of acetylcholine (ACh)-packed vesicles. These terminals lie in depressions called gutters in the postsynaptic sarcolemma.

The postsynaptic membrane at the NMJ is highly specialized; it is organized into deep transverse folds under the nerve terminal. The crests of these folds contain a high density of nicotinic ACh receptors (AChRs) (see Chap. 11). Acetylcholinesterase (AChE), the enzyme that terminates neurotransmitter action by hydrolyzing ACh to choline and acetate, is present in the basal lamina that coats the postsynaptic membrane. Voltage-dependent Na^+ channels are concentrated in the postsynaptic membrane, forming the troughs of the transverse folds.

The machinery for neurotransmitter release in the presynaptic terminal is also highly organized and is oriented with respect to the transverse folds of the postsynaptic membrane. A small fraction of the synaptic vesicles in the terminal are associated with regions of increased membrane density called release zones. These zones are located precisely over the infoldings of the postsynaptic membrane. Following nerve stimulation, vesicles at these sites fuse with the plasma membrane and release their content of ACh directly over the postsynaptic receptor molecules on the folds below.

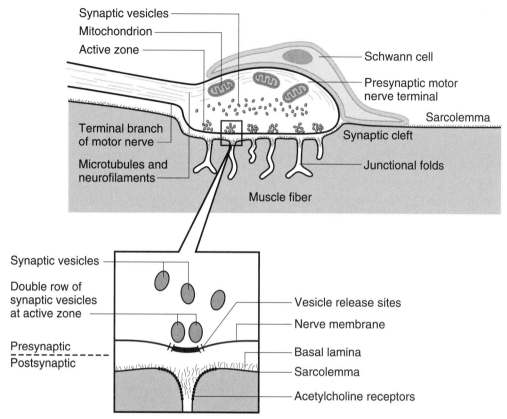

FIGURE 43-4.   Schematic representation of the key presynaptic and postsynaptic elements at the neuromuscular junction.

The muscle sarcolemma spreads the message

The muscle cell is surrounded by a plasma membrane that, together with the various connective tissue elements and collagen fibrils, forms the sarcolemma. The interior of the resting cell is maintained at an electrical potential about 80 mV more negative than the exterior by the combined action of pumps and channels in the plasma membrane. Unlike membranes of nerves, muscle membranes have a high conductance to chloride ions in the resting state; G_{Cl} accounts for about 70% of the total membrane conductance. Potassium ion conductance accounts for most of the remainder, and the membrane potential is normally close to the Nernst potential for these two ions (see Chap. 6). Asymmetrical concentration gradients for sodium and potassium ions are maintained at the cost of energy by the membrane Na,K-ATPase.

During the generation of an action potential, a rapid and stereotyped membrane depolarization is produced by an increase in sodium ion conductance mediated by voltage-dependent Na^+ channels [6]. The conductance increase is self-limited, and membrane repolarization is assisted by the delayed opening of a potassium ion conductance pathway. Action potentials originating at the NMJ spread in a nondecremental fashion over the entire surface of the muscle.

The transverse tubular system and sarcoplasmic reticulum combine to link electrical signals to Ca^{2+} release

Action potentials that originate in the sarcolemma penetrate the interior of the muscle cell along transverse (T) tubules that are continuous with the outer membrane (Fig. 43-5). These tubules are seen as openings on the surface of the muscle cell either at the level of the Z bands or at

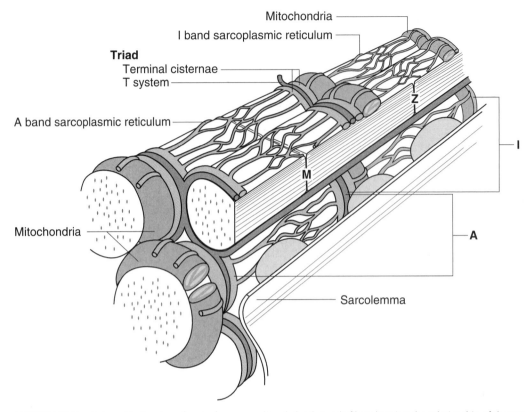

FIGURE 43-5.   Schematic drawing of part of a mammalian skeletal muscle fiber showing the relationship of the sarcoplasmic reticulum, terminal cisternae, transverse tubule (T) system and mitochondria to a few myofibrils.

the junction of the A and I bands, depending on the species, and the depolarization of this membrane system spreads activity to the center of the fiber. As this T-tubular network courses inward, close associations are formed with specialized terminal elements of the sarcoplasmic reticulum (SR). At the electron microscope level, the structure formed by a single tubule interposed between two terminal SR elements is called a *triad*. The SR stores Ca^{2+} in relaxed muscle and releases it into the sarcoplasm upon depolarization of the cell membrane and the T-tubular system.

A great deal of work has focused on the proteins present in the T-tubule/SR junction. These proteins may be the molecular counterpart of the so-called foot processes seen in electron micrographs by Franzini-Armstrong [7]. One protein, an integral component of the T-tubular membrane, is a form of L-type, dihydropyridine-sensitive, voltage-dependent calcium channel (see Box 23-1) [8]. Another, the ryanodine

receptor, is a large protein associated with the SR membrane in the triad that may couple the conformational changes in the Ca^{2+}-channel protein induced by T-tubular depolarization to the Ca^{2+} release from the SR [9].

A Ca^{2+}-channel protein is needed for coupling at the triad. The skeletal muscle T-tubular system contains a dihydropyridine-binding form of voltage-dependent Ca^{2+} channel. On biochemical analysis, this protein contains five subunits: a large α subunit, which contains the binding site for the dihydropyridines; a large, glycosylated β subunit; and smaller β, γ and δ subunits [6]. The α subunit bears strong sequence homology to the voltage-dependent Na^+ channel and by itself is capable of forming voltage-dependent ion channels when expressed in appropriate cell systems.

Skeletal muscle contains higher concentrations of this L-type Ca^{2+} channel that can be accounted for on the basis of measured voltage-dependent Ca^{2+} influx. It is now clear that much of the Ca^{2+}-channel protein in the T-tubular membrane does not actively gate calcium ion movement but, rather, acts as a voltage transducer that links depolarization of the T-tubular membrane to Ca^{2+} release through a receptor protein in the SR membrane.

The ryanodine receptor mediates sarcoplasmic reticulum Ca^{2+} release. The bar-like structures that connect the terminal elements of the SR with the T-tubular membrane in the triad are formed by a large protein that is the principal pathway for Ca^{2+} release from the SR [10]. This protein, which binds the plant alkaloid ryanodine with high affinity, is a huge homotetramer of 565-kDa polypeptide subunits. The purified complex, when incorporated into planar bilayers, exhibits Ca^{2+} channel activity that is modulated by ATP, Ca^{2+} and Mg^{2+}. The manner in which activation of the ryanodine receptor complex is coupled to events at the T-tubular membrane is not yet clear, although evidence now points to a direct mechanical linkage through a conformational change in the dihydropyridine receptor protein.

Ca^{2+} **reuptake** in the sarcoplasmic reticulum allows the relaxation of muscle and the maintenance of a low intracellular Ca^{2+} concentration in resting muscle by means of an ATP-dependent Ca^{2+} pump, the Ca^{2+}-ATPase, located in the SR membrane. The free energy of ATP hydrolysis is utilized for the concentrative uptake of Ca^{2+} into the SR vesicle through a phosphorylated enzyme intermediate (see Chap. 5). Other SR proteins assist in Ca^{2+} uptake and storage. Phospholamban is prominent in cardiac muscle and slow-twitch muscle, where its phosphorylation participates in the control of Ca^{2+}-ATPase and Ca^{2+}-uptake activity. Another protein, calsequestrin, contains numerous low-affinity Ca^{2+}-binding sites; it is present in the lumen of the SR and is thought to participate in the Ca^{2+}-storage function. Fast-twitch muscle contains a soluble Ca^{2+}-binding protein, parvalbumin, which is structurally related to troponin-C. Parvalbumin may play a role in regulating the Ca^{2+} concentration in the initial stages of relaxation (see Chap. 23).

DEFECTS IN NEUROMUSCULAR TRANSMISSION CAN INTERRUPT NORMAL MUSCLE FUNCTION

Since the NMJ represents the ultimate link between the CNS and the initiation of motor activity, diseases that affect its function can have profound clinical consequences. It also provides an "Achilles heel," an optimal target for toxins produced by predators whose intent is to immobilize their prey. An unusual number of plant products and animal toxins affect the NMJ (Table 43-1). In many cases, research into the pathophysiology of diseases and toxins affecting the junction has shed light on the underlying normal physiological mechanisms as well as on the clinical conditions themselves.

Events in synaptic transmission proceed in an orderly fashion from the depolarization of the presynaptic nerve terminal membrane through transmitter release and interaction with the postsynaptic membrane to the modulation of postsynaptic events (see Chap. 10). In considering pathological events at the NMJ, the same conceptual sequence is followed: toxins and disorders interfering with presynaptic mechanisms are considered first, followed by a discussion of those targeting events at the postsynaptic level.

TABLE 43-1.	**SOME TOXINS AND DISEASES AFFECTING THE NEUROMUSCULAR JUNCTION**[a]

Presynaptic action
  Botulinum toxin
  Black widow spider venom
  Snake β-neurotoxins
  Lambert-Eaton syndrome
Junctional action
  Inhibitors of AChE
  Congenital AChE deficiency
Postsynaptic action
  Snake α-neurotoxins
  Myasthenia gravis
  Congenital defects of ACh receptor structure

[a]AChE, acetylcholinesterase; ACh, acetylcholine.

Botulinum toxin blocks the release of synaptic vesicles from the presynaptic nerve terminal

Botulism is the clinical disorder that results from exposure to one of a family of exotoxins produced by strains of the bacterium *Clostridium botulinum* [11]. It usually results from the ingestion of foods contaminated with the anaerobic *Clostridium* organisms but can be produced by contamination of a deep penetrating wound with toxin-producing bacterium. The botulinum exotoxin is one of the most toxic substances known; a dose of less than 50 μg can be lethal in humans. This toxin specifically blocks neuromuscular transmission. If not treated rapidly, ingestion of the toxin can result in widespread weakness and ultimately death due to paralysis of the muscles of respiration. In addition, botulinum toxin interferes with transmission at cholinergic parasympathetic terminals, producing autonomic symptoms.

At least eight closely related forms of botulinum toxin have been identified (see Chap. 9). Although these toxins appear to be produced by the *Clostridium* bacteria, they are in fact the result of a lysogenic infection of the bacterium with a phage containing the genetic information encoding the toxin molecule. Individuals exposed to botulinum toxin develop progressive failure of neuromuscular transmission characterized by an abnormally small electrical response in muscle after maximal stimulation of the motor nerve, although activation and conduction in the motor nerve itself are normal. Repeated stimulation of the motor nerve leads to an increase in the amplitude of the muscle response, in contrast to the decremental response seen in patients with myasthenia gravis (see below). These clinical findings point to a defect in the release of ACh from the presynaptic terminal, which is overcome in part by the elevated levels of intraterminal Ca^{2+} that are produced by repetitive depolarizations.

Botulinum toxin is synthesized as an inactive protomer of ~150 kDa, which must be cleaved into two fragments of ~100 kDa and 50 kDa before it becomes biologically active [12]. These two components, designated the heavy

and light chains, are joined by a disulfide bridge; both are needed for toxicity.

The initial step in toxin action involves the binding of the disulfide-linked, light chain–heavy chain complex to specific receptors on the presynaptic membrane. Molecules of toxin bound to the surface membrane are then internalized in membrane vesicles, which ultimately discharge their contents into lysosomes. The toxin must then cross the lysosomal membrane and enter the cytoplasm before it can interfere with transmitter release. Here, the amino-terminal portion of the heavy chain plays a unique role (Fig. 43-6). It can form a transmembrane channel in a lipid bilayer that is large enough to

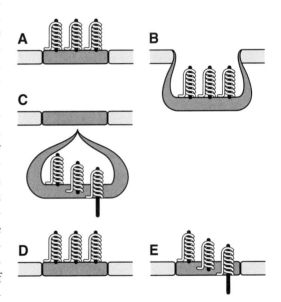

FIGURE 43-6. Proposed mechanism for the translocation of botulinum toxin into presynaptic nerve terminals. **A:** The toxin binds to a specific class of receptors on the plasma membrane of cholinergic nerve terminals. **B:** The toxin is then internalized by the process of receptor-mediated endocytosis. The endocytotic vesicles become progressively more acidic as they approach the lysosome, and the fall in pH triggers a conformational change in the toxin molecule. A portion of the molecule, probably the N terminus, partitions into the membrane and forms a channel. **C:** The light chain may then pass through this channel to reach the ultimate cytoplasmic site of action of the toxin. **D:** In an alternative mechanism, binding of the toxin complex to receptors on the cell surface may lead directly to endocytosis when the tissue is exposed to a medium with low pH and **E:** triggers pH-dependent channel formation in the plasma membrane. (From [11], with permission.)

allow an extended peptide chain to pass. In artificial bilayers, channel-forming activity is pH-dependent; it is most prominent when the side of the bilayer corresponding to the intralysosomal surface is at low pH, about 4.5, while the cytoplasmic face is neutral, pH 7.0, corresponding to the conditions that prevail *in vivo*.

The toxicity of botulinum toxin ultimately involves the action of the 50-kDa light chain after it is released into the cytoplasm of the presynaptic terminal. A very small number of toxin molecules, probably fewer than 20, are capable of completely blocking all stimulus-induced transmitter release from a synapse, suggesting that an amplification step is involved. The toxin light chains are specific proteases that cleave synaptobrevin, SNAP-25 or syntaxin, which form the trimolecular complex that acts in the priming and partial fusion of synaptic vesicles with plasmalemma prior to the Ca^{2+}-triggered release of ACh (see Chap. 9).

Black widow spider venom stimulates abnormal release of acetylcholine

The bite of the black widow spider initially produces an increase in neuromuscular activity that leads to painful skeletal muscle spasms and rigidity. This phase of hyperexcitability is rapidly followed by progressive failure of neuromuscular transmission and paralysis. The venom induces a transient but dramatic increase in spontaneous quantal release of ACh, followed by a progressive decline and failure of both spontaneous and induced transmitter release and depletion of presynaptic vesicles.

The toxic component of the venom of the female spider is a 130-kDa protein called α-latrotoxin; it has no known enzymatic activity [13]. When applied to planar lipid bilayers, purified latrotoxin forms an ion channel with a conductance in excess of 100 pS that is permeant to Na^+, K^+ and Ca^{2+} but not to anions [14]. If α-latrotoxin has a similar effect on the presynaptic membrane, the result will be membrane depolarization and Ca^{2+} influx; the depolarization alone could activate voltage-dependent Ca^{2+} channels, further adding to the influx of Ca^{2+}. The net effect would be the triggering of

synaptic vesicle fusion and transmitter release on a massive scale and eventually depletion of the neurotransmitter stores in the terminal. However, other mechanisms of action are also involved. It is necessary to explain how the activity of α-latrotoxin is confined so exquisitely to the presynaptic nerve terminal *in vivo* and how α-latrotoxin has both Ca^{2+}-dependent and Ca^{2+}-independent effects.

Two neuronal surface proteins that bind α-latrotoxin with nanomolar affinities have been found: neurexin-1α binds α-latrotoxin in a Ca^{2+}-dependent manner and latrophilin binds α-latrotoxin independently of Ca^{2+}. Latrophilin is also called calcium-independent receptor for latrotoxin (CIRL) [15]. Neurexins comprise a family of neuron-specific membrane proteins likely to be involved in axonal guidance, synaptogenesis and cell recognition. Neurexin-1α binds α-latrotoxin directly, with a K_d of about 4 nM, which is dependent on Ca^{2+} concentrations in the range of 30 mM [16]. Neurexin-1α also binds to synaptotagmin and syntaxin, presynaptic proteins involved in the fusion of synaptic vesicles with plasmalemma after priming (see Chap. 9), and this complex can be copurified on an α-latrotoxin affinity column. Although neurexin binding to synaptotagmin itself is independent of Ca^{2+} [17], antibodies against syntaxin and the neurexin coprecipitate [^{125}I]ω-conotoxin-binding sites, which reflects the association of this whole presynaptic molecular complex with Ca^{2+} channels [18].

Latrophilin is an *N*-glycosylated, single-polypeptide chain of 120 kDa that binds α-latrotoxin with a K_d of 0.5 to 0.7 nM and is differentially distributed among neuronal tissues. It is present in cerebral cortex at four times the amount found in cerebellum, and is highly enriched in synaptosomal membranes [19]. Molecular cloning and functional expression of the Ca^{2+}-independent receptor demonstrate that it is a member of the secretin receptor family and that it is coupled to a G protein. CIRL is copurified with syntaxin, a component of the synaptic vesicle fusion complex, on an α-latrotoxin affinity column and forms stable complexes with syntaxin *in vitro*, thus demonstrating that CIRL is a component of the synaptic vesicle fusion process in neurosecretion [20].

Knockout mice lacking the neurexin-1α gene demonstrate loss of Ca^{2+}-dependent binding of α-latrotoxin to brain membranes and major reductions in the [³H]glutamate release from synaptosomes that is triggered by α-latrotoxin in the presence of Ca^{2+}. Cultured hippocampal neurons derived from these animals, however, still show α-latrotoxin-activated neurotransmission in the absence of neurexin-1α. Thus, neurexin-1α, while not essential for α-latrotoxin action, does contribute to the action when Ca^{2+} is present. It has been proposed that α-latrotoxin action is mediated by two independent pathways: the CIRL/latrophilin path, which is sufficient for neurotransmitter release, and the neurexin-1α path, which contributes to the Ca^{2+}-dependent effects of α-latrotoxin [15]. The use of α-latrotoxin will assist in elucidating the processes of synaptic vesicle fusion and regulation of secretion and neurotransmitter release (see Chap. 9).

Some snake venoms contain β-toxins that interrupt presynaptic events

Many snake venoms contain polypeptide toxins that act on the NMJ. Some α-toxins act by interfering with the function of AChRs in the postsynaptic membrane; these toxins will be considered later in this chapter. A second group, the β-toxins, interferes with neuromuscular transmission through actions on the presynaptic nerve terminal. Although β-toxins are produced by a variety of crotalids, the β-bungarotoxin found in the venom of the snake *Bungarus multicinctus* is the best studied of this group.

β-Bungarotoxin, a protein of 20.5 kDa, is a heterodimer of a 13.5-kDa A chain and a 7-kDa B chain linked by at least one disulfide bond [21]. About 25 ng of this toxin is lethal to a mouse. The toxin inhibits the release of synaptic vesicles from motor nerve terminals and from some cholinergic autonomic terminals. Its onset of action is rather slow and involves a molecular rearrangement, not necessarily endocytosis, that abolishes immunobinding.

All of the presynaptically acting snake venoms exhibit phospholipase A_2 (PLA_2) activity [22] (see Chap. 3). This activity is abolished by treatment with *p*-bromophenacyl bromide

(BPB), which specifically modifies histidine residue 48 in the A chain. The A chain exhibits extensive sequence homology with other enzymes with PLA_2 activity, especially those from the porcine pancreas. The β-bungarotoxin B chain has sequence homology with a number of protease inhibitors.

After exposure of an isolated nerve–muscle preparation to β-bungarotoxin, there is first a slight reduction in end-plate potential (EPP) amplitude. This is followed over the next hour by an augmentation of EPP amplitude and, finally, by a slow but progressive decrease in amplitude that ends in complete block of stimulated transmitter release. During the second stage, there is also a transient increase in the frequency of miniature EPPs (MEPPs) consistent with an increase in intraterminal free Ca^{2+}. These effects require intact PLA_2 activity. Studies of a number of different PLA_2 neurotoxins indicate that these toxins bind at or near the cell surface and that their action, which is blocked by strontium ion, is on the plasma membrane [23]. The existence of a β-bungarotoxin-binding protein, called a presynaptic membrane receptor (PsMR), which may be involved in axon terminal slow K^+ currents and specifically reactive with subclasses of T and B cells in patients with myasthenia gravis (see later), is the subject of ongoing research [24,25].

Autoimmune diseases can interfere with neurotransmitter release

Some patients with carcinoma, especially small-cell carcinoma of the lung, develop an unusual syndrome of muscle weakness associated with autonomic dysfunction called the Lambert-Eaton myasthenic syndrome (LEMS). Complaints often begin with progressive proximal muscle weakness and fatigue; unlike myasthenia gravis, bulbar involvement is usually mild and respiratory compromise is unusual. Autonomic complaints can include dry mouth, impotence and orthostasis.

These patients demonstrate a remarkable reduction in the amplitude of the compound muscle action potential produced by single supramaximal stimulus to the motor nerve of a resting muscle [26]. Repeated stimulation of the same nerve, however, results in progressive improvement in response amplitude, often returning to nearly normal levels. These clinical findings are indicative of a defect in presynaptic neurotransmitter release.

When analyzed at the single cell level, LEMS is characterized by a dramatic reduction in the mean quantal content of the EPP, often to 10% or less of normal values. The amplitude of spontaneous MEPPs is normal, as is the MEPP frequency, but the MEPP frequency does not increase normally with increasing extracellular Ca^{2+}. Repetitive stimulation causes a progressive increase in quantal content of the EPP, consistent with the improvement seen in the compound muscle action potential.

LEMS is an autoimmune disease. The salient features of the disease can be passively transferred to mice by injection of IgG from patients who have the disorder. The autoantibodies in LEMS are heterogeneous and target a number of presynaptic proteins. Antibodies are most commonly observed against P/Q-type voltage-gated Ca^{2+} channels (VGCCs), but antibodies against L- and N-type VGCCs are also present (see Box 23-1). Antibodies against the synaptic vesicle protein synaptotagmin (see Chap. 9) have also been identified. A recent study with synthetic peptides suggests that the S5-6 loop in the VGCC α subunit is a particularly active target for LEMS autoantibodies.

In freeze-fracture images of presynaptic membranes (see Chap. 10), the normal organization of the large intramembranous particles that form the double rows of the active zones is disrupted. These particles are thought to represent Ca^{2+} channels associated with specific release sites for synaptic vesicles. The number of arrays is reduced, with many particles found instead in irregular aggregates. Mice treated with IgG from LEMS patients demonstrate the same changes in intramembranous particle distribution. In small-cell lung carcinoma, tumors express VGCCs on the surface, and Ca^{2+} currents in these cells are inhibited by LEMS serum. It seems likely that an immune response against the VGCC population in these cells causes the pathology in LEMS by cross-reacting with similar epitopes in presynaptic VGCCs in autonomic and neuromuscular junctions.

TOXINS AND DISEASES CAN ALSO BLOCK TRANSMISSION AT THE POSTSYNAPTIC LEVEL

ACh released from the nerve terminal interacts specifically with AChR molecules in the postsynaptic membrane (see Chap. 11). Molecules of AChE in the junctional basal lamina compete for the transmitter and inactivate it by hydrolysis, forming acetate and choline. Successful transmission requires that a significant proportion of the ACh in each quantum reaches receptors in the postsynaptic membrane prior to being hydrolyzed. This in turn depends on the relative number of functional AChR and AChE molecules present as well as their geometric organization in relation to the release zones of the motor nerve terminal. The safety margin of transmission can be adversely affected, and junctional transmission blocked, by factors that modify the number of AChRs, their functional ability or their organization in the synapse, as well as by factors that alter the properties of AChE.

α-Neurotoxins block the activation of nicotinic acetylcholine receptors

Toxins produced by snakes of the families Elapidae (cobras, kraits, coral snakes, mambas and so forth) and Hydrophidae (sea snakes) contain potent neuromuscular toxins. A major component in each of these toxins is a curarimimetic α-neurotoxin, which produces a nondepolarizing block of the postsynaptic AChR. When applied to the NMJ, these related small proteins block both EPPs and MEPPs. The frequency of MEPPs is not changed by pure α-toxin, although crude venom, which contains β-toxins as well, may have dramatic presynaptic effects. The LD_{50} for these toxins is typically 50 to 150 μg/kg in mice. Exposure of humans to low doses of toxin which induce partial blockade of junctional receptors can produce a clinical picture of weakness and fatigability that resembles acquired myasthenia gravis. Higher doses can lead to complete neuromuscular block, paralysis, respiratory failure and death. Scorpion venoms contain an insecticidal α-neurotoxin which binds to and slows the inactivation of axonal voltage-sensitive Na^+ channels (Chap. 6).

The α-toxins responsible for the postsynaptic curarimimetic activity are low-molecular-weight basic proteins of 7 to 8 kDa [27]. Chemically, they fall into two groups: the long toxins, which have 71 to 74 amino acids and five internal disulfide bonds, and the short toxins, with 60 to 62 amino acids and four internal disulfide bonds. All of the α-toxins have about the same equilibrium dissociation constant for the AChR, but they differ markedly in their binding kinetics. The short toxins bind to and dissociate from the AChR five to nine times faster than the long toxins. Because of this, the binding of the short toxins can be reversed by washing, while the long toxins bind essentially irreversibly. The relative irreversibility of the binding of the long α-neurotoxins to the AChR, especially that of α-bungarotoxin from the venom of *B. multicinctus,* has made them valuable tools for the purification and characterization of this ion-channel protein. Recently, α-bungarotoxin-sensitive nicotinic receptor currents have also been identified on interneurons in the hippocampus [28].

The α-toxins exhibit a high degree of homology when their primary sequences are aligned with respect to the cysteine residues. Several have been crystallized and their tertiary structure determined. The proteins are concave disks with a small projection at one end. Their elliptical dimensions are approximately 3.8 × 2.8 × 1.5 nm, and for the most part, the structure is only a single polypeptide chain thick. The reactive site of the protein is on the concave surface and involves the regions encompassed by residues 32 to 45 and 49 to 56 as well as isolated residues from other regions of the molecule.

The α-neurotoxins bind specifically to sites on the α subunits of the AChR; there is one binding site per subunit and, thus, two binding sites per receptor molecule (see Chap. 11). The binding site on the α subunit sterically overlaps that for ACh, and α-bungarotoxin binding prevents the interaction of ACh with the receptor. Binding of toxin to the α subunit of the nicotinic AChR may involve interactions at the interfaces between the α and other subunits [29,30].

Chronic treatment of rat diaphragm with α-bungarotoxin leads to upregulation of ACh quantal release from presynaptic terminals, which is apparently dependent on Ca^{2+}/calmodulin kinase II and tyrosine kinases in the presynaptic membrane [31]. Immunization with mixtures of several synthetic α-bungarotoxin peptide sequences has produced quite effective protection in mice later challenged with the whole toxin [32].

In myasthenia gravis, an autoimmune response against the acetylcholine receptor leads to neuromuscular failure

Myasthenia gravis (MG), the prototypic human disorder of neuromuscular transmission, is an acquired autoimmune disease affecting AChRs on the postsynaptic membrane. Clinically, the disorder is characterized by muscle weakness and abnormal fatigability. Most patients have circulating antibodies against the AChR in their serum.

Patients with MG typically show fluctuating symptoms; weakness and fatigability may be worse in the evenings and usually become more severe with exercise. Weakness may involve only the extraocular muscles, producing diplopia, or may be so extensive as to cause quadriparesis and respiratory compromise. Although spontaneous remissions can occur, the untreated disease is often progressive and can eventually lead to death from respiratory failure.

The classic electrophysiological observation in MG is a decremental response in the extracellularly recorded compound muscle action potential with repeated nerve stimulation (Fig. 43-7). Using intracellular electrodes, the amplitude of the MEPP is found to be decreased. The quantum content of the EPP is normal, although its amplitude is reduced consequent to a reduction in MEPP amplitude. The decrease in MEPP amplitude is due to a reduction in the number of AChR molecules present in the postsynaptic membrane combined with a pathological alteration in the architecture of the postsynaptic membrane.

The density of receptors in the myasthenic postsynaptic membrane may be as low as 20% of normal. In addition, the highly organized architecture of the postsynaptic membrane, with junctional folds immediately subjacent to presyn-

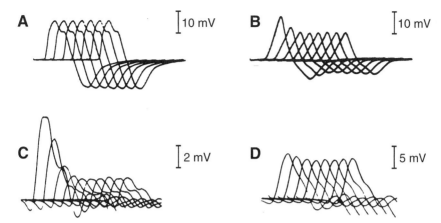

FIGURE 43-7. Compound muscle action potentials recorded from the abductor digiti minimi of human subjects during repetitive stimulation of the ulnar nerve at three stimuli per second. **A:** A recording from a normal individual shows no change in the amplitude of the muscle electrical response during the stimulation interval. **B:** In a patient with myasthenia gravis (MG), the same stimuli produce a 40% decrement in response amplitude over the first five stimuli, with a slow partial recovery during subsequent stimulation. Similar studies from a patient with severe MG before **(C)** and 2 min after **(D)** intravenous administration of 10 mg edrophonium, a short-acting acetylcholinesterase inhibitor. Note the change in amplitude scale between the two recordings and the reversal of the abnormal decrement by edrophonium.

aptic active zones and high densities of AChRs at the crests of these folds, is lost. The distance between pre- and postsynaptic membrane is often increased, and the postsynaptic membrane is highly simplified.

The destruction seen at the postsynaptic membrane is mediated by antibodies directed against the AChR [33]. Although it is attractive to postulate that functional block of AChRs by circulating antibodies is the primary mechanism through which transmission failure occurs, this does not seem to be the case. The major effects of anti-AChR antibodies seem to be twofold. First, antibodies cross-link receptor proteins and increase their rates of endocytosis and lysosomal degradation. In the absence of an increased rate of receptor synthesis, this results in a net decrease in receptor density in the postsynaptic membrane. Second, these antibodies target the postsynaptic membrane for complement fixation and activation of the lytic phase of the complement reaction cascade. The presence of lytic complement C9 in myasthenic postsynaptic membranes has been demonstrated both in humans and in animal models.

Although the mechanism of ongoing neuromuscular damage in this disease has been de-

fined, the nature of the initial triggering event is unclear. One hypothesis involves the role of myocytes, muscle-like cells that occur in the thymus gland. These cells express AChRs on their surface membranes. An initial inflammatory response in the thymus may trigger the generation of cross-reacting antibodies that subsequently target AChRs on muscle. This hypothesis would help to explain the beneficial role of thymectomy in patients with MG. The diversity of predisposing and associated factors, however, suggests that a number of different triggering events may lead to the development of a common clinical picture.

Genetic defects in receptor structure can produce clinical disease

Given the central role of the AChR in neuromuscular transmission, it is reasonable to expect that mutations that affect channel function will also interfere with normal neuromuscular transmission. Defects that render the channel nonfunctional would be lethal, but milder alterations might be compatible with life.

Recently, investigators have described several genetic disorders of neuromuscular transmission that in some ways resemble MG as it is seen in infants. In one of these, an abnormally low density of AChRs was found at the NMJ. In the other, the kinetics of channel opening appeared abnormal, with a marked prolongation of the EPP and MEPP, which was further increased by the addition of AChE inhibitors [34]. Although the quantum content of the EPP was normal, its amplitude was significantly reduced. Activity and kinetic properties of AChE were normal. It is postulated that the defect in this disorder is an abnormally slow closing rate for the channel.

Abnormalities in acetylcholinesterase activity can interfere with neuromuscular transmission

At the NMJ, the duration of neurotransmitter action on the postsynaptic membrane is controlled by the rate of hydrolysis of ACh by AChE (see Chap. 11). This enzyme is associated with the basal lamina between the presynaptic membrane and the muscle plasma membrane. Roughly one-third of the released ACh from each quantum is hydrolyzed before reaching the postsynaptic membrane. The remaining molecules interact with postsynaptic receptors but are rapidly inactivated before having an opportunity for significant lateral spread. Thus, the site of action of released ACh is focused at a small area under the point of release from the presynaptic active zone.

   Inhibition of AChE allows ACh to diffuse laterally out of the synapse and to interact with additional receptors along the way. The result is a marked prolongation of the EPP. Also, since receptors are desensitized after exposure to their transmitter, prolonged exposure to ACh eventually leads to reduced sensitivity and to block of neuromuscular transmission. Careful reduction of end-plate AChE activity following administration of AChEs can prolong the action of released ACh sufficiently to increase the amplitude of an abnormally low EPP above that required for successful neuromuscular transmission. It is this effect that allows these agents to be used in the treatment of MG. Too much medication, however, will produce long-term postsynaptic depolarization, receptor inactivation and trans-

mission block. Irreversible inhibitors of AChE are components of some nerve gases, and accidental poisoning by organophosphate insecticides can be fatal (see Chap. 11).

ABNORMAL EXCITABILITY OF THE SARCOLEMMA CAN AFFECT MUSCLE FUNCTION

Once a signal from a motor neuron has passed the NMJ, it must be spread throughout the muscle fiber as an action potential that is propagated along the sarcolemma and into the T-tubular system. The electrical activity of the sarcolemma must faithfully reproduce the activity of the innervating axon if the resulting contraction is to be of the intensity and duration dictated by the CNS. If the sarcolemma responds with multiple action potentials to a single stimulus at the NMJ, prolonged contractions will occur. Conversely, if the sarcolemma fails to respond to a postsynaptic potential of normal size, paralysis of the muscle will ensue. Both of these situations do occur: in the hyperexcitable states of the myotonic disorders and in the propagation failure of the periodic paralyses.

Normal excitability in the sarcolemma requires the integrated function of numerous ion channels

Like other excitable membranes, the muscle sarcolemmal membrane potential is produced by asymmetrical distributions of Na^+, K^+ and Cl^- ions in conjunction with varying conductances to these ions that are controlled by specific ion channels (Chap. 6). Action potentials result from a rapid but self-limited increase in Na^+ conductance mediated by voltage-dependent Na^+ channels, while activation of a delayed K^+ channel assists in membrane repolarization. Both channels function in muscle much as they do in nerve membranes (see Chap. 6).

   The T-tubular system in muscle, however, imposes some special constraints. Although the amount of K^+ moving outward with each action potential is normally inconsequential with respect to transmembrane concentration gradients when released into the extracellular space outside a neuron or muscle fiber, the same amount of K^+ released into the restricted volume of the tubule can increase the local K^+ concentration by as much as 0.4 mM with each impulse. This K^+ must diffuse out of the tubule, a process that occurs with a time constant of 20 msec or more.

With repeated stimulation of a muscle fiber, K^+ will accumulate in the T-tubular system. If K^+ conductance were the predominant ion conductance in the resting muscle surface membrane, this accumulation would ultimately cause depolarization of the sarcolemma, interfering with normal signal propagation. This effect is minimized in skeletal muscle by the presence of a high resting conductance to chloride ions (G_{Cl-}) in the sarcolemma. This shunting conductance normally damps out the effect of T-tubular potassium ion accumulation on the sarcolemmal membrane potential.

Abnormalities of membrane Cl^- conductance can induce repetitive firing in the sarcolemma

A number of human muscle diseases are characterized by an abnormality of muscle relaxation called myotonia. *Myotonia* is the persistent contraction of a skeletal muscle following voluntary activation that is associated with repetitive action potential generation in the surface membrane. The most common of these is myotonic muscular dystrophy, which is actually a multisystem disease in which the myotonic feature is a relatively minor component. In two other diseases, *myotonia congenita* and *recessive generalized myotonia*, however, myotonia is the major presenting symptom and is often the only abnormality found [35]. Patients afflicted with these inherited diseases have trouble relaxing their muscles normally: doorknobs and handshakes are difficult to release, clumsiness is a problem and falls often occur.

Years ago, an interesting disease similar to human myotonia congenita was described in a breed of goats. When studied electrically, muscle fibers from these goats generated multiple repetitive action potentials in response to a single stimulus; these persistent runs of action potentials caused a striking delay in relaxation of the

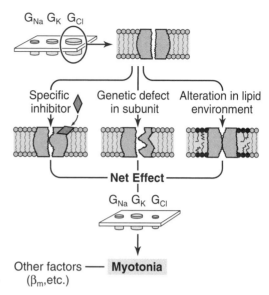

FIGURE 43-8. Myotonia can be produced in skeletal muscle by a variety of factors that block membrane chloride conductance *(G_{Cl})*. In normal muscle, this can result from exposure to specific inhibitors of the channel or from alterations in the lipid environment. Genetic defects in the channel protein underlie the most common inherited myotonic disorders.

muscle after a short stimulus to the motor nerve. Studies of these myotonic goats showed that the sarcolemma in affected animals had a remarkable reduction in membrane Cl^- conductance, often to less than 20% of normal. Blockade of Cl^- channels in normal goat muscle duplicated both the symptoms and the electrical abnormalities of the myotonic animals. Subsequently, a number of drugs and toxins that caused transient myotonia in animals and humans were found to act by blocking the sarcolemmal Cl^- channel, eventually leading to the hypothesis that many of the human myotonic disorders were also Cl^- channel defects (Fig. 43-8).

Mutations in the ClC1 muscle Cl^- channel produce human disease

Application of molecular genetic approaches to the human myotonic disorders has proven very fruitful. Myotonic dystrophy, which produces muscle weakness and wasting, mental retardation and skeletal and gonadal abnormalities in addition to myotonia, is associated with an expanded trinucleotide repeat mutation (see Chap. 40) at chromosome 19. The gene associated with this mutation appears to affect a form of kinase. The mechanism by which this mutation produces myotonia is as yet unknown. In myotonia congenita and recessive generalized myotonia, in which muscle myotonic symptoms are the principal expression of the disease, tight linkage has been found at chromosome 7q35. This site encodes the ClC1 skeletal muscle Cl^- channel family, whose members control anion flux in a number of tissues and are closely related in structure [36]. The ClC1 protein product is about 90 kDa, and four ClC1 monomers probably interact to form a single-channel homotetramer. Multiple mutations in the Cl^- channel coding sequence have now been identified in this gene in both the dominant and recessive forms of myotonia congenita (Fig. 43-9) [36].

A role for Cl^- channel mutations in producing human myotonia is also supported by work with the mouse mutants *mto* and *adr*. The phenotypes of both mutants resemble recessive generalized myotonia, and they show the same abnormal electrical activity and low Cl^- conduc-tance in the muscle membranes. The *adr* mutation is caused by a mutation in the skeletal muscle Cl^- channel (ClC1) gene that results from a transposon insertion [37]. The ClC1 gene is located on a portion of the mouse chromosome that is syntenic with the location of the defective human gene in myotonia congenita and recessive generalized myotonia.

The fact that mutations in the gene encoding ClC1 can produce either dominant or recessive effects was surprising. Mutants that introduce frameshifts of stop codons early in the coding sequence will produce a nonfunctional protein product. With one defective gene copy, wild-type channels encoded by the second gene copy should produce a net G_{Cl^-} about 50% of normal. When both gene copies carry the mutation, expression of the functional channels will be very low or absent and, as a recessive disorder, the myotonia can be severe. Point mutations can also lead to the alteration of a single amino acid in the primary structure of an otherwise full-length channel monomer, and channels formed from tetramers of this protein may not function normally. The possibility also exists that chan-

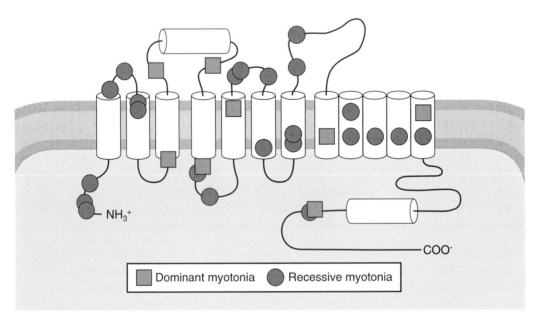

FIGURE 43-9. Approximate location of mutations reported in the skeletal muscle voltage-dependent chloride ion channel associated with either dominant or recessive myotonia. The secondary and tertiary structures of this channel remain largely unresolved; the model presented here is derived from that of Jentsch [48]. In particular, the topology of five potential transmembrane helices toward the carboxy terminus of the protein is unclear. The functional channel probably contains four of these monomeric subunits.

nels containing even a single mutant subunit may fail to function even though the other subunits are encoded by a normal copy of the gene. Such a dominant-negative effect, which has been demonstrated for a number of myotonia congenita mutations, leads to a dominant transmission of the disease phenotype. Since mixed tetramers containing different numbers of mutant subunits may have different levels of residual activity, the resulting membrane G_{Cl^-} may be more variable and the disease phenotype less severe than in the recessive form of the disease.

When the sarcolemma is not sufficiently excitable, weakness or paralysis can result

A fascinating group of inherited muscle diseases called the *periodic paralyses* is characterized by intermittent episodes of skeletal muscle weakness or paralysis that occur in people who usually appear completely normal between attacks. The periods of paralysis are often associated with changes in the serum K^+ concentration; while the serum K^+ concentration can go either up or down, the direction is usually consistent for a particular family and forms one basis for classifying these diseases as either *hyperkalemic* or *hypokalemic*. A variant of periodic paralysis, in which spells of weakness are less frequent and in which a form of myotonic hyperexcitability is often seen, is called *paramyotonia congenita*.

Recordings from muscle fibers isolated from patients during an attack of periodic paralysis have shown that the paralytic episodes are associated with acute depolarization of the sarcolemma. In all forms of the disease, this depolarization is due to an increase in membrane conductance to Na^+. In the case of hyperkalemic periodic paralysis and paramyotonia congenita, this abnormal conductance can be blocked by tetrodotoxin, a small polar molecule that is highly specific for the voltage-dependent Na^+ channel. Single-channel recordings in hyperkalemic periodic paralysis have revealed that some of the muscle membrane Na^+ channels show abnormal inactivation kinetics, intermittently entering a mode in which they fail to inactivate. These channels will produce a persistent, noninactivating Na^+ current that will in turn produce membrane depolarization. Since normal Na^+ channels enter an inactivated state after depolarization (see Chap. 6), the net result of long-term depolarization will be a loss of sarcolemmal excitability and paralysis.

Na$^+$ channel mutations cause periodic paralysis

The voltage-dependent Na^+ channel in skeletal muscle closely resembles those found in brain and cardiac muscle [38] (see Chap. 6). The purified protein contains one very large α subunit of ~260 kDa and one 38-kDa β subunit. Both subunits are heavily glycosylated. The α subunit, which has been cloned, sequenced and functionally expressed, contains all of the elements necessary for a normal ion-selective channel. This subunit has four large internal repeat domains, each encompassing 220 to 300 amino acids. Each domain contains six to eight transmembrane helices organized compactly in the plane of the membrane. Current models of channel structure propose that the four repeat domains are organized in a ring to form a central ion channel. One helix in each domain, the S4 helix, contains positively charged lysine or arginine residues at every third residue, separated by nonpolar amino acids. This positively charged helix plays a central role in the voltage-sensing function of the channel.

Several other regions of the sequence also play important functional roles. The extracellular loops that connect helices S5 and S6 in each domain fold back into the membrane to form the lining of the channel ion pore. Residues in this region control channel conductance and selectivity. The cytoplasmic loop joining the third and fourth repeat domains is also important; this region closes the channel during the inactivation process that follows voltage-dependent activation.

Once the voltage-dependent Na^+ channel had been cloned and sequenced from human skeletal muscle and its chromosomal localization determined, it was possible to test the involvement of this channel with the disease through genetic linkage analysis. Measurements in families with both hyperkalemic periodic paralysis and paramyotonia demonstrated a very tight linkage between the adult skeletal muscle Na^+ channel gene on chromosome 17q23.3–25.1 (SCN4A) and the phenotypic expression of the disease [39]. The hypokalemic form of periodic paralysis is not linked to this Na^+ channel gene.

When the sequences of the normal human skeletal muscle Na^+ channel and of the gene that encodes it became available, the door was opened to a direct analysis of defects in the coding sequence that might produce clinical disease. More than 20 different mutations have now been identified in the coding region of the SCN4A gene in different families with hyperkalemic periodic paralysis or paramyotonia congenita (Fig. 43-10) [39]. Although these mutations are distributed through a wide range of the channel coding region, a number are clustered in the ID3-4 region, known from biophysical studies to control inactivation. Others are located near the cytoplasmic ends of helices S5

and S6; these regions may contribute to the binding site for the ID3-4 inactivation gate when it closes. Mutations in these regions may destabilize this closed conformation, leading to abnormalities in channel inactivation. In addition to shedding light on the origin of the symptoms of the disease, each of these human mutations provides additional insight into the relationships between structure and function in the normal channel.

Most Na^+ channel mutations in periodic paralysis produce functional channels, but these channels have abnormalities in the kinetics of inactivation. Mutants associated with the paramyotonia congenita phenotype show a marked slowing in the major component of fast inactivation. In some cases, the voltage dependence of the inactivation rate constant, τ_h, is markedly reduced as well and the mutations appear to uncouple the inactivation process from the voltage-dependent events associated with inactivation.

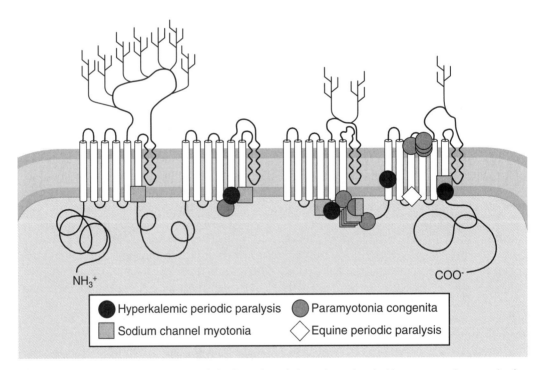

FIGURE 43-10. Mutations in the SkM1 skeletal muscle Na^+ channel associated with paramyotonia congenita, hyperkalemic periodic paralysis and atypical forms of myotonia. The Na^+ channel α subunit contains four repeat domains, each with six transmembrane segments. Most mutations are located in domains 3 and 4, with particular concentration in the interdomain 3–4 loop. The location of a mutation associated with equine periodic paralysis is also shown.

In some families with hyperkalemic periodic paralysis, the mutations cause a small, persistent inward Na^+ current at the macroscopic level that is the result of a shift in channel modal gating. Normal skeletal muscle Na^+ channels can shift between a fast and a slow inactivation gating mode. Usually, most of the channels are found in the fast inactivation mode. Channels with hyperkalemic periodic paralysis mutations spend a greater percentage of the time in the "slow" inactivation gating mode, and late openings associated with this slow gating mode contribute to the persistent inward macroscopic current seen with these mutations.

Under voltage-clamp conditions at the single-channel level, SkM1 channels with paramyotonia congenita mutations show multiple late openings and prolonged openings after depolarization. These late openings account for the slow inactivation observed at the macroscopic level. Hyperkalemic periodic paralysis mutations also show multiple late openings at the single-channel level, but these abnormal events are temporally clustered, consistent with an underlying shift in modal gating. Single-channel conductance is not altered by any of these mutations.

All sodium ion channel mutations in periodic paralysis produce dominant-negative effects. Although some mutant channels only intermittently exhibit abnormal inactivation, this small population of abnormally inactivating channels can modify the behavior of the remaining mutant and normal channels present in the membrane. Unlike the Cl^- channel mutations in myotonia congenita, which produce dominant-negative effects within a single channel multimer, these Na^+ channel mutations produce dominant-negative effects that reflect the relationship of normal channel inactivation to membrane potential. The persistent inward current carried by a small population of noninactivating channels, or the prolonged inward current resulting from mutant channels with slowed inactivation rates, results in a slight but long-lasting membrane depolarization. Since the relationship between voltage and inactivation in normal channels is very steep near the resting potential, this slight depolarization can produce inactivation of normal channels. If depolarization is sufficient, too few channels will remain in the noninactivated state to satisfy the requirements for a regenerative action potential and the muscle will become paralyzed.

Na^+ channel mutations also occur in heart and brain

While most attention has been focused on the SkM1 skeletal muscle Na^+ ion channel, mutations in other human Na^+ channel isoforms can also cause disease. Mutations in the cardiac Na^+ channel gene SCN5A, located on chromosome 3p21, produce the long QT syndrome [40]. In this disease, a short deletion in the ID3-4 region causes abnormal inactivation in this cardiac channel, leading to persistent depolarizing currents that can trigger fatal cardiac arrhythmias. Other forms of the same syndrome are associated with mutations in a cardiac potassium ion channel. Mutations in a brain Na^+ channel isoform, SCN8A, have recently been identified as the cause of several inherited mouse neurological disorders [41].

Ca^{2+} channel mutations produce hypokalemic periodic paralysis

Hypokalemic periodic paralysis, in which serum potassium drops during a paralytic episode, is the most common of the inherited periodic paralyses. Although paralysis is associated with membrane depolarization and increased resting Na^+ conductance, this conductance is not sensitive to tetrodotoxin. This disease is linked to a region of chromosome 1 (1q31-32) that encodes the α subunit of the skeletal muscle, dihydropyridine-sensitive Ca^{2+} channel, designated CACNL1A3. Although this channel in skeletal muscle contains at least five subunits, the channel-forming α subunit has a structure that bears strong sequence homology to the voltage-gated Na^+ channel. It is organized into four internal repeat domains, each containing six to eight transmembrane α helices. The fourth helix in each domain contains the identifying K/R-X-X repeating motif that is the signature of voltage-dependent ion channels. Three mutations have been identified in the Ca^{2+} channel gene in families with hypokalemic periodic paralysis [42]. Two of these are in locations where mutations in the homologous Na$^+$ channel residues also occur.

The pathophysiological mechanism linking these L-type muscle Ca^{2+} channel mutations to the depolarization seen during episodes of weakness in hypokalemic periodic paralysis is unclear. This dihydropyridine-sensitive Ca^{2+} channel is present in the T-tubular membrane at the triadic junction with the terminal elements of the SR. There, it is thought to provide the coupling between T-tubular depolarization and activation of the SR ryanodine-sensitive Ca^{2+} release channel with which it interacts. At the triad, this Ca^{2+} channel protein does not conduct ionic currents. Perhaps another uncharacterized form of the sarcolemmal Ca^{2+} channel, in which CACNL1A3 is complexed with different accessory subunits, is responsible for the abnormal Na$^+$ currents seen in this disorder.

DEFECTS AT THE TRIAD CAN ALSO AFFECT MUSCLE FUNCTION

A congenital absence of the L-type Ca^{2+} channel is fatal

An interesting hereditary disorder of mice called *muscular dysgenesis,* in which affected pups exhibit an absence of skeletal muscle movement and die from respiratory failure shortly after birth, has been described. Electrophysiological investigation of the defective muscle showed that the fault lay at the level of excitation–contraction coupling. When the muscle was analyzed biochemically, it was found to be deficient in the L-type voltage-dependent Ca^{2+} channel that is thought to link T-tubular depolarization to Ca^{2+} release from the terminal elements of the SR.

In an elegant experiment, Adams and Beam [43] restored excitation–contraction coupling to dysgenic muscle in culture by introducing a plasmid containing the full-length coding sequence for the dihydropyridine-sensitive Ca^{2+} channel from skeletal muscle into the nuclei of affected cells. Myotubes treated in this way showed normal contractions in response to electrical stimulation. While never described in humans, it seems likely that mutations affecting this

T-tubular protein could have similar profound effects on an affected fetus.

Malignant hyperthermia is linked to mutations in the ryanodine receptor protein

A rare complication of general inhalation anesthesia is a syndrome characterized by muscle stiffness and hyperpyrexia. If untreated, this syndrome, called malignant hyperthermia (MH), can be rapidly fatal. Although the inheritance pattern of the disease is difficult to trace, it is likely to be passed from generation to generation as an autosomal dominant trait. A similar disease occurs in a strain of pigs, and this experimental animal model has proven to be very useful in studying the physiology of the disease.

Measurements on isolated muscle from affected pigs or humans show that the defect is at the level of excitation–contraction coupling. Specifically, the muscles release Ca^{2+} when exposed to caffeine at concentrations much lower than that required for Ca^{2+} release from normal muscle. Once released, this Ca^{2+} produces persistent activation of tropomyosin and sustained contraction, which in turn leads to hypermetabolism and hyperpyrexia.

After the cDNA encoding the ryanodine receptor protein of the terminal SR had been cloned and sequenced, the gene encoding this protein was localized to the porcine chromosome 6 and to a syntenic region of human chromosome 19. Using restriction-length polymorphisms within this gene, linkage between the gene and expression of the MH phenotype could then be tested. It rapidly became apparent that in the porcine form of MH, as well as in many of the human families expressing the disease, the phenotype was indeed tightly linked to the ryanodine receptor gene [44].

Subsequent analysis of the ryanodine receptor gene sequence in affected individuals has uncovered seven mutations in the coding region of the protein that cosegregate with the MH phenotype [45]. These mutations cluster in a region of the protein that is thought to protrude into the space between the terminal SR and the T-tubule, perhaps in the region of interaction with the T-tubular Ca^{2+} channel. A mutation in the same region of the porcine ryanodine receptor has proven to be the cause of MH in animal models.

In many families with the MH phenotype, however, mutations in the ryanodine receptor gene have not yet been identified. Further work will be needed to determine whether the defect in these cases is also in this receptor or in another related but as yet unidentified protein.

REFERENCES

1. Pollard, T. D., and Cooper, J. A. Actin and actin-binding proteins. A critical evaluation of mechanisms and functions. *Annu. Rev. Biochem.* 55:987–1035, 1986.
2. Mondello, M. R., Bramanti, P., Cutroneo, G., Di Mauro, D., and Anastasi, G. Immunolocalization of the costameres in human skeletal muscle fibers: Confocal scanning laser microscope investigations. *Anat. Rec.* 245:481–487, 1996.
3. Harrington, W. F., and Rodgers, M. E. Myosin. *Annu. Rev. Biochem.* 53:35–74, 1984.
4. Hibberd, M. G., and Trentham, D. R. Relationships between chemical and mechanical events during muscular contraction. *Annu. Rev. Biophys. Biophys. Chem.* 15:119–161, 1986.
5. Zot, A. S., and Potter, J. D. Structural aspects of troponin–tropomyosin regulation of skeletal muscle contraction. *Annu. Rev. Biophys. Biophys. Chem.* 16:535–560, 1987.
6. Catterall, W. A. Structure and function of voltage-sensitive ion channels. *Science* 242:50–61, 1988.
7. Franzini-Armstrong, C. Studies of the triad. I. Structure of the junction of frog twitch fibers. *J. Cell Biol.* 47:488–499, 1979.
8. Catterall, W. A. Excitation–contraction coupling in vertebrate skeletal muscle: A tale of two calcium channels. *Cell* 64:871–874, 1991.
9. Campbell, K. P., Knudson, C. M., Imagawa, T., et al. Identification and characterization of the high affinity [^{3}H]ryanodine receptor of the junctional sarcoplasmic reticulum Ca^{2+} release channel. *J. Biol. Chem.* 262:6460–6463, 1987.
10. Wagenknecht, T., Grassucci, R., Frank, J., Saito, A., Inui, M., and Fleischer, S. Three-dimensional architecture of the calcium channel/foot structure of sarcoplasmic reticulum. *Nature* 338:167–170, 1989.
11. Sakaguchi, G. *Clostridium botulinum* toxins. *Pharmacol. Ther.* 19:165–194, 1983.
12. Simpson, L. L. Molecular pharmacology of botulinum toxin and tetanus toxin. *Annu. Rev. Pharmacol. Toxicol.* 26:427–453, 1986.
13. Howard, B. D., and Gunderson, C. B., Jr. Effects and mechanisms of polypeptide neurotoxins that act presynaptically. *Annu. Rev. Pharmacol. Toxicol.* 20:307–336, 1980.
14. Finkelstein, A., Rubin, L. L., and Tzeng, M. C. Black widow spider venom: Effect of purified toxin on lipid bilayer membranes. *Science* 193:1009–1011, 1976.
15. Geppert, M., Khvotchev, M., Krasnoperov, V., et al. Neurexin Iα is a major α-latrotoxin receptor that cooperates in α-latrotoxin action. *J. Biol. Chem.* 273:1705–1710, 1998.
16. Davletov, B. A., Krasnoperov, V., Hata, Y., Petrenko, A. G., and Sudhof, T. C. High affinity binding of α-latrotoxin to recombinant neurexin Iα. *J. Biol. Chem.* 270:23903–23905, 1995.
17. Perin, M. S. The COOH terminus of synaptotagmin mediates interaction with the neurexins. *J. Biol. Chem.* 269:8576–8581, 1994.
18. O'Connor, V. M., Shamotienko, O., Grishin, E., and Betz, H. On the structure of the "synaptosecretosome." Evidence for a neurexin/synaptotagmin/syntaxin/Ca^{2+} channel complex. *FEBS Lett.* 326:255–260, 1993.
19. Davletov, B. A., Shamotienko, O. G., Lelianova, V. G., Grishin, E. V., and Ushkaryov, Y. A. Isolation and biochemical characterization of a Ca^{2+}-independent α-latrotoxin-binding protein. *J. Biol. Chem.* 271:23239–23245, 1996.
20. Krasnoperov, V. G., Bittner, M. A., Beavis, R., et al. α-Latrotoxin stimulates exocytosis by the interaction with a neuronal G-protein-coupled receptor. *Neuron* 18:925–937, 1997.
21. Kondo, K., Narita, K., and Lee, C. Y. Amino acid sequences of the two polypeptide chains in β-bungarotoxin from the venom of *Bungarus multicinctus*. *J. Biochem.* 83:101–115, 1978.
22. Kondo, K., Toda, H., and Narita, K. Characterization of phospholipase A2 activity of β-bungarotoxin from *Bungarus multicinctus*. *J. Biochem.* 84:1291–1300, 1978.
23. Simpson, L. L., Lautenslager, G. T., Kaiser, I. I., and Middlebrook, J. L. Identification of the site at which phospholipase A2 neurotoxins localize to produce their neuromuscular blocking effects. *Toxicon* 31:13–26, 1993.
24. Shi, Y., Xu, Y., and Xu, K. Selective inhibition of the slow K^+ current at motor nerve ending by plasma from a myasthenia gravis patient. *J. Neurol. Sci.* 130:165–170, 1995.

25. Yi, Q., Pirskanen, R., and Lefvert, A. K. Presynaptic membrane receptor-reactive T lymphocytes in myasthenia gravis. *Scand. J. Immunol.* 43:81–87, 1996.

26. Lang, B., and Newsome-Davis, J. Immunopathology of the Lambert-Eaton myasthenic syndrome. *Springer Semin. Immunopathol.* 17:3–15, 1995.

27. Karlsson, E. Chemistry of protein toxins in snake venoms. In C. Y. Lee (ed.), *Snake Venoms.* Berlin: Springer-Verlag, 1979, pp. 159–204.

28. Frazier, C. F., Rollins, Y. D., Breese, C. R., Leonard, S., Freedman, R., and Dunwiddie, T. V. Acetylcholine activates an α-bungarotoxin-sensitive nicotinic current in rat hippocampal interneurons, but not pyramidal cells. *J. Neurosci.* 18:1187–1195, 1998.

29. Ackermann, E. J., and Taylor, P. Nonidentity of the α-neurotoxin binding sites on the nicotinic acetylcholine receptor revealed by modification in α-neurotoxin and receptor structures. *Biochemistry* 36:12836–12844, 1997.

30. Machold, J., Utkin, Y., Kirsch, D., Kaufmann, R., Tsetlin, V., and Hucho, F. Photolabeling reveals the proximity of the α-neurotoxin binding site to the M2 helix of the ion channel in the nicotinic acetylcholine receptor. *Proc. Natl. Acad. Sci. USA* 92:7282–7286, 1995.

31. Plomp, J. J., and Molenaar, P. C. Involvement of protein kinases in the upregulation of acetylcholine release at endplates of α-bungarotoxin-treated rats. *J. Physiol. (Lond.)* 493:175–186, 1996.

32. Dolimbek, B. Z., and Atassi, M. Z. Protection against α-bungarotoxin poisoning by immunization with synthetic toxin peptides. *Mol. Immunol.* 33:681–689, 1996.

33. Lindstrom, J. Immunobiology of myasthenia gravis, experimental autoimmune myasthenia gravis, and Lambert-Eaton syndrome. *Annu. Rev. Immunol.* 3:109–131, 1985.

34. Engel, A. G., Lambert, E. H., Mulder, D. M., et al. A newly recognized congenital myasthenic syndrome attributable to a prolonged open time of the acetylcholine-induced ion channel. *Ann. Neurol.* 11:553–569, 1982.

35. Barchi, R. L. The non-dystrophic myotonic syndromes. In R. N. Rosenberg, S. B. Prusiner, S. Di-Mauro, R. L. Barchi, and L. M. Kunkel (eds.), *The Molecular and Genetic Basis of Neurological Disease.*

Philadelphia: Butterworth, 1993, pp. 873–880.

36. Meyer-Kleine, C., Steinmeyer, K., Ricker, K., et al. Spectrum of mutations in the major human skeletal muscle chloride channel gene (ClC-1) leading to myotonia. *Am. J. Hum. Genet.* 57: 1325–1334, 1995.

37. Steinmeyer, K., Klocke, R., Ortland, C., et al. Inactivation of muscle chloride channel by transposon insertion in myotonic mice. *Nature* 354: 304–306, 1991.

38. Cohen, S., and Barchi, R. Voltage-dependent sodium channels. *Int. Rev. Cytol.* 137c:55–103, 1993.

39. Barchi, R. L. Ion channel mutations and diseases of skeletal muscle. *Neurobiol. Dis.* 4:254–264, 1997.

40. Wang, Q., Shen, J., Splawski, I., et al. SCN5A mutations associated with an inherited cardiac arrythmia, the long QT syndrome. *Cell* 80:805–811, 1995.

41. Kohrman, D., Smith, M., Goldin, A., Harris, J., and Meisler, M. A missense mutation in the sodium channel SCN8A is responsible for cerebellar ataxia in the mouse mutant jolting. *J. Neurosci.* 16:5993–5999, 1996.

42. Ptacek, L., Tawil, R., Griggs, R., et al. Dihydropyridine receptor mutations cause hypokalemic periodic paralysis. *Cell* 77:863–898, 1994.

43. Adams, B. A., and Beam, K. G. Muscular dysgenesis in mice: A model system for studying excitation–contraction coupling. *FASEB J.* 4: 2809–2816, 1990.

44. MacLennan, D. H., Duff, C., Zorzato, F., et al. Ryanodine receptor gene is a candidate for predisposition to malignant hyperthermia. *Nature* 343:559–561, 1990.

45. Mickelson, J. R., and Louis, C. F. Malignant hyperthermia: Excitation–contraction coupling, Ca^{++} release channel, and cell Ca^{++} regulation defects. *Physiol. Rev.* 76:537–592, 1996.

46. Huxley, H. E. The mechanism of muscle contraction. *Science* 164:1356, 1969.

47. Lowey, S., Slayter, H. S., Weeds, S. G., and Baker, H. Substructure of the myosin molecule. I. Subfragments of myosin by enzymatic degradation. *J. Mol. Biol.* 42:1, 1969.

48. Jentsch, T. J. Molecular physiology of anion channels. *Curr. Opin. Cell Biol.* 6:600, 1994.

44

Diseases of Amino Acid Metabolism

Marc Yudkoff

Basic Neurochemistry: Molecular, Cellular and Medical Aspects, 6th Ed., edited by G. J. Siegel et al. Published by Lippincott–Raven Publishers, Philadelphia, 1999. Correspondence to Marc Yudkoff, Children's Hospital of Philadelphia, 1 Children's Center, Philadelphia, Pennsylvania 19104.

Aminoacidopathies involve an inherited deficiency of an enzyme or transport system that mediates the metabolism of a particular amino acid (Table 44-1). As a result, the amino acid accumulates and evokes a toxicity syndrome that commonly extends to the CNS. The severity of the clinical picture depends on the amino acid involved, the duration of its accumulation and the supervention of other medical complications, for example, hypoglycemia [1,2].

Neurochemists have long been interested in the relationship between the biochemical derangement and brain injury since careful scrutiny of the latter may reveal the significance of the involved metabolic pathway to normal function. These relationships are still poorly understood for most amino acidurias.

BIOCHEMISTRY OF AMINO ACID DISORDERS

The metabolic fate of amino acids conforms to one or more of the following: (i) incorporation

TABLE 44-1.   DISORDERS OF AMINO ACID METABOLISM[a]

Disorder	Biochemical derangement	Classical findings[a]
Branched-chain amino aciduria (maple syrup urine disease)	Defective branched-chain amino acid breakdown (Fig. 44-1)	Coma, convulsions, vomiting, respiratory failure in neonate
Branched-chain organic acidurias	Failure of organic acid oxidation (Fig. 44-1), isovaleric, methylmalonic, propionic, etc.	Similar to above, may be metabolic acidemia and odd odor; often confused with sepsis of newborn; urine contains excessive amounts of different organic acids, depending on the nature of the defect; partial defects may present in later infancy or childhood
Glutaric acidurias	Type I: Primary defect of glutarate oxidation (Fig. 44-3)	Severe basal ganglia/cerebellar disease with macrocephaly, onset 1 to 2 years
	Type II: Defect of electron transfer flavoprotein (Fig. 44-3)	Fulminant neurological syndrome of the neonate, often with renal/hepatic cysts, usually fatal
Phenylketonuria (PKU)	Usually defect of phenylalanine hydroxylase. In rare cases, defect of biopterin metabolism (Fig. 44-4, reaction 1)	Normal at birth, mental retardation in untreated children, avoidable with early institution of diet therapy, prognosis less favorable in PKU secondary to defect of biopterin metabolism
Nonketotic hyperglycinemia	Defect of glycine-cleavage system (Fig. 44-5)	Intractable seizures in neonate, usually fatal in first few weeks of life
Homocystinuria	Usually a failure of cystathionine synthase (Fig. 44-2, reaction 5), rarely associated with aberrant vitamin B_{12} metabolism (Fig. 44-2)	Thromboembolic diathesis, marfanoid habitus, *ectopia lentis*; mental retardation is frequent
Urea cycle defects	Failure to convert ammonia to urea via urea cycle (Fig. 44-6)	Coma, convulsions, vomiting, respiratory failure in neonate; often mistaken for sepsis of the newborn; mental retardation, failure to thrive, lethargy, ataxia and coma in the older child; associated with hyperammonemia and abnormalities of blood aminogram
Defects of biotin metabolism	Failure to "activate" biotin, which is important in carboxylation of organic acids	Hypotonia, ataxia, acidosis, coma, dermatitis in the neonate; mental retardation and deafness in the older child
Disorders of glutathione metabolism	Defective synthesis of glutathione, the major intracellular antioxidant (Fig. 44-7)	Spinocerebellar degeneration, mental retardation, cataracts, hemolysis; severe acidosis in some cases
Disorders of GABA metabolism	Often an absence of succinic semialdehyde dehydrogenase	Hypotonia, ataxia, mental retardation in the older child; increased urine 4-OH-butyric acid
Canavan's disease	Absence of *N*-acetylaspartate acylase	Rapidly progressive demyelinating disease of infancy

[a] For disorders of carbohydrate metabolism and the primary lactic acidoses, see Chap. 42.

into protein; (ii) conversion into messenger compounds, such as neurotransmitters and hormones; and (iii) oxidation to form carbon dioxide, water and ammonia.

Congenital defects of protein synthesis have not yet been described. If they occur, they probably are lethal early in development. Inherited defects in the synthesis of messenger compounds are known, such as the formation of thyroid hormone from tyrosine, but so little amino acid flux is directed toward synthesis of these compounds that no amino acid accumulation is noted.

Almost all amino acidurias reflect derangements of amino acid oxidation, or conversion to CO_2, H_2O and NH_3. Before amino acids are so metabolized, they usually are converted to organic acids, that is, to relatively simple carboxylate anions, such as methylmalonic acid, which are transformed to tricarboxylic acid cycle (TCA) intermediates.

Many organic acidurias have been described (Table 44-1) [3,4]. These occur because of the absence of a specific enzyme of organic acid oxidation. In rare instances, the cause is a failure to activate or transport a water-soluble vitamin that serves as a cofactor for a pathway of organic acid metabolism.

The oxidation of amino acids gives rise to ammonia, which in high concentration is neurotoxic. Most organisms have developed mechanisms for the disposal of this metabolite. In mammals, the urea cycle serves this function, abetting the excretion of 10 to 20 g of ammonia per day in the healthy adult. Congenital deficiencies of the urea cycle (see below) cause hyperammonemia and other evidence of nitrogen accumulation, such as elevations in the plasma concentration of glutamine, which is formed from ammonia.

Various biochemical changes occur in experimental models of amino acid metabolism disorders, including compromised energy metabolism and depletion of ATP. Several underlying processes probably are involved, including an uncoupling of oxidative metabolism, impaired glucose homeostasis and alterations of the intracellular redox potential.

The pathophysiology also may involve competitive inhibition of amino acid transport across the blood–brain barrier. Many amino acids are transferred into the CNS via specialized transport systems, for example, the L system mediating the uptake of neutral amino acids. Excessive plasma concentrations of one amino acid, such as phenylalanine, may inhibit the transport of others. An increase in the ratio of the concentration of tryptophan to that of other amino acids, a phenomenon that occurs in patients who are treated with low-protein diets, may lead to greater tryptophan entry into the brain and increased synthesis of serotonin.

Decreases of lipids, proteolipids and cerebrosides have been noted in several of these syndromes, notably maple syrup urine disease. As noted above, pathological changes in brain myelin are common, especially in infants who die early in life. The fundamental lesion may involve a failure of myelin protein synthesis as a consequence of the imbalanced brain amino acid content.

Finally, in some instances, the injury may be caused by the formation of oxygen radicals or by disturbances of ion channel function. Indeed, the probability is high that disordered amino acid metabolism damages the brain by several independent mechanisms, each of which contributes to the final pathophysiology.

PATHOGENESIS OF CLINICAL FEATURES

Infants who succumb in the first days of life commonly manifest neuronal degeneration and reactive astrogliosis. Evidence of dysmyelination is common, particularly when the baby survives for a few weeks. Cortical atrophy is not unusual with long-standing disease. These findings are encountered in many other toxic encephalopathies [5,6].

BRANCHED-CHAIN AMINO ACID METABOLISM

Maple syrup urine disease was the first congenital defect of branched-chain amino acid catabolism to be described

Maple syrup urine disease (MSUD) is a deficiency of branched-chain ketoacid dehydrogenase (Fig. 44-1, reaction 2), a mitochondrial en-

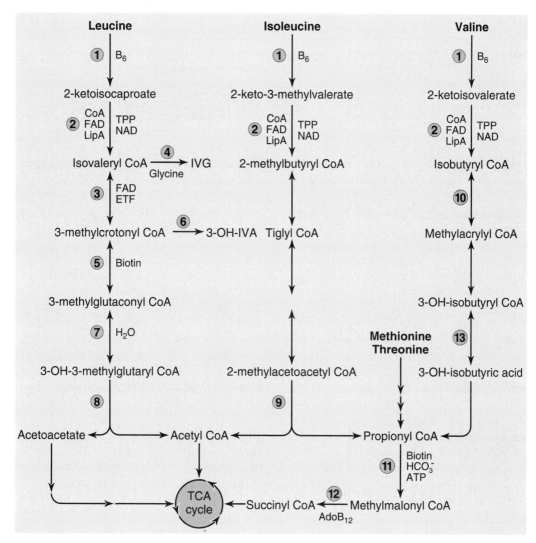

FIGURE 44-1. Major pathways of branched-chain amino acid metabolism. Maple syrup urine disease is caused by a congenital deficiency of reaction *2*. Many of the primary organic acidurias, for example, isovaleric acidemia and methylmalonic acidemia, are referable to inherited defects of enzymes involved in the oxidation of organic acids derived from the branched-chain amino acids. *Enzymes: 1,* branched-chain amino acid transaminase; *2,* branched-chain amino acid decarboxylase; *3,* isovaleryl-CoA dehydrogenase; *4,* glycine-*N*-acylase; *5,* 3-methylcrotonyl-CoA carboxylase; *6,* crotonase; *7,* 3-methylglutaconyl-CoA hydratase; *8,* 3-OH-3-methylglutaryl-CoA lyase; *9,* 2-ketothiolase; *10,* isobutyryl-CoA dehydrogenase; *11,* propionyl-CoA carboxylase; *12,* methylmalonyl-CoA mutase; *13,* 3-OH-isobutyryl-CoA deacylase. *TPP,* thiamine pyrophosphate; *LipA,* lipoic acid; *ETF,* electron transfer flavoprotein; *AdoB₁₂,* adenosylcobalamin; *IVA,* isovaleric acid; *IVG,* isovalerylglycine; *TCA,* tricarboxylic acid.

zyme. Decarboxylation of the branched-chain ketoacids, derived from transamination of branched-chain amino acids (BCAA), proceeds via a reaction for which the cofactors are thiamine pyrophosphate, lipoic acid, NAD, FAD and coenzyme A. The ketoacids are freely reaminated to the parent amino acids, the latter being

readily measured in the blood and urine. Ketoacids impart to the urine a distinct odor that sometimes is compared with maple syrup or burnt sugar.

The decarboxylase is composed of four subunits: E1-α, E1-β, E2 and E3. A specific kinase and phosphatase activate and deactivate, respectively, the enzyme complex. Most MSUD patients have mutations involving the E1-α subunit, which catalyzes the actual decarboxylation of the ketoacid, although defects of the E1-β protein have been described [7]. The E1-α mutation usually causes faulty assembly of the heterotetrameric ($\alpha_2\beta_2$) E1 protein. Lesions of either the E2 or E3 moiety are extremely rare. The E3 subunit is common to other decarboxylating systems, including pyruvate dehydrogenase and 2-oxyglutarate dehydrogenase. Hence, mutations in this protein can cause lactic acidosis and deranged TCA activity, as well as an accumulation of BCAA.

Infants are protected during gestation because the placenta clears most potential toxins. The classical form of the disease, therefore, does not become clinically manifest until a few days after birth. Initial periods of alternating irritability and lethargy progress over a period of days to coma and respiratory embarrassment. Irreversible brain damage is common in babies who survive, particularly those whose treatment is delayed until after the first week of life.

Survivors may suffer a metabolic relapse at any time. The most common cause of relapse is intercurrent infection, which often favors endogenous protein catabolism. As a consequence, the patient's limited capacity to oxidize BCAA is overwhelmed and these compounds, together with their cognate ketoacids, accumulate to a toxic level. Relapse also can occur in association with surgery, trauma and emotional upset.

Patients with partial enzymatic deficiencies may present later in life with intermittent ketoacidosis, prostration and recurrent ataxia. Plasma concentrations of BCAA are elevated during these episodes, but they may be normal or near normal during the periods when patients are metabolically compensated.

Rare patients respond to the administration of thiamine in large doses, 10 to 30 mg per day. In these patients, the clinical course is even more mild than in patients with intermittent disease. Thiamine is a cofactor for the branched-chain ketoacid dehydrogenase, and the presumed mutation in these patients involves faulty binding of the vitamin to the apoprotein.

In many localities, newborn screening has become standard for this disorder, which in the general population has an approximate incidence of 1 in 250,000 live births. Carrier detection is possible, either by measurement of enzymatic activity in cultured fibroblasts or by study of restriction endonuclease fragments of DNA via Southern blotting. Antenatal testing is possible.

Treatment entails continuous dietary restriction of the BCAA. This is accomplished by administration of a special formula from which these amino acids are removed. The outlook for intellectual development is favorable in youngsters whose diagnosis is made early and who do not suffer recurrent, severe episodes of metabolic decompensation [8].

Gene therapy for this metabolic defect may become available within the next few years. *In vitro* studies have demonstrated the feasibility of retrovirus-mediated gene transfer of both the E1-α and E2 subunits of the branched-chain decarboxylase complex [7,9].

DISORDERS OF ORGANIC ACID METABOLISM

The cause of isovaleric acidemia is a congenital deficiency of isovaleryl-CoA dehydrogenase, which mediates formation of 3-methylcrotonate

The dehydrogenase (Fig. 44-1, reaction 3) is a mitochondrial enzyme of approximately 175 kDa composed of four identical subunits that are coded on human chromosome 15. The enzyme first transfers electrons from isovaleryl-CoA to FAD and then to electron-transferring flavoprotein (ETF). A specific ETF dehydrogenase then shifts the electrons to coenzyme Q in the electron-transport chain.

Affected patients usually have <5% of control capacity to oxidize isovaleric acid. The clinical presentation includes both a fulminant syndrome of neonatal onset and an intermittent disorder that usually becomes manifest in the first year or two of life. In the former instance, the baby develops irritability, vomiting, convulsions and progressive loss of consciousness during the first week. The rancid odor of isovaleric acid, which often is apparent from the urine, saliva and ear cerumen, accounts for the unusual name, "sweaty socks syndrome." Patients frequently exhibit hyperammonemia, ketoaciduria, metabolic acidosis, pancytopenia and hypocalcemia.

Youngsters with intermittent disease usually present with the characteristic odor, lethargy, ataxia and vomiting in association with an intercurrent infection or the administration of a relatively large amount of protein. Hyperammonemia is common. A family may have children with both the neonatal and intermittent forms of the disease, suggesting that several phenotypes may be related to one genotype.

Glycine-*N*-acylase, a hepatic enzyme that mediates formation of hippuric acid from benzoyl-CoA and glycine, also catalyzes the synthesis of isovalerylglycine from glycine and isovaleryl-CoA, which has a K_m of approximately 0.6 mM (Fig. 44-1, reaction 4). Patients excrete isovalerylglycine even when clinically compensated, thereby facilitating diagnosis. Formation of isovalerylglycine also detoxifies isovaleric acid during periods of stress since the conjugate is hydrophilic and excreted into urine more efficiently than isovaleric acid itself. Indeed, supplementation of the diet with glycine is beneficial, especially during a crisis [10].

Patients usually fare well with a low-protein, that is, low-leucine, diet. Some suffer no relapses at all. The blood carnitine concentration usually is low, reflecting excessive excretion of isovalerylcarnitine. Carnitine therapy therefore has been suggested, but the utility of this approach still is uncertain.

3-Methylcrotonic aciduria is caused by defects in a biotin-dependent reaction that forms 3-methylglutaconic acid

Isolated carboxylase deficiencies (Fig. 44-1, reaction 5) are rare and should be distinguished from the syndrome of 3-methylcrotonic aciduria, which occurs secondarily to defects of biotin metabolism (see below). Some patients present in early infancy with vomiting, metabolic acidosis, hyperlactatemia, convulsions and coma. Others remain well for 2 to 5 years, when they develop recurrent vomiting, metabolic acidosis, hypoglycemia and progressive lethargy leading to coma.

The urine usually contains marked elevations of 3-hydroxyisovaleric acid, which is formed from 3-methylcrotonyl-CoA via crotonase (Fig. 44-1, reaction 6). It should be emphasized that 3-hydroxyisovaleric aciduria can be a nonspecific finding in ketotic patients. Excretion of 3-methylcrotonylglycine is elevated.

3-Methylglutaconic aciduria is caused by deficiencies of 3-methylglutaconyl-CoA hydratase, which mediates formation of 3-hydroxy-3-methylglutaryl-CoA

Defects in this enzyme (Fig. 44-1, reaction 7) are extremely rare. Patients may present only with delayed speech development or with relatively mild psychomotor retardation. The urine contains increased amounts of 3-methylglutaconate, 3-hydroxyisovalerate and 3-methylglutarate, the latter presumably being formed from hydrogenation of 3-methylglutaconic acid.

Several patients now have been described with an autosomal recessive disorder involving 3-methylglutaconic aciduria but with normal hydratase activity. Loading with oral leucine does not increase urinary excretion of 3-methylglutaconate. Most of these children have had a progressive course characterized by neurodegeneration, often beginning in the first few months of life, and death after a few months or years. These patients, unlike those with hydratase deficiency, do not excrete excessive amounts of 3-hydroxyisovaleric acid. The underlying biochemical defect is not yet known.

3-Hydroxy-3-methylglutaric aciduria is caused by a lack of 3-hydroxy-3-methylglutaryl-CoA lyase, which catalyzes conversion of 3-hydroxy-3-methylglutarate to acetoacetate and acetyl-CoA

Many patients with deficiency in this enzyme (Fig. 44-1, reaction 8) become ill as neonates. In others, the symptoms are inapparent until 6 to 12 months. The most prominent findings are vomiting, lethargy, coma, convulsions and metabolic acidosis. An important finding is hypoglycemia without significant ketoaciduria, reflecting the significance of 3-hydroxy-3-methylglutaryl-CoA lyase to the synthesis of ketone bodies. The hypoglycemia may be referable to excessive consumption of glucose in the absence of the capacity to utilize an alternate fuel such as acetoacetate. Hepatomegaly with increased serum transaminases and hyperammonemia can occur and may lead to confusion with Reye's syndrome.

The urine organic acid profile shows increased 3-hydroxy-3-methylglutarate even when patients are stable. Excretion of 3-methylglutaconic acid also is high because the hydratase reaction is reversible (Fig. 44-1, reaction 7).

Patients must avoid fasting, which predisposes them both to developing hypoglycemia and, by favoring the synthesis of ketones from fatty acids, to the accumulation of 3-hydroxy-3-methylglutaric acid. Restriction of dietary protein and fat also may have a therapeutic role.

β-Ketothiolase deficiency syndrome is caused by defects in 2-methylacetoacetyl-CoA thiolase, which mediates the conversion of 2-methylacetoacetyl-CoA to acetyl-CoA and propionyl-CoA

This thiolase (Fig. 44-1, reaction 9) is one of several 3-oxothiolases that catalyze formation of acetyl-CoA and the corresponding acyl-CoA. The reactions usually are reversible, and one such enzyme is a cytoplasmic protein that mediates the condensation of 2 mol of acetyl-CoA to form acetoacetyl-CoA, which then reacts with another mol of acetyl-CoA to generate 3-hydroxy-3-methylglutaryl-CoA in the pathway of cholesterol synthesis.

The mitochondrial thiolase is specific for 2-methylacetoacetyl-CoA. In the liver, this enzyme also abets ketogenesis by catalyzing synthesis of 3-hydroxy-3-methylglutaryl-CoA from aceto-acetyl-CoA and acetyl-CoA. It is a tetramer of approximately 170 kDa and is stimulated by potassium, unlike the cytosolic enzyme.

The inherited disorder, sometimes termed β-ketothiolase deficiency, causes recurrent acidosis, ketosis, vomiting and even death. Patients respond to intravenous glucose and bicarbonate. Mental retardation is not unprecedented, but it is exceptional.

Patients commonly excrete large amounts of 2-methyl-3-hydroxybutyric acid, formed via enzymatic reduction of 2-methylacetoacetyl-CoA.

Tiglyl-CoA, a precursor to 2-methylacetoacetyl-CoA in the pathway of isoleucine catabolism (Fig. 44-1), also accumulates and usually is excreted as tiglylglycine. The ketosis is referable to inhibition of acetoacetyl-CoA metabolism by 2-methylaceto-acetyl-CoA. Excretion of these metabolites is variable when patients are not acutely ill.

3-Hydroxyisobutyryl-CoA deacylase deficiency causes a block in valine catabolism by preventing the conversion of 3-hydroxybutyryl-CoA to 3-hydroxyisobutyric acid

Methylacrylyl-CoA, a valine metabolite proximal to the site of the metabolic block (Fig. 44-1, reaction 13), accumulates and forms ninhydrin-positive conjugates with cysteine and cysteamine, which can be detected with amino acid analysis. The urine organic acids are otherwise unremarkable. A single patient had multiple congenital anomalies, including tetralogy of Fallot, facial dysmorphism and dysgenesis of the brain. The infant died at 3 months of age. There is no treatment.

ORGANIC ACID METABOLISM

Propionate and methylmalonate are derived primarily from catabolism of the BCAA (Fig. 44-1). Additional sources are methionine and threonine, as well as odd-chain fatty acids and cholesterol. Methylmalonic acid (MMA) can be formed also from the catabolism of thymine.

Children with propionic acidemia and methylmalonic acidemia may manifest an intense hyperglycinemia. Indeed, these disorders once were known as "ketotic hyperglycinemia." As the underlying biochemistry became better understood, this description was discarded in favor of more specific terminology, that is, propionic acidemia and methylmalonic acidemia.

Propionyl-CoA carboxylase deficiency blocks the biotin- and ATP-dependent conversion of propionyl-CoA to methylmalonyl-CoA

The mitochondrial enzyme (Fig. 44-1, reaction 11) is a tetramer of 540 kDa composed of two α and two β subunits. The α subunit has been mapped to human chromosome 13 and the β subunit to chromosome 3. Leader peptides, facilitating transport of the propeptides into the mitochondria, also have been identified. The α subunit contains the biotin-binding site, at which a specific enzyme, holocarboxylase synthetase, mediates binding of this cofactor to the carboxylase.

Patients with a near-total enzyme deficiency become sick as neonates with dehydration, lethargy progressing to coma, vomiting, ketoaciduria and hypotonia. The toxicity may involve the bone marrow, resulting in neutropenia and thrombocytopenia. Hyperammonemia and death from hemorrhage are not unusual. Hyperglycinemia occurs in many cases. Acidosis is not an invariant feature of the syndrome [11].

Infants may relapse, particularly in association with an infection. Permanent brain damage, seizures and mental retardation are frequent. A poor outcome is common even in patients who have enjoyed ostensibly good metabolic control [12]. Some patients remain well until later infancy or childhood, when their developmental retardation and failure to thrive are first discovered.

A variety of neuropathological features have been noted [6], including vacuolization of the white matter and patchy neuronal degeneration. The basal ganglia are a special target of injury. Hemorrhagic lesions have been reported at autopsy in the caudate, putamen, globus pallidus and thalamus. Endothelial cells in these regions tended to be swollen and hyperplastic, perhaps indicating a breakdown of the blood–brain barrier. This type of injury has been termed a metabolic stroke [13].

Various mutations have been described. These were formerly classified into two groups, pccA and pccBC, depending upon the thermostability of the mutant enzyme, its affinity for the effector K^+ and the response to addition of avidin. The pccA group, which is more common, has little or no α chain and the pccBC mutants are defective in β chain activity. Inheritance is autosomal recessive.

Presumptive diagnosis requires demonstration of increased excretion of propionate derivatives, including propionylglycine, 3-hydroxypropionate, tiglylglycine and methylcitric acid, a condensation product of propionyl-CoA and oxaloacetate. Definitive diagnosis involves the measurement of enzymatic activity in peripheral blood leukocytes. Prenatal diagnosis is feasible. Hyperammonemia is a more common initial finding than metabolic acidemia.

Treatment entails the restriction of dietary protein to minimize propionate production. Most patients have growth failure. Propionyl-CoA carboxylase is stimulated by biotin, but supplementation with this vitamin is not of documented benefit. Blood carnitine is low, probably because of loss as propionylcarnitine, and some evidence points to clinical improvement with carnitine treatment. An important recent advance is orthotopic liver transplantation, which has been tried with some success in the most severe cases [14].

Methylmalonyl-CoA mutase deficiency prevents the isomerization of methylmalonyl-CoA to succinyl-CoA

The enzyme (Fig. 44-1, reaction 12) is a dimer of approximately 150 kDa made of two identical subunits bound to 1 mol of adenosylcobalamin (vitamin B_{12}). The gene has been mapped to the short arm of human chromosome 6. Patients can have a complete deficiency of the apoenzyme (mut^0), partial deficiency (mut^-) or various defects of vitamin B_{12} metabolism. The latter patients have homocystinuria and hypermethioninemia as well as methylmalonic aciduria.

Patients with the mut^0 lesion present as neonates with vomiting, acidosis, hyperammonemia, hepatomegaly, hyperglycinemia and hypoglycemia. Neutropenia and thrombocytopenia can occur. Growth failure is very common in children. Mortality is high and prognosis is poor in children with an early onset (<2 months) of disease. The outlook is somewhat improved in children with a late-onset syndrome, although even in this group morbidity tends to be quite high [15].

Examination of the brain with magnetic resonance imaging shows some white matter attenuation during the first month of life. This progresses to a failure of myelination as the infant grows. The globus pallidus may display a disproportionate degree of injury, although this may regress to a variable degree following institution of therapy to lower the toxic concentration of methylmalonic acid (MMA) [5].

The urine contains excessive MMA, even when patients are well. The concentration in the CSF equals or even exceeds that in the blood.

Treatment involves a diet that is low in the amino acid precursors to MMA. Medical attention should be sought whenever the patient develops an acute infection. There may be a role for L-carnitine supplementation.

High concentrations of MMA, or propionate, adversely affect oxidative metabolism, resulting in a depletion of ATP. Several enzyme systems, for example, pyruvate carboxylase, are inhibited by these organic acids. In addition, the sequestration of CoA as methylmalonyl-CoA or propionyl-CoA probably causes a depletion of the free CoA pool, which would adversely affect the synthesis of myelin, urea and glucose.

Vitamin B_{12} is ineffective in patients with either the mut^0 or mut^- lesions, but it may help infants with defects of cobalamin synthesis and/or transport (see below). There is no hazard associated with giving 1 to 2 mg per day of vitamin B_{12}, and this approach is warranted until the results of enzymatic studies are available.

Methylmalonic aciduria may be secondary to defects of cobalamin metabolism

Vitamin B_{12} is a cofactor for the MMA-CoA mutase reaction. Increased urinary methylmalonate is a common finding in patients with cobalamin deficiency, such as in pernicious anemia or congenital defects of cobalamin metabolism. Homocystinuria also is frequent because methylcobalamin is necessary for the remethylation of homocysteine to methionine (Fig. 44-2, reaction 4; also see below, section on disorders of sulfur-containing amino acids). Neurological symptoms, frequently severe and presenting in early infancy, are common to most of these syndromes.

Intestinal absorption of cobalamin requires intrinsic factor, a glycoprotein that is synthesized in the gastric parietal cells. The cobalamin–intrinsic factor complex is taken up by cells in the ileum, where the complex dissociates. Cobalamin enters the circulation bound to transcobalamin II (TC-II), which also abets uptake into tissues. Methylcobalamin is the major circulating form, but the major intracellular species, including in the brain, appears to be adenosylcobalamin. The cobalamin–TC-II complex is broken down by a specific lysosomal protease. The free cobalamin then is methylated in the cytoplasm, or it enters the mitochondrion, where, as adenosylcobalamin, it serves as cofactor for the MMA-CoA mutase reaction.

Several genetic defects have been identified, including anomalies involving either cobalamin absorption, cellular uptake or intracellular handling. Transport defects are represented by inherited deficiency of intrinsic factor in *juvenile pernicious anemia*, cobalamin malabsorption syndrome and TC-II deficiency. These patients usually have megaloblastic anemia, methylmalonic aciduria and homocystinuria. Neurological signs, especially in infants with TC-II deficiency, tend to be quite severe. The pathogenesis of the CNS lesions probably involves a failure to generate an adequate amount of S-adenosylmethionine, the major methyl donor in the developing brain. This pivotal compound is formed from methionine, which is regenerated from homocysteine in a reaction that is dependent upon methylcobalamin (see below, section on disorders of sulfur amino acid metabolism).

Primary defects in the synthesis of methylcobalamin and adenosylcobalamin have been described. Patients with methylmalonic aciduria secondary to deranged vitamin B_{12} metabolism can be distinguished from those with the mutase deficiency by their response to pharmacological doses of cyanocobalamin or adenosylcobalamin, which sharply reduce methylmalonate excretion. At least two distinct inherited forms of faulty adenosylcobalamin synthesis, known as *cbl*A and *cbl*B, have been identified from clinical findings and complementation analysis in skin fibroblasts. Unlike infants with the mutase deficiency, who present in the first 1 to 2 weeks of life, these patients do not become clinically ill until after the first month of life. They may have ketonuria and metabolic acidemia, as well as a severe neurological syndrome involving coma and convulsions. Survivors commonly have mental retardation and microcephaly. Evidence

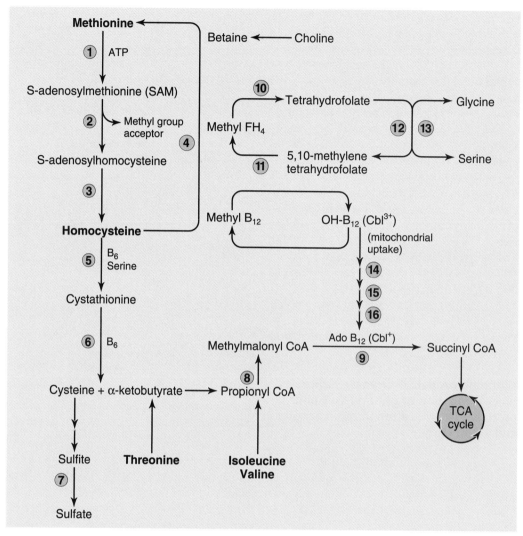

FIGURE 44-2. The trans-sulfuration pathway and related metabolic routes. Homocystinuria usually is caused by a congenital deficiency of cystathionine β-synthase (reaction 5). Sometimes homocystinuria is caused by a failure of the remethylation of homocysteine. This may occur because of a failure to generate methylfolate or methylcobalamin. If there is a generalized failure of cobalamin activation or absorption, methylmalonic aciduria as well as homocystinuria may result because cobalamin derivatives are essential to both pathways. *Enzymes:* 1, methionine-activating enzyme; 2, generic depiction of methyl group transfer from S-adenosylmethionine; 3, S-adenosylhomocysteine hydrolase; 4, homocysteine:methionine methyltransferase; 5, cystathionine β-synthase; 6, cystathionase; 7, sulfite oxidase; 8, propionyl-CoA carboxylase; 9, methylmalonyl-CoA mutase; 10, homocysteine:methionine methyltransferase, which is essentially the same as reaction 4, in which methyltetrahydrofolate (FH$_4$) is the methyl donor; 11, $N^{5,10}$-methylenetetrahydrofolate reductase; 12 and 13, glycine-cleavage system; 14 and 15, hydroxycobalamin reductases; 16, cobalamin adenosyltransferase. *OH-B$_{12}$*, hydroxocobalamin; *Ado B$_{12}$*, adenosylcobalamin; *Methyl-B$_{12}$*, methylcobalamin; *TCA*, tricarboxylic acid.

of pathology to the cerebellum and the dorsal columns of the spinal cord is common.

Patients with *cbl*A disease have defective adenosylcobalamin synthesis. The precise biochemical lesion is not yet known, although pa-tients have normal activity of the adenosyltransferase enzyme, which mediates the formation of adenosylcobalamin from ATP and hydroxocobalamin (Fig. 44-2, reaction 16). Patients may lack a specific mitochondrial cobalamin reductase (Fig. 44-2, reactions 14 and 15). Patients with *cbl*B disease are missing a functional adenosyltransferase enzyme (Fig. 44-2, reaction 16).

The diagnosis of defective adenosylcobalamin synthesis is suggested by methylmalonic aciduria without megaloblastic changes, homocystinuria or hypomethioninemia. The blood vitamin B_{12} concentration is normal. Prenatal diagnosis is feasible, either through study of the mutase reaction in amniocytes or by quantitation of MMA in amniotic fluid.

More than 90% of patients with the *cbl*A disease respond favorably to the administration of hydroxycobalamin, which reduces MMA excretion. They have a good prognosis, with most surviving into adulthood in an intact state. Only 40% of individuals with *cbl*B disease show a positive response. Their prognosis is less sanguine, with neurological impairment often noted among youngsters who survive the initial insult. Protein restriction, which minimizes production of MMA, is also indicated.

Glutaryl-CoA dehydrogenase deficiency blocks oxidation of glutaryl-CoA and produces degeneration in basal ganglia and white matter

Glutaric acid is an intermediate in the formation of crotonyl-CoA from α-ketoadipic acid, which is derived from the catabolism of lysine, hydroxylysine and tryptophan (Fig. 44-3). Patients with a congenital absence of glutaryl-CoA dehydrogenase (Fig. 44-3, reaction 3) seem normal at birth, although they may manifest macrocephaly. Normal development is common for the first 1 to 2 years, when they develop hypotonia, opisthotonus, seizures, rigidity, dystonia, facial grimacing and seizures. These signs may develop very abruptly, following an intercurrent illness, or in a more gradual manner. Developmental assessment is difficult because of severe motor involvement, but mental retardation may not occur. The neurological syndrome may be progressive, and death may occur during the first decade of life. The diagnostic hallmark is excretion of glutaric acid and 3-hydroxyglutaric acid. Imaging of the brain shows atrophy of the caudate and putamen and a loss of white matter in both frontal and occipital

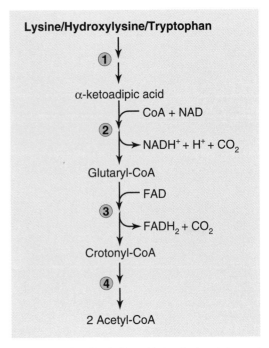

FIGURE 44-3. Catabolism of lysine, hydroxylysine and tryptophan. Glutaric aciduria is caused by a congenital absence of glutaryl-CoA dehydrogenase (reaction 3). *Enzymes: 1*, lysine-ketoglutarate dehydrogenase; *2*, NAD-dependent dehydrogenase; *3*, glutaryl-CoA dehydrogenase; *4*, crotonase.

horns. Pathological examination of the brain also shows degenerative changes in the basal ganglia and the cortical white matter. A special diet low in tryptophan and lysine will reduce excretion of glutaric acid, but it may not improve the clinical status.

Type II glutaric aciduria results from a deficiency in electron transfer proteins involved in mitochondrial respiration

Oxidation of glutaric acid (Fig. 44-3, reaction 3) involves transfer of electrons to FAD, in the process forming $FADH_2$. Glutaric aciduria type II usually is caused by a congenital deficiency of either ETF or ETF:ubiquinone reductase. These proteins, which are encoded by nuclear genes, mediate the transfer of electrons from flavoproteins to the respiratory chain in mitochondria. Other substrates that donate electrons to these proteins are dimethylglycine dehydrogenase and sarcosine dehydrogenase.

Patients often present as neonates with hepatomegaly, hypoglycemia without significant ketonemia, lipid storage myopathy with hypotonia, metabolic acidosis and a rancid urine odor similar to that of isovaleric acidemia (see above). The kidneys commonly are enlarged. Cystic changes of both the liver and kidney are frequent. Facial dysmorphism also can occur. Magnetic resonance imaging of brain typically suggests a leukodystrophy. The outlook is almost uniformly fatal, and the few babies who survive have severely compromised development and a cardiomyopathy that usually proves fatal. In rare cases, a patient stays asymptomatic until after the neonatal period, when hepatomegaly, vomiting, metabolic acidosis, hypoglycemia and a proximal myopathy become evident.

Pathological examination of the brain reveals dysplasias and other evidence of aberrant neural migration. The gyri of the cortex generally are reduced. ^{1}H-Magnetic resonance spectroscopy of the brain shows an increase of lactic acid concentration and of the choline:creatine ratio, suggesting dysmyelination. ^{31}P-Spectroscopy of muscle shows a severe compromise of energy metabolism [16]. Occasionally, patients have responded to riboflavin therapy [17], but there is no effective therapy.

PHENYLALANINE METABOLISM: PHENYLKETONURIA

Phenylketonuria is most commonly caused by a deficiency of phenylalanine hydroxylase, which converts phenylalanine into tyrosine

Phenylketonuria (PKU) is one of the most common aminoacidurias, with an occurrence of 1 in 20,000 live births. In addition to "classical" PKU (Fig. 44-4, reaction 1), many youngsters have hyperphenylalaninemia caused by a partial deficiency of the enzyme. They do not suffer mental retardation, but they may have more subtle neurological problems [18].

The hydroxylase is a trimer of approximately 150 kDa of identical subunits and is located predominantly in the liver. The enzyme has been mapped to human chromosome 12q22-24.1, where the gene comprises 13 exons extending over 90 kb of genomic DNA. Deletions in the gene are not common. A frequent cause among northern Europeans (~40%) is a G-to-A transition at the 5′ donor splice site in intron 12, resulting in absence of the C-terminus. Another relatively common (~20%) mutation in northern Europeans involves a C-to-T

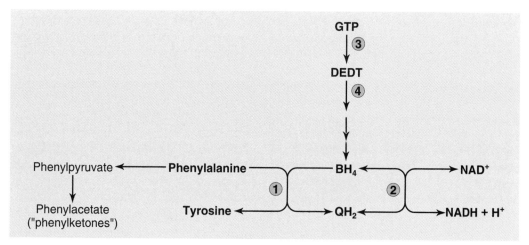

FIGURE 44-4.   The phenylalanine hydroxylase (PAH) pathway. Phenylketonuria usually is caused by a congenital deficiency of PAH (reaction 1), but it also can result from defects in the metabolism of biopterin, which is a cofactor for the hydroxylase. *Enzymes: 1,* phenylalanine hydroxylase; *2,* dihydropteridine reductase; *3,* GTP cyclohydrolase; *4,* 6-pyruvoyltetrahydrobiopterin synthase. *QH$_2$,* dihydrobiopterin; *BH$_4$,* tetrahydrobiopterin; *DEDT,* D-erythro-dihydroneopterin triphosphate.

transition in exon 12, resulting in substitution of a tryptophan for an arginine residue [19]. Over 70 different mutations have been described to date in the American population [20].

Mutations have been associated with specific haplotypes, the latter determined by analysis of restriction fragment length polymorphisms. This approach has been utilized for prenatal diagnosis. The study of haplotypes also has revealed that the majority (~75%) of northern European patients are compound PKU heterozygotes.

Affected babies are not retarded at birth, but almost all will be impaired if they are not treated by 3 months of age. Mass screening has largely eliminated the untreated PKU phenotype of eczema, poor growth, irritability, musty odor caused by phenylacetic acid and tendency to self-mutilation. Progressive motor dysfunction has been described in children with long-term hyperphenylalaninemia.

The clinical utility of dietary restriction of phenylalanine to 200 to 500 mg per day is clear. Well-controlled patients have normal intelligence, although there is an increased risk of perceptual learning disabilities, emotional problems and subtle motor difficulties [21]. Diet therapy is maintained throughout adolescence and, perhaps, indefinitely. Performance may deteriorate after the diet is discontinued.

Exposure to excessive (>1 mM) blood phenylalanine concentrations in early infancy can impair neuronal maturation and the synthesis of myelin. The responsible factor is excess phenylalanine, not a phenylalanine metabolite or tyrosine deficiency. One hypothesis suggests that excessive phenylalanine inhibits the transport of other neutral amino acids across the blood–brain barrier (see Chap. 32). Conversely, some have proposed that high intracerebral phenylalanine concentrations impair the transport of tyrosine from the brain to the blood. High brain phenylalanine concentrations can inhibit synaptosomal Na,K-ATPase activity and the synthesis of neurotransmitters. Excess phenylalanine also causes disaggregation of brain polysomes, which may explain the dysmyelination that has been described in the phenylketonuric brain. A loss of neurotransmitter receptors has been described in a murine model of hyperphenylalaninemia [22].

The genotypically normal offspring of an untreated mother may have microcephaly and irreversible brain injury, as well as cardiac defects. Scrupulous monitoring of dietary phenylalanine intake in these women has resulted in a much better outcome [23].

Phenylketonuria may also be caused by defects of biopterin metabolism

The electron donor for the phenylalanine hydroxylase is tetrahydrobiopterin (BH_4), which transfers electrons to molecular oxygen to form tyrosine and dihydrobiopterin (QH_2) (Fig. 44-4, reaction 2). BH_4 is regenerated from QH_2 in an NADH-dependent reaction (Fig. 44-4, reaction 2) that is catalyzed by dihydropteridine reductase (DHPR), which is widely distributed. In the brain, this enzyme also mediates hydroxylation of tyrosine and tryptophan. Human DHPR has been mapped to chromosome 4p15.1-p16.1 The coding sequence shows little homology to other reductases, for example, dihydrofolate reductase.

In rare instances, PKU is caused by defects in the metabolism of BH_4, which is synthesized from GTP via sepiapterin (Fig. 44-4, reactions 3 and 4) [24]. BH_4 functions also in the hydroxylation of tyrosine and tryptophan.

Even careful phenylalanine restriction fails to avert progressive neurological deterioration because patients are unable to hydroxylate tyrosine or tryptophan, the synthesis of which also requires BH_4. Thus, neurotransmitters are not produced in sufficient amount.

Patients sustain convulsions and neurological deterioration. The urine contains low concentrations of the metabolites of serotonin, norepinephrine and dopamine. The reductase also plays a role in the maintenance of tetrahydrofolate concentrations in brain, and some patients have had low folate in the serum and CNS. Treatment has been attempted with tryptophan and carbidopa to improve serotonin homeostasis and with folinic acid to replete diminished stores of reduced folic acid. This therapy sometimes is effective. Diagnosis involves assay of DHPR in skin fibroblasts or amniotic cells. Phenylalanine hydroxylase activity is normal.

Other causes of PKU secondary to defective BH_4 synthesis include GTP cyclohydrolase deficiency and 6-pyruvoyltetrahydrobiopterin synthase deficiency. Patients with either defect have psychomotor retardation, truncal hypotonia with limb hypertonia, seizures and a tendency to hyperthermia. Intravenous administration of BH_4 may lower blood phenylalanine concentrations, but this cofactor may not readily cross the blood–brain barrier. Treatment with synthetic pterin analogs or supplementation with tryptophan and carbidopa may prove more efficacious, particularly if treatment is started early in life.

GLYCINE METABOLISM: NONKETOTIC HYPERGLYCINEMIA

Nonketotic hyperglycinemia is caused by deficiencies in the glycine-cleavage system

Glycine is catabolized via the glycine-cleavage system (GCS), a group of mitochondrial proteins that mediate the interconversion of glycine and serine (Fig. 44-5, reaction 1). Pyridoxal phosphate and tetrahydrofolate are cofactors in this reaction. Glycine is the precursor to the "one-carbon pool" of folic acid intermediates that is pivotal to many synthetic reactions (Fig. 44-5, reaction 1) [25].

Affected infants become ill by the first or second day of life. Seizures are very prominent and even may occur *in utero*. EEG often displays a hypsarrythmia or a burst-suppression pattern. Patients display myoclonic jerks, hiccuping and a profound hypotonia. The few patients who survive past the first week of life usually sustain profound mental retardation and neurological disability. Brain imaging shows atrophy and a loss of myelin.

Rare patients present later in life with psychomotor retardation and growth failure. Others have had initially normal development followed by a progressive loss of developmental milestones. Some patients have manifested spinocerebellar degeneration and other symptoms of motor dysfunction [26].

Glycine is extremely high in the blood, often rising to >1 mM, with normal being 150 to 350 μM. The concentration in the CSF almost always exceeds 100 μM, with normal being ~10 μM. The CSF:blood ratio of glycine usually is five to ten times the control value of 0.02, especially with the classical form of the disease.

The GCS is composed of four distinct subunits: pyridoxal-dependent decarboxylase (P); heat-stable, lipoic acid-binding carrier of the aminoethyl group (H); tetrahydrofolate-requiring (T); and lipoamide dehydrogenase (L). Most infants with the classical disease have had defects either in the P or the T proteins.

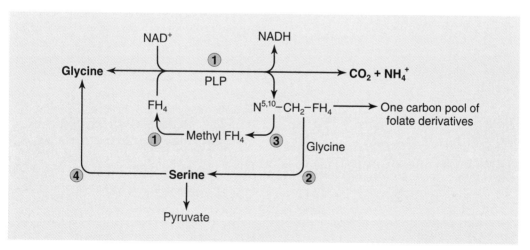

FIGURE 44-5.   Glycine-cleavage system and some related reactions. Glycine and serine are readily interchangeable. *Enzymes: 1,* glycine-cleavage system; *2,* and *4,* serine hydroxymethyltransferase; *3,* $N^{5,10}$-methylenetetrahydrolate reductase. $N^{5,10}CH_2$-FH_4, $N^{5,10}$-methylenetetrahydrolate; FH_4, tetrahydrofolic acid; *PLP,* pyridoxal phosphate.

A transient form of nonketotic hyperglycinemia (NKH), probably reflecting delayed maturation of the GCS, has been described in neonates with seizures but an otherwise normal neurological examination. The seizures ceased by 8 weeks of age and did not recur. Glycine concentrations in both the blood and the CSF were high. Urine organic acid analysis was normal.

There is no specific therapy. Exchange transfusion and dialysis usually do not alter the progressive neurological deterioration. Sodium benzoate has been administered in the hope that glycine would react with it to form hippuric acid, but this approach is not helpful. It may be that a combination of benzoate and carnitine therapy is more availing [27]. Similarly, the restriction of dietary protein and the administration of pyridoxine or choline have not proved useful.

Glycine is a neurotransmitter, having a postsynaptic inhibitory activity in the spinal cord and in some central neurons (see Chap. 16). Therapy with strychnine, which blocks the action of glycine at postsynaptic receptors, has been unhelpful. Treatment with diazepam has been attempted because this drug displaces strychnine from its binding sites. The combination of benzoate and diazepam may be more effective since high doses of the former reduce glycine concentrations in the CNS, thereby potentiating the ability of strychnine to block the glycine effect.

A few infants have been treated with antagonists of the N-methyl-D-aspartate (NMDA) receptor, an excitatory glutamatergic receptor which is potentiated by glycine (see Chap. 15) [28]. Ketamine and dextromethorphan have been used with inconclusive results. Some infants may have had an improvement of their irritability and EEG. One infant, treated with both benzoate and dextromethorphan, was seizure-free by 12 months of age and had only moderately delayed development. However, this favorable experience has not always been duplicated. Treatment with dextromethorphan at the recommended maximal dosage of 5 mg/kg/day seems to be well tolerated.

SULFUR AMINO ACID METABOLISM: HOMOCYSTINURIA

The trans-sulfuration pathway (Fig. 44-2) entails the transfer of the sulfur atom of methionine to serine with the ultimate formation of cysteine. The first step is activation of methionine, which reacts with ATP to form S-adenosylmethionine (SAM) (Fig. 44-2, reaction 1). This compound is a key methyl donor and plays a prominent role in the synthesis of several neurotransmitters and of creatine (Fig. 44-2, reaction 2). A portion of the carbon of spermidine and spermine is derived from SAM following the decarboxylation of that compound.

Transfer of a methyl group from SAM yields S-adenosylhomocysteine, which potently inhibits several methyltransferases, a phenomenon that may explain some of the pathology of homocystinuria (see below). Tissue concentrations of S-adenosylhomocysteine ordinarily are very low since this metabolite is rapidly cleaved by a specific hydrolase to homocysteine and adenosine (Fig. 44-2, reaction 3).

About half of the homocysteine so generated is remethylated to methionine, with either betaine or 5-methyltetrahydrofolic acid (methyl-FH$_4$) serving as methyl donor. The enzyme mediating remethylation, 5-methyltetrahydrofolate-betaine methyltransferase (Fig. 44-2, reaction 4), utilizes methylcobalamin as a cofactor. The kinetics of the reaction favor remethylation. One form of homocystinuria is caused by a defect of this remethylation process. Faulty remethylation can occur secondary to (i) dietary factors, such as vitamin B$_{12}$ deficiency; (ii) a congenital absence of the apoenzyme; (iii) a congenital inability to convert folate or vitamin B$_{12}$ to the methylated, metabolically active form (see below); or (iv) the presence of a metabolic inhibitor, for example, an antifolate agent that is used in an antineoplastic regimen.

The most common cause of homocystinuria is a deficiency of cystathionine β-synthetase

This enzyme (Fig. 44-2, reaction 5) is pyridoxine-dependent and converts homocysteine to cystathionine via condensation with serine. SAM potently stimulates the reaction in the forward direction [29]. This enzyme has been mapped to human chromosome 21. The equilibrium favors cystathionine synthesis. Thus, homocysteine concentrations normally are very low since both the remethylation pathway and the cystathionine synthetase route efficiently dispose of this amino acid.

Cleavage of cystathionine is accomplished by cystathionase, another pyridoxine-dependent enzyme, which is coded on human chromosome 16 (Fig. 44-2, reaction 6). The enzyme functions almost entirely to produce cysteine, there being virtually no reversal of the reaction.

A number of mutations that result in cystathionine synthetase deficiency have been described. The known mutations cause synthesis of an unstable enzyme; a protein that loosely binds either pyridoxal phosphate, serine or homocysteine; or an enzyme differing in size from the wild-type [30]. Cystathionine synthetase is present in many organs, including the brain, and homocystinuric patients typically manifest deficient enzyme activity in these tissues.

Blood homocysteine is elevated to 50 to 200 μM, with normal being <10 μM. The blood cysteine concentration tends to be low, reflecting the failure of cysteine synthesis. Increased remethylation of the homocysteine that is not converted to cystathionine results in elevated blood methionine, often in excess of 200 μM, with normal being 20 to 40 μM.

Some patients respond to the administration of pharmacological doses of pyridoxine, 25 to 100 mg daily, with a reduction of plasma homocysteine and methionine. Pyridoxine responsiveness appears to be hereditary, with siblings tending to show a concordant response. The clinical syndrome is milder in these individuals. Pyridoxine sensitivity can be documented by enzyme assay in skin fibroblasts. The precise biochemical mechanism of the pyridoxine effect is not well understood, but it may not reflect a mutation resulting in diminished affinity of the enzyme for cofactor because even high concentrations of pyridoxal phosphate do not restore mutant enzyme activity to a control level.

About half of the individuals who do not respond to pyridoxine (vitamin B$_6$) will sustain *ectopia lentis* by age 5 to 10 years. Indeed, the diagnosis commonly is made by an ophthalmologist to whom a child with bilaterally displaced lenses has been referred.

The median IQ scores for vitamin B$_6$-responsive and nonresponsive patients are 78 and 56, respectively. Some children may come to clinical attention at 1 to 2 years with psychomotor retardation. Other signs are convulsions, which occur in about 20% of patients, and psychiatric difficulties, notably depression and personality disorders, which occur in about half of cases.

The most striking feature is a thromboembolic diathesis. This can occur in virtually any vessel, with thrombi common in peripheral veins and arteries, the cerebral and renal vasculature and coronary arteries. Almost 25% of pyridoxine nonresponders sustain a major vascular insult during childhood. The comparable risk in untreated, pyridoxine-responsive subjects is 25% by age 20 years. Vascular insults sometimes occur in association with dehydration secondary to vomiting and diarrhea. The stress of major surgery and anesthesia increases the risk of thrombosis by ~5%. Homocystinuric patients who also have the relatively common Leiden mutation of clotting factor V are at sharply increased risk for developing a thrombosis [31].

Affected patients commonly manifest a marfanoid habitus with arachnodactyly, high-arched palate, tall stature and pes cavus. Bony abnormalities are common, with osteoporosis and scoliosis being frequent sources of clinical problems. The orthopedic findings are more common and more severe in patients who do not respond to pyridoxine treatment.

Demyelination and spongy degeneration of the white matter have been reported. Infarctions are relatively common in virtually all parts of the brain. The arterial wall shows thickening of the intima and splitting of the smooth musculature of the media. The changes are not dissimilar to those of atherosclerosis.

The probable cause of the pathology is excess homocysteine. Excess methionine is not thought to play an etiological role. The biochemical basis of homocysteine toxicity has been the subject of intense scrutiny. Homocysteine increases the adhesiveness of platelets *in vitro*, perhaps by favoring the synthesis of selected thromboxanes. Administration of homocysteine to rats or baboons can cause endothelial injury. Homocysteine may diminish the mean survival time of peripheral blood platelets, possibly by a direct toxic effect on the vascular endothelium, which becomes denuded and thereby provides an atherogenic nidus. A direct effect of homocysteine on the blood-clotting cascade also is possible. Thus, activation of factor V in cultured endothelial cells has been noted. This favors the conversion of prothrombin to thrombin.

Homocysteine also promotes accumulation of copper in the vascular endothelium. This induces the oxidation of ceruloplasmin and the concomitant release of sufficient H_2O_2 to injure endothelial cells. Supplementation of the medium with catalase protects against such an insult, thus confirming the role of oxidant injury.

High concentrations of homocysteine or one of its metabolites may directly affect brain function. Administration of homocysteine to rats induces grand mal convulsions, a phenomenon that is worsened by either methionine or pyridoxine. Homocysteine-induced blockade of the GABA receptor may be involved. In addition, brain can oxidize homocysteine to homocysteic acid, which has a glutamatergic activity.

A high intracerebral concentration of S-adenosylhomocysteine may inhibit methylation reactions involving SAM. The metabolic repercussions would be extensive, including deficient methylation of proteins and of phosphatidylethanolamine as well as an inhibition of catechol-O-methyltransferase and histamine-N-methyltransferase.

Patients who respond to large doses of vitamin B_6, 250 to 500 mg per day for several weeks, have the best prognosis. Efficacy of treatment usually is reflected in a reduction of blood homocysteine and methionine to normal or near-normal levels. Since supplementation with pyridoxine can cause a deficiency of folic acid, the latter should be given at 2 to 5 mg daily at the same time. Any patient receiving pyridoxine should be monitored carefully for any signs of hepatotoxicity and for a peripheral neuropathy.

Management of the pyridoxine-nonresponsive patient is difficult. Dietary restriction of methionine would seem logical, but this often is unpalatable, especially to an adult patient who has adapted to a diet that has not been purposefully restricted of protein.

A newer therapeutic approach is the administration of betaine, 6 to 12 g daily, which lowers homocysteine levels by favoring remethylation (Fig. 44-2, reaction 4) [32]. A theoretical hazard of betaine treatment is increasing the blood me-

thionine, sometimes to an extravagant degree, as high as 1 mM. Experience to date indicates that betaine administration is safe, with no major side effects except for a fishy odor to the urine.

Other therapeutic approaches have included the administration of salicylate and of dipyridamole to ameliorate the thromboembolic diathesis. Dipyridamole has been effective in animal studies at restoring platelet survival to a near-normal range. Patients also have been treated with dietary supplements of L-cystine since block of the trans-sulfuration pathway in theory could diminish the synthesis of this amino acid.

Remethylation deficiency homocystinuria is usually caused by aberrations in the metabolism of methylfolate or methylcobalamin

These are the cofactors for the remethylation reaction (Fig. 44-2, reaction 4). Patients often present early in life with lethargy, poor feeding, psychomotor retardation and growth failure. Hematological abnormalities are common, including megaloblastosis, macrocytosis, thrombocytopenia and hypersegmentation of the leukocytes. Occasional patients are clinically silent until later life, when seizures, dementia, hypotonia, mental retardation, spasticity or a myelopathy become evident.

Biochemical findings are variable. Interestingly, blood cobalamin and folate concentrations often are normal. Many have had homocysteinemia with hypomethioninemia, the latter helping to discriminate this group from homocystinuria secondary to cystathionine β-synthase deficiency. Urinary excretion of MMA may be high, reflecting the fact that vitamin B_{12} serves as a cofactor for the methylmalonyl-CoA mutase reaction (see above).

Methylenetetrahydrofolate reductase deficiency interferes with pteridine reduction and produces severe brain disease

5,10-Methylenetetrahydrofolate is reduced to methyltetrahydrofolate by a cytoplasmic, NADPH-dependent enzyme, methylenetetrahydrofolate reductase (Fig. 44-2, reaction 11).

SAM inhibits the reaction. The enzyme normally is present in human brain, where it may play a role in the reduction of dihydropteridines (see above, section on disorders of phenylalanine metabolism).

Patients typically present with severe developmental retardation, convulsions and microcephaly by age 6 to 12 months. A few individuals also have had psychiatric disturbances.

Homocysteinemia, usually ~50 μM, is the rule, with a relatively low blood methionine concentration of less than 20 μM. The blood concentration of vitamin B_{12} is normal, and, unlike individuals with defects of cobalamin metabolism, these patients manifest neither anemia nor methylmalonic aciduria. Blood folic acid is usually low.

A thromboembolic diathesis is not unusual, and thromboses have been reported in the brain vasculature. Other pathological changes have included microgyri, demyelination, gliosis and brain atrophy. Lipid-laden macrophages have been described.

A relatively large number of agents have been utilized to treat this intractable disorder: folinic acid (5-formyltetrahydrofolic acid), folic acid, methyltetrahydrofolic acid, betaine, methionine, pyridoxine, cobalamin and carnitine. Betaine, which provides methyl groups to the betaine:homocysteine methyltransferase reaction, appears to be a nontoxic approach that lowers blood homocysteine and increases methionine.

Methionine synthetase deficiency, also termed cobalamin-E disease, results in the inability to transfer a methyl group from methyltetrahydrofolate to homocysteine to yield methionine

A cobalamin group bound to the enzyme is converted to methylcobalamin prior to the final formation of methionine in this reaction (Fig. 44-2, reaction 4).

In cobalmin-E (*cbl*E) disease, there is a failure of methyl-vitamin B_{12} to bind to methionine synthetase. It is not known if this reflects a primary defect of methionine synthase or the absence of a separate enzymatic activity. Patients manifest megaloblastic changes with a pancytopenia, homocystinuria and hypomethionine-

mia. There is no methylmalonic aciduria. Patients usually become clinically manifest during infancy with vomiting, developmental retardation and lethargy. They respond well to injections of hydroxocobalamin.

The activity of methionine synthetase is restored to normal *in vitro* by addition of large amounts of thiols to the incubation mixture. In contrast, in *cbl*G disease, the enzymatic activity remains low even with thiol supplementation of the assay.

Cobalamin-C disease results from a defect in the activation of vitamin B_{12}

Complementation analysis allows the classification of patients with primary defects in the metabolism of vitamin B_{12} into one of three groups: *cbl*C, *cbl*D and *cbl*F. The most common variant is *cbl*C. Most individuals become ill in the first few months or weeks of life with hypotonia, lethargy and growth failure. Optic atrophy and retinal changes can occur. Methylmalonate excretion is excessive, although less than in methylmalonyl-CoA mutase deficiency. Patients do not display ketoaciduria or overwhelming metabolic acidosis.

Fibroblasts do not convert cyanocobalamin or hydroxocobalamin to methylcobalamin or adenosylcobalamin. The activities of both N^5-methyltetrahydrofolate:homocysteine methyltransferase and methylmalonyl-CoA mutase are consequently diminished. These biochemical lesions can be rectified by supplementation of the medium with hydroxocobalamin. The precise nature of the underlying defect remains obscure, although it appears to involve a step in the activation of B_{12}.

The diagnosis should be suspected in a child with homocystinuria, methylmalonic aciduria, megaloblastic anemia, hypomethioninemia and normal blood concentration of folate and vitamin B_{12}. A definitive diagnosis requires demonstration of these abnormalities in fibroblasts. Prenatal diagnosis is possible.

Treatment involves the administration of large doses (as much as 1 mg) of intramuscular hydroxocobalamin. Administration of folate and betaine (see above) may be helpful, as is a reduction of protein intake.

Cobalamin-D disease is an extremely rare variant

It may become clinically manifest only in later life with mild mental retardation and behavioral abnormality.

Hereditary folate malabsorption causes megaloblastic anemia, seizures and a syndrome of progressive neurological deterioration

Most patients have presented with megaloblastic anemia, seizures and a progressive syndrome of neurological deterioration. Folate, in both the blood and the CSF, is very low. The anemia is correctable with injections of folate or with the administration of large oral doses, but the concentration in the CSF remains low, suggesting

that a distinct carrier system mediates folate uptake into the brain and that this system is the same as that facilitating intestinal transport.

UREA CYCLE

The urea cycle (Fig. 44-6) mediates the removal of ammonia as urea in the amount of 10 to 20 g per day in the healthy adult. The absence of a fully functional urea cycle may result in hyperammonemic encephalopathy and irreversible brain injury in severe cases. A failure of ureagenesis occurs because of acquired disease, such as cirrhosis secondary to alcoholism, or secondary to an inherited defect, usually a congenital enzymopathy.

The initial two steps of the urea cycle are mitochondrial. Carbamyl phosphate synthetase

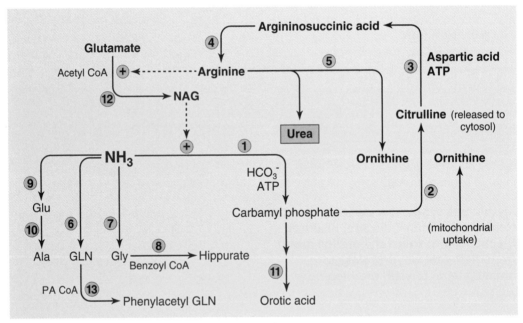

FIGURE 44-6.   The urea cycle and related reactions of ammonia metabolism. Congenital hyperammonemia syndromes usually are caused by a deficiency of one of the enzymes of the urea cycle. Ammonia also can be metabolized to glutamate, alanine, glutamine and glycine. Administration of phenylacetate or of benzoate favors the formation of phenylacetylglutamine and hippurate, respectively, thereby providing an effective "antidote" to ammonia toxicity. *Enzymes*: *1*, carbamyl phosphate synthetase; *2*, ornithine transcarbamylase; *3*, argininosuccinate synthetase; *4*, argininosuccinate lyase; *5*, arginase; *6*, glutamine synthetase; *7*, glycine-cleavage system; *8*, glycine-*N*-acylase; *9*, glutamate dehydrogenase; *10*, alanine aminotransferase; *11*, cytosolic pathway of orotic acid synthesis, which becomes prominent when there is a block at the level of reaction 2, thus resulting in increased orotic acid excretion; *12*, *N*-acetylglutamate synthetase; *13*, phenylacetyl-CoA:glutamine transferase. *NAG*, *N*-acetylglutamate; *PA-CoA*, phenylacetyl-CoA; *GLN*, glutamine. The + symbols denote that arginine and NAG are positive effectors for reactions 12 and 1, respectively.

(CPS), which has been mapped to human chromosome 2, mediates the formation of carbamyl phosphate from NH_3^-, HCO_3^- and ATP (Fig. 44-6, reaction 1). *N*-acetylglutamate (NAG), formed from glutamate and acetyl-CoA via NAG synthetase (Fig. 44-6, reaction 9), is an obligatory effector of CPS and an important regulator of ureagenesis. A variety of influences, including dietary protein, arginine and corticosteroids, augment the concentration of NAG in mitochondria.

Following condensation with ornithine, carbamyl phosphate is converted to citrulline in the ornithine transcarbamylase (OTC) reaction. OTC is coded on band p21.1 of the X chromosome, where the gene contains 8 exons and spans 85 kb of DNA. The activity of this enzyme is directly related to dietary protein. There may be "tunneling" of ornithine transported from the cytosol to OTC, with the availability of intramitochondrial ornithine serving to regulate the reaction.

Citrulline is released to the cytosol, where it condenses with aspartate to form argininosuccinate via argininosuccinate synthetase (AS) (Fig. 44-6, reaction 3). This enzyme is coded on human chromosome 9, where a 63-kb gene comprising 14 exons is located. The mRNA is markedly increased by starvation, treatment with corticosteroids or cAMP. Citrulline itself is a potent inducer of the mRNA.

Argininosuccinate is cleaved in the cytosol by argininosuccinate lyase (AL), which is coded on human chromosome 7 (Fig. 44-6, reaction 4). The products of the reaction are fumarate, which is oxidized in the TCA cycle, and arginine, which is rapidly cleaved to urea and ornithine via hepatic arginase. Both AL and arginase are induced by starvation, dibutyryl cAMP and corticosteroids. Several isozymes of arginase have been described.

Urea cycle defects cause hyperammonemia and may result in coma, convulsions and vomiting during the first few days of life

Clinical confusion with septicemia is common, and many infants are treated futilely with antibiotics. Hyperammonemia usually is severe, even in excess of 1 mM; normal in term infants is up to 100 μM.

Diagnosis usually is made from the blood aminogram. Plasma concentrations of glutamine and alanine, the major nitrogen-carrying amino acids, usually are high and that of arginine is low. Patients with citrullinemia, caused by a deficiency of AS, or argininosuccinic aciduria, caused by a deficiency of AL, will manifest marked increases of blood citrulline and argininosuccinate, respectively.

Urinary orotic acid generally is very elevated in babies with OTC deficiency and normal or even low in infants with CPS deficiency. Patients with OTC deficiency have increased excretion of orotic acid because carbamyl phosphate spills into the cytoplasm, where it enters the pathway of pyrimidine synthesis.

Diagnosis of the infant with either CPS or OTC deficiency may not always be apparent from the blood aminogram. Ornithine concentrations typically are normal in the latter disorder. The presence of hyperammonemia, hyperglutaminemia, hyperalaninemia and orotic aciduria in a critically ill infant affords strong presumptive evidence for OTC deficiency. Conversely, the presence of this pattern on the aminogram in the absence of an untoward orotic aciduria is suggestive of CPS deficiency.

Diagnosis of an urea cycle defect in the older child can be more problematic. Patients may present with psychomotor retardation, growth failure, vomiting, behavioral abnormalities, perceptual difficulties, recurrent cerebellar ataxia and headache. Thus, it is essential to monitor the blood ammonia in any patient with unexplained neurological symptoms. Measurement of blood NH_3 alone may not be sufficient for diagnosis since hyperammonemia can be an inconstant finding with partial enzymatic defects. In the latter group, quantitation of blood amino acids and of urinary orotic acid is indicated.

Hyperammonemia also occurs in some organic acidurias, particularly those that affect neonates. Thus, the urine organic acids should be quantitated in all patients with significant hyperammonemia.

A variety of biochemical changes in brain metabolism have been described in experimental models of hyperammonemia. High ammonia concentrations impair the malate–aspartate shuttle, which mediates the transport of NADH from the cytosol to mitochondria. Changes also occur in the rate of oxidation of glucose and/or pyruvate. The intracellular ATP pool may be depleted, especially in the reticular activating system.

Hyperammonemia also may affect brain volume control; cell swelling is sometimes observed, perhaps because of the marked increase of brain glutamine. This change probably is most prominent in the astrocytes, where it would be expected to have an osmotic effect. Glial swelling is a common pathological finding in hyperammonemic patients.

Hyperammonemia also affects neurotransmitter metabolism. Major effects on the handling of GABA and serotonin have been observed. In the latter instance, a possible mechanism may be increased passage of tryptophan across the blood–brain barrier and consequent increased synthesis of serotonin. Treatment of patients with blockers of serotonergic receptors may alleviate the anorexia that is common in this population. Extracellular glutamic acid tends to increase, and recent experimental evidence suggests excitotoxic injury. Ammonia also has been shown to affect ion flux, in particular that of Cl^-. This might cause hyperpolarization of membranes.

Surprisingly little is known about the changes in the brain of patients dying with hyperammonemia. Abnormal myelination with cystic degeneration of neurons has been described. Cell swelling, particularly of the astrocytes, is common. Cortical atrophy may occur in youngsters with long-standing disease.

Except for patients with argininosuccinic aciduria, who may demonstrate varying degrees of hepatic fibrosis, there is very little evidence of pathological changes outside of the CNS.

Carbamyl phosphate synthetase deficiency prevents the formation of carbamyl phosphate from ammonia

CPS deficiency is relatively rare. Neonates quickly develop lethargy, hypothermia, vomiting and irritability. The hyperammonemia typically is severe, even exceeding 1 mM. Occasional patients with partial enzyme deficiency have had a relapsing syndrome of lethargy and irritability upon exposure to protein. Brain damage can occur in both neonatal and late-onset groups.

N-Acetylglutamate synthetase deficiency leads secondarily to carbamyl phosphate synthetase deficiency

A deficiency of CPS activity also can arise because of the congenital absence of NAG synthetase, which catalyzes the formation of NAG from glutamate and acetyl-CoA. NAG is an obligatory effector of CPS. The few patients reported have had a malignant course of neonatal onset.

Ornithine transcarbamylase deficiency prevents the conversion of carbamyl phosphate to citrulline and is the most common of the urea cycle defects

Presentation is variable, ranging from a fulminant, fatal disorder of neonates to a schizophrenia-like illness in an otherwise healthy adult. Affected men characteristically fare more poorly than women with this X-linked disorder. This difference reflects the random inactivation of the X chromosome, termed Lyon's hypothesis. If the inactivation affects primarily the X chromosome bearing the mutant OTC gene, then a more favorable outcome can be anticipated. Conversely, if the wild-type X chromosome is inactivated, the woman is expected to have a much more active disease.

The human OTC gene spans 73 kb, comprising 10 exons and nine introns. In the mouse, a 750-bp promoter 5′ to the transcription initiation codon confers tissue specificity.

The diagnosis has been aided by the use of genetic markers based on intragenic restriction fragment length polymorphisms (RFLPs) (see also Chap. 40). More than 80% of carriers can be detected in this manner, and antenatal diagnosis is possible in many cases. Approximately one-third of the mothers of boys and two-thirds of the mothers of girls have been found to be noncarriers, reflecting the greater propensity for mutation in the male gamete.

Diagnosis of carriers can be made with protein-loading tests, in which the excretion of urinary orotic acid has been used as a marker. This approach detects 85 to 90% of carriers. A recent elaboration of these tests involves the administration of allopurinol to favor orotic acid excretion. Loading studies with $^{15}NH_4Cl$ as metabolic tracer indicate that symptomatic female carriers for OTC produce less ^{15}N urea compared with a control population. Asymptomatic heterozygotes form urea at a normal rate, but they produce excessive [5-^{15}N]glutamine. Thus, whole-body nitrogen metabolism is abnormal even in this group [33].

Animal models for OTC deficiency have been developed. These include the sparse fur *(spf)* mouse and the sparse fur–abnormal skin and hair *(spf-ash)* mouse. In the former model, a histidine residue replaces an asparagine at position 117 of the gene, resulting in an enzymatic activity that is 15% of control. The *spf-ash* mutation entails a base change in exon 4, resulting in a splicing mutation and a reduction of OTC activity to 5% of normal. Both kinds of mutant mice manifest hyperammonemia, orotic aciduria, growth failure and sparse fur.

OTC deficiency must be suspected in any patient, male or female, with unexplained neurological symptoms. The absence of hyperammonemia in a casual sample should not rule out the diagnosis, especially if the history is positive for protein intolerance or an untoward reaction to infections. Family history also may be suggestive. Blood amino acids and urinary orotic acid should be quantitated in such individuals.

Deficiencies in arginosuccinate synthetase cause citrullinemia

Neonates with AS deficiency (Fig. 44-6, reaction 3) usually die, and most survivors suffer major brain injury. Patients with a partial deficiency may have a milder course, and a few individuals with citrullinemia have been phenotypically normal.

The diagnosis usually is apparent from the hyperammonemia and the extreme hypercitrullinemia. The activity of AS can be deter-

mined in both fibroblasts and chorionic villus samples, thus simplifying the problem of antenatal diagnosis.

Argininosuccinic aciduria results from a deficiency in arginosuccinic lyase, preventing the formation of arginine

Patients with arginosuccinic aciduria excrete an enormous amount of argininosuccinate in their urine. The CSF also contains this polar molecule in high concentration. Neonates have a stormy clinical course, and almost all die or sustain severe brain injury. A peculiar finding in many cases is trichorrhexis nodosa, or dry brittle hair with nodular protrusions, which are best visible with light microscopy. The precise cause is unknown.

Arginase deficiency blocks the conversion of arginine to urea and ornithine and causes a progressive, spastic tetraplegia, especially in the lower extremities

Most patients are thought to have psychomotor retardation during the first year of life. Seizures and growth failure may occur, although some patients are of normal size. The motor dysfunction usually comes to clinical attention by age 2 to 3 years. Leukodystrophic changes are seen. Blood NH_3 is elevated less than in neonatal-onset disorders. The plasma arginine concentration usually is two to five times normal. Urine orotic acid excretion is extremely high, perhaps because arginine stimulates flux through the CPS reaction by favoring the synthesis of NAG.

Hyperornithinemia, hyperammonemia and hypercitrullinemia may also be caused by a failure of mitochondrial ornithine uptake

Electron microscopy of the liver has shown irregularities of mitochondrial shape. This results in a failure of citrulline synthesis and a consequent hyperammonemia. Urinary orotic acid is high, presumably because of underutilization of carbamyl phosphate. In contrast, excretion of creatine is low, reflecting the inhibition of glycine transamidinase by excessive concentrations of ornithine.

These conditions may result in growth failure and varying degrees of mental retardation. Sometimes symptoms are deferred until adulthood. Vomiting, lethargy and hypotonia are noted after protein ingestion. Recurrent hospitalizations for hyperammonemia are the rule. Some patients have manifested a bleeding diathesis and hepatomegaly.

Lysinuric protein intolerance is caused by defects in the transport of lysine, ornithine and arginine

The clinical course in neonates usually is not severe. After weaning or upon exposure to foods high in protein, the infants manifest growth failure, hepatomegaly, splenomegaly, vomiting, hypotonia, recurrent lethargy, coma, abdominal pain and, in rare instances, psychosis. Rarefaction of the bones is common, and both fractures and vertebral compression have been reported. Most patients are not mentally retarded, although this may occur. Some patients have died with interstitial pneumonia, which may respond to corticosteroid therapy.

The dibasic aminoaciduria reflects a failure of reabsorption of lysine, ornithine and arginine by the proximal tubule. There also is a failure to absorb these compounds by the intestinal mucosa. The transport defect occurs at the basolateral, rather than the luminal, membrane. Hyperammonemia reflects a deficiency of intramitochondrial ornithine. An effective treatment is oral citrulline supplementation, which corrects the hyperammonemia by allowing replenishment of the mitochondrial pool of ornithine.

Protein restriction is the mainstay of therapy for the management of urea cycle defects

In patients with very severe disease, tolerance for dietary protein may be so limited that it is not possible to support normal growth.

Treatment with sodium benzoate and sodium phenylacetate represents an important advance in the management of urea cycle defects. Benzoyl-CoA reacts rapidly in the liver with glycine to form hippurate, and phenylacetyl-CoA reacts with glutamine to yield phenylacetylglutamine. Thus, waste nitrogen is eliminated from the body not as urea but as amino acid conjugates of benzoate and phenylacetate [34–36]. Excretion of ammonia as phenylacetylglutamine is more efficient than excretion as hippurate because 2 mol of ammonia are excreted with each mole of phenylacetylglutamine. The clinical utility of phenylacetate is limited by its objectionable odor. Sodium phenylbutyrate, which is less malodorous and is converted in the liver to phenylacetate, has been used with success in place of phenylacetate. Acylation therapy has greatly improved the survival and morbidity for selected patients. Thus, the outlook is favorable for heterozygote girls with OTC deficiency treated from an early age [36].

Most patients who survive the neonatal period can be successfully maintained with a diet low in protein and treatment with sodium benzoate. A useful adjunct to treatment in cases of citrullinemia and argininosuccinic aciduria is supplementation of the diet with arginine, which enhances the ability to eliminate ammonia as either citrulline or argininosuccinate. In addition, maintenance of arginine concentrations in the normal range facilitates protein synthesis.

Liver transplantation has been utilized in children with urea cycle defects. The long-term utility is still uncertain. It appears to afford good metabolic correction, although some abnormalities of amino acid metabolism persist even after transplantation. The high morbidity of organ transplantation restricts the utility of this approach.

Dialysis, including hemodialysis and peritoneal dialysis, relieves acute toxicity during fulminant hyperammonemia. Exchange transfusions also have been performed, but this technique has not been equally useful in removing ammonia.

The possibility of gene therapy for these disorders has been a subject of intense scrutiny [37]. An adenoviral vector containing a cDNA for the OTC gene has been given to mice with a congenital deficiency of OTC. The result was complete correction of hepatic OTC activity over a 2-month period. Transient correction of serum glutamine and urine orotic acid was reported. This experimental approach holds enormous promise for the management of this enzymopathy and other inborn errors of intermediary metabolism.

BIOTIN METABOLISM

Biotin is a cofactor in two reactions involving amino acids: the carboxylation of 3-methyl-crotonyl-CoA in the pathway of leucine catabolism and the carboxylation of propionyl-CoA to form methylmalonyl-CoA (Fig. 44-1). Biotin also is a cofactor for the pyruvate carboxylase reaction in the gluconeogenic pathway and for acetyl-CoA carboxylase in the pathway of fatty acid synthesis. Hence, dietary deficiencies of biotin or congenital anomalies of biotin metabolism lead to the accumulation of several organic acids (Fig. 44-1, reactions 5 and 11).

Biotin is covalently bound to these enzymes via an amide linkage with ϵ-NH_2 groups of lysine residues. A specific enzyme, holocarboxylase synthetase, mediates this attachment. Another enzyme, biotinidase, cleaves biotinyl residues from enzymes, thereby facilitating the recycling of free biotin. Inherited defects of both biotinidase and holocarboxylase synthetase have been described. Prompt clinical recognition of these syndromes is essential because treatment with pharmacological doses of biotin dramatically improves outcome.

Holocarboxylase synthetase deficiency prevents biotinylation of holocarboxylase and results in metabolic acidosis, marked tachypnea, hypotonia, vomiting and seizures

Most patients become symptomatic early in life. The blood pH is typically quite low, often less than 7, and the blood lactate is high. Many infants also have hyperammonemia. Quantitation of urinary organic acids typically shows a marked ketoaciduria with excretion of lactate, 3-methylcrotonylglycine, tiglylglycine, 3-hydroxy-propionate, methylcitrate and 3-hydroxyiso-valerate, *inter alia*. If the disorder is not treated promptly, patients can develop a skin rash, alopecia and varying degrees of psychomotor retardation. Direct assay of holocarboxylase synthetase in fibroblasts is possible. Antenatal diagnosis is feasible, either by determination of enzyme activity or by quantitation of organic acids in the amniotic fluid.

Biotinidase deficiency prevents recycling of biotin and often causes developmental retardation, hypotonia, seizures, cerebellar signs, alopecia, dermatitis and conjunctivitis

Hearing loss is common. Quantitation of the urinary organic acids shows increased excretion of lactate, 3-hydroxyisovalerate, methylcitrate and 3-hydroxypropionate; however, these are not invariant findings, and the measurement of biotinidase activity in fibroblasts or peripheral blood cells may be necessary. Biotinidase activity in the serum of affected children usually is <10% that of control values. Antenatal diagnosis is possible.

Pathological lesions in the brain include cystic changes and demyelination. The cerebellum is especially vulnerable. A few patients have manifested changes suggesting meningoencephalitis. Virtually all patients respond favorably to oral biotin at a dose of 10 to 40 mg daily. Many of the clinical findings are reversible, even including some of the neurological abnormalities, although the hearing loss tends to persist.

GLUTATHIONE METABOLISM

The tripeptide glutathione (γ-glutamyl-cysteinyl-glycine), which serves as a coreactant in the glutathione peroxidase and glutathione transferase reactions, is the major intracellular antioxidant (Fig. 44-7).

The cycle is renewed after the cysteine formed in reaction 6 (Fig. 44-7) and the glutamate derived from reaction 5 are converted to γ-glutamylcysteine via γ-glutamylcysteine synthetase (Fig. 44-7, reaction 1). The most important congenital defects in glutathione metabolism are glutathione synthetase deficiency (Fig. 44-7, reaction 2), γ-glutamylcys-

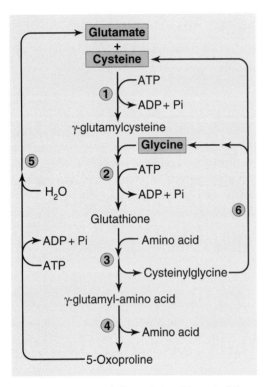

FIGURE 44-7. Metabolism of glutathione. Deficiency in reaction 2 leads to severe metabolic acidosis caused by excessive formation of 5-oxoproline from γ-glutamylcysteine in reaction 4. Deficiencies in reactions 1 and 3 also have neurological effects. Deficiencies in reaction 5 are known, but these patients have no significant neurologic symptoms. *Enzymes: 1,* γ-glutamylcysteine synthetase; *2,* glutathione synthetase; *3,* γ-glutamyltranspeptidase; *4,* cyclotransferase; *5,* 5-oxoprolinase; *6,* peptidase.

teine deficiency (Fig. 44-7, reaction 1), γ-glutamyltranspeptidase deficiency (Fig. 44-7, reaction 3) and 5-oxoprolinase deficiency (Fig. 44-7, reaction 5).

Glutathione synthetase deficiency leads to excessive formation of 5-oxoproline and may result in severe metabolic acidosis

Patients typically have a severe metabolic acidosis caused by excessive formation of 5-oxoproline, also termed pyroglutamic acid. This occurs because the diminution of intracellular glutathione relieves the feedback inhibition on the γ-glutamylcysteine synthetase pathway (Fig. 44-7, reaction 1), thereby augmenting the concen-

tration of γ-glutamylcysteine and the subsequent conversion of this dipeptide to cysteine and 5-oxoproline in the cyclotransferase pathway (Fig. 44-7, reaction 4).

This lesion has been diagnosed in a young adult with mental retardation, severe metabolic acidosis and evidence of a spastic quadriparesis and cerebellar disease. It also has been observed in patients who were first diagnosed in infancy, and who enjoyed a period of normal psychomotor development until late childhood, when a progressive loss of intellectual function became appreciated. Patients also may manifest a mild hemolysis. Pathological changes in the brain have included atrophy of the cerebellum and lesions in the cortex and thalamus. There is no specific therapy.

Patients with 5-oxoprolinase deficiency excrete increased amounts of oxoproline and have a somewhat elevated concentration. They do not have significant neurological problems.

γ-Glutamylcysteine synthetase deficiency is rare

Patients with this very rare disorder have displayed spinocerebellar degeneration, peripheral neuropathy, myopathy and an aminoaciduria secondary to renal tubular dysfunction. Psychosis and a hemolytic anemia have been features in some patients.

γ-Glutamyltranspeptidase deficiency blocks the major pathway for glutathione utilization and causes glutathionuria

These patients also have shown varying degrees of mental retardation. The precise relationship of the neurological signs to the biochemical lesion is problematic. The enzyme is present in the brain, primarily in the capillaries, where it may facilitate amino acid transport. No specific treatment is available.

GABA METABOLISM

GABA is formed via the action of glutamate decarboxylase (see Chap. 16). The metabolism of this neurotransmitter is mediated first by uptake into neurons and glia and second by transamination to succinic semialdehyde via GABA transaminase (GABA-T). The semialdehyde is oxidized to succinate via succinic semialdehyde dehydrogenase.

Pyridoxine dependency is characterized by severe seizure activity of early onset, perhaps even *in utero*

Patients respond dramatically to the parenteral administration of pyridoxine at a dose of 10 to 100 mg with a cessation of convulsions and a marked amelioration of the EEG. Speculation has centered on the possibility that the disease involves faulty binding of pyridoxine, a cofactor in the glutamate decarboxylase reaction, to the enzyme protein.

GABA-transaminase deficiency causes increased concentrations of GABA and β-alanine in the blood and cerebrospinal fluid

Patients with this very rare disorder have severe psychomotor retardation and hyperreflexia. Concentrations in the CSF and blood of GABA and β-alanine are much greater than normal, as is the concentration of homocarnosine in the CSF. GABA-T activity is much diminished in blood lymphocytes and in the liver. A curious finding is increased stature, perhaps reflecting the ability of GABA to evoke release of growth hormone.

Succinic semialdehyde dehydrogenase deficiency causes increased excretion of succinic semialdehyde and 4-hydroxybutyric acid

Affected patients have mental retardation, cerebellar disease and hypotonia. They excrete large amounts of both succinic semialdehyde and 4-hydroxybutyric acid. There is no known therapy.

N-ACETYLASPARTATE METABOLISM: CANAVAN'S DISEASE

Infants with Canavan's disease seem normal at birth, but a delay in development usually is apparent by 3 months of age. An increased head cir-

cumference that is greater than the 98th percentile is common, and hydrocephalus sometimes is suspected. Neurological function deteriorates rapidly over the next several months. Optic atrophy ultimately leads to blindness. These infants manifest minimal interest in their environment. Spasticity is frequent and seizures may occur. Imaging of the brain shows demyelination and brain atrophy with enlargment of the ventricles and widening of the sulci. Pathological examination shows swelling of the astrocytes with elongation of the mitochondria. Vacuoles appear in the myelin.

Excretion of *N*-acetylaspartate is grossly elevated, and the concentration of this amino acid in the CSF may be 50 times control values. The cause is a deficiency of aspartoacylase, which mediates the formation of aspartate and acetyl-CoA from *N*-acetylaspartate. Aspartoacylase normally is found primarily in the white matter, but *N*-acetylaspartate is most abundant in the gray matter. The defect is expressed in cultured skin fibroblasts. *N*-acetylaspartate is among the most abundant amino acids in the brain, although its precise function remains elusive. Putative roles have included osmoregulation and the storage of acetyl groups that subsequently are utilized for myelin synthesis. The relationship of the enzyme defect to the clinical findings remains problematic. No specific therapy is yet available.

REFERENCES

1. Nyhan, W. L. *Diagnostic Recognition of Genetic Disease.* Philadelphia: Lea & Febiger, 1987.
2. Scriver, C. R., Beaudet, A. L., Sly, W. S., and Valle, D. *The Metabolic Basis of Inherited Disease.* New York: McGraw-Hill, 1989.
3. Chalmers, R. A., and Lawson, A. M. *Organic Acids in Man, The Analytical Chemistry, Biochemistry and Diagnosis of the Organic Acidurias.* London: Chapman and Hall, 1982.
4. Goodman, S. I., and Markey, S. P. *Diagnosis of Organic Acidemias by Gas Chromatography-Mass Spectrometry. Laboratory and Research Methods in Biology and Medicine.* New York: Alan R. Liss, 1981.
5. Brismar, J., and Ozand, P. T. CT and MR of the brain in disorders of the propionate and methylmalonate metabolism. *Am. J. Neuroradiol.* 15:1459–1473, 1994.

6. Hamilton, R. L., Haas, R. H., Nyhan, W. L., Powell, H. C., and Grafe, M. R. Neuropathology of propionic acidemia: A report of two patients with basal ganglia lesions. *J. Child Neurol.* 10:25–30, 1995.

7. Chuang, D. T., Davie, J. R., Wynn, R. M., Chuang, J. L., Koyata, H., and Cox, R. P. Molecular basis of maple syrup urine disease and stable correction by retroviral gene transfer. *J. Nutr.* 125:1766S–1772S, 1995.

8. Kaplan, P., Mazur, A., Field, M., et al. Intellectual outcome in children with maple syrup urine disease. *J. Pediatr.* 119:46–50, 1991.

9. Mueller, G. M., McKenzie, L. R., Homanics, G. E., Watkins, S. C., Robbins, P. D., and Paul, H. S. Complementation of defective leucine decarboxylation in fibroblasts from a maple syrup urine disease patient by retrovirus-mediated gene transfer. *Gene Ther.* 2:461–468, 1995.

10. Yudkoff, M., Cohn, R. M., Puschak, R., and Segal, S. Glycine therapy in isovaleric acidemia. *J. Pediatr.* 92:813–817, 1978.

11. Walter, J. H., Wraith, J. E., and Cleary, M. A. Absence of acidosis in the initial presentation of propionic acidaemia. *Arch. Dis. Child.* 72:F197–F199, 1995.

12. North, K. N., Korson, M. S., Gopal, Y. R., et al. Neonatal-onset propionic acidemia: Neurologic and developmental profiles, and implications for management. *J. Pediatr.* 126:916–922, 1995.

13. Haas, R. H., Marsden, D. L., Capistrano-Estrada, S., et al. Acute basal ganglia infarction in propionic acidemia. *J. Child. Neurol.* 10:18–22, 1995.

14. Leonard, J. V. The management and outcome of propionic and methylmalonic acidaemia. *J. Inherit. Metab. Dis.* 18:430–434, 1995.

15. Depondt, E., Rapoport, D., Rabier, D., et al. Clinical outcome of long-term management of patients with vitamin B_{12}-unresponsive methylmalonic acidemia. *J. Pediatr.* 125:903–908, 1995.

16. Shevell, M. I., Didomenicantonio, G., Sylvain, M., Arnold, D. L., O'Gorman, A. M., and Scriver, C. R. Glutaric acidemia type II: Neuroimaging and spectroscopy evidence for developmental encephalomyopathy. *Pediatr. Neurol.* 12:350–353, 1995.

17. Uziel, G., Garavaglia, B., Ciceri, E., Moroni, I., and Rimoldi, M. Riboflavin-responsive glutaric aciduria type II presenting as a leukodystrophy. *Pediatr. Neurol.* 13:333–335, 1995.

18. Bickel, H. Differential diagnosis and treatment of hyperphenylalaninemia. *Prog. Clin. Biol. Res.* 177:93–98, 1985.

19. Eisensmith, R. C., and Woo, S. L. Phenylketonuria and the phenylalanine hydroxylase gene. *Mol. Biol. Med.* 8:3–10, 1991.

20. Guldberg, P., Levy, H. L., Hanley, W. B., et al. Phenylalanine hydroxylase gene mutations in the United States: Report from the Maternal PKU Collaborative Study. *Am. J. Hum. Genet.* 59:84–94, 1996.

21. Diamond, A., and Herzberg, C. Impaired sensitivity to visual contrast in children treated early and continuously for phenylketonuria. *Brain* 119:523–538, 1996.

22. Hommes, F. A. Loss of neurotransmitter receptors by hyperphenylalaninemia in the HPH-5 mouse brain. *Acta Paediatr. Suppl.* 407:120–121, 1994.

23. Levy, H. L., and Ghavami, M. Maternal phenylketonuria: A metabolic teratogen. *Teratology* 53:176–184, 1996.

24. Kaufman, S. Hyperphenylalaninaemia caused by defects in biopterin metabolism. *J. Inherit. Metab. Dis.* 8(Suppl 1):20–27, 1983.

25. Kikuchi, G. The glycine cleavage system: Composition, reaction mechanism and physiological significance. *Mol. Cell. Biochem.* 1:169–175, 1973.

26. Steiner, R. D., Sweetser, D. A., Rohrbaugh, J. R., Dowton, S. B., Toone, J. R., and Applegarth, D. A. Nonketotic hyperglycinemia: Atypical clinical and biochemical manifestations. *J. Pediatr.* 128:243–246, 1996.

27. Van Hove, J. L., Kishnani, P., Muenzer, J., et al. Benzoate therapy and carnitine deficiency in nonketotic hyperglycinemia. *Am. J. Med. Genet.* 59:444–453, 1995.

28. Alemzadeh, R., Gammeltoft, K., and Matteson, K. Efficacy of low-dose dextromethorphan in the treatment of nonketotic hyperglycinemia. *Pediatrics* 97:924–926, 1996.

29. Kluijtmans, L. A., Boers, G. H., Stevens, E. M., et al. Defective cystathionine beta-synthase regulation by *S*-adenosylmethionine in a partially pyridoxine responsive homocystinuria patient. *J. Clin. Invest.* 98:285–289, 1996.

30. Kraus, J. P. Komrower Lecture. Molecular basis of phenotype expression in homocystinuria. *J. Inherit. Metab. Dis.* 17:383–390, 1994.

31. Mandel, H., Brenner, B., Berant, M., et al. Coexistence of hereditary homocystinuria and factor V Leiden—effect on thrombosis. *N. Engl. J. Med.* 334:763–768, 1996.

32. Dudman, N. P., Guo, X. W., Gordon, R. B., Dawson, P. A., and Wilcken, D. E. Human homocysteine catabolism: Three major pathways and their relevance to development of arterial occlusive disease. *J. Nutr.* 126(Suppl. 4):295s–300s, 1996.

33. Yudkoff, M., Daikhin, Y., Nissim, I., Jawad, A., Wilson, J., and Batshaw, M. B. *In vivo* nitrogen metabolism in ornithine transcarbamylase deficiency. *J. Clin. Invest.* 98:2167–2173, 1996.

34. Brusilow, S., Tinker, J., and Batshaw, M. L. Amino acid acylation: A mechanism of nitrogen excretion in inborn errors of urea synthesis. *Science* 207:659, 1980.

35. Maestri, N. E., Hauser, E. R., Bartholomew, D., and Brusilow, S. W. Prospective treatment of urea cycle disorders. *J. Pediatr.* 119:923, 1991.

36. Maestri, N. E., Brusilow, S. W., Clissold, D. B., and Bassett, S. S. Long-term treatment of girls with ornithine transcarbamylase deficiency. *N. Engl. J. Med.* 335:855–859, 1996.

37. Ye, X., Robinson, M. B., Batshaw, M. L., Furth, E. E., Smith, I., and Wilson, J. M. Prolonged metabolic correction in adult ornithine transcarbamylase-deficient mice with adenoviral vectors. *J. Biol. Chem.* 271:3639–3646, 1996.

45

Neurotransmitters and Disorders of the Basal Ganglia

J. Sian, M. B. H. Youdim, P. Riederer and M. Gerlach

Basic Neurochemistry: Molecular, Cellular and Medical Aspects, 6th Ed., edited by G. J. Siegel et al. Published by Lippincott–Raven Publishers, Philadelphia, 1999. Correspondence to J. Sian, Division of Clinical Neurochemistry, Department of Psychiatry, University of Würzburg, 97080 Würzburg, Germany.

BIOCHEMICAL ANATOMY OF THE BASAL GANGLIA AND ASSOCIATED NEURAL SYSTEMS

The basal ganglia consist of several large, anatomically distinct masses of gray matter situated in the core of the cerebral hemispheres among ascending and descending tracts of white matter and astride the brainstem. These constitute the striatum, comprised of the caudate and putamen, and the pallidum, comprised of the internal and external portions of the globus pallidus. The striatopallidal system is a complex, integrated unit that has many afferent and efferent connections to other parts of the brain and, with several other subcortical structures, constitutes an extrapyramidal system regulating sensorimotor activity, including tone and posture. It is also a part of a frontal cortical–subcortical system implicated in schizophrenia (Chap. 51). The neurotransmitters present in various regions of the brain have been identified, the enzymes involved in the biosynthesis and degradation of many of these transmitters have been described and the presence of uptake sites for inactivation of transmitters as well as receptors mediating their effects on neuronal activity has been demonstrated. To better understand the functional role of the relevant neurotransmitters and neuromodulators, it is important to consider also the neuronal circuits and connections of the basal ganglia.

Neurotransmitter systems involving catecholamines, serotonin and GABA have been identified in the basal ganglia

A number of important techniques for precise cellular localization of neurotransmitters, enzymes involved in their synthesis or degradation, receptors and their subtypes and transporters have been applied to studies of the various neuronal pathways projecting to or arising from the basal ganglia. Catecholamines (CAs), including dopamine (DA), norepinephrine (NE) and epinephrine, as well as serotonin (5-HT), can be converted to fluorescent derivatives, which can then be used to delineate their distribution in neurons and their processes. Antibodies to neurotransmitters such as GABA and peptides, as well as against specific proteins, are useful for their immunohistological demonstration in brain. Radiolabeled neurotransmitters and ligands or blockers of transporters and receptors have been used for autoradiographic localization of uptake sites and receptor subtypes. The application of *in situ* hybridization using cDNA probes for mRNAs that encode peptide precursors, receptors, transporters, biosynthetic enzymes and specific neuronal proteins has provided a wealth of information regarding neuronal pathways throughout the brain, including the basal ganglia. These techniques provide quantitative as well as anatomical information, and together with biochemical assays, neurophysiologically monitored responses and behavioral studies have enormously enhanced our understanding of the basal ganglia, associated structures and the involved neurotransmitters (Fig. 45-1).

The basal ganglia are heterogeneous structures

In the striatum, differences in the intensity of staining with several neuronal markers show that the populations of cells in various regions are not uniform. Compartmentalization was first suggested by differences in the intensity of staining for acetylcholinesterase (AChE). Whereas most of the striatum stains heavily for this enzyme, AChE-poor islands, termed *striasomes* or patches, constitute 10 to 20% of the striatum. The striasomes constitute a labyrinthine mesh embedded in a matrix of AChE-rich striatal tissue. In addition to differences in AChE content, these areas have been found to differ quantitatively from the remainder of the striatum with respect to the concentration of several other substances (see below); furthermore, the neurons in the striasomes appear to receive distinct cortical input and to project differently from those in the matrix [1,2].

Excitatory amino acids provide afferent input to the basal ganglia

Glutamate and aspartate are excitatory amino acid neurotransmitters present in many neurons throughout the brain (Chap. 15). They are involved in basal ganglia afferent, connecting and efferent pathways, which together with thalamic and subthalamic nuclei constitute feedback circuits that modulate cerebral cortical function. The major afferent neuronal pathways to the striatum are from the sensorimotor and other cortical areas and from the thalamus; these fibers release excitatory amino acids, mostly glutamate, in synapses with dendrites on striatal neurons. Glutamate is also the excitatory neurotransmitter released from terminals of the subthalamic neurons projecting to the pallidum, particularly to the internal layer of the globus pallidus, and from the axon terminals of thalamic neurons that send fibers mainly to the cortex.

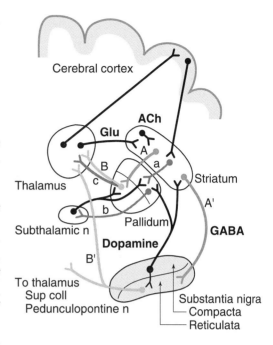

FIGURE 45-1. The direct pathway contains two inhibitory GABAergic synapses: *A* or *A' (dark orange)* is between the striatum and the medial pallidum, or the substantia nigra pars reticulata (SNr); *B* or *B' (light orange)* is between the medial pallidum or SNr and the ventroanterior and ventrolateral nuclei of the thalamus. Activation of this pathway produces disinhibition of the excitatory glutamatergic thalamic input to the sensory, motor and associated areas of the cortex. The indirect pathway, *a, b, c (gray)*, includes one excitatory glutamatergic and three inhibitory GABAergic synapses: *a* is between the striatum and the lateral pallidum; *b* is between the lateral pallidum and the subthalamic nucleus, and the subthalamic nucleus projects excitatory fibers to the medial pallidum; and *c* is between the medial pallidum and the thalamus. In contrast to the direct pathway, the three inhibitory synapses *(a, b, c)* result in net inhibition (inhibition of disinhibition) of the thalamic-cortical projections when the indirect circuit is activated. The activity in the two pathways depends, among other factors, on the balance of excitatory and inhibitory receptors activated on the striatal GABAergic neurons. D1 excitatory receptors are found mainly on the direct pathway and D2 inhibitory receptors, mainly on the indirect path. The dopaminergic innervations of the striatum from the substantia nigra pars compacta and the intrastriatal cholinergic neurons are among the most important modulators of these circuits. In addition, a number of peptides, variably colocalized with the four major neurotransmitters, modulate basal ganglia function (see text). *ACh*, acetylcholine; *Sup coll*, superior colliculus; *Glu*, glutamate; *n*, nuclei.

In the striatum, release of the excitatory transmitters is modulated by presynaptic receptors for acetylcholine (ACh), DA, GABA, opioids and adenosine. Also present are many peptides and other neuromodulators (Table 45-1), which may have modulatory effects similar to those of the cotransmitters. Nitric oxide (NO) is a prime example of a neuromodulator (see Chap. 10). It is a small, gaseous, lipophilic molecular mediator, which readily diffuses across cellular membranes. Thus, it can elicit both anterograde and retrograde signaling at the synapses. In addition, it plays a vital role in N-methyl-D-aspartate (NMDA)-mediated transmission. NO is synthesized from L-arginine by a family of NO synthases (NOS). NOS is found in both glia and neurons, particularly in the medium aspiny neurons of the striatum and other brain regions.

Ionotropic and metabotropic excitatory amino acid receptors are localized on striatal neurons

The excitatory amino acids glutamate and aspartate are unevenly distributed in the basal ganglia thalamocortical circuits (Fig. 45-2A). The receptors that respond to excitatory amino acids, particularly to glutamate, may be ionotropic or metabotropic (see Chap. 15). There are at least three types of ionotropic glutamate receptors that can be distinguished in the striatum by their responses to selective agonists. These are NMDA, kainate (KA) and α-amino-3-hydroxy-5-methyl-4-isoxazolepropionic acid (AMPA). It is believed that NMDA receptors reside mainly

TABLE 45-1.	PEPTIDES AND NEURO-MODULATORS FOUND IN THE BASAL GANGLIA
Substance P (S)[a]	Somatostatin (M)[a]
Substance K	Dynorphin (S)[a]
Cholecystokinin	Enkephalin (M)[a]
Neurotensin (S)[a]	Galinin
Neurokinin B	Nitric oxide
Lys[8]-Asn[9]-neurotensin (8–13)	Carbon monoxide
Neuropeptide Y	Phenylethylamine

[a]Preferentially localized in striosomes (S) or matrix (M) as indicated in text.

on the GABAergic efferent neurons of the striatonigral pathway. NMDA receptors are associated with ligand-gated Ca^{2+} channels, whereas KA and AMPA receptors are associated with ligand-gated K^+/Na^+ channels. Since decortication of rats does not diminish significantly the binding of radiolabeled NMDA, KA or AMPA in the striatum whereas destruction of striatal neurons with the excitotoxin quinolinic acid does strikingly decrease binding of these ligands, it appears that most of these receptors are postjunctional. Four subtypes of excitatory amino acid metabotropic glutamate receptors have also been identified in the striatum, mGluR1–mGluR4.

GABA is the neurotransmitter of most striatal efferent neurons

High concentrations of GABA are found in the substantia nigra, globus pallidus and subthalamic nucleus (Fig. 45-2). The striatum is reputed to contain a population of GABAergic aspiny interneurons. In addition, a vast number of medium spiny neurons release GABA as a neurotransmitter. This was first demonstrated by use of an antibody specific for the enzyme responsible for GABA formation, glutamic acid decarboxylase (GAD) and, later, with antibodies to GABA (Chap. 16). Antibodies to peptide neurotransmitters or probes for mRNA encoding the peptides or their precursors have been used to demonstrate colocalization of these peptides in subpopulations of GABAergic neurons. Some peptides that have been found in the striatum are listed in Table 45-1. GABAergic efferent neurons of the striatum project to the external and internal layers of the pallidum and to the substantia nigra; the latter constitute the striatonigral path (Fig. 45-1). Those that project to the external layer of the globus pallidus often contain enkephalin as a cotransmitter. They synapse on GABAergic neurons which project from the external layer of the globus pallidus to the glutamatergic neurons in the subthalamic nucleus; these form the indirect pathway (Fig. 45-1). The GABAergic striatal neurons that project to the internal layer of the globus pallidus and substantia nigra pars reticulata often contain substance P and/or dynorphin; these form the direct pathway

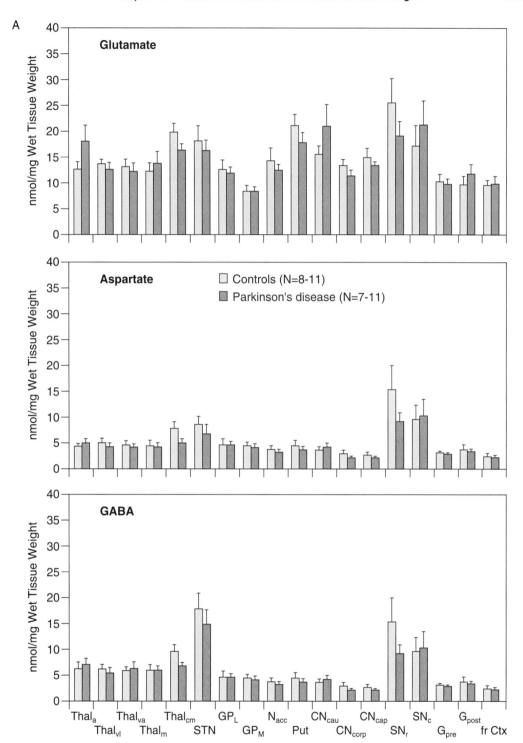

FIGURE 45-2. Concentrations in the basal ganglia of control and Parkinson's disease human brains. **A:** Glutamate, aspartate and GABA. Values are presented as mean ± SEM. $Thal_a$, anterior thalamus; $Thal_{vl}$, ventral lateral thalamus; $Thal_{va}$, ventral anterior thalamus; $Thal_m$, medial thalamus; $Thal_{cm}$, centromedial thalamus; STN, subthalamic nucleus; GP_L, lateral globus pallidus; GP_M, medial globus pallidus; N_{acc}, nucleus accumbens; Put, anterior putamen; CN_{cau}, tail of caudate nucleus; CN_{corp}, body of the caudate nucleus; CN_{cap}, head of caudate nucleus; SN_r, substantia nigra pars reticulata; SN_c, substantia nigra pars compacta; G_{pre}, precentral gyrus; G_{post}, postcentral gyrus; *fr Ctx*, frontal cortex. (Modified from [32], with permission.) (*Figure continues on next page.*)

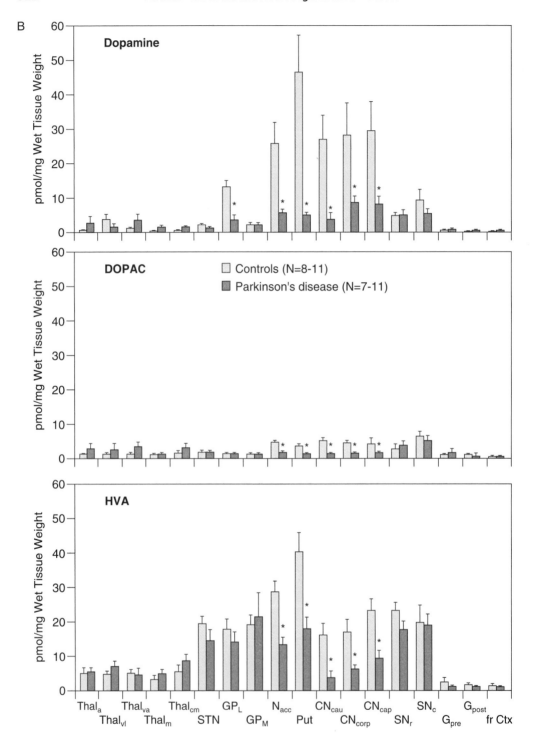

FIGURE 45-2. *(Continued)* **B:** Dopamine and its metabolites 3,4-dihydroxyphenylacetic acid *(DOPAC)* and homovanillic acid *(HVA)*. Values are presented as mean ± SEM. *Thal*$_a$, anterior thalamus; *Thal*$_{vl}$, ventral lateral thalamus; *Thal*$_{va}$, ventral anterior thalamus; *Thal*$_m$, medial thalamus; *Thal*$_{cm}$, centromedial thalamus; *STN*, subthalamic nucleus; *GP*$_L$, lateral globus pallidus; *GP*$_M$, medial globus pallidus; *N*$_{acc}$, nucleus accumbens; *Put*, anterior putamen; *CN*$_{cau}$, tail of caudate nucleus; *CN*$_{corp}$, body of the caudate nucleus; *CN*$_{cap}$, head of caudate nucleus; *SN*$_r$, substantia nigra pars reticulata; *SN*$_c$, substantia nigra pars compacta; *G*$_{pre}$, precentral gyrus; *G*$_{post}$, postcentral gyrus; *fr Ctx*, frontal cortex. (Modified from [32], with permission.)

(Fig. 45-1). GABAergic neurons in the stria-somes appear to project to the substantia nigra pars compacta. Many of these neurons contain neurotensin; tachykinins, including substance P or K; and/or dynorphin.

GABA receptors are abundant in the basal ganglia, hypothalamus, hippocampus and dorsal horn of the spinal cord. Two GABA receptor subtypes have been characterized, GABA$_A$ and GABA$_B$ (see Chap. 16). The postsynaptic GABA$_A$ receptor executes the inhibitory effects of the neurotransmitter, primarily by altering the membrane permeability to chloride ions. In contrast, the presynaptic GABA$_B$ receptor modulates the release of GABA.

Acetylcholine is the neurotransmitter of striatal interneurons

ACh is the neurotransmitter contained in many of the large spiny neurons that make up about 5% of the striatal neurons. These neurons, which are distinguished by immunoreactivity to choline acetyltransferase (ChAT), the enzyme responsible for synthesis of ACh, receive several types of synaptic input: (i) glutamatergic fibers from the cerebral cortex; (ii) tyrosine hydroxylase (TH)-immunoreactive, presumably dopaminergic, fibers which form small, symmetrical synapses on the soma and proximal dendrites; and (iii) substance P/GAD-immunopositive boutons, believed to be axon collaterals from medium spiny neurons. These cholinergic interneurons have relatively short axons that are confined to the striatum and that innervate predominantly the medium spiny neurons.

Both muscarinic and nicotinic cholinergic receptors are found in the striatum (see Chap. 11). Muscarinic receptors on glutamatergic terminals are thought to inhibit release of the excitatory transmitter, acting as a modulator of glutamatergic stimulation of striatal neurons, whereas nicotinic receptor activation enhances transmitter release.

Dopamine is the neurotransmitter of the nigrostriatal pathway

DA is widely distributed throughout the brain, but, as shown in Figure 45-2, particularly high concentrations are found in the striatal areas [3]. Indeed, although DA accounts for about half of the total CAs in the brain, over 80% of DA in the brain is in the basal ganglia and its concentration in the striatum is much greater than that of NE. Such differences in distribution were the first indication of its role as a neurotransmitter. Histofluorescence techniques for visualizing DA and immunohistological localization of TH, the rate-limiting enzyme for its biosynthesis, have been used to map DA-containing neurons and the pathways of their axons to the terminal arborizations at their target regions (Chap. 12).

The principal dopaminergic fiber systems in brain are the *nigrostriatal,* from the substantia nigra pars compacta to the caudate nucleus and putamen; the *mesolimbic,* from the ventral tegmental area to the nucleus accumbens; the *mesocortical,* from the ventral tegmental area to the cerebral cortex; and the *tuberoinfundibular,* from the arcuate nucleus to the median eminence. There are also DA-containing neurons and terminals in other brain regions, in the retina and in the spinal cord. These neurons store DA in vesicles within varicosities of the nerve terminals. Intravesicular concentrations of DA are maintained at high concentrations, 1 to 20 mg/g fresh weight.

DA in the striatum is contained in a dense aborization of the fine terminals derived from the DA-containing neurons of the substantia nigra pars compacta. These structures contain TH so that DA can be synthesized directly at the terminal varicosities. TH requires iron and tetrahydropteridine in order to oxidize tyrosine to 3,4-dihydroxyphenylalanine (levodopa, L-DOPA) (Chap. 12). Only small amounts of L-DOPA are found in the tissue; however, it is readily decarboxylated by aromatic amino acid decarboxylase (AADC). This enzyme is present in many tissues, including serotonergic neurons, where it decarboxylates 5-hydroxytryptophan (5-HTP) to form serotonin (see Chap. 13). Like other amino acid decarboxylases, AADC requires pyridoxyl phosphate as its coenzyme. AADC is inhibited by many compounds, a few of which have been used therapeutically. The chemical structures of some decarboxylase inhibitors are shown in Figure 45-3. DA synthesis in the nerve terminals is accelerated during depolarization-induced re-

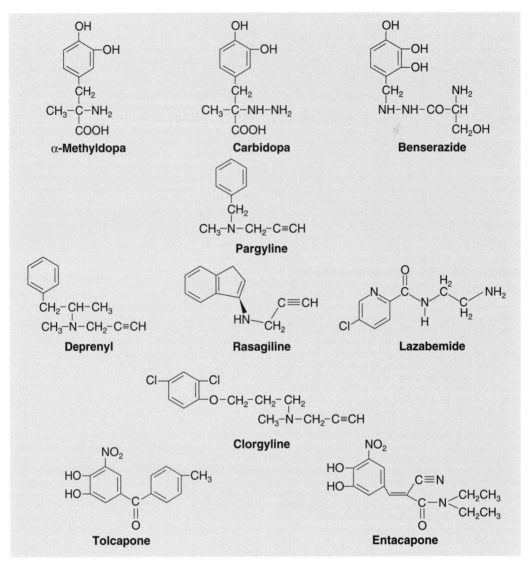

FIGURE 45-3.   Inhibitors of enzymes involved in the metabolism of levodopa and of dopamine. Aromatic amino acid decarboxylase *(AADC)* is inhibited by α-methyldopa, carbidopa and benserazide. Pargyline inhibits both monoamine oxidase *(MAO)* subtypes, whereas deprenyl, rasagiline and lazabemide are selective for MAO type B and clorgyline for MAO type A. Tolcapone and entacapone inhibit catechol-*O*-methyltransferase.

lease of the neurotransmitter. This is the result of rapid activation of TH. Enhanced release of DA results in elevated levels of its metabolites in the tissues and in the surrounding fluids.

Both D1 and D2 receptors have been defined pharmacologically; thus, there are specific ligands for these receptors (see Chap. 12 for receptor classification). D1 receptors contain D1 and D5 receptor gene products and D2 receptors are comprised of D2, D3 and D4 gene products.

However, the more recent identification of D3, D4 and D5 is chiefly based on findings from molecular genetic studies; therefore, the classical pharmacological nomenclature is still often adopted. D1 receptors are present on dynorphin/substance P-containing medium spiny neurons, and both D1 and D2 receptors are present on a subpopulation of striatal neurons. There are D2 receptors on the terminals of corticostriatal projections, on enkephalin-containing medium spiny neurons and cholinergic interneurons and, as autoreceptors, on dopaminergic neurons on the substantia nigra pars compacta.

There is considerable evidence that there are important functional distinctions and interactions between the D1 and D2 families of receptors. D1 and D5 receptors are excitatory; they stimulate adenylyl cyclase activity and, possibly, phosphoinositide hydrolysis. D2, D3 and D4 receptors are inhibitory, and they reduce adenylyl cyclase activity (see Chaps. 12 and 22). D1 and D2 receptors, which are both abundant in the striatum, are the principal DA receptors involved in the pathophysiology of Parkinson's disease. D1 is the main type of DA receptor on the striatal neurons of the direct pathway, while D2 is the main type in the indirect pathway (Fig. 45-1). Combined administration of D1 and D2 agonists appears to have synergistic biochemical and behavioral effects. Functional studies related to the basal ganglia demonstrate that, for the im-

plementation of motor behavior, the synergistic action of both D1 and, mainly, D2 receptors is required.

Dopamine is primarily metabolized by *O*-methylation and oxidative deamination

The major metabolites of DA are products of *O*-methylation and/or oxidative deamination. Major products include 3-methoxytyramine (3-MT), 3,4-dihydroxyphenylacetic acid (DOPAC) and 4-hydroxy-3-methoxyphenylacetic acid, or homovanillic acid (HVA) (Fig. 45-2). These are depicted in Figure 45-4, which also shows the alternative pathways of metabolism of DA. Some of the compounds shown in Figure 45-4 are conjugated with sulfate or glucuronate before excretion in the urine or bile.

The amine and its *O*-methyl derivative are both subject to the action of monoamine oxidase (MAO), a flavoprotein present in the outer

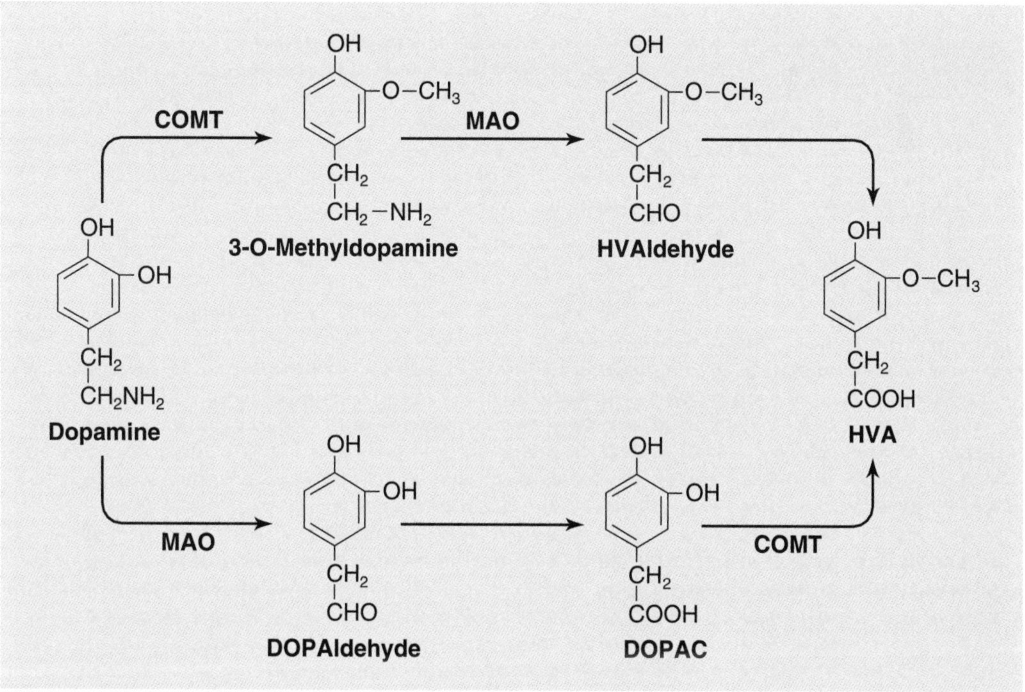

FIGURE 45-4. Dopamine and its major metabolites. Dopamine is sequentially deaminated and *O*-methylated or vice versa, depending on the site of metabolism (see text). *MAO*, monoamine oxidase; *COMT*, catechol-*O*-methyltransferase; *HVA*, homovanillic acid; *DOPAC*, 3,4-dihydroxyphenylacetic acid.

membrane of the mitochondria. MAO exists in two forms: MAO type A (MAO-A) is especially sensitive to inhibition by clorgyline and is present in catecholaminergic neurons and their axons, whereas MAO type B (MAO-B) is inhibited selectively by deprenyl and predominates in serotonin-containing neurons and in astrocytes. Pargyline irreversibly inhibits both MAO-A and MAO-B. The chemical structures of these three propargylamine inhibitors are shown in Figure 45-3.

Products of the MAO reaction include the aldehyde corresponding to the amine substrate, hydrogen peroxide and ammonia. Most of the aldehyde undergoes further dehydrogenation to form, in the case of DA, DOPAC, which is the substrate for catechol-O-methyltransferase (COMT), an enzyme that catalyzes the transfer of the methyl group from S-adenosylmethionine to the m-hydroxyl group. This process appears to be very efficient in human brain because normally there are only very small quantities of DOPAC in the striatum but substantial amounts of HVA. A portion of the aldehyde undergoes reduction catalyzed by alcohol dehydrogenase or a similar enzyme, with the participation of nicotinamide coenzyme. The alcoholic products that are formed are far less abundant than the acidic metabolites of DA but are major metabolites of NE.

The black pigment neuromelanin, which accumulates in the neurons of the substantia nigra pars compacta with aging (see Chap. 30), is derived from polymerization of quinones formed from catechols, mostly L-DOPA and DA. The function, if any, of neuromelanin is unknown. It may be related to the vulnerability of these neurons to toxic damage or degenerative processes, including the release of iron from ferritin. These factors may relate to Parkinson's disease (see below).

The circuits of the basal ganglia are regulated by feedback systems and modulatory peptide cotransmitters

The two principal intrinsic basal ganglia circuits presently recognized consist of the direct and indirect pathways between the striatum and the thalamus, as depicted in Figure 45-1. The direct path is composed of GABAergic inhibitory fibers from the striatum to the internal or medial globus pallidus (GPm) and to the substantia nigra pars reticulata (SNr), the main efferent nuclei of the basal ganglia. From these nuclei, another set of GABAergic inhibitory fibers extends to the ventroanterior (VA) and ventrolateral (VL) nuclei of the thalamus. The thalamic VA and VL nuclei project excitatory glutamatergic fibers to the cortex, where these fibers modulate cortical outflows back to the striatum, to the spinal cord and elsewhere. DA fibers from the substantia nigra pars compacta (SNc) stimulate the direct path through D1 receptors on the GABAergic striatal neurons, which results in disinhibition of the thalamus and net activation of the cortex. The indirect path is formed of GABAergic inhibitory fibers from the striatum to the external or lateral globus pallidus (GPl), which extends GABAergic inhibitory fibers to the subthalamic nucleus (STN); the latter, in turn, projects excitatory glutamatergic fibers to the efferent stage, GPm and SNr. Thus, excitation of the indirect path would lead to inhibition of the thalamus. The interposition in the indirect circuit of additional excitatory and inhibitory synapses has the dual effect of delaying an impulse in the indirect relative to the direct circuit and, when activated, of producing net inhibition rather than stimulation of cortical neurons. However, there is a critical difference in the DA effects on these two routes. The indirect circuit is inhibited by SNc DA fibers through inhibitory D2 receptors, leading to disinhibition by these DA fibers as in the direct path. The striatal neurons are modulated normally by both excitatory and inhibitory transmitters and receptors. Loss of the nigrostriatal DA input from the SNc, as in Parkinson's disease (see below), results in complicated patterns of imbalance in these circuits and generally a greatly increased inhibitory striatal outflow through the GPm and SNr with net reductions in thalamocortical activation.

Cholinergic and substance P axons terminate on the proximal portions of the dendrites of the medium spiny neurons in the striatum. The extensive axon collaterals of these spiny neurons release GABA, and probably their peptide cotransmitters, into synapses near or on the cell bodies of other spiny neurons. Interneurons that release ACh also contain somatostatin and neuropeptide Y (NPY), which may modulate striatal neuron activity. Best known and perhaps most important, dopaminergic fibers from the SNc that synapse on the medium spiny neurons, as well as fibers that synapse on the more distal parts of their dendritic tree, modulate striatal efferent GABAergic output.

As indicated above, dopaminergic neurons project mainly from the SNc to innervate the striatum, and 80% of the DA content in the brain is found in the basal ganglia. DA plays a multifunctional role in the basal ganglia. It regulates cortically initiated basal ganglia–thalamic conduction. DA released in the striatum can act at any of several receptor sites to modulate outflow of GABAergic neuronal activity to the globus pallidus or substantia nigra. The complexity of interconnections via neuronal networks, feedback circuits and D1 and D2 receptors on the same cell defies simple analysis, but it is evident that the net effects of DA deficiency are responsible for the striking motor abnormalities seen in parkinsonian syndromes (Table 45-2). Conversely, conditions that cause overactivity of DA or the systems normally activated by DA result in an array of involuntary dyskinesias. These sometimes appear in association with the hy-pokinetic features of parkinsonism and are generally attributed to disorders of the basal ganglia and its output pathways. Thus, basal ganglia disorders are associated with parkinsonian hypokinetic, as well as a variety of hyperkinetic, conditions.

PARKINSON'S DISEASE

Parkinson's disease was first described in a classic monograph, "The Shaking Palsy," published in 1817 by the London physician James Parkinson. The cardinal features of Parkinson's disease are (i) tremor, mainly at rest; (ii) muscular rigidity, which leads to difficulties in walking, writing, speaking and masking of facial expression; (iii) bradykinesia, a slowness in initiating and executing movements; and (iv) stooped posture and instability. Many of these clinical features are also manifested by other basal ganglia disorders and, thus, often referred to as parkinsonian syndromes (Table 45-3). Parkinsonian symptoms may occur with any disorder that causes damage to the nigrostriatal DA neurons or that results in an imbalance diminishing the disinhibition in the indirect circuit. SNc DA fibers would normally increase the total disinhibition

TABLE 45-2.	STRIATAL DOPAMINE CONCENTRATION IN PARKINSON'S DISEASE, PARKINSONIAN SYNDROMES AND OTHER NEURODEGENERATIVE DISORDERS		
		% Normal control values	
Disease		**Caudate nucleus**	**Putamen**
Parkinson's disease		31	22
		10	4
		18	2
Postencephalitis parkinsonism		6	6
		1.5	0.6
Parkinsonian syndromes			
Striatonigral degeneration		<0.4	<0.4
Steele-Richardson-Olszewski disease		20	27
Hallervorden-Spatz disease		1.4	0.9
Olivopontocerebellar atrophy		0.3	0.01
AIDS		43	—
Huntington's disease		86 (NSC)	99 (NSC)
Alzheimer's disease		61 (NSC)	50 (NSC)
Alzheimer's + Lewy body pathology		16	5

NSC, nonsignificant change.
From [34] with permission.

TABLE 45-3.	CLASSIFICATION OF THE VARIOUS FORMS OF PARKINSONISM, BASED ON DIFFERENTIAL ETIOLOGY
Parkinson's disease	Idiopathic Parkinson's disease
Parkinsonian syndromes	Steele-Richardson-Olszewski disease
	Striatonigral degeneration
	Corticobasal degeneration
	Hallervorden-Spatz disease
	Wilson's disease
	Shy-Drager syndrome
	Olivopontocerebellar atrophy
Symptomatic parkinsonism	Toxin-induced (e.g., MPTP, carbon monoxide, manganese)
	Drug-induced (e.g., reserpine, calcium antagonists, neuroleptics)
	Infectious (e.g., encephalitis lethargica, luetic)
	Vascular trauma
	Brain carcinomas

From [20] with permission.

of the thalamus through both the excitatory D1 receptors in the direct circuit and the inhibitory D2 receptors in the indirect circuit (Fig. 45-1). Thus, lesions of the pallidum, as well as those of the SNc, result in the appearance of parkinson-like movement disorders [4].

Neurological disorders such as progressive supranuclear palsy, multiple system atrophy and the Parkinson–amyotrophic lateral sclerosis (ALS)–dementia complex that include parkinsonian movement abnormalities in addition to other neurological deficits are termed "parkinsonism-plus" syndromes (Table 45-3) [5]. Infectious disease, tumors, metabolic disturbances and toxins may also produce forms of parkinsonism. Parkinson's disease progresses slowly but may ultimately produce akinesia and complete helplessness. Although the clinical features were well described, the pathological basis of the disease remained unknown for over 100 years. The frequent occurrence of parkinsonism as a sequel to von Economo's encephalitis lethargica, which reached epidemic proportions in 1918 to 1921, led to the discovery that depigmentation of the substantia nigra is a constant feature of

parkinsonism, whether as a result of a virus, exposure to toxins or unknown causes. In view of widespread changes elsewhere, there was, however, hesitancy in attributing to so small a brain lesion so extensive a movement disorder.

The chemical pathology of Parkinson's disease includes degeneration of the dopaminergic nigrostriatal tract and reduction in striatal dopamine

Nearly two generations elapsed before the next major advances in understanding Parkinson's disease. In 1958, Carlsson and coworkers [6] reported on the distribution of DA in the brain, its highest concentrations in the striatum, its depletion by reserpine and the dramatic effect of L-DOPA in reversing reserpine-induced tranquilization, impoverished motor activity and ptosis in mice and rabbits. They showed also that pretreatment with an MAO inhibitor potentiated the effects of L-DOPA in reversing the effects of reserpine. The uneven distribution of DA in the brain suggested that this substance may function as a neurotransmitter. Two years later, Ehringer and Hornykiewicz [7] noted the greatly reduced DA concentrations, to about one-tenth of normal, in the caudate, putamen and substantia nigra in brains from parkinsonian patients (Fig. 45-2B). Shortly thereafter, newly developed histofluorescence techniques demonstrated the previously unknown nigrostriatal DA-containing tract with cell bodies in the SNc and axonal projections to the striatum. These techniques also showed that the striatal DA deficit was not due to a reduction in the activity of TH, the dopaminergic rate-limiting enzyme, but rather to loss of the nigrostriatal dopaminergic neurons. Similarly, DA depletions were also found in all of the parkinsonian syndromes. The DA deficit appeared to be confined to disorders exhibiting striatal pathology (Table 45-2).

Diminished formation and metabolism of DA in Parkinson's disease are reflected in low postmortem concentrations of DA, DOPAC and HVA in the caudate nucleus and putamen (Table 45-4). Very small amounts of DA are detectable in the CSF. In contrast, some HVA normally diffuses, in particular from the caudate nucleus into the CSF, where it is readily de-

TABLE 45-4.   NEUROBIOCHEMICAL CHANGES IN THE DOPAMINERGIC SYSTEM IN THE NIGROSTRIATAL PATHWAY IN PARKINSON'S DISEASE

	Brain region	% Normal control values
Concentration of dopamine and its metabolites		
Dopamine	Substantia nigra	17
	Caudate nucleus	10
	Putamen	4
DOPAC	Substantia nigra	2
	Putamen	10
HVA	Substantia nigra	48
	Putamen	29
Activity of dopamine-related enzymes		
Tyrosine hydroxylase	Substantia nigra	46
	Caudate nucleus	60
	Putamen	16
Aromatic amino acid decarboxylase	Caudate nucleus	9
	Putamen	4
Catechol-*O*-methyl transferase	Substantia nigra	82
	Caudate nucleus	70
	Putamen	78
Monoamine oxidase-B	Substantia nigra	125
Presynaptic dopamine uptake	Caudate nucleus	32
	Putamen	16

DOPAC, 3,4-dihydroxyphenylacetic acid; HVA, homovanillic acid.
From [33] with permission.

tectable [8]. In Parkinson's disease, particularly in more severely affected patients, the CSF concentrations of HVA are far below those found in patients with neurological disorders not involving the basal ganglia. Because HVA is a substrate for the active transport mechanism that removes acidic compounds into the circulation, there is a steep gradient in CSF concentrations of HVA, with the highest concentrations in the lateral ventricles and the lowest in the lumbar CSF. This acid-transport system is inhibited in a dose-dependent manner by probenecid (*p*-dipropylsulfamylbenzoic acid). Probenecid has been used to differentiate low concentrations of HVA in CSF in other disorders of the CNS from those found in Parkinson's disease. Parkinsonian patients given probenecid show a lower increase in HVA than do patients with other neurological disorders. Also, it is now possible, using positron-emitting analogs of L-DOPA such as [^{18}F]6-fluorodopa, to demonstrate the deficiency in forming and storing DA in living parkinsonian patients (see Chap. 54). Parkinsonian syndromes that primarily involve the DA system may benefit from therapies aimed at DA replacement, whereas those involving other pathways are generally unresponsive to such treatments.

L-DOPA is used to treat Parkinson's disease

L-DOPA treatment was first advocated by Birkmayer and Hornykiewicz (intravenously) [9] and Barbeau and colleagues (orally) [10] in 1961. Both of these groups found highly favorable responses of most of the motor deficits associated with Parkinson's disease, and the findings from these studies established the contention that most of the clinical signs and symptoms of Parkinson's disease are a result of DA deficiency.

There is also marked loss of norepinephrinergic neurons in the locus ceruleus. In addition, there appears to be a dysfunction in the serotonergic system in Parkinson's disease. This contention is reflected by reduced concentrations of serotonin metabolites in the CSF of parkinsonian patients, particularly in depressed patients. There has been a strong suggestion of dysfunction of both the norepinephrinergic and serotonergic systems in Parkinson's disease-related depressive psychosis.

Although there are other biochemical abnormalities in the parkinsonian brain, such as diminished concentrations of serotonin, NE, GABA and GAD, these are not as striking as the loss of DA, which appears to be crucial. Strategies were then focused on enhancing the efficacy of L-DOPA treatment to improve its access to the brain and to reduce its peripheral side effects.

L-DOPA treatment is potentiated by inhibition of peripheral decarboxylation

Passage of ingested L-DOPA into the brain parenchyma entails its absorption from the intestine, passage through the hepatic circulation and transfer to the brain from blood through the endothelial cells lining the capillaries. Considerable AADC activity is present in the intestinal wall, the liver, the kidneys and the brain capillary endothelium; DA formed by decarboxylation of L-DOPA at these sites is excluded from the brain. Selective inhibition of extracerebral AADC was therefore explored as a means of enhancing L-DOPA efficacy. The first compound found to inhibit AADC was α-methyldopa (Fig. 45-3). This drug inhibits the decarboxylation of L-DOPA but is itself a substrate for the enzyme and is converted to α-methyldopamine and α-methylnorepinephrine, which can replace the physiological neurotransmitters. Since they are not as effective at activating receptors, these "false transmitters" reduce catecholaminergic activity. Although α-methyldopa proved useful in treating hypertension, it occasionally results in the appearance of parkinsonian symptoms by diminishing brain DA.

It has long been known that DA does not penetrate the blood–brain barrier, while its amino acid precursor, L-DOPA, readily enters the brain, where it is decarboxylated to form DA. This has been shown through behavioral and biochemical studies. However, brain DA replacement with L-DOPA was greatly limited because of severe side effects, particularly nausea and vomiting. Thus, the discovery and introduction by Birkmayer and Mentasti [11] of the decarboxylase inhibitor benserazide proved to be highly useful in the potentiation of centrally mediated L-DOPA effects. Consequently, this allowed the gradual decrease in oral doses of L-DOPA to achieve symptomatic improvement without loss of efficacy. More importantly, reduction of the L-DOPA dose resulted in curtailing the notorious adverse peripheral side effects of the drug [12]. Carbidopa and benserazide (Fig. 45-3) can be administered in doses that affect only extracerebral AADC, including that of the brain capillaries, and both have been found to be useful adjuncts to L-DOPA treatment [13].

When L-DOPA has crossed the blood–brain barrier, aided by an active transport mechanism, it must be converted to DA. Some question arises as to the source of the decarboxylase for this since many of the dopaminergic neurons, including the AADC found in them, are absent in the disease. Studies of postmortem striatum, however, have not yet revealed any cases with a total deficiency of AADC in the striatum; there has always been at least a residue of enzyme activity (Table 45-4). Moreover, cells of the striatum receive connections from many sources, including serotonin-producing raphe nuclei. Hence, L-DOPA could also be converted to DA by the decarboxylase within those neurons. The DA formed would then be available in brain tissue, although its path of diffusion to sensitive receptors might be longer than usual. Untreated parkinsonian patients have elevated densities of D2 receptors in the striatum, presumably reflecting a "supersensitive" state in which responses could be elicited by lower DA concentrations. Treatment with L-DOPA lowers the density of D2 receptors to that in control tissue.

Chronic L-DOPA treatment induces other complications, such as dyskinesia, or involuntary movement, and dystonia. These complications associated with long-term L-DOPA treatment led to the quest for alternative pharmacological approaches to ameliorate the undesirable actions of L-DOPA. Consequently, the actions of MAO and COMT inhibitors were explored.

L-DOPA treatment is potentiated by monoamine oxidase or catechol-*O*-methyltransferase inhibition

The revelation that the striatal DA deficit elicits the motor symptoms in Parkinson's disease gave rise to another strategy to potentiate the effects of endogenous DA. This strategy was based on blocking two key enzymes involved in the catabolism of DA, namely, MAO and COMT. The inhibition of DA catabolism was suggested to be an adjunct to L-DOPA to enhance its availability at postsynaptic receptor sites [14]. DA is a substrate for both forms of MAO; however, in the human brain, it exhibits a preference for MAO-B. Since it was observed that inhibitors of this enzyme potentiate the effects of L-DOPA in reversing reserpine-induced tranquilization, it was apparent that this might also be true for L-DOPA used in treating Parkinson's disease. However, the use of nonselective MAO inhibitors produced a distinct untoward reaction, referred to as the "cheese effect." This revelation was precipitated in depressed patients treated with MAO inhibitors who ingested foods rich in tyramine, such as cheese and wine, and consequently developed acute severe hypertensive reactions. Since similar reactions could occur with concurrent use of L-DOPA and MAO inhibitors then in use, these drugs were contraindicated in parkinsonian patients being treated with L-DOPA.

However, after the discovery that the hypertensive reactions were due to inhibition of MAO-A, it was found that deprenyl, or selegiline, an irreversible inhibitor of MAO-B, is devoid of the "cheese effect" (Fig. 45-3). Birkmayer and colleagues [14] found that the use of deprenyl as an adjunct to L-DOPA therapy, including a peripheral decarboxylase inhibitor, not only enhanced the efficacy of L-DOPA but appeared to stabilize fluctuations in response and to prolong the effects of L-DOPA [14]. Deprenyl has a twofold beneficial role as an adjunct in L-DOPA therapy. First, it inhibits the metabolism of DA, thereby allowing the preservation of DA in the basal ganglia and, thus, allowing lower L-DOPA doses without loss of efficacy. Additionally, it delays starting L-DOPA treatment by at least 1 year, thereby reducing the occurrence of L-DOPA-related adverse effects, including "on–off" plasma fluctuations, dyskinesia and dystonia. Deprenyl monotherapy is usually administered in the early, mild stages of the disease since it appears to have only a modest beneficial effect on the clinical deficits.

The clinical benefits of another, but reversible, MAO-B inhibitor, labazemide, appear similar to those of deprenyl. Rasagiline, an irreversible MAO-B inhibitor similar to deprenyl, may be marginally superior in comparison with the other inhibitors in so far as it is not metabolized to amphetamine. Indeed, there is evidence suggesting that the L-amphetamine produced from deprenyl may be detrimental to the beneficial actions of the drug itself. Moclobamide, a MAO-A inhibitor, has been shown to produce both alleviation of parkinsonian clinical symptoms and depression. L-DOPA is a substrate for COMT, and when decarboxylation is blocked, plasma levels of 3-O-methyldopa (3-OMD) are elevated. Because both L-DOPA and 3-OMD are absorbed from the intestine and transported into the brain by the same saturable carrier system for which many large neutral amino acids (LNAAs) are substrates, 3-OMD and dietary amino acids influence the efficacy of L-DOPA treatment. Furthermore, 3-O-methylation contributes to the rapid metabolism of L-DOPA. Clinical assessment of the COMT inhibitors (Fig. 45-3) tolcapone and entacapone has shown that these drugs enhance the efficacy of L-DOPA; in addition, they appear to reduce the fluctuations related to "wearing-off," a period when the plasma levels of L-DOPA decline. Thus, these drugs are beneficial as adjunct therapy. In preclinical studies, tolcapone has been shown to enhance the effects of L-DOPA by virtue of its dual action, including inhibition of L-DOPA metabolism in the periphery and DA breakdown in the brain. Entacapone primarily acts peripherally.

There are other alternatives and adjuncts to L-DOPA treatment of Parkinson's disease

Unfortunately, chronic L-DOPA treatment manifests some clinical and pharmacological complications, including dyskinesia, "on–off" and "wearing-off" syndromes and psychosis. Regardless of the L-DOPA regimen, it has been reported that more than 50% of patients develop "on–off"-induced dyskinesias after a period of 5 years of treatment. The "on" and "off" periods have been ascribed to adaptations in receptor or neuronal responses to variations in brain or plasma concentrations of L-DOPA or DA. Therefore careful titration of L-DOPA doses may be warranted, to maintain more steady plasma L-DOPA concentrations.

The actions of L-DOPA in Parkinson's disease or of DA at receptor sites in the CNS are mimicked by a number of compounds. Apomorphine, a semisynthetic ergot alkaloid, has a brief dopaminergic action (Fig. 45-5) and affects both D1 and D2 receptors. It is chiefly administered, usually by subcutaneous infusion, in the event of abrupt "off" attacks. It acts both pre- and postsynaptically, and the presynaptic autoreceptors are particularly sensitive to this drug. Its best recognized action is at the DA receptor sites making up the area postrema. Like L-DOPA, apomorphine affects certain neuroendocrine systems. In humans, subemetic doses provoke striking increases in concentration of growth hormone in the plasma, presumably by acting on cells producing the appropriate releasing factor. In many species, it depresses the concentration of serum prolactin by a direct action

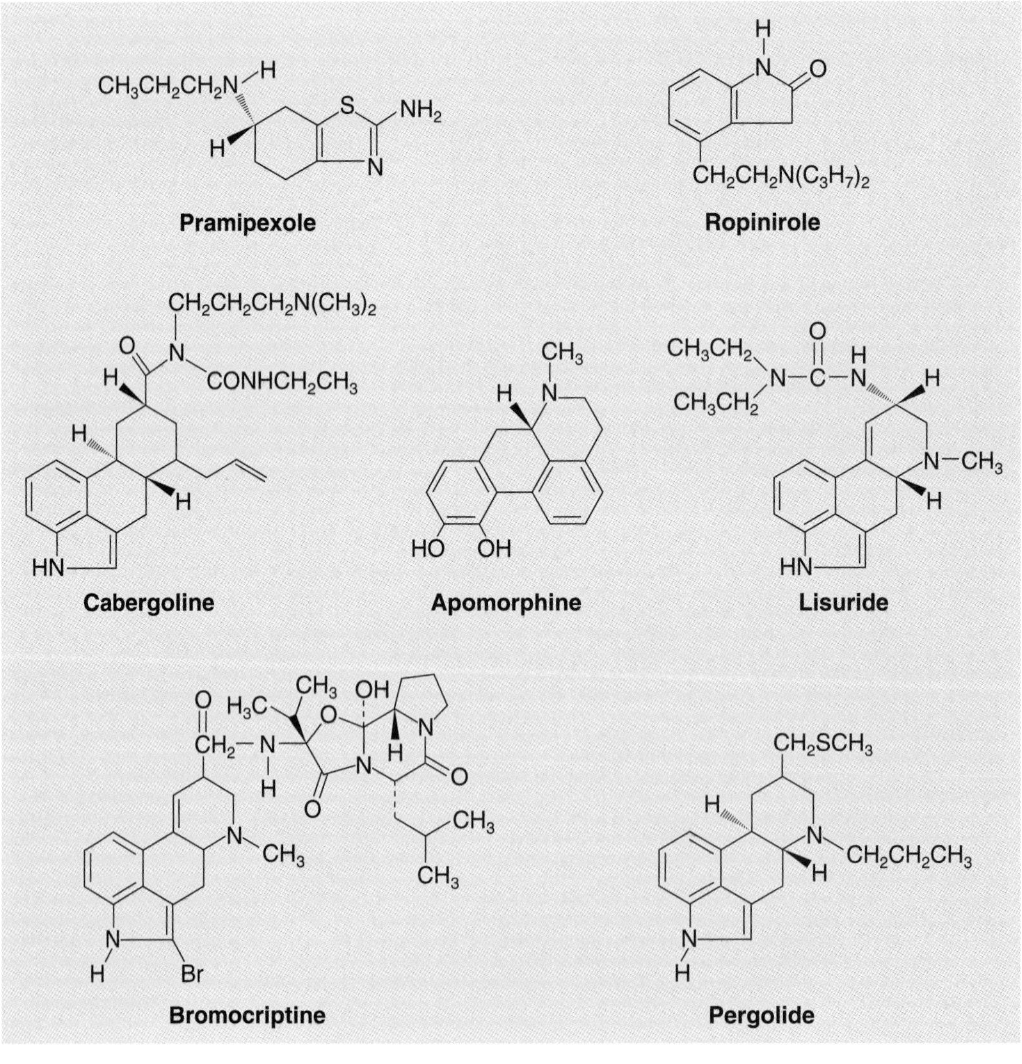

FIGURE 45-5. Dopamine receptor agonists.

on D2 receptors. More importantly, it has potent iron-chelating properties, which may explain its antioxidant abilities.

Three other DA agonists (Fig. 45-5), bromocriptine (D2), lisuride (D1 and D2) and pergolide (D1 and D2), all of which are ergoline derivatives and act predominantly as D2-receptor agonists, have found some practical use in the treatment of early symptoms of Parkinson's disease or as adjuncts to L-DOPA/carbidopa or L-DOPA/benserazide in later stages [15]. Long-term studies have revealed that the efficacy of L-DOPA is enhanced when it is administered in combination with DA agonists, including bromocriptine, lisuride or pergolide. It has been reported that a combination of bromocriptine and L-DOPA in early Parkinson's disease appears to be more effective at reducing the onset of development of L-DOPA-related dyskinesias. In addition, it can be employed as monotherapy in early Parkinson's disease. Lisuride is significantly more potent than bromocriptine; unfortunately, it is relatively short-acting, which may severely limit its clinical use. Similar to deprenyl, it may delay starting L-DOPA treatment by at least 1 year. The newly launched DA agonists ropinirole (D2) and pramipexole (mainly D3 but also D1, D2L and D4), both of which are devoid of the ergot structure, and long-acting cabergoline (Fig. 45-5), may also reduce the incidence of dyskinesia, probably by decreasing the required dose of L-DOPA. Therefore, effective pharmacological management of Parkinson's disease appears to involve direct and constant stimulation of the dopaminergic system.

Before the advent of L-DOPA, anticholinergic agents were among the most commonly used drugs and were the therapeutic mainstay in the treatment of Parkinson's disease. Anticholinergics such as trihexyphenidyl and benztropine may offer marginal clinical benefit to the parkinsonian tremor. They appear to restore the balance that is disturbed when striatal cholinergic neurons are released from the inhibitory action of DA fibers that synapse with them. Nevertheless, they are contraindicated in parkinsonian patients with dementia since administration of anticholinergics in these patients would aggravate the cognitive dysfunction.

The noncompetitive NMDA receptor antagonist memantine has shown modest advantage in curtailing Parkinson's disease motor deficits, particularly akinesia. In contrast, budipine, which is also an NMDA antagonist, is particularly effective at alleviating tremor, akinesia and rigidity.

There may be an involvement of the serotonergic inhibitory pathway from the raphe nucleus to the nigrostriatal pathway in the etiology of parkinsonian tremor (see above). Indeed, this notion is supported by the marked improvement of tremor demonstrated in parkinsonian patients treated with the 5-HT$_2$ receptor antagonist ritanserin.

Parkinson's disease can also be treated surgically

The surgical technique of pallidotomy was first employed in Parkinson's disease in the early 1950s [16]. It was later superseded by thalamotomy, which appeared to be more effective at relieving tremor. However, in the wake of the highly successful L-DOPA treatment, the utilization of surgical treatment in Parkinson's disease gradually waned. Currently, the focus on surgical intervention in Parkinson's disease has awakened once again. This is chiefly due to the beneficial effects of ventrolateral medial pallidotomy demonstrated by Laiten and colleagues [17] in advanced Parkinson's disease, which rekindled worldwide interest in this procedure and reinforced its potential in the management of the disease.

Pallidotomy is primarily engineered to reduce the hyperactivity in the internal segment of the GPm caused by an excessive input from the STN. Indeed, the overactivity of the globus pallidus has been implicated in the motor disabilities associated with Parkinson's disease. This is in accordance with the suggestion that striatal DA deficit results in the overactivity of the GPm as a result of disinhibition of glutamatergic innervations from the STN to the globus pallidus (Fig. 45-1). This technique has proven particularly effective in advanced Parkinson's disease.

Some other dramatic effects of pallidotomy include the almost complete abolition of L-DOPA-induced dyskinesia contralateral to the side of the lesion and enhancement of the efficacy of dopaminergic drugs. It also reduces motor fluctuations associated with the "on" states, as well as both the severity and occurrence of the "off" periods. In addition, pallidotomy appears to be more beneficial than thalamotomy, which is highly effective at eliminating tremor and rigidity only. The progression of the disease is largely governed by the course of bradykinesia, which does not appear to be grossly altered by thalamotomy. However, the mechanism(s) underlying the effect of surgery on the rate of degenerative process is not clearly understood.

A pertinent observation is reflected by the impressive reduction in tremor achieved in parkinsonian patients by high-frequency stimulation of the STN. This is achieved by implanting a microstimulating device in this region [18]. This procedure allows the functional inhibition of specific brain regions without the application of a lesion. Therefore, it is considered to be safer than and superior to pallidotomy or thalamotomy. Another advantage of subthalamic stimulation is that, by virtue of its attenuation of tremor, it consequently reduces both the required dose of L-DOPA and L-DOPA-related dyskinesias.

MPTP-INDUCED PARKINSONIAN SYNDROME

Although many toxins and neurological insults that damage the basal ganglia and/or the substantia nigra result in neurological disorders which include parkinsonian features (see below), one toxin, 1-methyl-4-phenyl-1,2,3,6-tetrahydropyridine (MPTP), appears to target relatively specifically those neurons that are involved in Parkinson's disease. MPTP has been used to develop animal models for testing new therapies in the human disease. Investigations of the mechanisms of MPTP toxicity have also provided insights regarding the possible pathogenesis of Parkinson's disease.

MPTP toxicity was discovered after inadvertent self-administration by drug abusers

These people had ingested a compound produced during illicit synthesis of a narcotic related to meperidine. The users rapidly developed a movement disorder that closely resembles Parkinson's disease, including low concentrations of HVA in the CSF. Similarly, MPTP induces most of the biochemical, pathological and clinical features akin to Parkinson's disease in nonhuman primates.

The mechanisms implicated in MPTP toxicity [19] are depicted in Figure 45-6. MPTP, which is lipid-soluble, readily penetrates the blood–brain barrier and enters the brain cells. Because it is amphiphilic, it is captured into acidic organelles, mostly lysosomes, of astrocytes. MPTP itself does not appear to be toxic, but its oxidized product, 1-methyl-4-phenylpyridinium (MPP$^+$), is toxic. Astrocytes and serotonergic neurons contain MAO-B, which converts MPTP to MPP$^+$. The toxic oxidation product reaches the extracellular fluid and then is transported by the DA transporter into DA nerve terminals. Inhibition of either MAO-B or the DA transporter protects against MPTP-generated MPP$^+$ toxicity.

Although the precise mechanism(s) underlying the mode of MPP$^+$ toxicity is unknown, it has been suggested that the toxicity of MPP$^+$ is dependent on a mitochondrial concentrating mechanism via selective uptake. Energy-driven mitochondrial uptake of MPP$^+$ results in sufficiently high concentrations of the toxin to interfere with mitochondrial respiration. The site at which MPP$^+$ acts, complex I, appears to be at or near the region where several other agents, such as rotenone, act to block mitochondrial oxidation. Blockade of mitochondrial respiration has two cytotoxic consequences. First, it impairs ATP formation, resulting in the inhibition of energy-dependent processes such as ion transport. A recent study suggests that inhibition of complex I is not solely involved in eliciting cell death. Indeed, disruption of calcium ion homeostasis plays a vital role in MPP$^+$ toxicity. This results in an elevation of intracellular Ca^{2+}, leading to the activation of Ca^{2+}-dependent enzymes, for example, protein kinase and calpains I and II, which disturbs the normal cell function, resulting in cellular damage (see Chaps. 23 and 34). Second, MPP$^+$ appears to support the occurrence of oxidative stress. This notion is demonstrated by the generation of reactive oxygen radicals and free iron. MPP$^+$ and mitochondrial

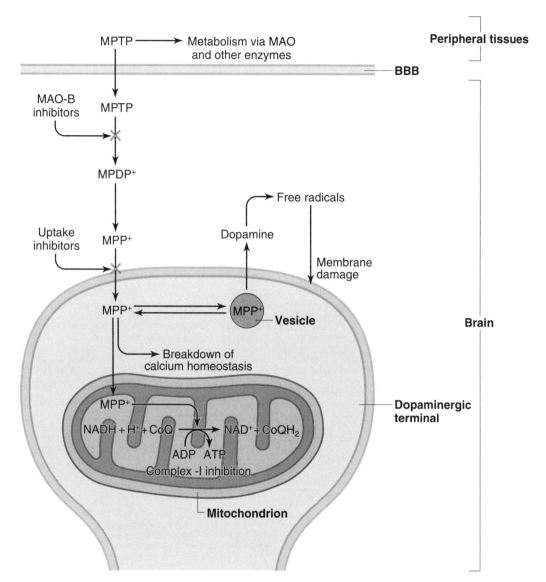

FIGURE 45-6.   Schematic representation of the mechanisms involved in toxicity of 1-methyl-4-phenyl-1,2,3,6-tetrahydropyridine (MPTP). *BBB,* blood–brain barrier; *MPDP$^+$,* 1-methyl-4-phenyl-2,3-dihydropyridinium; *MPTP,* 1-methyl-4-phenyl-1,2,3,6-tetrahydropyridine; *MPP$^+$,* its four-electron oxidation product 1-methyl-4-phenylpyridinium; *MAO,* monoamine oxidase. (From [33], with permission.)

NADH dehydrogenase have been suggested to yield toxic hydroxyl radicals derived from hydrogen peroxide. In monkeys, MPP$^+$ has been shown to release toxic iron (II) (Fe^{2+}), which in turn may react with hydrogen peroxide via the Fenton reaction and, thus, yield hydroxyl radicals ($^•$OH) (see Chap. 34). Hydroxyl and other free radical species and Fe^{2+} have been strongly implicated in the pathogenesis of Parkinson's disease. More importantly, MPTP mimics another fundamental nigral biochemical change in Parkinson's disease, that is, a reduction of glutathione content, as observed in rodents.

However, there are some fundamental changes found in Parkinson's disease that are not induced by MPTP. Consequently, this has raised some doubts about the involvement of some MPTP-like toxins in Parkinson's disease. Indeed, in nonhuman primates and rodents, there has been no evidence for the occurrence of the pathological hallmark of Parkinson's disease, namely, Lewy bodies. In some older, MPTP-treated primates, eosinophilic inclusions were observed in the substantia nigra and locus ceruleus; however, the identity of these features remains largely unresolved. Resting tremor, which is one of the most prominent clinical features of Parkinson's disease, is seldom observed in MPTP-induced parkinsonism. The neurodegeneration of the nigral neurons and the manifestation of Parkinson's disease clinical symptoms are progressive. In contrast, the development of Parkinson's disease-like symptoms subsequent to MPTP exposure is acute. In Parkinson's disease, the cholinergic cells of the substantia innominata exhibit evidence for neuronal loss and Lewy body pathology, whereas MPTP does not elicit these changes. Some of these diversities may be based on species differences; however, they do seem to suggest a divergence in the mechanism(s) evoking cell death in Parkinson's disease and MPTP.

Nevertheless, MPTP remains the "best" model for investigating Parkinson's disease to date, although many other dopaminergic neurotoxins have evolved, which are being actively employed. In addition, the MPTP scenario had a great impact on the quest to unravel the putative pathogenesis underlying the disease. It furnished a possible mechanism(s) by which the dopaminergic neurons in Parkinson's disease may degenerate. Additionally, it triggered the search for some endogenous or exogenous neurotoxin which may be involved in eliciting the nigral cell death characteristic of the disease. Some of these neurotoxins include 6-hydroxydopamine (6-OH-DA), iron and methamphetamine.

MPTP provides clues to the pathogenesis of Parkinson's disease

The selective vulnerability of nigrostriatal DA neurons to MPTP toxicity and the resemblance of the resulting clinical syndrome to Parkinson's disease refocused attention on determining the etiological factors that contribute to the development of Parkinson's disease. Three separate, but not necessarily exclusive, hypotheses have been explored [20].

The first hypothesis suggests that there are one or more toxic substances acquired from the environment or produced in the brain, at least for some vulnerable persons. A genetic component may ultimately determine the predisposition of those individuals to the particular toxin, although the familial coincidence of the disease is low.

The second hypothesis suggests that oxidative stress may play a pivotal role in dopaminergic cell death (Table 45-5). However, it remains debatable as to whether oxidative stress represents a cause or a consequence of the disease. Oxidative stress is a condition in which reactive oxygen-derived free radical species comprise the chief factor leading to cell degeneration (see Chap. 34). The catabolism of DA itself, via both enzymatic deamination and auto-oxidation, is reputed to generate toxic superoxide and hydroxyl radicals, which may in turn trigger a self-amplifying cell-destruction cycle. The postmortem evidence for the occurrence of oxidative stress is vast and highly supportive of its involvement in the pathogenesis of Parkinson's disease (Table 45-5). The first documentation of oxidative stress was provided by the nigral depletion of the antioxidant glutathione in Parkinson's disease. Other antioxidants, such as catalase, were also found to be depleted in the substantia nigra in Parkinson's disease. This reflects a general reduced state of cellular defenses in the disease, perhaps due to "consumption" of antioxidant molecules by active, free radical-generating processes. The mitochondrial dysfunction in Parkinson's disease, as reflected by the decrease of respiratory complex I activity, may generate superoxide radicals, which may elicit cell destruction and exacerbate the complex I defect. Also, the shift in the Fe^{2+}: Fe^{3+} ratio from 2:1 in the normal substantia nigra to 1:2 in that of Parkinson's disease may generate hydroxyl radicals from hydrogen peroxide through the iron-dependent Fenton reaction. Thus, the elevation of mitochondrial Mn^{2+}-dependent superoxide dismutase activity found in Parkinson's disease perhaps represents a compensatory mechanism to curtail the effects of excess superoxide radical formation. These free radical species may ultimately induce cell death via disruption of normal cellular Ca^{2+} homeostasis (Chap. 34).

TABLE 45-5. EVIDENCE FROM POSTMORTEM FINDINGS FOR THE OCCURRENCE OF OXIDATIVE STRESS IN PARKINSON'S DISEASE

	Brain region	% Normal control values
Antioxidants/antioxidant enzymes		
Glutathione		
GSH	Substantia nigra	↓ 40
		↓ 46
GSSG	Substantia nigra	NSC
		NSC
γ-Glutamyl transpeptidase	Substantia nigra	↑ 76
Glutathione peroxidase	Substantia nigra	↓ 61
Catalase	Substantia nigra	↓ 36
	Putamen	↓ 33
Superoxide dismutase	Substantia nigra	↑ 33
Iron homeostasis		
Total iron	Substantia nigra	↑ 77
	Globus pallidus	↑ 20
$Fe^{2+} : Fe^{3+}$ ratio	Substantia nigra	↓ 57
Ferritin	Substantia nigra	↑ 29
Lipid peroxidation		
Polyunsaturated fat	Substantia nigra	↓ 15
Thiobarbituric acid-reactive substances	Substantia nigra	↑ 35
DNA damage		
8-Hydroxy-2'-deoxyguanosine	Substantia nigra	↑ 38
	Putamen	↑ 50
	Caudate nucleus	↑ 75

NSC, nonsignificant change, GSH, reduced glutathione; GSSG, oxidized glutathione.
From [33] with permission.

Intracerebral administration of the neurotoxin 6-OHDA provides an acute animal model for Parkinson's disease. This is a particularly important model because this toxin also induces oxidative stress and, thus, allows the possibility of investigating biochemical parameters affected by this cytotoxic process. Moreover, the biochemical alterations that 6-OHDA induces are very similar to those reported in Parkinson's disease and, thus, support the occurrence of oxidative stress in the latter. The neurotoxicity of 6-OHDA is believed to be related to production of hydrogen peroxide-derived hydroxyl radicals, which probably induce destruction of nigral neurons. In addition, 6-OHDA initiates the release of iron from ferritin, which may account for its ability to generate hydroxyl radicals via the Fenton reaction. It is supposed that 6-OHDA is more effective than MPP^+ at inhibiting mitochondrial complex I activity and may also generate other toxic free radicals, such as superoxide radicals. Consequently, the reductions in the activity of superoxide dismutase and in glutathione content in the striatum may represent compensatory actions against a 6-OHDA-elicited toxic mechanism(s).

The third hypothesis suggests a putative association between oxidative stress and other free radical-generating processes, such as excitatory and immune pathways (see Chap. 34). Immune-related mechanisms may also be conducive to selective regional cell death in Parkinson's disease. Indeed, microgliosis is most marked in the ventral tier of the SNc of Parkinson's disease, an area blighted by the degenerative processes of the disease. It has been shown that reactive microglia can mediate secondary cell destruction by releasing cytotoxic species, such as hydroxyl radicals, superoxide radicals, NO and glutamate. Furthermore, the fact of elevated concentrations of interleukin-6 in the CSF of *de novo* parkinsonian patients confirms the occurrence of immunologically mediated processes in the disorder.

Although the cause(s) of Parkinson's disease has not yet been elucidated, reactive oxygen species appear to play a salient role in the degenerative process. Therefore, neuroprotection represents one of the strategies evolved to combat some of these active degenerative processes.

Neuroprotective strategies have some benefits in Parkinson's disease

Neuroprotective drugs that have demonstrated some benefit in experimental animal models of Parkinson's disease and have fulfilled the safety requirements were subsequently assessed in parkinsonian patients. Deprenyl and α-tocopherol were the first two compounds to be clinically evaluated as potential candidates for neuroprotective treatment in Parkinson's disease [21]. Deprenyl effects a triad of cellular protective mechanism(s). These include neuroprotection, neurorescue and neurorestoration. Its neuroprotective effects are exerted by inhibiting the degradation of DA or other MPTP-like neurotoxins and, thus, the production of potential cytotoxic metabolites, including hydrogen peroxide, via MAO-mediated deamination, and DA quinones, via auto-oxidation. *In vivo* experiments for oxidative stress have clearly shown protective actions of the drug in nigrostriatal neurons of animals treated with haloperidol or reserpine. In addition, deprenyl affords neuroprotection against other dopaminergic toxins, including 6-OHDA and *N*-(2-chloroethyl)-*N*-ethyl-2-bromobenzylamine. Its neuroprotective ability may also be related to the attenuation of the neurotoxic actions of the endogenous toxins β-carbolines and tetrahydroisoquinolines.

The neurorescuing actions of deprenyl are clearly demonstrated by the protection it affords to dopaminergic neurons after the administration of MPTP at a time when most of the latter is metabolized to toxic MPP$^+$. It has been suggested that the mode of neurorescue in this case may involve an interaction of deprenyl or its metabolites with some cellular antiapoptotic factors. Deprenyl also has been reported to promote the production of neurotrophic factors; this may explain its role as a neurorestorative agent. This particular feature may be of importance in the preservation of the nigral neurons in

a progressive and degenerative disorder such as Parkinson's disease. Although not proven, these attributes may explain its described ability to increase life expectancy in parkinsonian patients [22].

There has been some implication that the MAO-A inhibitor moclobemide (*p*-chloro-*N*-[2morpholinoethyl]benzamide) may also provide cellular protection by inhibition of MAO-A-derived hydrogen peroxide generation. α-Tocopherol treatment may exert some neuroprotective effect, probably by scavenging free radicals and, thus, inhibiting cytotoxic processes such as lipid peroxidation. However, no clinical benefit was demonstrated by oral ingestion of 2 g per day of α-tocopherol in the DATATOP clinical study [23]. The absence of protective clinical effect from ingestion may be due to insufficient brain concentrations of α-tocopherol. Little is known about vitamin transport into the brain (see Chap. 33).

Findings from *in vitro* and *in vivo* studies suggest that some DA agonists may afford neuroprotection by scavenging reactive free radical species, although this attribute has not yet been clinically proven. Pergolide is currently being evaluated for potential neuroprotective activity in Parkinson's disease (Fig. 45-5). Other DA agonists also believed to afford some neuronal protection by virtue of their ability to scavenge free radicals include ropinirole, bromocriptine and pramipexole. Positron emission tomography may be used to assess the neuroprotective actions of ropinirole, which is advocated in early Parkinson's disease (see Chap. 54).

Amantadine possibly provides some protective activity in Parkinson's disease. These cellular protective effects are believed to be based on the ability of amantadine to block the excitatory amino acid NMDA receptor. If present in intact human brain, such an action may confer an ability to increase life expectancy in the parkinsonian patient.

Multiple synergistic pathways have been suggested to play crucial roles in the cell death cascade. Therefore, it would be an effective therapeutic strategy to employ a combination of compounds to affect multiple "target sites" in the cell-destruction pathway(s). Drugs such as budipine, an NMDA receptor antagonist; the dihydropyridine type of Ca^{2+} channel antagonists;

N-nitro-L-arginine, an NO inhibitor; and iron chelators represent candidates for Parkinson's disease treatment. Perhaps the most effective mode of cell-protective therapy would be a combination of these compounds as opposed to monotherapy. However, for these drugs to implement their neuroprotective actions effectively, they would have to be administered in the early stages of the disease. This therapeutic requirement highlights the need to elucidate a marker for asymptomatic, or early, Parkinson's disease. Furthermore, this contention is emphasized by the fact that it is difficult to demonstrate the neuroprotective benefit of these drugs in clinical trials involving advanced disease since they do not produce instant clinical improvement or restoration of neurons.

Both experimental and clinical studies suggest that neurotrophic factors may play significant roles in the survival, growth and differentiation of dopaminergic neurons. These observations provide support for potential roles of these factors, to some degree, in neuroprotection and regeneration of the denervated neuronal network in Parkinson's disease. It appears that the trophic factors exert their beneficial effect by supporting differentiation of the neuronal phenotype rather than survival, but a reduction in their availability or in the receptors for neurotrophic factors may exert serious consequences on both cellular function and survival. However, a deficit in neurotrophic factors is not known to cause Parkinson's disease or any other neurological disease. Neurotrophic factors, such as nerve growth factor, brain-derived neurotrophic factors or glial-derived neurotrophic factors, do not effectively cross the blood–brain barrier and, therefore, need to be administered either directly into the ventricles or into the striatum. This may prove to be cumbersome and a hindrance to the use of these factors in the long-term management of the disease.

DRUG- OR TOXIN-INDUCED MOVEMENT DISORDERS

In addition to MPTP, other drugs that alter the availability of DA or that affect its actions at receptors may induce movement disorders with parkinsonian features. Some drugs have an opposite effect, producing hyperactive states with involuntary, abnormal movements. Indeed, an important and distressing adverse effect of L-DOPA is the appearance of dyskinesias in some parkinsonian patients. Furthermore, the neurons of the basal ganglia and associated structures are uniquely vulnerable to the effects of a variety of toxins, and this sensitivity is a critical factor in the neurological complications that accompany these substances. Generally, toxins produce more extensive neurological damage and a greater variety of clinical deficits than are found in Parkinson's disease. Damage to the nigrostriatal dopaminergic neurons appears to be responsible for the parkinsonian features that occur after exposure to these toxins, whereas involvement of other basal ganglia or associated systems may be responsible for the development of involuntary dyskinesias.

Pharmacological dopamine depletion induces parkinsonism

Reserpine, a natural alkaloid that blocks vesicular transport of monoamines, depletes stored monoamines, including DA. DA depletion is associated with emergence of a form of parkinsonism. This effect of reserpine and its reversal by treatment with L-DOPA and/or an MAO inhibitor are among the first clues that parkinsonism is the result of DA deficiency (see above). Generally, the parkinsonism resulting from reserpine is reversible.

As indicated earlier, α-methyldopa treatment of hypertension sometimes results in the appearance of parkinsonian symptoms. This is presumed to be a consequence of DA depletion by replacement of DA with the relatively inactive false transmitter α-methyldopamine, as well as by inhibition of AADC.

Neuroleptics may induce parkinsonism or dyskinesias

Antipsychotic drugs, also termed neuroleptics, used in the treatment of schizophrenia frequently produce parkinsonian symptoms as unwanted effects [24]. The neuroleptics block the action of DA on its receptors, and their therapeutic effect seems to be related to this action. Although these drugs act on DA systems without distinction, some are more selective. Thioridazine, clozapine and molindone, for example, have electrophysiological effects in the limbic region of the brain but little action in the nigrostriatal area. This selectivity may be related to receptor subtype specificity (see Chaps. 12 and 51).

Patients who have received neuroleptics for long periods of time may develop a hyperkinetic disorder of the extrapyramidal system characterized by involuntary, purposeless movements affecting many parts of the body. This is known as *tardive dyskinesia*. Most commonly, these are manifested in a syndrome involving abnormal movements of the tongue, mouth and masticatory muscles. There are also choreoathetoid movements of the extremities. The mechanism of neurotransmitter disturbance in tardive dyskinesias remains unknown.

Chronic heavy metal and industrial toxin exposure can cause movement disorders

Manganese. A small proportion of miners exposed to manganese dust develop manganism. Manganese is absorbed from the intestine as well as through the pulmonary epithelium, and once in the systemic circulation, it readily enters the brain. After a relatively short interval, that is, several months of exposure to high doses of the dust, the disease is ushered in by self-limited psychiatric problems. "Manganese madness" is characterized by emotional lability, hallucinations, irritability and aggressiveness. When the exposure is to low amounts of manganese, the behavioral changes may be mild and reversible. After more prolonged exposure, behavioral symptoms are replaced by signs of neurological damage. The manifestations are those of extrapyramidal disease and respond in some measure to treatment with L-DOPA. The dyskinetic features that do not respond to L-DOPA treatment are likely to be the result of more diffuse brain pathology [25]. In contrast to Parkinson's disease, the globus pallidus and SNr are the sites of greatest damage; but the striatum, STN, frontal and parietal cortex, cerebellum and hypothalamus may also be involved. Furthermore, epidemiological studies have shown no risk for the development of Parkinson's disease from drinking of well water rich in manganese. This discrepancy demonstrates the need for further research into the mechanism(s) of manganese-induced movement disorders.

Iron. In accordance with a recent study, exposure only to iron does not pose a great risk or threat in the occurrence or precipitation of parkinsonian clinical features. This fact, coupled with the marked nigral elevation in both Fe^{3+} and total iron in Parkinson's disease, suggests that the increase of this metal is not a consequence of an external condition, such as exposure. Although the true mechanism(s) underlying the elevation of iron content in substantia nigra and other areas of the basal ganglia is undefined, it is likely to be related to some alteration in iron homeostasis rather than exposure [26].

Iron serves a biphasic role. During development and growth it plays a vital role. Additionally, it is an important factor in many metabolic reactions, including protein synthesis as a cofactor of both heme and nonheme enzymes, and in the development of neuronal processes. However, free iron, particularly Fe^{2+}, is highly toxic by virtue of its ability to trigger cellular deleterious effects, including the Fenton reaction, which generates free radical species and lipid peroxidation (Chap. 34). The Fe^{3+} rat model is particularly useful for investigating oxidative stress in Parkinson's disease; the mode of Fe^{3+} neurotoxicity is proposed to be exerted via the reduced form, Fe^{2+}, coupled with the oxidation of endogenous ascorbate. The benefit of this model rests on its ability to mimic some important features of the disease, including DA deficit, akinesia and loss of tyrosine-immunoreactive neurons. Another advantage of employing iron is that the changes induced are chronically progressive and, therefore, more relevant to the neurodegenerative process occurring in Parkinson's disease.

Carbon disulfide (CS_2) is a volatile, lipid-soluble industrial solvent that enters the body by inhalation or absorption through the skin. The early symptoms of CS_2 poisoning resemble those of manganese; subsequently, neurological deficits are widespread and include peripheral neuropathy as well as encephalopathy with memory loss, incoordination and parkinsonism. Relatively little is known about the pathological changes in humans, but in monkeys exposed to CS_2, damage to the globus pallidus and substantia nigra suggest that similar pathological changes may account for the parkinsonian features of toxicity in humans. Other sulfur compounds, such as sulfuric acid and sulfur hydride, have also been implicated in inducing parkinsonian-like clinical features.

Carbon monoxide. Inhalation of carbon monoxide, which binds avidly to hemoglobin and to cytochromes, is one of the most fatal forms of poisoning or suicide. Survivors of acute carbon monoxide poisoning may develop, over several days or weeks, a delayed encephalopathy with memory loss, personality changes and some parkinsonian movement deficits, presumably associated with damage to the globus pallidus, which has been reported among the pathological features of this syndrome at autopsy. In spite of all of these detrimental effects, CO is also a putative neurotransmitter (see Chap. 10).

HEPATOLENTICULAR DEGENERATION: WILSON'S DISEASE

This is a rare, inherited, autosomal recessive metabolic disorder. The disease presents itself between the first and the third decade. It is characterized by deposition of copper in organs, particularly in the brain, liver and cornea. The deposition of copper in the basal ganglia results in the clinical manifestations of tremor, dyskinesias and rigidity. Other CNS symptoms include behavioral abnormalities and mental deterioration.

Whereas copper is essential for the normal functioning of a number of enzymes, for example, as a prosthetic group to tyrosinase, cytochrome oxidase and superoxide dismutase, excess free copper ions, similar to Fe^{2+}, are toxic. Adult humans require about 1 to 2 mg of copper daily. Copper metabolites are regulated by en-

terohepatic circulation, with excess copper excreted in the bile and feces. Most copper in plasma is present in ceruloplasmin, which is low in Wilson's disease, and normally only about 5% is present as copper ions bound to protein. In Wilson's disease, toxic accumulations of copper in the liver cause acute fulminant hepatitis or recurrent hepatitis with hepatic cirrhosis of the course type. Excess copper in the brain produces lesions of the lenticular nucleus, including the putamen and pallidum, and other brain regions, which result in progressive rigidity, intention tremor and, ultimately, mental deterioration. The persistence of extrapyramidal symptoms after surgical procedures, such as orthotopic liver transplantation, suggests that the destruction to the basal ganglia is irreversible. Rings of copper pigment, known as the Kayser-Fleisher phenomenon, may be exhibited in the cornea.

In animals administered an excess of copper, the metal is deposited in the liver, kidney and other organs, while the brain is spared. Similarly, in genetic disorders of copper metabolism in animals, copper accumulation in peripheral organs is not accompanied by brain copper toxicity. In Wilson's disease, excessive deposition of copper in the basal ganglia presumably is one of the factors causing the neurological syndrome, but it is not known how the metal breaks through the blood–brain barrier and what specific neuronal or metabolic functions it damages. Now that the mutated gene for Cu-ATPase has been identified in affected subjects with Wilson's disease, the molecular basis for the disorder may become clear (see Box 45-1).

Transition metals, such as copper (I) and Fe^{2+}, are believed to induce hydroxyl radical formation via the Fenton reaction (see Chap. 34). This initiates a cascade of cellular cytotoxic events, including mitochondrial dysfunction, lipid peroxidation, disruption of calcium ion homeostasis and, finally, cell death. The liberation of oxidant radicals may result in part from the reduced ability of metallothionein to bind and detoxify copper.

The involvement of the DA system in Wilson's disease is reflected by a depletion of striatal DA and TH [27]. L-DOPA offers little or no therapeutic benefit, thereby illustrating the dysfunction of postsynaptic D_2 receptors. For treatment of the

BOX 45-1

LINKAGE OF COPPER AND IRON METABOLISM IN BASAL GANGLIA DISORDERS

Copper, about 1 mg daily, is absorbed in the gastrointestinal (GI) tract, and equivalent amounts are normally excreted into the GI tract through the bile. Absorbed copper is bound to albumin and transported to the liver, where it is distributed throughout the hepatocytes. Ceruloplasmin (Cp), a glycoprotein, is synthesized in the liver and incorporates six atoms of copper prior to its secretion into the plasma, by which means the copper is delivered to various organs for incorporation into other holoproteins and enzymes, such as cytochrome oxidase, superoxide dismutase, dopamine β-hydroxylase, tyrosinase and lysyl oxidase. Normally, Cp binds about 95% of the plasma copper. However, Cp, contrary to earlier beliefs, is not essential for copper transport but, rather, for iron transport and metabolism. Cp is necessary for ferroxidase activity: $Cp\text{-}Cu^{2+}$ is reduced to $Cp\text{-}Cu^{+}$ as Fe^{2+} is oxidized to Fe^{3+}. Fe^{3+} is then bound by transferrin (TF) for transport. A cell-surface receptor (TFR) binds $TF\text{-}Fe^{3+}$ for endocytosis, acidification and release of the iron into an acid endosome. Knowledge of the copper and iron cycles has been advanced by the elucidation of mutations in genes for Cp synthesis (see below) and for two P-type, copper-transporting ATPases (see Chap. 5), one found mutated in Wilson's disease [1,2] and the other in Menkes' disease [3]. The two P-type ATPase genes are 65% homologous, but the Menkes' gene is X-linked and expressed in most tissues other than liver, while the Wilson's gene is at locus 13q14.3 and is expressed predominantly in the liver. The Menkes' ATPase gene mutation results in deficient placental copper transport and intestinal absorption, producing a copper-deficient, or *hypocupremic,* state with onset before birth. The disease manifests as decreased liver copper, abnormal (kinky) hair, gray matter degeneration and early death. Wilson's disease (see text), however, begins late in childhood with severe basal ganglia dysfunction and is associated with increased liver copper and decreased biliary copper excretion. In the current model, both P-type Cu-ATPases are localized in the late secretory pathway of cells [4]. The Wilson's disease ATPase transports copper from the cytosol into the Golgi secretory pathway, where it is available for incorporation into Cp and then sequestered into endosomes for transport into bile. The decreased copper transport from the cytosol into the secretory pathway in Wilson's disease leads to accumulation of cellular copper ions, or a *hypercupremic* state, and the synthesis of abnormal Cp, which is unstable and lacking in oxidase activity, presumably owing to the lack of copper incorporation. The instability results secondarily in low serum concentrations of Cp despite increased turnover rates.

The actual function of Cp is suggested by studies of another group of patients with mutations in the gene for Cp (3q23–35) [5]. These studies identify aceruloplasminemia as

disease, a low-copper diet and copper-chelating agents, including *d*-penicillamine (3,3-dimethylcysteine) and triethylenetetramine dihydrochloride, or zinc acetate, which prevents copper absorption from the gastrointestinal tract, are recommended. It has been suggested that zinc acetate also induces the synthesis of liver metallothionein, which sequesters copper in a nontoxic pool.

AMYOTROPHIC LATERAL SCLEROSIS–PARKINSONISM–DEMENTIA OF GUAM

The Chamorro people of Guam have had a very high incidence of a syndrome resembling amyotrophic lateral sclerosis (ALS), with strong elements of parkinsonism and dementia. Positron

Box 45-1 (Continued)

an autosomal recessive disorder of iron metabolism. These patients, with adult onset of disease, have diabetes mellitus, dementia, extrapyramidal symptoms, retinal degeneration, greatly decreased serum Cp and normal hepatic copper concentrations but elevated liver iron stores. T2-magnetic resonance images show basal ganglia densities indicative of iron deposition. Although the patients have iron deficiency-type anemia, their iron stores are increased and treatment is restriction of dietary iron with administration of Cp. Free iron is quite toxic, particularly in the basal ganglia and when the ratio of $Fe^{2+}:Fe^{3+}$ is increased (see text). While having aceruloplasminemia, these patients have exhibited no abnormalities in copper metabolism. Thus, Cp is not essential for copper transport.

Animal studies have shown that copper is essential for hemoglobin synthesis and that copper deficiency results in liver iron overload that can be mobilized with Cp. In yeast, a homologous copper oxidase has a role in iron metabolism. These observations taken together indicate that Cp and copper are critical to iron metabolism. It is believed that Cp, functioning as a ferroxidase, links ferrous iron release from storage sites to ferric iron uptake and transport by transferrin. Thus, the tertiary effect in Wilson's disease may be abnormal iron metabolism due to decreased Cp, in turn owing to decreased Cu-ATPase in the Golgi apparatus. However, increased iron

stores alone cannot account for the basal ganglia pathology since hemochromatosis is not associated with the type of dysfunction seen in these Cu-ATPase or Cp disorders. The precise role of the P-type ATPases in copper transport and the mechanisms of brain injury from alterations in copper and iron metabolism or accumulation, although apparently linked, are still not completely understood.

—*George J. Siegel*

REFERENCES

1. Bull, P. C., Thomas, G. R., Rommens, J. M., Forbes, J. R., and Cox, D. W. The Wilson disease gene is a putative copper transporting P-type ATPase similar to the Menkes gene. *Nat. Genet.* 5:327–337, 1993.
2. Tanzi, R. E., Petrukhin, K., Chernov, I., et al. The Wilson disease gene is a copper transporting ATPase with homology to the Menkes disease gene. *Nat. Genet.* 5:344–350, 1993.
3. Vulpe, C., Levinson, B., Whitney, S., Packman, S., and Gitschier, J. Isolation of a candidate gene for Menkes disease and evidence that it encodes a copper-transporting ATPase. *Nat. Genet.* 3:7–13, 1993.
4. Harris, Z. L., and Gitlin, J. D. Genetic and molecular basis for copper toxicity. *Am. J. Clin. Nutr.* 63:836S–841S, 1996.
5. Harris, Z. L., Takahashi, Y., Miyajima, H., Serizawa, M., MacGillivray, R. T. A., and Gitlin, J. D. Aceruloplasminemia: Molecular characterization of this disorder of iron metabolism. *Proc. Natl. Acad. Sci. USA* 92:2539–2543, 1995.

emission tomographic studies have shown that patients with prominent parkinsonism have greater reductions in striatal [^{18}F] 6-fluorodopa uptake than those with mainly ALS [28]. This disease apparently developed prominently during the second World War, when seeds of *Cycas circinalis,* also known as false sago, came into use as a food source. These seeds contain

β-*N*-methylamino-L-alanine (BMAA), an amino acid with an affinity for NMDA receptors. On chronic administration to monkeys, BMAA reproduces some of the features of ALS–parkinsonism–dementia. Studies of the content of BMAA in flour prepared from the seeds have made it seem very unlikely that sufficient quantities of BMAA could be ingested to cause the widespread neurofibrillary degeneration of nerve cells observed in this disease [29]. Interestingly, Guamanian men with ALS–parkinsonism–dementia who joined the U.S. army as young adults, and thus had minimal exposure to Guamanian life, nevertheless developed progressive neurodegeneration similar to that of the inhabitants of Guam. This suggests that exposure to a particular toxin during early life may subsequently manifest progressive syndromes in later life. Other possible causes are being sought, but fortunately, the disease seems to be disappearing.

HUNTINGTON'S DISEASE

Huntington's disease is characterized by abnormal movements, personality changes and progressive dementia. These movements embody elements of chorea, athetosis and dystonia. Abnormalities of the conjugated gaze may also be observed. This progressive, autosomal dominant disorder usually starts in early adulthood, although juvenile cases have been reported. The highest prevalence of the disease has been reported in the Western European population. The gene abnormality is on the short arm of chromosome 4. The gene product, huntingtin, is not involved in transcriptional regulation. Immunostaining studies indicate that huntingtin, is localized in both neuronal and nonneuronal structures. The relevance of this gene product to the disease is still not understood since it has been detected in brain regions other than the striatum. It has been suggested that huntingtin may be related to the apoptotic mechanism(s) of cell death. Alternatively, huntingtin may bind to some neuronal protein, such as glyceraldehyde-3-phosphate dehydrogenase, forming a cytotoxic complex which induces cell death. This finding may have important implications for the pathogenesis of the disease.

In Huntington's disease, the pathology exhibits a preference for particular striatal areas, such as the ventral tier of this region. Similarly, the large aspiny cholinergic neurons are relatively well preserved. In contrast, there is marked destruction and gliosis of GABAergic, enkephalin- and substance P-containing medium spiny neurons in the caudate nucleus and putamen. The caudate nucleus appears to be more severely affected compared to the putamen. Indeed, computed tomography and magnetic resonance images display flattening of the normally rounded medial surface of the caudate nuclei. Thus, the consequent GABA deficit may induce hyperactivity of the thalamocortical feedback pathway and, finally, chorea. Receptors, including muscarinic, cholinergic, dopaminergic and others, associated with these neurons are also depleted. There is a marginal, insignificant depletion in DA in the caudate nucleus (Table 45–2). Also, there is a 50% reduction in the activity of ChAT in the striatum. This may subsequently account for the disruption of compensatory DA turnover in the caudate nucleus. It has been suggested that there is a marked decrease in the activities of mitochondrial respiratory chain enzymes, complexes II, III and IV, in the caudate nucleus in Huntington's disease. This deficit in mitochondrial activity supports the involvement of oxidative stress in the disease pathogenesis.

A reduction of striatal NMDA receptor density has been reported in the disease [30]. This change is coupled with an elevation of astrocytes, probably as a protective mechanism against glutamate-related cell death. Furthermore, simulation of Huntington striatal pathology by the administration of NMDA receptor agonists, such as quinolinic acid, in animal models affirms the evidence for the involvement of an excitotoxic mechanism(s) in the pathogenesis of the disorder. Therefore, both excitotoxic and oxidative mechanisms appear to operate in the cell-destruction pathway. These two processes may function in a synergistic fashion, as postulated in Parkinson's disease, or independently. However, the cause of the disease remains obscure. Therapy usually involves palliative treatment with dopaminergic antagonists, such as haloperidol, or drugs that affect dopaminergic uptake, including reserpine and tetrabenazine (see also Chap. 12).

Excitotoxin-induced lesions in animals mimic Huntington's disease

Direct injection of excitatory neurotoxins, such as kainic acid, a rigid analog of glutamate, into the striatum causes destruction of intrinsic GABA-containing and cholinergic neurons but spares glia and afferent axons [31]. Affected neurons are those which possess receptors for excitatory amino acid neurotransmitters, including NMDA, AMPA and KA receptors. Quinolinic acid, a tryptophan metabolite found in brain and other tissues, has a more restricted neurotoxicity. Although quinolinic acid lowers cerebral GABA and substance P, unlike kainic acid, it does not alter amounts of somatostatin and NPY. Thus, quinolinic acid-treated animals appear to mimic the chemical pathology of Huntington's disease more precisely. However, the presence of receptors for excitatory amino acid neurotransmitters is insufficient to account for the death of these neurons as neurons bearing such receptors are dispersed widely throughout the unaffected regions of the brain. Factors that have been considered but have not been demonstrated to be significant include excess release of excitatory amino acid neurotransmitters and impaired ability to maintain homeostasis of ions, such as Ca^{2+}, when there is increased excitatory activity or deficient sequestration of intracellular Ca^{2+}.

The neurotoxin 3-nitropropionic acid is an irreversible inhibitor of succinate dehydrogenase (complex II of the mitochondria respiratory chain described in Chap. 42) and induces selective striatal degeneration similar to that observed in Huntington's disease. Indeed, it has been shown that chronic administration of 3-nitropropionic acid to nonhuman primates mimics some of the clinical features and biochemical changes characteristic of Huntington's disease.

KERNICTERUS

Erythroblastosis fetalis is secondary to rhesus and blood group incompatibilities between the mother and the fetus during the neonatal period. This results in a consequential increase in bilirubin in the brain. The tendency of bilirubin to be concentrated in the STN and basal ganglia cells may result in kernicterus, or jaundice of the nuclei of the brain. Affected babies initially have decreased muscle tone, which after several weeks increases to rigidity and the gaze palsies. Children who survive often develop choreoathetosis, dystonia and/or tremors in addition to the persistent rigidity. Although there is considerable knowledge regarding bilirubin metabolism, the primary molecular target in the brain is not known.

Kernicterus appears when the rate of entry of unconjugated bilirubin into the brain exceeds the capacity of the brain bilirubin oxidase system to dispose of bilirubin. This may result from hemolysis, a low albumin reserve, low pH or administration of displacing drugs so that excess free bilirubin is present in plasma and enters the brain or, if the brain bilirubin oxidase system is ineffective because of immaturity, birth asphyxia or other forms of CNS injury. Although the mechanism of bilirubin toxicity is not known, removing bilirubin is beneficial and therapy is directed at prevention of high concentrations of bilirubin by exchange transfusion or photoinactivation therapy with blue light.

ACKNOWLEDGMENTS

We would like to express our appreciation to Dr. I. Kopin and Dr. T. Sourkes for permission to incorporate sections from previous editions into our manuscript. In addition, we would like to convey our gratitude to Dr. G. Siegel for his contribution to this chapter. The preparation of this manuscript was supported by a grant provided by the Bundesministerium for Bildung und Forschung.

REFERENCES

1. Graybiel, A. M. Neurotransmitters and neuromodulators in the basal ganglia. *Trends Neurosci.* 13:244–253, 1990.
2. Gerfen, C. R. The neostriatal mosaic: Multiple

levels of compartmental organization in the basal ganglia. *Annu. Rev. Neurosci.* 15:285–320, 1992.

3. Palkovits, M., and Brownstein, M. Catecholamines in the central nervous system. In U. Trendelenberg and N. Weiner (eds.), *Catecholamines II.* Berlin: Springer, 1989, pp. 1–26.

4. McGeer P. L., McGeer S, Itagak S, et al. Anatomy and pathology of the basal ganglia. *Can. J. Neurol. Sci.* 14:363–372, 1987.

5. Fahn, S. Secondary parkinsonism. In E. S. Goldenson and S. H. Appel (eds.), *Scientific Approaches to Clinical Neurology.* Philadelphia: Lea & Febiger, 1977, pp. 1159–1189.

6. Carlsson, A., Lindquist, M., Magnusson, T., and Waldeck, B. On the presence of 3 hydroxytyramine in brain. *Science* 127:471–472, 1958.

7. Ehringer, H., and Hornykiewicz, O. Distribution of noradrenaline and dopamine (3-hydroxytyramine) in the human brain and their behavior in diseases of the extrapyramidal system. *Klin. Wochenschr.* 38:1236–1239, 1960.

8. Sourkes, T. L. On the origin of homovanillic acid in the cerebrospinal fluid. *J. Neural Transm.* 34:153–157, 1973.

9. Birkmayer, W., and Hornykiewicz, O. Der L-3,4-dioxyphenyl-alanin (L-dopa). Effekt bei der Parkinson-Akinesia. *Wien Klin. Wochenschr.* 73:787–788, 1961.

10. Barbeau A. Dopamine and basal ganglia disease. *Arch. Neurol.* 4:97–102, 1961.

11. Birkmayer, W., and Mentasi, M. Weitere experimentelle Untersuchungen uber den Catecholaminostoffwechsel bei extrapyramidalen Erkrankungen. *Arch. Psychiatr. Nervenkr.* 210:29–35, 1967.

12. Cotzias, G. C., Papavasilious, P. S., and Gellene, R. Modification of parkinsonism—chronic treatment with L-dopa. *N. Engl. J. Med.* 280:337–345, 1969.

13. Yahr, M. D., and Duvoisin, R. C. Drug therapy of parkinsonism. *N. Engl. J. Med.* 287:20–24, 1972.

14. Birkmayer, W., Riederer, P., Youdim, M. B. H., and Linauer, W. Potentiation of antikinetic effect after L-dopa treatment by an inhibitor of MAO B, L-deprenyl. *J. Neural Transm.* 36:303–323, 1975.

15. Goetz, C. G. Dopamine agonists in the treatment of Parkinson's disease. *Neurology* 40 (Suppl. 3):50–54, 1990.

16. Hassler, R., and Riechert, T. Indikationen und lokalisationsmethode der gezielten Hirnoperationen. *Nervenarzt* 25:441–448, 1954.

17. Laiten, L. V., Bergenheim, A. T., and Hariz, M. I. Leksell's postero-ventral pallidotomy in the treatment of Parkinson's disease. *J. Neurosurg.* 76:53–61, 1992.

18. Dostrovsky, J. O., Davis, K. D., Lee, L. et al. Electrical stimulation-induced effects in the human thalamus. *Adv. Neurol.* 63:219–229, 1993.

19. Kopin, I. J. Features of the dopaminergic neurotoxin MPTP. *Ann. N. Y. Acad. Sci.* 648:96–104, 1992.

20. Gerlach, M., and Riederer, P. Theories concerning the aetiology and pathogenesis of Parkinson's disease. *J. Neural. Transm.* (in press), 1998.

21. Gerlach, M., Youdim, M. B. H., and Riederer, P. Pharmacology of selegiline. *Neurology* 47: S137–S145, 1996.

22. Birkmayer, W., Knoll, J., Riederer, P., Youdim, M. B., Hars, V., and Marton, J. Increased life expectancy resulting from addition of L-deprenyl to Madopar treatment in Parkinson's disease: A long-term study. *J. Neural Transm.* 64:113–127, 1985.

23. The Parkinson Study Group. Effects of tocopherol and deprenyl on the progression of disability in early Parkinson's disease. *N. Engl. J. Med.* 328:176–183, 1993.

24. Baldessarini, R. J., and Tarsy, D. Dopamine and the pathophysiology of dyskinesias induced by antipsychotic drugs. *Annu. Rev. Neurosci.* 3:23–41, 1980.

25. Mena, I. Manganese poisoning. In P. J. Vinkeh and G. W. Broyh (eds.), *Handbook of Clinical Neurology.* New York: Elsevier, 1977, vol. 21, pp. 217–327.

26. Gerlach, M., Ben-Shachar, D., Riederer, P., and Youdim, M. B. H. Altered brain metabolism of iron as a cause of neurodegenerative diseases? *J. Neurochem.* 63:795–807, 1994.

27. Nyberg, P., Gottfries, C. T. G., Holmgreen, G., et al. Advanced catecholaminergic disturbances in the brain in case of Wilson's disease. *Acta. Neurol. Sci.* 65:71–75, 1982.

28. Snow, B. J., Peppard, R. F., Guttman, M., et al. Positron emission tomographic scanning demonstrates a presynaptic dopaminergic lesion in Lytico-Bodig. The amyotrophic lateral sclerosis–parkinsonism–dementia complex of Guam. *Arch. Neurol.* 47:870–874, 1990.

29. Duncan, M. W., Steele, J. C., Kopin, I. J., and Markey, S. P. 2-Amino-3-(methylamino)-propanoic acid (BMAA) in cyad flour: An unlikely cause of amyotrophic lateral sclerosis and parkinsonism–dementia of Guam. *Neurology* 40:767–772, 1990.

30. Young, A. B., Greenmayre, Z., and Hollingsworth, R. NMDA receptor losses in putamen from patients with Huntington's disease. *Science* 241:981–983, 1988.

31. DiFiglia, M. Excitotoxic injury of the neostriatum: A model for Huntington's disease. *Trends Neurosci.* 13:286–289, 1990.

32. Gerlach, M., Gsell, W., Kornhuber, J., et al. A post mortem study on neurochemical markers of dopaminergic, GABA-ergic and glutamatergic neurons in basal ganglia–thalamocortical circuits in Parkinson's syndrome. *Brain Res.* 741: 142–152, 1996.

33. Gerlach, M., and Riederer, P. Animal models of Parkinson's disease: An empirical comparison with the phenomenology of the disease in man. *J. Neural Transm.* 103:987–1041, 1996.

34. Gerlach, M., and Riederer, P. Pathobiochemische Befunde bei extrapyramidal motorischen Erkrankungen. In G. Huffmann, H.-J. Braune, and K.-H. Henn (eds.), *Extrapyramidalmotorische Erkrankungen.* Einhorn Presse Verlag, 1994, pp. 49–59.

46

Biochemistry of Alzheimer's and Prion Diseases

Dennis J. Selkoe and Peter J. Lansbury, Jr.

Basic Neurochemistry: Molecular, Cellular and Medical Aspects, 6th Ed., edited by G. J. Siegel et al. Published by Lippincott–Raven Publishers, Philadelphia, 1999. Correspondence to Dennis J. Selkoe and Peter Lansbury, Department of Neurology and Program in Neuroscience, Harvard Medical School and Center for Neurologic Diseases, Brigham and Women's Hospital, Boston, Massachusetts 02115.

ALZHEIMER'S DISEASE IS THE MOST COMMON NEURODEGENERATIVE DISORDER

The intense scientific interest that Alzheimer's disease (AD) has generated in recent years is in considerable part a reflection of the commonness of this progressive neurodegenerative disorder. Since the pioneering work of Blessed, Tomlinson and Roth in the 1960s, neuropathologists have increasingly recognized that the clinicopathological syndrome which the Bavarian psychiatrist Alois Alzheimer originally described in a 51-year-old woman is also the most common basis for late-life cognitive failure. Many autopsy studies of patients with senile dementia have shown that the amyloid plaques and neurofibrillary tangles (NFTs) to which Alzheimer called attention in 1907 appear to be the pathological substrate for some 50 to 70% of cases. Senile dementia is defined as the progressive loss of memory and other cognitive functions occurring after the age of 65 years; if the same clinical syndrome occurs prior to age 65, it is referred to as presenile dementia (see also Chap. 30).

Estimates of the prevalence of senile dementia and AD have varied considerably among population surveys conducted in different countries. A representative example for the United States comes from the Framingham, Massachusetts epidemiological study, in which about 2.5% of subjects aged 65 to 74 years had a clinical diagnosis of senile dementia compared to 4% of those aged 75 to 79, 11% of those aged 80 to 84 and 24% of those aged 85 to 93 [1]. In this study, about 55% of all cases of senile dementia were felt to have probable AD. These and other figures from similar surveys lead to a projection of some 3 to 4 million patients with probable AD in the United States. The soci-

etal costs are estimated at upward of $100 billion annually in the United States alone. AD affects individuals in all races and ethnic groups, and it occurs slightly more commonly in women than in men, even taking into account the greater longevity of women in our society.

Amyloid-bearing plaques, neurofibrillary tangles and neuronal dystrophy and loss characterize the pathology of Alzheimer's disease

It is becoming increasingly clear that AD represents a syndrome with well-defined clinical and neuropathological hallmarks but with an array of specific molecular defects which can initiate the pathology. Despite this etiological heterogeneity, growing evidence suggests that there is a common and rather stereotyped pathogenetic cascade which can result from distinct gene defects and/or as yet unknown environmental factors. External examination of the brains of AD patients usually reveals considerable cortical atrophy, particularly in the limbic and association cortices, together with enlargement of the lateral ventricles. However, the hallmarks of the disorder that confirm the diagnosis are observed on microscopic examination, usually with the aid of a silver stain (Fig. 46-1). These include loss of neurons, particularly medium- and large-sized pyramidal cells, and the presence of intraneuronal NFTs and extracellular deposits of amyloid filaments surrounded by altered neuritic processes and glia. These are termed senile plaques and are not specific for AD. Senile plaques can be seen in many functionally normal individuals beginning after age 60 years in small numbers and in limited topographic distribution, particularly in the hippocampus, amygdala and other limbic structures.

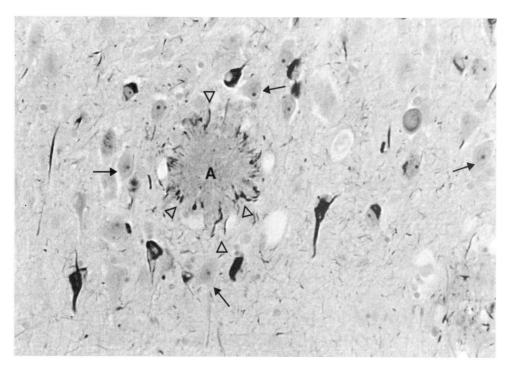

FIGURE 46-1.   The classical histopathological lesions of Alzheimer's disease demonstrated by the modified Bielschowsky silver stain. A 6-μm paraffin section of the amygdala from a 69-year-old man with a 6-year history of progressive dementia. Darkly staining neurofibrillary tangles occupy much of the cytoplasm of selected pyramidal neurons, in contrast to the clear cytoplasm of adjacent cytologically normal neurons *(arrows)*. In the center, a senile plaque consists of a large, compacted deposit of extracellular amyloid *(A)* surrounded by a halo of dilated, structurally abnormal, or dystrophic, neurites *(open arrowheads)*. Altered axons and dendrites are both present in such neuritic plaques. Reactive microglia and fibrillary astrocytes associated with such plaques are not well visualized here. The edge of a second neuritic plaque is seen in the *lower right corner*.

Senile plaques are structurally complex lesions, the temporal development of which is only partially understood. Many, if not all, senile plaques probably begin as amorphous, largely nonfilamentous aggregates of a 40- to 42-residue protein, the amyloid β protein (Aβ). After a period of time, the length of which is not known, some of these "diffuse" Aβ deposits become increasingly fibrillar and gradually acquire the classical features of amyloid plaques, namely, relatively compacted bundles of ∼8-nm filaments which bind certain histochemical dyes, such as Congo red and thioflavin, and have principally a β-pleated sheet protein conformation. Compacted or mature amyloid plaques are frequently associated with numerous dystrophic axons and dendritic processes that lie within or immediately around the fibrous amyloid deposit. These neurites are often thickened and intensely silver-positive. Such mature plaques also display activated microglia intimately associated with the central amyloid deposit and fibrous astrocytes rimming the plaque. The finding of large numbers of such senile or neuritic plaques in limbic and association cortices is probably the single most reliable neuropathological marker of the diagnostic entity of AD.

In the large majority of AD brains, senile plaques are accompanied by argyrophilic bundles of intraneuronal cytoplasmic fibers, the NFTs. Electron microscopy of such neurons demonstrates that the tangles are generally composed of masses of paired, helically wound, ∼10-nm filaments (PHFs), often intermixed with ∼15-nm straight filaments. Anatomical studies have shown that NFTs are frequently present in the cell bodies of neurons whose axons project to the sites of neuritic plaques, for example, the entorhinal → hippocampal perforant pathway and the basal forebrain → hippocampal/neocortical pathway. NFTs are a less specific histological marker of AD than are neuritic plaques. They can occur in the absence of neuritic plaques in a number of etiologically diverse neurological disorders, such as subacute sclerosing panencephalitis, Kufs' disease and Hallervorden-Spatz disease. Moreover, a minority of AD brains, perhaps 10 to 15%, show abundant amyloid-bearing neuritic plaques but few or no NFTs in the neocortex. Thus, there can be a clear dissociation of plaques and tangles under some circumstances. The wide variety of neuropathological disorders in which NFTs occur suggests that PHF formation is a relatively nonspecific marker of certain kinds of neuronal injury.

In addition to a variety of morphological types of Aβ protein deposits present in the brain parenchyma, the cortical and meningeal arteries, arterioles, capillaries and, to a lesser extent, venules may contain multifocal deposits of amyloid filaments composed of Aβ. The amyloid deposits appear to be preferentially localized to the abluminal basement membrane of these microvessels. The number of amyloid-bearing cortical vessels can vary dramatically among AD cases having relatively similar densities of amyloid plaques. The association of microvascular amyloidosis with parenchymal amyloidosis in AD has aroused interest in view of the discovery of missense mutations in the β-amyloid precursor protein (βAPP) in both families with AD and families with severe amyloid angiopathy causing cerebral hemorrhages (see below).

Neurons in the limbic and association cortices and the subcortical nuclei that project to them are particularly vulnerable to neurofibrillary tangle formation

In most cases of AD, the innumerable NFTs found in the limbic and association cortices are accompanied by NFTs in neurons of subcortical nuclei that project to these regions. These nuclei include the cholinergic basal forebrain complex, the locus ceruleus and the median raphe nuclei. NFTs are very rarely found in regions of brain that are only minimally involved, both pathologically and clinically, in AD, for example, the cerebellum. In such largely unaffected areas, diffuse

or "preamyloid" forms of Aβ deposits (see below) may occur but there is little surrounding neuritic dystrophy and usually no NFT formation.

In addition to containing NFTs, neurons in the limbic and association cortices and in the subcortical nuclei that project to them often undergo perikaryal shrinkage and actual cell death. It is likely that some or many neurons which shrink and die in AD do not pass through a stage of actual NFT formation.

Most cases of AD that have extensive NFTs also show widespread dystrophic neurites, sometimes called neuropil threads or curly fibers, that are scattered in the cortical neuropil and not specifically localized to amyloid plaques. An abundance of dystrophic neurites in the cerebral cortex has been correlated to some extent with both the presence of NFTs and the occurrence of clinical dementia. Such dystrophic neurites are not specific for AD and have been found in other neurological disorders in which NFTs occur in the absence of amyloid plaques.

Multiple neurotransmitter systems are affected in a pattern that correlates with the cellular pathology

The topographically widespread and cytologically heterogeneous populations of neurons affected in the AD brain are associated with a complex array of neurotransmitter deficits. The first transmitter alteration to be defined was a marked decline in the activities of choline acetyltransferase and acetylcholinesterase, indicating dysfunction and loss of basal forebrain cholinergic neurons and their cortical projections. Although the decline in these cholinergic markers has been correlated with both the degree of dementia and the number of neuritic plaques, cholinergic loss should not be considered the preeminent neurotransmitter alteration in AD because many neurons releasing monoamine or neuropeptide transmitters also become morphologically abnormal and undergo attrition. These neurons include, for example, noradrenergic and serotonergic cells in the brainstem, cells producing somatostatin or corticotropin-releasing factor in the neocortex and neurons which release glutamate, GABA, substance P and/or neuropeptide Y. The degrees of decline in the concentrations of these transmitters and their biosynthetic and catabolic enzymes vary markedly among AD brains. This heterogeneity of neurotransmitter alterations together with possible involvement of their second-messenger systems helps to explain why attempts at replacement therapy aimed at just one of these neurotransmitters, most commonly the use of cholinergic agents, have met with very limited success in terms of measurable and sustained improvement in objective cognitive tests. It is clear that AD does not follow the patterns of certain other neurodegenerative disorders, such as Parkinson's disease (Chap. 45), which are more specific in their neurotransmitter profile.

The search for etiologies has resulted in a focus on genetic factors

Ever since the original description of the disorder by Alzheimer, there has been a lively debate as to what factor or factors could initiate this complex, multicellular degeneration. Although AD shows limited parallels with the infectious/inherited spongiform encephalopathies, such as Creutzfeldt-Jakob disease and Gerstmann-Straussler-Scheinker syndrome (see below, "Prion Diseases"), no compelling evidence that AD is caused by an infectious pathogen has been presented. The possibility that an environmental toxin could precipitate the disorder has revolved largely around the role of metal ions, particularly aluminum. Aluminum initially became a candidate simply because it was found to induce silver-positive bundles of neurofilaments in neurons upon injection into rabbit CNS. However, these filamentous lesions are now known to be distinct from Alzheimer-type NFTs, both structurally and biochemically. Some investigators have reported elevated concentrations of aluminum in cortical regions affected by Alzheimer pathology, particularly within the NFTs themselves. However, equal or greater aluminum accumulation has been found in the NFTs of Guam Parkinson dementia complex and certain variants of Hallervorden-Spatz disease, disorders in which few or no amyloid plaques or amyloid angiopathy of the Alzheimer type appear. This ob-

servation suggests that aluminum deposition is not unique to AD but, rather, that aluminum can associate secondarily with NFTs, regardless of the specific disease that causes the tangle formation.

Investigators who have demonstrated aluminum within NFTs have sometimes reported abnormal concentrations of other metals, particularly magnesium, calcium and iron, in AD neurons. The presence of aluminum in amyloid plaque cores has been reported, but this association has been less clearly confirmed than that with NFT. It should also be noted that some investigators have reported no substantial elevation of aluminum in the AD brains which they examined. The pathological role of neuronal aluminum deposition in AD remains unclear, and there is little compelling evidence that it serves as a primary toxin which can initiate the disease. In this regard, it is worth noting that aluminum is ubiquitous in our environment, including in the drinking water of many communities. There are currently no rigorous data indicating an unusual or specific source of aluminum, such as antacids, aluminum containers or deodorants, as a risk factor for AD in the general population.

It has been known for decades that some cases of AD occur in an autosomal dominant Mendelian pattern, and this has turned out to be a fruitful clue for the etiological study of the disorder. The percentage of all AD cases that clearly shows such a pattern has often been reported as 10 to 15%, but a much higher percentage of patients has a clinical history of one or more first-degree relatives with a highly similar dementing syndrome. Because of the late onset of most AD cases, it has been difficult to ascertain whether members of previous generations were actually afflicted with the disease. Mounting evidence suggests that a high percentage of subjects, although by no means all, have inherited some type of genetic predisposition to the disease. In a growing number of families, specific DNA mutations have now been identified.

Support for the hypothesis that AD could be genetically based came initially from the observation that virtually all subjects with trisomy 21, also termed Down's syndrome, develop typical histopathological lesions of AD if they survive into their 40s and beyond. This single clini-copathological clue has been perhaps the most significant factor in unraveling the mechanism of AD. Numerous important discoveries about the causation and biochemical mechanism have derived from the link between trisomy 21 and AD lesions. Of particular interest in this regard has been the realization, since the mid-1980s, that subjects with Down's syndrome dying in their teens or 20s may show low to moderate densities of diffuse Aβ deposits in the limbic and association cortices in the absence of detectable surrounding neuronal or glial changes, neuritic dystrophy or NFTs. This important observation has strengthened the concept that deposition of Aβ is a very early event in the disease, preceding other histological changes.

Clues to the mechanisms of familial Alzheimer's disease have arisen from biochemical analyses of the neuropathological phenotype

Although early attempts to purify and chemically analyze pathological structures in AD brain tissue focused on the study of NFTs (see next section), these have not yet led to clues about the molecular etiology of this disease. Instead, the purification of amyloid deposits from meningeal blood vessels by Glenner and Wong in 1984 [2] provided the seminal biochemical information that led both to the identification of the first specific molecular cause of AD and to a plausible model for the pathogenetic cascade. Prior to the study of the cerebral amyloid, widespread doubts had been expressed as to whether biochemical analysis of the histopathological lesions would lead to useful insights about early events in the disease. However, knowledge of other human amyloidoses suggested that extracellular deposits of amyloid-forming proteins could cause local cytopathology and organ dysfunction. Particularly in cases where there were genetic defects in the amyloidogenic protein, such as transthyretin in familial amyloidotic polyneuropathy, these deposits could explain the etiology of the disease in which the amyloid appeared. This scenario has now proven to be the case in AD. As the study of the disease continues,

it is becoming apparent that it follows in considerable part the rules of systemic amyloidoses, while in other respects the β-amyloid process is distinct from these disorders.

Neurofibrillary tangles and dystrophic cortical neurites contain post-translationally modified forms of tau proteins

Biochemical analysis of the PHFs which accumulate as perikaryal NFTs and within dystrophic cortical neurites, both in neuritic plaques and outside of plaques in the cortical neuropil, began well before the characterization of the amyloid. A large number of immuno-chemical and biochemical experiments have led to the conclusion that the principal protein subunit of PHFs is an altered form of the microtubule-associated protein tau (Chap. 8). Tau normally copurifies with tubulin during repetitive cycles of assembly and disassembly of microtubules, and it is known to bind to tubulin and promote the assembly and stability of microtubules. The identification of tau as the major antigenic constituent of PHF was made using antibodies both to purified PHF and to tau (see, for example [3]). Subsequently, harsh methods were used to extract and sequence fragments of tau from purified PHF, many of which are highly insoluble in strong detergents and solvents. These studies demonstrated that tau, particularly portions from the carboxyl third of the molecule containing its microtubule-binding domains, were incorporated into PHF. A separate line of investigation came to a similar conclusion, that the tau protein is the major or sole component of PHF. Wolozin and Davies [4] raised monoclonal antibodies to particulate fractions of AD brain and identified a particular antibody, designated Alz 50, that bound to NFTs, to a large number of dystrophic cortical neurites and to some abnormal neuronal cell bodies that did not contain NFTs. In extracts of AD cortex, Alz 50 recognized a group of proteins having electrophoretic mobility slightly slower than normal tau; these were designated A68 because their relative migration clustered around 68 kDa [4]. The subsequent use of Alz 50 to probe protein fractions from normal brain demonstrated that the antibody recognized normal tau proteins, both in their phosphorylated state (see Chap. 24) and following their *in vitro* dephosphorylation [5]. These results suggested that A68 proteins represent an altered phosphorylation state of tau that causes its slower electrophoretic mobility on gels. This conclusion was supported by the development of a method to purify a subset of PHFs that were soluble in ionic detergents and the demonstration that such PHFs were solely composed of the A68 forms of tau [6]. Analyses of purified A68, also designated PHF-tau, from AD cerebral cortex have demonstrated that the altered tau molecules contain additional phosphate groups beyond those normally present on tau. The mechanism by which the hyperphosphorylated tau arises may include the increased activities of several kinases which can putatively phosphorylate tau as well as the decreased activities of certain cellular phosphatases (see Chap. 24).

There has been considerable speculation about polypeptides besides tau that may contribute to the PHF structure. Presently, the most clear and reproducible data have suggested that tau is the principal, if not the sole, structural constituent of the filaments. However, like a variety of neuronal inclusions in diseases other than AD, such as Lewy bodies in dopaminergic neurons in Parkinson's disease, NFTs contain ubiquitin. In addition, glycosaminoglycans (GAGs) have been detected in NFTs and in adjacent neurons not bearing tangles per se, and these have been shown to be capable of enhancing the polymerization of tau into PHF structures *in vitro* [7]. On this basis, it has been postulated that GAGs or proteoglycans bearing them may serve as a critical nidus for the initiation of PHF formation in neurons.

Amyloid in Alzheimer's disease plaques is composed of a 40- to 42-amino-acid portion of an integral membrane glycoprotein, the β-amyloid precursor protein

The initial sequence of the Aβ protein, obtained from the meningovascular amyloid deposits by Glenner and Wong, [2] extended to 24 residues and was not homologous with previously described proteins. Shortly after this observation, the partial purification of the amyloid plaque cores and their solubilization in high concentrations of formic acid or guanidine thiocyanate demonstrated that their subunit protein had an amino acid composition indistinguishable from meningovascular Aβ, although there appeared to be considerable heterogeneity of the amino terminus, including blocked species [8,9]. The sequence of the vascular amyloid was later extended to 40 residues, whereas that of the plaque amyloid was found to be heterogeneous but principally 40 or 42 residues in length [10].

Because of the difficulty of purifying the highly self-aggregating amyloid protein from postmortem cerebral tissue, only a limited number of biochemical analyses have been published. It is likely that even more heterogeneity than is currently recognized, that is, the presence of various truncated Aβ fragments, occurs in many amyloid deposits. Nonetheless, the major species identified to date appear to be $A\beta_{1-40}$ and $A\beta_{1-42}$. There are reproducible biochemical differences between meningovascular and plaque core amyloid; for example, the former, but not the latter, is soluble in 6 M guanidine hydrochloride, and the former is composed in very large part of Aβ peptides ending at residue 40, whereas the latter contains both $A\beta_{40}$ and $A\beta_{42}$ species.

The establishment of the amino-terminal sequence of the Aβ protein led to the cloning of its precursor polypeptide by four laboratories independently in 1987 [10,11]. The first full-length cDNA which was isolated encoded βAPP, a 695-residue protein that contained a single domain with a hydrophobic, putative transmembrane sequence near its carboxy terminus (Fig. 46-2). Subsequent studies of βAPP itself in human tissues and cultured cells demonstrated that it comprised a heterogeneous group of polypeptides ranging from ~105 to 140 kDa [12] and that the protein underwent *N*- and *O*-glycosylation as well as tyrosine sulfation during its posttranslational maturation in the secretory pathway [13].

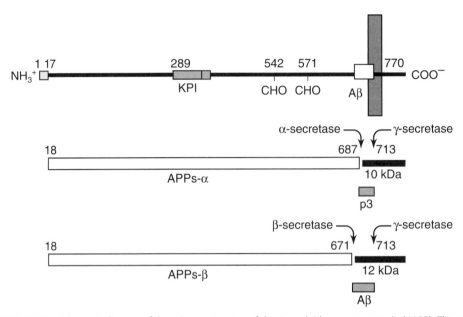

FIGURE 46-2. Schematic diagram of the primary structure of the β-amyloid precursor protein (βAPP). The molecule depicted here is the largest of the known alternate transcripts, comprising 770 amino acids. Several regions of interest are indicated at their correct relative positions. A 17-residue signal peptide occurs at the N terminus. Two alternatively spliced exons of 56 and 19 amino acids are inserted at residue 289; the first contains a serine protease inhibitor domain of the Kunitz type (KPI). Two sites of *N*-glycosylation are found at residues 542 and 571. In the **top diagram,** a single membrane-spanning domain at amino acids 700–723 is indicated by the vertical orange bar. The amyloid β protein (Aβ) fragment *(white box)* includes 28 residues just outside the membrane plus the first 12 to 14 residues of the transmembrane domain. In the **middle diagram,** the *arrow* indicates the site, after residue 687, of a constitutive proteolytic cleavage made by an unknown protease(s), designated α-secretase, that enables secretion of the large, soluble ectodomain of APP (APPs-α) into the medium and retention of the 83-residue carboxy-terminal fragment (~10 kDa) in the membrane. The 10-kDa fragment can undergo cleavage by an unknown protease(s), γ-secretase, at residue 711 or residue 713 to release the p3 peptides. The **lower diagram** depicts the alternative proteolytic cleavage after residue 671 by an unknown enzymes(s) called β-secretase that results in the secretion of a truncated APPs (APPs-β) molecule and the retention of a 99-residue (~12 kDa) carboxy-terminal fragment. The 12-kDa fragment can also undergo cleavage by γ-secretase to release the Aβ peptides.

The cloning of βAPP led immediately to the localization of its gene to the long arm of chromosome 21. This finding offered an explanation for the long-standing neuropathological observation that patients with trisomy 21 develop amyloid-bearing plaques and other lesions of AD. Subsequent cloning of βAPP cDNAs from other mammals demonstrated a high degree of evolutionary conservation of this gene. Indeed, the 695-amino-acid isoform, βAPP$_{695}$, is 100% conserved between the cynomologus monkey and human, while rat and mouse show more than 95% conservation. Gene products with considerable homology to βAPP occur in *Drosophila* and *Caenorhabditis elegans;* these molecules do not, however, contain the Aβ sequence.

cDNA and genomic cloning demonstrated that βAPP polypeptides arise by alternative exon splicing. The initially cloned isoform, βAPP$_{695}$, is almost exclusively expressed in brain, primarily in neurons. Alternate transcripts of 751 and 770 amino acids that have an inserted exon encoding a Kunitz-type serine protease inhibitor (KPI) motif are the major expressed isoforms in virtually all peripheral cells and are expressed in brain cells. Additional alternative transcripts of low abundance have been identified. Examination of the exon/intron structure of the βAPP gene reveals that the 40- to 42-amino-acid Aβ fragments contain portions of two adjacent exons and, thus, must arise by proteolytic processing rather than by alternative splicing.

Deposition of amyloid β protein precedes the lesions of Alzheimer's disease and arises from alternative proteolytic processing of β-amyloid precursor protein

The fact that some subjects with Down's syndrome dying in their teens show amorphous deposits of Aβ, termed diffuse plaques, in the absence of any other cytological lesions of AD has supported the concept that Aβ deposition can occur prior to AD-type neuronal or glial alteration. It is not possible to establish a precise temporal sequence of pathological changes directly in AD because the brain can be examined only at the end of the disease. However, the presence of large numbers of diffuse plaques, outnumbering compacted, neurite-containing plaques, in AD brains and the fact that the amyloid lesions of Down's syndrome are indistinguishable from those of AD support the notion that diffuse plaques represent the earliest discernible morphological change also in AD. As will be discussed shortly, strong support for this hypothesis has come from the identification of point mutations in the βAPP gene, which segregate with the AD phenotype in certain autosomal dominant pedigrees.

Normal cellular processing of βAPP has been shown to include a pathway that involves maturation of the protein in the Golgi apparatus (Chap. 2), trafficking to the plasma membrane and cleavage at residue 16 within the Aβ domain (residue 687 of $βAPP_{770}$), liberating the large amino-terminal hydrophilic portion of the precursor into the medium [13] and retaining an ~10-kDa membrane-associated carboxy-terminal fragment [12] inside the cell (Fig. 46-2). This so-called α-secretory processing, which appears to occur primarily at or near the cell surface, precludes the formation of intact Aβ. There is evidence that α-secretory processing also occurs in intracellular organelles [14]. βAPP contains an Asn-Pro-Thr-Tyr motif in its cytoplasmic tail that resembles a consensus sequence for the internalization of cell-surface receptors via clathrin-coated vesicles (see Chap. 9). Based on this knowledge, experiments have demonstrated an alternative processing route which involves the reinternalization of holo-βAPP from the cell

surface and its trafficking to endosomes and lysosomes. When late endosomes/lysosomes are purified from cultured cells, an array of carboxy-terminal fragments of βAPP can be detected. Indeed, such Aβ-containing fragments have been directly identified in human tissues.

The high degree of insolubility of Aβ isolated from senile plaque and meningovascular deposits and the fact that Aβ is derived from an integral membrane sequence led to the widely held assumption that Aβ must arise from aberrant proteolysis of βAPP following membrane injury. It was therefore surprising to discover that small amounts of Aβ are released continuously from a variety of cultured cells under normal metabolic conditions and that this Aβ in the media is entirely soluble [15–17] (Fig. 46-2). Moreover, soluble Aβ has also been detected in normal and AD cerebrospinal fluid and plasma [16–18]. These data indicate that the Aβ peptide is a normal metabolic product of βAPP throughout life. Furthermore, the findings suggest that cultured human cells can be used as simple *in vitro* screening systems to identify compounds which decrease Aβ production. Drugs that inhibit the still unidentified protease(s) that creates the C terminus of Aβ, termed γ-secretase, are now being prepared for therapeutic trials in patients. Another outcome of the discovery of soluble Aβ in spinal fluid and plasma has been the development of sensitive ELISA assays, which reveal that many, but not all, AD patients have a lower CSF concentration of the soluble $Aβ_{42}$ peptide than do normal elderly subjects. To what extent this finding and analogous assays in plasma will be useful in establishing risk for the disease in elderly humans and monitoring the efficacy of anti-amyloid drug therapy in affected patients will soon become clear.

The normal generation of Aβ by cultured cells has enabled studies of the mechanisms of Aβ production. Considerable evidence has emerged that early endosomes, which internalize and recycle βAPP to the cell surface as if it were a receptor, are a principal site for the formation of the 40-residue form of Aβ (Table 46-1). It is currently not clear whether and to what extent the more amyloidogenic 42-residue form is made during endocytic recycling. However, there is mounting evidence that $Aβ_{42}$ can be gen-

TABLE 46-1.	DATA SUPPORTING EARLY EN-DOSOMES AS THE PRINCIPAL SITE OF Aβ GENERATION

Deleting β-amyloid precursor protein (βAPP) cytoplasmic domain (GYENPTY) lowers amyloid β protein (Aβ) production

Mild alkalinization lowers Aβ production

Altering vesicular H^+ transport lowers Aβ production

Late endosome/lysosome fractions do not contain Aβ

Endocytosis of surface-labeled βAPP molecules leads directly to release of labeled Aβ

Kinetics of labeled Aβ release are slightly slower than those of APP_s and consistent with those of recycling endosomes

Depleting cellular K^+ inhibits clathrin-mediated endocytosis and lowers Aβ production

erated early during the secretory trafficking of βAPP, namely, in the endoplasmic reticulum and Golgi [19]. Therefore, the proteases referred to as β- and γ-secretases are apparently distributed to several subcellular compartments.

The 99-residue C-terminal fragment of βAPP, which is the product of β-secretase action, may be cleaved by distinct γ-secretases at either residue 40 or residue 42 of the Aβ region. Ongoing work should reveal more details about precisely where in the cell the $Aβ_{40}$ and $Aβ_{42}$ peptides are made and the identity of the responsible enzymes.

A rare form of autosomal dominant Alzheimer's disease is caused by point mutations in the gene that encodes β-amyloid precursor protein

The genetic linkage to AD of DNA markers on the long arm of chromosome 21 in some autosomal dominant pedigrees raised the likelihood that βAPP itself could be a disease-causing gene. In 1991, two families were identified in which affected members had a point mutation at codon 717 of $βAPP_{770}$ (Fig. 46-3) [20]. This observation provided the first specific molecular cause

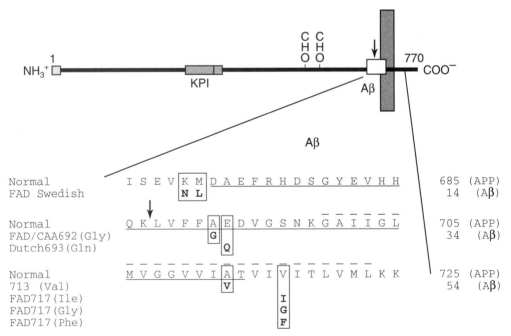

FIGURE 46-3.   The sequence of β-amyloid precursor protein (βAPP) containing the amyloid β protein (Aβ) and transmembrane region is expanded and shown by the single-letter amino acid code. The *underlined residues* represent the $Aβ_{1-43}$ peptide. The *broken line* indicates the location of the transmembrane domain. The *boxed residues* depict the currently known missense mutations identified in certain patients with familial Alzheimer's disease (FAD) or hereditary cerebral hemorrhage with amyloidosis of the Dutch type (Dutch). *CAA* indicates that the family with a 692 Gly mutation can display congophilic amyloid angiopathy as well as Alzheimer's disease as the phenotype. Three-digit numbers refer to the residue number according to the $βAPP_{770}$ isoform. Two-digit numbers refer to the Aβ sequence ($Asp_{672} = 1$).

of AD and suggested that alterations in βAPP could initiate β-amyloidosis in the absence of any pre-existing pathological events. Even prior to this discovery, a mutation at codon 693 of βAPP$_{770}$ had been found in individuals with the Aβ deposition disease hereditary cerebral hemorrhage with amyloidosis of the Dutch type (HCHWA-D) [21]. This rare disorder is marked by severe Aβ deposition in meningeal and cerebral vessels plus large numbers of diffuse plaques. Very few or no mature neuritic plaques or NFTs are observed, and no Alzheimer-like dementia has been described in these patients. It appears that HCHWA-D is closely related to AD, both genotypically and phenotypically, although the clinical outcome is multiple cerebral hemorrhages rather than dementia.

Since these discoveries, a few other point mutations in the βAPP gene have been found in affected members of families with autosomal dominant, or familial, AD (see Fig. 46-3). In addition to the original familial AD mutation at codon APP$_{717}$, Val → Ile, two other missense mutations at the same codon have been discovered: Val → Gly and Val → Phe. Also, a missense mutation changing codon 692 from Ala to Gly has been discovered in a Flemish family having both congophilic angiopathy with hemorrhage and progressive dementia as the clinical phenotypes. A double missense mutation immediately preceding the Aβ region has been found in an extended Swedish kindred with familial AD: APP$_{670}$ Lys → Asn plus APP$_{671}$ Met → Leu. Importantly, all of the βAPP mutations discovered to date in AD pedigrees cluster in the Aβ region

of the precursor. Indeed, the fact that they are at or near the α-, β- or γ-secretase-cleavage sites strongly supports the hypothesis that they alter the proteolytic processing of βAPP in ways that enhance the production of Aβ, especially its highly amyloidogenic 42-residue form. Such enhancement has been demonstrated in both cultured cells and transgenic mouse models [22,23] (Table 46-2).

Mutations in the presenilin 1 and 2 genes represent the most common cause of early-onset, autosomal dominant Alzheimer's disease

Shortly after the discovery of the βAPP mutations, a sizable portion of early-onset AD families was linked to an unknown gene on chromosome 14. Further linkage analyses and positional cloning led to the identification of the responsible gene product as a polytopic membrane protein of 467 amino acids currently designated presenilin 1 (PS1) [24]. A large number of missense mutations (close to 45 at this writing) and one exon deletion in PS1 have been found in families of diverse ethnic origins. Immediately after the cloning of PS1, a highly homologous gene called presenilin 2 (PS2) was identified on chromosome 1, and just two missense mutations have been discovered to date in these familial AD kindreds [25]. The presenilins are in turn homologous to the *sel-12* gene in *C. elegans*, a facilitator of the function of the lin-12/Notch proteins that are involved in cell–cell recognition and specification of cell fate during embryogenesis. These

TABLE 46-2.   **β-AMYLOID PRECURSOR PROTEIN MUTATIONS: GENOTYPE-TO-PHENOTYPE CONVERSIONS**

Codon	Mutation	"Name"	Effects on Aβ *in vitro*
670/671	KM → NL	Swedish	↑ in Aβ production
692	A → G	Flemish	↑ Aβ/p3
			↑ Alternative Aβ N-termini
693	E → Q	Dutch	↑ Aβ/p3
			↑ Aβ fibrillogenesis (synthetic peptide)
	V → I		
717	V → G	London	↑ Long Aβ (42 residues)
	V → F		

discoveries have led to a rapidly growing number of studies of the functional activities of the presenilins in worms and mammals [26], as well as attempts to understand whether these functions are affected by the mutations in PS1 and PS2 which cause early-onset AD.

It is clear that PS1 expression is required for proper mammalian embryogenesis and survival, but it appears that mutant human PS1 can convey these vital developmental functions as well. Rather than conferring a fundamental loss of function of presenilin, the PS1 and PS2 mutations linked to familial AD seem to lead to a gain of toxic function: the disregulation of γ-secretase(s) in a way that selectively enhances the proteolysis of βAPP at Aβ_{42}. A roughly twofold increase in relative Aβ_{42} production has been documented in transfected cells and transgenic mouse brains harboring PS1 or PS2 mutations [27,28], and this elevation has been directly demonstrated in the plasma, skin fibroblast media and brains of humans with such mutations [18,29]. How presenilin mutations increase Aβ_{42} generation is not yet known, but the effect may involve the formation of complexes between presenilin and βAPP, and perhaps additional polypeptides, and may occur in the endoplasmic reticulum and/or Golgi apparatus.

The ϵ4 allele of apolipoprotein E is a major genetic risk factor for late-onset Alzheimer's disease

Biochemical studies searching for CSF proteins capable of binding to Aβ identified apolipoprotein E as one such protein [30]. Subsequent genetic analyses showed that the naturally occurring ϵ4 polymorphism of the ApoE gene was substantially over-represented in sporadic AD subjects compared to age-matched controls and, thus, appeared to represent a major risk factor for the development of the disease [30]. It has since been confirmed that inheritance of one or two ApoE ϵ4 alleles significantly increases the likelihood of developing late-onset sporadic AD and decreases its age of onset. Conversely, inheritance of the infrequent ApoE ϵ2 allele appears to confer a decreased risk of developing the disorder compared to that seen in humans harboring the common ϵ3 allele.

The ApoE4 protein, which lacks cysteines and therefore cannot undergo intramolecular or intermolecular disulfide crosslinking, increases the likelihood of AD whereas the ApoE3 and ApoE2 proteins, which do contain cysteines, do not; however, the molecular mechanism remains unclear. A major clue to the mechanism has come from the observation, now confirmed in numerous laboratories, that AD subjects with two ϵ4 alleles have a significantly higher number and density of Aβ deposits in the brain than subjects with no ϵ4 alleles, while subjects with one ϵ4 allele generally fall in between [31]. *In vitro* biochemical studies have suggested that the ApoE4 protein may be less effective in retarding the aggregation of Aβ into amyloid fibrils than ApoE2 or ApoE3. Alternative hypotheses for the effect of ApoE4 in AD have been proposed. These are based on evidence that (i) ApoE4 does not support neurite outgrowth *in vitro* and is less salutary for normal neuronal structure and function than ApoE3 and (ii) ApoE4 may permit tau to become dissociated from microtubules and participate in enhanced PHF formation. However, the latter hypothesis is inconsistent with the observation that amyloid plaque density, not NFT density, correlates with ApoE4 gene dosage in AD patients [31].

TABLE 46-3.	GENETIC FACTORS PREDISPOSING TO ALZHEIMER'S DISEASE: RELATIONSHIPS TO THE β-AMYLOID (Aβ) PHENOTYPE		
Chromosome	**Gene defect**	**Age of onset**	**Aβ phenotype**
21	βAPP mutations	50s	↑ production of total Aβ peptides or of Aβ_{42} peptides
19	ApoE4 polymorphism	60s and older	↑ density of Aβ plaques and vascular deposits
14	Presenilin 1 mutations	40s and 50s	↑ production of Aβ_{42} peptides
1	Presenilin 2 mutations	50s	↑ production of Aβ_{42} peptides

Additional chromosomal loci exist but are not yet specifically identified.

Genotype-to-phenotype relationships implicate β-amyloidosis as an early and necessary factor in all known forms of familial Alzheimer's disease

To summarize at this juncture, four genes that are unequivocally associated with the development of AD have been identified to date, and linkage analyses of other families make it clear that additional genes can be responsible (Table 46-3). Three of the known genes, *APP, PS1* and *PS2*, can be said to be causative of AD in the respective families in which mutations in these genes occur. In each of these three cases, there is now compelling evidence that the pathogenic mechanism involves altered APP catabolism to generate increased amounts of Aβ peptides, particularly the highly aggregation-prone, 42-residue form (Table 46-3). In the case of the ApoE gene on chromosome 19, its ε4 allele is a major genetic risk factor for the development of AD, perhaps contributing to the development of the disorder in some 30 to 40% of all patients. However, ApoE4 is not causative per se because some patients with one or two ApoE4 alleles show no signs of the clinical disease even late in life and, conversely, more than half of all AD patients do not bear an ε4 allele.

Our discussion thus far has emphasized the possible role of APP metabolism and the gradual accumulation of insoluble Aβ deposits in the pathogenesis of the disease. However, many other biochemical and structural abnormalities have also been observed in the brains of AD patients. Although it is impossible to determine a precise temporal sequence of progression, the outlines of a pathogenic cascade are emerging (Fig. 46-4). Insights into the temporal course of the disorder in its preclinical phase derive primarily from three sources: (i) the study of the accrual of AD-type brain changes in patients with trisomy 21 who have died of other causes at various ages from early childhood to late adulthood; (ii) similar analyses of the development of AD-type lesions during the normal aging process in humans, other primates, dogs and cats; and (iii) studies of transgenic mice which overexpress mutant forms of human APP that cause early-onset AD in humans [22,23].

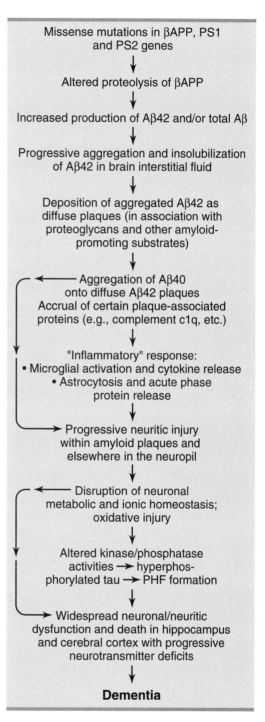

FIGURE 46-4.   A hypothetical sequence of the molecular pathogenesis of familial forms of Alzheimer's disease.

Analyses of Down's syndrome (DS) brains have provided perhaps the most relevant information about how AD may progress. Numerous investigators have reported that the earliest AD-like morphological change found in very young DS brains, 12 to 15 years old, is the accrual of amorphous, largely nonfibrillar forms of Aβ deposits, the diffuse plaques. Some or many such deposits are found in limbic and association cortices and often in striatum, cerebellum and elsewhere in trisomic individuals dying after age 12 years or so. Importantly, such diffuse plaques also accumulate in the brains of nontrisomic people with normal cognition who have died of other causes after the age of 60 years. Diffuse plaques are also abundantly present in typical AD brains at the end of the disease.

Light and electron microscopic studies of diffuse plaques in AD and in DS demonstrate very little or no structural alteration of axons, dendrites, astrocytes and microglia within and immediately surrounding these amorphous Aβ deposits. This lack of cytopathology appears to correlate with a relative dearth of fibrillar amyloid in the diffuse deposits. When the brains of DS patients of increasing age are examined, fibrillar plaques with surrounding neuritic and glial dystrophy are detected increasingly after approximately age 30. At about the same time, NFTs also begin to appear. Although such temporal correlation is imprecise in the relatively limited number of DS patients reported to date, a consensus has emerged that diffuse Aβ plaques clearly precede the other AD-type changes that occur in DS. The early accumulation of diffuse plaques is assumed to be caused by the elevated APP gene dosage and the consequent increase in APP expression and Aβ concentrations documented in these patients.

APP transgenic mice experience high brain expression of APP from birth and are thus analogous in some respects to patients with DS. However, the mice reported to date have the additional influence of familial AD-linked missense mutation flanking the Aβ region of APP [22,23]. Although such animals have high neuronal expression of the APP transgene as well as high amounts of soluble Aβ within their brains from birth, they develop diffuse and compacted Aβ plaques resembling those of AD beginning at

around 5 to 8 months (mice normally live about 2 to 2.5 years). During the next several months, the transgenic mice show increasing numbers of Aβ deposits, many of which are now Congo red-positive, suggesting that they contain fibrillar amyloid; and electron microscopy clearly reveals filamentous amyloid cores. Moreover, after Aβ plaques develop, the mice show morphologically and immunocytochemically abnormal neurites intimately associated with the amyloid plaques [22,23]. Cytoskeletal proteins such as the microtubule-associated protein 2 (MAP2), the neurofilament protein and even the tau protein can show abnormal immunoreactivity in these dystrophic neurites and in some nearby neuronal cell bodies [22,23], although the formation of human-type NFT has not been reported to date. A brisk reactive astrocytosis occurs within and around the Aβ plaques, and activated microglial cells occur near the centers of many of the plaques. Confocal microscopy of the mouse plaques and immunostaining for synaptic proteins indicate that degeneration and loss of synapses is occurring, particularly in the vicinity of the plaques [22]. The extent of behavioral impairment is not yet clear [22,23].

Although the rather rapid acquisition of AD-like lesions in transgenic mice, resulting from high expression of APP from birth, cannot be considered an ideal model of human AD, these mice clearly provide a highly useful and manipulatable representation of the AD process.

Assuming that studies of disease progression in DS and in transgenic mice are relevant to the mechanism of AD, one may postulate that the gradual accrual of Aβ peptides in the form of first diffuse and then fibrillar plaques may result in local cellular effects that include activation of microglial cells, reactive astrocytosis and alterations of nearby axons and dendrites. A hypothetical sequence of the pathogenic cascade leading to clinical cascade is shown in Figure 46-4. The extent to which these cytotoxic events derive from properties of the aggregated Aβ protein itself or from the numerous β-amyloid-associated proteins that have been detected in plaques is yet unclear.

These associated polypeptides, some of which have been referred to as "pathological chaperones" because of their putative role in enhancing the aggregation, deposition and toxicity of Aβ, include the normally secreted proteins α1-antichymotrypsin, ApoE, serum amyloid P component, heparan sulfate proteoglycans and various components of the classical complement pathway. Activated microglia, which become associated with maturing plaques, are capable of releasing a number of well-characterized cytokines that can, in turn, stimulate local astrocytes to release yet other proteins, including α1-antichymotrypsin and ApoE. The serum amyloid P protein, which is associated with all forms of central and peripheral amyloid deposits, is not expressed in the brain and thus must come to the plaque via passage across the blood–brain barrier. To what extent other circulating molecules, including Aβ itself, breach the blood–brain barrier to contribute to the pathological changes is unclear.

It can be concluded that many proteins potentially capable of exerting biological activity on surrounding neurons and glia accumulate within the amyloid plaque. We thus face an embarrassment of riches in terms of potential effectors of AD cytopathology. At exactly which point axons and dendrites in the vicinity, as well as their cell bodies of origin, undergo an activation of kinases, deactivation of phosphatases or both, resulting in the hyperphosphorylation of tau proteins underlying tangle formation, is difficult to say [32]. In all probability, the multiple molecular and cellular alterations found in the AD cortex develop at varying rates but in reasonable proximity to each other.

Biochemical and morphological changes can presumably also occur in cortical and subcortical neurons and their processes, which are not intimately associated with amyloid deposits. Subcortical neurons in regions such as the cholinergic nucleus basalis of Meynert, the noradrenergic locus ceruleus and the serotonergic median raphe nuclei, whose axons all project into plaque-rich cortical areas, often show shrinkage, NFT formation and cell loss. The complex array of plaque-associated and non-plaque-associated cytopathology observed by the end stage of AD may ultimately be very difficult to order into a precise sequence of temporal evolution.

The multiple neurotransmitter alterations in AD brain that were uncovered beginning in the late 1970s are now known to include several monoaminergic and neuropeptide deficiencies beyond the loss of cholinergic function that was first described. In the context of the complex, multicellular pathogenic cascade discussed above, it comes as no surprise that AD does not affect a single neurotransmitter system. Indeed, morphological studies have demonstrated that any one amyloid-bearing neuritic plaque may contain altered neurites derived from neurons of multiple neurotransmitter specificities. These considerations provide one explanation for the general lack of robust symptomatic improvement in patients given cholinergic replacement therapy, such as acetylcholinesterase inhibitors.

The fact that NFTs arise in a variety of etiologically unrelated diseases in the absence of Aβ deposits suggests that they represent a response of neurons to a range of insults and are not specific for the amyloidotic process. The same may also be true of the tau-positive neuropil threads in the cortex, which can also occur in certain other degenerative diseases bearing tangles but lacking amyloid. However, the neuritic plaque, with its severe microglial and astrocytic cytopathology, is more specific for AD and DS. The abundant Aβ deposits that can be found in some cognitively normal elderly subjects are predominantly of the diffuse type, lacking neuritic and glial alteration. This distinction may explain why they are not associated with clinical dysfunction.

Therapeutic strategies arise from understanding the molecular basis of Alzheimer's disease

The development of therapies expected to slow or arrest the progression of a disease requires as true and detailed an understanding of the molecular pathogenesis as possible. The tools for screening a wide array of compounds for possible efficacy in AD include cell culture systems and the transgenic mouse models. These are used to test an array of potential therapeutic targets, which are discussed in the following section.

The inhibition of Aβ secretion from neuronal and non-neuronal cells has been actively pursued. One way this can be accomplished is by designing specific inhibitors of the β- and γ-secretases after these proteases are identified and cloned. However, there may be other ways of lowering Aβ production that do not involve direct inhibition of these enzymes. In any event, the testing of potentially therapeutic chemicals on cells that continuously secrete Aβ has already led to the identification of compounds which lower the production of the peptides. One question regarding this general approach relates to whether chronic treatment with cholinergic agonists will result in increased processing of APP molecules by the α-secretase pathway and, thus, in diminished production of Aβ. Such a possibility can initially be examined in transgenic mice, in which both cerebral and CSF Aβ concentrations can be measured, but it must then be confirmed in treated patients by measuring CSF Aβ concentrations. A number of other first messengers that affect intracellular regulation (see Chaps. 20–22) could turn out to be at least as effective as cholinergic agonists in shifting APP processing from the β- to the α-secretase pathway.

A therapeutic approach that seems particularly attractive is to attempt to slow the aggregation of the secreted Aβ peptide into its fibrillar, putatively cytotoxic form. *In vitro* studies indicate that certain small molecules, including the amyloid-binding dye Congo red, can retard the aggregation of synthetic Aβ peptides into high-molecular-weight aggregates. Compounds which interfere with Aβ assembly into amyloid fibrils could act in the extracellular space of the brain and, thus, avoid interference with the metabolism of APP and other molecules inside cells. Full-length APP and its various metabolites, including APP_s and perhaps even Aβ, have normal functions, whereas the aggregated forms of Aβ that plaques are composed of are believed to represent solely pathological moieties. Thus, interfering with Aβ aggregation, if it can be done in a selective fashion, could avoid effects on the metabolism of APP and other molecules. The transgenic mouse models, which have fibrillar amyloid plaques, should be a reasonable system

in which to evaluate the efficacy and safety of such compounds.

Yet another therapeutic approach based on the growing understanding of presymptomatic events in AD is the use of anti-inflammatory drugs that could interfere in part with the microglial activation, cytokine release and acute phase responses that occur in maturing amyloid plaques. Epidemiological evidence suggests that individuals who have been on nonsteroidal anti-inflammatory drugs may have a lower likelihood of developing the pathological and clinical features of AD. One may assume that the inflammatory process which appears around amyloid plaques is sufficiently distinct from peripheral forms of inflammation that it will require specialized anti-inflammatory compounds, which could again be identified and characterized in transgenic mice.

The devastating impairment of higher cortical functions which characterizes AD must ultimately be attributed to profound neuronal dysfunction and degeneration. Therefore, a variety of neuroprotective strategies can be envisioned in this disorder. One relatively specific approach would be to attempt to design compounds that interfere with any altered signal-transduction pathways that are proven to mediate the effects of extracellular amyloid filaments and their closely associated molecules on neuronal homeostasis. However, no single cell-surface receptor for Aβ in its monomeric or aggregated form has yet been found to fully mediate the toxicity. Agents that could hypothetically interfere with Aβ toxicity would include compounds that coat the amyloid aggregates in a way that makes them "invisible" to the cell and molecules which inhibit a downstream effector pathway inside the neuron.

In addition to such approaches directed at the specific neurotoxic cascade putatively induced by amyloid, general therapies could be applied that might be equally applicable to AD and to other neurodegenerative disorders. Such strategies might include the use of inhibitors of excitotoxicity, agents that block calcium entry into cells, free radical scavengers and antioxidant treatments (see Chap. 34). Evidence is mounting from *in vitro* studies that aggregated Aβ induces multiple features of oxidative injury in cultured neurons.

Another general approach to retarding neurodegeneration that might also be applicable to AD would be neurotrophic therapy. However, technical hurdles must be overcome to chronically deliver neurotrophic peptides to the appropriate sites in the brains of elderly subjects. In addition, more must be learned about all of the effects of trophic factors on APP expression and on the complex effects of upregulation of trophic influences.

The combined power of genetics, molecular biology and biochemistry has produced remarkable advances in our understanding of the causes and mechanisms of AD, and all of these sciences are required for therapeutic approaches.

PRION DISEASES

The brain pathology of prion diseases, like Alzheimer's disease, involves neurodegeneration and abnormal protein aggregates

The prion diseases, originally designated transmissible spongiform encephalopathies (TSEs), are, like AD, slow-onset, progressive, neurodegenerative diseases. In contrast to AD, sporadic TSE disease is very rare and the majority of cases are familial. Symptoms can vary widely but often involve ataxia and progressive dementia [33,34]. Brains from cases of human, livestock and experimental animal TSEs exhibit similar pathology. Spongiform neurodegeneration is accompanied by aggregates of protease-resistant fibrils and occasional amyloid plaques, sometimes adjacent to dystrophic neurites. Prion plaques show some histochemical properties of AD amyloid: birefringent staining with Congo Red and immunoreactivity for ubiquitin and heparan sulfate proteoglycans. However, prion plaques do not react with antibodies raised against the AD Aβ protein. The prion diseases also differ from AD in that they are transmissible via infected tissue.

Prion diseases were originally described in sheep

Scrapie, in sheep, was the first of the prion diseases to be described. This disease was found to be transmissible via infected brain tissue. Subsequently, a group of TSEs have been described in other animal populations, including bovine spongiform encephalopathy (BSE), also termed mad cow disease; transmissible mink encephalopathy; and chronic wasting disease of mule deer and elk. Scrapie has also been transmitted to mice and hamsters for experimental studies. This advance has allowed biochemical studies of the infectious agent (see below). The first human example of TSE arose from the discovery of the infectious etiology of kuru in the indigenous tribes of Papua New Guinea. Kuru was spread by ritual cannibalism; it has since been determined that human TSE can also be spread by corneal transplants with infected tissue or by contaminated cadaver-derived human growth hormone. The experimental transmission of TSE diseases between species has been demonstrated in laboratory animals, although this transmission is much less effective than transmission within a species. This fact has led to speculation that the TSEs of livestock, scrapie and BSE could be transmitted into the human population via infected meat. This speculation was fueled in 1996 by the report of an unusual human TSE, designated a new variant of Creutzfeldt-Jakob disease (CJD) (see below).

The infectious agent may contain only the prion protein

The transmission of scrapie into experimental animals allowed the transmissible agent to be studied in detail. Although it was originally thought to be a virus, the agent proved to be much smaller and more chemically stable than a typical virus. This led to the proposal, in 1967, that the scrapie agent contained only protein and was devoid of nucleic acid [35]. Several mechanisms to explain how a protein could behave like a virus were proposed. Later, the major protein constituent of the infectious agent was sequenced and named the prion protein (PrP), to reflect the possibility that it was the sole necessary constituent of the infectious agent, designated the prion, for proteinaceous infectious particles [36]. Prions were originally defined as "small proteinaceous infectious particles that resist inactivation by procedures which modify nucleic acids." Although a large amount of indirect evidence has accumulated which supports the proposal that the infectious agent is a single protein, direct proof is lacking. Since a single infectious unit contains 10^5 scrapie prion protein (PrP^{Sc}) molecules, it is extremely difficult to rule out definitively the possibility that a small amount of nucleic acid or other cofactor may be an integral part of the infectious agent. However, since an unusual scrapie virus with unprecedented chemical properties has not been isolated, the possibility of a protein-only infectious agent is being seriously investigated.

The prion protein is a normal host protein that is required for scrapie infection

Unexpectedly, PrP is encoded by a single-copy normal chromosomal gene on chromosome 20. PrP is a cell-surface protein, anchored to the membrane through a glycoinositol phospholipid (see Chap. 3). The normal function of PrP is unknown. Mice in which the PrP gene has been removed are qualitatively normal, although some groups have reported slight abnormalities with respect to long-term potentiation and circadian rhythms. Significantly, these mice are "immune" to infection with scrapie, suggesting that this protein plays a key permissive role in the disease process, although the normal form of PrP is innocuous [37]. The normal PrP (PrP^C) and the PrP associated with the infectious agent (PrP^{Sc}) are indistinguishable at the level of covalent chemical structure, but their physical and biochemical properties are very different, suggesting that they are structural isomers [35]. For example, PrP^C is sensitive to proteolysis and is soluble, while PrP^{Sc} is relatively resistant to proteolysis and is relatively insoluble. PrP^C and PrP^{Sc} also differ with respect to their spectroscopic properties. Thus, the conversion of PrP^C to PrP^{Sc}, which may be "catalyzed" in some way by the PrP^{Sc} in the infectious agent, seems to be critical to the disease process [34,35].

Mutations in the prion protein cause human prion diseases

The conversion of PrP^C to PrP^{Sc} also occurs in the absence of the infectious agent. In rare cases of sporadic human TSE and in inherited human disease, it is caused by mutations in PrP^C. Three inherited human TSEs have been traced to mutations in PrP: familial CJD, Gerstmann-Straussler-Scheinker (GSS) syndrome and fatal familial insomnia. Transgenic mice harboring a GSS mutation in the PrP gene, a leucine substitution at codon 102, have been shown to develop scrapies-like neurodegeneration [38].

Elucidation of the infectious mechanism and of normal prion protein conversion to scrapie prion protein is necessary to design compounds for therapeutic intervention

The protein-only hypothesis holds that the conversion of PrP^C to PrP^{Sc} is induced by infectious PrP^{Sc}. In order to elucidate the mechanism of this process, a cell-free system has been developed, which behaves like the infectious process with respect to species barriers [39]. The cell-free conversion of PrP^C to PrP^{Sc} requires oligomeric PrP^{Sc}, supporting the hypothesis that PrP^{Sc} is an ordered oligomer of PrP that acts as a polymerization seed for cellular PrP [40]. At the mechanistic level, this process may resemble the *in vitro* generation of Aβ amyloid fibrils. Congo red, which is known to bind to Aβ amyloid and PrP amyloid and to inhibit the formation of Aβ amyloid fibrils *in vitro,* slows the onset of scrapie in infected animals. This finding suggests a common therapeutic strategy against prion disease and AD, that is, the inhibition of protein polymerization.

The mechanism of prion neurotoxicity is unknown

As is the case in AD, the precise mechanism whereby ordered protein aggregates lead to neuronal death is unclear. Fibrils comprising peptides derived from PrP are neurotoxic in culture. However, PrP^{Sc} produced in a brain graft of mice lacking PrP does not cause spongiform degeneration of surrounding PrP^- tissue. This finding suggests that *in vitro* neurotoxicity and *in vivo* neurotoxicity may differ and that PrP^C is critical for the latter. The elucidation of this process should provide another target for therapeutic intervention.

REFERENCES

1. Bachman, D. L., et al. Prevalence of dementia and probable senile dementia of the Alzheimer type in the Framingham study. *Neurology* 42:115–119, 1992.
2. Glenner, G. G., and Wong, C. W. Alzheimer's disease: Initial report of the purification and characterization of a novel cerebrovascular amyloid protein. *Biochem. Biophys. Res. Commun.* 120:885–890, 1984.
3. Grundke-Iqbal, I., et al. Microtubule-associated protein tau: A component of Alzheimer paired helical filaments. *J. Biol. Chem.* 261:6084–6089, 1986.
4. Wolozin, B. L., et al. A neuronal antigen in the brains of Alzheimer patients. *Science* 232:648–650, 1986.
5. Nukina, N., et al. The monoclonal antibody, Alz 50, recognizes tau protein in Alzheimer's disease brain. *Neurosci. Lett.* 87:240–246, 1988.
6. Lee, V. M.-Y., et al. A major subunit of paired helical filaments and derivatized forms of normal tau. *Science* 251:675–678, 1991.
7. Goedert, M., et al. Assembly of microtubule-associated protein tau into Alzheimer-like filaments induced by sulphated glycosaminoglycans. *Nature* 383:550–553, 1996.
8. Masters, C. L., et al. Amyloid plaque core protein in Alzheimer disease and Down syndrome. *Proc. Natl. Acad. Sci. USA* 82:4245–4249, 1985.
9. Selkoe, D. J., et al. Isolation of low-molecular-weight proteins from amyloid plaque fibers in Alzheimer's disease. *J. Neurochem.* 146:1820–1834, 1986.
10. Kang, J., et al. The precursor of Alzheimer's disease amyloid A4 protein resembles a cell-surface receptor. *Nature* 325:733–736, 1987.
11. Goldgaber, D., et al. Characterization and chromosomal localization of a cDNA encoding brain amyloid of Alzheimer's disease. *Science* 235:877–884, 1987.
12. Selkoe, D. J., et al. β-Amyloid precursor protein of Alzheimer disease occurs as 110–135 kilodalton membrane-associated proteins in neural and nonneural tissues. *Proc. Natl. Acad. Sci. USA* 85:7341–7345, 1988.
13. Weidemann, A., et al. Identification, biogenesis and localization of precursors of Alzheimer's disease A4 amyloid protein. *Cell* 57:115–126, 1989.
14. Sambamurti, K., et al. Evidence for intracellular cleavage of the Alzheimer's amyloid precursor in PC12 cells. *J. Neurosci. Res.* 33:319–329, 1992.
15. Haass, C., et al. Amyloid β-peptide is produced by cultured cells during normal metabolism. *Nature* 359:322–325, 1992.
16. Seubert, P., et al. Isolation and quantitation of soluble Alzheimer's β-peptide from biological fluids. *Nature* 359:325–327, 1992.
17. Shoji, M., et al. Production of the Alzheimer amyloid β protein by normal proteolytic processing. *Science* 258:126–129, 1992.
18. Scheuner, D., et al. Secreted amyloid β-protein similar to that in the senile plaques of Alzheimer's disease is increased *in vivo* by the presenilin 1 and 2 and APP mutations linked to familial Alzheimer's disease. *Nat. Med.* 2:864–870, 1996.
19. Wild-Bode, C., et al. Intracellular generation and accumulation of amyloid β-peptide terminating at amino acid 42. *J. Biol. Chem.* 272:16085–16088, 1997.
20. Goate, A., et al. Segregation of a missense mutation in the amyloid precursor protein gene with familial Alzheimer's disease. *Nature* 349:704–706, 1991.
21. Levy, E., et al. Mutation of the Alzheimer's disease amyloid gene in hereditary cerebral hemorrhage, Dutch-type. *Science* 248:1124–1126, 1990.
22. Games, D., et al. Alzheimer-type neuropathology in transgenic mice overexpressing V717F β-amyloid precursor protein. *Nature* 373:523–527, 1995.
23. Hsiao, K., et al. Correlative memory deficits, Aβ elevation and amyloid plaques in transgenic mice. *Science* 274:99–102, 1996.
24. Sherrington, R., et al. Cloning of a novel gene bearing missense mutations in early onset familial Alzheimer's disease. *Trends Neurosci.* 20:154–159, 1997.
25. Levy-Lehad, E., et al. A familial Alzheimer's disease locus on chromosome 1. *Science* 269:970–973, 1995.
26. Shen, J., et al. Skeletal and CNS defects in presenilin-1 deficient mice. *Cell* 89:629–639, 1997.
27. Duff, K., et al. Increased amyloid Aβ42(43) in brains of mice expressing mutant presenilin 1. *Nature* 383:710–713, 1996.
28. Borchelt, D. R., et al. Familial Alzheimer's disease-linked presenilin 1 variants elevate Aβ1-42/1-40 ratio *in vitro* and *in vivo*. *Neuron* 17:1005–1013, 1996.
29. Lemere, C. A., et al. The E280A presenilin 1 Alzheimer's mutation produces increased Aβ42 deposition and severe cerebellar pathology. *Nat. Med.* 2:1146–1148, 1996.
30. Strittmatter, W. J., et al. Apolipoprotein E: High-avidity binding to β-amyloid and increased fre-

quency of type 4 allele in late-onset familial Alzheimer disease. *Proc. Natl. Acad. Sci. USA* 90:1977–1981, 1993.

31. Schmechel, D. E., et al. Increased amyloid β-peptide deposition in cerebral cortex as a consequence of apolipoprotein E genotype in late-onset Alzheimer disease. *Proc. Natl. Acad. Sci. USA* 90:9649–9653, 1993.

32. Lee, V. M.-Y. Disruption of the cytoskeleton in Alzheimer's disease. *Curr. Opin. Neurobiol.* 5:663–668, 1995.

33. Horwich, A. L., and Weissman, J. S. Deadly conformation-protein misfolding in prion disease. *Cell* 89:499–510, 1997.

34. Prusiner, S. B. Molecular biology of prion disease. *Science* 252:1515–1522, 1991.

35. Griffith, J. S. Self-replication and scrapie. *Nature* 215:1043–1044, 1967.

36. Prusiner, S. B. Novel proteinaceous infectious particles cause scrapie. *Science* 216:136–144, 1982.

37. Bueler, H., et al. Mice devoid of PrP are resistant to scrapie. *Cell* 73:1339–1347, 1993.

38. Hsiao, K. K., et al. Spontaneous neurodegeneration in transgenic mice with mutant prion protein. *Science* 250:1587–1590, 1990.

39. Kocisko, D. A., et al. Cell-free formation of protease-resistant prion protein. *Nature* 370:471–474, 1994.

40. Caughey, B., et al. Aggregates of scrapie-associated prion protein induce the cell free conversion of protease-sensitive prion protein to the protease resistant state. *Chem. Biol.* 2:807–818, 1995.

Neural Processing and Behavior

Molecular Biology of Vision

Hitoshi Shichi

Basic Neurochemistry: Molecular, Cellular and Medical Aspects, 6th Ed., edited by G. J. Siegel et al. Published by
Lippincott–Raven Publishers, Philadelphia, 1999. Correspondence to Hitoshi Shichi, Department of Ophthalmology, Wayne
State University School of Medicine, Detroit, Michigan 48201.

PHYSIOLOGICAL BACKGROUND

Light-absorbing pigments differentiate rod cells for black–white vision and three types of cone cells for color vision

The eye, a remarkable photosensor, can detect a single photon and transmit its signal to the brain. The receptors for light in the vertebrate eye are the visual, photoreceptor, cells of the retina. Each visual cell comprises two principal parts: the outer segment, which contains light-absorbing visual pigments, and the inner segment, which contains the nucleus, mitochondria and other subcellular organelles and which metabolically supports the functions of the outer segment (Fig. 47-1). The segments are connected by the ciliary process, or cilium. The inner segments of visual cells have terminals that synapse with horizontal cells and bipolar cells. The bipolar cells, in turn, form synapses with ganglion and amacrine cells.

Visual cells are of two types. Rod cells, which have elongated outer segments, contain rhodopsin, with a light wavelength for maximal absorption (λ_{max}) of ~500 nm, the visual pigment responsible for dim-light vision, also termed black-and-white or scotopic vision. Cone cells, possessing cone-shaped outer segments, are the photoreceptors for daylight vision, also termed color or photopic vision. In the human retina, there are three types of cone cells, each containing one of three pigments: λ_{max} 420, 530 and 560 nm. According to one estimate, the human eye contains 120 million rod cells in the peripheral region of the retina and 6.5 million cone cells concentrated mainly in the central, or foveal, region.

Absorption of light causes inhibition of vertebrate photoreceptor cells, which then initiate programs of responses among retinal neurons

The plasma membrane of each rod outer segment possesses several thousand Na^+ channels, through which Na^+ enters the cell at a rate of about 2.6×10^{-4} Na^+ per channel per second. Na^+ ions also enter the outer segment by Na^+-Ca^{2+} exchange. In contrast, the plasma membrane of the rod inner segment has ATP-dependent Na^+/K^+ pumps that pump Na^+ out of the cell (Chap. 5). The Na^+ permeability of the outer segment is higher in the dark than in the light. Thus, the plasma membrane of the vertebrate rod cell shows a membrane poten-

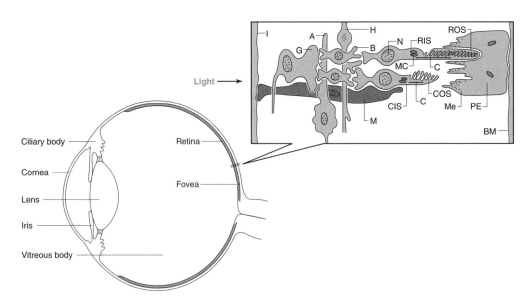

FIGURE 47-1. The vertebrate retina: *A*, amacrine cell; *B*, bipolar cell; *BM*, Bruch's membrane; *C*, ciliary process (cilium); *CIS*, cone inner segment; *COS*, cone outer segment; *G*, ganglion cell; *H*, horizontal cell; *I*, inner limiting membrane; *M*, Müller cell (glial cell); *Me*, melanin granule; *MC*, mitochondrion; *N*, nucleus; *PE*, retinal pigmented epithelium; *RIS*, rod inner segment; *ROS*, rod outer segment.

tial of 35 to 45 mV (inside negative) and is depolarized in the dark. Light reduces the Na^+ permeability of the outer segment and hyperpolarizes the membrane. Therefore, "visual excitation" in the vertebrate photoreceptor means hyperpolarization, or inhibition, of the visual cell plasma membrane. The release of a chemical transmitter, glutamate, at the synaptic terminal of a visual cell in the dark is also inhibited by light. The retina, which is part of the CNS, contains numerous neurotransmitters, including acetylcholine, dopamine, GABA, glycine, glutamate, aspartate and neuropeptides [1]. For a given substance to be a neurotransmitter, it must be present in sufficient quantities in, and synthesized by, a specific neuron; be released in response to a stimulatory signal; evoke a postsynaptic response; and be rapidly inactivated (see Chap. 10).

Glutamate, an excitatory transmitter, has been identified as a neurotransmitter of the photoreceptors. Both rod and cone bipolar cells have glutamate receptors. GABA and its synthesizing enzyme, glutamate decarboxylase, have been found in horizontal cells. Both horizontal cells and bipolar cells possess GABA receptors. The inhibitory transmitter glycine is found in the cone bipolar cells. Amacrine cells are diverse and contain GABA and glycine, as well as acetylcholine, dopamine and serotonin. Amacrine cells also contain various neuropeptides, including substance P, enkephalin, glucagon, somatostatin, neurotensin, neuropeptide Y, vasoactive intestinal polypeptide and cholecystokinin, which colocalize with other neurotransmitter substances and function as neuromodulators. The effects of neuromodulators generally are slower and last longer than those of neurotransmitters (Chap. 18). Elucidation of the mechanism by which retinal neurons are regulated by neurotransmitters and modulators, especially molecular characterization of their receptors, is a subject of active research.

Retinal responses to different light frequencies are encoded in the retina and conveyed to the thalamus and visual cortex

Absorption of photons by visual cells triggers a series of events that result in a particular pattern of retinal stimulation and, eventually, stimulation of cerebral neurons. In dim-light vision, the magnitude of the neural response in rod cells is directly related to the perception of brightness. In color vision, absorption of light by at least two cone cell pigments with different absorption maxima is essential to discriminate color. The ratio of the magnitudes of the induced photoresponses determines the color perceived. The arrays of visual signals generated by the photoreceptor cells and programmed by retinal neurons, principally bipolar cells, are transmitted to the lateral geniculate bodies via ganglion cell axons, which make up the optic nerves and tracts. Impulses are conveyed by the geniculocalcarine radiations to the visual cortex of the brain, where the signals representing light intensity and wavelength are decoded separately by different neurons. The coding and decoding of visual signals, an important area of neurophysiology, is not covered here. This chapter deals primarily with the structure and function of photoreceptors and the molecular events that take place after photon absorption by the visual cells [2–5].

PHOTORECEPTOR MEMBRANES AND VISUAL PIGMENTS

Rod outer segment membranes are arranged in stacks of disks containing rhodopsin

The outer segment of a rod cell consists of a stack of several hundred disks encased in a sack of plasma membrane. It is presumed that the disks are formed by evagination of the plasma membrane in the proximal region of the outer segment, followed by fusion of two adjacent evaginates and detachment from the plasma membrane. This is probably controlled by the ciliary process. The effect of this repeated evagination and disk formation is to increase greatly the area of rod cell membrane and, thus, the amount of visual pigment, a membrane-bound protein, that is exposed to light. As new disks are formed, older disks are pushed toward the apex of the outer segment. Disks that eventually reach the apex are shed from the tip and phagocytized by the pigmented epithelial cells. In

```
MESFAVAAQLGPHFAPLSNGSVVDKVTPMMAHLI---SPYWNQFPAMDPI (fly)
MNGTEGPNFYVPFSNATGVV----------------RSPFEYPQYYLAEP (rod)
MRKMSEEQFYLFKNISSV-----------------GPWDGPQYHIAPV   (b)
MAQQWSLQRLAGRHPQDSYEDSTQSSIFTYTNSNSTRGPFEGPNYHIAPR (r)
MAQQWSLQRLAGRHPQDSYEDSTQSSIFTYTNSNSTRGPFEGPNYHIAPR (g)


W_AKILTAYMIMIGMISWCGNGVVIYIFATTKSLRTPANLLVINLAISDF (fly)
WQFSMLAAYMFLLEVLGFPINFLTLYVTVQHKKLRTPLNYILLNLAVADL (rod)
WAFYLQAAFMGTVFLIGFPLNAMVLVATLRYKKLRQPLNYILVNVSFGGF (b)
WVYHLTSVWMIFVVTSAVFTNGLVLAATMKFKKLRHPLNWILVNLAVADL (r)
WVYHLTSVWMIFVVISAVFTNGLVLAATMKFKKLRHPLNWILVNLAVADL (g)
    ←—————————1—————————→      ←—————————2———
GIMITNTPMMGINLYFETWVLGPMMCDIYAGLGSAFGCSSIWSMCMISLD (fly)
FMVLGGFTSTLYTSLHGYFVFGPTGCNLEGFFATLGGFIALQSLVVLAIE (rod)
LLCIFSVFPVFVASCNGYFVFGRHVCALEGFLGTVAGLVTGWSLAFLAFE (b)
AETVIASTISIVNEVSGWFVLGHPMCVLEGYTVSLCGITGLWSLAIISWE (r)
AETVIASTISVVNQVYGYFVLGHPMCVLEGYTVSLCGITGLWSLAIISWE (g)
   ——2——→              ←—————————3—————————→
RYQVIVKGMAGRPMTIPLALGKIAYIWFMSSIWCLAPAFGWSRYVPEGNL (fly)
RYVVVCKPMSNRFRFGENHAIMGVAFTWVMALACAAPPLAGWSRYIPEGLQ (rod)
RYIVICKPFGNRFSSKHALTVVLATWTIGIGVSIPPFFGWSRFIPEGLQ (b)
RWLVVCKPFGNVRFDAKLAIVGIAFSWIWSAVWTAPPIFGWSRYWPHGLK (r)
RWMVVCKPFGNVRFDAKLAIVGIAFSWIWAAVWTAPPIFGWSRYWPHGLK (g)
-3—→               ←—————————4—————————→
TSCGIDYLERDWNPRSYLIFYSIFV--YYIPLFLICYSYWFIIAAVSAHE (fly)
CSCGIDYYTLKPEVNNESFVIYMFVVHFTIPMIIIFFCYGQLVFTVKEAA (rod)
CSCGPDWYTVGTKYRSESYTWFLFIFCFIVPLSLICFSYTQLLRALKAVA (b)
TSCGPDVFSGSSYPGVQSYMIVLMVTCCIIPLAIIMLCYLQVWLAIRAVA (r)
TSCGPDVFSGSSYPGVQSYMIVLMVTCCITPLSIIVLCYLQVWLAIRAVA (g)
                 ←—————————5—————————→
KAMREQAKKMNV-------------------------------------- (fly)


KSLRSSEDAEKSAEGKLAKVALVTITLWFMAWTPYLVINCMGLFKFEG_LT (fly)
AQQQESATTQKAEKEVTRMVIIMVIAFLI_CWVPYASVAFYIFTHQGSNFG (rod)
AQQQQSQTTQKAEREVSRMVVVMVGSFCV_CYVPYAAFAMYMVNNRNHGLD (b)
KQQKESESTQKAEKEVTRMVVVMIFAYCV_CWGPYTFFACFAAANPGYAFH (r)
KQQKESESTQKAEKEVTRMVVVMVLAFCF_CWGPYAFFACFAAANPGYPFH (g)
       ←—————————6—————————→
PLNTIWGACFAKSAACYNPIVYGISHPKYRLALKEKCPCCVFGKVDDGKS (fly)
PIFMTIPAFFAKSAAIYNPVIYIMMNKQFRNCMLTTICCGKNPLGDDEAS (rod)
LRLVTIPSFFSKSACIYNPIIYCFMNKQFQACIMKMVCEKAMTDESDTCS (b)
PLMAALPAYFAKSATIYNPVIYVFMNRQFRNCILQLFGKKVDDGSELSSA (r)
PLMAALPAFFAKSATIYNPVIYVFMNRQFRNCILQLFGKKVDDGSELSSA (g)
  ←—————7—————→
SDAQSEATASEAE---SKA    378                    (fly)
ATVSKTETS_____QVAPA    348                    (rod)
S__QKTEVSTVSSTQVGPN    348                    (b)
S___KTEVSSVSS__VSPA    364                    (r)
S___KTEVSSVSS__VSPA    364                    (g)
```

higher-order animals, rod disk shedding follows a circadian rhythm: shedding is minimal in the dark, and a burst of shedding occurs soon after the onset of light [6]. The life cycle of a single disk may last from a few days to months, depending on the species. Disk membrane components, such as proteins, carbohydrates and lipids, are synthesized in the inner segment and then transported to the basal region of the ciliary process, where membrane assembly occurs. In contrast to rod disks, cone disks generally remain continuous with the plasma membrane and shedding occurs in the dark rather than in the light.

Rod outer segment membranes, which are comprised of >95% disk membranes and <5% plasma membrane, consist of 60% protein and 40% phospholipid. In vertebrate photoreceptors, phosphatidylethanolamine and phosphatidylcholine account for about 80% of the phospholipid. The most abundant polyunsaturated fatty acid is docosahexaenoic acid, consisting of 22 carbons and six unsaturated bonds, linked to the middle carbon of the glycerol moiety of phospholipids. High concentration of polyunsaturated fatty acids make rod membranes as fluid as olive oil at physiological temperatures, allowing the integral membrane protein rhodopsin to rotate freely and diffuse within the membrane. This fluidity may be important in allowing photoactivated rhodopsin to collide quickly with so many molecules of the peripheral membrane proteins, such as G proteins.

Rhodopsin is a transmembrane protein linked to 11-*cis*-retinal, which, on photoabsorption, decomposes to opsin and all-*trans*-retinal

Rhodopsin has a molecular weight of about 40,000. Its C-terminus is exposed on the cytoplasmic surface of the disk, and its sugar-containing N-terminal sequence is exposed on the intraluminal surface. Half of the mass is embedded in the hydrophobic region of the membrane lipid bilayer, with the remaining half distributed equally on both surfaces of the membrane. The primary structures of visual pigment proteins are known for many visual pigments, including human rhodopsin and cone pigments (Fig. 47-2) [7]. All visual pigments possess seven segments of hydrophobic sequences separated by segments of hydrophilic sequences. It has been hypothesized that the seven hydrophobic sequences, designated helices 1–7 (see bovine rhodopsin shown as an example in Fig. 47-3), are in α-helical conformation and form a bundle that spans the membrane from one side to the other. Two sugar moieties, each composed of three mannoses and three N-acetylglucosamines, are linked to asparagine-2 and asparagine-15 in bovine rhodopsin. Cysteine-322 and cysteine-323 carry palmitoyl groups which probably penetrate the membrane, thereby forming an additional polypeptide loop. The C-terminal sequence contains a cluster of serine and threonine residues that serve as phosphorylation sites.

The chromophore 11-*cis*-retinal is linked to the ε-amino group of lysine-296 by a protonated Schiff base. Protonated Schiff bases usually absorb light maximally at around 440 nm, but the λ_{max} of rhodopsin is near 500 nm. The 60-nm "red" shift of λ_{max} toward the longer wavelength side can be explained by the strength of interaction of the positive charge of the protonated Schiff base with a counter ion. The more the counter ion is removed from the Schiff base, the greater is the red shift. The counter ion is the carboxylate group of glutamic acid-113 (Fig. 47-3). When the helices are bundled together, the acidic residue may move in the vicinity of the chromophore and donate the necessary negative charge. On absorption of light, rhodopsin is decomposed to the opsin

FIGURE 47-2. The primary structures of visual pigments. The fly sequence is from *Drosophila*. All other sequences are human. The lower three are the sequences of cone pigments deduced from cDNA sequences: b, blue-sensitive; r, red-sensitive; and g, green-sensitive. The single-letter amino acid code used here is defined in the Glossary. Residues identical in all sequences are shown in boldface. Gaps necessary to maintain the alignment are connected by *dashed lines*. The transmembrane segments shown in Figure 47-3 are indicated by the *numbered arrows* below the corresponding sequences. The lysine to which retinal is linked to form the chromophore is indicated as *K* near the center of transmembrane segment 7.

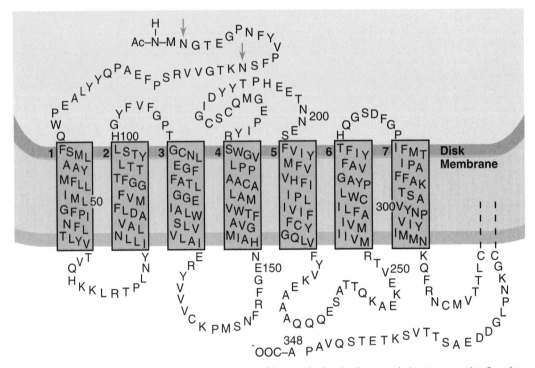

FIGURE 47-3. Proposed transmembrane disposition of bovine rhodopsin. Sugar moieties at asparagine-2 and asparagine-15 are shown with *orange arrows*. Palmitoyl groups at cysteine-322 and cysteine-323 are indicated with *broken lines*. Hydroxyamino acid residues that may be phosphorylated by rhodopsin kinase are clustered in a C-terminal domain of the molecule.

protein and all-*trans*-retinal. The reaction occurs through several spectrally distinct intermediates (Fig. 47-4). The formation of bathorhodopsin involves photoisomerization of the 11-*cis*-retinylidene chromophore to a constrained all-*trans* form and takes place within a few picoseconds after light absorption at physiological temperature. Bathorhodopsin then undergoes thermal relaxation, giving rise first to lumirhodopsin and then to *meta*-rhodopsin I. The formation of *meta*-rhodopsin II is of particular importance because it is presumably this intermediate that transmits the photosignal to a G protein (Chap. 20).

Bleached rhodopsin must be regenerated to maintain normal vision

Regeneration of rhodopsin occurs by several mechanisms. The major mechanism involves isomerization of all-*trans*-retinal to the 11-*cis*

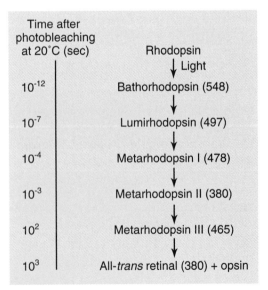

FIGURE 47-4. Intermediates formed after photic bleaching of vertebrate rhodopsin. Numbers in parentheses are wavelengths of light (in nanometers) absorbed maximally by the individual intermediates.

form in the retinal pigmented epithelium, transport of 11-*cis*-retinal to the outer segment and recombination with opsin [8]. According to a current hypothesis, all-*trans*-retinyl ester is isomerized to the 11-*cis* form and quickly hydrolyzed. Thus, the free energy of hydrolysis of the ester coupled to isomerization drives the isomerization process. The shuttle of retinoids between the photoreceptor and pigmented epithelium may involve several retinoid-binding proteins. A second mechanism is photoconversion of thermal intermediates, such as *meta*-rhodopsins, to rhodopsin. For example, regeneration of squid rhodopsin occurs mainly by photoisomerization of opsin-linked retinal at pH 10 and subsequent dark adaptation [9]. In a third mechanism, the photoisomerization of all-*trans*-retinal to the 11-*cis* form may take place within the rod outer segment. For example, all-*trans*-retinylidene phospholipid is photoisomerized to the 11-*cis* form within the disk membrane and reacts with opsin [10].

Cone-cell pigments contain different opsins that have high sequence homology

The primary structures of the three human cone pigments were deduced from analysis of the genomic and complementary DNA clones encoding them [11] (Fig. 47-2). The sequences of cone pigments show 41% identity with rhodopsin. Red and green pigments show high sequence homology: only 15 of 364 residues are different. Genetic analysis locates the rhodopsin gene on chromosome 3 and the blue pigment gene on chromosome 7. Although none of the human cone pigments has been isolated, the chicken cone pigment iodopsin has been purified and characterized. The primary structure of this pigment is known [12]. Iodopsin (λ_{max} 571 nm) forms bathoiodopsin on light absorption at $-196°C$. This intermediate reverts back to iodopsin on warming. If illuminated by 600-nm light at $-183°C$, iodopsin is converted to lumi-iodopsin, which thermally decays to *meta*-iodopsin I and *meta*-iodopsin II.

PHOTOTRANSDUCTION

Light absorption by rhodopsin leads to closure of Na$^+$-conductance channels via a chemical messenger system

Light is known to close the Na$^+$ channels on the outer segment plasma membrane and to induce hyperpolarization of the membrane within 100 msec. The magnitude of light response reaches a maximum by absorption of several hundred photons per rod cell. Below the saturation light intensity, the relationship between the magnitude of light response (*I*) and the energy of irradiating light (*A*) is given by

$$I = I_{max} A/(A + K)$$

where I_{max} is the magnitude of response at the saturation light intensity and K is light energy required for 50% of the maximum response [13]. This equation has the same form as the Michaelis-Menten equation of enzyme kinetics. By analogy to enzyme kinetics, we may assume that rhodopsin reacts with light to form a complex, photoactivated rhodopsin, probably *meta*-rhodopsin II, which gives rise to an intracellular messenger, X, that links the photochemical reaction of rhodopsin to the plasma membrane. It is logical to postulate such a messenger because the disk membrane, where rhodopsin is localized, is not continuous with the plasma membrane that contains the Na$^+$ channels.

The messenger compound must satisfy at least two properties. First, its concentration in the outer segment cytoplasm must change rapidly on light irradiation and return to the original value after light is turned off. Second, when the compound is introduced into the outer segment cytoplasm in the dark, it must mimic the effect of light. The first candidate proposed for messenger X was Ca^{2+} [14]. The Ca^{2+} hypothesis assumes that a large number of Ca^{2+} ions are sequestered within the disk in the dark and are released into cytoplasm when a single rhodopsin molecule in the disk membrane absorbs a photon. Ca^{2+} has been assumed to close the Na$^+$ channels in the plasma membrane. In support of the hypothesis, injection of

Ca^{2+} into the outer segment in the dark suppresses Na^+ permeability and induces membrane hyperpolarization; however, several findings contradict this hypothesis. Cytoplasmic Ca^{2+} concentration in the outer segment does not increase on light illumination but decreases instead. There is no evidence that the disks can actively accumulate Ca^{2+} in the dark, and in patch-clamp experiments in which a small piece of outer segment plasma membrane is attached by suction to the tip of an electrode, exposure of the cytoplasmic surface of the membrane to Ca^{2+} does not inhibit Na^+ conductance of the membrane fragment [15]. Thus, the Ca^{2+} hypothesis fails to explain the phototransduction process in vertebrate eyes.

A G-protein/cGMP system in outer segments is responsive to photoactivated rhodopsin

Another candidate for messenger X is cGMP. According to the cGMP hypothesis, the Na^+ channel is kept open by cGMP and closes when cGMP is hydrolyzed in light. The cGMP-gated channel protein of rod photoreceptors consists of two distinct subunits, α and β [16,17]. Exposure of an outer segment membrane fragment to cGMP in patch-clamp experiments increases its Na^+ conductance in the dark [15]. This effect is reversible. The concentration of cGMP in dark-adapted rod outer segments is high and decreases rapidly when the rod is irradiated at low Ca^{2+} concentrations. The decrease of cGMP is proportional to the log of light intensity. Hence, the amount of messenger X that is expected to "accumulate" in light is represented by the amount of cGMP hydrolyzed. cGMP phosphodiesterase (PDE), the enzyme that hydrolyzes cGMP to 5'-GMP, is indirectly activated by light. The activation is mediated by a G protein ($G_{\alpha\beta\gamma}$) called transducin, which is activated by photoactivated rhodopsin (R*) (Fig. 47-5). According to the cGMP hypothesis, a single R* molecule may produce hundreds of active G-protein molecules. This is the rate-limiting step in rod vision. The polypeptide loops between helices 3 and 4 and helices 5 and 6 and a loop between helix 7 and the palmitoyl anchors of R* (Fig. 47-3) are probably involved in binding to the G protein. The G protein consists of

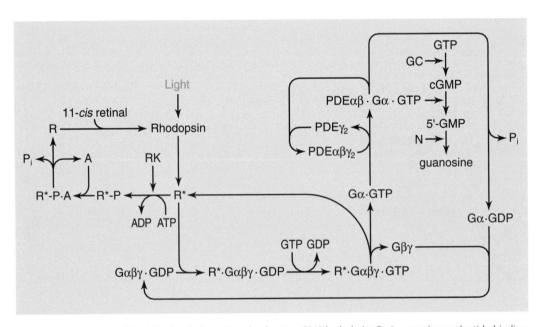

FIGURE 47-5.   Light-elicited biochemical reactions leading to cGMP hydrolysis: *G$\alpha\beta\gamma$*, guanine nucleotide-binding protein (transducin); *PDE$\alpha\beta\gamma$2*, phosphodiesterase; *GC*, guanylyl cyclase; *N*,5'-nucleotidase; *P$_i$*, inorganic phosphate; *RK*, rhodopsin kinase; *R**, photoactivated rhodopsin; *R*, inactive form of rhodopsin; *A*, arrestin. cGMP binds to the cation channel protein of the plasma membrane and opens the channel.

three subunits, α, β and γ, and has GDP bound to the α subunit in the inactive form. The R* catalyzes exchange of GTP for GDP, and the G_α-GTP thus formed dissociates from the β and γ subunits. Two G_α-GTP molecules then activate one PDE molecule ($PDE_{\alpha\beta\gamma2}$) by dissociating the two γ subunits in succession. The γ subunits are internal inhibitors of the PDE. The G_β subunit is common to G proteins associated with various receptors, but G_α is specific to the individual receptors (see Chap. 20). Rod and cone outer segments have different α subunits. The primary structure of rod G-protein subunits has been elucidated (references are found in Sugimoto et al. [18]).

The cGMP hypothesis can explain many aspects of phototransduction in vertebrate photoreceptors, including the effect of Ca^{2+}. Ca^{2+} plays an important role in the regulation of light adaptation [3,19]. A decrease in free intracellular Ca^{2+} in the light causes rapid deactivation of cGMP-PDE and stimulation of guanylyl cyclase [4]. A Ca^{2+}-binding protein called recoverin inhibits rhodopsin kinase at high Ca^{2+}. At low Ca^{2+} concentrations, the inhibition is relieved and accelerated rhodopsin phosphorylation results in the deactivation of cGMP-PDE. Guanylyl cyclase activation involves Ca^{2+}-binding proteins which are distinct from recoverin and inhibit the cyclase at high Ca^{2+} [20,21]. A point to be noted is that the Ca^{2+} and cGMP concentrations in the photoreceptors are reciprocally related. Phototransduction for color vision proceeds very much like that for rod vision, involving cone pigments, GTP-binding protein, cGMP-PDE and cGMP-gated cation channels.

Although growing evidence supports the importance of the cGMP hypothesis for vertebrate vision, it remains unresolved whether cGMP plays a key role in invertebrate vision. Because invertebrate visual cells depolarize in light, a rise in cGMP is expected upon light absorption. However, light does not increase cGMP in invertebrate photoreceptors [22], and a different mechanism may exist. A mechanism proposed for invertebrate phototransduction involves light-stimulated hydrolysis of phosphatidylinositol-4,5-bisphosphate (PIP_2). Reception of an external signal by a variety of receptors is known to evoke hydrolysis of PIP_2 to diacylglycerol (DAG) and inositol-1,4,5-trisphosphate (IP_3) by activating phospholipase C (see Chap. 21). In this mechanism, both IP_3 and DAG can serve as intracellular messengers: IP_3 increases intracellular Ca^{2+}, and DAG stimulates protein kinase C. Injection of IP_3 into *Limulus* ventral photoreceptors in the dark mimics the light effect, evoking membrane depolarization without latency and an increase in intracellular Ca^{2+} [23,24]. Injection of IP_3 into salamander rod outer segments induces membrane hyperpolarization in the dark.

Whatever mechanism is involved in phototransduction, the process must be regulated to reset the system. In the cGMP-cascade mechanism, hydrolysis of G protein-bound GTP to GDP inactivates G protein. Thermal decay of R*, presumably *meta*-rhodopsin II, to opsin and all-*trans*-retinal terminates activation of G protein; R* is also inactivated by phosphorylation [25] and binding of arrestin, a protein with a molecular weight of 48,000, to phosphorylated R* [26]. As described above, Ca^{2+} concentrations regulate guanylyl cyclase activation.

Regulation of G protein-mediated membrane receptors by phosphorylation, as exemplified by phosphorylation of R*, may be of general importance. Different G protein-mediated membrane receptors have structural similarities. For example, the mammalian β-adrenergic receptor and the muscarinic acetylcholine receptor show significant amino acid sequence homology with rhodopsin [27], and a β receptor-specific protein kinase phosphorylates rhodopsin [28]. An arrestin-like protein modulates the β receptor. Similarities between the photoreceptor system and other G protein-mediated membrane receptor systems suggest that they are evolutionarily related (Chap. 20).

COLOR BLINDNESS

Red–green color blindness is explained by unequal intragenic recombination between a pair of X chromosomes

Amino acid sequences of the three cone pigments of human retina (Fig. 47-2) indicate that red and green pigments are very similar, showing 96% homology, but blue pigment is different. The blue pigment gene is located on chromosome 7, whereas the red and green pigment genes reside on the X chromosome [11]. Peculiarly, each X chromosome has one red pigment gene and either one, two or three green pigment genes in color normals. A hypothesis to explain the variability of the green pigment gene is that the red pigment gene occurs upstream of the 5′ end of the green pigment gene and a pair of homologous red–green gene arrangements has undergone unequal recombinations during evolution. Red–green color blindness is explained by abnormalities in the unequal intragenic recombination as described below.

Approximately 8% of Caucasian men inherit a color abnormality: dichromats, who require only two primary wavelengths to match all colors, and anomalous trichromats, who require three primary wavelengths but make color matches different from the normal. Loss of one of the three color pigments or systems explains dichromats, while a shift in the spectral sensitivity of one of the three pigments or systems may be responsible for anomalous trichromatism. Blue cone abnormalities are inherited as autosomal traits and are rare. Therefore, abnormalities in the red and green cone systems have been most extensively studied. From psychophysical studies, defects in the red and green cone systems are mapped to two tightly linked loci on the X chromosome and most likely to the loci of red and green pigment genes.

What are the underlying genetic mechanisms that produce dichromats and anomalous trichromats? Nathans [29] hypothesizes that visual abnormalities are caused by alterations in red and green pigment genes by unequal intragenic recombination. Red and green pigment genes are similar and tightly linked on the X chromosome, as described above. If, during the development of ova and sperm cells, a pair of chromosomes joins by crossing over in the region encoding red and green pigments and breaks between the two genes of one of the chromosomes, one chromosome may lose the green pigment gene and the other chromosome may have two. However, breaking within a gene may result in a hybrid gene composed of part of the green pigment gene and part of the red pigment gene. If the X chromosome lacking the green pigment gene is inherited, the carrier is a true dichromat. Depending on the location of breakpoints, a variety of hybrid genes are generated; a man with a hybrid gene producing a

nonfunctional pigment similar to the normal pigment will be a dichromat. However, the carriers of hybrid genes producing pigments with spectral sensitivities intermediate between those of red and green pigments will be anomalous trichromats.

RETINITIS PIGMENTOSA

Mutations in rhodopsin and other photoreceptor proteins are linked to retinitis pigmentosa

Retinitis pigmentosa (RP) is a group of inherited retinopathies that affects about 1 in 4,000 humans [30]. RP may be classified into four types: autosomal dominant (19%), autosomal recessive (19%), X-linked (8%) and allied diseases (54%). RP is characterized by loss of night vision in the early stage, followed by loss of peripheral vision.

The first gene suspected to be linked to dominant-type RP was located on the long arm of chromosome 3, and its mutant product was found to be a rhodopsin: replacement of proline 23 by histidine [30]. More than 60 point mutations within the rhodopsin gene have so far been reported, including mutations causing autosomal recessive RP and congenital stationary night blindness. Another gene of dominant-type RP, localized on the short arm of chromosome 6, was recently identified to be peripherin, a structural protein with an M_r of 35,000, present in the rim of disks of rod outer segments [31]. A defect in the peripherin gene is involved in a hereditary retinopathy of the mouse, termed retinal degeneration slow, or rds [32]. In another form of mouse retinopathy, rd, a defect is in the β subunit of cGMP-PDE. These findings suggest that defects causing photoreceptor degenerations in different forms of RP could be in any structural and functional proteins associated with rod outer segments. Very little is known about how mutations in these proteins bring about degenerations of the rod cells. It is possible that various elements released into the subretinal space via the retinal vasculature normally protect the photoreceptors and that mutations forfeit the protection. In RCS rats, a strain with inherited retinal dystrophy, in which the ability of the retinal pigmented epithelium to phagocytize photoreceptor outer segments is impaired, subretinal or intravitreal injection of basic fibroblast growth factor causes a significant delay in retinal degeneration [33].

Choroideremia can be classified, broadly, as an X-linked form of RP. A recent study of lymphoblasts from subjects with this disorder has disclosed deficient activity of geranylgeranyl transferase (Chap. 3) [34]. This enzyme catalyzes the transfer of geranylgeranyl groups to guanine nucleotide-binding proteins. This modification is necessary for these proteins to participate in membrane fusion processes. Both the biogenesis of photoreceptor disks and their subsequent phagocytosis by the pigmented epithelial cells involve very active membrane fusion and turnover (Figs. 47-2–47-5). Thus, it is quite possible that the pathology of RP may arise from an enzyme deficiency of this type.

AGE-RELATED MACULAR DEGENERATION

A genetic defect leads to macular degeneration among the elderly

Age-related macular degeneration is a common cause of central vision impairment in the elderly, affecting more than 11 million people in the United States. A juvenile form of macular degeneration, called Stargardt's disease, is caused by mutations in a gene encoding an ATP-binding cassette transporter protein (ABCR) expressed in the retina (see Chap. 5). Environmental factors, such as cigarette smoking and diet, as well as genetic factors contribute to age-related macular degeneration. In order to examine whether ABCR mutations are associated with the disease, 167 unrelated patients were recently screened [35]. Alterations in the ABCR gene were found among as high as 16% of patients. Age-related macular degeneration is clinically subdivided into "dry" and "wet" forms. The dry form is characterized by the accumulation of cellular debris, called drusen, in and under the retinal pigmented epithelium, and the wet form involves choroidal neovascularization. ABCR gene mutations were found to be more frequent among patients with dry than those with wet macular degeneration. Cell debris and other waste materials accumulate in the pigmented epithelium due to combined effects of aging and environmental factors. If the ABCR protein is defective and not able to transport these materials across the cell membrane, the buildup of waste materials may become toxic and cause retinal degeneration.

REFERENCES

1. Pourcho, R. G. Neurotransmitters in the retina. *Curr. Eye Res.* 15:797–803, 1996.
2. Stryer, L., Dowling, J., and Wiesel, T. (organizers) A collection of papers presented at a colloquium entitled "Vision From Photon to Perception." *Proc. Natl. Acad. Sci. USA* 93:557–639, 1996.
3. Yau, K. W. Phototransduction mechanism in retinal rods and cones. *Invest. Ophthalmol. Vis. Sci.* 35:9–32, 1994.
4. Yarfitz, S., and Hurley, J. B. Transduction mechanisms of vertebrate and invertebrate photoreceptors. *J. Biol. Chem.* 269:14329–14332, 1994.
5. Rao, V. R., and Oprian, D. D. Activating mutants of rhodopsin and other G protein-coupled receptors. *Annu. Rev. Biophys. Biomol. Struct.* 25:287–314, 1996.
6. Bok, D. Retinal photoreceptor–pigment epithelium interactions. *Invest. Ophthalmol. Vis. Sci.* 26:1659–1694, 1985.
7. Hargrave, P. A., and McDowell, J. H. Rhodopsin and phototransduction: A model system for G protein-linked receptors. *FASEB J.* 6:2323–2331, 1992.
8. Crouch, R. K., Chader, G. J., Wiggert, B., and Pepperberg, D. R. Retinoids and the visual process. *Photochem. Photobiol.* 64:613–621, 1996.
9. Suzuki, T., Sugahara, M., and Kito, Y. An intermediate in the photoregeneration of squid rhodopsin. *Biochem. Biophys. Acta* 275:260–270, 1972.
10. Shichi, H., and Somers, R. L. Possible involvement of retinylidene phospholipid in photoisomerization of all-*trans* to 11-*cis* retinal. *J. Biol. Chem.* 249:6570–6577, 1974.
11. Nathans, J., Thomas, D., and Hogness, D. S. Molecular genetics of human color vision: The genes encoding blue, green, and red pigments. *Science* 232:193–202, 1986.
12. Yoshizawa, T., and Kuwata, O. Iodopsin, a red-sensitive cone visual pigment in the chicken retina. *Photochem. Photobiol.* 54:1061–1070, 1991.
13. Korenbrot, J. I. Signal mechanisms of phototransduction in retinal rod. *CRC Crit. Rev. Biochem.* 17:223–256, 1985.
14. Hagins, W. A. The visual process: Excitatory

mechanisms in the primary receptor cells. *Annu. Rev. Biophys. Bioeng.* 1:131–158, 1972.

15. Fesenko, E., Kolesnikov, S. S., and Lyubarsky, A. L. Induction by cyclic GMP of cationic conductance in plasma membrane of retinal rod outer segment. *Nature* 313:310–313, 1985.

16. Kaupp, U. B., Niidome, T., Tanabe, T., et al. Primary structure and functional expression from complementary DNA of the rod photoreceptor cyclic GMP-gated channel. *Nature* 342:762–766, 1989.

17. Koerschen, H. G., Illing, M., Seifert, R., et al. A 240 kDa protein represents the complete β subunit of the cyclic nucleotide-gated channel from rod photoreceptor. *Neuron* 15:627–636, 1995.

18. Sugimoto, K., Nukada, T., Tanabe, T., et al. Primary structure of the β-subunit of bovine transducin deduced from the cDNA sequence. *FEBS Lett.* 191:235–240, 1985.

19. Torre, V., Matthews, H. R., and Lamb, T. D. Role of calcium in regulating the cyclic GMP cascade of phototransduction in retinal rods. *Proc. Natl. Acad. Sci. USA* 83:7109–7113, 1986.

20. Gorczyca, W. A., Polans, A., Surgucheva, I. G., Subbaraya, I., Baehr, W., and Palczewski, K. Guanylyl cyclase activating protein: A calcium-sensitive regulator of phototransduction. *J. Biol. Chem.* 270:22029–22036, 1995.

21. Dizhoor, A. M., Olshevskaya, E. V., Henzel, W. J., et al. Cloning, sequencing, and expression of a 24-kDa Ca^{2+}-binding protein activating photoreceptor. *J. Biol. Chem.* 270:25200–25206, 1995.

22. Brown, J. E., Faddis, M., and Combs, A. Light does not induce an increase in cyclic-GMP content of squid or *Limulus* photoreceptors. *Exp. Eye Res.* 54:403–410, 1992.

23. Brown, J. E., Rubin, L. J., Ghalayini, A. J., et al. Myo-inositol polyphosphate may be a messenger for visual excitation in *Limulus* photoreceptors. *Nature* 311:160–163, 1984.

24. Fein, A. Excitation and adaptation of *Limulus* photoreceptors by light and inositol 1,4,5-triphosphate. *Trends Neurosci.* 9:110–114, 1986.

25. Liebman, P. A., and Pugh, E. N. ATP mediates rapid reversal of cyclic GMP phosphodiesterase activation in visual receptor membranes. *Nature* 287:734–736, 1980.

26. Kuehn, H., Hall, S. W., and Wilden, U. Light-induced binding of 48-kDa protein to photoreceptor membranes is highly enhanced by phosphorylation of rhodopsin. *FEBS Lett.* 176:473–478, 1984.

27. Kubo, T., Fukuda, K., Mikami, A., et al. Cloning, sequencing and expression of complementary DNA encoding the muscarinic acetylcholine receptor. *Nature* 232:411–416, 1986.

28. Benovic, J. L., Mayor, F., Somers, R. L., Caron, M. G., and Lefkowitz, R. J. Light-dependent phosphorylation of rhodopsin by β-adrenergic receptor kinase. *Nature* 321:869–872, 1986.

29. Nathans, J. Molecular biology of visual pigments. *Annu. Rev. Neurosci.* 10:163–194, 1987.

30. Berson, E. L. Retinitis pigmentosa. *Invest. Ophthalmol. Vis. Sci.* 34:1659–1676, 1993.

31. Humphries, P., Kenna, P., and Farrar, G. J. On the molecular genetics of retinitis pigmentosa. *Science* 256:804–808, 1992.

32. Arikawa, K., Molday, L. L., Molday, R. S., and Williams, D. S. Localization of peripherin/rds in the disk membranes of cone and rod photoreceptors: Relationship to disk membrane morphogenesis and retinal degeneration. *J. Cell Biol.* 116:659–667, 1992.

33. Faktorovich, E. G., Steinberg, R. H., Yasumura, D., Matthes, M., and La Vail, M. M. Photoreceptor degeneration in inherited retinal dystrophy delayed by basic fibroblast growth factor. *Nature* 347:83–86, 1990.

34. Seabra, M. C., Brown, M. S., and Goldstein, J. L. Retinal degeneration in choroideremia: Deficiency of rat geranylgeranyl transferase. *Science* 259:377–381, 1993.

35. Allikmets, R., Shroyer, N. F., Singh, N., et al. Mutation of the Stargardt disease gene (ABCR) in age-related macular degeneration. *Science* 277:1805–1807, 1997.

Box 47-1

MECHANOSENSORY TRANSDUCTION: HAIR CELLS

Hair cells are the sensory cells of the internal ear, essential both for our appreciation of sound and for our sense of balance [1]. The hair cell's transduction apparatus, the molecular machinery that converts forces and displacements into electrical responses, can respond to mechanical stimuli of less than 1 nm in amplitude, and of tens or even hundreds of kilohertz in frequency. Indeed, our hearing is ultimately limited by Brownian motion of water molecules impinging on the transduction apparatus.

Although cells exhibiting mechanical transduction are found throughout the body, hair cells of the inner ear remain the best characterized and the model for all others. Even though well characterized at a biophysical level, the mechanical transduction mechanism of hair cells is still not understood in molecular terms. This discrepancy is in part due to the extreme scarcity of hair cells; instead of the millions or even hundreds of millions of receptor cells that the olfactory and visual systems possess, only a few tens of thousands of hair cells are found in the internal ears of most vertebrate species. The small number of hair cells and the direct transduction mechanism has greatly impeded molecular biological and biochemical characterization. Molecular description of hair-cell transduction has consequentally lagged behind description of vision and olfaction.

A comprehensive model for hair-cell transduction has emerged, derived primarily from biophysical and morphological investigations. Residing in the mechanoreceptive organelle of a hair cell, the hair bundle, the transduction apparatus consists of at least three components: the *transduction channel,* a mechanically gated ion channel; the *tip link,* an extracellular filament that transmits force to the channel's gate; and the *adaptation motor,* a mechanism that maintains an optimal tension in the tip link so that the channel can respond to displacements of atomic dimensions (Figure). The tip link appears to be the anatomical correlate of the *gating spring,* an elastic element through which stimulus energy can affect the transduction channel. Although highly specialized for the internal ear, these elements are likely to be general requirements for any mechanical transduction apparatus; detailed characterization of the transduction apparatus of the hair cell may therefore eventually illuminate other transduction systems.

Because they could generate the forces required for adaptation, move processively, and operate with the appropriate polarity, a cluster of myosin molecules has been hypothesized to constitute the adaptation motor. Hair cells express a variety of myosin isozymes. Although mice with mutations in the myosin-VI or -VIIa genes are deaf, these isozymes apparently mediate essential hair-cell functions besides adaptation [2]. Because it is located at the tips of the stereocilia, near the tip-link anchors, another isozyme, myosin-Iβ, is the best candidate for the adaptation motor [3]. At present, no strong candidate families have been advanced for the tip link, which appears to consist of two or three braided glycoprotein filaments.

Although the transduction channel has attracted much attention, it too has yet to be identified. This channel passes cations, including Ca^{2+}, and can be inhibited by aminoglycoside antibiotics and amiloride derivatives. Unless controlled by tension applied through the gating spring, the channel remains shut. One suggestion is that this channel belongs to the epithelial sodium-channel family; if so, immunolocalization suggests that the transduction channel may be located at a site different from that proposed above

(Box continues on next page)

Box 47-1 *(Continued)*

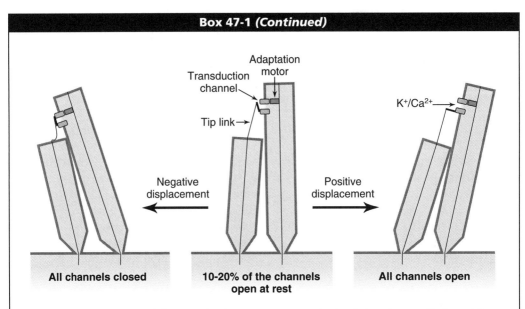

FIGURE.   Components of the transduction apparatus. A pair of actin-based stereocilia (out of 60 or so in a hair bundle) are shown. An excitatory stimulus stretches the tip link; the increased tension is transmitted to the gate of the transduction channel, which opens. The adaption motor relieves the increased tension by slipping down the actin cytoskeleton. An inhibitory stimulus reduces tip-link tension and the channels close.

[4]. One of the more compelling reasons to consider this hypothesis is the observation that genes that control touch sensation in the worm *C. elegans* include several proteins related to the epithelial sodium channel family. Although not well described at a biophysical level, nearly all of the genes mediating touch sensation in *C. elegans* have been identified and have been incorporated into a model that strikingly resembles the vertebrate hair cell model [5]. Comparing and contrasting vertebrate and invertebrate mechanical transduction systems is likely to continue to provide insight in both.

—*Peter Gillespie*

REFERENCES

1. Hudspeth, A. J. How the ear's works work. *Nature* 341:397–404, 1989.
2. Hasson, T., Gillespie, P. G., Garcia, J. A., et al. Unconventional myosins in inner-ear sensory epithelia. *J. Cell Biol.* 137:1287–1307, 1997.
3. Gillespie, P. G., and Corey, D. P. Myosin and hair-cell adaptation. *Neuron* 19:955–958, 1997.
4. Hackney, C. M., and Furness, D. N. Mechanotransduction in vertebrate hair cells: Structure and function of the stereociliary bundles. *Am. J. Physiol.* 268:C1-C13, 1995.
5. Garcia-Anoveros, J., and Corey, D. P. The molecules of mechanosensation. *Ann. Rev. Neurosci.* 20:567–94, 1997.

48

Molecular Biology of Olfaction and Taste

Stuart J. Firestein, Robert F. Margolskee and Sue Kinnamon

Basic Neurochemistry: Molecular, Cellular and Medical Aspects, 6th Ed., edited by G. J. Siegel et al. Published by Lippincott–Raven Publishers, Philadelphia, 1999. Correspondence to Stuart J. Firestein, Department of Biological Sciences, Columbia University, New York, New York 10027.

In recent years, enormous strides have been made in understanding the molecular mechanisms which underlie olfaction and taste in vertebrates. The application of innovative physiological, biochemical and molecular biological techniques has allowed for the identification and characterization of molecules involved in the initial events in perception in these two sensory systems and has provided fresh insight into the processes by which olfactory and gustatory discriminations are achieved.

OLFACTION

The mammalian olfactory system possesses enormous discriminatory power

It is claimed that humans can perceive many thousands of different odorous molecules, termed odorants, and that they can discriminate at least two to three thousand of these. It is also well known that even slight alterations in the structure of an odorant can lead to profound changes in perceived odor quality. One commonly cited example is carvone, whose L- and D-stereoisomers are perceived as spearmint and caraway, respectively. However, more subtle molecular alterations can also generate striking changes in perception.

The fine discriminatory power of the mammalian olfactory system is likely to derive from information-processing events that occur at several distinct anatomical sites: the olfactory epithelium of the nasal cavity, where odors are first sensed by olfactory sensory neurons; the olfactory bulb, where information received from the sensory neurons is presumably processed; and the cortex, where information received from the olfactory bulb is thought to be further refined to allow for the discrimination of thousands of different odors [1].

The initial events in olfaction occur in a specialized olfactory neurepithelium

In mammals, this structure lines the posterior nasal cavity (Fig. 48-1). The olfactory epithelium contains three predominant cell types: the olfac-

tory sensory neuron; the supporting, or sustentacular, cell; and the basal, or stem, cell. Olfactory neurons are the only mammalian neurons that are known to turn over throughout life. They are continuously replaced from the basal layer of stem cells. Two morphologically distinguishable types of dividing basal cell have been identified in mammals, the horizontal basal cell and the globose basal cell. At present, it is not clear what lineage relationship these two cell types bear to each other, but both have been proposed as stem cell precursors to the olfactory neuron.

The olfactory neuron is a bipolar cell that extends a single dendrite to the epithelial surface (Fig. 48-1). From the dendritic terminus, nu-

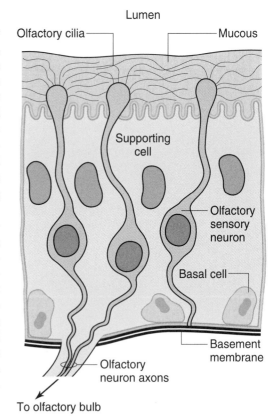

FIGURE 48-1. A schematic diagram of the olfactory epithelium. The initial events in odor perception occur in the olfactory epithelium of the nasal cavity. Odorants interact with specific odorant receptors on the lumenal cilia of olfactory sensory neurons. The signals generated by the initial binding events are transmitted along olfactory neuron axons to the olfactory bulb of the brain.

merous fine cilia extend into the layer of mucus that lines the nasal lumen. The cilia are the loci of the molecular transduction machinery, as has been shown by physiological [2] and biochemical [3] experiments. The details of signal generation and propagation will be discussed in a later section.

Each olfactory neuron projects an unbranched axon to the olfactory bulb, where it forms synapses within specialized regions of neuropil, called glomeruli, with periglomerular interneurons and the two major output neurons of the bulb, the mitral and tufted cells. The bulbar neurons, in turn, project to the olfactory cortex.

Odor discrimination is likely to depend upon the ability of different olfactory sensory neurons to recognize different odorants

However, electrophysiological studies of olfactory sensory neurons exposed to different odorants indicate that most neurons recognize multiple odorants or sets of odorants [4,5]. It is thought that the patterns of synapses formed in the olfactory bulb by olfactory neurons that recognize different odorants might constitute elementary odor codes. It is not clear how many different types of odorant receptor would be required in such a coding scheme nor is it obvious how narrowly or broadly tuned they might be or how their expression might be organized to achieve a high level of sensory discrimination.

Odor discrimination could involve a very large number of different odorant receptors, each highly specific for one or a small set of odorants

At the other extreme, there could be a relatively small number of different odorant receptors, each of low specificity and capable of interacting with a wide assortment of different odorous ligands. Individual olfactory neurons could each express only a single odorant-receptor type or multiple different odorant receptors.

The recent identification and cloning of genes encoding odorant receptors [6] has made it possible to begin to address these questions. By assuming that odorant receptors would be encoded by a multigene family and that the odorant receptors would belong to a large superfamily of receptors that transduce signals via interaction with heterotrimeric G proteins, Buck and Axel [6] were able to identify a novel multigene family in rat which appears to code for hundreds of diverse odorant receptors. Northern blot analyses and cDNA library screens demonstrated that the members of this family are expressed in the olfactory epithelium but not in a variety of other neural or non-neural tissues and that within the olfactory epithelium they are expressed exclusively by olfactory neurons. In a series of Southern blotting and genomic library screening experiments, they further showed that the odorant receptor multigene family contains nearly 1,000 separate genes, making this one of the largest, if not the largest, multigene family in the genome.

The amino acid sequences encoded by ten cDNAs sequenced in these initial experiments are shown in Figure 48-2 [6]. As expected, the odorant receptors belong to the G protein-coupled receptor superfamily. Like other G protein-coupled receptors, the odorant receptors all display seven hydrophobic domains, which are likely to serve as membrane-spanning regions, giving rise to a molecule that transverses the membrane seven times (Fig. 48-3). The odorant receptors also contain several limited sequence motifs which are commonly seen in members of the G protein-coupled superfamily, such as the NP pair in transmembrane domain 7 (TM7). However, the odorant receptors share extensive sequence motifs with one another that are not seen in other G protein-coupled receptors (Fig. 48-2) (see Chap. 20).

There are two striking features of the odorant receptors that may be relevant to the role of these molecules in odor discrimination [6]. Although the odorant receptors, as a group, display a number of conserved sequence motifs, they also display an impressive degree of diversity in the nonconserved regions. Detailed studies involving *in vitro* mutagenesis and domain swapping have been performed with the β-adrenergic receptor and several other members of the G protein-coupled superfamily in order to ascer-

```
                                    I                                                    II
F3    MDSSNRTRVSEFILLGFVENKDLQPLIYGLFLSMYLVTTVIGNISITVAIISDPCLHTPMYFFLSNLSFVDICFISTTVPKML     82
F5    MSSTNQSSVTEFILLGLSROPOQQOLFLLFIIMYLATVIGNLLLILAIGTDSRLHTPMYFFLSNLSFVDVCFSSTTVPKVL      82
F6    MAWSTGQNLSTPGPFILLGFPGPRSMRIGLFLLFIIFALFLSMYLVTVIGNLLIIMAIITOSHLHTPMYFFLANLSFVDICFTSTTIPKML  85
F12   MN--NQTFITOFILLGLPIPEEHQHLFYALFLVMYLTTLGNLLIIIVLVQLDSOLHTPMYLFLSNLSFDLCFSSVTMPKML       83
I3    MESGNSTRRFSSFFLLGFTENPQLHFIIFALFLSMYLVTVIGNLLIIMAIITOSHLHTPMYFLANLSFVDICFTSTTIPKML      80
I7    MERRNHSGRVSEFVLLGFPAPAPLRVLFFLSLLXYVLVLTENMLIIIAIRNHPTLHKPMYFFLANMSFLEIWYVTVTIPKML      83
I8    MN--NKTVITHFLLLGLPIPPEHQOLFFALFLIMYLTTPLGNLLIVVLVQLDSHLHTPMYLFLSNLSFSDLCFSSVTMLKLL      80
I9    MTRRNQTAISQFFLLGLPLPPPEYQHLFYALFLAMYLTTLIGNLIIILILLDSHLHTPMYLFLSNLSFADLCFSSVTMPKLL      82
I14   MTGNNQTILEFLLLGLPIPSEYHLLFYALFLAMYLTILIGNLLIIVLVRLDSHLHHPMYLFLSNLSFSDLCFSSVTMPKLL       82
I15   MTEENQTVISQFLLLFLPIPSEHQHVFYALFLSMYLTTVIGNLIIILIHLDSHLHTPMYLFLSNLSFSDLCFSSVTMPKLL       82

                                    III                                                   IV
F3    ----VNIQTQNNVITYAGCITQIYFFLLFVELDNFLLTIMAYDRYVAICHPMHYTVIMNYKLCGFLVLVSWIVSVLHALFQSLMM    163
F5    ----ANHILGSQAISFSGCLTQLYFLAVFQNMDNFLLAVMSYDRFVAICHPLHYTTKMTRQLCVLLVSGWVVANMNCLLHILLM     163
F6    ----ATFAPRGGVISLAGCATQMYFVFSLGCTEYFLLAVMAYDRYLAICLPLRYGGIMTPGLAMRLALGSWLCGFSAITVPATLI    166
F12   ----VNIYTQSKSITYEDCISQMCVFLVFAELGNFLLAVMAYDRYVAXCHPLCYTVIVNHRLCILLLLSWVISIFPHAFIQSLIV    164
I3    ----QNMRSQDTSIPVGGCLAQTYFMVFGDMESFLLVAMAYDRYVAICHPLHYPVVSSRLCVQMAAGSWAGGFGISMKVFLI       161
I7    AGFIGSKENHGQLISFEACMTQLYFLGLGCTECVLLAVMAYDRYVAICHPLHYPVVSSRLCVQMAAGSWAGGFGISMKVFLI      168
I8    ----QNIQSQVPSISYAGCLTQIPFFLLFGYLGNFLLVAMAYDRYVAICFPLHYTNIMSHKLCTCLLLVFWIMTSSHAMMHTLLA    161
I9    ----QNMQSQVPSIPVAGCLAQIYFFLFFGDLGNFLLVAMAYDRYVAICFPLHYMSIMSPKLCVSLVVLSWVLTTPHAMLHTLLM    163
I14   ----QNMQSQVPSISYTGCLTQLYFFMVFGDMESFLLVMAYDRYVAICFPLRYTTIMSTKFCASLVLLLWMLTWTHALLHTLLI     163
I15   ----QNMQSQVPSIPFAGCLTQLYFLYFADLESFLLVAMAYDRYVAICFPLHYMSIMSPKLCVSLVVLSWVLTTPHAMLHTLLM     163

                                    V                                                     VI
F3    LALPFCTHLEIPHYFCEPNQVIOLTCSDAFLNDLVIYFTLVLLATVPLAGIFYSYFKIVSSICAISSVHGKYKAFSTCASHLSVV    248
F5    ARKSFCADNMIPHFFCDGTPLLKLSCSDTHLNELMILTEGAVVMVTPFVCILISYIHITCAVLRVSSPRGGWKSFTCGSHLAVV     248
F6    ARLSFCGSRVINHFFCDISPWIVLSCTDTQVVELVSFGIAFCVILGSCGITLVSYAYIITTIKIPSARGRHRAFSTCSSHLTVV     251
F12   LQLTFCGDVKIPHFFCELNQLSQLTCSDNFPSHLIMNLVPVMLAAISFSGILYSYFKIVSSIHSISTVQGKYKAFSTCASHLSIV    249
I3    ARLSFCENNVLNFFCDLFVLLKLACSDTYINELMIFIMSTLLIIPFFLIVMSYARIISSILKVPSTQICKVFSTCGSHLSVV      246
I7    SRLSYCGPNTNHFFCDVSPLLNLSCTDMSTAELTDFVLAIFIILGPLSVVGASYMAITGAVMRIPSAAGRHKAFSTCASHLTVV    253
I8    ARLSFCENNVLLNFFCDLFVLLKLACSDTYVNELMIHIMGVIIIYFVLIVISYAKIISSILKVPSTQSIHKVFTCGSHLSVV      246
I9    ARLSFCEDSTYFCMSTLLKVACSDTHDNELAIFILGGPIVVLPFLLIIVSYARIVSSIFKVPSSQSIHKAFSTCGSHLSVV       248
I14   ARLSFCEKNVIIHFFCDISALLKLSCSDIYVNELMIYIILGGLIIIIPFLLIVMSYVRIFFSILKFPSIQDIYKVFSTCGSHLSVV   248
I15   ARLSFCADNMIPHFFCDISPLLKLSCSDTHVNELVIFVMGGLVIVIPFVLIIVSYARVVASILKVPSVRGIHKIFSTCGSHLSVV    248

                                    VII
F3    SLFYCTGLGVLSSAANNSSQASATASVMYTVVTPMVNPFIYSLRNKDVKSVLKKTLCEEVIRSPPSLLHFFLVLCHLPCFIFCY    333
F5    CLFYGTVIAVVFNPSSSHLAGRDMAAAVMVAVTPMLNPFIYSLRNSDMKAALRKVLAMRFPSKQ                        313
F6    LIWYGSTIFLHVRTSVESSLDLTKAITVLNTIVTPVLNPFIYTLRNKDVKEALRRTVKGK                            311
F12   SLFYSTGLGVYVSSAVVQSSHSAASASVMYTVTPMLNPFIYSLRNKDVKRALERLLEGNCKVHHWTG                     317
I3    SLFYGSTLGLYLCPAGNNSTVKRNRDMRALIRVICSMKITL                                               310
I7    IIFYAASIFIYARPKALSAFDTNKLVSVLYAVIVPLFNPIIYCLRNQDVKRALRRTLHLAQDQEANTNKGSKIG              327
I8    SLFYGTIIGLYLCPSGDNFSLKGSAMAMMYTVVTPMLNPFIYSLRNRDMKQALIRVTCSKKISLPW                      312
I9    SLFYGTVIGLYILCPSANNSTVKETVMSLMYTMVTPMLNPFIYSLRNRDIKDALEKIMCKKQIPSFL                     314
I14   TLFYGTIFGIYLCPSGNNSTVKEIAMAMMYTVVTPMLNPFIYSLRNRDMRALIRVICTKKISL                         312
I15   SLFYGTIIGLYLCPSANNSTVKETVMAMMYTVVTPMLNPFIYSLRNRDMKEALIRVLCKKKITFCL                      312
```

FIGURE 48-2. The protein sequences encoded by ten odorant receptor cDNA clones. *Shaded* residues are those conserved in 60% or more of the proteins. The presence of seven hydrophobic domains (*I–VII*), as well as short conserved motifs shared with other members of the superfamily, indicates that these molecules are members of the seven transmembrane-domain, G protein-coupled receptor superfamily. The presence of extensive shared sequence motifs unique to the olfactory proteins indicates that these proteins are members of a novel receptor family within the superfamily. The pronounced sequence diversity evident in transmembrane domains III, IV and V is likely to allow different members of the odorant receptor family to bind to structurally diverse odorous ligands. (From [6], with permission.)

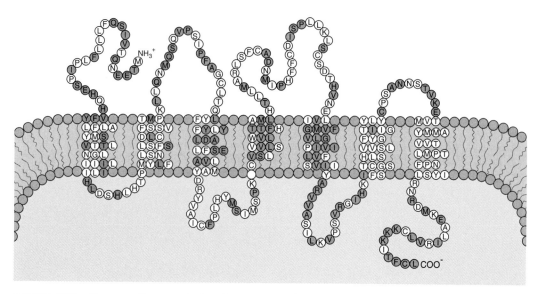

FIGURE 48-3.   Sequence divergence in the odorant receptor family. In this schematic, the protein encoded by one rat cDNA clone (I15) is shown traversing the plasma membrane seven times. The N-terminus is located extracellularly and the C-terminus, intracellularly. The vertical cylinders indicate the seven putative membrane-spanning regions. Positions at which 60% or more of the ten receptors shown in Figure 48-2 share the same residue as I15 are shown as *white balls*. More variable positions are shown as *orange balls*. The extensive variability observed within several of the transmembrane domains is evident.

tain what regions of these molecules are involved in ligand binding [7]. These studies indicate that many G protein-coupled receptors bind to ligand via a ligand-binding pocket, which is formed in the plane of the membrane by a combination of the transmembrane domains. The importance of the transmembrane domains in ligand binding is further stressed in alignments of members of small families of G protein-coupled receptors that bind to the same ligand, such as the adrenergic receptor family or the muscarinic acetylcholine receptor family. These comparisons reveal that sequence conservation among receptors that bind the same ligand is highest in the transmembrane domains. In contrast, the odorant receptor family exhibits extensive sequence divergence in several transmembrane domains (TM3, TM4 and TM5) (Figs. 48-2 and 48-3). This diversity in potential ligand-binding regions within the odorant receptor family is consistent with an ability of this family to interact with a large number of structurally diverse odorous ligands.

A second interesting feature of the odorant-receptor family that may be important in odor discrimination is the presence of subfamilies [6]. As already mentioned, TM5, which could be involved in ligand binding, is highly divergent in members of the odorant receptor family. However, as shown in Figure 48-4, members of the odorant receptor-family appear to fall into subfamilies whose members can be almost identical in this divergent region. It is tempting to propose that the members of divergent subfamilies recognize different structural classes of odorants. The highly related members of a subfamily might either recognize the same odorants or detect subtle differences between structurally related odorants.

Interestingly, Southern blotting experiments indicate that subfamilies are a characteristic feature of the odorant receptor multigene family [6,8,9]. When different members of the multigene family are hybridized to Southern blots of restriction enzyme-digested genomic DNA, distinct patterns of hybridizing species are seen, each of which is likely to represent a different member of the subfamily. The individual subfamilies appear to range in size from one to 20 members but on average have about seven to ten members.

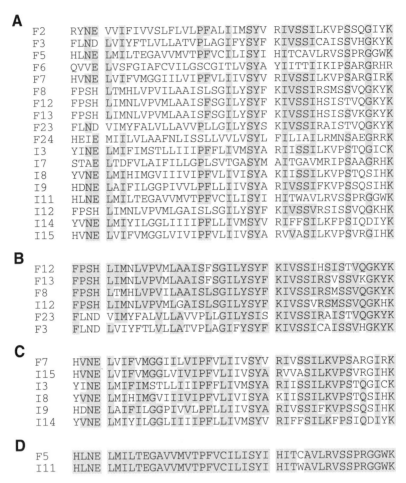

A

F2	RYNE	VVIFIVVSLFLVLPFALIIMSYV	RIVSSILKVPSSQGIYK
F3	FLND	LVIYFTLVLLATVPLAGIFYSYF	KIVSSICAISSVHGKYK
F5	HLNE	LMILTEGAVVMVTPFVCILISYI	HITCAVLRVSSPRGGWK
F6	QVVE	LVSFGIAFCVILGSCGITLVSYA	YIITTIIKIPSARGRHR
F7	HVNE	LVIFVMGGIILVIPFVLIIVSYV	RIVSSILKVPSARGIRK
F8	FPSH	LTMHLVPVILAAISLSGILYSYF	KIVSSIRSMSSVQGKYK
F12	FPSH	LIMNLVPVMLAAISFSGILYSYF	KIVSSIHSISTVQGKYK
F13	FPSH	LIMNLVPVMLAAISFSGILYSYF	KIVSSIHSISSVKGKYK
F23	FLND	VIMYFALVLLAVVPLLGILYSYS	KIVSSIRAISTVQGKYK
F24	HEIE	MIILVLAAFNLISSLLVVLVSYL	FILIAILRMNSAEGRRK
I3	YINE	LMIFIMSTLLIIIPFFLIVMSYA	RIISSILKVPSTQGICK
I7	STAE	LTDFVLAIFILLGPLSVTGASYM	AITGAVMRIPSAAGRHK
I8	YVNE	LMIHIMGVIIIVIPFVLIVISYA	KIISSILKVPSTQSIHK
I9	HDNE	LAIFILGGPIVVLPFLLIIVSYA	RIVSSIFKVPSSQSIHK
I11	HLNE	LMILTEGAVVMVTPFVCILISYI	HITWAVLRVSSPRGGWK
I12	FPSH	LIMNLVPVMLGAISLSGILYSYF	KIVSSVRSISSVQGKHK
I14	YVNE	LMIYILGGLIIIIPFLLIVMSYV	RIFFSILKFPSIQDIYK
I15	HVNE	LVIFVMGGLVIVIPFVLIIVSYA	RVVASILKVPSVRGIHK

B

F12	FPSH	LIMNLVPVMLAAISFSGILYSYF	KIVSSIHSISTVQGKYK
F13	FPSH	LIMNLVPVMLAAISFSGILYSYF	KIVSSIRSVSSVKGKYK
F8	FPSH	LTMHLVPVILAAISLSGILYSYF	KIVSSIRSMSSVQGKYK
I12	FPSH	LIMNLVPVMLGAISLSGILYSYF	KIVSSVRSMSSVQGKHK
F23	FLND	VIMYFALVLLAVVPLLGILYSIS	KIVSSIRAISTVQGKYK
F3	FLND	LVIYFTLVLLATVPLAGIFYSYF	KIVSSICAISSVHGKYK

C

F7	HVNE	LVIFVMGGIILVIPFVLIIVSYV	RIVSSILKVPSARGIRK
I15	HVNE	LVIFVMGGLVIVIPFVLIIVSYA	RVVASILKVPSVRGIHK
I3	YINE	LMIFIMSTLLIIIPFFLIVMSYA	RIISSILKVPSTQGICK
I8	YVNE	LMIHIMGVIIIVIPFVLIVISYA	KIISSILKVPSTQSIHK
I9	HDNE	LAIFILGGPIVVLPFLLIIVSYA	RIVSSIFKVPSSQSIHK
I14	YVNE	LMIYILGGLIIIIPFLLIVMSYV	RIFFSILKFPSIQDIYK

D

F5	HLNE	LMILTEGAVVMVTPFVCILISYI	HITCAVLRVSSPRGGWK
I11	HLNE	LMILTEGAVVMVTPFVCILISYI	HITWAVLRVSSPRGGWK

FIGURE 48-4.   Evidence for subfamilies within the odorant receptor family. The deduced protein sequences of 18 different cDNA clones in and around transmembrane domain V are shown. **A:** Residues shared by 60% or more of the proteins at a given position are *shaded*. Transmembrane domain V appears to be highly variable in members of the odorant receptor family (see Figs. 48-2 and 48-3). **B–D:** These proteins can be grouped into subfamilies in which the individual members share considerable homology in this divergent region. (From [6], with permission.)

The remarkable size and diversity of the odorant receptor multigene family in mammals suggests that odor discrimination relies heavily on the initial event in olfactory perception, the interaction of odorant receptor with odorant. In this respect, olfaction contrasts sharply with color vision, where signals derived from only three peripheral receptor types, the three color opsins, are processed to allow the perception of a multitude of different hues. The extremely large number of odorant receptor genes further suggests that individual receptors could be fairly specific, each one recognizing only one or a small set of structurally similar odorants.

The information generated by hundreds of different receptor types must be organized to achieve a high level of olfactory discrimination

Most sensory systems localize environmental information in space and possess neural topographical maps of that spatial information. The olfactory system does not perceptually localize environmental information in external space. However, it could use spatial determinants within the nervous system to encode information. If so, topographical maps or spatial codes for odors might be evident within the olfactory epithelium or olfactory bulb. For example, olfactory neurons that express a particular odorant receptor gene, and therefore recognize the same odorants, might be clustered in one region of the olfactory epithelium or might all form synapses at a discrete site in the olfactory bulb. On the other hand, neurons that express the same odorant receptor gene could be broadly distributed in the olfactory epithelium or form synapses at many different bulbar sites, encoding information by a nontopographical strategy.

Zonal organization in the olfactory epithelium.

To address these questions, Ressler et al. [8] and Vassar et al. [9] analyzed the patterns of expression of different odorant receptor genes within the olfactory epithelium of the mouse. They found that different odorant receptors are expressed in distinct topographical patterns within the nasal cavity. It appears that the olfactory epithelium is divided into a limited series of expression zones. These zones exhibit bilateral symmetry in the two nasal cavities and are virtually identical in different individuals. Within each zone, many different members of the odorant receptor gene family are expressed. However, each individual gene may be expressed only within a single zone. Although the zonal assignment of each gene appears to be strictly regulated, within each zone neurons that express a particular receptor gene are broadly distributed. It thus appears that when an olfactory neuron or its progenitor chooses which odorant-receptor gene(s) to express, it is restricted to a single zonal gene set but may choose a receptor gene or set of genes to express from among the zonal set via a stochastic mechanism.

Organization in the epithelium to bulb projection.

The odorant receptor expression zones in the olfactory epithelium exhibit a pronounced dorsal-ventral and medial-lateral organization [8]. Interestingly, the axonal projection from the olfactory epithelium to the olfactory bulb is also organized along the dorsal-ventral and medial-lateral axes [10]. Comparisons of the locations of the expression zones with the topography of projections between the olfactory epithelium and olfactory bulb indicate that the organization of odorant receptor gene expression in the epithelium is preserved in the axonal projection to

the olfactory bulb [8]. Indeed, the map is even more specific than this. For reasons that remain obscure, mRNA for receptors can be found at low levels in the synaptic terminals of olfactory axons. With *in situ* hybridization using receptor probes it has been possible to visualize specific glomeruli that are "hot spots" for each receptor gene type. That is, each of the 1,900 glomeruli in a rat is dominated by inputs from cells expressing the same receptor. In an even more remarkable set of experiments on transgenic mice [11], the marker gene *lacz* was placed under the control of a specific, odor receptor promoter such that all of the cells expressing that receptor would be a dark blue color. Several thousand cells, scattered throughout a single expression zone in the epithelium, could be seen sending their axons to two glomeruli in each bulb. Thus, it appears that all of the cells expressing a particular receptor are somehow targeted to one or two among approximately 1,900 glomeruli in the mouse olfactory bulb.

These results suggest that an initial organization of olfactory sensory information occurs in the olfactory epithelium and that this organization is maintained in the patterns of signals transmitted to the olfactory bulb [12]. This conclusion is consistent with the results of recent electrophysiological studies which showed that responses in mitral cells to odors applied to the epithelium are narrowly tuned and that sensitivity to particular types of odor, determined by either functional group or carbon chain length, is spatially organized in the bulb [13]. Thus, the organization of receptors into broad zones in the epithelium is further refined in the bulb, where receptors find common targets.

The reputed sensitivity of the olfactory system is likely to derive from the capacity of the olfactory transduction apparatus to effectively amplify and rapidly terminate signals

The olfactory system is thought to respond to extremely low concentrations of odorants and to have a fast recovery of perceptual sensitivity. In recent years, significant advances have been made in the understanding of the signal-transduction events that take place when an olfactory sensory neuron is exposed to an odorant. Before discussing the biochemical events involved in the signal-transduction process, it is instructive to consider the sensitivity of the olfactory system at the level of perception versus the individual neuron.

Although olfactory perception is believed to be extremely sensitive, the degree of sensitivity is controversial. Some reports, especially in insects, have suggested that odors involved in sexual attraction could be detected by male animals at the level of the single molecule, that is, concentrations as low as 10^{-14} M. Human olfactory thresholds of 10^{-11} M have been measured by psychophysical methods. In such studies, however, the actual concentration of odorant at the odorant receptor cannot be known definitively. Due to factors such as odor molecule interactions, diffusion, adsorption into mucus, and anatomical structures which may trap and concentrate odor molecules, these estimates could be as much as two to four orders of magnitude too low.

Physiological recordings from single receptor neurons suggest somewhat lower sensitivities, with $K_{1/2}$ values between 1 and 50 μM [14]. These values could allow for broad specificity and rapid termination of odorant responses. For example, since $K_d = k_{off}/k_{on}$ and the on rate, approximately 10^8 $M^{-1}\cdot sec^{-1}$, is ultimately limited by diffusional encounters between ligand and receptor, the K_d is limited by the range of acceptable off rates. A K_d of 10^{-6} would result in molecular encounters lasting a few hundred milliseconds, whereas a K_d of 10^{-11} would result in dwell times of more than 5 min.

It can be shown from the law of mass action that with significant amplification mechanisms, such that occupation of only a few receptors would be sufficient to elicit a response, thresholds as much as five or six orders of magnitude lower than the K_d can be attained. Thus, K_d values of 10^{-6} could, in theory, produce threshold responses at odor concentrations as low as 10^{-11}, permitting the olfactory system to maintain the broad specificity seen in physiological recordings [5] and the high threshold sensitivity measured in psychophysical experiments. Several amplification mechanisms that could serve this purpose are described below.

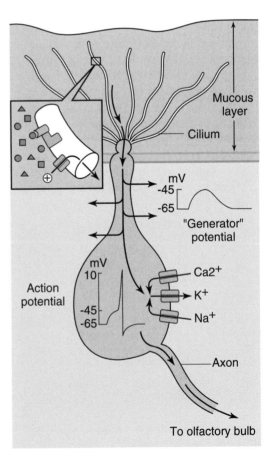

FIGURE 48-5. Schematic drawing of an olfactory neuron showing the single bipolar morphology, with a single thick dendrite ending in a knob-like swelling and an unbranched axon projecting from the proximal soma centrally to the olfactory bulb. The cell is highly compartmentalized into transduction and signaling regions. Transduction occurs in the cilia, which extend from the distal dendritic knob into the mucous layer. A receptor-coupled second-messenger system (see Fig. 48-6) results in the opening of a cation-selective channel in the ciliary membrane. The influx of cations depolarizes the cell membrane from its resting level near −65 to −45 mV, in a graded manner. This depolarization spreads by passive current flow through the dendrite to the soma. A depolarization that reaches −45 mV is sufficient to activate voltage-gated Na^+ channels and initiate impulse generation. This Na^+ current along with several varieties of voltage-dependent K^+ currents and a small Ca^{2+} current produce one or more action potentials that are propagated down the axon to the brain.

Odorant recognition initiates a second-messenger system leading to the depolarization of the neuron and the generation of action potentials

Recordings of the electrical activity of single olfactory receptor neurons show that exposure to odorants causes the membrane to depolarize, leading to the generation of action potentials [2]. Underlying the initial depolarization is the influx of cations through a conductance in the specialized cilia extending from the distal end of the cell into the mucous lining of the nasal cavity (Fig. 48-5). The biochemical elements coupling odorant receptor binding to the opening of a cation channel are now understood in some detail [15]. A consensus view is presented in Figure 48-6.

The second-messenger cascade of olfactory transduction is a classic cyclic nucleotide-based system with one or two interesting modifications. A G protein that is likely to couple odorant receptors to other intracellular elements of the cascade, G_{olf}, was identified by Reed [15] and shown to be an isoform of G_s specific to olfactory neurons. It has been shown that high concentrations of G_{olf} are present in olfactory cilia. Since G_{olf} can interact with G protein-coupled receptors other than odorant receptors, it has been proposed that the existence of a separate gene for G_{olf} may, in some manner, permit the specific and high level of expression of this protein observed in olfactory neurons (Chaps. 20, 23).

An adenylyl cyclase has been identified in olfactory neurons which also appears to be specific to these cells and is biochemically distinct from other known isoforms of this enzyme. Also cloned and characterized by Reed, it has been termed adenylyl cyclase type III [15]. An important characteristic of this isozyme is that, when

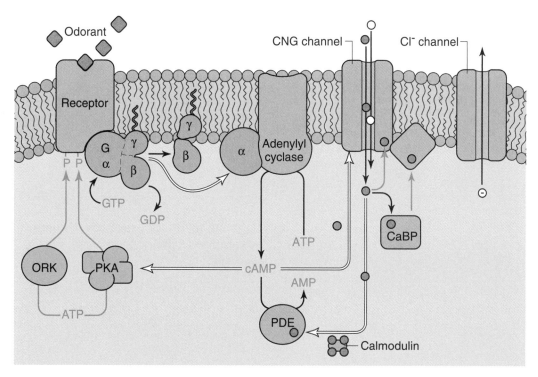

FIGURE 48-6. A model for the operation of the cAMP-based second-messenger system in olfactory neurons. The individual steps are detailed in the text. Note that there are several feedback loops that modulate the response. These include inhibition of the channel by Ca^{2+} ions that permeate the channel, a cAMP-dependent protein kinase (PKA) that may phosphorylate the receptor and a receptor kinase (ORK) that selectively phosphorylates occupied receptors. Sites of action are shown by *white arrows*, indicating stimulatory effects, and *orange arrows*, indicating inhibitory effects. *ORK*, putative olfactory receptor kinase; *PKA*, protein kinase A; *PDE*, phosphodiesterase; *CNG*, cyclic nucleotide-gated channel; *CaBP*, putative calcium-binding protein.

expressed in a mammalian cell line, its basal activity is extremely low, while in its stimulated state, it has a catalytic rate higher than other known cyclases. These properties could confer a high signal-to-noise ratio on the system, being quiescent in the absence of stimulus but able to rapidly generate large amounts of cAMP upon odor exposure.

Consistent with this idea are the kinetics of cAMP accumulation, which have been followed on a sub-second time scale by Breer [3] using a rapid quench technique. When odorants were added to an olfactory cilia preparation, cAMP increased linearly with odorant concentration up to a level fourfold greater than baseline. The increase peaked within 50 msec of exposure to the odor stimuli and returned to baseline levels within about 300 msec, suggesting that odorant stimulates the pulsatile production of cAMP.

In 1987, Nakamura and Gold [16] recorded ion currents from a ciliary conductance that was activated directly by cAMP, without an intervening phosphorylation step. This was the final link between the biochemical cascade and the electrical signal. The channel was subsequently cloned and characterized in several species [15]. The channel is selective for cations; is curiously sensitive to both cAMP, with a K_d of 20 μM, and cGMP with a K_d of 5 μM; and requires at least three molecules of cyclic nucleotide to bind for activation. It shares 65% similarity with the cGMP-activated channel found in photoreceptors, and, most interestingly, it bears strong homology with voltage-sensitive channels, such as K^+ and Ca^{2+} channels.

The activation of tens to hundreds of these channels and the subsequent influx of cations, including both Na^+ and Ca^{2+}, lead to depolarization of the cell membrane. Olfactory neurons have one additional level of amplication that is rather unusual. A Ca^{2+}-activated Cl^- channel is also present on the cilia and is opened during the odor response by the Ca^{2+} ions flowing into the cilia through the cAMP-gated channel [17]. Curiously, olfactory neurons maintain a very high intracellular Cl^- concentration, perhaps as high as 125 mM, so that the driving force for Cl^- ions is *outward* and, therefore, further *depolarizes* the cell. This additional current may be important for pre-serving ionic driving forces across a membrane in a compartment that is not highly regulated, that is, the mucus. Changing ion concetrations in the mucus could affect the driving forces on ions, so the olfactory neuron supplies its own driving force by maintaining a high intracellular concentration of Cl^-.

Some of the important physiological characterics of the odor response can be seen in recordings of currents through the cAMP-sensitive channels in response to pulses of odor stimuli (Fig. 48-7) [14]. There is a long, concentration-dependent latency between the binding of odor molecules and the activation of the current, lasting 150 to 450 msec. The peak current amplitude is a sigmoidal function of the log odor concentration that can be fit by the Hill equation with a Hill coefficient of between 2 and 4. The cooperativity in the response appears to emanate from the requirement of the cAMP channel for cooperative activation by cAMP and from activation of the Cl^- current by Ca^{2+} ions [17]. There is no indication that odorant receptors bind odorant ligands cooperatively.

This pathway provides several amplification steps between odorant binding and signal generation. Due to the electrically compact structure of the cell, it is possible for the activation of only a few tens of channels to drive the membrane to threshold for action potential generation. Thus, it is theoretically possible that the limit of olfactory detection is the single molecule, although this has not yet been conclusively demonstrated.

Negative feedback processes mediate adaptation in the odor-induced response

Upon application of a sustained odor stimulus to an olfactory neuron, the current response is transient, falling back to baseline within 4 to 5 sec [2]. The termination of a response in the continued presence of agonist is characteristic of many signaling systems and is variously known as adaptation or desensitization, depending on the putative site of the off mechanism. Typically, a negative feedback process is at work such that accumulation of a product of the agonist response serves to turn off an upstream link in the signal-generating cascade. In the olfactory neuron, two feedback messengers have been identified, and, as might be expected, they are Ca^{2+} and cAMP.

The ion channel activated by cAMP is permeable to cations, including Ca^{2+} [18]. Thus, increased channel activation results in influx of

Ca^{2+} and a transient rise in the intracellular concentration of Ca^{2+}. Intracellular Ca^{2+} concentrations of 1 to 3 μM have been found to lead to a decrease in the open probability of the ion channel, even in the presence of high concentrations of cAMP [19]. The mechanism could involve a direct effect of Ca^{2+} on the channel or be mediated via an intermediate Ca^{2+}-binding protein. In either case, this is an attractive mechanism for mediating a rapid but short-lasting form of adaptation since it is dependent on the influx of Ca^{2+} during the response to an odor. It has been shown that virtually all short-term adaptation could indeed be accounted for in this way. Comparing adaptation to odors with that induced by the photolytic release of cAMP in the cell, it was found that adaptation to both was identical. That is, the rise in cAMP and the consequent opening of cAMP-gated channels alone was enough to cause the cell to adapt to further stimulation, suggesting that this last step in the transduction cascade was the primary site of adaptation.

A second pathway, utilizing a phosphorylation step, resembles desensitization mechanisms described for the β-adrenergic receptor and rhodopsin [3,7,20]. cAMP, in addition to opening the ion channel, appears to activate a form of cAMP-dependent protein kinase (PKA), which inactivates some earlier step in the transduction process. Addition of a peptide fragment of the Walsh inhibitor protein (WIPTIDE), a PKA antagonist, prolongs the odorant-induced production of cAMP [3]. Studies of desensitization of the β-adrenergic receptor and rhodopsin have

A

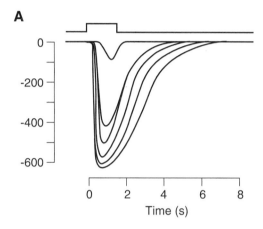

B

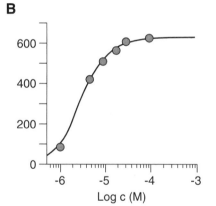

C

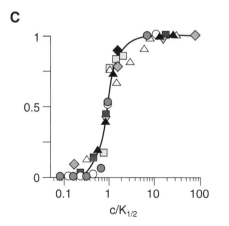

FIGURE 48-7.   Responses of single neurons to varying concentrations of odorant. **A:** A family of responses in a single olfactory neuron to the odor cineole at concentrations varying from 1 to 100 μM. *Downward deflections* represent inward ionic currents whose peak amplitudes range from 50 to 600 pA. Note the latency, rapid rise and slow decay. The stimulus bar **(top)** shows the time course of the odor ligand. **B:** Dose-response relation for the peak current versus the odor concentration. **C:** Dose-response relations for five different cells, showing the narrow operating range characteristic of olfactory neurons. (From [14], with permission.)

revealed two specialized but closely related kinases, β-adrenergic receptor kinase (βARK) (Chap. 24) and rhodopsin kinase (Chap. 47), respectively, that phosphorylate the activated receptor. Interestingly, a recently characterized isoform of βARK has been shown to be highly enriched in olfactory sensory neurons [20]. Odorant-induced phosphorylation of ciliary proteins by both PKA and protein kinase C (PKC) has been demonstrated, but the phosphorylated proteins have not been conclusively identified. Thus, it is possible that the cAMP generated in response to odor stimulation activates negative-feedback pathways that act to truncate an ongoing response.

Alternative second-messenger pathways may be at work in olfactory transduction

The role of cAMP in olfactory transduction is well established. Are there alternative pathways, such as those involving phospholipids and Ca^{2+}? Breer and his colleagues [3] have assayed for inositol 1,4,5,-trisphosphate (IP_3) production in the rat using odorants that failed to produce cAMP in biochemical assays. They found rapid and significant increases in IP_3, and that a given odorant led to the production of either cAMP or IP_3, never both. More recently, they have found evidence for two pathways for adaptation, one utilizing PKA and the other PKC, and have shown that the responses to odors using one or the other pathway are completely additive. Utilizing cultured mammalian olfactory neurons, Ronnett and her colleagues have found evidence that many odorants can stimulate both IP_3 and cAMP production but that the ratio of IP_3 to cAMP varies according to odorant.

In contrast to these data, a mouse in which the cAMP-gated channel was knocked out was determined to be completely anosmic, that is, incapable of smelling, indicating that there is only one second-messenger pathway and it utilizes cAMP [21]. This is also consistent with most physiological data, which show that exogenous application of IP_3 to intact olfactory neurons does not affect the odor-transduction system. It may still be determined that IP_3 may have a modulatory role, but it appears unlikely to be a

signal-transduction pathway in vertebrate olfaction. It should be noted, however, that among invertebrates there is good evidence that IP_3, as well as cAMP, play important roles in olfactory signal transduction [22].

The vomeronasal organ is an accessory chemosensing system devoted to detecting conspecific chemical cues, also known as pheromones

These cues are important in rearing, territorial, courtship and, in particular, sexual behaviors. The vomeronasal organ (VNO) is separate from the main epithelium in mammals, comprising a thin epithelial tissue within a bony capsule in the lateral wall of the nasal cavity. At least two populations of chemosensory neurons share this tissue, as determined by the differential expression of the G proteins G_i or G_o. Aside from this single fact, little is known of the transduction pathway in the VNO neurons, but it appears to be neither cyclic nucleotides nor phospholipids.

A family of G protein-coupled receptors was cloned in the VNO and apparently represents the pheromone receptors [23]. These receptors are in the seven-transmembrane domain family of receptors but are only weakly similar to the odor receptors of the main epithelium. There appear to be at least 50 to 100 different receptors specific to the VNO, and it remains a possibility that this is not the only family of pheromone receptors since all of these receptors are expressed in only one of the two classes of VNO neuron.

TASTE

Taste perception can be reduced to primary stimuli

Our total perception of food is a complex experience based upon multiple senses: taste per se, which includes sweet, sour, salty and bitter; olfaction, which includes aromas; touch, also termed "mouth feel," that is, texture and fat content; and thermoreception and nociception, for example, that caused by pungent spices and irritants. Taste proper is commonly divided into four categories of primary stimuli: sweet, sour, salty and bitter. One other primary taste, savory, termed umami, is controversial. Mixtures of these primaries can mimic the tastes of more complex foods.

The chemical complexity of taste stimuli suggests that taste receptor cells utilize multiple molecular mechanisms to detect and distinguish among these compounds. Our sense of taste can detect and discriminate various ionic stimuli, for example, Na^+ as salty, H^+ as sour, sugars as sweet and alkaloids as bitter. Sweet and bitter compounds display great structural diversity, suggesting the presence of multiple discriminatory receptors.

Taste receptor cells are organized into taste buds

The chemical detection of taste agents resides in specialized epithelial cells, taste receptor cells, which in vertebrates are present as ovoid clusters, or taste buds (Fig. 48-8), each containing 50 to 100 cells. The taste buds are embedded within the nonsensory lingual epithelium of the tongue, and they are housed within connective tissue specializations called papillae, which are fungiform, foliate and circumvallate. Taste buds are also found in the palate, pharynx and upper portion of the esophagus.

The taste bud is a polarized structure with a narrow apical opening, termed the taste pore,

and basolateral synapses with afferent nerve fibers. Solutes in the oral cavity make contact with the apical membranes of the taste receptor cells via the taste pore. There is a significant amount of lateral connectedness between taste cells within a bud: both electrical synapses between taste receptor cells and chemical synapses between taste receptor cells and Merkel-like basal cells have been demonstrated to occur [24]. Furthermore, there are symmetrical synapses between taste receptor cells and Merkel-like basal cells [24]. In addition, Merkel-like basal cells synapse with the afferent nerve fiber, suggesting that they may function in effect as interneurons [24]. The extensive lateral interconnections within a bud along with the branching of afferent fibers to synapse with several receptor cells within a given bud suggest that much signal processing occurs peripherally within the taste bud itself [24].

Sensory afferents within three cranial nerves innervate the taste buds

The sensory fibers that innervate the taste buds travel in cranial nerves VII, IX and X. The chorda tympani carries fibers from VII to innervate taste buds on the anterior portion of the tongue, within the fungiform papillae and the anterior portion of the foliate papillae. Buds

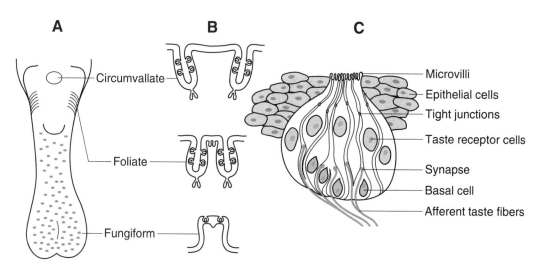

FIGURE 48-8.   Rat tongue, taste papillae and taste buds. **A:** Surface of the rat tongue showing location of the taste papillae. **B:** Cross-section of the three main types of taste papillae: fungiform, foliate and circumvallate. **C:** The taste bud contains 50 to 100 taste cells, including receptor cells and basal cells.

within the circumvallate papillae and the posterior portion of the foliate papillae are innervated by the lingual branch of the glossopharyngeal nerve (IX). Taste buds of the epiglottis and the esophagus are innervated by the superior laryngeal branch of the vagus (X).

Projections from the afferent taste fibers synapse in the medulla within the gustatory portion of the nucleus of the solitary tract (Fig. 48-9). The more rostral portion of the nucleus of the solitary tract contains the gustatory nucleus, whereas the caudal portion receives afferent input from visceral organs. The visceral inputs to the solitary tract relay their information to more rostral brainstem nuclei. Neurons from the gustatory nucleus project to the thalamus via the central tegmental tract and terminate in the small-cell (parvocellular) region of the ventral posterior media nucleus (VPMpc).

Information coding of taste is not strictly according to a labeled line

Two different models have been proposed to account for information coding in the gustatory system: (i) labeled line and (ii) across-fiber pattern code. The labeled-line model predicts that individual taste receptor cells will respond to only a single taste quality. Information about each taste quality is then transmitted by separate afferent pathways to the gustatory cortex via the medulla and the thalamus [25]. Thus, in the labeled-line model, the function of any one neuron in an afferent pathway is to signal its particular encoded taste quality. The across-fiber pattern-coding model proposes that individual taste cells respond to different taste qualities. Information about taste quality is then transmitted to the brain by afferent fibers that have broadly overlapping response spectra [26]. Thus, the code for a particular quality is determined by the pattern of activity across all of the afferent nerve fibers, rather than by activity in any single nerve fiber.

Experimental results argue against a strict labeled-line model. However, gustatory information coding may utilize both types of mechanisms. For example, in the hamster, single chorda tympani fibers respond to multiple taste qualities, such as salt and sour or sour and bitter. This im-

plies that some type of pattern-recognition processing must occur since multiple taste qualities are carried centrally by the same fiber. However, it is likely that some selectivity occurs within the fibers themselves with a preferential response to a given taste quality, for example, salt > sour or sour > bitter. Hence, an across-fiber pattern code could make use of several types of taste quality-preferred fiber such as salt best or sweet best.

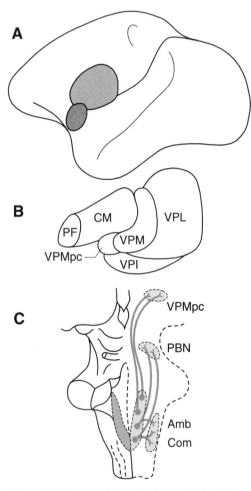

FIGURE 48-9. Central projections of taste information. **A:** Cortical taste projections. **B:** Thalamic taste projections. **C:** Medullary taste nuclei. *CM*, centromedian; *PF*, parafasicular; *VPM*, ventral posteromedial; *VPL*, ventral posterolateral; *VPMpc*, ventral posteromedial parvocellular part; *VPI*, ventral posterior inferior; *PBN*, pontine parabrachial nucleus; *Amb/Com*, ambiguous nucleus complex.

Taste cells have multiple types of ion channels

Taste receptor cells are electrically excitable and capable of generating action potentials: voltage-dependent channels for Na^+, Ca^{2+} and K^+, similar to those in neurons, have been detected in vertebrate taste cells (for a recent review, see [27]). The surface distribution of these ion channels may reflect differences in their functional activities. The taste cell of the amphibian mudpuppy *Necturus maculosus* has a prominent voltage-gated K^+ conductance concentrated on its apical surface, whereas Na^+ and Ca^{2+} channels are distributed through its surface [28]. Mammalian taste cells do not display this prominent apical K^+ channel: no significant apical K^+ conductance could be found in the fungiform taste buds of the hamster. Mammalian foliate- and circumvallate-derived taste buds have not yet been tested for this apical K^+ conductance, nor has it been determined if the distribution of Na^+ and Ca^{2+} channels differs between apical and basolateral surfaces. Multiple types of K^+ channel have been found in vertebrate taste cells: (i) a voltage-independent K^+ channel of ~40 pS conductance in frog; (ii) a 90-pS, delayed rectifier K^+ conductance in rat; and (iii) a 225-pS, Ca^{2+}-dependent K^+ channel in rat. In mammals, at least two types of Na^+ conductance occur: (i) a tetrodotoxin-blockable, voltage-dependent Na^+ channel, similar to neuronal Na^+ conductances, and (ii) an amiloride-blockable, voltage-independent Na^+ channel, similar to to epithelial Na^+ conductances.

Salts and acids are transduced by direct interaction with ion channels

Several lines of evidence suggest that salt taste in mammals is mediated, at least in part, by the voltage-independent, amiloride-blockable, apical Na^+ channel. These Na^+ channels are of a type commonly found in epithelial cells involved in solute transport, such as renal epithelial cells. Micromolar concentrations of amiloride block this Na^+ conductance in isolated taste cells and reduce Na^+ salt stimulation of gustatory nerve fibers [29]. The presumed mechanism for taste cell response to salt is direct influx of Na^+ through this amiloride-blockable channel, leading to taste cell depolarization, action potential generation and neurotransmitter release (Fig. 48-10). Other mechanisms must contribute to the transduction of Na^+ salt since about 20% of the afferent nerve response to NaCl is amiloride-insensitive. One of these mechanisms is believed to involve permeation of Na^+ through the tight junctions that connect taste cells at the apex of the taste bud; the Na^+ presumably enters taste cells through basolateral Na^+ channels [30]. Whether these basolateral Na^+ channels are amiloride-sensitive is not known since amiloride would not permeate the tight junctions. Recent studies suggest that basolateral Na^+ channels may be more important for NaCl transduction in humans since amiloride applied to the human tongue has little effect on the saltiness of NaCl [31].

Sour taste is a function of the acidity of a solution, depending primarily on the proton concentration and to a lesser extent on the particular anion involved. As with salty taste, sour taste is perceived as a result of the direct interaction of protons with ion channels of taste cells (Fig. 48-10). Several mechanisms have been found to contribute to sour transduction. One of these mechanisms, in hamsters, involves influx of protons through the amiloride-sensitive Na^+ channel, the same channel that is involved in Na^+ transduction. In the absence of Na^+, protons permeate the channel, depolarizing taste receptor cells [32]. Clearly, other mechanisms must be involved or we could not distinguish salts from acids. In the mudpuppy, K^+ channels are concentrated in the apical surface of the taste cell, and this apical K^+ conductance dominates the resting potential of the taste cell [28]. Protons block this K^+ conductance, leading to taste-cell depolarization. Patch-clamp recording of excised patches from the mudpuppy taste cell demonstrated H^+ blockade of a 100-pS K^+ channel. Other mechanisms of acid transduction include a proton-gated cation channel, in frog taste cells, and proton permeation of the tight junctions at the apex of the taste bud. The basolateral targets of protons have not been identified.

Taste cells contain receptors, G proteins and second-messenger-effector enzymes

Research on the biochemistry and molecular biology of taste has been hindered by the relative inaccessibility of taste receptor cells and the lack

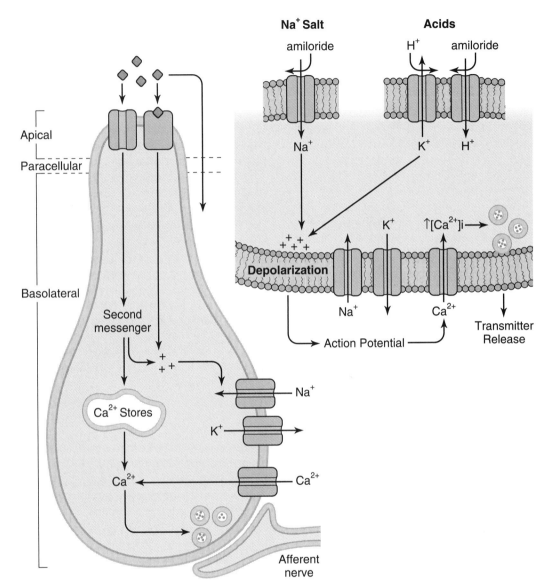

FIGURE 48-10.   Proposed mechanisms for transduction of ionic taste stimuli. Salty stimuli (Na$^+$) enter taste cells via amiloride-sensitive Na$^+$ channels present in the apical membrane. Sour stimuli (H$^+$) permeate the amiloride-sensitive Na$^+$ channels (mammals) or block apical K$^+$ channels (mudpuppy). In addition to these mechanisms, both Na$^+$ and H$^+$ permeate the paracellular pathway and enter ion channels in the basolateral membrane. These ion channels have not been identified.

of high-affinity ligands specific for taste receptors. Biochemical and histological analyses of mammalian taste tissue demonstrate high concentrations of adenylyl cyclase, phosphodiesterase and IP$_3$ receptors. The catfish *Ictalurus punctatus* provides a very rich source of taste tissue: immunological and biochemical analyses demonstrate the presence of G$_s$-like and G$_i$-like G proteins in catfish taste membranes [33]. PCR

has been used to molecularly clone the components of receptor/G protein pathways from a taste cell-specific cDNA library (see below).

Sweet, bitter and umami involve receptor-coupled second-messenger pathways

Sweet taste utilizes G protein-dependent, receptor-mediated transduction pathways (Fig. 48-11).

Sugars and artificial sweeteners bind to the taste cell surface and to taste cell membrane fractions. Biochemical studies with rat anterior tongue membranes enriched in fungiform papillae, or intact taste buds from rat circumvallate papillae show that sugars activate adenylyl cyclase, which in turn elevates intracellular cAMP concentrations [34]. A competitive sugar antagonist inhibited sweet-induced elevation of cAMP, and in membrane extracts adenylyl cyclase activation by sucrose is GTP-dependent. These results argue for the presence of a receptor(s) that upon activation by sugars activates G_s or a G_s-like protein, which in turn activates adenylyl cyclase

to generate cAMP as the intracellular second messenger.

Electrophysiological studies of rodent taste cells have shown that sucrose causes taste cell depolarization along with decreased K^+ conductance [35]. Injection of cAMP or cGMP into taste cells also elicits depolarization with decreased K^+ conductance. These results argue for sweet pathway-generated cyclic nucleotides as the mediator of taste-cell depolarization via K^+ channel closure. There is molecular biological and electrophysiological evidence for the existence in taste cells of a cyclic nucleotide-regulated channel such as is present in olfactory and

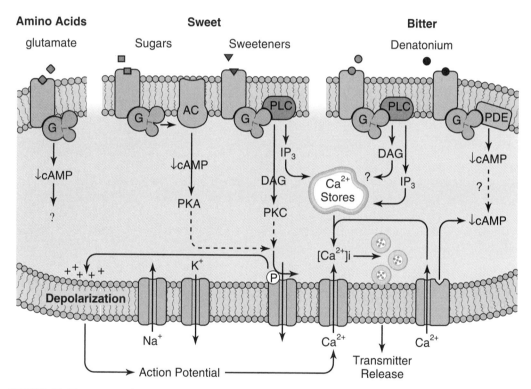

FIGURE 48-11. Proposed receptor-mediated transduction mechanisms. Sugars bind to specific receptors coupled to a G protein ($\alpha\beta\gamma$): activation of this pathway leads to adenylyl cyclase *(AC)* generation of cAMP, which is proposed to activate protein kinase A *(PKA)* and to lead to phosphorylation *(P)* and closure of basolateral K^+ channels. Closure of K^+ channels leads to taste-cell depolarization. Synthetic sweeteners bind to specific receptors that are coupled to a G-protein stimulation of phospholipase C *(PLC)*. Activation of PLC produces inositol 1,4,5-trisphosphate *(IP₃)* and diacylglycerol *(DAG)*; IP_3 elicits a release of Ca^{2+} from intracellular stores, while DAG activates protein kinase C *(PKC)*. It is expected that PKC and PKA converge on the same K^+ channels to depolarize taste cells. Bitter stimuli are thought to bind to specific receptors coupled to G proteins. Two bitter-transduction mechanisms are proposed. In one pathway, a G_q-like G protein activates PLC, leading to generation of IP_3. IP_3 causes Ca^{2+} release from internal stores, which leads to neurotransmitter release onto gustatory afferents. A second pathway for bitter transduction is for gustducin to activate cAMP phosphodiesterase *(PDE)*, leading to decreased intracellular cAMP. The decreased cAMP would relieve block of a cyclic nucleotide-blocked Ca^{2+} channel, resulting in taste-cell depolarization. Umami taste transduction involves binding of glutamate to a metabotropic glutamate receptor, mGluR4. Activation of mGluR4 is thought to cause a decrease of cAMP, but neither the G protein nor the target ion channels have been identified.

photoreceptor cells. However, based on electrophysiology of frog taste receptor cells, it was proposed that the primary action of cAMP is to activate PKA to phosphorylate and thereby close the 40-pS basolateral K^+ channel. It was further proposed that sugars lead to taste-cell depolarization via this mechanism [36].

Recent evidence suggests that synthetic sweeteners utilize a different second-messenger pathway for transduction. Biochemical measurements and Ca^{2+} imaging have shown that sucrose stimulated cAMP, while synthetic sweeteners such as saccharin stimulated IP_3 and diacylglycerol, eliciting the release of Ca^{2+} from intracellular stores [37]. These two second-messenger pathways must ultimately converge to act on the same K^+ channels to depolarize taste cells since synthetic sweeteners and cyclic nucleotides show cross-adaptation [38].

Bitter agents are very structurally diverse, suggesting multiplicity of receptors and/or multiplicity of detection pathways (Fig. 48-11). Many bitter compounds are lipophilic and membrane-permeant. It has been proposed that these compounds directly act on intracellular taste cell phosphodiesterases. Other models for bitter have suggested non-receptor-mediated physical effects upon the lipid bilayer. However, it is unclear what specificity, if any, would be provided by taste cell membranes versus any other type of membrane.

The intensely bitter compound denatonium chloride is membrane-impermeant: using fura-2 imaging of intracellular Ca^{2+}, it was shown that denatonium caused a release of Ca^{2+} from internal stores [39]. Presumably, this effect is elicited by bitter receptor activation of a G_q-like G protein, which in turn activates phospholipase C to generate IP_3 (Chaps. 21, 23). Immunological and histochemical evidence has demonstrated the presence of the IP_3 receptor in taste cells along with other components of the phosphatidylinositol-signaling pathway. A recent study has demonstrated the presence of a G_q-like G protein in taste cells [40]: $G_{\alpha 14}$ was shown to be specifically expressed in taste cells (see below).

Amino acids are potent taste stimuli in several species (Fig. 48-11). L-Glutamate is believed to elicit a unique taste sensation in mammals, which is called umami. A recent study utilizing molecular cloning strategies has identified a metabotropic glutamate receptor, mGluR4, that is expressed in taste buds but not in surrounding lingual epithelium [41]. Evidence that mGluR4 is involved in glutamate taste comes from a behavioral study showing that the specific ligand for mGluR4, L-amino-4-phosphonobutyrate, evokes a taste similar to that of monosodium glutamate in rats. Electrophysiological experiments will be necessary to confirm that mGluR4 mediates umami taste transduction.

Expression of some G proteins is elevated in taste cells

Several known G protein α subunits, α_s, α_{12}, α_{14}, α_{i-2} and α_{i-3}, were cloned from a rat taste tissue-specific cDNA library (Table 48-1) [40]. RNA expression of α_s, α_{14} and α_{i-3} is elevated in taste buds versus the surrounding nonsensory epithelium. G_s or a G_s-like G protein has been proposed to mediate transduction of sugars; the elevated expression of G_s in taste buds is consistent with G_s itself playing a role in sweet transduction. Furthermore, the α subunit of the G_s-like G_{olf} protein is not expressed in taste tissue, ruling out any role for G_{olf} in taste transduction. G_{14} is a G_q-like G protein which can generate IP_3 via phospholipase C activation; G_{14} may play a role in denatonium generation of IP_3 and subsequent Ca^{2+} release. G_{i-3} presumably inhibits adenylyl cyclase in taste cells; it may have a role in the termination of sweet responses or in bitter transduction via decreased concentrations of cAMP.

Gustducin is a taste cell-specific G protein closely related to the transducins

A novel G protein α subunit, α-gustducin, was cloned from rat taste tissue [40] and shown to be expressed in taste buds of the circumvallate, foliate and fungiform papillae. Gustducin is not expressed in nonsensory portions of the tongue or in liver, heart, kidney, muscle, brain, retina or olfactory epithelium. Recently, gustducin has been found in apparent chemosensory cells of the stomach and duodenum [42]. Gustducin is most closely related to the transducins, the rod and cone photoreceptor G proteins, which have also been found in taste cells. At the amino acid level, gustducin is 79 to 80% identical and 90%

TABLE 48-1. ISOLATES OF G PROTEIN α SUBUNIT CLONES FROM RAT TASTE TISSUE

	5′KWIHCF 3′FLNKKD	5′DVGGQR 3′FLNKKD	5′HLFNSIC 3′VFDAVTD	5′TIVKQM 3′FLNKQD
α_{i-2}	4	—	—	—
$\alpha_{i-1,3}$	5	—	—	—
α_{q-1}	—	1	—	—
α_{q-2}	—	1	—	—
α_{s}	—	—	—	1
α_{gust}	5	—	4	1

Degenerate polymerase chain reaction (PCR) primers corresponding to conserved amino acids of G proteins were made and used pairwise in PCR to amplify DNA corresponding to G proteins. The G protein α subunit isolates cloned from PCR-amplified rat taste tissue cDNA are listed in the left-hand column. The heading above each column lists the upstream (5′) and downstream (3′) primers. The numbers in each column represent independent clonal isolates from the particular PCR amplification.
From [40], with permission.

similar to the transducins. This is about the same level of relatedness between rod and cone transducins, which are 81% identical and 90% similar. An alignment of the protein sequences of α-gustducin and the α-transducins reveals that these three proteins are highly homologous throughout their entire length (Fig. 48-12). The C-terminal 38 amino acids of α-gustducin and of the α-transducins are identical. This C-terminal region of transducin has been implicated in

```
Gustducin   MGSGISSESK ESAKRSKELE KKLQEDAERD ARTVKLLLLG AGESGKSTIV KQMKIIHKNG 60
Bovinecone  MGSGASAEDK ELAKRSKELE KKLQEDADKE AKTVKLLLLG AGESGKSTIV KQMKIIHQDG 60
Bovinerod   MGAGASAEEK ....HSRELE KKLKEDAEKD ARTVKLLLLG AGESGKSTIV KQMKIIHQDG 56
Consensus   MGSGASAE-K E-AKRSKELE KKLQEDADKD ARTVKLLLLG AGESGKSTIV KQMKIIHQDG 60

Gustducin   YSKQECMEFK AVVYSNTLQS ILAIVKAMTT LGIDYVNPRS REDQQLLLSM ANTLEDGDMT 120
Bovinecone  YSPEECLEYK AIIYGNVLQS ILAIIRAMPT LGIDYAEVSC VDNGRQLNNL ANSIEEGTMP 120
Bovinerod   YSLEECLEFI AIIYGNTLQS ILAIVRAMTT LNIQYGDSAR QDDARKLMHM ANTIEEGTMP 116
Consensus   YS-EECLEFK AIIYGNTLQS ILAIVRAMTT LGIDY----- -DD-R-L--M ADTIEEGTMP 120

Gustducin   PQLAEIIKRL WGDPGIQACF ERASEYQLND SAAYYLNDLD RLTAPGYVPN EQDVLHSRVK 180
Bovinecone  PELVEVIRKL WKDGGVQACF DRAAEYQLND SASYYLNQLD RITAPDYLPN EQDVLRSRVK 180
Bovinerod   KEMSDIIQRL WKDSGIQACF DRASEYQLND SAGYYLSDLE RLVTPGYVPT EQDVLRSRVK 176
Consensus   PEL-EII-RL WKD-GIQACF DRASEYQLND SA-YYLNDLD RLTAPGYVPN EQDVLRSRVK 180

Gustducin   TTGIIETQFS FKDLNFRMFD VGGQRSERKK WIHCFEGVTC IIFCAALSAY DMVLVEDEEV 240
Bovinecone  TTGIIETKFS VKDLNFRMFD VGGQRSERKK WIHCFEGVTC IIFCAALSAY DMVLVEDDEV 240
Bovinerod   TTGIIETQFS FKDLNFRMFD VGGQRSERKK WIHCFEGVTC IIFIAALSAY DMVLVEDDEV 236
Consensus   TTGIIETQFS FKDLNFRMFD VGGQRSERKK WIHCFEGVTC IIFCAALSAY DMVLVEDDEV 240

Gustducin   NRMHESLHLF NSICNHKYFA TTSIVLFLNK KDLFQEKVTK VHLSICFPEY TGPNTFEDAG 300
Bovinecone  NRMHESLHLF NSICNHKFFA ATSIVLFLNK KDLFEEKIKK VHLSICFPEY DGNNSYEDAG 300
Bovinerod   NRMHESLHLF NSICNHRYFA TTSIVLFLNK KDVFSEKIKK AHLSICFPDY NGPNTYEDAG 296
Consensus   NRMHESLHLF NSICNHKYFA TTSIVLFLNK KDLF-EKIKK VHLSICFPEY -GPNTYEDAG 300

Gustducin   NYIKNQFLDL NLKKEDKEIY SHMTCATDTQ NVKFVFDAVT DIIIKENLKD CGLF 354
Bovinecone  NYIKSQFLDL NMRKDVKEIY SHMTCATDTQ NVKFVFDAVT DIIIKENLKD CGLF 354
Bovinerod   NYIKVQFLEL NMRRDVKEIY SHMTCATDTQ NVKFVFDAVT DIIIKENLKD CGLF 350
Consensus   NYIK-QFLDL NMRKDVKEIY SHMTCATDTQ NVKFVFDAVT DIIIKENLKD CGLF 354
```

FIGURE 48-12. Alignment of amino acid sequences of α subunits of rat gustducin, bovine rod transducin and bovine cone transducin. Consensus sequence matches, that is, at least two out of the three proteins match, are denoted by *dark orange shading*. Conservative changes are denoted by *light orange shading*. Nonconservative changes are depicted by *unshaded regions*. The consensus line shows positions where at least two of the three proteins match; *dashes* in the consensus sequence correspond to nonconserved positions. *Dots* in the rod transducin sequence correspond to gaps to align it with the other sequences. Note the high degree of conservation of the three sequences throughout their length. The last 38 amino acids of all three proteins are identical; this region has been implicated in receptor interaction. (From [40], with permission.)

its interaction with rhodopsin, suggesting that the taste receptor(s) which interacts with gustducin may have structural similarity to the opsins.

It was proposed that the role of gustducin in taste transduction would be similar to that of transducin in phototransduction [40]. In the retina, transducin relays activation of rhodopsin into activation of phosphodiesterase (PDE) by binding to the inhibitory subunit of PDE. A 22-amino-acid-long portion of rod transducin was recently shown to activate PDE. This effector-activation region is adjacent to the C-terminal receptor-interaction site of transducin: this region of rod and cone transducin is well conserved, 86% identical, 95% similar and, similar to the analogous region of gustducin, 91% similar, consistent with the presumptive role of gustducin as a PDE activator.

It was speculated originally that the role of gustducin in taste transduction is in the bitter pathway [40]. In this model, bitter receptor activation would lead to gustducin activation, which in turn would activate taste cell cAMP PDE and lead to decreased concentrations of taste cell cAMP. This is consistent with the known high concentrations of taste cell PDE, and with the correlation between PDE activators and bitter compounds. Direct evidence for this model has now been obtained from biochemical studies [43], in which it was shown that denatonium and quinine activate gustducin or transducin in the presence of bovine taste cell membranes, suggesting that a bitter receptor couples to gustducin or transducin in taste cells. Further studies identified a taste cell PDE responsive to activation by gustducin or transducin. Spielman and coworkers [44] have shown that denatonium, sucrose octa-acetate and other bitter compounds lead to IP_3 generation in mouse taste tissue. It is presently unclear if this involves gustducin, either its α or $\beta\gamma$ subunits or another G protein, such as G_i or G_{14}.

The gustducin gene has now been "knocked out" by targeted gene replacement [45]. These gustducin null mice had normal responses to salts and acids but reduced responses to bitter stimuli. These data were expected since denatonium activated gustducin in biochemical assays.

What was unexpected was that the null mice also had reduced responses to sweet stimuli. Further studies will be required to determine the role of gustducin in the sweet transduction cascade.

ACKNOWLEDGMENTS

We thank S. K. McLaughlin and R. F. Margolskee for data on G-protein expression.

REFERENCES

1. Shepherd, G. M. Discrimination of molecular signals by the olfactory receptor neuron. *Neuron* 13:771–790, 1994.
2. Firestein, S., Shepherd, G. M., and Werblin, F. S. Time course of the membrane current underlying sensory transduction in salamander olfactory receptor neurones. *J. Physiol.* 430:135–158, 1990.
3. Breer, H. Odor recognition and second messenger signaling in olfactory receptor neurons. *Semin. Cell Biol.* 5:25–32, 1994.
4. Sicard, G., and Holley, A. Receptor cell responses to odorants: Similarities and differences among odorants. *Brain Res.* 292:283–296, 1984.
5. Firestein, S. Electrical signals in olfactory transduction. *Curr. Opin. Neurobiol.* 2:444–448, 1992.
6. Buck, L., and Axel, R. A novel multigene family may encode odorant receptors: A molecular basis for odor recognition. *Cell* 65:175–187, 1991.
7. Dohlman, H. G., Torner, J., Caron, M. G., and Lefkowitz, R. J. Model systems for the study of seven-transmembrane-segment receptors. *Annu. Rev. Biochem.* 60:653–688, 1991.
8. Ressler, K. J., Sullivan, S. L., and Buck, L. B. A zonal organization of odorant receptor gene expression in the olfactory epithelium. *Cell* 73:597–609, 1993.
9. Vassar, R., Ngai, J., and Axel, R. Spatial segregation of odorant receptor expression in the mammalian olfactory epithelium. *Cell* 74:309–318, 1993.
10. Astic, L., Saucier, D., and Holley, A. Topographical relationships between olfactory receptor cells and glomerular foci in the rat olfactory bulb. *Brain Res.* 424:144–152, 1987.
11. Mombaerts, P., Wang, F., Dulac, C., et al. Visualizing an olfactory sensory map. *Cell* 87:675–686, 1996.
12. Axel, R. The molecular logic of smell. *Sci. Am.* 273:154–159, 1995.

13. Mori, K., and Yoshihara, Y. Molecular recognition and olfactory processing in the mammalian olfactory system. *Prog. Neurobiol.* 45:585–619, 1995.

14. Firestein, S., Picco, C., and Menini, A. The relation between stimulus and response in olfactory receptor cells of the tiger salamander. *J. Physiol.* 468:1–10, 1993.

15. Reed, R. R. Signalling pathways in odorant detection. *Neuron* 8:205–209, 1992.

16. Nakamura, T., and Gold, G. H. A cyclic-nucleotide gated conductance in olfactory receptor cilia. *Nature* 325:442–444, 1987.

17. Kurahashi, T., and Yau, K.-W. Tale of an unusual chloride current. *Curr. Biol.* 4:256–258, 1994.

18. Frings, S., Seifert, R., Godde, M., and Kaupp, U. B. Profoundly different calcium permeation and blockage determine the specific function of distinct cyclic nucleotide-gated channels. *Neuron* 15:169–179, 1995.

19. Chen, T.-Y., and Yau, K.-W. Direct modulation by Ca^{2+}-calmodulin of cyclic nucleotide-activated channel of rat olfactory receptor neurons. *Nature* 368:545–548, 1994.

20. Dawson, T. M., Arriza, J. L., Jaworsky, D. E., et al. β-Adrenergic receptor kinase-2 and β-arrestin-2 as mediators of odorant-induced desensitization. *Science* 259:825–829, 1993.

21. Brunet, L. J., Gold, G. H., and Ngai, J. General anosmia caused by a targeted disruption of the mouse olfactory cyclic nucleotide-gated cation channel. *Neuron* 17:681–693, 1996.

22. Fadool, D. A., and Ache, B. W. Plasma membrane inositol 1,4,5-trisphosphate-activated channels mediate signal transduction in lobster olfactory receptor neurons. *Neuron* 9:907–918, 1992.

23. Dulac, C., and Axel, R. A novel family of genes encoding putative pheromone receptors in mammals. *Cell* 83:195–206, 1995.

24. Roper, S. D. The microphysiology of peripheral taste organs. *J. Neurosci.* 12:1127–1134, 1992.

25. Frank, M., and Pfaffmann, C. Taste nerve fibers: A random distribution of sensitivities to four tastes. *Science* 164:1183–1185, 1969.

26. Pfaffmann, C. Gustatory afferent impulses. *J. Cell. Comp. Physiol.* 17:263–258, 1941.

27. Kinnamon, S. C., and Margolskee, R. F. Mechanisms of taste transduction. *Curr. Opin. Neurobiol.* 6:506–513, 1996.

28. Kinnamon, S. C., Dionne, V. E., and Beam, K. G. Apical localization of K^+ channels in taste cells provides the basis for sour taste transduction. *Proc. Natl. Acad. Sci. USA* 85:7023–7027, 1988.

29. Heck, G. L., Mierson, S., and DeSimone, J. A. Salt taste transduction occurs through an amiloride-sensitive sodium transport pathway. *Science* 223:403–405, 1984.

30. Ye, Q., Heck, G. L., and DeSimone, J. A. The anion paradox in sodium reception: Resolution by voltage clamp studies. *Science* 254:724–726, 1991.

31. Ossebaard, C. A., and Smith, D. V. Effect of amiloride on the taste of NaCl, Na-gluconate and KCl in humans: Implications for Na^+ receptor mechanisms. *Chem. Senses* 20:37–46, 1995.

32. Gilbertson, T. A., Avenet, P., Kinnamon, S. C., and Roper, S. D. Proton currents through amiloride-sensitive Na channels in hamster taste cells: Role in acid transduction. *J. Gen. Physiol.* 100:803–824, 1992.

33. Bruch, R. C., and Kalinoski, D. L. Interaction of GTP-binding regulatory proteins with chemosensory receptors. *J. Biol. Chem.* 262:2404, 1987.

34. Striem, B. J., Pace, U., Zehavi, U., Naim, M., and Lancet, D. Sweet tastants stimulate adenylate cyclase coupled to GTP binding protein in rat tongue membranes. *Biochem. J.* 260:121–126, 1989.

35. Tonosaki, K., and Funakoshi, M. Cyclic nucleotides may mediate taste transduction. *Nature* 331:354–356, 1988.

36. Avenet, P., Hofmann, F., and Lindemann, B. Transduction in taste receptor cells requires cAMP-dependent protein kinase. *Nature* 331:351–354, 1988.

37. Bernhardt, S. J., Naim, M., Zehavi, U., and Lindemann, B. Changes in IP_3 and cytosolic Ca^{2+} in response to sugars and non-sugar sweeteners in transduction of sweet taste in the rat. *J. Physiol.* 490:325–336, 1996.

38. Cummings, T. A., Daniels, C., and Kinnamon, S. C. Sweet taste transduction in hamster: Sweeteners and cyclic nucleotides depolarize taste cells by reducing a K^+ current. *J. Neurophysiol.* 75:1256–1263, 1996.

39. Akabas, M. H., Dodd, J., and Al-Awqati, Q. A bitter substance induces a rise in intracellular calcium in a subpopulation of rat taste cells. *Science* 242:1047–1050, 1988.

40. McLaughlin, S. K., McKinnon, P. J., and Margolskee, R. F. Gustducin is a taste-cell-specific G protein closely related to the transducins. *Nature* 357:563–569, 1992.

41. Chaudhari, N., Yang, H., Lamp, C., et al. The taste of MSG: Membrane receptors in taste buds. *J. Neurosci.* 16:3817–3826, 1996.

42. Hoefer, D., Pueschel, B., and Drenckhahn, D. Taste receptor-like cells in the rat gut identified by

expression of alpha-gustducin. *Proc. Natl. Acad. Sci. USA* 93:6631–6634, 1996.

43. Ruiz-Avila, L., McLaughlin, S. K., Wildman, D., et al. Coupling of bitter receptor to phosphodiesterase through transducin in taste receptor cells. *Nature* 376:80–85, 1995.

44. Spielman, A. I., Nagai, G., Sunavala, G., et al. Rapid kinetics of second messenger production in bitter taste. *Am. J. Physiol.* 270:C926–C931, 1996.

45. Wong, G. T., Gannon, K. S., and Margolskee, R. F. Transduction of bitter and sweet by gustducin. *Nature* 381:796–800, 1996.

49

Endocrine Effects on the Brain and Their Relationship to Behavior

Bruce S. McEwen

Basic Neurochemistry: Molecular, Cellular and Medical Aspects, 6th Ed., edited by G. J. Siegel et al. Published by Lippincott–Raven Publishers, Philadelphia, 1999. Correspondence to Bruce S. McEwen, Laboratory of Neuroendocrinology, Rockefeller University, 1230 York Avenue, New York, New York 10021.

The brain undergoes changes in its chemistry and structure in response to changes in the environment. Circulating hormones of the adrenals, thyroid and gonads play an important role in this adaptation because the endocrine system is controlled by the brain through the pituitary gland (Fig. 49-1). This control allows environmental signals to regulate hormonal secretion. Furthermore, circulating hormones act on the brain as well as on other tissues and organs of the

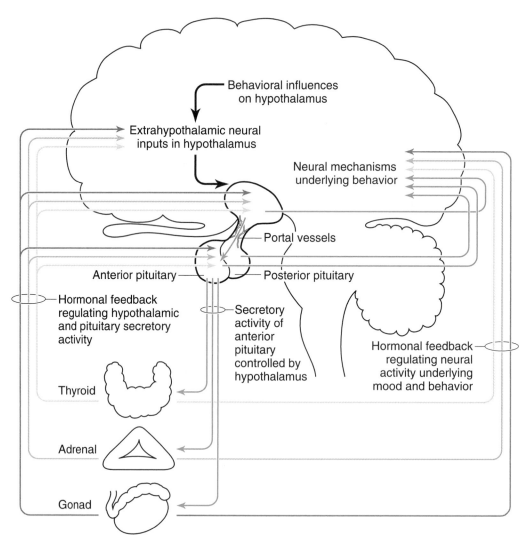

FIGURE 49-1. Schematic representation of possible and known reciprocal interactions among hypothalamic, pituitary, thyroid, adrenal and gonadal hormones.

body to modify their structure and chemistry via two mechanisms: (i) intracellular receptors that bind to DNA and alter gene expression and (ii) cell-surface receptors that modulate ion channels and second-messenger systems.

Hormonal actions occur during sensitive periods in development, in adult life during natural endocrine cycles and in response to experience as well as during the aging process (see Chap. 30). As a result of their fundamental actions on cellular processes and genomic activity and of the control of their secretion by environmental signals, steroid and thyroid hormone actions on the brain provide unique insights into the plasticity of the brain and behavior (see also Chap. 50).

Awareness of endocrine influences on brain function is as old as endocrinology itself. In 1849, Berthold described striking behavioral changes resulting from castration of roosters and the reversal of these changes after testes had been transplanted into the castrated animals (see [1]). Nearly 100 years later, Beach published *Hormones and Behavior* (see [1]), which has served to instruct generations of investigators and to motivate them to explore in depth the interactions of hormones and brain. Spectacular growth of the field of neuroendocrinology (see also Chap. 18) offers the present generation of neurobiologists unparalleled opportunities to explore with great sophistication the influence of neural activity on endocrine secretion and the effect of hormones, in turn, on neural activity and behavior.

This chapter focuses on the neurochemical and molecular aspects of the influences of hormones on the nervous system and behavior, after first considering the chemical signals, behavioral events and underlying neural activity that regulate hormonal secretion.

BEHAVIORAL CONTROL OF HORMONAL SECRETION

The hypothalamic releasing factors regulate release of the anterior pituitary trophic hormones

As summarized in Figure 49-1, the releasing factors are produced in various neuronal groups within the hypothalamus and are transported to the median eminence for release into the portal circulation to the anterior pituitary. Neurons in the hypothalamus also produce the hormones oxytocin and vasopressin, which are released by the posterior pituitary into the blood. Therefore, it is not surprising that behavior and experience, which influence the hypothalamus, sometimes alter the secretion of these hypothalamic releasing factors and hormones.

Secretion of pituitary hormones is responsive to behavior and effects of experience

Consider, for example, the phenomenon of lactation, in which the sucking stimulus to the nipple triggers the release of oxytocin, which facilitates milk ejection, and of prolactin, which helps the mammary gland to replenish the supply of milk [2]. The phenomenon of stress also illustrates the behavioral and emotional control of anterior pituitary hormone secretion. Conditions associated with tissue injury and surgical trauma, as well as the so-called psychic stresses of fear, novelty and even joy, can activate the release of adrenocorticotropic hormone (ACTH), which in turn stimulates the secretion of adrenal glucocorticoids [2]. The behavioral–emotional stimuli are mediated by neural pathways that can be modified readily by learning.

In the female rabbit, copulation activates spinal reflex pathways that stimulate the secretion of luteinizing hormone (LH), which leads to ovulation [3]. In the male rabbit, copulation also activates the secretion of LH and increases plasma testosterone [3]. Social stimuli also modify gonadotropin secretion. Olfactory cues between female mice can interrupt normal estrous cycles and lead to pseudopregnancies or to periods of prolonged diestrus, termed the *Lee-Boot effect*; olfactory cues from male mice can shorten the estrous cycle and either cause rapid attainment of estrus, termed the *Whitten effect,* or terminate pregnancy in a newly impregnated mouse, termed the *Bruce effect* [3]. In male rhesus monkeys, sudden, decisive defeat by other males leads to prolonged reduction in plasma testosterone, which can be reversed in the defeated male by the introduction of a female companion [3]. In men, the anticipation of sexual intercourse has been reported to increase beard growth, a process under the control of circulating androgen [3], although this finding has not been documented.

Hormones secreted in response to behavioral signals act in turn on the brain and on other tissues

Functional changes caused by hormones secreted in response to behavioral signals include modifications of behavior. With the sex hormones, these changes strengthen and guide the reproductive process. Thus, aggressive encounters between male birds or mammals in defense of territory during the mating period stimulate gonadotropin and testosterone secretion. Increases in these hormones further increase readiness for sexual activity by enhancing supplies of sperm and seminal fluid. This analysis was taken further by Lehrman (see [1]), who showed that among doves the behavioral sequence of courtship, mating, nest building and parenting involves complex behavioral interplay between the partners that triggers further hormonal secretion, which unfolds the next phase of behavior and hormonal secretion.

Regarding the adrenal steroids, the behavioral activation of hormonal secretion in stress is part of a mechanism for restoring homeostatic balance. For example, an encounter with a predator may require rapid evasive action in which neural activity and rapidly mobilized hormones such as epinephrine play a role. Adrenal steroid secretion is slower, reaching a peak minutes after the stressful event, and as such is not expected to play a role in coping with the immediate situation. If the evasive action is successful and the animal survives, it will have to re-establish homeostasis; presumably, it also will learn from the experience to minimize the chances of another such encounter. Adrenal steroids facilitate such long-term adaptation; that is, they facilitate the extinction of a conditioned avoidance response [4]. Suppose an animal has learned to avoid a certain place where previously it was punished; it later discovers that being in that place no longer results in punishment. If, for example, that place also contains a food or water supply, it is in the best interest of the animal to

extinguish the avoidance response in order to take advantage of the available food or water. Adrenal steroids have, in fact, been found to facilitate such extinction and, thus, can be said to facilitate a form of behavioral adaptation [4]. Adrenal steroids also appear to play a role in both selective attention and consolidation of a variety of learned information related to episodes or events in daily life [5]. Another aspect of adaptation in which stress-induced secretion of adrenal steroids participates concerns the ability of the organism to cope with a repeated stressful event through a variety of neurochemical changes [6].

Besides stress, adrenal steroids are secreted in varying amounts according to the time of day, and in this capacity they perform an important role in coordinating daily activity and sleep patterns with food-seeking and processing of information [3]. In nocturnally active animals, such as the rat, adrenal steroids are secreted at the end of the light period prior to onset of darkness. In humans and monkeys, adrenal steroid secretion precedes waking in the morning to begin daily activity. In both rats and primates, adrenal steroid secretion precedes the waking period and appears to contribute, during waking, to optimal synaptic efficacy in the hippocampus for long-term potentiation, a correlate of learning. It is this aspect of adrenal steroid action that contributes to enhanced attention and improved retention of episodic memories [5] (see Chap. 50). Moreover, adrenal steroid elevation prior to waking also increases food-seeking behavior and enhances appetite for carbohydrates [6].

Cyclic changes in hormonal secretion, which are under the control of daily and seasonal light–dark rhythms, are important not only for the adrenals but for the gonads as well. Estrous cycles, menstrual cycles and seasonal breeding patterns represent adaptations of individual species to climatic conditions of the environment. The feedback actions of gonadal and adrenal hormones, which are secreted in response to rhythmic output of hypothalamic and pituitary hormones, prime or activate the nervous system to perform the appropriate behavioral responses. It is important to stress that hormones themselves do not cause behaviors; rather, hormones induce chemical changes in particular sets of neurons, making certain behavioral outcomes more likely as a result of the strengthening or weakening of particular neural pathways.

CLASSIFICATION OF HORMONAL EFFECTS

Hormonal actions on target neurons are classified in terms of cellular mechanisms of action

Hormones act either via cell-surface or intracellular receptors. Peptide hormones and amino acid derivatives, such as epinephrine, act on cell-surface receptors that do such things as open ion channels, cause rapid electrical responses and facilitate exocytosis of hormones or neurotransmitters. Alternatively, they activate second-messenger systems at the cell membrane, such as those involving cAMP, Ca^{2+}/calmodulin or phosphoinositides (see Chaps. 20–24), which leads to phosphorylation of proteins inside various parts of the target cell (Fig. 49-2A). Steroid hormones and thyroid hormone, on the other hand, act on intracellular receptors in cell nuclei to regulate gene expression and protein synthesis (Fig. 49-2B). Steroid hormones can also affect cell-surface events via receptors at or near the cell surface.

The various modes of hormonal action summarized in Figure 49-2 may be distinguished from each other by time course. The fastest effects, in both latency and duration, are those involving direct opening of ion channels and stimulation of exocytosis. Intermediate effects involve phosphorylation of enzymes, ion channels, receptors or structural proteins, which may last for minutes or even hours. The slowest and most enduring effects are those that alter gene expression and lead to induction or repression of enzyme or receptor proteins, growth responses and even the structural remodeling of tissues.

As summarized in Figure 49-3, steroid/thyroid hormone receptors bind to other proteins as well as to DNA [7–9]. In the simplest type of action (Fig. 49-3A), the steroid/thyroid hormone receptor becomes activated after the hormone binds to it; activation results in conformational changes that include shedding of other proteins, such as heat-shock proteins, and exposing the DNA-binding domain. The receptor then binds to the specific sequence of DNA, called a "hormone-response element" or enhancer, located on the coding strand of DNA;

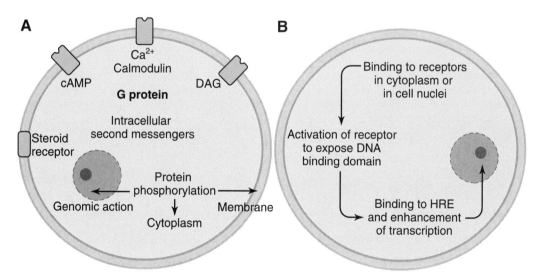

FIGURE 49-2. There are two modes of hormonal action. **A:** Activation of cell-surface receptors and coupled second-messenger systems, with a variety of intracellular consequences. **B:** Entry of hormone into the target cell, binding to and activation of an intracellular receptor and binding of the receptor–hormone complex to specific DNA sequences to activate or repress gene expression. *DAG*, diacylglycerol; *HRE*, hormone-response element.

A

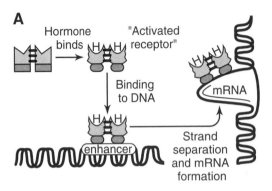

B

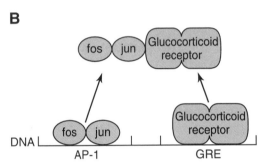

C

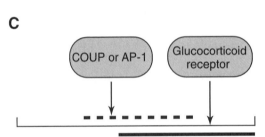

FIGURE 49-3. Intracellular receptors mediate at least three distinct types of actions on gene expression. **A:** Binding of the hormone–receptor complex to a hormone-response element, a DNA sequence that is placed in a position where receptor binding to it can enhance unwinding of the double helix and attachment of other transcription factors. **B:** Binding of the steroid receptor to another protein transcription factor, for example, the *fos–jun* complex through protein–protein interactions, removing both transcription factors from binding to DNA. *GRE,* glucocorticoid response element. **C:** Binding of the hormone receptor to a hormone-response element located in the middle of a site for binding of another transcription factor-response element, such as the adaptor protein-1 (AP-1) or chicken ovalbumin upstream promoter-transcription factor (COUP) sites, resulting in inhibition of transcription normally activated by transcription factors acting on these response elements (see [6–8]).

this enhances transcription by permitting other transcription factors as well as the RNA polymerase to bind to the promoter region [7–9]. A second scheme (Fig. 49-3B) is for the hormone receptor to bind with high affinity to another protein transcription factor, in this case the c-fos–c-jun complex, removing both protein complexes from binding to DNA [7–9]. Such a result also blocks the enhancement of transcription by either agent, although it also could reduce inhibitory effects produced by the hormone receptor through the scheme shown in Figure 49-3C. A variant on this theme, not shown in the figure, is "squelching," in which multiple transcription factors compete with each other for a limited supply of soluble ligands that enhance their activities [7–9]. A third scheme, shown in Figure 49-3C, is for the steroid receptor to compete with another transcription factor for binding sites in the promoter regions. These other factors may be COUP or the cAMP-dependent transcription factors that bind to the adapter protein-1 (AP-1) response element. The result of this competition is inhibition of transcription since, in this situation, the other transcription factor enhances transcription, whereas the hormone receptor does not do so when it binds to the coding DNA strand [7–9].

As we have noted, second-messenger systems, through phosphorylation of nuclear proteins, can influence gene expression. There is evidence that even the classical steroid receptors are subject to regulation by phosphorylation and that phosphorylations promoted by a neurotransmitter such as dopamine (Chap. 12) are able to cause nuclear translocation of a steroid receptor in the absence of the steroid [10].

So far, the best understood examples of genomic regulation of neuronal function stem from the actions of gonadal and adrenal steroids and thyroid hormone, and many of these actions are involved in the plasticity of behavior that results from hormonal secretion, such as changes in aggressive and reproductive behavior and adaptation to repeated stress. In fact, hormonal actions that involve the genome are pervasive throughout the life cycle.

We can distinguish four major types of hormonal actions on the nervous system: (i) *developmental actions,* such as those involved in sexual differentiation and the effects of thyroid hormone and retinoic acid; (ii) *reversible, and often cyclical, effects* on the structure and function of neurons and glial cells that underlie corresponding cyclical changes in behavior, such as in reproduction and the daily rhythms of sleep and waking; (iii) *experiential effects* involving environmentally induced changes in hormonal secretion that evoke adaptive or maladaptive changes in the brain, as in stress; and (iv) *effects that protect neurons or potentiate damage* and lead to cell death.

It will be seen below that, in addition to genomic actions, there are nongenomic effects of steroids that modulate neurotransmitter release as well as ion traffic across the cell membrane and do so frequently in coordination with genomic actions.

BIOCHEMISTRY OF STEROID AND THYROID HORMONE ACTIONS

Steroid hormones are divided into six classes, based on physiological effects: estrogens, androgens, progestins, glucocorticoids, mineralocorticoids and vitamin D

As shown in Figures 49-2 and 49-3, steroid hormone action on the brain and on other target tissues involves intracellular receptor sites that interact with the genome [1]. There are also important metabolic transformations of certain steroids, occurring in the nervous system, that either generate more active metabolites or result in the production of less active steroids. Such transformations are particularly important for the actions of androgens, of lesser importance for estrogens and progestins and of practically no importance for glucocorticoids and mineralocorticoids. For vitamin D, the principal transformation to an active metabolite occurs in the kidney and liver [11]. Some metabolites, such as allopregnanolone and allotetrahydrodeoxycorticosterone, produce nongenomic effects on the $GABA_A$ receptor.

Some steroid hormones are converted in the brain to more or less active products that interact with receptors

The brain, like the seminal vesicles, is able to reduce testosterone to 5α-dihydrotestosterone (DHT); and, like the placenta, the brain aromatizes testosterone to estradiol (Fig. 49-4). Neither conversion occurs equally in all brain regions. The aromatization reaction is discussed below. Regional distribution of 5α-reductase activity toward testosterone in rat brain reveals that the highest activity is found in midbrain and brainstem, intermediate activity is found in the hypothalamus and thalamus and the lowest activity is found in the cerebral cortex [12]. The pituitary has higher α-reductase activity than any region of the brain, and its activity is subject to changes as a result of gonadectomy, hormone replacement and postnatal age [3,12]. 5α-DHT has been implicated in the hypothalamus and pituitary as a potent regulator of gonadotropin secretion, but it is relatively inactive toward male rat sexual behavior [3]. Labeled metabolites with Rf values of 5α-DHT have been detected in extracts of hypothalamic and pituitary tissue after [³H]-testosterone administration in both adult and newborn rats. It is interesting that progesterone inhibits 5α-reductase activity toward [³H]testosterone and that [³H]progesterone is converted to [³H]5α-dihydroprogesterone (Fig. 49-4). Progesterone competition for 5α-reductase may explain some of the antiandrogenicity of this steroid [3,12]. 5β-DHT is a metabolite of testosterone formed in the avian CNS, as is 5αDHT. 5β-DHT is inactive toward sexual behavior and is believed to represent an inactivation pathway for testosterone.

The aromatization of testosterone to form estradiol, and of androstenedione to form estrone (Fig. 49-4), has been described in brain tissue *in vitro* and *in vivo* [12]. Aromatization is higher in hypothalamus and limbic structures than in cerebral cortex or pituitary gland, and, in noncastrated animals, it is higher in the male than in the female brain. Aromatization has been found in reptile and amphibian brain as well as in mammalian brain [12]. The capacity to aromatize testosterone and related androgens, therefore, may be a general property of vertebrate

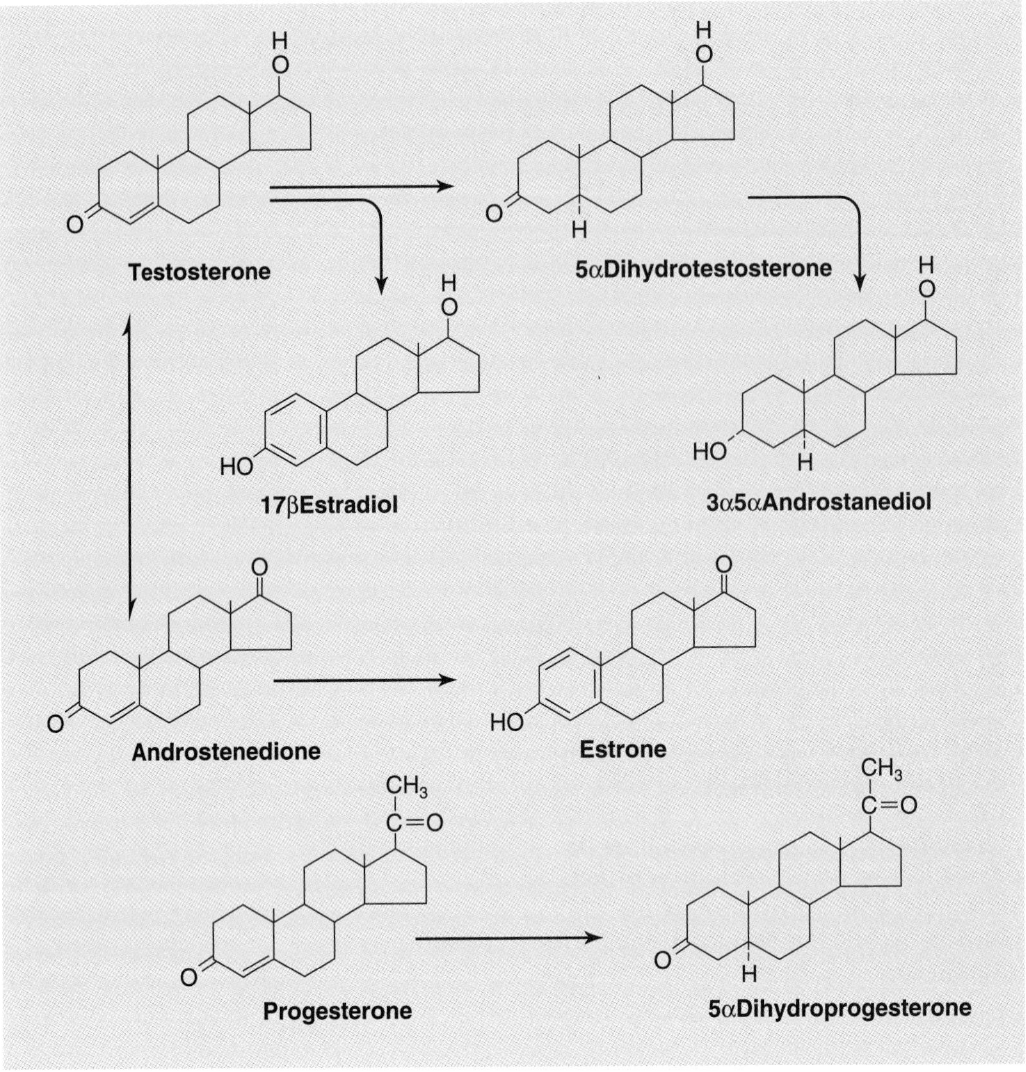

FIGURE 49-4.   Some steroid transformations that are carried out by neural tissue.

brains. The functional role of aromatization has been studied most extensively in the rat. Male sexual behavior is facilitated by estradiol [13], and testosterone facilitation of male sexual behavior can be blocked by a steroidal inhibitor of aromatization [3,12,13]. There are indications that a similar situation exists in birds, amphibians and reptiles; that is, testosterone and estradiol can stimulate male and female heterotypical sexual behavior. Curiously, not all mammals are like the rat; for example, male sexual behavior of guinea pig and rhesus monkey is restored by the nonaromatizable androgen DHT [3,13].

Both aromatization and 5α-reductase are regulated by gonadal steroids. In mammals such as the rat, it is principally the neural aromatase activity that is upregulated by androgens acting via neural androgen receptors [14]. In birds, both neural aromatase and 5α-reductase are induced by testosterone, and this regulation provides a way by which androgens can regulate CNS hormone sensitivity without regulating receptor number [15].

Both estrogens and glucocorticoids appear to act on brain cells without first being metabolized because both [³H]estradiol and [³H]corti-

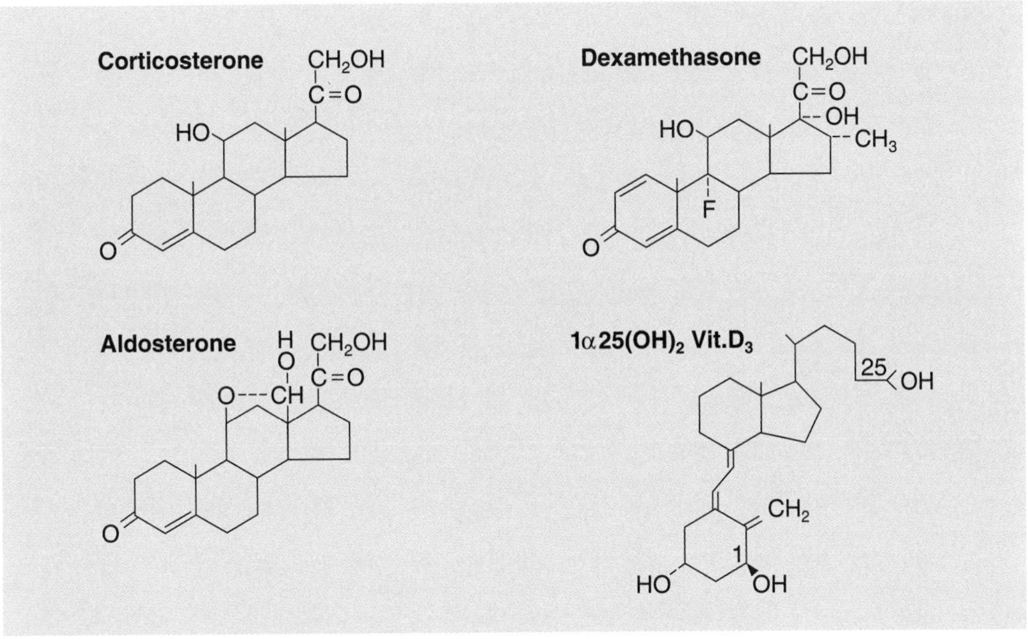

FIGURE 49-5.   Formulas of four steroid hormones.

costerone are recovered unchanged from their cell nuclear binding sites in brain [3]. However, estradiol is subject to conversion to the catechol estrogen 2-hydroxyestradiol, and this metabolite is both a moderately potent estrogen via intracellular estrogen receptors as well as an agent capable of interacting with cell-surface receptors such as those for catecholamines, albeit at fairly high concentrations [16] (see Chap. 12).

Vitamin D, prior to acting in the brain, is converted to an active metabolite, 1,25-dihydroxy vitamin D_3, by enzymes in liver and kidney [11] (see Fig. 49-5). The nervous system also is capable of cleaving the side chain from cholesterol to generate the same initial series of steroids [17] that are produced by the adrenals and gonads, namely, pregnenolone, dehydroepiandrosterone and progesterone (Fig. 49-6). In addition, neural tissue converts progesterone via reduction of the Δ4-5 double bond and reduction of the 3 keto group to 3α,5α-pregnanolone, which is active on the chloride channel of the $GABA_A$ receptor [18] (Fig. 49-7). Glial cells are believed to be the primary sites of both cholesterol side-chain cleavage and generation of pregnanolone from progesterone [17]. While steroids generated in

the brain have been referred to as "neurosteroids," a more useful term is "neuroactive steroids" to refer to all steroids that affect brain function via any mechanism and irrespective of site of formation. The term *neuroactive steroid* also has been used to describe neuroactive steroid drugs.

Genomic receptors for steroid hormones have been clearly identified in the nervous system

The detection of intracellular, DNA-binding steroid receptors became possible with the introduction of tritium-labeled steroid hormones of high specific radioactivity: 20 to 25 Ci/mmol at each labeled position. The limited number of these sites had escaped detection using steroids labeled with ^{14}C at a much lower specific radioactivity. Tritium labeling also permitted histological localization of steroid receptors because the high spatial resolution of ^{3}H, 1 to 2 μm in light-microscopic autoradiography, allows cellular and even cell nuclear localization of the radioactivity.

Cell fractionation procedures were fundamental to the biochemical identification of

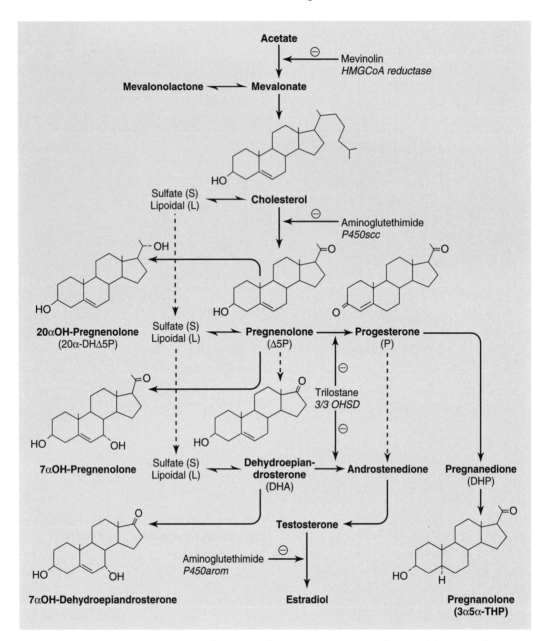

FIGURE 49-6.   Biosynthesis/metabolism of steroids in the CNS. The conversion of Δ5P to dehydroepiandrosterone (DHA) is postulated but not demonstrated. Δ5P and DHA inhibit and 3α,5α-THP potentiates GABA_A receptor function, as summarized in Figure 49-7. *Solid arrows* indicate demonstrated pathways; *dotted arrows* indicate possible pathways. Metabolic inhibitors of enzymes are indicated by ⊖. (Redrawn from [40], with permission.)

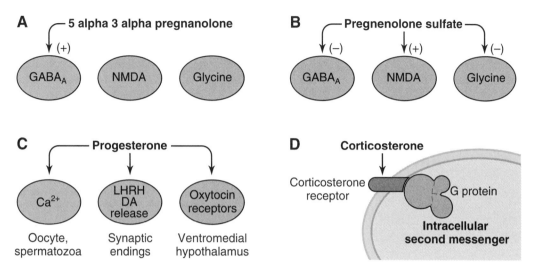

FIGURE 49-7. Schematic summary of four ways in which steroids affect cell surface-mediated events and neuronal activity by nongenomic mechanisms. **A:** Activation of GABA$_A$ receptor by 5α,3α-pregnanolone. **B:** Activation of NMDA receptor and inhibition of GABA$_A$ and glycine receptors by pregnenolone sulfate. **C:** Activation of Ca^{2+} mobilization in oocytes and spermatozoa by progesterone; the same is postulated to happen in certain synaptic endings and may be involved in the rapid, direct effect of progesterone on the oxytocin receptor. **D:** Corticosterone binds to a cell surface receptor linked to a G protein, and presumably through it to a second-messenger system, in some brain cells. *DA*, dopamine; *LHRH*, luteinizing hormone releasing hormone; *NMDA*, N-methyl-D-aspartate.

steroid and thyroid hormone receptors in brain as well as in other tissues. Isolation of highly purified cell nuclei from small amounts of tissue from discrete brain regions generally is accomplished with the aid of a nonionic detergent, such as Triton X-100 [19]. Cytosolic fractions of brain tissue, prepared by centrifugation of homogenates at 105,000 g for 60 min, contain the soluble steroid hormone-binding proteins, and a variety of methods intended to separate bound from unbound steroid have been used for measuring their binding activity [3,19]. The most commonly employed are gel filtration chromatography and sucrose density gradient centrifugation. Dextran-coated charcoal or Sephadex LH20 are frequently used because they effectively absorb unbound steroid and leave intact the complexes between steroid and putative receptor. Other methods, such as gel electrophoresis and precipitation of putative receptor material with protamine sulfate, have more restricted uses.

The objective of such studies is to measure the affinity, capacity and specificity of the hormone–receptor interaction [3,19]. Measure-

ments of affinity and capacity are accomplished with equilibrium binding analysis. Specificity is based on competition between the labeled and various unlabeled ligands for binding sites.

Because the nervous system is highly heterogeneous from the standpoint of many neurochemical characteristics, including steroid and thyroid hormone receptors, the most useful techniques for mapping these receptors have been histochemical. Steroid autoradiography was the first such method. With purification of receptors and generation of antibodies, immunocytochemistry has been added as a tool. Cloning of steroid and thyroid receptors has opened the way to mapping of receptor mRNAs via *in situ* hybridization histochemistry.

Several criteria determine whether a steroid hormone-binding site is a putative receptor. First, the steroid hormone-binding site must be present in hormone-responsive tissues or brain regions and absent from nonresponsive ones. Second, it should bind steroids that are either active agonists or effective antagonists of the hormone effect and should not bind steroids that are inactive in either sense.

There is an ongoing controversy regarding intracellular localization of steroid and thyroid hormone receptors in cells. With the exception of thyroid hormone receptors, which are exclusively nuclear in location, cell fractionation studies have revealed that in the absence of hormone, steroid receptors are extracted in the soluble or cytosolic fraction. However, when steroid is present in the cell, many occupied receptors are retained by purified cell nuclei. Histological procedures, such as immunocytochemistry, have confirmed the largely nuclear localization of occupied receptors, but they also have revealed a nuclear localization of receptors in the absence of hormone in the tissue. This is true for estrogen, progestin and androgen receptors, but the mineralocorticoid and glucocorticoid receptors show a cytoplasmic localization in the absence of hormone. Thus, steroid receptors may exist in nuclei in a loose association that is disrupted during cell fractionation. This is not an uncommon situation for many constituents of cell nuclei [19].

INTRACELLULAR STEROID RECEPTORS: PROPERTIES AND TOPOGRAPHY

Steroid hormone receptors are phosphoproteins that have a DNA-binding domain and a steroid-binding domain

All steroid receptors have a molecular weight of 55,000 to 120,000. The state of phosphorylation appears to influence functional activity.

Estradiol. The first neuroactive steroid receptor type to be recognized was that for estradiol [1]. *In vivo* uptake of [^{3}H] estradiol and binding to cell nuclei isolated from hypothalamus, pituitary and other brain regions revealed steroid specificity closely resembling that of the uterus, where steroid receptors were first discovered [1]. Cytosolic estrogen receptors isolated from pituitary and brain tissue closely resemble those found in uterus and mammary tissue. A hallmark of the estrogen receptor is its existence as an aggregate of subunits that dissociate during steroid-in-

duced transformation to the DNA-binding nuclear form of the receptor. This part of the estrogen receptor complex was cloned from human breast cancer cells and consists of a 65- to 70-kDa hormone and DNA-binding subunit [6,20]. The dissociation constant of estradiol binding is approximately 0.2 nM.

Estrogen receptors are found in the adult pituitary, hypothalamus, preoptic area and amygdala. They are principally in neurons, although glial cells also may express these receptors in some brain regions [1]. The developing rat brain expresses estrogen receptors in cerebral cortex and hippocampus, but these receptors largely disappear as the brain matures [21]. A newly described second form of the estrogen receptor, the β-estrogen receptor, is similar to the α form in affinity and specificity but different in tissue distribution [22].

Progesterone receptors in brain were detected using the synthetic progestin R5020 (promegestrone; 17α, 21-dimethyl-19-nor-pregna-4,9-diene-3,20-dione), which has a high affinity for the progestin receptor, with a K_d of 0.4 nM [23]. The progestin receptor, cloned from chick oviduct, consists of a steroid- and DNA-binding subunit of 108 kDa, although one 79-kDa subunit has also been described [6,20]. Progestin receptors with similar properties are found in pituitary, reproductive tract and most estrogen receptor-containing brain regions; these receptors are inducible by estrogen treatment [23]. There are also progestin receptor sites in brain areas lacking estrogen receptors, such as the cerebral cortex of the rat; these receptors are not induced by estradiol treatment. Nevertheless, such receptors resemble those induced by estradiol [23]. Another inducer of progestin receptors in brain is testosterone, which works through its conversion to estradiol via aromatization [23]. Progesterone acts rapidly to induce feminine sexual behavior, termed lordosis, in female rats that have been primed with estradiol to induce progestin receptors [23]. The principal site of estradiol and progesterone action is the ventromedial nucleus of the hypothalamus [1].

Androgen receptors have a steroid-binding subunit estimated to be 120 kDa [6,20]. The estimated K_d for active androgens is approximately 1 to 2 nM [1]. Androgen receptors are widely distributed in brain and pituitary tissue, although highest concentrations are found in hypothalamus, preoptic area and limbic brain tissue [24]. Androgen receptors are deficient in the androgen-insensitivity (Tfm) mutation, and animals with this mutation show defects in sexual behavior, juvenile rough-and-tumble play behavior and certain aspects of neuroendocrine function, thus indicating the actions of testosterone that are mediated by androgen receptors, as opposed to those mediated by aromatization of testosterone to estradiol (see above) and estrogen receptors [12].

Glucocorticoid. Adrenal steroid receptors have been subdivided into two categories, one of which is the classical glucocorticoid receptor [4]. This receptor, cloned from human and rat sources, consists of a steroid- and DNA-binding subunit of 95 kDa [6,20]. Such receptors, which have dissociation constants of 4 to 5 nM for glucocorticoids, are widely distributed across brain regions and are found in neurons and glial cells [4].

Mineralocorticoid. The other type of glucocorticoid receptor is similar to the mineralocorticoid receptor originally described in the kidney [4]. In the brain, receptors of this type bind the glucocorticoid corticosterone with high affinity, having a K_d of approximately 1 nM, and they are responsible for the high uptake of tracer levels of [^{3}H]-corticosterone by the hippocampus [4]. These corticosterone receptors, which are found in high concentrations in the hippocampus but are also widely distributed in other brain regions at lower concentrations, may be involved in mediating the effects of diurnally varying concentrations of corticosterone [5]. Uptake of [^{3}H]aldosterone by brain tissues reveals two types of binding sites: those in the hippocampus, which can be occupied preferentially by corticosterone, and those more diffusely distributed in the brain, which appear to retain [^{3}H]aldosterone preferentially in the presence of the normally higher concentrations of corticosterone [4]. The reasons for this selectivity of an enzyme, 11β-hydroxysteroid dehydrogenase, are that, at least in the kidney-

collecting tubules, it converts corticosterone to an inactive metabolite and allows aldosterone access to the mineralocorticoid receptors [24].

Vitamin D is a steroid hormone, production of which by the body requires the action of light. Therefore, it is often necessary to provide some vitamin D in the diet [11] (see Chap. 33). Moreover, vitamin D is converted by the kidney and liver to the active metabolite 1,25-dihydroxyvitamin D_3 (Fig. 49-5) [11]. Vitamin D_3 receptors consist of a hormone- and DNA-binding subunit of 55 kDa [7,20]. Receptor sites for 1,25-dihydroxyvitamin D_3 are found in pituitary and brain, especially in the forebrain, hindbrain and spinal cord neurons [25]. In the brain, one site containing vitamin D_3 receptors, the bed nucleus of the stria terminalis, responds to exogenous 1,25-dihydroxyvitamin D_3 with an induction of choline acetyltransferase, even though the calcium-binding protein that is regulated by vitamin D_3 in the intestine is not regulated by this hormone in the brain [26]. Moreover, vitamin D_3 also corrects deficiencies in serum testosterone and LH in vitamin D-deficient male rats [26]. It is not clear, however, whether this represents a major effect of vitamin D_3 in the pituitary gland or brain or both.

IDENTIFICATION OF MEMBRANE STEROID RECEPTORS

The known rapid effects of some steroid hormones on neuronal excitability are difficult to explain in terms of genomic action [18]. Instead, some type of membrane receptor interaction is inferred. Indeed, several types of interaction between neuroactive steroids and neural membranes have been described. Direct binding assays have revealed membrane sites for glucocorticoids and gonadal steroids and one instance of a membrane receptor coupled to a G protein (Fig. 49-7). Additionally, indirect binding assay results have implied interaction of the catechol estrogens with dopamine and with adrenergic receptors [18].

There are now indications for the interaction of progesterone metabolites with the Cl$^-$ channel of the GABA$_A$ receptor (Fig. 49-7). The A-ring-reduced steroids, especially those with the $5\alpha,3\alpha$ configuration, are particularly active on the $GABA_A$ receptor [18]. By facilitating chloride channel opening, these steroids produce anesthetic, anxiolytic and sedative–hypnotic effects (see Chap. 16).

Another "neurosteroid" (Fig. 49-6), pregnenolone sulfate (PS), produces effects that in many ways antagonize those of the steroids that open the $GABA_A$ receptor Cl^- channel [17,18]. PS in micromolar concentrations inhibits the $GABA_A$ receptor and the inhibitory glycine receptor and facilitates activity of the excitatory *N*-methyl-D-aspartate (NMDA) receptor (Fig. 49-7). It is unclear, however, whether these effects are physiologically relevant, since the PS concentration needed to produce them is rather high. However, PS is produced locally in the brain and may reach sufficiently high concentrations in some compartments within the nervous system.

Progesterone also produces direct membrane effects [18]. These include actions that promote maturation of spermatozoa as well as oocytes and facilitation of the release of neurotransmitters such as dopamine and LH-releasing hormone (LHRH) (Fig. 49-7). Membrane actions of progesterone also activate oxytocin receptors in the hypothalamus in a way that enables oxytocin to turn on sexual behavior in the estrogen-primed female rat [1].

None of these findings undermines the importance of the intracellular genomic actions of steroids. Rather, they increase the richness of the cellular actions of steroid hormones and raise the possibility that there may be connections between genomic and nongenomic actions of steroids. For example, genomic action may induce receptors that mediate nongenomic effects. Moreover, the activation of oxytocin receptors by progesterone is dependent on the ability of estrogen priming to induce the formation of new oxytocin receptors via a genomic mechanism; these receptors are then transported along dendrites to sites where the progesterone action occurs at the membrane level [1].

BIOCHEMISTRY OF THYROID HORMONE ACTIONS ON BRAIN

Like steroid hormones, thyroid hormones interact with receptors to alter genomic activity and affect the synthesis of specific proteins during development [27]. As with testosterone and progesterone, metabolic transformation of thyroxine (T_4) is critical to its action [27]. Moreover, as with steroid hormones, thyroid hormones alter brain functions in adult life in ways that both resemble and differ from their action during development [27,28].

The initial step after cellular uptake of T_4 is metabolic transformation to 3,5,3'-tri-iodothyronine (T_3) (Fig. 49-8), which interacts with cytosolic and nuclear receptors, as well as with synaptosomal membrane binding sites of unknown function [27]. Cytosolic receptors are proteins of 70 kDa that do not appear to undergo translocation to cell nuclei, nor do they appear to be nuclear proteins that have leaked out of cell nuclei during cell rupture; nuclear receptors are proteins of 50 to 70 kDa that have both DNA- and hormone-binding domains [27]. Evidence points to homology between the nuclear T_3 receptor and the *c-erb-A* gene, the cellular counterpart of the viral oncogene v-*erb-A* [7,20].

Nuclear T_3 receptors are present in higher levels during neural development than they are in adult life [27]. In human fetal brain, nuclear T_3 receptors increase in concentration from 10 weeks of gestation to the 16th week, when neuroblast multiplication is high [29]. Glial cells as well as neurons contain nuclear T_3 receptors [29]. Functionally, many neurons develop prior

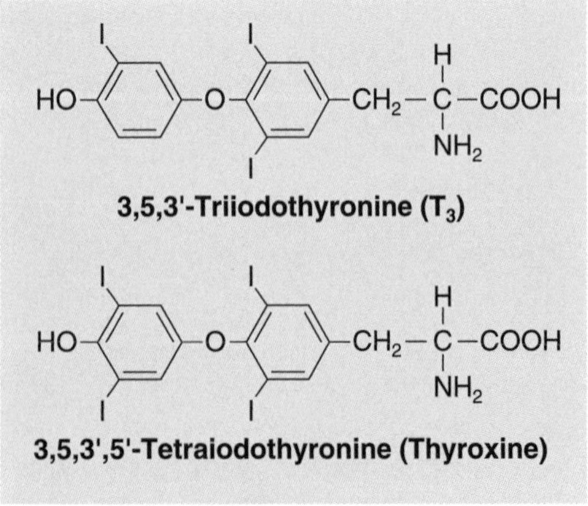

FIGURE 49-8. Structures for thyroxine (T_4) and triiodothyronine (T_3).

to the appearance of significant T_3 receptor levels and, therefore, appear to be independent of large-scale thyroid influence [30]. Other neurons, such as those in the cortex and cerebellum, show a more profound dependence on thyroid function [27]. Although thyroid hormone affects the number of replicating cells in the external granular layer of the developing cerebellum, it is not possible to conclude that T_3 directly affects the mechanism of cell replication [27]. Rather, the most pronounced effect of hypothyroidism is a hypoplastic neuropil, with shortened dendrites and fewer spines. It has been shown that a major effect of T_3 involves development of the neuronal cytoskeleton [27]. Proteins, such as microtubule-associated protein (MAP2) and tau (see Chap. 27), which are polymorphic and affect microtubular assembly, are differentially affected by T_3 absence or excess [27].

Developmentally, thyroid hormones interact with sex hormones such that hypothyroidism prolongs the critical period for testosterone-induced defeminization (see below) [3]; in contrast, the hyperthyroid state prematurely terminates the sensitivity to testosterone [3]. Undoubtedly, an important link in these and other effects is synapse formation. Hypothyroidism increases synaptic density, at least transiently [3]. Interesting parallels with synapse formation are reported for learning behavior in rats; neonatal hypothyroidism impairs learning ability, whereas hyperthyroidism accelerates learning initially, followed by a decline later in life [3].

The adult brain is endowed with nuclear as well as cytosolic and membrane T_3 receptors that have been visualized by autoradiography and studied biochemically [27,30]. Both neurons and neuropil are labeled by $[^{125}I]T_3$, and the labeling is selective across brain regions. Functionally, one of the most prominent features of neural action of thyroid hormone in adulthood is subsensitivity to norepinephrine as a result of a hypothyroid state [28]. These changes may be reflections of loss of dendritic spines in at least some neurons of the adult brain (see [27]). Clinically, thyroid hormone deficiency increases the probability of depressive illness, whereas thyroid excess increases the probability of mania (Chap. 52) in susceptible individuals [28].

DIVERSITY OF STEROID HORMONE ACTIONS ON THE BRAIN

Steroid hormone effects on the brain link the environment surrounding the organism with the genome of target brain cells through the process of variable genomic activity [25]. By this we mean that an organism experiences light, dark, heat, cold, fear and sexual excitement. These experiences influence hormonal secretion, and these hormones in turn act on the genome of receptor-containing brain cells to alter their functional state. The genome of brain cells, like that of other cells of the body, is continually active from embryonic life until death and continually responsive to intra- and extracellular signals. This activity can be seen from the high rates of RNA metabolism in neurons. The differential influence of steroid hormones on variable genomic activity is evident from studies showing rapid and brain region-specific induction of ribosomal and mRNA, as well as changes in cell nuclear diameter and chromatin and structure [1]. However, variable genomic activity changes qualitatively with the state of differentiation of the target cells: embryonic neurons show growth responses that result in permanent changes in circuitry, whereas adult neurons show impermanent responses. Under other circumstances, the same hormonal signals can promote damage and even neuronal loss; under still other conditions, adult neurons can be stimulated by treatment with hormones to grow and repair the damage.

During development, steroid hormone receptors become evident in target neurons of the brain

These receptors appear within several days of final cell division [13]. Whether some receptors are also present in dividing neuronal precursors is not clear. After they have appeared, these receptors mediate a variety of developmental actions. For example, glucocorticoids direct differentiation of adrenergic/cholinergic neurons of the autonomic nervous system to develop in the adrenergic direction [4]. Glucocorticoids also increase the number of epinephrine-containing, small, intensely fluorescent cells, often referred to as SIF, in autonomic ganglia and are required for the normal postnatal ontogeny of serotonin neurons in the forebrain [4]. These effects may not all be direct but may involve hormonal modulation of growth factors produced by other cells surrounding the developing neurons.

Gonadal hormones, however, are involved in sexual differentiation of the reproductive tract and brain [13]. Mammals, among which animals have X and Y chromosomes, undergo sexual differentiation under the impetus of testosterone secreted by the testes during a period of perinatal life; in humans, this period is in mid-gestation, while in rats it is from the end of gestation into neonatal life. Key features of sexual behavior in birds are determined in the reverse manner, in keeping with the fact that the female has the chromosomal heterogeneity: females produce either estradiol or testosterone, either of which feminizes the brain, which otherwise would develop a masculine pattern in the absence of gonadal steroids [13,31].

As for the mechanisms of sexual differentiation, we must consider the metabolism of the hormone receptor types involved and the primary receptor-mediated events. Testosterone, as noted above, is a prohormone that is converted into either 5α-DHT or estradiol within the brain; these products exert effects on brain sexual differentiation via androgen and estrogen receptors, respectively [13,31]. Masculinization of sexual and aggressive behavior involves either 5α-DHT alone or a combination of 5α-DHT and estradiol acting on different cells. Besides masculinization, there is in some mammals a process of defeminization, in which feminine responses that would develop in the absence of testosterone are suppressed by its presence during the critical period. Conversion to estradiol appears to be involved in this process [13,31]. Progesterone plays no major role in brain sexual differentiation, but it does have the ability to antagonize actions at both androgen and estrogen receptors and, thus, can moderate the degree of masculinization and defeminization.

As to the primary developmental actions of testosterone, growth and differentiation appear to be involved. Testosterone or estradiol stimulates outgrowth of neurites from developing hypothalamic neurons that contain estrogen receptors [13]. This is believed to be one of the principal aspects of testosterone action that increases the number and the size of neurons within specific hypothalamic nuclei in males, compared to females [32]. 5α-DHT may have a similar effect on androgen-sensitive neurons. Differentiation of target neurons also occurs; in adult brain tissue, hormones like estradiol can evoke responses that differ between adult male and female rats [1,32].

The response of neural tissue to damage involves some degree of structural plasticity, as in development

Collateral growth and reinnervation of vacant synaptic sites is facilitated in some cases by steroid hormones [32]. In the hypothalamus, estrogen treatment after knife cuts that destroy certain inputs promotes increases in the number of synapses. In the hippocampus, glucocorticoid treatment promotes homotypical sprouting of serotonin fibers to replace damaged serotonin input. It has also been noted that androgens enhance the regrowth of the severed hypoglossal nerve [32]. One interpretation of these steroid effects is that injury reactivates programs of steroid-responsive genomic activity that normally operate during the phase of synaptogenesis in early development [32].

Another aspect of steroid action is stabilization of neurons against death and replacement. In the dentate gyrus of both the neonate and the adult rat, neurons are born and die; rates of both birth and death are increased by adrenalectomy, and these increases are prevented by low doses of adrenal steroids acting via mineralocorticoid receptors [4,6,33] (Fig. 49-9). Regulation of the turnover rate of dentate gyrus neurons may provide the hippocampal formation of the adult with the potential to increase and decrease its volume and functional capacity, as occurs in relation to seasonal or other long-term changes in the environment. This process also occurs in the developing dentate gyrus [33].

Activation and adaptation behaviors may be mediated by hormones

Hormonal secretion by the adrenals and gonads is controlled by endogenous oscillators that can

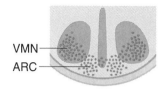

The ventrolateral ventromedial nuclei (VMN) and arcuate nuclei (ARC) contain estrogen-sensitive neurons in which estradiol induces receptors for progesterone. Dots indicate approximate location of estrogen-sensitive neurons.

VMN
ARC

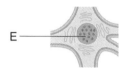

E

The VMN responds more rapidly and extensively to estradiol (E) than ARC. VMN neurons respond to E within 2h; cell body and nuclear diameters are increased; nucleolar size increases and rough endoplasmic reticulum and ribosomal RNA increase in the cytoplasm.

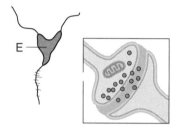

E

One of the consequences of this rapid increase in protein synthetic capacity in VMN neurons is that E increases the number of spines on dendrites and increases the density of synapses in the VMN. These events occur cyclically during the estrous cycle of the female rat. Dots indicate presynaptic vesicles containing neurotransmitter.

FIGURE 49-9. Summary of adrenal steroid effects on neurons of the hippocampus, illustrating their ability to protect and stabilize the population of the dentate granule neurons and to potentiate damage caused by excitatory amino acid release upon pyramidal neurons. *E*, estrogen. (From [32], with permission.)

be entrained by environmental cues such as light and dark. The actions of cyclically secreted hormones on behavior and brain function are referred to as activational effects. In addition to the cyclic mode, there is another mode of secretion initiated by such experiences as stress, fear and aggressive and sexual encounters. In this case, actions of adrenal steroid hormones secreted in response to experience lead to adaptive brain responses, which help the animal cope with stressful situations [4,6]. The activational and adaptational effects are largely reversible and involve a variety of neurochemical changes, most of which appear to be initiated at the genomic level. For example, estradiol is secreted cyclically during the estrous cycle in the female rat and triggers the surge of LH, which induces a surge of progesterone from the ovary. Progesterone, in turn, stimulates sexual responsiveness to the male rat [1].

Estradiol action to promote feminine sexual behavior in the rat involves a cascade of induced protein synthesis in specific hypothalamic neurons accompanied by morphological changes indicative of increased genomic activity [1]. Among the induced proteins are receptors for progesterone (see above), crucial for activat-

ing sexual behavior; receptors for acetylcholine and oxytocin that are active in enabling the hypothalamic neurons to respond to afferent input; proteins that are axonally transported from the hypothalamus to the midbrain, where they may be involved in neurotransmission; and structural proteins that contribute to formation of new synapses that come and go during the estrous cycle [1] (Fig. 49-10).

Adrenal steroids secreted in the diurnal cycle are reponsible for reversibly activating exploratory activity, food-seeking behavior, carbohydrate appetite and synaptic efficacy. These appear to do so by acting on the hippocampus, where there are many mineralocorticoid and glucocorticoid receptors (see above). Adaptational effects of adrenal steroids that result from stress appear to operate via the classical glucocorticoid receptor found not only in hippocampus but also in other brain regions [3,4]. Changes in synaptic vesicle proteins, high-affinity GABA transport, neurotransmitter-stimulated cAMP formation and central serotonin and noradrenergic sensitivity accompany repeated glucocorticoid elevations [3,4]. One view of these changes induced by glucocorticoids is that they

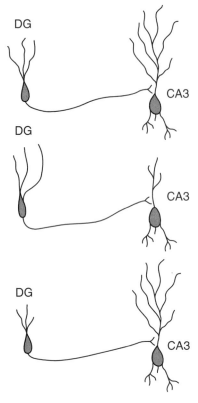

CA3 pyramidal neurons receive the mossy fiber input from the granule neurons of the dentate gyrus. This connection is part of the 3-cell circuit of the hippocampus that is believed to be involved in learning and memory.

Chronic corticosterone treatment or repeated restraint stress promotes atrophy of apical dendrites of CA3 pyramidal neurons.

Adrenalectomy causes neurons of the dentate gyrus to die and to be replaced by new neurons, whereas pyramidal neurons are unaffected. Low levels of adrenal steroids prevent this and stabilize the dentate granule neuron population; they do this via Type I adrenal steroid receptors.

FIGURE 49-10.   Summary of estrogen effects on the ventromedial nuclei related to its activation of female sexual behavior in the rat. *DG,* dentate gyrus. (From [32], with permission.)

counter-regulate some of the immediate and persistent neural effects of stress and are, therefore, part of the mechanism of adaptation [3,4,6]. This and other aspects of adaptation protect the organism; without adrenal secretions, the body likely would not survive many events in daily life.

The price of adaptation often includes some wear and tear and damage, called allostatic load [34]. *Allostasis,* meaning to achieve stability through change, is another word to describe adaptation. The wear and tear is the result of the inefficiency or overactivity of allostatic systems, including those like the adrenal cortex and autonomic nervous system, which respond to challenge and promote adaptation. This takes three forms: (i) repeated activation by many stressful events; (ii) failing to shut off after the challenge is over; and (iii) inability to be activated adequately, allowing other systems that are normally counter-regulated to become overactive,

for example, inflammatory cytokines. In each of these situations, there is a cumulative as well as an immediate effect on many organs, including the heart and brain, as well as on the immune system.

Enhancement of neuronal atrophy and cell loss during aging by severe and prolonged psychosocial stress are examples of allostatic load

Repeated psychosocial stress in primates and rodents causes pathological changes in various body organs, including neuronal loss in the hippocampus [6,35]. Shorter exposure of rats to restraint stress, psychosocial stress or corticosterone causes atrophy of neurons in the hippocampus, particularly in the CA3 region, which receives heavy input from the dentate gyrus mossy fiber system (Fig. 49-9). The mossy fiber input is also responsible for kainic acid-

and seizure-induced damage of the CA3 region and strongly suggests the importance of excitatory amino acids.

Indeed, the stress-induced atrophy is blocked by NMDA receptor blockers and by an anticonvulsant drug, phenytoin. The presence of elevated glucocorticoids at the time of hypoxic damage or kainic acid lesions (Chaps. 34 and 35) to the brain potentiates the necrosis produced by these treatments, especially in the hippocampus. Adrenalectomy reduces such damage and retards loss of neurons with age [6,35]. Thus, adrenal steroids operate in conjunction with neural excitability to produce damage, and it has been suggested that they do so by compromising the ability of the brain to obtain nutrients to support ATP generation [35].

The concept of allostatic load implies that there is a paradox in the actions of adrenal steroids: they exert protection in the short run and have the potential to cause damage in the long run if the allostatic, that is, the adaptation-promoting, responses are not managed efficiently. "Good stress" is therefore the efficient management of an allostatic response, whereas "bad stress" involves the persistence or otherwise inefficient operation of these normally adaptive responses.

There are gradients of health status across socioeconomic status that are not explained by access to health care or other simple explanations [36]. Therefore, it may be of great relevance in the future to understand the role of such factors as sense of control, helplessness, persistent fear and anxiety, diet, exercise and the impact of the living and social, for example, family and work, environments in regulating the allostatic systems; these factors could cause allostatic systems to operate inefficiently.

Gonadal hormones, like adrenal steroids, can produce both protection and damage. High-dose estrogen treatment of adult female rats induces hypothalamic disconnection syndrome by activating low-level persistent ovarian estrogen secretion. This persistent ovarian secretion induces morphological changes in the hypothalamus associated with dysfunction of the cyclic gonadotropin-releasing mechanism [37]. Persistent effects of estrogen secretion occurring naturally throughout the life span are believed to facilitate termination of cyclic hypothalamic function with regard to ovulation [37]. In the opposite sense, the suppression of gonadal function by repeated stress is likely to deprive the brain and cardiovascular system of protective actions of gonadal hormones and, thus, increase allostatic load [38,39].

REFERENCES

1. McEwen, B. S., Coirini, H., Danielsson, A., et al. Steroid and thyroid hormones modulate a changing brain. *J. Steroid Biochem. Mol. Biol.* 40:1–14, 1991.
2. Ganong, W. F. *Review of Medical Physiology,* 14th Ed. Norwalk, CT: Appleton and Lange, 1991.
3. McEwen, B. S. Endocrine effects on the brain and their relationship to behavior. In G. J. Siegel, R. W. Albers, B. W. Agranoff, and R. Katzman (eds.), *Basic Neurochemistry,* 3rd Ed. Boston: Little Brown and Co., 1981, pp. 775–799.
4. McEwen, B. S., DeKloet, R., and Rostene, W. Adrenal steroid receptors and actions in the nervous system. *Physiol. Rev.* 66:1121–1188, 1986.
5. Lupien, S. J., and McEwen, B. S. The acute effects of glucocorticoids on cognition: Integration of animal and human model studies. *Brain Res. Rev.* 24:1–27, 1997.
6. McEwen, B. S., Albeck, D., Cameron, H., et al. Stress and the brain: A paradoxical role for adrenal steroids. *Vitam. Horm.* 51:371–402, 1995.
7. Fuller, P. The steroid receptor superfamily: Mechanisms of diversity. *FASEB J.* 5:3092–3099, 1991.
8. Miner, J., and Yamamoto, K. Regulatory crosstalk at composite response elements. *Trends Biochem. Sci.* 16:423–426, 1991.
9. Drouin, J., Sun, Y.-L., and Nemer, M. Glucocorticoid repression of pro-opiomelanocortin gene transcription. *J. Steroid Biochem.* 34:63–69, 1989.
10. Power, R. F., Mani, S. K., Codina, J., Conneely, O. M., and O'Malley, B. W. Dopaminergic and ligand-independent activation of steroid hormone receptors. *Science* 254:1636–1639, 1991.
11. Norman, A., and Henry, H. Vitamin D to 1,25-dihydroxycholecalciferol: Evolution of a steroid hormone. *Trends Biochem. Sci.* 5:414–418, 1979.
12. Celotti, F., Naftolin, F., and Martini, L. (eds.), *Metabolism of Hormonal Steroids in Neuroendocrine Structures.* New York: Raven Press, 1984.

13. Goy, R., and McEwen, B. S. (eds.), *Sexual Differentiation of the Brain*. Cambridge, MA: MIT Press, 1980.

14. Roselli, C., Horton, L., and Resko, J. Distribution and regulation of aromatase activity in the rat hypothalamus and limbic system. *Endocrinology* 117:2471–2477, 1985.

15. Schumacher, M., and Balthazart, J. Testosterone-induced brain aromatase is sexually dimorphic. *Brain Res.* 370:285–293, 1986.

16. Merriam, G. R., and Lipsett, M. B. (eds.), *Catechol Estrogens*. New York: Raven Press, 1983.

17. Robel, P., Bourreau, E., Corpéachot, C., et al. Neuro-steroids: 3β-Hydroxy-Δ5-derivatives in rat and monkey brain. *J. Steroid Biochem.* 27:649–655, 1987.

18. McEwen, B. S. Nongenomic effects of steroids on neural activity. *Trends Pharmacol. Sci.* 12: 141–147, 1991.

19. McEwen, B. S., and Zigmond, R. Isolation of brain cell nuclei. In N. Marks and R. Rodnight (eds.), *Research Methods in Neurochemistry*. New York: Plenum Press, 1972, Vol. 1, pp. 140–161.

20. Parker, M. The expanding family of nuclear hormone receptors. *J. Endocrinol.* 119:175–177, 1988.

21. O'Keefe, J., and Handa, R. Transient elevation of estrogen receptors in the neonatal rat hippocampus. *Dev. Brain Res.* 57:119–127, 1990.

22. Kuiper, G. G. J. M., Carlsson, B., Grandien, K., et al. Comparison of the ligand binding specificity and transcript tissue distribution of estrogen receptors alpha and beta. *Endocrinology* 138:863–870, 1997.

23. McEwen, B. S., Davis, P., Gerlach, J., et al. Progestin receptors in the brain and pituitary gland. In C. W. Bardin, P. Mauvais-Jarvis, and E. Milgrom (eds.), *Progesterone and Progestin*. New York: Raven Press, 1983, pp. 59–76.

24. Edwards, C. R. W., Burt, D., McIntyre, M. A., et al. Localization of 11β-hydroxysteroid dehydrogenase tissue specific protector of the mineralocorticoid receptor. *Lancet* 2:986–989, 1988.

25. Stumpf, W., Sar, M., and Clark, S. Brain target sites for 1,25-dihydroxy vitamin D3. *Science* 215:1403–1405, 1982.

26. Sonnenberg, J., Luine, V., Krey, L., and Christakos, S. 1,25-Dihydroxyvitamin D3 treatment results in increased choline acetyltransferase activity in specific brain nuclei. *Endocrinology* 118:1433–1439, 1986.

27. Nunez, J. Effects of thyroid hormones during brain differentiation. *Mol. Cell. Endocrinol.* 37:125–132, 1984.

28. Whybrow, P., and Prange, A. A hypothesis of thyroid–catecholamine receptor interaction. *Arch. Gen. Psychiatry* 38:106–133, 1981.

29. Bernal, J., and Pekonen, F. Ontogenesis of the nuclear 3,5,3′-triiodothyronine receptor in the human fetal brain. *Endocrinology* 114:677–680, 1984.

30. Mellstrom, B., Naranjo, J. R., Santos, A., Gonzalez, A. M., and Bernal, J. Independent expression of the alpha and beta c-erbA genes in developing rat brain. *Mol. Endocrinol.* 5:1339–1350, 1991.

31. Adler, N. (ed.), *Neuroendocrinology of Reproduction, Physiology and Behavior*. New York: Plenum Press, 1981.

32. McEwen, B. S. Our changing ideas about steroid effects on an ever-changing brain. *Semin. Neurosci.* 4:497–507, 1991.

33. Cameron, H. A., and Gould, E. The control of neuronal birth and survival. In C. A. Shaw (ed.), *Receptor Dynamics in Neural Development*. Boca Raton, FL: CRC Press, 1996, pp. 141–157.

34. McEwen, B. S., and Stellar, E. Stress and the individual: Mechanisms leading to disease. *Arch. Intern. Med.* 153:2093–2101, 1993.

35. Sapolsky, R. M. *Stress, the Aging Brain and the Mechanisms of Neuron Death*. Cambridge, MA: MIT Press, 1992.

36. Adler, H., Boyce, T., Chesney, M. A., et al. Socioeconomic status and health: The challenge of the gradient. *Am. Psychol.* 49:15–24, 1994.

37. Brawer, J., Schipper, H., and Naftolin, F. Ovary-dependent degeneration in the hypothalamic arcuate nucleus. *Endocrinology* 107:274–279, 1980.

38. Mizoguchi, K., Kunishita, T., Chui, D. H., and Tabira, T. Stress induces neuronal death in the hippocampus of castrated rats. *Neurosci. Lett.* 138:157–160, 1992.

39. Shively, C. A., and Clarkson, T. Social status incongruity and coronary artery atherosclerosis in female monkeys. *Atherosclerosis Thrombosis* 14:721–726, 1994.

40. Baulieu, E-E. Neurosteroids: A function of the Brain. In Costa, S. M. Paul (eds.) *Neurosteroids and Brain Function*. New York: Thieme Medical Publishing, 1991, Vol. 8, pp. 63–73.

50

Learning and Memory

Bernard W. Agranoff, Carl W. Cotman and Michael D. Uhler

Basic Neurochemistry: Molecular, Cellular and Medical Aspects, 6th Ed., edited by G. J. Siegel et al. Published by Lippincott–Raven Publishers, Philadelphia, 1999. Correspondence to Bernard W. Agranoff, Mental Health Research Institute, University of Michigan, 1103 E. Huron, Ann Arbor, Michigan 48104-1687.

How do biochemists study behavior?

In the nineteenth century, it was proposed that the brain is to the mind as a violin is to music. Today, more apt metaphors for brain and mind are the computer and its programs. The computer's hard-wired circuitry is analogous to the genetically determined brain, while its software programs are akin to inferred modifications of the brain resulting from behavioral experience. Much has been learned about how the genes that determine brain development are expressed (Chap. 27). Cellular differentiation and migration, neurite outgrowth, synaptogenesis and even growth cone retraction and cell death all play crucial roles in development. A growing network of neurons and glia in the developing brain are known to respond to growth factors and chemical gradients in a highly integrated and selective program that is largely complete at birth. We know further that the newborn animal brain is not a blank slate. There are hardwired behaviors we refer to as instincts. For example, a fish will recognize and flee from a conspecific predator upon its first visual encounter, and a hungry infant will cry. One question that arises is whether some of the same cellular and molecular processes that are active during development but reduced or absent in the mature brain can be induced regionally to serve as the physical basis of learning and memory, as defined below. Alternatively, the elusive physical manifestations of learning and memory, sometimes referred to as the engram, might be mediated by neurobiological mechanisms that are completely unique for the acquisition and storage of new behaviors.

Learning can be defined as an adaptive change in response to an environmental input

It can be argued that learning and memory exist outside of the nervous system, for example, in the immunological response, but we will here consider only the brain and behavior. Learning is quantified experimentally as the probability that an organism will respond to the same stimulus differently upon retesting. This altered probability is based on the organism's memory of what it has learned. It is thus not possible to consider learning without memory or, conversely, memory without learning. We can, however, distinguish between the memory necessary for learning, termed acquisition, or short-term memory, and that required to demonstrate a learned behavior over longer periods of time. For example, an animal might demonstrate acquisition of a conditioned response following repetitive trials during an initial training session, indicating the occurrence of learning and the attendant short-term memory of the training task. Evocation of the newly learned behavior in a second training session hours to weeks later constitutes evidence for long-term memory formation. Thus, during and shortly after a training session, performance by the subject of a learned behavior is considered to be based on short-term memory; at later times, it is believed to be mediated by retrieval of long-term memory. That short-term and long-term memory are distinct processes was inferred from studies employing interventive agents (Fig. 50-1) [1]. It is important to remember that although we conceive of learning and memory as intrinsic biological processes or states, our behavioral measures are based entirely on the experimental subject's performance. When a previously trained animal does not demonstrate an acquired behavior under a specified set of conditions, such as in a drug-induced state, it will then depend on the skill of the experimenter to determine whether the absent behavior is suppressed or whether the subject is truly amnesic.

Studying neurochemical correlates of learning and memory is a compromise between meeting behavioral criteria and the accessibility of the system employed to molecular and cellular biological approaches

Simple experimental systems such as sensitization and habituation, in which a repetitive stimulus produces a decreased or an augmented behavioral response, respectively, have proven useful. These responses are employed in studies of primitive organisms, such as invertebrates, the neural circuits of which are believed to be simpler and more experimentally accessible than those of a vertebrate brain. Another reductionist approach uses *in vitro* preparations of brain tissue slices, which permit direct examination of lasting alterations in synaptic transmission following a brief sequence of nerve stimulation, in the belief that the electrical inputs mimic events occurring in the intact brain during learning. Thus, the experimenter may compromise the direct relevance of a behavioral paradigm in order to measure a neural transmission model of learning and memory using a simpler model system or, alternatively, to study conventionally defined behavior in an intact, functioning laboratory animal but with less than ideal cellular, biochemical and molecular measurements. More complex behaviors in intact animals, usually vertebrates, including humans, are discussed below.

Investigation of learning and memory in intact behaving animals generally involves one of two strategies: interventive or correlative

Antibiotic inhibitors of macromolecular synthesis and various pharmacological agents, such as neurotransmitter agonists and antagonists, are examples of interventive agents. Administered systematically or even intracranially, they gener-

A

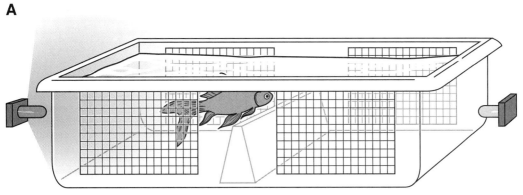

FIGURE 50-1. Effects of administration of agents that block long-term memory of a multitrial task. **A:** A goldfish (*Carassius auratus*) is shown in a shuttle box used for training of a shock-avoidance task. Goldfish are transferred from home tanks to one side of a training apparatus termed a shuttle box, which is divided into halves by a submerged barrier. A trial begins with the onset of a light signal, the conditioned stimulus, on the end of the shuttle box nearest the fish. This is followed 20 sec later by a mild electrical shock, the unconditioned stimulus, administered through the water. Naive fish respond to the unconditioned stimulus by swimming over the barrier at the onset of shock to the dark, and presumably safe, end of the shuttle box. This escape response is eventually replaced after many trials by the learned avoidance response, in which the fish swims over the barrier before the onset of the punishing shock. Whether the fish demonstrates the conditioned response or the unconditioned response, it will end up on the side of the shuttle box opposite its position at the beginning of the trial. The next trial begins with a light signal at the fish's end of the apparatus. The location of the fish in the shuttle box is determined by photodetectors, and its avoidance or escape scores are recorded automatically. (*Figure continues on next page.*)

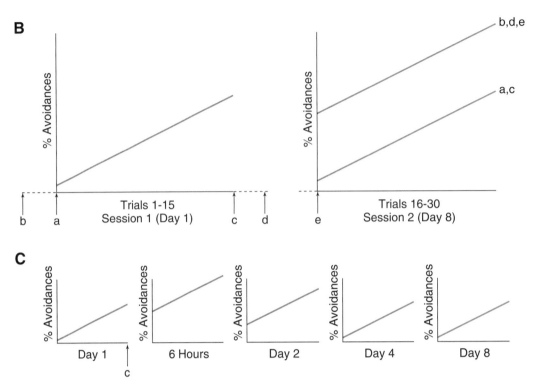

FIGURE 50-1. (Continued) **B:** The probability of an avoidance response during 15 trials (session 1) increases progressively, indicating that short-term memory is formed. Fish returned immediately to their home tanks and, retrained 1 week later, demonstrate their prior learning and show additional improvement in session 2. If an amnestic agent is injected intracranially just before the session (time *a*), normal acquisition is seen but there is a profound deficit in performance upon retraining 1 week later. If the agent is administered sufficiently in advance of session 1 (time *b*), normal retention is seen on day 8 since the effects of the injection will have worn off by the time of the training session. By varying the time of injection before training, the duration of a given agent's amnestic effect can be established. Intracranial injection of the protein synthesis inhibitor puromycin is effective when given 24, but not 72, hr before session 1. An injection immediately after session 1 *(c)* results in profound deficits upon retraining 1 week later (session 2). The process is time-dependent since fish return to their home tanks and, given the injection a few hours later *(d)*, show no deficit upon retraining in session 2. In fact, fish not treated previously and given the amnestic agent just before retraining on day 8 *(e)* still show the learned response. This time dependence of the treatment rules out both chronic, or lingering, and acute toxic effects of the amnestic agents as possible explanations for the observed reduced responding rates and indicates that the agent produces a specific memory loss. **C:** The decay of short-term memory. Injection of a blocking agent just after, or before, session 1 results in failure to form long-term memory. In this experiment, individual groups of animals so treated and retrained at various times earlier than 8 days or 6, 48, or 96 hr after session 1 demonstrate gradual loss of the learned response. The experiments thus constitute evidence for the decay of short-term memory (see text). (From [1], with permission.)

ally do not provide anatomical localization and usually affect multiple metabolic sites. Nevertheless, much can be gained from experiments utilizing such substances; they can point the way to subsequent correlative studies to confirm or refute conclusions drawn from the intervention. Thus, radioisotopic studies may investigate whether a specific metabolic process thought to be crucial to memory formation is indeed altered by behavioral manipulation in the absence of the interventive agent. Genetic approaches that use mutation, knockouts or transgenic procedures are by their nature interventive. Noninvasive measures of brain activity such as functional positron emission tomography (PET) and functional magnetic resonance imaging (fMRI) are promising correlative approaches, particularly useful for studying human learning and memory (see below). The various correlative and interventive strategies and model systems prove to be most useful when they can be integrated into a consistent hypothesis that leads to further critical experiments or when constraints can be added to theoretical models of how the brain processes and stores behavioral information.

BASIC ASSUMPTIONS

Current hypotheses concerning the neurochemical basis of memory are based on a number of premises, which are enumerated here. The remainder of this chapter relies on their validity.

The generally accepted basic behavioral paradigm for studying learning and memory is the conditioned response

What we mean by learning and memory encompasses a wide variety of adaptive responses in greatly different species. Pavlov's characterization of conditioning [2] has served as a standard template for acceptable criteria in intact animals and, by analogy, in cellular and subcellular models of learning and memory. He emphasized temporal requirements for optimal learning: in order for learning to occur, the conditioned, or neutral, stimulus (CS), such as a tone, must precede the unconditioned stimulus (US), such as food presentation, which results in the response, salivation. Similarly, a punishing electrical shock that results in altered heart rate or a puff of air that results in an eye blink can serve as unconditioned stimuli to be paired with neutral light or sound stimuli. The contingency criteria, that is, that the CS precedes the US and that there be an optimal latency, or CS–US interval, must be met in true associative learning. These criteria can be applied to simple systems, such as the invertebrate nervous system, where identified neurons appear to mediate behavior, or to mammalian brain slice preparations, in which performance is measured electrophysiologically, as described later.

Protein synthesis is required to form long-term, but not short-term, memory

Studies in fish, rodents, birds and invertebrates have indicated that the formation of short-term and long-term memory can be distinguished on the basis of susceptibility to antibiotic agents that block brain protein synthesis, such as puromycin, cycloheximide and anisomycin [1]. Consideration of the temporal aspects of learning and memory and knowledge of the temporal scale of biochemical processes have led to the prediction that learning and short-term memory formation, which can occur within milliseconds and last for minutes to hours, are mediated by post-translational modification at the synapse. Biochemical processes that could mediate short-term memory are discussed below. Long-term memory, which may take longer to form and can last a lifetime, is predicted to be mediated by a process that (i) requires *de novo* protein synthesis, and (ii) is therefore dependent on the neuronal genome, and (iii) thus, must require that there be communication between the cell surface and nucleus, presumably by axonal transport (see Chap. 28).

Behavioral information is ultimately stored in synaptic connections

This concept can be traced to Ramón y Cajal, who first recognized the enormous complexity of the neuronal networks in the brain. Although it may seem self-evident that an organism's most complex function resides in its most complex structures, the premise remains inferential. It is supported by many indications that synaptic complexity increases with development and environmental input (see SYNAPTIC PLASTICITY, below). Alternative hypotheses, such as that memory resides in glia, have not been pursued sufficiently to warrant further consideration here. It was once proposed that memory is not based on altered chemical states but rather on reverberating electrical circuits or charge distributions, yet there is ample evidence that memory survives seizures as well as periods of electrical silence in the brain. Neurochemists generally adopt the premise that long-lived biological phenomena are ultimately preserved and protected in the form of covalent chemical bonds, but this cannot lead to a simple accretion hypothesis in which new synaptic connections are "soldered," because while memories can last a lifetime, brain proteins turn over at measurable rates of hours, days or weeks. Altered synaptic relationships that underlie stored long-term memory, which can last for years, must then depend on feed-forward loops generated in the cell nucleus. There is ample independent evidence that the genome regulates phenotypic expression throughout the lifetime of the cell, and in the case of neurons, this means the lifetime of the individual. It remains to be demonstrated which of the events that occur during learning at the presynaptic and postsynaptic membrane surfaces are communicated to their neuronal nuclei, as is discussed next.

These three assumptions serve as a framework for evaluating the diverse experimental neurochemical approaches to attaining an understanding of learning and memory that follow in this chapter.

SYNAPTIC PLASTICITY AS A MODEL FOR LEARNING AND MEMORY RESEARCH

During early development there is continuous growth and modification of connections between neurons and their targets. As noted above, it is increasingly apparent that environmental input contributes to the shaping and tuning of neuronal circuitry during development and continues throughout life. Neuronal connectivity is not fixed once development is complete but continues to change throughout life. Remodeling of synaptic connectivity can occur in response to general environmental manipulations, sensory stimulation or learning a specific new task and may even be associated with cyclic changes in the physiological status of the organism. These remodeling events are discussed below.

Changes in environment can evoke plastic neuronal responses

A prime purpose of learning is to adapt successfully to an ever-changing environment. It is now clear that changes in the environment and the organism's interactions with it can produce dramatic changes in cellular morphology in the brain. Experiments supporting this claim involve placement of rats in an enriched environ-

ment and comparison of their brains with those of rats maintained in an impoverished environment. The impoverished condition consists of animals living in solitary housing in plain, small cages with minimal ambient stimulation. The enriched environment usually consists of group housing in large cages with toys, ladders, mazes and social interactions. These conditions can profoundly influence learning, as well as the chemical and anatomical structure of the brain.

Exposing young rats to such an enriched environment results in better performance on spatial learning tasks as adults compared with rats housed under impoverished conditions. In addition, the behavioral effects of environmental enrichment are complemented by physical changes in the brain [3,4]. Exposing rats to enriched conditions for 30 days increases the number of synapses and the complexity of dendritic branching in the frontal and occipital cortex. Not only are neurons affected but there are also increases in the surface area of astrocytes and in the vascularization of the brain. The effects can be of sufficient magnitude to generate an increase in the overall cortical thickness. An increase in neurotrophins may be one of the contributing molecular mechanisms to these impressive effects. While these general adaptive responses are most pronounced in the brain of young rats, environmental stimulation produces effects in the aging rat brain as well. Aging rats, 25 to 30 months, housed in enriched conditions for several months show enhanced learning performance, accompanied by increases in cortical thickness, angiogenesis and dendritic fields [5,6]. Observations on the effects of environmental enrichment in rodents further emphasize the importance of physical activity and mental stimulation on brain function and brain plasticity. However, such general environmental experiences do not define the key contributing factors.

Motor learning can modify synaptic connectivity

In complex learned tasks in animal models, there are usually repetitive learning and activity components. Is the repetitive task or is the learning more critical for structural changes in the brain, or are both essential? It might be anticipated that the brain structure is more responsive to the learning process than to motor activity and performance. In an experiment designed to determine the relative contributions of each condition [7], a group of rats was trained in an aerobic learning condition, which required extensive motor learning plus activity. Another group exercised in a voluntary wheel-running, or exercise, condition, which had only a small learning component in it. These two groups were compared to each other and to rats that were inactive. The aerobic condition consisted of training on an elevated obstacle path, which had balance beams, see-saws, rope bridges and other obstacles. The course was made progressively longer and more challenging over a 30-day training period. After the training, animals showed improvements in the rate at which they traversed the course. At the end of the 30-day period, the cerebellar cortex, which participates in learned motor skills, was analyzed for the number of synapses per Purkinje cell and the density of blood vessels. The results showed that the aerobic learning condition led to an increase in synapses, whereas the exercise condition produced an increase in blood vessel density (Fig. 50-2) [7].

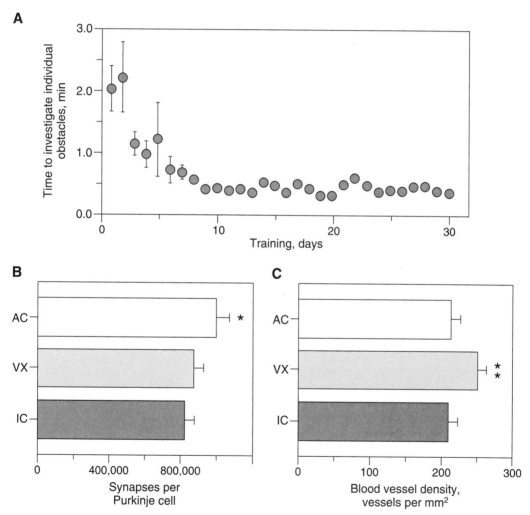

FIGURE 50-2. Effects of various motor tasks on brain microanatomical measures. Groups of rats were subjected to training of a novel acrobatic skill *(AC)* or voluntary wheel-running exercise *(VX)* or were caged in an inactive condition *(IC)*. The AC group learning curve **(A)** is compared with increases in synapses per cerebellar Purkinje cell **(B)** and blood vessel density **(C)**. It can be seen that AC is associated with increased synaptic number, while voluntary exercise elicits an increase in vascularity. (Modified from [7], with permission.)

Thus, it appears that when the environment presents a need for skilled movements, there is an increase in synapses. However, when the environment demands extensive repetition, the vascular density is increased to provide for increased metabolic demand. Exercise itself can initiate molecular changes in the brain and, in turn, influence learning and memory mechanisms. Rats exposed to daily treadmill running have enhanced performance in various learning tasks, including spatial learning [8]. Relative to sedentary control rats, long-term treadmill running produces changes in high-affinity choline uptake, a marker of cholinergic function, in hippocampus and parietal cortex; increases muscarinic receptor density; prevents age-related declines in hippocampal muscarinic receptor density; and increases hippocampal immunoreactivity for select neuropeptides [9]. Only a few days of voluntary running increases expression of trophic factors, such as brain-derived neurotrophic factor (BDNF), in the hippocampus [10].

In addition, environmental stimulation can facilitate recovery after brain damage; exposure to enriched conditions following brain injury appears to improve performance on learning and motor tasks. It is generally accepted that this involves axon sprouting and reactive synaptogenesis (see Chap. 29) in combination with use-dependent plasticity mechanisms directed by the environment. Exercise reportedly also renders the brain more resistant to injury [11]. Increased brain activity may induce neurotrophins such as BDNF, which can in turn influence synaptic plasticity and neuronal resistance to insult.

There is, thus, evidence from both animal and human studies that environmental enrichment and physical fitness may be related to cognitive and memory functions. These plasticity mechanisms may fine-tune neural circuitry and evoke essential support systems. Such changes are further layered upon a background of other plasticity mechanisms controlled by the endocrine system.

Endogenous hormones cause structural changes in the nervous system

It is well established that circulating hormones in the body elicit specific behaviors (see also Chap. 49). Recent evidence demonstrates that changes in hormone concentrations induce changes in neuronal morphology in the CNS. For example, in the normal rodent brain, the development of the synaptic density in the CA1 region of the hippocampus depends on the availability of androgens. In addition, it appears that removal of circulating gonadal steroids by ovariectomy causes a decrease in dendritic spine density in the CA1 region of the female adult rat. These changes are observed shortly after treatment, raising the possibility that there are hormone-induced changes in synaptic density during the normal estrous cycle. Quantitative electron microscopic analysis has confirmed that dendritic spines on neurons in the CA1 hippocampal region and the ventromedial hypothalamus undergo cyclic changes during the estrous cycle of the rat. Specifically, during estrus the spine density is significantly lower than during proestrus. It might be anticipated that such changes would be translated to learning and memory mechanisms that involve the hippocampus, and this is a topic of active investigation.

Nerve regeneration serves as a model of neuroplasticity in learning and memory formation

Nerve regeneration, like synaptic remodeling, inferred to occur in learning and memory formation, occurs within the scaffolding of the postmitotic adult brain. The regenerating visual system of cold-blooded vertebrates has been of particular interest in that it can occur entirely within the CNS, whereas CNS regeneration does not occur in warm-blooded vertebrates, that is, birds and mammals. As a consequence, the axotomized goldfish optic nerve has been studied extensively for the presence of novel proteins induced during regeneration. An example of such a protein is the growth-associated protein GAP-43, which has been identified as a component of the growth cone of the regenerating axon. GAP-43 is expressed in the rat hippocampus, and its phosphorylation is enhanced under conditions which induce long-term potentiation (LTP) [12]. Hence, GAP-43 serves as one example of a protein first characterized as playing a role in regeneration but later shown to participate in other forms of neuronal plasticity. Such proteins may also prove to be useful probes of synaptic plasticity induced by behavioral inputs, as occurs in learning and memory formation.

INVERTEBRATE LEARNING AND MEMORY

Invertebrates offer a number of advantages as model systems for learning and memory. Foremost among these advantages is the simplicity of the neuronal networks, which are often organized into several discrete ganglia rather than a CNS. In addition, the genome is typically less complex in invertebrates than in vertebrates so that the number of genes involved in a learning response is likely to be smaller as well.

Aplysia provides a cellular model of learning and memory

Kandel and co-workers [13] pioneered the use of the sea snail *Aplysia californica* as a model system for the study neuronal events associated with learning. *Aplysia* has a relatively simple nervous system, consisting of approximately 10,000 neurons, many of which are sufficiently large to allow them to be manipulated directly within defined neuronal circuits.

Three behaviors, each of which has adaptive value, have been studied in *Aplysia:* habituation, sensitization and classical conditioning. *Habituation* describes a learned response in which a decrease is observed in a specific behavioral response after repeated stimulation. In *Aplysia*, habituation serves as a rudimentary model that shares some aspects of regulation relevant to learning. A snail ordinarily withdraws its gill after gentle tactile stimulation of the siphon. Upon repeated stimulation, the gill-withdrawal reflex diminishes in both magnitude and duration. If the habituation experience consists of one training session of relatively few stimulations, say, less than ten, over a short period of time, less than 1 hr, then the habituation lasts for only a few hours after the training. If, however, four or more individual training ses-

sions are given, the habituation response can last for several weeks. These two forms of habituation have been interpreted as models of short- and long-term memory.

There is a difference in how short-term and long-term memory are measured in *Aplysia* experiments and in behavior in vertebrates such as the goldfish. In *Aplysia*, short-term memory refers to a fleeting memory resulting from few training trials. With additional trials, memory appears to be more robust and to last longer. In experiments with goldfish and rats, the same training session is thought to give rise to both a short- and long-term form of memory. Short-term memory is formed during the training session, while long-term memory proceeds by a consolidation process that takes place after the training session. In both fish and *Aplysia*, it appears that the short-term memory formation does not require ongoing protein synthesis, while the long-term form does.

The relatively simple neuronal circuitry involved in habituation of the gill-withdrawal reflex is shown in Figure 50-3. Stimulation of a sensory neuron innervating the siphon causes stimulation of motor neurons that innervate the gill muscle. As habituation proceeds, the number of postsynaptic potentials produced in the motor neuron decreases. When completely habituated, the motor neuron does not depolarize and there is no gill withdrawal, while depolarization of the sensory neuron in response to siphon stimulation is unaffected. Kandel and co-workers [13] have shown that habituation is the result of a decrease in synaptic efficacy between the sensory neuron and the motor neuron due to altered permeability of the Ca^{2+} required for neurotransmitter release at the presynaptic terminal. The Ca^{2+} enters the presynaptic terminal through voltage-sensitive Ca^{2+} channels, and during habituation, Ca^{2+} channels in the presynaptic terminal become inactivated. Although specific mechanisms for this inactivation have been postulated, its nature in the synaptic terminal of the sensory neurons is unknown. Furthermore, since the long-term habituation appears to involve protein synthesis, the known mechanisms for inactivation of Ca^{2+} channels do not suffice to explain it.

A second form of learning in *Aplysia*,

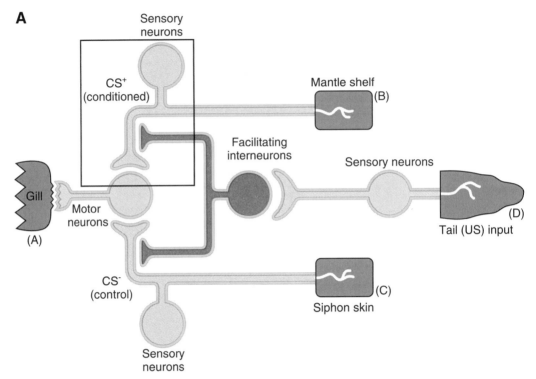

FIGURE 50-3.   A: A simplified diagram of the circuitry involved in sensitization, habituation and classical condition-ing in *Aplysia*. Sensory neurons, motor neurons and facilitating interneurons are indicated. Sensory neurons from the mantle shelf *(B)* and siphon skin *(C)* innervate the motor neurons, which control gill withdrawal *(A)*, while sensory neu-rons from the tail *(D)* innervate facilitating interneurons. The facilitating interneurons form the axo-axonic synapse, which is modified during sensitization and conditioning. *CS*, conditioned stimulus, *US*, unconditioned stimulus.

known as sensitization, involves a more complex learning paradigm and depends on a more com-plicated cellular regulatory mechanism. In one type of sensitization experiment, a mild tail shock is given to the animal shortly preceding tactile stimulation of the siphon. The prior tail shock sensitizes the animal so that the normal gill-withdrawal reflex associated with siphon stimulation is increased in magnitude and dura-tion. Like habituation, sensitization can be either short-term or long-term in nature, depending on the duration and number of training sessions involved.

The neuronal pathway involved in the tail-shock-sensitization experiment is schematized in Figure 50-3A. Stimulation of sensory neurons in the tail causes generation of an action poten-tial in the specific interneurons that facilitate sensitization. These facilitating interneurons form a specific synaptic connection with axons of the sensory neuron that innervate the siphon. The synapses of the facilitating interneurons are positioned so that release of neurotransmitter from their axons is targeted to the axons of the sensory neuron, forming an axo-axonic synapse. In tail shock sensitization, the facilitating in-terneurons release serotonin onto the axonal ter-minals of the sensory neurons. Specific sero-tonin receptors on the sensory axons respond to the serotonin and increase axonal cAMP con-centrations (Fig. 50-3B). The elevated cAMP then activates cAMP-dependent protein kinase (PKA), which has multiple substrates in the sen-sory neuron. Initially, PKA phosphorylates K^+ channels in the sensory axon. The resulting de-crease in K^+ influx prolongs the action potential and increases the duration of Ca^{2+} influx through voltage-sensitive Ca^{2+} channels. The net effect of this phosphorylation event is that more Ca^{2+} flows into the axon, and since Ca^{2+} is

B

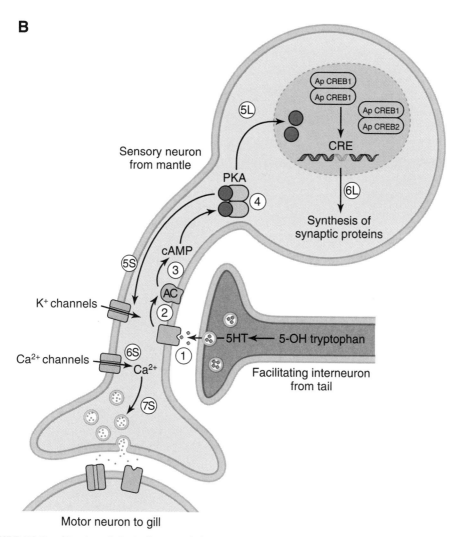

FIGURE 50-3. (Continued) **B:** A diagram of the inset in **A,** focusing on biochemical events at the axo-axonic synapse. ① Serotonin *(5HT)* released from the facilitating interneuron binds to ② its receptor on the sensory neuron and ③ elevates cAMP, which in turn activates ④ cAMP-dependent protein kinase *(PKA)*. During short-term learning, K⁺ channels are phosphorylated *(5S)*, leading to longer depolarization, greater influx of Ca²⁺ through voltage-sensitive Ca²⁺ channels *(6S)* and increased neurotransmitter release *(7S)*. During long-term learning, the catalytic subunit of PKA translocates to the nucleus *(5L)* and stimulates gene transcription through the cAMP response element–binding *(CREB)*, and now protein synthesis follows *(6L)*. *CRE,* cAMP response element; *Ap, Aplysia.*

required for synaptic vesicle fusion with the membrane, greater neurotransmitter release is observed when the neuron is depolarized following activation of the serotonin receptor. The greater release of neurotransmitter from sensory axons onto the motor neurons results in increased contraction of muscles involved in gill withdrawal. This mechanism, involving only phosphorylation of existing proteins, is suffi-

cient to account for most of the changes seen during short-term sensitization.

Long-term sensitization can last for days to weeks and has been shown to result in morphological changes which suggest that the conversion from short-term to long-term memory involves the translation of synaptic transmission efficiency into morphological changes of the synapse. Long-term sensitization requires RNA and protein synthesis in order to allow the growth of new synaptic contacts between pre- and postsynaptic cells. The basic mechanism for long-term sensitization relies on the same serotonergic activation of PKA; however, during the repeated training sessions required for long-term sensitization, the persistent activation of PKA causes nuclear translocation of the catalytic subunit of the kinase (Fig. 50-3B). In the nucleus, the catalytic subunit phosphorylates transcription factors, which regulate transcription from specific genes. One class of transcription factor binds to enhancer sequences which are responsible for increasing transcription after activation of PKA. These cAMP response element (CRE) enhancer sequences generally conform to the consensus sequence TGACGTCA and have been characterized in mammals as well as in *Aplysia* (see Chap. 26). The CRE-binding (CREB) protein specifically recognizes the CRE sequences near the promoter of responsive genes and mediates the increase in transcription only when it is phosphorylated by PKA. Microinjection of a synthetic CRE oligonucleotide into the nucleus of the sensory neuron has been shown to abolish long-term sensitization, presumably by diverting CREB protein away from the target genes required for long-term changes in gene expression. Two forms of CREB have been described in *Aplysia*: ApCREB1, which acts as a positive mediator of cAMP regulation of transcription, and ApCREB2, which shows homology to ApCREB1 but lacks the PKA phosphorylation site. Experiments suggest that ApCREB2 acts as a repressor of long-term sensitization and that phosphorylation by other kinases may be required to relieve this repression [14,15].

Some of the events following activation of ApCREB1 have been defined [13]. One of the genes which is downstream of the initial phosphorylation of CREB has been identified as the *Aplysia* CCAAT enhancer-binding protein (ApC/EBP). This protein is a homologue of a mammalian transcription factor known to regulate the immediate early gene c-*fos*. It is likely that the induced ApC/EBP protein is responsible for a secondary induction of a number of genes responsible for the formation of new synaptic connections. A second gene induced directly by ApCREB1 is a ubiquitin hydrolase. This enzyme

has been implicated in the proteolytic degradation of the regulatory subunit of PKA, resulting in the prolonged activation of the catalytic subunit seen during long-term sensitization. The ubiquitin hydrolase may also play a role in the degradation of *Aplysia* cell adhesion molecule (ApCAM). Degradation of the ApCAM has been postulated to allow the activation of endocytosis required for growth of new synapses [13].

The most complex form of learning which can be studied conveniently in *Aplysia* is classical conditioning. In this paradigm, tail shock results in withdrawal of the gill, and if the siphon is stimulated shortly before (<1 sec) the tail shock, the animal eventually learns to associate siphon stimulation with the tail shock. In contrast, if the mantle is stimulated shortly after the tail response, there is no learned response. The cellular mechanisms underlying classical conditioning in *Aplysia* are similar to those involved in sensitization, but the crucial difference lies in the strict temporal dependence found in classical conditioning. At the same axo-axonal synapse where serotonin release from the sensory neuron stimulates cAMP production during sensitization, prior depolarization of the conditioned stimulus pathway (siphon stimulation in Fig. 50-3 above) results in depolarization of the presynaptic terminal. This depolarization results in elevated concentrations of Ca^{2+} in the presynaptic terminal as a result of influx through voltage-sensitive Ca^{2+} channels. The increase is transient, and Ca^{2+} eventually returns to resting intracellular concentrations as it is pumped out through plasma membrane Ca^{2+} pumps. If, however, the presynaptic terminal is stimulated with serotonin while the Ca^{2+} concentration is elevated within the presynaptic terminal, the effects of serotonin on generation of cAMP are potentiated by the elevated Ca^{2+}. This effect appears to be due to a Ca^{2+}-sensitive form of adenylyl cyclase, which shows greater stimulation of cyclase activity by serotonin in the presence of high Ca^{2+} concentration. Thus, if serotonin release triggered by the US closely follows activation of the CS pathway, the potentiation of the cyclase activity results in higher concentrations of cAMP, greater activation of PKA, greater phosphorylation of the same K^+ channels involved in sensitization and increased release of

A

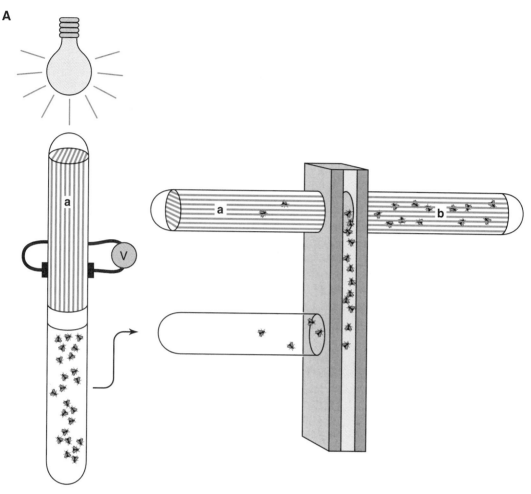

FIGURE 50-4.   A: The training and testing paradigm for *Drosophila* learning and memory. Flies are first trained to avoid an odorant, such as cyclohexanol, on an electrified grid. After training, the flies are allowed to choose between two chambers, one *(a)* containing the training odorant and one *(b)* containing a neutral odorant. The distribution of flies in the two chambers is then analyzed. (*Figure continues on next page.*)

neurotransmitter from the presynaptic terminal. This then constitutes a synaptic model of conditioning, regulated at the molecular level.

Drosophila are useful as a genetic system for studying learning and memory

Seymour Benzer and his associates pioneered the use of genetics to study learning and memory in *Drosophila* [16,17]. These researchers have identified a number of mutant strains that appear normal except for the inability to learn or to store memory of a specific training task. Some

forms of sensitization, habituation and classical conditioning paradigms have been demonstrated in *Drosophila*. Furthermore, behavioral screens have been devised for the detection of strains defective in these behaviors. One of the commonly used screening strategies for characterization of *Drosophila* mutants involves operant conditioning and olfactory cues (Fig. 50-4). Flies are exposed to an odorant, such as 4-methylcyclohexanol, spread onto an electrified wire grid. Eventually, normal flies learn to associate the electric shock with the odorant and avoid it. After this type of training, learning can be quantitated by exposing the flies to two cham-

B

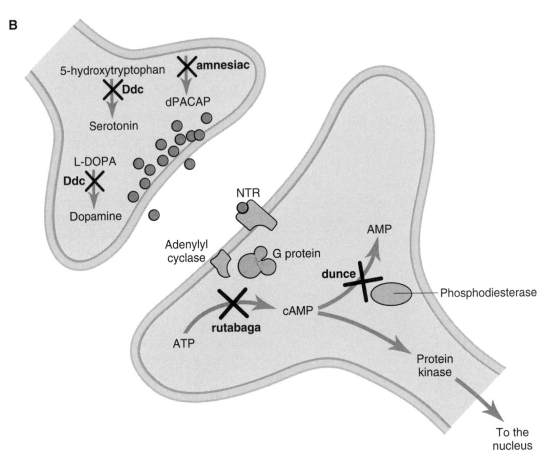

FIGURE 50-4. (Continued) **B:** The nature of various *Drosophila* mutations known to affect learning or memory include dopa decarboxylase *(Ddc); rutabaga,* a Ca^{2+}/calmodulin-sensitive adenylyl cyclase; *dunce,* a cAMP phosphodiesterase; and *amnesiac,* a pituitary adenylyl cyclase–activated peptide *(dPACAP).* Generic postsynaptic neurotransmitter receptors are designated NTR.

bers that have different odorants and determining the percentage of flies that have learned to avoid the conditioning odorant. This percentage is known as the avoidance index. Fly stocks can be mutagenized, and mutant flies that are altered in their ability to associate the electric shock with the odorant selected. Avoidance indices of 0.9 are common for wild-type *Drosophila,* while mutant strains may have avoidance indices of 0.3 or less.

One of the best-documented behavioral mutants is *dunce (dnc),* in which a deficiency in the structural gene for a cAMP phosphodiesterase (PDE) has been established (Fig. 50-4B) [18]. These PDEs specifically hydrolyze cAMP to 5'-AMP and are responsible for returning cellular concentrations of cAMP to resting values following stimulation of adenylyl cyclase. Many isoforms of PDE have been characterized that are differentially regulated and expressed in a tissue-specific manner (Chap. 22). The *dnc* gene organization is extremely complex and is distributed over at least 150 kb of the *Drosophila* genome. Multiple RNA transcripts from this gene encode several different PDE protein isoforms. Antibodies generated to a conserved region of these isoforms have been used to show that the *dnc* PDE is concentrated within a region of the *Drosophila* nervous system known as the mushroom body. The mushroom body has been implicated as the anatomical site of olfactory learning and memory on the basis of many experiments. The relatively restricted expression of the *dnc* PDE to this region suggests that the dnc protein plays a direct role in mediating memory formation. How the PDE gene defect is translated into a behavioral deficit is not known. The behavioral deficit does not seem to be due to a generalized developmental defect in the nervous system since the brains of *dnc* flies appear morphologically normal and the flies are able to form memory, albeit extremely short-term.

A related *Drosophila* behavioral mutant is *rutabaga (rut)*. Like *dnc* mutants, memory forms in the *rut* mutant but decays rapidly. Adenylyl cyclase from *rut* flies has an increased K_m for ATP. Two forms of adenylyl cyclase activity can be distinguished in normal *Drosophila*, based on sensitivity to calmodulin. The *rut* mutants appear to be deficient in calmodulin-stimulated adenylyl cyclase. Mammalian cDNA clones for adenylyl cyclase have been used to isolate the *Drosophila* homologues. The *rut* gene product encodes a calmodulin-stimulated adenylyl cyclase [19]. The *rut* mutants contain a single base change, which results in an amino acid substitution of arginine for the glycine normally found at residue 1026 of the adenylyl cyclase. This single amino acid substitution is sufficient to completely abolish cyclase activity. These observations suggest that, in *Drosophila*, complex behaviors such as learning can be drastically altered by relatively simple alterations to the genome.

Mutant flies producing defective enzymes required for neurotransmitter metabolism, such as DOPA decarboxylase, have been reported to be deficient in olfactory and behavioral learning paradigms. DOPA decarboxylase is necessary for the synthesis of dopamine, serotonin and octopamine. Because this enzyme is essential not only for neurotransmitter synthesis but also for synthesis of the cuticle, these mutants are impaired in their exoskeletal development and the phenotype is complex [17]. This problem has been overcome by use of temperature-sensitive alleles of the mutation. These alleles function normally and permit normal development at 25°C. Subsequent induction of the neural phenotype can be brought about by relatively brief exposure of the adult flies to an elevated temperature which inhibits the mutant enzyme.

The *amnesiac (amn)* mutant has been characterized at a molecular level, and the gene responsible has been identified as a neuropeptide precursor which contains two peptides related to the mammalian pituitary adenylyl cyclase-activating peptide (PACAP) [20]. As the name implies, PACAP elevates cAMP levels by activating adenylyl cyclase. However, it has not yet been demonstrated that any of the neuropeptides derived from the *amn* precursor elevate cAMP in *Drosophila* neurons.

In addition to these behavioral mutant fly strains obtained by forward-genetic screening, a number of reverse-genetic experiments have demonstrated that all of the following play essential roles in learning and memory: the α subunit of G_s, both the regulatory and catalytic subunits of PKA and a fly homologue of CREB designated dCREB2. Interestingly, different transcripts of the same dCREB2 gene can be formed by alternative splicing to produce both an activator and a repressor of gene transcription, much like the mammalian CRE modulator gene (see Chap. 26).

Other invertebrates are being developed as model systems for experimental studies of memory

In the marine invertebrate *Hermissenda crassicornis*, the CS is a positive phototaxis that is paired with high-speed rotation, the US, which leads to suppression of the unconditioned response [21]. Daily sessions of 50 to 100 pairings for a few days result in retention of the learned response for over 2 weeks. Of a number of cellular changes found following conditioning, a reduced K^+ current in type B photoreceptors has been pursued experimentally. From experiments involving various drugs and microinjections of enzymes, it has been inferred that Ca^{2+}/calmodulin-activated protein kinases and PKA mediate associative learning in *Hermissenda*. However, in *Hermissenda*, unlike *Aplysia*, Ca^{2+} influx is the result of depolarization, as is proposed in hippocampal LTP, whereas in *Aplysia*, it is neurotransmitter-mediated. Inhibitors of protein synthesis prolong the altered biophysical correlates of conditioning in *Hermissenda*. It has been speculated that this seemingly paradoxical result is related to short-term, rather than long-term, memory formation. Microinjection experiments and the application of phorbol esters indicate that protein kinase C (PKC) and the phosphoinositide pathway may also play an important role in associative learning, as is further discussed below, in relation to LTP.

Caenorhabditis elegans represents another species which has been subjected to genetic analysis in order to identify the molecular components of neural development and, ultimately, of learning and memory [22]. Mutant animals which show defects in both short-term and long-term memory have been isolated, but identification of the genes affected has not been completed. Although *C. elegans* is less impressive than the fruit fly in terms of its behavioral repertoire, it has the anatomical advantage of possessing only a few hundred neurons. Thus, if altered phenotypic expression in the morphology of the nervous system occurs, it can be more readily correlated with altered behavior.

STUDIES OF LEARNING AND MEMORY IN VERTEBRATES

Rodents, particularly the mouse and rat, have been by far the most favored experimental vertebrate animals for behavioral study. The mouse is appropriate for genetic studies because of the availability of inbred populations, including many mutant strains, and for available transgenic techniques for manipulation of genomic sequences. The rabbit has been useful for studies on classical conditioning, employing the eye blink response. The avian brain has proven attractive for the study of behavioral imprinting, in which newborn chicks and ducklings follow a moving object to which they are first exposed following hatching. Neurochemical correlates such as increased macromolecular synthesis have been investigated extensively [23]. Changes in macromolecular synthesis in the roof of the avian telencephalon have been correlated with successful imprinting of a taste aversion. Acquisition of birdsong has been associated with immediate early gene encoding in the forebrain of zebra finches and canaries. Lower primates are of special interest because of the similarity in

their CNS structure to that of the human. The concept that higher brain function can be localized receives support from studies on human learning and memory employing PET and fMRI (see below).

Long-term potentiation leads to structural changes at the synapse

Learning and memory formation are thought to involve structural changes in the brain, specifically at the synapses, but the mechanisms underlying these processes remain elusive. One of the goals of neuroscience research has been to identify and understand these synaptic correlates of mammalian learning and memory. As previously discussed, learning involves an adaptive change in response to a stimulus. In the mammalian brain, LTP is a useful synaptic correlate of learning and memory [24]. As a function of an increase in the frequency of action potentials or of stimulus history, some presynaptic pathways can generate a long-lasting potentiation in the magnitude of the synaptic potential. After a series of short, high-frequency synaptic bursts, 100 per second, the amplitude of the synaptic response increases and can be maintained *in vivo* at the increased level for days or weeks. LTP is particularly robust in higher cortical structures such as the hippocampus. Detailed studies have shown that development of LTP requires a stimulus threshold determined by complex interactions between the frequency and the strength of the electrical stimulation to the afferent pathway. This requirement correlates with both a release of neurotransmitter from the presynaptic cells and a strong depolarization of the postsynaptic cells. LTP can be elicited *in vitro* (see below). It should be noted, however, that LTP has not been clearly associated with any behavioral modification observed in an intact animal.

As shown in Figure 50-5, the anatomical arrangement of synaptic connections within the hippocampus renders this structure particularly amenable to experiment. Furthermore, these pathways are preserved in a hippocampal slice, a section of the hippocampus which can be experimentally studied for many hours. Three distinct classes of hippocampal synaptic connections

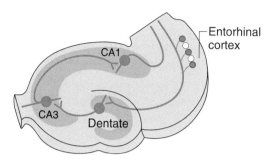

FIGURE 50-5. Diagram of the hippocampal network of neurons involved in long-term potentiation (LTP). Neurons of the entorhinal cortex innervate the dentate granule cells, which send "mossy fiber" tracts to the pyramidal cells of the CA3 region, which in turn synapse with the CA1 neurons, forming the Schaffer collateral pathway. LTP can be induced at the perforant–dentate, the mossy fiber–CA3 and the Schaffer collateral–CA1 synapses.

have been studied: the "perforant path" consists of axons from the entorhinal cortex that synapse with granule cells of the dentate gyrus; axons designated as "mossy fibers" of these dentate granule cells in turn synapse with pyramidal cells of the CA3 region; and the CA3 pyramidal cells synapse with CA1 neurons and form the "Schaffer collateral pathway." Although each of these three pathways may develop LTP, the mossy fiber pathway to CA3 neurons is unique in several ways. The Schaffer collateral pathway is the most widely studied and best understood of these synaptic pathways.

One of the most impressive aspects of LTP is "synapse specificity." For example, although a given CA1 neuron may receive many afferent synapses from distinct CA3 pyramidal cells, LTP generally will be observed only in the synapses of afferents that have received the tetanic stimulation. There is considerable evidence to indicate that glutamate plays a key role as the excitatory neurotransmitter in LTP formation [25]. Since antagonists of the *N*-methyl-D-aspartate (NMDA) receptor, such as 4-amino-5-phosphonovaleric acid (see Chap. 17), can prevent induction of LTP, it has been proposed that postsynaptic receptors activated during LTP are of the NMDA type. This is true for LTP observed in both the dentate and CA1 neurons. The metabotropic glutamate receptor (mG1uR) plays a key

role in induction of LTP, whether or not NMDA receptors are additionally activated. When stimulation conditions are optimal for LTP formation, there appears to be a significant increase in postsynaptic Ca^{2+}. This Ca^{2+} increase is required for LTP in CA1 neurons since injection of EGTA and other Ca^{2+}-chelating agents into postsynaptic neurons prevents LTP. It remains uncertain precisely how the elevation of postsynaptic Ca^{2+} leads to LTP. The most strongly favored hypotheses involve Ca^{2+} activation of one or more protein kinases, but the identity of these kinases is unclear. PKC activation has been shown to occur following induction of LTP, and this activation is required for LTP formation, as determined by studies of mice deficient in PKCγ [25]. It has even been postulated that phosphorylation of GAP-43 by PKC may be required. PKC is activated by Ca^{2+} as well as by diacylglycerol (DAG) released in the breakdown of the phosphoinositides (see Chap. 21). A second protein kinase implicated in LTP is Ca^{2+}/calmodulin-dependent protein kinase II (CaMKII), which may constitute up to 20% of the protein in postsynaptic density preparations. When activated by Ca^{2+}, CaMKII is autophosphorylated. This prolongs its activity in the absence of Ca^{2+}. Many of the *in vitro* properties of this enzyme can be correlated with events known to occur in LTP. Homozygous mice deficient in a major form of CaMKII have been derived using gene-ablation techniques (see Chap. 40), and these mutant mice have been shown to be perturbed in the development of LTP [26]. Gene-ablation experiments can be complicated by the fact that the deficient protein may be required for proper differentiation and development of the nervous system, so these results do not necessarily implicate a direct role of CaMKII in LTP. However, no gross abnormalities in CNS development were noted in these mutant mice.

A number of proteins in addition to CaMKII and PKC have been implicated in LTP [26]. Gene ablation of the tyrosine kinase fyn has been shown to impair LTP of CA1 neurons, although effects on other forms of LTP were not examined. Mice deficient in mGluR1 are deficient in CA1 LTP but not in LTP at mossy fiber–CA3 synapses. PKA-deficient mice also show deficits in LTP at mossy fiber–CA3 synapses, specifically in the late phase of LTP, and individual isoforms of the regulatory and catalytic subunits of PKA are involved. Overall, these results indicate that the major neuronal signaling pathways involved in LTP may differ for various neuronal populations.

It has become clear that many critical aspects of LTP can be mediated by the postsynaptic neuron. If the increase in neurotransmitter release from the presynaptic cells underlies LTP formation, then the postsynaptic cell must communicate in some fashion with the presynaptic cell surface. Much effort is currently focused on identification of the postulated chemical messenger released from the postsynaptic cell that regulates presynaptic neurotransmitter release. The putative retrograde messenger from the postsynaptic neuron has not been clearly identified, and it is possible that several substances may be involved. Candidate molecules include prostanoids and nitric oxide, among other substances. The key question is: What is the process that converts a transient response to a lasting one? Several lines of evidence suggest that LTP can induce the formation of additional synapses, a hypothesis that has remained elusive in its documentation.

Studies of hippocampal slices, complemented by hippocampal cell culture electrophysiology, reveal a potent effect of BDNF on synaptic plasticity and LTP [27]. Within minutes of bath application of BDNF to hippocampal cultures, the spontaneous presynaptic firing rate increases dramatically and the amplitude of postsynaptic currents is increased [28]. Furthermore, in hippocampal slices from BDNF knockout mice, LTP is impaired: both homo $(-/-)$ and heterozygous $(-/+)$ mutant mice show significantly reduced LTP in the CA1 area of the hippocampus, and bath application of BDNF to hippocampal slices completely reverses deficits in LTP [29]. Further, and importantly, re-expression of BDNF in the CA1 of BDNF mutant mice by virus-mediated gene transfer restores LTP as well [30]. This evidence strongly suggests that BDNF plays a functional role in the expression of hippocampal LTP. Additional evidence for BDNF involvement in learning and memory is provided by the observation that learning increases BDNF mRNA in the hippocampus [31],

and direct injection of BDNF antisense oligonucleotides into the hippocampus before task assimilation markedly impairs retention performance, reduces hippocampal BDNF mRNA and impairs LTP [31].

The precise mechanism by which BDNF modulates synaptic plasticity probably involves both presynaptic and postsynaptic effects. BDNF has been postulated to be a selective retrograde messenger [29]. High K^+, glutamate or carbachol results in the activity-mediated release of BDNF from both soma and neurites, particularly dendrites, of cultured hippocampal neurons [32]. Thus, BDNF may serve as another modulator of presynaptic activity. BDNF enhances the release of classic transmitter substances, such as glutamate and acetylcholine, from neurons, such as hippocampal neurons, which express the BDNF receptor trkB, and promotes the release of neurotrophins, including BDNF [33]. BDNF-induced neurotransmitter and neurotrophin release are likely to be two mechanisms by which BDNF modulates synaptic plasticity.

Behavioral measures of learning and memory define types of memory

With the growing number of available mutant mice deficient in individual gene products, a concept of the role of individual neuronal pathways in learning and memory is forming [34]. A major conclusion is that multiple types of learning exist in vertebrate animals and that distinct behavioral tests can be derived to examine them. Spatial learning is often measured using the Morris water maze, in which the location of a platform submerged under opaque liquid is learned by repeated trials in the tank. Another type of learning, contextual fear conditioning, has been localized to the amygdala. The PKCγ mutant mouse shows defects in both of these forms of learning, and this has been used to argue for the role of the CA1 synapses since other forms of LTP in the hippocampus are unaffected in these mice. Work with PKA-deficient mice supports this notion since, in these animals, CA1 synapses are unaffected and both spatial and contextual learning are intact. As additional behavioral paradigms are developed, the role of dentate LTP and mossy fiber LTP in other forms of learning may be more clearly elucidated.

STUDIES OF LEARNING AND MEMORY IN HUMANS

In the foregoing sections of this chapter, we have identified key molecular events in learning and memory formation in invertebrates and subprimate vertebrates. We have learned the importance of protein synthesis in long-term, but not in short-term, memory formation and the role of intracellular and intranuclear biochemical signaling in long-term memory formation. Studies on the biological basis of human memory formation have until recently been confined to inferences from purely behavioral approaches, such as interference with rote learning, reaction times and more complex tasks involving cognitive skills. In addition, much has been learned from the behavioral deficits seen following localized trauma to the brain, including that produced by surgical procedures, such as have been deemed necessary in the treatment of intractable epilepsy. From studies on these patients, as well as on subhuman species, primarily monkeys, a classification of memory into declarative, or *explicit,* and nondeclarative, or *implicit,* has evolved. Explicit memory in humans deals with facts, including specific times and places, for example, the recollection of an event in the past and of persons who were present. Explicit memory formation requires the hippocampus and associated cortical regions. Once formed, long-term explicit memory appears to be broadly distributed in the brain. Implicit memory includes acquisition of skills of which we are usually not conscious, such as riding a bicycle or driving a car. For a human subject with bilateral hippocampal damage, time has stopped. The subject can be taught a motor skill, such as putting x's into circles. While there is daily improvement in this task, for the subject, each training session is the first. Implicit memory appears to be formed in a variety of brain loci and may be task-specific. Cerebellum and neocortex are among the implicated brain regions. These categories have been extended to other species and tasks. For example, learning of a swimming maze in the rat is considered to be explicit on the basis of the spatial specificity of the task and its demonstrated dependence on the hippocampus.

Metabolic correlates of behavior can be localized noninvasively in brain

More recently, noninvasive techniques have made it possible to investigate metabolic correlates of learning and memory in the human brain. Since increased regional metabolic activity is accompanied by increased regional cerebral blood flow (CBF), single photon emission computerized tomography (SPECT) and PET have proven useful in studies of normal and pathological human behavior (see Chaps. 31 and 54). A particularly useful probe is $[^{15}O]H_2O$. Its entry into the brain is diffusion-limited and dependent on the rate of CBF (Fig. 50-6). The short half-life of ^{15}O, 2 min, is useful in the design of test–retest experiments: the subject is presented with condition I, under which it is known that memory will form. After 10 min, which is five half-lives later, the subject is presented with condition II, in which the same sensorimotor sequences are used but the experimental design is such that no memory will be formed. The two digitized images are superimposed, and the control value for each pixel is subtracted from the anatomically corresponding experimental pixel, leaving a pattern of CBF increase attributable to memory formation. This approach is illustrated in Figure 50-6B. fMRI promises to be a useful tool for further cognitive studies. It is based on the blood oxygenation level-dependent (BOLD) technique. Deoxyhemoglobin has a strong paramagnetic signal, while oxyhemoglobin does not. It is claimed that the enhanced CBF associated with increased local metabolism secondary to increased nerve activity leads to increased oxyhemoglobin and lowered deoxyhemoglobin. This results in an elevated BOLD signal. The advantages of fMRI over PET are the reduced radiation dose to the subject, the higher spatial resolution and the convenience of getting a conventional, or structural, MRI scan in the same scanner at the same time. PET has the advantages that the CBF measurement is based on a physiological model that quantitatively measures CBF rates and that the scan, unlike MRI scans, is quiet and,

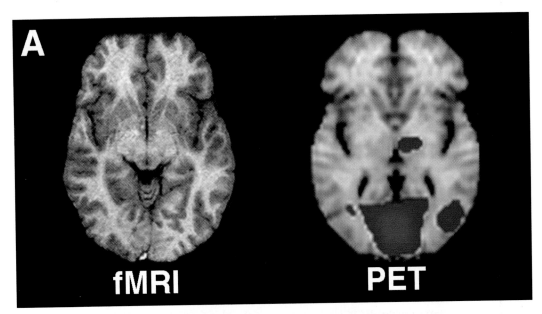

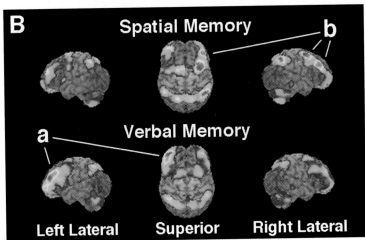

FIGURE 50-6. Functional brain imaging. **A:** Comparison of functional magnetic resonance imaging (fMRI) and [^{15}O]H$_2$O scans of human brain during visual stimulation. In the fMRI scan, the colored region represents increases in the paramagnetic signal from oxyhemoglobin, obtained by subtracting signal generated during presentation of an alternating annular checkerboard pattern to subjects from that recorded in their brains at rest. Increases are seen in the primary visual reception and association areas of the occipital cortex (color) and are displayed superimposed on a structural tomographic MRI, based on proton signaling, primarily from tissue water. The scan on the **right** is an average of several positron emission tomographic (PET) scans of subjects injected with [^{15}O]H$_2$O and then exposed to the same conditions of visual stimulation and rest used for the fMRI. The emitted radioactivity was localized tomographically by means of a PET scanner (see Chap. 54). The color represents averaged quantitative differences in pixels of the pooled digitized images that reached a specified level of significance, superimposed on an averaged structural MRI image (see text). The increases in radioactivity can be quantitatively related to rates of cerebral blood flow (CBF) (Chap. 31 and 54). (fMRI images are courtesy of Drs. T. Chenevert, B. Kim and C. Meyer, Department of Radiology, University of Michigan; PET scans are from Drs. S. Taylor, Department of Psychiatry, and R. Koeppe, Department of Internal Medicine, University of Michigan.) **B:** PET images from a memory task. [^{15}O]H$_2$O scans of human brain during performance of two memory tasks, one "spatial" and the other "verbal." The color scale in this instance represents quantitative differences in CBF associated with increased local metabolism (see Chap. 31). In both tasks, alphabetic characters (letters) appear in different spatial locations once every 3 sec on a video monitor. In the spatial task, subjects press one of two buttons to indicate whether a displayed item is or is not in the same location as it was

thus, less distracting to the subject. While fMRI potentially has higher temporal resolution than PET, the limiting factor in these noninvasive experiments is the physiological delay between nerve stimulation and increased CBF, which appears to take many seconds.

The Sokoloff deoxyglucose technique (Chap. 31) has proven useful in elucidating regional changes in brain metabolism but has not been used extensively in memory studies. In human experiments with ^{18}F-fluorodeoxyglucose, $t_{1/2} = 110$ min, or even with ^{11}C-deoxyglucose, $t_{1/2} = 20$ min, only one PET brain scan per session can be planned because at least three half-lives must pass before a scan can be repeated, to avoid interference of the radionuclide used in the first scan with the second. Thus, the strength of a test–retest paradigm is lost. The use of ^{14}C- or ^{3}H-labeled deoxyglucose to study regional metabolic differences in experimental animals offers the potential advantage of high anatomical resolution, but since the animal must be sacrificed for autoradiography, a test–retest paradigm is not possible in this case either. A possible solution for animal experiments is to use a double-label approach, in which radioactivity from each of two isotopic forms of deoxyglucose, which have been sequentially injected, can be analyzed in the same autoradiogram [35]. Indications that deoxyglucose might be used successfully to study learning and memory have been reported in the rat, in a classical conditioning paradigm in which the US is cardiac slowing produced by stimulation of reticular formation. Coupling this stimulation to an auditory tone, which serves as the CS, leads to classical conditioning. Presentation of the tone after learning is correlated with increased labeling of the molecular layer of the hippocampus [36].

REMAINING QUESTIONS AND FUTURE DIRECTIONS

There are many kinds of learning and memory

We have advanced, in the past few years, from the implication of macromolecular synthesis in long-term memory formation to putative candidate messenger systems that could mediate the requisite feed-forward loops posited in the introduction to this chapter. What then is the molecular basis of short-term memory formation, that is, learning? This too requires a perseverating process but one not requiring *de novo* protein synthesis. Post-translational processes such as phosphorylation could alter synaptic properties for minutes to hours, or even a few days. It has been proposed that there are several stages of short-term memory formation, one of which may represent maintained ion gradients [37]. The lipid peroxidation product 4-hydroxynonenol has been proposed to play such a role [38]. Metabolic oscillatory behavior has been proposed as a candidate model for perseveration of signals initiated by biochemical reactions (see Box 50-1).

It may be useful at this point to distinguish "memory" and "memories." Although there is considerable evidence that specific regions in the mammalian brain, such as the hippocampus and amygdala, play key roles in memory formation, there is also evidence that, once formed, stored memories are broadly distributed in the brain.

---

three trials previously, whether or not it is the same letter. In the verbal task, buttons are pressed to indicate whether or not the item is the same letter as presented three trials previously, whether or not it is in the same spatial location. This is termed a verbal task because it evokes silent rehearsal of the name of the letter by the subject. For both the spatial and verbal tasks, appropriate nonmemory control trials were also administered so that CBF changes related to sensorimotor aspects of the tasks could be subtracted. It can be seen that performing the spatial task leads to a greater increase in regional CBF in right dorsolateral prefrontal cortex and right premotor regions *(b)*, while the verbal task pattern is more lateralized, with greater increases in the left dorsolateral prefrontal cortex and Broca's region *(a)*. These surface images are reconstructed from PET CBF images, in *color,* superimposed on MRI structural images, in *gray.* (PET images are courtesy of Drs. E. Smith, J. Jonides, Department of Psychology and R. Koeppe, Department of Internal Medicine, University of Michigan.)

Given the capacity of the brain to store seemingly limitless quantities of detailed information, a distributed network, in which combinations of neuronal ensembles are employed, would seem more likely than a point-by-point, "one association per structural element" system. Thus, with approaches that seek out brain regions in which metabolic correlates of memory are localized, one does not search for the locus of a specific memory but for the site of a process that "fixes," or "prints," memory of many different experiences.

Furthermore, while the rule of parsimony in scientific discovery demands that we invoke a single mechanism for memory formation, it is clear that many kinds of memory may have evolved through selective pressure. "Bait-shyness" [38] serves as an example. It is a special kind of memory of an ingested noxious substance that results in its future avoidance, obviously an advantage to the animal. The time between eating a poisonous food and illness might be hours, indicating a much longer CS–US interval than is compatible with most other forms of conditioning, and the underlying molecular basis for its formation may prove to be different as well.

Can human memory formation or storage be enhanced?

Neurological and psychiatric diseases are associated with specific behavioral deficits that selectively affect learning and memory. For example, memory loss is striking in Alzheimer's disease (Chap. 46), but it is also a common characteristic and complaint in otherwise healthy aged subjects.

The idea that a pharmacological agent could enhance memory has long intrigued neuropharmacologists, but effective agents have not yet been described. Many screening programs for cognition activators have employed animals in which a behavioral decrement produced by one agent is reversed by the test drug. For example, scopolamine-induced amnesia can be relieved by cholinergic agonists in a screening assay. Because of the artifactual nature of the approach, results of such studies must be interpreted cautiously. More recently, molecular genetic screens have become available and drugs based on the CREB switch, for

example, have been proposed. Evidence for participation of CREB proteins in consolidation of a spatial memory task in the rat hippocampus [40] may add to the inferences for such a role from studies in invertebrates and LTP discussed earlier in this chapter. In the 1960s, there was a flurry of claims for memory improvement and of drugs actually on the market that were purported to achieve this. Given recent advances in our knowledge, this is predicted to become an active field of investigation again in the next decade.

We have seen then, in this chapter, evidence from several experimental systems derived from a variety of species beginning to converge on protein synthesis-dependent synaptic mechanisms that mediate the formation of long-term memory.

REFERENCES

1. Agranoff, B. W. Biochemical events mediating the formation of short- and long-term memory. In Y. Tsukada and B. W. Agranoff (eds.), *Neurobiological Basis of Learning and Memory.* New York: Wiley, 1980, pp. 135–147.

2. Pavlov, I. P. In G. V. Anrep (ed.), *Conditioned Reflexes: An Investigation of the Physiological Activity of the Cerebral Cortex.* London: Oxford University Press, 1940.

3. Escorihuela, R. M., Tobena, A., and Fernandez, T. Environmental enrichment reverses the detrimental action of early inconsistent stimulation and increases the beneficial effects of postnatal handling on shuttlebox learning in adult rats. *Behav. Brain Res.* 61:169–173, 1995.

4. Falkenberg, T., Mohammed, A. K., Henriksson, B., Persson, H., Winblad, B., and Lindefors, N. Increased expression of brain-derived neurotrophic factor mRNA in rat hippocampus is associated with improved spatial memory and enriched environment. *Neurosci. Lett.* 138:153–156, 1992.

5. Diamond, M. C., Johnson, R. E., Protti, A. M., Ott, C., and Kajisa, L. Plasticity in the 904-day-old male rat cerebral cortex. *Exp. Neurol.* 87:309–317, 1985.

6. Greenough, W. T., McDonald, J. W., Parnisari, R. M., and Camel, J. E. Environmental conditions modulate degeneration and new dendrite growth in cerebellum of senescent rats. *Brain Res.* 380:136–143, 1986.

7. Black, J. E., Isaacs, K. R., Anderson, B. J., Alcantara, A. A., and Greenough, W. T. Learning causes synaptogenesis, whereas motor activity causes angiogenesis, in cerebellar cortex of adult rats. *Proc. Natl. Acad. Sci. USA* 87:5568–5572, 1990.

8. Fordyce, D. E., and Wehner, J. M. Physical activity enhances spatial learning performance with an associated alteration in hippocampal protein kinase C activity in C57BL/6 and DBA/2 mice. *Brain Res.* 619:111–119, 1993.

9. Bucinskaite, V., Theodorsson, E., Crumpton, K., Stenfors, C., Ekblom, A., and Lundeberg, T. Effects of repeated sensory stimulation (electro-acupuncture) and physical exercise (running) on open-field behaviour and concentrations of neuropeptides in the hippocampus in WKY and SHR rats. *Eur. J. Neurosci.* 8:382–387, 1996.

10. Neeper, S. A., Gomez, P. F., Choi, J., and Cotman, C. W. Physical activity increases mRNA for brain-derived neurotrophic factor and nerve growth factor in rat brain. *Brain Res.* 726:49–56, 1996.

11. Stummer, W., Weber, K., Tranmer, B., Baethmann, A., and Kempski, O. Reduced mortality and brain damage after locomotor activity in gerbil forebrain ischemia. *Stroke* 25:1862–1869, 1994.

12. Routtenberg, A., Lovinger, D. M., and Steward, O. Selective increase in phosphorylation of a 47 kDa protein (Fl) is directly related to long-term potentiation. *Behav. Neural Biol.* 43:3–11, 1986.

13. Bailey, C. H., Bartsch, D., and Kandel, E. R. Toward a molecular definition of long-term memory storage. *Proc. Natl. Acad. Sci. USA* 93:13445–13452, 1996.

14. Abel, T., Martin, K. C., Bartsch, D., and Kandel, E. R. Memory suppressor genes: Inhibitory constraints on the storage of long-term memory. *Science* 279:338–341, 1998.

15. Michael, D., Martin, K. C., Seger, R., Ning, M. M., Baston, R., and Kandel, E. R. Repeated pulses of serotonin required for long-term facilitation activate mitogen-activated protein kinase in sensory neurons of *Aplysia*. *Proc. Natl. Acad. Sci. USA* 95:1864–1869, 1998.

16. Hotta, Y., and Benzer, S. Mapping behaviour in *Drosophila* mosaics. *Nature* 240:527–535, 1972.

17. Belvin, M. P., and Yin, J. C. *Drosophila* learning and memory: Recent progress and new approaches. *Bioessays* 19:1083–1089, 1997.

18. Davis, R. L. Physiology and biochemistry of *Drosophila* learning mutants. *Physiol. Rev.* 76:299–317, 1996.

19. Levin, L. R., Han, P.-L., Hwang, P. M., Feinstein, P. G., Davis, R. L., and Reed, R. R. The *Drosophila* learning and memory gene *rutabaga* encodes a Ca^{2+}/calmodulin-responsive adenylyl cyclase. *Cell* 68:479–489, 1992.

20. Feany, M. B., and Quinn, W. G. A neuropeptide gene defined by the *Drosophila* memory mutant amnesiac. *Science* 268:869–873, 1995.

21. Frysztak, R. J., and Crow, T. J. Synaptic enhancement and enhanced excitability in presynaptic and postsynaptic neurons in the conditioned stimulus pathway of *Hermissenda*. *J. Neurosci.* 17:4426–4433, 1997.

22. Wen, J. Y., Kumar, N., Morrison, G., et al. Mutations that prevent associative learning in *C. elegans*. *Behav. Neurosci.* 111:354–368, 1997.

23. Rose, F. D., al-Khamees, K., Davey, M. J., and Attree, E. A. Environmental enrichment following brain damage: An aid to recovery or compensation? *Behav. Brain Res.* 56:93–100, 1993.

24. Bliss, T. V. P., and Lomo, T. Long-lasting potentiation of synaptic transmission in the dentate gyrus of the rat following selective depletion of monoamines. *J. Physiol. (Lond.)* 232:331–356, 1973.

25. Cain, D. P. LTP, NMDA, genes and learning. *Curr. Opin. Neurobiol.* 7:235–242, 1997.

26. Chen, C., and Tonegawa, S. Molecular genetic analysis of synaptic plasticity, activity-dependent neural development, learning, and memory in the mammalian brain. *Annu. Rev. Neurosci.* 20:157–184, 1997.

27. Lindholm, D. Neurotrophic factors and neuronal plasticity: Is there a link? *Adv. Neurol.* 73:1–6, 1997.

28. Levine, E. S., Dreyfus, C. F., Black, I. B., and Plummer, M. R. Brain-derived neurotrophic factor rapidly enhances synaptic transmission in hippocampal neurons via postsynaptic tyrosine kinase receptors. *Proc. Natl. Acad. Sci. USA* 92:8074–8077, 1995.

29. Griesbeck, O., Korte, M., Staiger, V., et al. Combination of gene targeting and gene transfer by adenoviral vectors in the analysis of neurotrophin-mediated neuronal plasticity. *Cold Spring Harb. Symp. Quant. Biol.* 61:77–83, 1996.

30. Korte, M., Griesbeck, O., Gravel, C., et al. Virus-mediated gene transfer into hippocampal CA1 region restores long-term potentiation in brain-derived neurotrophic factor mutant mice. *Proc. Natl. Acad. Sci. USA* 93:12547–12552, 1996.

31. Ma, Y. L., Wang, H. L., Wu, H. C., Wei, C. L., and Lee, E. H. Y. Brain-derived neurotrophic factor antisense oligonucleotide impairs memory retention and inhibits long-term potentiation in rats. *Neuroscience* 82:957–967, 1998.

32. Tongiorgi, E., Righi, M., and Cattaneo, A. Activity-dependent dendritic targeting of BDNF and TrkB mRNAs in hippocampal neurons. *J. Neurosci.* 17:9492–9505, 1997.

33. Canossa, M., Griesbeck, O., Berninger, B., Campana, G., Kolbeck, R., and Thoenen, H. Neurotrophin release by neurotrophins: Implications for activity-dependent neuronal plasticity. *Proc. Natl. Acad. Sci. USA* 94:13279–13286, 1997.

34. Keverne, E. B. An evaluation of what the mouse knockout experiments are telling us about mammalian behaviour. *Bioessays* 19:1091–1098, 1997.

35. Olds, J. L., Frey, K. A., and Agranoff, B. W. Sequential double label deoxyglucose autoradiography for determining cerebral metabolic change: Origins of variability within a single brain. *Neuroprotocols* 5:12–24, 1994.

36. Gonzalez-Lima, F., and Scheich, H. Classical conditioning of tone-signaled bradycardia modifies 2-deoxyglucose uptake patterns in cortex, thalamus, habenula, caudate-putamen and hippocampal formation. *Brain Res.* 363:239–255, 1986.

37. Tully, T. Regulation of gene expression and its role in long-term memory and synaptic plasticity. *Proc. Natl. Acad. Sci. USA* 94:4239–4241, 1997.

38. Mattson, M. P. Modification of ion homeostasis by lipid peroxidation: Roles in neuronal degeneration and adaptive plasticity. *Trends Neurosci.* 21:53–57, 1998.

39. Palmerino, C. C., Rusiniak, K. W., and Garcia, J. Flavor-illness aversions: The roles of odor and taste in memory for poison. *Science* 208:753–755, 1980.

40. Guzowski, J. F. and McGaugh, J. L. Antisense oligonucleotide-mediated disruption of hippocampal cAMP response element binding protein levels impairs consolidation of memory for water maze training. *Proc. Natl. Acad. Sci. USA* 94:2693–2698, 1997.

GENERAL REFERENCES

Kandel, E. R., Schwartz, J. H., and Jessell, T. M. Cellular mechanisms of learning and memory. In *Essentials of Neural Science and Behavior*. Norwalk, CT: Appleton and Lange, 1995, pp. 667–694.

Levitan, I. B., and Kaczmarek, L. K. Learning and memory. In *The Neuron*. New York: Oxford University Press, 1997, pp. 475–507.

National Academy of Sciences Colloquium on Memory: Recording experience in cells and circuits. *Proc. Natl. Acad. Sci. USA* 93:13435–13551, 1996.

BOX 50-1

THE BIOCHEMICAL BASES OF OSCILLATORY PHENOMENA AND THEIR POSSIBLE FUNCTIONS IN BRAIN PLASTICITY

Biologically important oscillations occur with periods ranging from milliseconds to hours. Rhythmic activity of longer periodicity often involves neural networks and, at the molecular level, regulation of gene transcription. However, such activity can occur in single cells and even in cell-free systems. A much studied biochemical example of oscillation is anaerobic glycolysis in cell extracts [1] (see Fig. 31-2). Although of uncertain physiological significance, this example illustrates, for an open, nonequilibrium system, the minimum requirements for oscillatory behavior. These are (i) a sustaining energy source (glucose) and (ii) a rate-controlling molecular event that is nonlinearly (allosterically) regulated (phosphofructokinase, PFK).

ADP strongly accelerates the PFK reaction and is a product of the same reaction. ATP depletion in turn slows the PFK reaction. This occurs because the pool of adenine nucleotides is essentially constant relative to the time scale of cycling (minutes). ATP regeneration by the downstream glycolytic reactions progressively restores the PFK reaction rate. Of course, there is net ATP production by glycolysis, but this is mostly utilized by other reactions, categorized as ATPases in the cell-free extracts. Downstream reactions also produce a periodic reduction and reoxidation of NAD, which provides an optical signal that oscillates in phase with ADP levels (see Figure).

Nerve impulses (Chap. 6) and cytoplasmic Ca^{2+} waves (Chap. 23) have the same basic requirements of an energy source and a nonlinear feedback process that controls some type of molecular switch. The immediate energy sources in these cases are ion gradients generated by membrane pumps, and the molecular switches are ion-gating do-

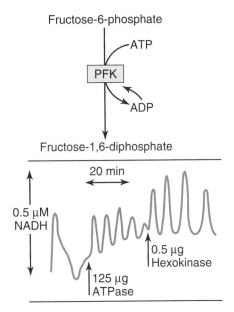

FIGURE. Top: Phosphofructokinase (PFK) activation by ADP is essential for oscillatory behavior of glycolysis **(bottom)**. Amplitude and period of glycolytic oscillations vary as rate of utilization and production is changed. (From [9], with permission.)

mains of membrane channels. The Hodgkin-Huxley equations that describe nerve impulses (Chap. 6) are mathematically analogous to kinetic equations that describe the spatiotemporal propagation of cytoplasmic Ca^{2+} waves [2]. Regulation of channel gating takes many forms, including transmembrane voltages, ligand binding, covalent modifications and intrinsic hysteresis. Further complexity can arise when multiple oscillating systems interact with each other. For example, voltage-dependent ion channel responses can be modulated by oscillations of cytoplasmic Ca^{2+}, as occurs in cardiac myocytes and pancreatic β cells [1].

Neurons must precisely compare and integrate varied synaptic inputs to derive use-

(Box continues on next page)

Box 50-1 (Continued)

ful information. Synchronized oscillations of the membrane potentials of arrays of neurons are thought to mediate these processes. Fields of neurons several millimeters in extent can manifest synchronous 30 to 70 Hz "γ oscillations" of membrane potentials that are evoked by synaptic input to sensory cortex or hippocampus [3]. In visual cortex, "chattering neurons" that emit bursts of extremely high-frequency spikes, <1 msec duration, at γ frequencies are thought to be generators of γ oscillations [4]. Inhibitory interneurons may be involved in the recruitment into functionally synchronized arrays of excitatory pyramidal neurons [5].

Neuronal field potentials at lower θ frequencies, <10 Hz, appear to mediate sensory detection by "phase locking," for example, to the "active touch" input from rat whiskers [6]. At the synaptic level, long-term potentiation (LTP) and long-term depression (LTD) are molecular switching mechanisms that determine whether a given input will be "recorded" at a synapse. Experimentally, application of a cholinergic agonist induces θ oscillations in hippocampal slices. The phase of these oscillations in relation to the timing of synaptic stimuli determines the type of neuronal response: LTP occurs if stimulation coincides with a θ peak, whereas LTD occurs if it coincides with a θ trough [7].

A major component of the postsynaptic complex that appears to mediate LTP and LTD is Ca^{2+}/calmodulin-dependent protein kinase. Because of its autophosphorylation properties, this kinase may act as a frequency detector, acquiring different levels of activity in response to the local patterns of Ca^{2+} oscillations that are produced by postsynaptic depolarizations [8]. A current hypothesis is that the level of activity of this kinase regulates the probability of glutamatergic AMPA-channel opening.

—*R. Wayne Albers*

REFERENCES

1. Goldbeter, A. *Biochemical Oscillations and Cellular Rhythms, Revised.* Cambridge: Cambridge University Press, 1996.
2. Li, Y. X., and Rinzel, J. Equations for InsP$_3$ receptor-mediated $[Ca^{2+}]_i$ oscillations derived from a detailed kinetic model: A Hodgkin-Huxley like formalism. *J. Theor. Biol.* 166:461–473, 1994.
3. Cobb, S. R., Halasy, K., Vida, I., et al. Synaptic effects of identified interneurons innervating both interneurons and pyramidal cells in the rat hippocampus. *Neuroscience* 79:629–648, 1997.
4. Gray, C. M., and McCormick, D. A. Chattering cells: Superficial pyramidal neurons contributing to the generation of synchronous oscillations in the visual cortex [see comments]. *Science* 274:109–113, 1996.
5. Cobb, S. R., Buhl, E. H., Halasy, K., Paulsen, O., and Somogyi, P. Synchronization of neuronal activity in hippocampus by individual GABAergic interneurons. *Nature* 378:75–78, 1995.
6. Ahissar, E., Haidarliu, S., and Zacksenhouse, M. Decoding temporally encoded sensory input by cortical oscillations and thalamic phase comparators. *Proc. Natl. Acad. Sci. USA* 94:11633–11638, 1997.
7. Huerta, P. T., and Lisman, J. E. Bidirectional synaptic plasticity induced by a single burst during cholinergic theta oscillation in CA1 in vitro. *Neuron* 15:1053–1063, 1995.
8. Dosemeci, A., and Albers, R. W. A mechanism for synaptic frequency detection through autophosphorylation of CaM kinase II. *Biophys. J.* 70:2493–2501, 1996.
9. Frenkel, R. Control of reduced diphosphopyridine nucleotide oscillations in beef heart extracts. *Arch. Biochem. Biophys.* 125:151–156, 1968.

51

Neurochemistry of Schizophrenia

Herbert Y. Meltzer and Ariel Y. Deutch

CLINICAL ASPECTS OF SCHIZOPHRENIA 1054

ETIOLOGY 1056

CELLULAR AND PHARMACOLOGICAL STUDIES 1059

Basic Neurochemistry: Molecular, Cellular and Medical Aspects, 6th Ed. edited by G. J. Siegel et al. Published by Lippincott–Raven Publishers, Philadelphia, 1999. Correspondence to Herbert Y. Meltzer, Department of Psychiatry, Vanderbilt University School of Medicine, Nashville, Tennessee 37232.

CLINICAL ASPECTS OF SCHIZOPHRENIA

Schizophrenia, manic-depressive illness, psychotic depression and organic psychoses of known etiology, such as the alcoholic and senile psychoses, are the major forms of psychotic disorders

At some level of neural function, they share the ability to produce characteristic clinical features: (i) delusions or false beliefs; (ii) hallucinations or false perceptions, usually without insight into their pathological nature; and (iii) disorganization of thought, for example, incoherence. These are sometimes accompanied by bizarre behavior. Abnormalities in the structure or function of neurons are central to the various forms of psychosis. This chapter focuses on schizophrenia as an example of psychosis. It is chosen because of the challenge it represents to neurochemistry and because it is a devastating disease which affects about 1% of the population, has a 9 to 13% suicide rate and leads to annual costs, in the United States alone, for 1995, of about 65 billion dollars for medical expenses and indirect costs, such as lost income.

The current view of schizophrenia began with the pioneering clinical observations of Emil Kraepelin, a German psychiatrist, who in 1896 identified a group of psychotic patients with an early age at onset, usually at the end of the second or beginning of the third decade of life, which permanently impaired cognition and usually ended in poor outcome. The characteristic age at onset and impairment in cognition led him to designate this illness as dementia praecox. The term schizophrenia was coined by Eugen Bleuler about one decade later because of his view that many patients with the same hallucinations and delusions present in dementia praecox did not, in fact, develop severe dementia. Schizophrenia was intended to reflect the splitting of affect, or feelings, and cognition. It does not refer to split personality. Bleuler emphasized four types of symptoms: autism, ambivalence, flat affect and disturbances in volition, or will. The current view of schizophrenia is an integration of both Kraepelin's and Bleuler's views, emphasizing characteristic symptoms and cognitive disturbance in a disorder which generally comes on between the ages of 16 and 45. The pendulum has swung back to the view that cognitive impairment, which consists of deficits in attention; vigilance; working, semantic and storage memory; and executive function, is central to the illness [1]. Diagnostic criteria for schizophrenia may be found in the *Diagnostic and Statistical Manual-IV* of the American Psychiatric Association.

The psychopathology of schizophrenia is usually described in terms of three somewhat independent syndromes, or symptom clusters

These are positive, disorganized and negative symptoms [2]. Positive symptoms consist of the florid psychotic symptoms, mainly delusions and hallucinations. The delusions in patients with schizophrenia are usually paranoid, that is, delusions of persecution. Other characteristics are delusions of control, thoughts being inserted or removed from one's mind, grandiosity, somatic and tactile delusions and other bizarre ideas, from the perspective of normal people. Hallucinations are usually auditory in nature and may be experienced as coming from internal or external sources. Recent studies have shown abnormal temporal lobe activity in auditory sensory areas during the experience of auditory hallucinations. Disorganization as a syndrome of schizophrenia includes incoherence, illogicality, loose associations, inappropriate affect and poverty of thought content. Negative symptoms include withdrawal, impoverished emotional state, motivational difficulties, lack of energy, affective flattening, loss of spontaneity and lack of initiative. Depression and anxiety are also frequently present in schizophrenia and are independent of the three syndromes described above, which are core features of the diagnosis of schizophrenia.

Not all of these symptoms are present at any one time. They also vary in severity over time. Neurochemical studies of schizophrenia are, thus, carried out on heterogeneous populations of patients from the point of view of psychopathology. Such studies must distinguish between so-called *state* characteristics, such as transient increases in positive symptoms which respond to treatment, and *trait* characteristics, such as negative symptoms and cognitive impairment which are relatively stable. Even negative symptoms may be variable. So-called primary negative symptoms are stable and not related to positive symptoms, depression or side effects of antipsychotic drugs, while secondary negative symptoms are, as the name implies, believed to be the results of other disease processes in schizophrenia [3]. As current therapies are differentially effective in treating various components of schizophrenia (see below), it is most important to understand the neurochemical underpinnings of these components whose etiology may be only partially overlapping.

When mood symptoms are a major feature of a patient with otherwise characteristic schizophrenia, the diagnosis of schizoaffective disorder is made. Various genetic studies have established that this mixed syndrome is more closely related to schizophrenia than to mood disorders, although there is considerable support for the hypothesis that these two groups of psychoses share some genes. From the point of view of genetic and neurochemical studies, it is also important to be aware of the concept of schizophrenic spectrum disorders. These include schizoid and schizotypal personality disorders. Schizoid individuals have mainly the negative symptoms of schizophrenia without positive symptoms or disorganization, while schizotypal personality disorders manifest mild forms of positive symptoms and disorganization that do not reach the threshold of being considered psychotic.

Cognitive impairment in schizophrenia may be present to a minor extent in childhood and early adolescence but is relatively modest at that time compared with the degree of dysfunction present at the time the diagnosis of schizophrenia is made following the emergence of positive symptoms. The importance of cognitive impairment in schizophrenia is underlined by the findings that it, rather than positive symptoms, is most important for the impaired work function [4]. It is believed that during the prodromal periods prior to the emergence of delusions and halluci-

nations, neural abnormalities at a functional and perhaps structural level develop, producing cognitive impairment. These abnormalities are most likely quite diffuse in nature, but the functions that are predominantly localized to the frontal cortex and temporal lobe rather than the parietal lobe are the most compromised. There is also increasing evidence of a role for the basal ganglia in cognitive function. Deficits in connectivity between regions may be as important as or more important than abnormalities confined to specific brain regions. Functional magnetic resonance imaging is making it possible to study the sequence of activation of specific brain regions recruited during the performance of specific types of cognitive tasks (see Fig. 50-6) and to demonstrate whether patients with schizophrenia have the capacity to modulate the activity of various brain regions in the same fashion as normal controls. The nature of the cognitive deficits in schizophrenia varies considerably from one patient to the next, suggesting that complex neurochemical processes that evolve differently in patients with this illness are involved. Compensatory mechanisms may make it possible for some patients to perform within the normal range on specific tasks. The overall IQ is important in this regard. The neurochemistry of cognition probably involves many neurotransmitters; acetylcholine (ACh), dopamine (DA), serotonin (5-HT), GABA and glutamate, all of which have been implicated in schizophrenia, are believed to be of the greatest importance for cognition.

The cornerstone of the treatment of schizophrenia is a group of antipsychotic drugs which are of value for most forms of psychosis

The serendipitous discovery of the antipsychotic effects of chlorpromazine in 1953 by Laborit, Delay and Denicker in France and the subsequent demonstration by Arvid Carlsson of Sweden that their antipsychotic action was due to the blockade of DA receptors opened up the modern era of schizophrenia treatment and research. Chlorpromazine was followed by the introduction of many other DA receptor blockers of different chemical classes, aided by the demonstration that a specific type of DA receptor, the D2 receptor, negatively coupled to adenylyl cyclase, was their apparent target of action. These agents are called neuroleptics because they impair motor function in animals and humans. These motor effects, which are due to impairment of the extrapyramidal system, are similar to the symptoms of Parkinson's disease: rigidity, difficulty in initiating movements and tremor. In addition, antipsychotic drugs may produce dystonias and result in a very disturbing type of restlessness and agitation called *akathisia*. They can also produce a long-term, sometimes irreversible, impairment of motor function; because this condition is usually delayed in onset, it is called *tardive dyskinesia* (see Chap. 45). Tardive dyskinesia consists of abnormal involuntary movements, usually involving the facial muscles, the tongue, and sometimes the limbs and diaphragm. The rate of development of tardive dyskinesia is 4 to 5% per year of continuous exposure to neuroleptics, but for reasons unknown, less than 25% of patients will develop this side effect. Because of their ability to block D2 receptors in the anterior pituitary gland, neuroleptics also stimulate prolactin secretion, especially in females. This may produce milk secretion, termed galactorrhea.

Among the commonly used neuroleptics are haloperidol, fluphenazine, molindone, thiothixene, sulpiride and thioridazine. There is little evidence that these drugs are differentially effective in schizophrenia, but they differ in potency and side effects, including motor side effects.

Because of the many negative consequences of unwanted blockade of dopaminergic function in the basal ganglia, agents which can achieve an antipsychotic action without causing motor side effects were sought from the earliest period of drug discovery in this area. The first such agent was clozapine [5]. Although chemically related to the neuroleptic loxapine, clozapine did not produce catalepsy in rodents nor did it produce acute or subacute extrapyramidal dysfunction or tardive dyskinesia in humans. Furthermore, low doses of clozapine have been shown to be tolerable to Parkinson's disease patients, who are given the drug to block psychotic symptoms produced by dopamine replacement therapy. Clozapine produces agranulocytosis in 1% of patients, which has limited its usefulness to pa-

tients who are neuroleptic-intolerant or do not respond adequately to the neuroleptics. Independent of its lack of motor side effects, clozapine is more effective than the neuroleptics in the control of positive and negative symptoms in patients who fail to respond adequately to neuroleptics [6]. Since the discovery of clozapine, other agents which are antipsychotic and have reduced motor side effects have been discovered: iloperidone, melperone, olanzapine, ORG 5222, quetiapine, risperidone, sertindole and ziprasidone. These agents are usually referred to as atypical antipsychotics because they cause less of the characteristic motor side effects of neuroleptics at clinically effective doses. They do not necessarily share any of the other characteristics of clozapine and differ among themselves in important ways. Clozapine, olanzapine and risperidone appear to improve cognitive function more so than typical neuroleptic drugs, although the pattern of changes produced by each drug is different. All of these agents also seem to have advantages for negative symptoms. It is debated whether these advantages are true for both primary and secondary negative symptoms or only for secondary negative symptoms. Risperidone produces marked increases in prolactin secretion, which the others do not. As will be discussed, one feature all these drugs share is a high affinity for the 5-HT_{2a} receptor relative to the D2 receptors [5].

Other pharmacological profiles may also produce atypical antipsychotic drugs. Remoxipride has selective antagonism for D2 receptors (see below). It was dropped from clinical use because it produced aplastic anemia. Recent studies suggest that drugs which are 5-HT_{1a} agonists as well as D2 antagonists may also have atypical properties.

ETIOLOGY

Schizophrenia affects 0.75 to 1.5% of the adult population. The incidence depends on the specific criteria and reliability of case finding; when corrected for such factors, the incidence is comparable in all societies that have been studied. Individuals in lower socioeconomic classes are reported to have higher rates of schizophrenia as a result of the markedly impaired work function of patients with this illness.

Schizophrenia is slightly more common in men than women. The impairment in men is, on average, greater than in women because their response to neuroleptic treatment tends to be worse. The age at onset of positive symptoms of some types of schizophrenia is gender-related. Women, especially the paranoid subtype, have an age at onset that averages 5 years later than that in men. The mean age at onset for women is 23 to 28 years, with 19 to 32 being the most common. For men, mean age at onset ranges from 20 to 26 years. Patients with poor responses to currently available therapies have an earlier age at onset than those who are more responsive. There are both childhood and late-life (past the age of 45 years) forms of the illness which have psychopathology and courses comparable to typical schizophrenia.

The view that schizophrenia is the result of specific disturbances in child-rearing received considerable attention up until 1960. In particular, communication deviance between parents and schizophrenic offspring was considered to be a sufficient cause by some. This view has been rejected, although there is evidence that environmental factors, including family dynamics, may contribute to stress and coping skills, which can strongly influence the onset of psychosis, response to drug treatment and compliance with treatment. Nevertheless, there is little evidence to support a primary causal effect of nongenetic familial influences. The view of schizophrenia as a brain disease supplanted this concept as the evidence for a genetic basis for schizophrenia emerged [7].

It is generally accepted, despite the absence of evidence, that schizophrenia is a group of disorders with a common overlapping phenotype rather than a single disease entity

It has a complex mode of inheritance and variable expression. Adoption, twin and family studies carried out in the 1960s established that the vulnerability to develop schizophrenia is largely genetic. What is inherited is an increase in the risk of becoming schizophrenic rather than a gene or genes that absolutely predict the occurrence of schizophrenia. Thus, about half of monozygotic (MZ) twins are concordant for schizophrenia compared to less than 20% of dizygotic (DZ) twins, using psychosis as the phenotype. It is therefore clear that environmental as well as genetic factors are important in the development of the disorder.

The high rate of discordance between MZ twins indicates that what is inherited is a predisposition but not a certainty of developing schizophrenia. In first-degree relatives, percent lifetime expectancy to develop schizophrenia is about 10% if one parent or a sibling has schizophrenia and 45 to 50% for offspring of two schizophrenic parents. In second-degree and third-degree relatives, the expectancy drops to 3.3% and 2.4%, respectively. Furthermore, adoption studies show a lifetime prevalence of 9.4% in the adopted-away offspring of schizophrenic parents and a lifetime prevalence of 1.2% in control adoptees [8].

The distribution of schizophrenia in families indicates a complex inheritance since the risk to relatives declines markedly as the relationship becomes more distant. Studies of extended pedigrees with multigenerational schizophrenia have ruled out single dominant genes as the cause of the illness in the majority of cases. However, there may be a small proportion of cases in which a single major gene, acting either alone or in concert with multiple small genetic and environmental factors, accounts for the vulnerability to become schizophrenic. It is likely that additive effects of several genes of modest effect, termed *oligogenic inheritance*, or many genes of small effect, termed *polygenic inheritance*, are the basis for the vulnerability.

Epidemiological studies of the genetics of schizophrenia are well established and have led to numerous studies using diverse methods to identify specific genes. Many studies reporting the involvement of specific genes in schizophrenia have failed replication. One reason for this is differences in the criteria for the phenotype. Linkage results vary greatly as to whether criteria based on symptomatology are restrictive or broad, for example, excluding schizoaffective patients and/or schizophrenia spectrum patients. Additionally, so-called logarithm of odds (lod) scores must be substantially higher than 3, that is, one chance in 1,000, in a complex disorder such as schizophrenia. Early studies accepted lod scores of 2 or 3 as proof of linkage.

Current major strategies to identify the genes in schizophrenia involve genome scanning through linkage and association studies and candidate gene analysis, for example, D2, D4 and 5-HT$_2$ receptor genes [9]. The latter strategy ruled out the involvement of various genes that are part of the DA system, such as the genes for tyrosine hydroxylase and the D1, D2 and D4 receptors. However, several studies have suggested an association between exon 1 of the D3 receptor and schizophrenia. Despite some nonreplications, this possibility is still the subject of considerable research. Although DA is the main neurotransmitter implicated in schizophrenia, there is also keen interest in 5-HT. Associations between a T to C polymorphism at nucleotide 102 in the 5-HT$_{2A}$ receptor and schizophrenia, and between a Ser-to-Tyr polymorphism at nucleotide 452 and response to clozapine have been reported in several studies [9]. Positional cloning is most likely to be successful when applied to large families containing multiply affected members, when the disease gene has a major effect, when the mode of inheritance of the phenotype is known and when there are few diagnostic errors. These features are not characteristic of schizophrenia and have led to a number of reports of linkage or association that have not been replicated. For these reasons, the currently favored strategy is based on identity by descent involving the analysis of affected siblings. Evidence of linkage is provided when affected sibling pairs share loci more often than would be expected by chance alone. This method does not require knowledge of the mode of transmission, has the power to detect genes of modest effect, is not very sensitive to misdiagnosis and can be readily applied to schizophrenia.

Using the affected sibling pair method, there have been several replications of a locus on chromosome 6p24-p22 for schizophrenia [8]. This region contains the human leukocyte antigen (HLA) locus, which has been postulated to be relevant to schizophrenia. There is limited and controversial evidence that schizophrenia may be one of a group of disorders in which expanded trinucleotide repeats of variable length

are present (see Chap. 40). Advances in the molecular genetics of schizophrenia in the future may lead to identification of the group of genes that convey vulnerability to this syndrome.

The neurodevelopmental hypothesis suggests that the etiology of schizophrenia may involve pathological processes during brain development

This hypothesis is based on the demonstration of behavioral and cognitive disturbances in childhood and adolescence that are eventually diagnosed as schizophrenic [10]. The absence of marked neurodegenerative changes in the schizophrenic brain together with findings suggestive of cortical maldevelopment are consistent with this hypothesis.

According to this hypothesis, the etiology of schizophrenia may involve pathological processes which begin *in utero* or perinatally and continue to unfold until the brain approaches its adult anatomical state as a result of extensive neuronal loss and synaptic pruning during early and late adolescence. These neurodevelopmental abnormalities are proposed to lead to the activation of pathological neural circuits during adolescence or young adulthood, perhaps due to severe stress, leading to the emergence of positive or negative symptoms or both. Some cases with the phenotype of schizophrenia may be due to embryonic maldevelopment, especially of the corpus callosum and temporal lobe, for example, temporal lobe epilepsy. The emergence of evidence for cortical maldevelopment in schizophrenia and the development of several plausible animal models, which are based on neonatal lesions that produce behavioral abnormalities or altered sensitivity to dopaminergic drugs only in adolescent or adult animals [11], have made the link between maldevelopment and schizophrenia more tenable.

A consistent finding in schizophrenia is cerebral ventricular enlargement [12]. A large number of computed tomography (CT) and magnetic resonance imaging (MRI) studies indicate lateral and third ventricular enlargement and widening of cortical fissures and sulci; these are present at the onset of the illness, progress very slowly if at all and are, therefore, unrelated to the duration of illness or the treatment received. Affected MZ twins discordant for schizophrenia have larger ventricles than unaffected twins. The loss of gray matter is correlated with poor premorbid social and educational adjustment during early childhood as well as obstetric complications. These findings are not specific for schizophrenia, however, as they are also found to almost the same extent in manic-depressive illness.

Despite extensive efforts to discover a neuropathological basis for schizophrenia, no consistent characteristic lesions, at either the micro- or the macroscopic level, have yet been identified

However, various abnormalities in the temporohippocampal and frontal lobes, the two brain regions most likely to be abnormal in schizophrenia, are currently being studied. There is extensive evidence that gliosis is not present, indicating that there is no neuronal death due to traumatic, inflammatory processes or infection in schizophrenia. However, an abnormality of programmed cell death, that is, apoptosis, has not been ruled out. Increased density of neurons in the prefrontal cortex, loss of interneurons in the cingulate and prefrontal cortices and abnormalities in migration of cells from the cortical plate to the gray matter of the cortex are among the most interesting recent findings. However, they are based on a small number of samples and have not been shown to be specific for schizophrenia.

Since the mid-1980s, there has been an increasing reliance on anatomical methods to reveal neurochemical changes in postmortem studies of schizophrenia. This has been due in large part to a growing appreciation of the diversity of neurons within what were once considered by most neurochemists, and indeed most neuroscientists, to be single classes of neurons. For example, studies of the gene encoding the GABA biosynthetic enzyme glutamic acid decarboxylase (GAD), as a marker of cortical GABA cells treat these interneurons as a unitary class of cells. However, well over a dozen different types of interneurons can be distinguished morphologically, and the morphological distinctions are paralleled by physiological and neurochemical distinctions. Anatomical methods have proven very useful since they allow subpopulations of interest to be distinguished.

Recent studies have revealed various neuropathological changes in the brain, particularly in the prefrontal cortices, including the pregenual anterior cingulate cortex, and the medial temporal lobe, including the hippocampus, parahippocampal gyrus and entorhinal cortex. Unfortunately, the types of changes reported (ranging from cell loss and changes in cell density in the absence of cell loss to changes in neuronal size, position or orientation) are inconsistent. With increasingly rigorous application of quantitative, computer-assisted, neuroanatomical methods, a greater degree of consistency may emerge. It is clear that representative samples of adequate size must be studied and the comparison groups (such as bipolar disorder and major depression) be included in such studies.

Since schizophrenia typically first occurs in late adolescence or early adulthood, developmental processes are considered key to its pathogenesis. The developmental hypotheses of schizophrenia implicitly assume that changes in neurochemical and neuroanatomical markers represent the culmination of a process and that such end points may be indirect or direct.

CELLULAR AND PHARMACOLOGICAL STUDIES

The dopamine hypothesis has dominated schizophrenia research since the mid-1960s

This is due in large part to the fact that antipsychotic drugs block DA receptors, suggesting that overactivity of central DA systems underlies schizophrenia. However, several other hypotheses have recently been advanced or reformulated to account for the pathophysiology of schizophrenia; most pay homage to the DA hypothesis by incorporating secondary changes in central DA systems that are due to some other putative primary defect.

Several types of studies have attempted to test the hypothesis that there is a primary change in central DA function in schizophrenia. These include examination of (i) differences in concentrations of DA or its metabolites in various brain sites, (ii) the ability of chronic administration of high doses of amphetamine to induce a paranoid form of schizophrenia, (iii) the relationship between the ability of antipsychotic drugs to block D2 receptors and their specific responses and (iv) changes in other types of DA receptors. Unfortunately, the pattern of changes in the various studies is not consistent.

It is important to remember that all classification schemes for schizophrenia emphasize that there are different subtypes. In addition, a substantial body of data demonstrates age-related changes in the DA system; such changes may interact with the number of psychotic episodes and drug treatment to yield different specific symptoms of schizophrenia. It is, therefore, not unexpected that there might be comparable heterogeneity in various markers of DA function.

Dopamine and dopamine metabolite concentrations. Despite considerable effort to detect changes in concentrations of DA or its acidic metabolite homovanillic acid (HVA) in the striatum and other relevant brain areas, most findings have been negative; studies reporting changes, which in some cases are lateralized, have generally been difficult to replicate. Studies of HVA concentrations in cerebrospinal fluid (CSF) and plasma have also been disappointing. While many studies have reported increases in plasma concentrations of HVA in schizophrenia, other reports have found no differences or even decreases relative to normal controls. There is a consistent observation that neuroleptics increase CSF HVA concentrations, although the relationship of such changes to symptomatic improvement remains unclear. Part of the difficulty in obtaining reliable CSF HVA data appears to be technical in nature since in many of the studies no attempt was made to control for the contribution of peripheral sources of HVA, as can be accomplished using debrisoquin, a peripheral monoamine oxidase inhibitor, or by employing probenecid treatment to prevent blood–CSF ex-

change of HVA. However, even in those studies using such methods to eliminate the contribution of peripheral DA, the precise sources of CSF HVA are unclear. In one study of nonhuman primates, CSF HVA and tissue DA concentrations showed a significant correlation in only one brain area, and that accounted for only about 10% of the variance. Because the relationship between central DA function and CSF and plasma HVA concentrations is unclear, these measures do not provide strong support for a primary or major dopaminergic dysfunction in schizophrenia.

Dopamine receptors. Since the mid-1960s, striking similarities between the psychosis seen in certain subjects taking high doses of amphetamine and the symptoms of patients with paranoid schizophrenia have been noted and placed into the context of increased catecholaminergic neurotransmission. Subsequent studies emphasized the contribution of the central dopaminergic, rather than noradrenergic, systems to psychosis. The ability to treat psychosis with D2 receptor antagonists was consistent with the idea of an overactivity of central DA function.

The most compelling of the data marshaled to support the DA hypothesis of schizophrenia is the clear relationship between antipsychotic drug efficacy and affinity for D2 receptors [13]. All known drugs with broad antipsychotic efficacy disrupt DA transmission. With the exception of reserpine, which acts by depleting vesicular stores of DA and is no longer used in the treatment of schizophrenia in Western medicine, antipyschotic drugs block the D2 receptor. An almost linear relationship between the D2 receptor affinity of an antipsychotic drug and some index of the drug's action, such as the average daily dose or plasma or CSF concentrations, has emerged. The exception to this picture has been clozapine; some of the newer atypical antipsychotic drugs also diverge modestly from this relationship. The affinity of these newer atypical antipsychotic drugs for the D2 receptor is relatively low. However, most studies have focused on the affinity of the parent compound for the D2 receptor, without considering active metabolites. Hepatic metabolism of clozapine yields active metabolites that achieve high brain concentrations; one of these, desmethyl-clozapine, has a higher affinity for the D2 receptor than clozapine. Nevertheless, it is unlikely that D2 receptor blockade is the sole basis for the effectiveness of these atypical agents (see below).

The ability of antipsychotic drugs to block D2 receptors has led to attempts to measure the density of DA receptors in the brains of schizophrenic subjects. The genes for five DA receptors have now been cloned and designated as D1, D2, D3, D4 and D5 [14]. The D1 and D5 receptors are positively coupled to adenylyl cyclase, with current pharmacological probes unable to distinguish between these two D1-type receptors. The two receptors have different regional patterns of expression in the brain, with the D5 receptor transcript being much more restricted in its distribution [15]. The other three DA receptors belong to the D2 family and are negatively coupled to adenylyl cyclase. Again, the CNS distributions of these receptors differ considerably, both within and across different species [15].

The D2-like receptors have been the major target of investigations aimed at uncovering changes in DA receptors in schizophrenia. The D2 receptor is the most widely distributed of the D2 family receptors and has a high affinity for typical antipsychotic drugs but lower affinity for atypical antipsychotic drugs. Atypical antipsychotic drugs, of which clozapine is the best known, have antipsychotic efficacy but lack or have a much reduced, ability to elicit extrapyramidal (parkinsonian-like) side effects (EPS) [16]. The ability of atypical antipsychotic drugs to reduce symptomatology without accompanying motor side effects may be due to their relatively low degree of occupancy, as well as reduced affinity, of striatal D2 receptors. In contrast to typical antipsychotic drugs, which result in virtually complete occupancy of dorsal striatal D2 receptors, clozapine occupancy of D2 receptors is variable across patients but almost never exceeds 70% as measured by positron emission tomography (PET) (see Chap. 54) [17]. Given the remarkable functional compensation of the striatal DA system, which may be depleted by 70% or more before giving rise to the symptoms of Parkinson's disease, the rela-

tively low occupancy of striatal D2 receptors may be sufficient to avoid EPS. However, there are other actions of clozapine, such as the ability to treat patients who do not respond to conventional antipsychotic drugs and better efficacy in reducing certain symptoms of schizophrenia [16], which have been suggested to be due to full D2 occupancy by clozapine in cortical regions [18].

Despite a generation of studies on the involvement of D2 receptors in schizophrenia, a strong data-based argument in support of this is difficult to sustain. Most autoradiographic and *in vitro* assessments of D2 receptor density have not uncovered consistent evidence of an increase in the density of D2 receptors in the striatum or other brain sites. Early PET studies suggested that striatal D2 receptor density was increased in schizophrenia, but subsequent PET and single photon emission computerized tomographic (SPECT) studies using several different radioligands have failed to observe such an increase in D2 receptor density in nonmedicated schizophrenic subjects [19].

Other CNS areas examined, such as the prefrontal cortex, have also shown no dramatic changes in D2 receptor density. A recent autoradiographic study of D2 receptor-binding sites in the temporal lobe reported differences in the pattern of D2 receptor expression, with opposite directions of change in the supragranular and granular layers of temporal cortices [20].

Autoradiographic binding studies of receptors are often plagued by technical difficulties owing to the relatively long interval between death and the collection of brain tissue. The susceptibility of receptor-binding studies to long postmortem intervals can be overcome to some degree by studying receptor gene expression, since the mRNAs encoding for the receptors are more stable than the encoded proteins. However, the few studies of D2 gene expression that have been reported do not suggest a change in D2 gene expression in schizophrenia [21].

The D3 receptor has a more restricted distribution than the D2 receptor, with high expression in the ventral striatum, including nucleus accumbens, and moderate expression in some cortical regions in primate, but not rodent, species [15]. The D3 receptor exhibits considerably less affinity for clozapine than for typical antipsychotic drugs, and the precise intracellular transduction pathways through which D3 receptor occupancy is translated into intracellular events are not clear [14]. D3-binding sites in the nucleus accumbens have been reported to be increased in patients who did not receive antipsychotic drug treatment in the month prior to death [20]. In those patients receiving antipsychotic drugs within 72 hr of death, the density of D3 receptor sites was the same as seen in control subjects. These data suggest that D3 receptors are increased by the disease but paradoxically decreased by administration of DA receptor antagonists; the latter point has been confirmed in rodent studies.

In contrast to the increase in D3 receptor-binding sites reported in the ventral striatum of schizophrenics, D3 receptor mRNA levels in the cortex appear to be lower in schizophrenic subjects. However, the levels of a truncated form of the D3 receptor are not changed, suggesting that abnormal splicing of a D3 gene may lead to decreased levels of the D3 receptor with a relative accumulation of the truncated receptor [22].

The D3 receptor has several alleles. Relative abundance of one of the D3 allelic variants is associated with an increased risk for development of tardive dyskinesia after antipsychotic drug treatment.

The D4 receptor differs from the D2 and D3 receptors by displaying a very high affinity for the atypical antipsychotic drug clozapine as well as conventional neuroleptics such as haloperidol. The D4 receptor is relatively enriched in cortical regions, including the hippocampus, of primates but present in very low abundance in the striatum [15]. In view of the high affinity of the D4 receptor for clozapine, there has been considerable effort expended on studying the expression of this receptor in schizophrenia.

Despite the low density of the D4 receptor in the striatum, several groups have used the difference between the density of striatal DA receptor sites as revealed by [³H]raclopride binding, which labels D2 and D3 receptors, and [³H]YM-09151 binding, which labels D2, D3 and D4 receptors, as an indirect index of D4 receptor density. Using this approach, most studies have found a significant increase in the density of D4-like DA receptors in the striatum [23]. The development of specific D4 receptor antagonists lagged behind the cloning of the receptor and hampered the direct assessment of D4 receptor density in schizophrenics. Several specific antagonists are now available, and studies of D4 receptor density in the schizophrenic brain are in progress.

Despite the apparent increase in D4 receptor-binding sites, as revealed by the subtractive autoradiographic method, studies using polymerase chain reaction amplification to detect D4 receptor transcripts have failed to detect any change from normal in D4 gene expression in the striatum or several cortical regions of schizophrenic subjects. More recently, however, an *in situ* hybridization study reported that D4 mRNA is increased in the orbitofrontal, but not other prefrontal, cortical regions [21], emphasizing that regional differences may be striking. The development of selective D4 receptor antagonists has recently culminated in clinical trials. However, the open trials reported to date have not found antipsychotic efficacy of these D4 antagonists.

Several physiological and pharmacological studies in rodents have noted that the actions of DA and certain D2-like agonists, such as, quinpirole, cannot be fully accounted for by binding to one of the five cloned DA receptors. This seems to be particularly true in cortical regions, such as the prefrontal and entorhinal cortices. The genes encoding some D2-like DA receptors, including those present in the renal medulla and brown adipose tissue of rodents, have not been cloned. Molecular biological studies of striatal DA receptors have been interpreted to suggest that the reported striatal D4 receptor differs from the cloned D4 receptor. While it remains to be determined to what degree this site corresponds to the D4 receptor, there are sufficient data to suggest that other D2-like DA receptors may be identified and found to contribute to the pathophysiology of schizophrenia [24].

Less attention has focused on potential changes in D1 receptors than on D2-like receptors, primarily due to the high correlation between antipsychotic efficacy and D2, but not D1, receptor affinities. Those data that have been reported do not offer much support for the involvement of D1 receptors in schizophrenia. A relatively large number of antipsychotic drugs lack appreciable affinity for the D1 receptor *in vivo*. Moreover, selective D1 antagonists, all of which target D5 receptors as well, have not been shown in clinical studies to have antipsychotic effects. In addition, there does not appear to be any change in the density of D1 receptor-binding sites in the striatum. However, a recent PET study of D1 receptor occupancy in schizophrenic patients has suggested that D1, but not D2, receptors are decreased in the prefrontal cortex; this report awaits independent confirmation.

Prefrontal cortical dopaminergic hypoactivity. The past decade has marked a turn from the view that hyperactivity of central DA systems is the major defect in schizophrenia. In addition, recent technical advances have allowed investigators to probe the dynamic function of the DA system rather than relying on static measures. Studies on the neurochemical basis of schizophrenia have focused on uncovering increases in concentrations of DA or its metabolites or concentrations of DA receptors. However, awareness of trans-synaptic regulation of striatal DA systems led investigators to consider the possibility of an increase in striatal DA function being secondary to, or accompanied by, a decrease in functional DA tone in cortical regions that project onto the striatum.

A series of studies a generation ago reported that rats sustaining experimental depletions of DA in the prefrontal cortex showed increases in dopaminergic function in the striatal complex. Although it has proven difficult to replicate exactly the original reports, subsequent studies have consistently found that depletion of prefrontal cortical DA leads to an enhanced responsiveness of striatal DA systems in response to various challenges; these effects are observed primarily in the nucleus accumbens [25]. Among the challenges that evoke such changes in striatal DA function are stress, psychostimulant drugs and DA receptor antagonists [25]. Behavioral studies also have shown that changes in DA in the prefrontal cortex lead to behavioral changes that can be linked to the cognitive deficits present in schizophrenia. Interestingly, several behavioral studies have suggested that deviation in either direction from some ideal level of DA function in the prefrontal cortex may be deleterious.

Most animal studies examining corticostriatal relationships after cortical DA depletions have used indirect measures of trans-synaptic changes in downstream targets, such as the striatum, as the dependent measure. However, there are few direct data in human studies that indicate a decrease in DA levels in the prefrontal cortex. As noted earlier, one report has suggested that D1 receptor density may be decreased in the prefrontal cortex. In addition, recent immunohistochemical data have suggested a decrease in the density of both tyrosine hydroxylase– and DA transporter–immunoreactive axons in the prefrontal cortex of schizophrenic subjects [26].

The concept of concurrent cortical hypodopaminergic state and subcortical hyperdopaminergic tone has profound implications for our current understanding of schizophrenia and the treatment of the disorder [25,27]. As noted earlier, symptomatology in schizophrenia can be viewed as positive or negative. Positive symptoms, such as hallucinations and delusions, are typically sensitive to antipsychotic drug treatment, whereas negative symptoms, such as motivational difficulties, impoverished emotional state and withdrawal, are difficult to treat with conventional antipsychotic drugs but in many cases respond relatively well to clozapine [28]. Negative symptoms have been linked to a decrease in cortical DA tone, while positive symptoms are thought to reflect excessive dopaminergic tone in subcortical sites such as the nucleus accumbens [25,27]. The ability of clozapine to target negative symptoms may be related to its ability to sharply increase extracellular DA levels in the prefrontal cortex [29] or to its relatively high 5-HT_2:D2 receptor affinity [5].

Changes in evoked dopamine release. Studies of changes in receptor density or concentrations of DA or DA metabolites are static measures, providing a snapshot of the status of DA systems at a given point in time. However, many systems exhibit normal baseline function but are dysfunctional when tested under conditions that perturb the system. Until recently it has not feasible to study dynamic neurochemical changes in the schizophrenic brain.

The availability of contemporary *in vivo* imaging techniques has led to recent studies specifically aimed at uncovering abnormalities in the dynamic function of central DA systems (see Chap. 54). By monitoring D2 receptor occupancy with a radioligand that is readily displaced from the DA receptor by endogenous DA, it is possible to monitor changes in release of DA. Two recent studies, using $[^{11}C]$raclopride and $[^{123}I]$iodobenzamide for PET and SPECT, respectively, have found that amphetamine-evoked DA release is increased in the striatum of schizophrenic subjects [30,31]. These data strongly suggest a change in phasic DA release under demand conditions. Since several stimuli, including stress as well as psychostimulants, can transiently increase DA release in the forebrain, examination of the effects of behavioral or pharmacological challenges to the DA system will be a major focus of investigation of neurobiological studies of schizophrenia.

Serotonin has been implicated in a variety of behaviors and somatic functions which are disturbed in schizophrenia

These include hallucinations, cognition, sensory gating, mood, aggression, sexual drive, appetite, motor activity, pain threshold, endocrine function and sleep [32]. It also has an important role in neurodevelopment. Many of these functions are clearly relevant to the etiology of positive and negative symptoms and of the cognitive impairment, which constitute the core abnormalities of schizophrenia. The biochemical and anatomical complexity and diversity of the serotonergic system and its extensive interactions with multiple neurotransmitters provide the physiological substrate for the ability of 5-HT to influence all of these behaviors. There are 14 known 5-HT receptor subtypes, two presynaptic and 12 postsynaptic, that mediate the multiple actions of 5-HT. Serotonin has potent influences on dopaminergic and glutamatergic neurotransmission via its action on 5-HT_{1A}, 5-HT_{2A} and 5-HT_3 receptors, in particular. These interactions occur at the level of DA neurons in the ventral tegmentum and sub-stantia nigra and of 5-HT neurons in the medial and dorsal raphe, as well as at various projection fields of these nuclei. Serotonin may have an overall inhibitory effect on dopaminergic neuro-transmission in the basal ganglia and prefrontal cortex. However, stimulatory effects have also been reported, depending on the nature of the influences on dopaminergic neurotransmission (Chap. 13).

The first hypothesis of an involvement of 5-HT in the etiology of schizophrenia was based on the psychotomimetic effect of lysergic acid diethylamide (LSD), which was found to be an antagonist at brain 5-HT receptors. This led to the hypothesis that decreased serotonergic activity was related to the positive symptoms of schizophrenia [32]. It was subsequently found that this effect of LSD was due to its 5-HT_{2A} agonist properties, not 5-HT antagonism, since the ability to produce visual hallucinations of a large number of indolealkylamine drugs with agonist activity is highly correlated with their affinity for this receptor [32]. Furthermore, the primary effect of LSD in humans is visual hallucinations, which are relatively rare in schizophrenia. None of the other core symptoms of schizophrenia or the cognitive dysfunction described previously are reliably produced by LSD and related drugs. Decreasing serotonergic activity with the 5-HT synthesis inhibitor parachlorophenylalanine does not exacerbate schizophrenia or produce psychosis in normals [32,33]. As discussed below, some studies indicate decreased 5-HT_{2A} receptor density in the cortex of schizophrenics.

The 5-HT deficiency hypothesis was followed by the hypothesis that endogenous production of psychotomimetic indoleamines, such as *N,N*-dimethyltryptamine or psilocybin, might be etiological in schizophrenia. However, the concentrations of such compounds in the brain, plasma and urine of patients with schizophrenia are not increased nor has an increase in the *N*-methyltransferase enzyme required for the synthesis of some of these compounds been found [32]. However, the decrease in the density of 5-HT_{2A} receptors in schizophrenia is consistent with downregulation secondary to an increase in stimulation of this receptor by 5-HT or related compounds.

The major hypothesis concerning the role

of 5-HT in schizophrenia is based, in part, on the interest in the role of 5-HT in the mechanism of action of drugs such as clozapine, olanzapine, risperidone, ziprasidone, sertindole and M 100907, formerly MDL 100907. As previously mentioned, these drugs are called atypical antipsychotic drugs because they produce no (clozapine) or diminished motor side effects at clinically effective doses. Furthermore, they have varying advantages for treating the cognitive dysfunction and positive and negative symptoms of patients with schizophrenia. Clozapine is effective in treating the positive symptoms of up to 60% of those patients with schizophrenia whose positive symptoms fail to respond to typical neuroleptic drugs. The basis for this advantage has been the subject of intensive research interest. One feature which they share is potent $5\text{-}HT_{2A}$ receptor antagonism relative to weak D2 receptor antagonism, which contrasts with the typical neuroleptic drugs [34]. The selective $5\text{-}HT_{2A}$ antagonist M 100907 has been reported to be effective for both positive and negative symptoms in early clinical trials; these results need to be confirmed by further controlled study. There is considerable evidence that $5\text{-}HT_{2A}$ receptor antagonism can modulate dopaminergic and glutamatergic neurotransmission. This is consistent with the hypothesis that there is increased $5\text{-}HT_{2A}$-mediated neurotransmission in schizo-phrenia which may be normalized by these agents [28]. This, in turn, may contribute to decreased glutamatergic activity via the recently discovered $5\text{-}HT_{2A}$ receptors on the apical dendrites of pyramidal neurons in the frontal cortex, which project to the mesolimbic regions implicated in schizophrenia. They may also contribute to the decreased dopaminergic activity in the prefrontal cortex which has been suggested to be a factor in the etiology of negative symptoms. There are also strong influences of 5-HT on the cholinergic system which may be relevant to the cognitive impairment in schizophrenia. Clozapine has been shown to increase the extracellular concentration of ACh in the frontal cortex of rats [35]. This may explain its ability to improve cognition because it is also a potent antimuscarinic agent which would be expected to lead to impaired memory function.

The serotonin system and its interactions. No major differences in CSF concentrations of 5-hydroxyindoleacetic acid (5-HIAA), the major metabolite of 5-HT, between schizophrenic patients and controls have been reported. However, a significant inverse relationship between CSF 5-HIAA concentrations and brain atrophy, as determined by CT, has been found [32]. Consistent with the hypothesis that the interaction between 5-HT and DA is most relevant to schizophrenia, neither CSF HVA nor 5-HIAA concentrations alone correlated with ventricular brain ratio, a measure of white matter loss, which is often increased in schizophrenia, whereas the ratio of HVA to 5-HIAA was negatively correlated with ventricular brain ratio [32,35]. This suggests that structural brain abnormalities in schizophrenia might be associated with a relative increase in serotonergic, compared to dopaminergic, activity.

The 5-HT hypothesis of schizophrenia predicts that patients should have abnormal responses to serotonergic challenge agents. Thus, it has been shown that the temperature and hormone response to MK-212, a $5\text{-}HT_{2A/2C}$ agonist, and MCPP, a $5\text{-}HT_{2C}$ agonist, are blunted in unmedicated schizophrenic patients. These results are consistent with the hypothesis that $5\text{-}HT_{2A/2C}$ responsivity is diminished in schizophrenia and the postmortem data of decreased $5\text{-}HT_{2A}$ receptor densities in schizophrenia [36]. Enhanced response to the $5\text{-}HT_{1A}$ agonist ipsapirone has also been reported.

A number of studies have found a decrease in $5\text{-}HT_{2A}$ receptor binding in various cortical areas [36]. Decreased $5\text{-}HT_{2A}$ receptor mRNA was also found in the dorsolateral prefrontal, superior temporal, anterior cingulate and striate cortices of patients with schizophrenia. These decreases could be due to downregulation of $5\text{-}HT_{2A}$ receptors. Since $5\text{-}HT_{2A}$ receptor density is decreased by $5\text{-}HT_{2A}$ receptor stimulation, this may be the result of increased $5\text{-}HT_{2A}$ receptor activity. However, the possibility that antipsychotic drug treatment is the cause of these decreases in $5\text{-}HT_{2A}$ receptor density has not been fully excluded.

There is also evidence for an increase in the density of $5\text{-}HT_{1A}$ receptors in the prefrontal, orbital and temporal cortex and in the hippocampus in postmortem specimens in patients with schizophrenia [36]. 5-HT_{1A} receptors are located pre- and postsynaptically on glutamatergic neurons. Increased glutamate-uptake sites, kainate, N-methyl-D aspartate (NMDA) and 5-HT receptors have been found in the same individuals, leading to the suggestion that the abnormalities in these two neurotransmitters are linked. It was suggested that 5-HT_{1A} modulation of glutamatergic activity might be abnormal in schizophrenia [37].

5-HT_{1A} agonists and 5-HT_{2A} antagonists usually have synergistic, but sometimes opposite, effects on a variety of biochemical systems [38]. It is noteworthy that both decreased 5-HT_{2A} and increased 5-HT_{1A} receptor-binding sites have been reported in the dorsolateral prefrontal cortex in schizophrenia. These two abnormalities together might produce synergistic influences on cortical processes, for example, glutamate outflow to subcortical areas such as the nucleus accumbens. An imbalance in the 5-HT_{1A} to 5-HT_{2A} receptor ratio could also contribute to abnormalities in the function of cortical association pathways.

Derangements in central nervous system GABA systems have long been suspected in schizophrenia

Although several reports have suggested that CSF concentrations of GABA are decreased in schizophrenia, there are as many negative reports as positive ones. Early reports suggested that the activity of GAD is decreased in several brain regions in schizophrenia and that high-affinity GABA uptake is altered in medial temporal lobe structures. However, these studies have also been difficult to replicate.

The dual role of GABA as a transmitter and as an integral part of intermediary metabolism have clouded the significance of changes in GABA concentration in post-mortem samples from schizophrenia. Despite long-standing speculation concerning the role of GABA in schizophrenia, conflicting biochemical data in various postmortem studies have dampened enthusiasm for its importance in the pathophysiology of the disease. However, recent anatomical studies, focusing on cortical areas, have led to a resurgence in interest in the role of GABA in the pathophysiology of schizophrenia. The different types of cortical GABAergic interneurons have dictated an emphasis on chemical neuroanatomy of the GABAergic system rather than neurochemical studies of GABA synthesis and metabolism. Specifically, reports of a lamina-specific decrease in the number of small (presumptive) interneurons in the pregenual anterior cingulate and prefrontal cortices of schizophrenic patients have been most influential [39]. In addition, several reports have suggested an upregulation of benzodiazepine binding in the cortex in a regionally specific fashion [40]; these reports fit well with clinical literature documenting the benefits of benzodiazepine augmentation of conventional neuroleptic treatment.

The number of GAD55 mRNA-expressing neurons in the dorsolateral prefrontal cortex in schizophrenia have been reported to be decreased, but a corresponding decrease in the number of small (presumptive) interneurons in the same cortical region was not observed [41]. Moreover, the number of prefrontal cortical neurons expressing NADPH diaphorase, which is a marker for nitric oxide synthase–containing cortical neurons representing a small subset of GABAergic interneurons, was sharply decreased in prefrontal cortical gray matter but markedly increased in the underlying white matter [42]. This observation suggests a failure of specific interneurons to migrate to their normal cortical targets. Finally, recent data suggest that expression of the GABA transporter GAT-1 is decreased in GABAergic terminals in the prefrontal cortex.

The difficulties in obtaining consistent data concerning the numbers of interneurons as reflected by measurements of cell size or markers for all interneurons, such as GAD protein or transcripts, may be due to these markers identifying all of the several different types of cortical interneurons. Such global measures would hamper the ability to detect a consistent significant change in a discrete subpopulation of interneurons. Accordingly, attention has recently shifted to studies of markers of subpopulations of interneurons. Cortical interneurons can be categorized on the basis of expression of three different calcium-binding proteins: parvalbumin, calbindin and calretinin. Their distributions in the cortices are largely nonoverlapping, and there are morphological and physiological distinctions that are correlated with particular calcium-binding, protein-containing interneurons. Most studies have reported no changes in the number, density or laminar distribution of parvalbumin-containing prefrontal cortical interneurons; there also does not appear to be a change in the number of calretinin-containing interneurons. However, a single report has indicated an increase in the density of calbindin-containing interneurons. Despite the utility of defining interneurons on the basis of calcium-binding proteins, it should be recognized that each of the three classes of interneurons divided in this fashion can be further subdivided. Thus, further studies will be required to define changes in specific interneurons.

Any changes in GABAergic systems in schizophrenia, particularly changes observed in the cortex, may be a direct manifestation of some dysfunction of GABA neurons, such as derangement in the normal development and migration of GABA neurons. Alternatively, GABA dysfunction may be secondary to primary changes in afferents that regulate GABA neurons. Dopaminergic axons in the cortex synapse with both interneurons and pyramidal cells in the cortex and appear to excite certain GABAergic interneurons. If there is a decrease in the dopaminergic innervation of the prefrontal cortex in schizophrenia, it follows that certain changes in interneurons, such as a decrease in GAD67 mRNA, may be secondary to a primary dysfunction of the cortical DA innervation. Obviously, in studies of postmortem tissue aimed at uncovering possible GABA interactions with DA, it will be necessary to exclude any contribution of antipsychotic drugs. 5-HT axons synapse with and drive cortical interneurons, some of which express the 5-HT$_{2A}$ receptor, and may, therefore, also trans-synaptically regulate interneurons.

Excitatory amino acids may play a role in the pathophysiology of schizophrenia

It has been two decades since the initial report of a decrease in CSF concentrations of glutamate and the elaboration of an hypothesis that schizophrenia may be due to decreased glutamatergic tone. During the period since publication of this paper, there has been an explosion of interest in the role of excitatory amino acids in neurodegeneration. More recently, two series of studies, one clinical and one preclinical, have led to an intense interest in derangements of excitatory amino acid systems as contributors to the pathogenesis of schizophrenia.

Several clinical studies have reported that the NMDA receptor antagonists phencyclidine (PCP) and, to a lesser extent, ketamine can evoke mental changes that resemble the negative and positive symptoms of schizophrenia in normal subjects and that exacerbate these symptoms in schizophrenics [43]. The reported ability to elicit both positive and negative symptoms is different from the response to chronic high-dose amphetamine administration, which produces mainly positive symptoms. However, it must be noted that the negative symptoms produced by PCP and ketamine, such as withdrawal and lack of motivations, are secondary to the disorganization and depersonalization produced by these drugs. Moreover, positive symptoms produced by amphetamines are rarely the classic paranoia and auditory hallucinations of schizophrenia. More interesting is the cognitive impairment produced by ketamine and PCP. A counterpoint to the findings that NMDA antagonists can result in a schizophreniform psychosis has been the attempt to pharmacologically modify a presumed hypoglutamatergic tone, as suggested by the PCP and ketamine studies, by administering drugs that act at the glycine modulatory site of the NMDA receptor. Several reports indicate that administration of glycine and *d*-cycloserine, usually as neuroleptic augmentation strategies, improves symptomatology in schizophrenic subjects [44].

Concurrent with studies examining the consequences of NMDA receptor antagonists in humans were studies of the effects of these antagonists in laboratory animals. Acute administration to adult, but not neonatal, rats of competitive and noncompetitive NMDA antagonists results in a circumscribed loss of neurons but does not induce gliosis; the pattern of neuronal, but not glial, involvement is the hallmark of pathological studies of schizophrenia. NMDA antagonist-elicited neurotoxicity can be blocked by administration of clozapine and other atypical antipsychotic drugs [45]. The number of neurons that undergo degeneration after NMDA receptor antagonist treatment is quite small, and the areas most impacted are the posterior cingulate and retrosplenial cortices, with a very limited degeneration in other cortical regions, including the hippocampus and amygdala. Unfortunately, this distribution of neurodegenerative changes does not mirror the pathological changes that have been reported in schizophrenia. A recent study has followed dopaminergic markers and cognitive function in nonhuman primates subchronically treated with PCP and reported persistent decreases in DA utilization in the prefrontal cortices paired with specific cognitive deficits; the latter were reversed by administration of clozapine [46].

The endogenous processes that might lead to NMDA receptor-dependent degeneration are not known. Among the potential endogenous ligands that may occupy the NMDA receptor or regulate the function of NMDA receptors is *N*-acetylaspartyl glutamate (NAAG), which is found in neurons and antagonizes NMDA receptor-mediated events. NAAG is metabolized to glutamate and *N*-acetylaspartate by *N*-acetyl α-linked acidic dipeptidase (NAALADase). NAAG concentrations have been reported to be increased in the hippocampus of schizophrenic subjects, and NAALADase activity is decreased in the hippocampus and prefrontal cortex [47]. Either an increase in NAAG by blocking NMDA receptor-mediated events or the associated decrease in glutamate and aspartate would lead to the glutamatergic hypofunction.

There are a variety of complex interactions between excitatory amino acid systems and central DA systems. Since neuroleptics markedly alter various indices of glutamatergic function, it is difficult to eliminate their contribution to various postmortem measurements of amino acids. The use of tissue obtained from non-schizophrenic patients who are maintained on antipsychotic drugs is one strategy, but even this strategy cannot eliminate an interaction between medication and diagnosis. The difficulty in obtaining tissue from untreated patients or patients in whom neuroleptic treatment had been discontinued for a reasonable period of time prior to death continues to make it difficult to dissect state- and trait-dependent differences in excitatory amino acid metabolism.

While NMDA receptors have figured most prominently in hypotheses of the pathogenesis of schizophrenia, several studies have reported changes in various non-NMDA, α-amino-3-hydroxy-5-methyl-4-isoxazole propionic acid (AMPA) and kainic acid receptors as well. Among the most consistent findings are a decrease in AMPA and kainate receptor subunit mRNAs in neurons of the medial temporal lobe, especially the hippocampus. In addition, kainic acid receptor binding has been reported to be decreased in the prefrontal cortex of schizophrenic patients.

Neuropeptides that function as neurotransmitters may play a role in schizophrenia

Neuropeptides are usually colocalized with conventional transmitters; in many cases, two or more peptides and a classical transmitter may be present in certain cells (see Chap. 18). Thus, it is not surprising that neuropeptides have been the focus of considerable attention in studies of psychoses such as schizophrenia. Of the large number of known neuroactive peptides, neurotensin, cholecystokinin (CCK), neuropeptide Y (NPY) and somatostatin have been implicated in schizophrenia, to date.

Neurotensin is a tridecapeptide found in a large number of brain regions that are typically associated with schizophrenia, including medial temporal lobe structures, the prefrontal cortices, basal ganglia structures and the amygdala. In addition, neurotensin in the rodent is colocalized with DA in ventral tegmental area neurons that project to the prefrontal cortex and ventral striatum; colocalization of neurotensin and DA is much more restricted in midbrain neurons of primate species, including humans.

Several studies have reported decreased CSF neurotensin concentrations in schizophrenic patients, although there are negative reports as well. It has been suggested that decreased concentrations of neurotensin define those patients with prominent negative symptoms, and antipsychotic drug treatment tends to normalize CSF concentrations of neurotensin [48]. However, neuroleptics have minimal effect on negative symptoms. There have been few studies of neurotensin receptors, of which two have been cloned and at least one additional neurotensin receptor postulated on the basis of physiological and pharmacological data. [^{125}I] Neurotensin binding has been reported to be decreased in the entorhinal cortex of schizophrenic patients.

Part of the continued interest in neurotensin in schizophrenia is due to a large body of literature that has found that central administration results in changes very similar to those observed with atypical antipsychotic drugs [49]. Moreover, neurotensin and DA are colocalized in certain midbrain neurons, and in the striatum neurotensin expression in medium spiny neurons is regulated by antipsychotic drugs through a D2 receptor mechanism. However, it has been difficult to study the role that neurotensin may play in antipsychotic drug actions because of a paucity of pharmacological tools. The development of neurotensin agonists and antagonists that enter the CNS should help this situation.

Cholecystokinin (CCK) is colocalized with virtually all midbrain DA neurons in the rat and is present in neurons in other regions (including the entorhinal and prefrontal cortices, hippocampus and the amygdala) that have been suggested to undergo structural changes in schizophrenia. A fairly large number of clinical trials of the effects of CCK or CCK analogues, such as ceruletide, in schizophrenia have been performed. However, despite an initial flush of optimism, the great majority of placebo-controlled studies reported no significant effect of CCK, either alone or as an adjunct to conventional antipsychotic drugs. Similarly, controlled studies of small numbers of patients on the CCK antagonist proglumide failed to show efficacy.

Despite the overall lack of success in clinical trials, certain preclinical and postmortem studies suggest that CCK may play a role in the pathophysiology of schizophrenia. CCK is present in most, if not all, midbrain DA neurons of the rat, and CCK-B receptor antagonists have

electrophysiological effects on these DA neurons that are strikingly similar to those of antipsychotic drugs.

There have been very few postmortem studies of CCK gene expression or CCK receptors in schizophrenia. One interesting series of studies noted that although midbrain DA neurons of the rat typically contain CCK, studies of human substantia nigra have failed to observe CCK mRNA-containing cells in this region. Strikingly, however, CCK mRNA-containing substantia nigra neurons were relatively abundant in samples from most schizophrenic subjects; this increase in CCK gene expression does not appear to be due to neuroleptic treatment. A single study has reported the number of CCK mRNA-containing cells in the entorhinal cortex to be decreased in schizophrenia.

Neuropeptide Y (NPY) and somatostatin concentrations have been found to be decreased, in several postmortem studies of schizophrenia, in the cortex [50], where these peptides are found in interneurons. In addition, decreased CSF concentrations of NPY have been reported. Cortical concentrations of NPY and somatostatin are markedly decreased in Alzheimer's disease and related dementias [50], and these decreases in schizophrenia are most often seen in studies of elderly patients or those with a marked cognitive decline. More studies are clearly warranted to define the contribution of changes in NPY and somatostatin to the cognitive dysfunction that is present in schizophrenia.

Acetylcholine has also been suggested to play a role in schizophrenia

This is based on the observation that extrapyramidal side effects elicited by treatment with antipsychotic drugs are often treated by administration of anticholinergic drugs. The rationale for anticholinergic treatment to reduce EPS is based on the fact that ACh is the transmitter of striatal interneurons that impinge on medium spiny neurons. Because of the intricate interrelationship between striatal DA and ACh, early hypotheses emphasized an imbalance between DA and ACh in tardive dyskinesia and schizophrenia.

Early studies focused on measures of ACh function in the striatum and reported that choline acetyltransferase (ChAT) activity was decreased in the nucleus accumbens of schizophrenics. Early studies also reported changes in acetylcholinesterase (AChE) activity in red blood cells and the nucleus accumbens of schizophrenic patients. There have been no controlled studies of such changes in unmedicated schizophrenics.

Several contemporary studies have implicated the prefrontal cortex as a potential site at which cholinergic dysfunction is manifested. This focus was dictated in part by the cognitive dysfunction seen in schizophrenia. Both ChAT and AChE activity are decreased in the cortex of schizophrenic patients who do not meet the pathological criteria for Alzheimer's disease. In addition to these neurochemical studies, recent postmortem studies have reported an increase in the number of pedunculopontine tegmental nucleus cells containing NAPDH diaphorase, which is present in pontine cholinergic cells, in schizophrenic subjects [51]. However, the level of pontine ChAT protein as measured by immunoblotting was decreased. The observation of an increase in the number of NADPH diaphorase neurons may be due to the use of this marker rather than a specific cholinergic marker such as ChAT. Nonetheless, in view of the function of these pontine reticular formation cholinergic neurons in attention and cognition, it will be important to unravel specific changes in the pontine cholinergic neurons. Recent studies have found that clozapine can increase extracellular concentrations of ACh in rat prefrontal cortex.

Schizophrenic subjects and unaffected relatives show a decrease in the P50 auditory evoked response to the second of two sequential tone presentations. Freedman et al. [52] found that the P50 deficit was linked to a locus on the long arm of chromosome 15. This appears to be the locus of the α7 nicotinic receptor subunit, which forms homomeric functional nicotinic ACh receptors that are characterized by their ability to bind α-bungarotoxin. Since deficits in the P50 evoked response had previously been linked to deficits in bungarotoxin binding in the interneurons of the hippocampus and since nicotine nor-

malizes the deficit in sensory gating, deficits in α7 nicotinic ACh receptors on interneurons of the hippocampal complex have been suggested to be a predisposing factor to the development of schizophrenia.

REFERENCES

1. Saykin, A. J., Gur, R. C., Gur, R. E., et al. Neuropsychological function in schizophrenia. Selective impairment in memory and learning. *Arch. Gen. Psychiatry* 48:618–624, 1991.

2. Liddle, P. F., Barnes, T. R., Morris, D., and Haque, S. Three syndromes in chronic schizophrenia. *Br. J. Psychiatry Suppl.* 7:119–122, 1989.

3. Carpenter, W. T., Jr., Heinrichs, D. W., and Wagman, A. M. Deficit and nondeficit forms of schizophrenia: The concept. *Am. J. Psychiatry* 145:578–583, 1988.

4. Green, M. F. What are the functional consequences of neurocognitive deficits in schizophrenia? *Am. J. Psychiatry* 153:321–330, 1996.

5. Fatemi, H. S., Meltzer, H. Y., and Roth, R. H. Atypical antipsychotic drugs: Clinical and preclinical studies. In J. G. Csernansky (ed.), *Antipsychotics*. Berlin: Springer, 1996, pp. 77–115.

6. Kane, J., Honigfeld, G., Singer, J., Meltzer, H. Y., and the Clozaril Collaborative Study Group. Clozapine for the treatment-resistant schizophrenic: A double-blind comparison with chlorpromazine. *Arch. Gen. Psychiatry* 45:789–796, 1988.

7. Kendler, K. S. The genetics of schizophrenia: A current perspective. In H. Y. Meltzer (ed.), *Psychopharmacology: The Third Generation of Progress*. New York: Raven Press, 1987, pp. 705–714.

8. Murphy, K. C., Cardon, A. G., and McGuffin, P. The molecular genetics of schizophrenia. *J. Mol. Neurosci.* 7:147–157, 1996.

9. O'Donovan, M., and Owen, M. The molecular genetics of schizophrenia. The Finnish Medical Society DUODECIM. *Ann. Med.* 28:541–546, 1996.

10. Weinberger, D. R. Schizophrenia as a neurodevelopmental disorder. In S. R. Hirsch and D. R. Weinberger (eds.), *Schizophrenia*. Oxford: Blackwell Science, 1995, pp. 293–323.

11. Lipska, B. K., Jaskiw, G. E., and Weinberger, D. R. Postpubertal emergence of hyperresponsiveness to stress and to amphetamine after neonatal excitotoxic hippocampal damage: A potential animal

model of schizophrenia. *Neuropsychopharmacology* 9:67–75, 1993.

12. Elkis, H., Friedman, L., Wise, A., and Meltzer, H. Y. Meta-analyses of studies of ventricular enlargement or cortical sulcal prominence in mood disorders—Comparison to controls or patients with schizophrenia. *Arch. Gen. Psychiatry* 52:735–746, 1995.

13. Seeman, P., and Van Tol, H. H. *Trends Pharmacol. Sci.* 15:264–270, 1994.

14. Hartman, D., Monsma, F., and Civelli, O. Interaction of antipsychotic drugs with dopamine receptor subtypes. In J. G. Csernansky (ed.), *Antipsychotics*. Berlin: Springer, 1996, pp. 43–75.

15. Mansour, A., and Watson, S. J., Jr. Dopamine receptor expression in the central nervous system. In F. E. Bloom and D. J. Kupfer (eds.), *Psychopharmacology*. New York: Raven Press, 1996, pp. 207–219.

16. Meltzer, H. Y., and Fatemi, S. H. The role of serotonin in schizophrenia and the mechanism of action of antipsychotic drugs. In J. M. Kane, H. J. Möller and F. Awouters, (eds.), *Serotonin in Antipsychotic Treatment: Mechanisms and Clinical Practice*. New York: Marcel Dekler, 1996, pp. 77–107.

17. Farde, L., and Nordstrom, A. L. PET examination of central D2 dopamine receptor occupancy in relation to extrapyramidal syndromes in patients being treated with neuroleptic drugs. *Psychopharmacol. Ser.* 10:94–100, 1993.

18. Pilowsky, L. S., Mulligan, R. S., Acton, P. D., Ell, P. J., Costa, D. C., and Kerwin, R. W. Limbic selectivity of clozapine. *Lancet* 350:490–491, 1997.

19. Nordstrom, A. L., Farde, L., Eriksson, L., and Halldin, C. No elevated D2 dopamine receptors in neuroleptic-naive schizophrenic patients revealed by positron emission tomography and [^{11}C]*N*-methylspiperone. *Psychiatry Res.* 61:67–83, 1995.

20. Joyce, J. N., Goldsmith, S. G., and Gurevich, E. V. Limbic circuits and monoamine receptors: Dissecting the effects of antipsychotics from disease process. *J. Psychiatr. Res.* 31:197–217, 1997.

21. Meador-Woodruff, J. H., Haroutunian, V., Powchick, P., Davidson, M., Davis, K. L., and Watson, S. J. Dopamine receptor transcript expression in striatum and prefrontal and occipital cortex: Focal abnormalities in orbitofrontal cortex in schizophrenia. *Arch. Gen. Psychiatry* 54:1089–1095, 1997.

22. Schmauss, C. Enhanced cleavage of an atypical intron of dopamine D3-receptor pre-mRNA in chronic schizophrenia. *J. Neurosci.* 16:7902–7909, 1996.

23. Seeman, P., Guan, H. C., and Van Tol, H. H. Dopamine D4 receptors elevated in schizophrenia. *Nature* 365:441–445, 1993.

24. Deutch, A. Y. Sites and mechanisms of action of antipsychotic drugs as revealed by immediate-early gene expression. In J. G. Csernansky (ed.), *Antipsychotics*. Berlin: Springer, 1996, pp. 117–161.

25. Deutch, A. Y. The regulation of subcortical dopamine systems by the prefrontal cortex: Interactions of central dopamine systems and the pathogenesis of schizophrenia. *J. Neural Transm. Suppl.* 36:61–89, 1992.

26. Akil, M., and Lewis, D. A. Reduced dopamine innervation of the prefrontal cortex in schizophrenia. *Soc. Neurosci. Abstr.* 22:1679, 1996.

27. Davis, K. L., Kahn, R. S., Ko, G., and Davidson, M. Dopamine in schizophrenia: A review and reconceptualization. *Am. J. Psychiatry.* 148:1474–1486, 1991.

28. Meltzer, H. Y. Clozapine: Clinical advantages and biological mechanisms. In S. C. Schultz and C. Tamminga (eds.), *Schizophrenia: A Scientific Focus.* New York: Oxford University Press, 1989, pp. S18–S27.

29. Youngren, K. D., Moghaddam, B., Bunney, B. S., and Roth, R. H. Preferential activation of dopamine overflow in prefrontal cortex produced by chronic clozapine treatment. *Neurosci. Lett.* 165:41–44, 1994.

30. Laurelle, M., Abi-Dargham, A., van Dyck, C. H., et al. Single photon emission computerized tomography imaging of amphetamine-induced dopamine release in drug-free schizophrenic subjects. *Proc. Natl. Acad. Sci. USA* 93:9235–9240, 1996.

31. Breier, A., Su, T. P., Saunders, R., et al. Schizophrenia is associated with elevated amphetamine-induced synaptic dopamine concentrations: Evidence from a novel positron emission tomography method. *Proc. Natl. Acad. Sci. USA* 94:2569–2574, 1997.

32. Roth, B. L., and Meltzer, H. Y. The role of serotonin in schizophrenia. In C. B. Nemeroff and D. Kupfer (eds.), *Psychopharmacology: The Fourth Generation of Progress.* New York: Raven Press, 1995, pp. 1215–1227.

33. Bleich, A., Brown, S. L., Kahn, R., and van Praag, H. M. The role of serotonin in schizophrenia. *Schizophr. Bull.* 14:297–315, 1988.

34. Meltzer, H. Y., Matsubara, S., and Lee, J. C. Classification of typical and atypical antipsychotic drugs on the basis of dopamine D1, D2 and serotonin$_2$ pKi values. *J. Pharmacol. Exp. Ther.* 251:238–246, 1989.

35. Parada, M. A., Hernandez, L., Puig De Parada, M., Rada, P., and Murzi, E. Selective action of acute systemic clozapine on acetylcholine release in the rat prefrontal cortex by reference to the nucleus accumbens and striatum. *J. Pharmacol. Exp. Ther.* 281:582–588, 1997.

36. Abi-Dargham, A., Laruell, M., Aghajanian, G. K., Charney, D., and Krystal, J. The role of serotonin in the pathophysiology and treatment of schizophrenia. *Neuropsychiatry Clin. Neurosci.* 9:1–17, 1997.

37. Simpson, M., Lubman, D., Slater, P., and Deakin, J. F. Autoradiography with [^{3}H]8-OH-DPAT reveals increases in 5-HT$_{1A}$ receptors in ventral prefrontal cortex in schizophrenia. *Biol. Psychiatry* 39:919–928, 1996.

38. Meltzer, H. Y., Maes, M., and Lee, M. A. The cimetidine-induced increase in prolactin secretion in schizophrenia: Effect of clozapine. *Psychopharmacology* 112:S95–S104, 1993.

39. Benes, F. M., McSparren, J., Bird, E. D., SanGiovanni, J. P., and Vincent, S. L. Deficits in small interneurons in prefrontal and cingulate cortices of schizophrenic and schizoaffective patients. *Arch. Gen. Psychiatry* 48:996–1001, 1991.

40. Benes, F. M., Vincent, S. L., Marie, A., and Khan, Y. Up-regulation of GABA$_A$ receptor binding on neurons of the prefrontal cortex in schizophrenic subjects. *Neuroscience* 75:1021–1031, 1996.

41. Akbarian, S., Kim, J. J., Potkin, S. G., et al. Gene expression for glutamic acid decarboxylase is reduced without loss of neurons in prefrontal cortex of schizophrenics. *Arch. Gen. Psychiatry* 52:258–266, 1995.

42. Akbarian, S., Bunney, W. E., Jr., Potkin, S. G., et al. Altered distribution of nicotinamine-adenine dinucleotide phosphate-diaphorase cells in frontal lobe of schizophrenics implies disturbances of cortical development. *Arch. Gen. Psychiatry* 50:169–177, 1993.

43. Krystal, J. H., Karper, L. P., Seibyl, J. P., et al. Subanesthetic effects of the noncompetitive NMDA antagonist, ketamine, in humans. Psychotomimetic, perceptual, cognitive, and neuroendocrine responses. *Arch. Gen. Psychiatry* 51:199–214, 1994.

44. Javitt, D. C., Zylberman, I., Zukin, S. R., Heresco-Levy, U., and Lindenmayer, J. P. Amelioration of negative symptoms in schizophrenia by glycine. *Am. J. Psychiatry* 151:1234–1236, 1994.

45. Olney, J. W., and Farber, N. B. Glutamate receptor dysfunction and schizophrenia. *Arch. Gen. Psychiatry* 52:998–1007, 1995.

46. Jentsch, J. D., Redmond, D. E., Jr., Elsworth, J. D., Taylor, J. R., Youngren, K. D., and Roth, R. H. Enduring cognitive deficits and cortical dopamine dysfunction in monkeys after long-term administration of phencyclidine. *Science* 277: 953–955, 1997.

47. Tsai, G., Passani, L. A., Slusher, B. S., et al. Abnormal excitatory neurotransmitter metabolism in schizophrenic brains. *Arch. Gen. Psychiatry* 52:829–836, 1995.

48. Sharma, R. P., Janicak, P. G., Bissette, G., and Nemeroff, C. B. CSF neurotensin concentration and antipsychotic treatment in schizophrenia and schizoaffective disorder. *Am. J. Psychiatry* 154: 1019–1021, 1997.

49. Nemeroff, C. B., Levant, B., Myers, B., and Bissette, G. Neurotensin, antipsychotic drugs, and schizophrenia: Basic and clinical studies. *Ann. N. Y. Acad. Sci.* 668:146–156, 1992.

50. Gabriel, S. M., Davidson, M., Haroutunian, V., et al. Neuropeptide deficits in schizophrenia vs. Alzheimer's disease cerebral cortex. *Biol. Psychiatry* 39:82–91, 1996.

51. Garcia-Rill, E., Biedermann, J. A., Chambers, T., et al. Mesopontine neurons in schizophrenia. *Neuroscience* 66:321–335, 1995.

52. Freedman, R., Coon, H., Miles-Worseley, M., et al. Linkage of a neurophysiological deficit in schizophrenia to a chromosome 15 locus. *Proc. Natl. Acad. Sci. USA* 94:587–592, 1997.

52

Biochemical Hypotheses of Mood and Anxiety Disorders

Jack D. Barchas and Margaret Altemus

Basic Neurochemistry, Molecular, Cellular and Medical Aspects, 6th Ed., edited by G. J. Siegel et al. Published by Lippincott–Raven Publishers, Philadelphia, 1999. Correspondence to Jack D. Barchas, Department of Psychiatry, Cornell University Medical College, 525 East 68th Street, New York, New York 10026.

The neurochemistry of psychiatric conditions has been a very active and fruitful field, and despite the limitations of current assumptions, biological hypotheses of mental disorders have been of enormous value in focusing research efforts on the link between psychological states and the biological sciences. Many of the biological hypotheses of mental disorders initially came from observations of relief of psychiatric symptoms by diverse pharmacological agents which came into use either by serendipitous discovery or by deliberate design. Studies of the mechanisms of action of such substances in humans and animals have provided important knowledge of the fundamental neurochemical processes of the brain.

The goal of research related to mental disorders has been to identify circumscribed biochemical mechanisms that are involved in clinical pathology and thus are potential targets for therapeutic intervention. For most conditions, progress has been exceedingly slow. For some illnesses, however, key neuroregulatory systems that may be involved are becoming clearer. The knowledge thus gained offers the potential of novel treatments directed at these systems. Two groups of illnesses representing the most common of all psychiatric conditions, the mood and anxiety disorders, are now moving into the latter category.

DEPRESSION AND MANIC-DEPRESSIVE ILLNESS: TWO MAJOR CATEGORIES OF MOOD DISORDERS

Mood disorders refer to a group of mental illnesses that include various forms of depression, mania and manic-depressive disorder. They are characterized by disturbances of affect severe enough to alter cognition, judgment and interpersonal relationships [1–7]. Appetite, energy level and sleeping patterns can also be profoundly disturbed.

Everyone goes through periods of feeling sad, discouraged, lonely or disappointed, but these feelings normally pass and do not impair day-to-day functioning. In contrast, patients with clinically significant depression undergo such profound changes in the way they perceive themselves and the world that their lives are greatly disrupted. The symptoms vary from patient to patient, and not all have the same pattern. Typically, patients feel sad or empty, and attitudes may be marked by a sense of hopelessness and helplessness. Most depressed patients tend to express little interest or enjoyment in activities previously judged pleasurable. Patients frequently have fatigue; energy levels can plummet to the point where the simple act of speaking becomes slow and labored. A diminished ability to think or concentrate and indecisiveness often become apparent. Overwhelming feelings of worthlessness or excessive or inappropriate guilt may appear. Attempts at suicide are not uncommon.

The changes that develop during depression disrupt interpersonal relationships and can exacerbate social losses that may be occurring in the life of the patient. Some depressions seem to be related to obvious social losses, while others are not. Nonetheless, depression can impact on all of the activities of the individual, including employment and the full range of social life.

In its most extreme form, depressed patients become psychotic. Such patients distort or misperceive reality, experience hallucinations or develop bizarre beliefs and behaviors.

Although mania can be intuitively thought of as the opposite of depression, the two syndromes share several characteristics [2,7]. Manic patients initially feel elated, carefree, overconfident and euphoric. They often overestimate their attractiveness, intelligence and abilities. They seem to have limitless energy and feel little need for sleep or sustenance. Some feel that they can literally conquer the world; however, euphoria often quickly changes to irritability and hostility. As in depression, cognition and judgment may become significantly impaired, leading to catastrophic consequences. In severe forms, psychosis develops, manifested by delusional beliefs of omnipotence, paranoia and "flight of ideas," which is the occurrence of thoughts so rapid and complex that verbalizations are often difficult to follow.

Patients who have only recurrent bouts of depression are said to have *unipolar* depression, whereas those having both depression and mania are considered to have *bipolar* disorder. Patients with chronic milder depressive symptoms have the diagnosis of *dysthymia*. Multiple combinations of these problems are seen. Many patients who experience one depressive episode will unfortunately suffer recurrences. Others will not only experience repeated depressions but also have episodes of mania or near-mania, also called *hypomania*, interspersed among their depressions. A few patients experience intermittent bouts of mania without marked depressive episodes. Depression and mania can coexist with a number of other psychiatric disorders, including anxiety disorders and substance abuse (see Chap. 53). An unwarranted assumption has been that unipolar depression and bipolar disorder are discrete syndromes; however, clinical studies have shown that unipolar depression and bipolar disorder may each be divided into subtypes. For example, late-onset depression tends to be associated with vascular changes in the brain and is more independent of family history of depression.

Epidemiological studies have been extremely important in the study of depression [8] and have demonstrated that it is found in a wide range of cultures. Recognition that its incidence is increasing in various cultures suggests that depression represents an interaction between biological and psychosocial processes. Depression impacts an enormous number of people: at any one time 3 to 4% of the population of the United States suffer from an affective disorder, and the lifetime risk for having at least one major depressive episode is 10 to 15% in the general population. There are over 30,000 deaths by suicide each year in the United States, making it a leading cause of death. Understanding the pathophysiological mechanisms underlying mood disturbances is thus of the utmost importance.

BIOLOGICAL CONCOMITANTS OF MOOD DISORDERS

A number of physiological changes occur in mood disorders

In addition to alterations in mood and perception, a variety of basic physiological parameters are frequently altered in depression and mania [1,3,4,6,7]. Patients may gain or lose significant quantities of weight when not attempting diet alteration. Some individuals experience changes in circadian rhythms: some have great difficulty obtaining a normal night's sleep, while others sleep 12 to 18 hours per day. Either agitation or retardation of movement may predominate. Melancholic depression is characterized by the hyperaroused symptom profile of insomnia, anorexia and agitation, while "atypical" depression is characterized by symptoms of hypoarousal including hypersomnia, hyperphagia and lethargy. Physical symptoms such as dizziness, headaches, backaches, tightness in the chest or dry mouth often accompany depression and can be the presenting complaints, masking the underlying psychiatric illness.

Anatomical and metabolic changes in the brain are associated with depression

A number of different approaches to the functional anatomical changes that may be associated with mood disorders are now being taken. One of these involves investigation of the pattern of mood disorders following various types of cerebral vascular disease [9]. Mood disorders occur in 30 to 50% of stroke patients and can last more than a year if left untreated. Major depression is most often associated with left frontal or left basal ganglia lesions. Such empirical studies are a first step in developing the functional and biochemical neuroanatomy associated with mood disorders.

Studies using magnetic resonance imaging (MRI) and positron emission tomography (PET) (see Chap. 54) are also providing information regarding anatomical changes that relate to depression [10,11]. PET studies indicate decreased prefrontal cortical metabolism, especially in the orbital cortex, anterior cingulate and basal ganglia associated with depression [12,13]. PET studies with evoked imagery [14] as well as investigation of psychotic processes [15] and receptor ligand tracers (see Chap. 54) hold the promise of further defining the localization of neurochemical changes in depression and mania.

Genetic factors are likely to play a role in mood disorders

Family and twin studies with epidemiological methods have indicated that mood disorders (i) cluster within families, (ii) are most likely to occur in first-degree relatives of those with the disorder and (iii) are more prevalent among monozygotic than dizygotic twins. Manic-depressive illness has provided particularly strong epidemiological evidence for genetic factors.

However, to date, it has been difficult to demonstrate a specific gene or set of genes associated with bipolar or unipolar depression. One replicated finding has been the association of several polymorphic markers in the pericentromeric region of chromosome 18 with bipolar disorder [16]. These findings point to a gene or genes with relatively minor effects on the illness at this site. There also have been several reports of linkage of bipolar disorder to a site on chromosome 21 [17]. Many other reports of linkage and candidate gene findings in bipolar and unipolar depression have been negative or could not be replicated. Thus, while there is strong evidence for an inherited contribution to the mood disorders, the mode of genetic transmission and the genes involved remain unclear. It is likely that a number of genetic factors contribute to increase vulnerability to the illness, and that these factors vary among families, greatly increasing the difficulty of identifying genetic factors. In addition, environmental factors also play a critical etiologic role, further complicating genetic and epidemiologic analyses.

Pharmacological treatments are effective for mood disorders

A variety of pharmacological agents have substantial effects on mood and behavior [18–21]. A common assumption has been that if an agent modifies a psychiatric symptom for better or worse, then the cellular or neurochemical action of the drug may be directly related to the biological dysfunction causing the symptom. This assumption may be flawed. The psychopharmacological agent may act at a site that is independent of the neurochemical abnormality causing the illness yet produce changes in brain function that compensate for the abnormality. Another common assumption underlying much of the work in this area is that many of the medications useful for the treatment of depression work via shared mechanisms; it is more likely that there are several distinct processes associated with symptom relief.

Patients with affective disorders vary greatly in their responses to medication. Some are markedly improved; others obtain minimal benefit. Some respond equally well to psychosocial treatments, and in many cases there appear to be substantial benefits from combining pharmacological and psychological treatments [2–7]. Much effort has gone into determining the variables that predict or explain differences in medication responses among patients, thus far without success. Variations in treatment response are likely to be linked to the as yet poorly understood heterogeneity of affective illness. Affective illnesses are likely to encompass multiple disorders with different etiologies but apparently similar presentation.

MONOAMINE HYPOTHESES OF MOOD DISORDERS

Biogenic amines have been important in hypotheses of mood disorders

The catecholamine hypothesis of depression was an important organizing step that helped to define modern biological research in psychiatry [22–24]. It states that depression is caused by a functional deficiency of catecholamines, particularly norepinephrine (NE), whereas mania is caused by a functional excess of catecholamines at critical synapses in the brain. This hypothesis was based on a correlation of the psychological and cellular actions of a variety of psychotropic agents. Other biogenic amines in the brain have also been linked to depression and mania with the development of monoamine or biogenic amine hypotheses. These amines have included the indolamine serotonin (5-hydroxytryptamine [5-HT]) and two catecholamines in addition to NE, dopamine (DA) and epinephrine.

A number of strategies are used to investigate neuroregulators in mood disorders

Several strategies have been used to examine the role of monoamines in the mood disorders. Precursor loading entails administering precursors of biogenic amines to subjects to raise monoamine concentrations in the brain. The serotonin precursors L-tryptophan and 5-hydroxytryptophan (5-HTP), with or without concomitant antidepressant medication, and the

catecholamine precursors tyrosine and levodopa have been attempted as therapeutic regimens. None of these compounds is in routine clinical use for mood disorders. Blockers of neurotransmitter degradation, such as monoamine oxidase (MAO) inhibitors, have also been employed, as described below. See Chapters 12 and 13 regarding the metabolism and synaptic effects of these amines.

Another approach has been to deplete amines by dietary means or by administering inhibitors of enzymes involved in the formation of biogenic amines. Although dietary depletion of tryptophan, the serotonin precursor amino acid, does not change mood in unmedicated depressed subjects, this procedure produces a relapse of depression in recovered subjects who have been treated with antidepressant medication or light therapy. Dietary tryptophan depletion also can induce depressive symptoms in subjects with a family history of depression but not in control subjects. Similarly, para-chlorophenylalanine (PCPA), an inhibitor of tryptophan hydroxylase, lowers levels of 5-HT and has been found to reverse the antidepressant effects of imipramine but to have no effect on mania. A competitive inhibitor of tyrosine hydroxylase, α-methyl-para-tyrosine (AMPT), which lowers levels of catecholamines, also has been reported to worsen depression in some previously depressed patients treated with antidepressant medication. In addition, AMPT appears to improve mania in some patients. These intriguing findings are the subject of ongoing research.

Another important strategy has involved studies of the metabolites of the neuroregulators by determination of their concentrations in cerebrospinal fluid (CSF), blood or urine. There has generally been considerable inconsistency in such studies, but this may reflect not only the fact that such methods involve a summation of many events in many areas of the brain but also that the bulk of monoamine transmitters released at synapses does not spill over into the CSF or peripheral circulation. Techniques have been developed, based on radiolabeled tracers, to more accurately estimate synaptic spillover of catecholamines under different conditions. These studies have shown enhanced plasma noradrenergic activity in patients with severe agitated depression. Additional difficulties arise from the necessarily small number of subjects in these sampling studies and the likelihood of substantial clinical heterogeneity with possibly multiple disorders presenting as common syndromes.

Catecholamine hypotheses remain important for depression and mania

The norepinephrine-deficiency hypothesis of depression had several roots: one observation concerned the natural alkaloid reserpine. Treatments involving reserpine had been used in India for centuries as a treatment for mental illness. Beginning in the 1950s, reserpine was used more widely for the treatment of hypertension and schizophrenia. It was noted that, in some patients, reserpine caused a syndrome resembling depression. Animals given reserpine also developed a depression-like syndrome, consisting of sedation and motor retardation. Subsequently, it was demonstrated that reserpine caused the depletion of presynaptic stores of NE, 5-HT and DA. While it is now recognized that depression is relatively uncommon following reserpine administration, the drug had a key role in the development of psychopharmacology and was a powerful impetus to the study of the biochemistry of neuroregulators in the brain.

In contrast to reserpine, iproniazid, a compound synthesized in the 1950s for the treatment of tuberculosis, was reported to produce euphoria and hyperactive behavior in some patients. It was found to increase brain concentrations of NE and 5-HT by inhibiting the metabolic enzyme MAO. Iproniazid as well as other MAO inhibitors were soon shown to be effective in alleviating depression.

The clinical and cellular actions of tricyclic antidepressants, such as amitriptyline, were considered to support the monoamine hypothesis of mood disorders. These drugs, resulting from a modification of the phenothiazine nucleus, were found to alleviate depression consistently, as did the MAO inhibitors. Their major cellular action is to block the reuptake by presynaptic terminals of monoamine transmitters, thereby, presumably, increasing the concentration of mono-amines available to interact with synaptic receptors. Thus, the actions of reserpine, MAO inhibitors and tricyclics were initially thought to be consistent in supporting the monoamine hypothesis.

Inconsistencies arose, however. The pharmacological activities of several other clinically effective compounds are difficult to reconcile with the monoamine hypothesis. Several antidepressant agents do not significantly inhibit MAO or block the reuptake of monoamines. The antimanic agent lithium (discussed below) can also be used to treat depression, yet it does not chronically increase synaptic concentrations of monoamines. Conversely, cocaine, a potent inhibitor of monoamine reuptake, has no antidepressant activity.

More detailed examination of the actions of reserpine, MAO inhibitors and tricyclics also reveals inconsistencies among their actions. Reserpine induces depression in only about 6% of patients, an incidence quite similar to the estimated incidence of depression in the general population. More importantly, the cellular effects of MAO inhibitors and tricyclic antidepressants on catecholamines are immediate, yet their clinical antidepressant effects develop quite slowly, generally over 2 to 6 weeks.

Attempts to directly measure changes in brain monoamine concentrations in the mood disorders have provided intriguing but inconsistent results. Initially, investigators concentrated on measuring the catecholamine metabolite 3-methoxy-4-hydroxyphenylglycol (MHPG), in urine and CSF. Early evidence suggested that there were decreased urinary MHPG concentrations in depressed patients and increased levels in manic patients but later reports did not bear this out. This is not entirely surprising as it is now known that urinary MHPG is a poor indicator of CNS NE turnover because the CNS contributes as little as 20% of urinary MHPG content. In addition, MHPG concentrations are substantially affected by physical activity, which was often not well controlled in research studies. Concentrations of MHPG in the CSF, which may represent a more direct measure of brain NE function, have generally been found to be unaltered in mood disorders, although this remains a controversial area (see Chap. 12).

Dopamine mechanisms may be important in some forms of depression and mania

DA may also be involved in depression, and a body of literature suggests that there may be a subgroup of mood disorders in which the neuroregulator is altered [18–21]. DA receptor agonists have been reported to have some antidepressant effects in at least subgroups of patients. A number of antidepressant drugs also have DA agonist activities. Furthermore, patients in the DA-depleted state of Parkinson's disease (see Chap. 45) often develop a concomitant depression, although that may be for other reasons. Conversely, there is evidence linking DA to mania in certain patients. Several drugs that increase available amounts of DA produce behaviors that simulate some aspects of mania. Administration of levodopa (L-DOPA), the metabolic precursor of DA, can induce hypomania in some patients, a finding particularly noted in persons with bipolar disorder. In addition, DA antagonists are useful pharmacological treatments for mania, and there is evidence that DA synthesis inhibitors may also be effective. Neuroleptic drugs are also important agents for resolution of psychotic symptoms that occur in severe cases of both mania and depression [18]. However, there are problems with postulating a primary role for DA in the mood disorders. Most notably, neuroleptic medications that are known to block DA receptors and used to treat psychosis (Chap. 51) are not generally associated with the induction of depression. It is more likely that other, primary pathophysiological processes impact on dopaminergic systems, especially in more severe, psychotic forms of affective illness.

Studies of the major metabolite of DA in CSF, homovanillic acid (HVA), have been somewhat inconsistent, suggesting decreased concentrations in at least some patients with depression. Comparison between studies has been difficult due to small sample size and differences among clinical populations, including age differences. A number of studies have suggested elevated concentrations of the metabolite in the CSF of manic individuals. However, metabolites for other transmitters were also elevated in some of these studies.

Serotonin has a role in some forms of depression

A major hypothesis is that some forms of mood disorder may be due to a relative deficiency of serotonin [18–21,25]. The efficacy of several new antidepressant medications that have a high specificity as serotonin-reuptake blockers has been taken as a form of proof of the existence of such a subtype of patients. Preclinical studies indicate that chronic administration of these drugs increases the efficiency of serotonergic neurotransmission. Further support for this hypothesis comes from repeated findings of precipitation of depression during serotonin depletion in vulnerable individuals, as described above. In addition, cerebral metabolic responses to the 5-HT-releasing agent fenfluramine (see Chap. 13) are reduced in patients with depression.

One of the most consistent findings in biological research dealing with mental disorders has been that some patients with low CSF 5-hydroxyindoleacetic acid (5-HIAA) are prone to commit suicide [26]. The lower concentrations of 5-HIAA are not specific to depression; there has also been a correlation between decreased 5-HIAA and aggressive behavior in some individuals.

ACETYLCHOLINE MECHANISMS HAVE BEEN IMPLICATED IN MOOD DISORDERS

The cholinergic hypothesis [27] suggests that hyper- and hypocholinergic states induce depression and mania, respectively. Support for this hypothesis comes from the finding that acetylcholinesterase inhibitors and cholinomimetics produce depressive symptoms under certain conditions. Conversely, anticholinergic agents have some antidepressant and euphorigenic properties and anticholinergic toxicity can induce a state resembling mania. However, agents that act on cholinergic receptors are not very effective in the treatment of mood disorders. In an attempt to reconcile the data on the involvement of cholinergic and monoaminergic systems in the mood disorders, it has been proposed that an abnormal balance between cholinergic and monoaminergic systems might be critical in the development of depression and mania. Clinical studies of acetylcholine and its metabolites are limited by the current methodological difficulties involved in studying these systems. Investigation of cholinergic mechanisms has therefore focused on pharmacological challenge studies. Cholinergic transmission is discussed in Chapter 11.

RECEPTOR HYPOTHESES OF MOOD DISORDERS

β-Adrenergic and serotonergic receptors may mediate the clinical effects of antidepressant drugs

During the search for neurochemical events that occur over the same time course as antidepressant actions, investigators found that in experimental animals, long-term (>2 weeks) antidepressant treatment caused a reduction in NE- or isopro-terenol-stimulated cAMP accumulation in the brain [28] (see Chap. 22). Thus, antidepressant treatment dampens the ability of adrenergic agents to stimulate second-messenger signaling inside the cell. One mechanism underlying this effect of chronic antidepressant administration has been shown to be a decrease in the density of β-adrenergic receptors. This decrease in receptor density may be due to the antidepressant-induced increase in synaptic availability of NE and a consequent downregulation of β-adrenergic receptors. Notably, the decrease in estimated cAMP accumulation has been shown to occur not only with MAO inhibitors and tricyclic antidepressants but also with iprindole, mianserin and electroconvulsive therapy (ECT), all of which are effective in the treatment of depression in humans.

Downregulation of the 5-HT$_2$ receptor, a subtype of the 5-HT receptor, has also been demonstrated to occur following long-term, but not acute, antidepressant treatment (see Chap. 13). Lesioning the serotonergic system can prevent the downregulation of β-adrenergic receptors produced by antidepressants, a finding that suggests a possible strong link between serotonergic and noradrenergic systems in mediating the actions of antidepressants.

A corollary of the neurotransmitter-receptor hypothesis is that some forms of depression and mania may be caused by an abnormality in the regulation of postsynaptic β-adrenergic, and possibly serotonergic, receptors. In the past, it was difficult to test this hypothesis in humans because to do so required obtaining unfixed brain tissue shortly after death from a large number of affected individuals and controls. Nonetheless, studies with a limited number of autopsy samples tend to show a significant increase in the number of β-adrenergic and 5-HT$_2$ receptors in the brains of suicide victims compared with controls [29]. There is also some indication from studies of lymphocytes and skin fibroblasts that β-adrenoreceptor agonist-induced downregulation of protein kinase A (see Chap. 24) is impaired in patients with major depression. The advent of molecular biological methods will facilitate postmortem brain studies. In addition, the development of PET, which allows *in vivo* quantitation of neurotransmitter receptors, should make it possible to extend these studies noninvasively (see Chap. 54).

Other receptor mechanisms have been implicated in mood disorders

Attention has also been focused on glucocorticoid receptors in mood disorders since they play a critical role in feedback regulation of stress responses. Chronic treatment with a number of antidepressant agents upregulates brain glucocorticoid receptors. This effect is seen in hippocampal cell culture as well as in intact animals, suggesting that it occurs independently of monoamine-reuptake blockade.

Postreceptor intracellular transduction systems may play a role in mood disorders

G proteins play an important role in postreceptor signal transduction by modulating a number of second messenger systems within the cell, including adenylyl cyclases, phospholipases and phosphoinositide-mediated systems [21] (see Chap. 20 for a detailed discussion of G proteins). Almost all monoamine neurotransmitter receptors are linked to G proteins. Changes in G protein synthesis and activity have been noted after several weeks of antidepressant treatment, mirroring the time of onset of antidepressant drug efficacy. Recent studies have shown that binding of GTP is also inhibited by lithium ions (Li^+) and that both Li^+ and antidepressant drugs modulate both the expression of particular G protein subunits in the brain and G protein activation of adenylyl cyclase. In addition there have been reports of decreases in the G_s protein function in patients with depression. In patients with bipolar disorder, there have been several reports of increased G_s protein activation in lymphocytes and postmortem brain samples. Further research on G proteins and intracellular mechanisms involved in antidepressant action may point to novel targets for drug development.

Li^+ AND ANTICONVULSANTS ARE IMPORTANT IN THE TREATMENT OF MOOD DISORDERS

Li^+ is effective in treating mania and depression

Until recently (see below), Li^+ was universally accepted as the treatment of choice for bipolar disorder [3–5,7]. Well-controlled clinical studies have shown it to decrease the severity, length and recurrence of manic episodes. Li^+ also has significant antidepressant properties in both bipolar disorder and unipolar depression.

The discovery of the clinical effectiveness of Li^+ in treating mania was serendipitous. In 1949, John Cade, an Australian, injected the urine of manic patients into guinea pigs to test for a toxic substance that might cause illness. The procedure often killed the animals because of the toxicity of urea. While attempting to determine how uric acid modified urea toxicity, he administered Li^+ urate, the most soluble urate salt, and observed that the animals often became sedated. By performing appropriate controls, Cade discovered that Li^+ was the sedative agent. After finding that self-administration produced no significant adverse effects, Cade administered Li^+ to manic patients, fortuitously in a dose that turned out to be clinically optimal. All of the patients responded positively. Soon after, in a series of clinical trials in Denmark, Schou proved that Li^+ was an effective agent in treating mania and in preventing the recurrence of manic episodes. Li^+ was in common use in Europe by the mid-1960s and was approved for clinical use in the United States in 1969.

Li^+ has a number of effects on neuroregulatory systems

Li^+ has a wide range of biological actions [30], involving enzymes, ion pumps, ion channels and membrane-transport mechanisms. Li^+ inhibits adenylyl cyclase, alters certain types of protein phosphorylation, changes the expression of some G proteins and subtypes of adenylyl cyclase and alters the coupling of some neurotransmitter receptors to G proteins (see Chaps. 20 and 22).

Li^+ also has a variety of effects on brain monoamine mechanisms, with the change depending upon the specific measure and chronicity of treatment. Li^+ blocks the release associated with stimulation of NE from brain slices and may increase reuptake of the transmitter from the synapse. Li^+ also has effects on monoamine receptors; some of these actions are consistent with a stabilizing role. For example, Li^+ has been reported to prevent the development of neuroleptic-induced DA receptor supersensitivity and, like the antidepressants, can inhibit the β-adrenergic receptor stimulation of adenylyl cyclase.

Li^+ has important effects on the phosphatidylinositol system

Over the past decade, an area of intense research has been the effect of Li^+ on phosphoinositide (PPI) systems in the brain [21,30,31]. PPI turnover is increased by a variety of putative neurotransmitters and has second-messenger activity analogous to that of the adenylyl cyclase–cAMP cascade (see Chap. 21).

The "inositol depletion hypothesis" is based on its uncompetitive inhibition of inositol monophosphate (Chap. 21) [31]. It has several attractive aspects, including the prediction that the ability of Li^+ to antagonize PPI turnover is dependent on activation of receptor-stimulated PPI turnover (see Chap. 21). Such a mechanism might explain how Li^+ is able to treat both mania and depression successfully, behavioral states that probably reflect the activation of distinct neuronal systems. Furthermore, a variety of transmitters, all with the common property of being coupled to PPI turnover, would be affected by Li^+.

Although both tricyclic antidepressants and Li^+ alter the sensitivity of the adenylyl cyclase–cAMP cascade, only Li^+ additionally affects PPI turnover. These two second-messenger systems are now known to be involved in the actions of a large and growing number of neurotransmitter receptor systems (see Chap. 10). It is possible that the basic biological defects underlying some mood disorders lie not with neurotransmitter synthesis or metabolism nor with their receptors but, rather, with the regulation of one or both of these intracellular biochemical cascades. Protein kinases A and C, the kinases activated by cAMP and PPI turnover, respectively, can phosphorylate and thereby modulate receptors, synthetic enzymes and G proteins, the proteins that couple receptors to effector systems (see Chap. 24). In addition, these protein kinases can modulate gene expression through alterations in nuclear transcription regulatory factors. Chronic administration of Li^+ has been associated with altered expression of immediate early genes and genes coding for other substances, including the glucocorticoid receptor, G proteins and adenylyl cyclases. The relationship of these changes in gene expression to the clinical efficacy of Li^+ remains to be clarified.

An abnormality at one step in the second-messenger cascade could have appreciable consequences for a variety of cellular processes and could help explain the diverse results from clinical studies and the variety of reported actions of antidepressants and Li^+. There are a number of questions regarding the specific effects of Li^+ on PPI-related systems and which physiological processes are consequently activated or inhibited by Li^+.

In summary, the relationship between the biochemical effects of Li^+ and its therapeutic activity in mania and depression is an area of active investigation. Li^+ has broad actions within the cell; further understanding of the mechanisms of its action may lead to new conceptions of affective illnesses and to still more specific pharmacological treatments.

Anticonvulsants and electroconvulsive shock therapy are effective in the treatment of mood disorders

Anticonvulsant medications have emerged as powerful agents for the treatment of bipolar disorder [2–5,7]. These drugs are particularly effective for treatment of states of mixed mania and depression and for treatment of rapid cycling bipolar disorder. Although the mechanism of action of these agents is not clear, this is an active area of investigation. In a similar vein, for many decades, it has been recognized that ECT, which also generates an anticonvulsant effect after the induced seizure, can result in marked and rapid improvement of individuals with mood disorders who may be refractory to other forms of treatment. In many cases, the treatment can be life-saving. Studies of the biochemical effects of ECT have revealed a wide range of changes, although there is not yet agreement as to the critical process. Clarification of the mechanisms of these effects could lead to new hypotheses of mood disorders.

ENDOCRINE, CIRCADIAN AND BEHAVIORAL PROCESSES IN MOOD DISORDERS

Several endocrine systems are implicated in the pathophysiology of mood disorders

A variety of endocrine disturbances, particularly thyroid disorders and adrenal disorders, may have profound psychiatric manifestations [6]. More subtle changes in these systems have been identified in patients with mood disorders, with most studies focused on patients with major depression. In addition, clinical observations indicate that fluxes in reproductive hormones can influence the course of mood disorders.

There is a consistent finding that during major depression, but not after recovery, a significant subpopulation of depressed patients hypersecrete cortisol [32]. Studies converge to describe hypersecretion of hypothalamic corticotropin-releasing hormone (CRH) and inadequate glucocorticoid feedback at multiple levels of the hypothalamic-pituitary-adrenal axis [33] (see in Chaps. 18 and 49). Findings in depressed subjects include increased postmortem hypothalamic CRH peptide and mRNA, increased blood and urine cortisol levels, hypertrophy of adrenal glands and impaired suppression of the axis in response to exogenous glucocorticoid administration. These abnormalities seem to be state-related, reversing after recovery from the depressive episode. The behavioral effects of central CRH administration to animals, hyperarousal, insomnia and decreased feeding and sexual behavior mirror the symptom profile of some forms of severe depression and suggest that CRH inhibitors may have antidepressive effects. Preliminary studies showing beneficial effects of cortisol synthesis inhibitors in depressed patients suggest that cortisol itself may contribute to depressed mood.

Thyroid hormone has also been linked to depression, and its administration seems to be an effective adjunctive treatment for many patients with unipolar and bipolar depression. Increased blood concentrations of thyroid-stimulating hormone, an indicator of low thyroid hormone function, have been associated with reductions in cerebral blood flow and cerebral metabolism in depressed patients.

In addition, several clinical syndromes point to a major influence of reproductive hormones on mood. The immediate postpartum period is a time of greatly increased risk for the onset and relapse of mood disorders. In addition, recurrent depressive symptoms can be limited to the premenstrual period, and more enduring depression is typically exacerbated premenstrually. It is also clear that women have an increased incidence of both unipolar depression and the rapid cycling form of bipolar illness. Further work is necessary to determine the validity of recent reports suggesting that estrogen may be an effective treatment for postpartum and menopausal depression and that dihydroepiandrosterone (DHEA), an adrenal androgen, may have antidepressant effects in older men. Identification of the physiological processes underlying the effects of reproductive hormones and sex differences in mood disorders should provide a window into understanding the pathophysiology of mood disorders.

The study of sleep and circadian mechanisms and of seasonal affective disorder provides insights into mood disorders

Sleep and circadian rhythm disturbances are common in mood disorders [34]. Patients have a decreased need for sleep during manic episodes, and the onset of mania is often preceded by a lack of sleep. Patients with major depression have a shortened latency to onset of rapid eye movement (REM) sleep and increased REM duration. They also have elevated core body temperature and abnormalities in the nocturnal secretion of cortisol, growth hormone and prolactin. In addition, sleep deprivation can produce a transient elevation in mood in depressed patients and may hasten the relief of symptoms during antidepressant treatment. These findings and those of local metabolic changes in the brain during sleep depression have a number of implications for the neurochemistry of mood disorders.

A new dimension in depression research has come from studies of seasonal affective disorder, in which depression seems to be triggered by changes in light [35]. Patients with this form of depression have symptoms of hypoarousal, including fatigue, increased appetite and weight gain. There is evidence that this form of depression may be related to the pineal gland and to the secretion of melatonin (see Chap. 13). This form of depression can be treated by exposure to light, as an alternative to standard antidepressant treatments. While light therapy was first developed in response to the identification of seasonal affective disorder, there is some evidence that light may also be helpful in other forms of depression. In addition, other forms of depression may show seasonal changes. Epidemiological studies indicate that depression and suicide are most common in the spring and fall and that mania occurs more often in the summer.

Behavioral neurochemistry provides ways to study depression in animal models

A wide range of behavioral models with direct relevance for the study of neurochemical changes associated with mood disorders have been developed. Common features of the models have been described, including the roles of separation and loss of behavioral control. In the relatively few studies conducted to date, there are also commonalities in aspects of the biochemical findings, including changes in NE and 5-HT systems as well as in endocrine function.

Among the most intensely studied paradigms have been stress-induced models of depression. A psychological mechanism that can be considered in specific physiological terms has been inferred from the "learned helplessness" model. It has taken a special place as insights derived from the psychological aspects of the paradigm have been applied in the clinical treatment situation. Pharmacological studies have suggested that components of the learned helplessness behavior involve several neuroregulatory systems thought to be involved in depression.

Studies of an electrophysiological kindling model suggest that episodes of affective illness could themselves cause a variety of changes in gene expression and thereby further alter behavioral processes. These changes may result in increased future vulnerability through a variety of mechanisms [36]. Animal studies have also shown profound effects of rearing conditions and early separation stress on adult brain function and neurochemistry. A variety of other environmental conditions, including social dominance hierarchies in rats and primates, have also been utilized for neurochemical, endocrine and pharmacological studies relevant to the mood disorders. Investigation of these reciprocal relationships involving the interactions between behavior and biology may prove key to the development of behavioral neurochemistry. See Chapter 49 for a discussion of steroid hormone relationships to stress, behavior and adaptation.

ANXIETY DISORDERS

Anxiety is the apprehension of danger or something unpleasant. Whereas fear is a response to current, tangible threats, anxiety occurs in anticipation of a threat not yet present and often not clearly defined. Anxiety is a familiar part of every-

day human life, and something akin to anxiety, or conditional fear, occurs in most vertebrate species. Anxiety has clear adaptive value, and in humans, it must certainly be considered normal. Yet in some of us, anxiety reaches a level that is counterproductive or even incapacitating [1,3–5]. Anxiety disorders are among the most common of all psychiatric conditions. In addition, anxiety is a prominent symptom in almost all other psychiatric illnesses. Various studies have found that from about 3 to 8% of the population has clinically significant anxiety at any one time. This prevalence is surprisingly consistent from culture to culture throughout the world. Because of the tremendous costs to society, anxiety and anxiety disorders have been the subject of intense study. For many years, this study was confined to the psychological realm, and the knowledge gained remains central to a full understanding of anxiety and the treatment of its disorders. Since the late 1960s, however, a picture of the biology and chemistry of anxiety has begun to emerge; although far from complete, it is changing our perception of anxiety and leading to new approaches for therapy.

Anxiety is recognized as one of the most important emotional processes with firm neurobiological roots. It can be studied in humans and other species. The fundamental neurochemical mechanisms are important for a wide range of mental disorders as well as substance abuse, and progress is being made in understanding them. The evidence used to determine the neurochemical bases of anxiety has been similar to that for the mood disorders. Most information has come from studying the action of anxiety-reducing, or anxiolytic, drugs. This has been aided by the existence of several animal models of anxiety. These models are probably closer to the human condition than are animal models of mood disorders. The four major thrusts of current work dealing with anxiety disorders have centered around the GABA mechanisms, the serotonergic system, noradrenergic mechanisms and neuropeptides.

There are distinct forms of anxiety disorders

Disorders in which the level of anxiety becomes pathological are divided according to their characteristic clustering of symptoms [1,3–5]. The standard reference for categorization of mental disorders is the *Diagnostic and Statistical Manual* (DSM-IV) of the American Psychiatric Association [1]. The following materials, derived in part from this source, highlight the emerging classification of anxiety disorders, many of which are now recognized as profoundly disabling.

Panic attacks can be associated with many anxiety disorders and are characterized by discrete episodes, typically lasting a few minutes, with symptoms such as accelerated or more forceful heart action, sweating, trembling, shortness of breath, chest pain, abdominal distress, dizziness and a fear on the part of the patient that he or she is "going crazy" or will die. Some persons have multiple episodes of panic attacks without another concomitant mental disorder; such problems are recognized as panic disorder. A substantial number of individuals who are subject to panic attacks, but usually not normal controls, can have panic episodes precipitated by physical challenges such as lactate infusions, CO_2 inhalation or infusion of the peptide cholecystokinin (CCK). The relationships of these challenge agents to anxiety generation are not yet well understood. Family and twin studies suggest that there may be a genetic component.

Specific phobias involve excessive fear that is cued by specific stimuli, such as heights, enclosed places or other situations. The phobic individual may experience full panic attacks when exposed to such stimuli. Social phobia is a marked and persistent fear of social situations.

Obsessive-compulsive disorder is a particularly important form of anxiety disorder. Obsessions include recurrent thoughts that may not be about real-life problems and which the person fails to ignore or suppress. Compulsions are repetitive behaviors that the person feels driven to perform in response to an obsession. The compulsive behaviors attempt to reduce the distress from the obsessions. Patients realize that the thoughts and behaviors are unreasonable, yet they cause marked distress and can consume considerable time.

Post-traumatic stress disorder stems from a serious threat to oneself or another with a response of fear or horror. The traumatic event is persistently re-experienced, and there is avoidance of stimuli associated with the trauma. Patients have persistent symptoms of increased arousal, including difficulty sleeping, irritability, difficulty concentrating, hypervigilance or exaggerated startle response. The disorder can continue for a sustained period of time with marked impairment in functioning.

Acute stress disorder has many of the same type of starting points as post-traumatic stress disorder, but the duration of the clinical manifestations is less than 4 weeks. Typically, individuals have dissociative problems, with symptoms such as numbing or detachment, reduction in awareness or loss of memory for aspects of the event. In acute stress disorder there are re-experiences of the event, avoidance of stimuli that arouse its recollection and marked symptoms of anxiety or increased arousal.

Generalized anxiety disorder involves a broad presentation of anxiety. Patients experience ongoing excessive anxiety and worry for over 6 months about a number of aspects of their lives. They have a difficult time controlling the worry. The pattern of symptoms will vary from patient to patient, but typical symptoms include some of the following: restlessness, fatigue, difficulty concentrating, irritability, muscle tension and sleep disturbances. The focus of the psychological sense of worry in these patients can be quite broad, and the symptoms may cause considerable distress and impairment.

The distinct types can be classified with good reproducibility and with a high degree of agreement among trained raters. There is strong pharmacological and chemical evidence that the underlying neurochemistry and neurobiology are different between types. For example, while almost all forms of anxiety can be blunted by benzodiazepines, only the specific serotonin-reuptake inhibitors are very effective in the treatment of obsessive-compulsive disorder, and the 5-HT_{1A} serotonin receptor partial agonists, such as buspirone, seem particularly effective in the treatment of generalized anxiety disorders.

BIOCHEMICAL ASPECTS OF ANXIETY

Benzodiazepines have revolutionized the treatment of anxiety disorders

The introduction of benzodiazepines has also set the stage for greatly increasing our understanding of the biochemistry of anxiety. Anxiolytic drugs can be considered to be among the earliest effective pharmaceutical agents devised since one of the most prominent effects of ethanol is its tendency to obliterate anxiety, which is a major reason for its continuing popularity. Opiate alkaloids and belladonna derivatives also have long been known to have potent anxiolytic activities, as do barbiturates. Propanediol carbamates, such as meprobamate, were used extensively in the past for the relief of anxiety; their discovery and use was an important step conceptually. The use of each of these drugs is limited by several side effects, most notably their serious toxicity at high doses and, with the exception of belladonna, their high liability for addiction.

The benzodiazepines are highly effective for the relief of anxiety [3–5,18–21]. They have a lower potential for addiction than many other drugs that were used earlier and are less likely to cause death or serious, lasting harm when taken in overdoses. There are now several dozen benzodiazepine drugs in clinical use worldwide, although use has become less popular because of side effects, including dependence. The various compounds appear to differ primarily in their pharmacokinetics, that is, the speed with which they are taken up and eliminated by the body, rather than in differences in their clinical effects.

The clinical effects of the benzodiazepines are fourfold: anxiolytic, sedative or sleep-inducing, anticonvulsant and muscle relaxant. It was thought at first that the benzodiazepines might have a different mechanism of action for each of these effects. For example, it was noted that tolerance to sedation, but not anxiolytic action, quickly develops in patients taking benzodiazepines. While the mechanisms of these differences are not fully understood, all clinical effects of benzodiazepines appear to be mediated centrally.

Receptors for the benzodiazepines relate to their behavioral effects

In 1977, two groups independently discovered high-affinity binding sites for diazepam in the brain. The affinities of a variety of benzodiazepines for these sites correlated well with their clinical potency. Correlations with potency in animal models of anxiety were also sought. The most common animal model for anxiety involves pairing a reward for which the animal must perform some behavior, such as lever pressing, with an aversive stimulus, such as a mild electric shock. A conflict is thus produced. Agents that appear to reduce this conflict and to increase the rate of responses punished with the shock, termed punished-responding agents, generally act as anxiolytics in humans.

Benzodiazepines that were most potent in releasing punished-responding behavior had the highest affinity for benzodiazepine-binding sites. These binding sites were found in highest density in areas of the brain that developed later in evolution, for example, in cerebral cortex, and are thought to be concerned with the production of emotional responses such as anxiety. The interaction of the benzodiazepines with their receptors is quite specific, and benzodiazepines have not demonstrated high affinity for any other neurotransmitter receptors in competitive binding assays. These studies were taken as evidence that it was the binding to these sites that mediated the action of the benzodiazepines [37].

Central nervous system benzodiazepine-binding sites are associated with the GABA_A receptor

Much effort has gone into determining the nature of benzodiazepine-binding sites. For some time, it was suspected that benzodiazepine action might be closely associated with GABAergic mechanisms; electrophysiological studies demonstrated that diazepam facilitated GABAergic synaptic transmission. Based on responsiveness to agonist stimulation, GABA receptors were divided into two major classes, $GABA_A$, which is bicuculline-sensitive, and $GABA_B$, which is baclofen-sensitive.

It is now known that the benzodiazepines interact with the GABA$_A$ subtype of GABA receptor, which is widely distributed in the CNS, primarily postsynaptically, and which mediates changes in neuronal membrane potential by opening Cl$^-$ channels. The GABA$_A$ receptor, the benzodiazepine-binding site and the Cl$^-$ ionophore are part of a single large macromolecular complex that is believed to be a critical key to the action of the drugs. The receptor has been cloned and consists of several distinct subunits. GABA and the benzodiazepines each allosterically modulate the binding of the other to this macromolecular complex: the benzodiazepines act by binding to the α subunit and GABA by binding to the β subunit (see Chap. 16).

In vitro, Cl$^-$ increases benzodiazepine receptor affinity, and it is necessary for the reciprocal regulation of GABA and benzodiazepine binding. Benzodiazepines facilitate GABAergic transmission primarily by increasing the frequency of Cl$^-$ channel opening in response to occupancy of the GABA$_A$ receptor by GABA. There is also a distinct benzodiazepine-binding site in the periphery that is not associated with GABA receptors.

Barbiturates also mediate at least some of their important actions via binding to some portion of this complex closely associated with the Cl$^-$ ionophore (see Chap. 16). Like benzodiazepines, they facilitate GABA-dependent Cl$^-$ flux in brain slices and cultured neurons. In addition, barbiturates enhance benzodiazepine and GABA agonist binding to their respective sites in *in vitro* binding assays; however, the exact mechanism appears to be somewhat different from that of the benzodiazepines. First, barbiturates are not competitive inhibitors of ligands for either GABA$_A$- or benzodiazepine-binding sites. Second, unlike benzodiazepines, barbiturates decrease the frequency of opening of GABA-activated Cl$^-$ channels but still potentiate GABA responses by increasing the mean open time of the ionophore.

GABA agonists have anxiolytic effects

The GABA agonist muscimol has anxiolytic activity in animal models, and picrotoxin, a drug that potentially inhibits GABA-promoted Cl$^-$ flux, has the opposite effect. The experimental and clinical utility of GABAergic drugs is restricted, however, by their toxicity and in some cases by their limited ability to cross the blood–brain barrier. There is some evidence that ethanol and the propanediol carbamates also produce some of their anxiolytic effects by acting at the GABA–benzodiazepine receptor–Cl$^-$ ionophore complex.

Several classes of compounds act as benzodiazepine antagonists

Compounds that act as benzodiazepine antagonists have also been called inverse agonists because they have behavioral actions opposite to those produced by benzodiazepines; that is, they increase sleeplessness and in higher doses cause seizures. The first type of benzodiazepine antagonists described were esters of β-carbolines. These compounds were first studied as possible ligands for the benzodiazepine-binding site. Several candidate endogenous ligands for the receptor, including peptides, have been suggested. The existence and physiological function of these endogenous ligands have yet to be established in humans, but research continues. Inverse agonist drugs have proven medically useful in the reversal of benzodiazepine-induced anesthesia, such as following endoscopic procedures.

Multiple benzodiazepine receptors are involved in differential pharmacological actions

Considerable progress in understanding the structure of the receptors is facilitating the understanding of benzodiazepine actions. Molecular biological investigations of the subunits of the benzodiazepine receptor have revealed that there is substantial heterogeneity. At least five classes of subunits have been identified, which can be coexpressed in varying combinations to create a GABA$_A$ receptor (see Chap. 16). The initial classification of benzodiazepine receptors into the BZ-1 form, found throughout the brain with highest concentrations in the cerebellum, and the BZ-2 form, found primarily in the cortex and hippocampus, has now been shown to be determined by different receptor subunit combinations.

Experiments with recombinant receptors have allowed analysis of the various forms with the demonstration of differential affinities of the subunit forms for various ligands. Behavioral and physiological effects of pharmacological agents can be differentiated. The anatomical pattern of gene expression in rat brain has been determined for six forms of the α subunit using *in situ* hybridization, with dramatic differences in localization observed. Information regarding these different receptor subtypes is being used by chemists to design more specific pharmacological agents, some of which are based upon partial agonist actions.

Neurosteroids may modulate anxiety symptoms

Several steroid hormones are thought of as neurosteroids because they can be synthesized within the CNS by neurons and glial cells (Chap. 49). Neurosteroids seem to modulate neurotransmission both by acting directly on the neuronal membrane and by affecting gene transcription. There is good evidence that, among other actions, neurosteroids modulate DA release from striatal neurons and modulate function of the nicotinic acetylcholine, GABA$_A$ and NMDA receptors [38]. Some neurosteroids have excitatory and others inhibitory effects on neuronal activity and behavior. One of the best studied effects of a neurosteroid is the potent facilitation of GABA action at GABA$_A$ receptors by 3α,5α-pregnan-3α-ol-20-one (THPROG). This steroid has anesthetic, hypnotic and anxiolytic effects. Many of the neurosteroid hormones are produced both in the brain and in the periphery, by the gonads and adrenal glands, from which they pass easily into the brain. Thus, the action of these steroid hormones may be tied to fluctuations in peripheral hormone and hormone precursor concentrations which occur during pregnancy, across the menstrual cycle and during stress (see Chap. 49). The therapeutic potential of synthetic steroids that may be anxiolytic without sedative effects is under active investigation.

Mechanisms involving catecholamine function may be important in anxiety

An important hypothesis of anxiety mechanisms has centered about brain NE systems, particularly those in the locus ceruleus. The locus ceruleus is the nucleus for 80% of brain noradrenergic neurons. This nucleus projects to multiple brain areas, including the limbic system, hypothalamus and cortex. Activation of the locus ceruleus and the peripheral autonomic nervous system are major components of the normal stress response. Stress increases the turnover of NE in the brain, and this can be inhibited by antianxiety agents. The locus ceruleus receives a wide range of inputs and, thus, can integrate information from a variety of sources. There are particularly strong connections between the locus ceruleus and the amygdala, a well-known site of integration of danger stimuli. In addition, multiple neuroregulatory systems, including GABA, opioid peptides, CRH and serotonin, to mention a few, interact at the level of the locus ceruleus.

Evidence linking the locus ceruleus to anxiety is based upon pharmacological as well as physiological studies. Drugs that increase activity in the locus ceruleus increase anxiety, while those that decrease this activity decrease anxiety. In freely moving animals, fear-inducing stimuli produce a rapid increase in the firing of neurons in the locus ceruleus. Many of the somatic signs of anxiety, such as tachycardia, increased blood pressure and shortness of breath, are mediated by the autonomic nervous system. Noradrenergic mechanisms have been related to both panic attacks and post-traumatic stress disorder [39]. Some of the somatic symptoms associated with phobias and panic, for example, can be reversed in humans by behavioral training [40].

Further evidence for the importance of catecholamine systems in the generation of anxiety comes from challenge studies in humans using adrenergic receptor agonists and antagonists. In addition, as described above, antidepressant agents, which are also effective treatment for panic and other anxiety disorders, downregulate β-adrenergic receptors.

Serotonin has been linked to anxiety processes

Aside from the GABA–benzodiazepine receptor complex, no neurotransmitter system has received as much attention in relation to anxiety disorders as has serotonin (5-HT) [41]. It has long been known that depletion of 5-HT with PCPA or lesioning of the dorsal raphe nucleus, the site of most CNS 5-HT neuronal bodies, with 5,7-dihydroxytryptamine produces an anxiolytic-like state in rodents (Chap. 13). It is also known that in some cases serotonergic agonists increase anxiety; however, some 5-HT antagonists tend to change punished-responding behavior in animals or reduce anxiety in humans, whereas others have the opposite effect. Confidence in a serotonergic role in anxiety has also been tempered by the fact that the lesioning procedures produce a number of alterations in neurotransmitter systems other than those utilizing 5-HT. It has long been suspected that many serotonergic drugs are nonspecific, and this has been borne out by the demonstration of multiple distinct CNS 5-HT receptor subtypes. Brain serotonin receptors have been divided into a wide range of subtypes based on their pharmacological specificities, anatomical distribution and function (see Chap. 13). Activation of the 5-HT$_2$ and 5-HT$_3$ postsynaptic receptors seems to produce anxiogenic effects, while activation of 5-HT$_{1a}$ postsynaptic receptors seems to have a more anxiolytic effect. In humans, the 5-HT$_2$ agonist *m*-chlorophenylpiperazine (mCPP) has been shown to generate anxiety in control subjects and in patients with a variety of anxiety disorders.

The compound buspirone has been introduced as the first anxiolytic agent whose clinical effects are probably mediated primarily by effects on the 5-HT system. Buspirone and related compounds may both alter the treatment of anxiety and offer new tools for its study, just as the benzodiazepines did a generation ago. In contrast to the benzodiazepines, buspirone has a delayed onset of action in that it must be administered for up to several weeks before a significant reduction of anxiety is observed. This delay raises interesting questions as to the mode of action and cascade of effects beyond impacting on the 5-HT$_{1a}$ receptor. The drug has almost no sedative, anticonvulsant or muscle-relaxant activity and no significant addiction liability. These last considerations make this type of drug an advance in the treatment of anxiety in many patients. Buspirone is useful in the treatment of generalized anxiety disorder but not in the treatment of panic.

Buspirone has no direct effect on the GABA$_A$–benzodiazepine receptor system and only a weak effect on DA receptors. Several additional 5-HT$_{1A}$-active compounds also have demonstrated anxiolytic activity in animals. The 5-HT$_{1A}$ receptor is linked via G$_i$ proteins to either inhibition of adenylyl cyclase or the opening of potassium channels (Chap. 20). It is widely distributed as a postsynaptic receptor in the forebrain and serves as a somatodendritic autoreceptor on raphe neurons. Drugs believed to act as partial agonists at 5-HT$_{1a}$ autoreceptors may decrease the firing of the serotonergic raphe neurons.

Important hypotheses of panic disorder and obsessive-compulsive disorder come from findings that serotonin-reuptake inhibitors have proven useful. The finding that a number of drugs that are useful in panic disorder are not useful in generalized anxiety disorder, and vice versa, suggest that the fundamental mechanisms of these processes are different.

Neuropeptides function in anxiety processes

Many neuropeptides and neuropeptide receptor agonists and antagonists have been shown to have anxiogenic or anxiolytic effects when administered centrally to animals. Opiates have long been used for that purpose. CRH, vasopressin, oxytocin, somatostatin, neuropeptide Y, CCK and other peptides have been studied (Chap. 18) [42]. Behavioral effects of these peptides also have been studied using molecular biological techniques, including central administration of antisense sequences that block translation of peptides or peptide receptor proteins, overexpression of peptides in intact animals and generation of knockout mice lacking particular peptides or peptide receptors [43]. Changes in anxiety behaviors have been demonstrated using these techniques with several neuropeptides.

Only a fraction of the neuropeptides that may act as critical neuroregulators have been identified. Some neuropeptides may be coreleased with other neuroregulators and have important transmitter and regulatory roles (see Chap. 18). Changes in CSF concentration of several neuropeptides, particularly CRH and somatostatin, have been noted in patients with anxiety disorders.

An important question is whether there may be new approaches to the understanding and treatment of anxiety in humans using neuropeptide agonists or antagonists. Currently, this approach is limited since peptides cannot be given orally and have limited penetration of the blood–brain barrier. However, nonpeptide agonist and antagonist compounds have the potential to overcome such limitations. Several nonpeptide compounds are currently under active development and should prove useful in further study and possible treatment of anxiety disorders.

Obsessive-compulsive disorder has neurobiological concomitants

The pharmacological therapy of obsessive-compulsive disorder centers on specific serotonin-reuptake inhibitors, which were originally developed as antidepressant agents [18,20]. Most antidepressant drugs are not active in obsessive-compulsive disorder, but those that are show a striking specificity and are of benefit in patients with obsessive-compulsive disorder but not depression. Compared to use of these agents in depression, the effectiveness in obsessional states occurs at higher doses, requires longer treatment and usually results in a lessening of symptoms rather than a total remission. There is frequently a relapse following discontinuation of the drugs.

A particularly useful animal model of obsessive-compulsive behavior may have been found in a naturally occurring disorder in dogs, canine acral lick, involving excessive licking of paws or flanks. The canine problem can produce ulcers and infections. The investigators who found the model have demonstrated in an experimentally controlled manner that serotonin-reuptake blockers are a specific treatment. This model should permit further pharmacological and neurochemical investigation [44]. The finding in humans of a genotype linking low catechol-*O*-methyltransferase (COMT) to obsessive-compulsive disorder may open another avenue of study [45].

DA antagonists are useful adjunctive treatment agents in a subgroup of patients with ob-

sessive-compulsive disorder. Response to treatment may help to define biological subtypes of patients with obsessive-compulsive disorder.

Another new line of research suggests that childhood-onset cases of obsessive-compulsive disorder may be triggered by an autoimmune reaction to streptococcal infection, in a manner similar to the etiology of Sydenham's chorea, a variant of rheumatic fever. Sydenham's chorea is often accompanied by obsessive-compulsive symptoms. Both patients with childhood-onset obsessive-compulsive disorder and patients with Sydenham's chorea have increased expression of the B-cell marker D8/17, which was previously thought to be associated only with rheumatic fever [46].

Panic disorder has specific biochemical characteristics

Patients with panic disorder have enhanced sensitivity to several challenge agents compared to healthy controls and patients with other anxiety disorders. These sensitivities may provide clues to the pathophysiology of panic disorder. Panic disorder patients are particularly sensitive to CO_2 inhalation, caffeine, other xanthines and the α_2-adrenergic receptor antagonist yohimbine. A suffocation alarm hypothesis [47] has been proposed to explain the enhanced sensitivity to CO_2, but the neurobiological substrates of this sensitivity remain to be determined.

Brain mapping and imaging are being applied to the study of anxiety disorders

Brain mapping and functional imaging methods can add a new dimension to the understanding of anxiety disorders by identifying brain areas involved in the generation of anxiety disorders. Intense interest is now focused on the use of various forms of brain imaging for the study of anxiety disorders, with particular attention to obsessive-compulsive disorder. Most baseline and symptom provocation studies of obsessive-compulsive disorder patients using PET, single photon emission computed tomography (SPECT) and functional MRI show relative activation in the caudate, thalamus, amygdala and paralimbic areas, including the anterior cingulate and orbitofrontal cortex. Anatomical and functional evidence suggests that these areas are part of a circuit or loop which is hyperactive in obsessive-compulsive disorder [48]. Evidence that behavior can influence neurochemistry comes from studies showing normalization of the functional imaging abnormalities when obsessive-compulsive disorder patients are treated with either behavior therapy or with pharmacotherapy [49]. Although caudate and lenticular activation seems to be specific to obsessive-compulsive disorder, activation of paralimbic areas and the amygdala is also seen in post-traumatic stress disorder, panic disorder and simple phobia. Limbic and paralimbic areas are also activated in healthy control subjects by internally generated emotions and autonomic stimulation [50]. There are many differences among studies, and the technologies and methodologies are undergoing rapid change.

One can anticipate, in the near future, new systems of diagnosis for severe mental disorders based on enhanced understanding that will be gleaned from the combination of several technologies, such as more sophisticated clinical assessments, new neurochemical imaging techniques and the use of genetic markers. Improved and more specific pharmacotherapies will be developed as a result of the enormous advances in our understanding of the molecular biology and genetics of neuroregulatory mechanisms, including the neurotransmitter receptors and transporters as well as associated second messenger systems [51].

REFERENCES

1. *Diagnostic and Statistical Manual (DSM-IV)*, 4th ed. Washington, D.C.: American Psychiatric Association, 1996.
2. *Practice Guideline for Major Depressive Disorder in Adults.* Washington, D.C.: American Psychiatric Association, 1993.
3. Andreasen, N. C., and Black, D. W. *Introductory Textbook of Psychiatry.* Washington, D.C.: American Psychiatric Press, 1995.
4. Kaplan, H. I., and Saddock, B. J. (eds.) *Comprehensive Textbook of Psychiatry.* Baltimore: Williams and Wilkins, 1995.
5. Gabbard, G. O. (ed.) *Treatments of Psychiatric Disorders.* Washington, D.C.: American Psychiatric Press, 1995.
6. Gold, P. W., Goodwin, F. K., and Chrousos, G. P. Clinical and biochemical manifestations of depression (two parts). *N. Engl. J. Med.* 319:348–420, 1988.
7. Goodwin, F. K., and Jamison, K. R. *Manic-Depressive Illness.* New York: Oxford University Press, 1990.
8. Gershon, E. S., Cloninger, C. R., and Barrett, J. E. (eds.) *Genetic Approaches to Mental Illness.* Washington, D.C.: American Psychiatric Press, 1994.
9. Alexopoulos, G. S., Meyers, B. S., Young, R. C., Campbell, S., Silbersweig, D., and Charlson, M. The "vascular depression" hypothesis. *Arch. Gen. Psychiatry* 54:915–922, 1997.
10. Elkis, H., Friedman, L., Wise, A., and Meltzer, H. Y. Meta-analysis of studies of ventricular enlargement and cortical sulcal prominence in mood disorders. *Arch. Gen. Psychiatry* 52:735–746, 1995.
11. Dupont, R. M., Jernigan, T. L., Heindel, W., et al. Magnetic resonance imaging and mood disorders. *Arch. Gen. Psychiatry* 52:747–755, 1995.
12. Baxter, L. R., Guze, B. H., Schwartz, J. M., Phelps, M. E., Mazziotta, J. C., and Szuba, M. P. PET studies of cerebral function in major depression and related disorders. In N. A. Lassen, D. H. Ingvar, M. E. Raichle, and L. Frebery (eds.), *Brain Work and Mental Activity.* Copenhagen: Munksgaard, 1991, pp. 403–418.
13. Drevets, W. C., Videnn, T. O., Price, J. L., Preskorn, S. H., Carmichael, S. T., and Raicle, M. E. A functional anatomical study of unipolar depression. *J. Neurosci.* 12:3628–3641, 1992.
14. George, M. S., Ketter, T. A., Parekh, P. I., et al. Blunted left cingulate activation in mood disorder subjects during a response interference task (the Stroop). *J. Neuropsychiatry Clin. Neurosci.* 9:55–63, 1997.
15. Silbersweig, D. A., Stern, E., Frith, C., et al. A functional neuroanatomy of hallucinations in schizophrenia. *Nature* 378:176–179, 1995.
16. Berrettini, W. H., Ferraro, T. N., Goldin, L. R., et al. Pericentromeric chromosome 18 DNA markers and manic-depressive illness: Evidence for a susceptibility gene. *Proc. Natl. Acad. Sci. USA* 91:5918–5921, 1994.
17. Detera-Wadleigh, S. D., Badner, J. A., Goldin, L. R., et al. Analysis of linkage to bipolar illness on chromosome 21q. *Am. J. Hum. Genet.* 1996.
18. Bloom, F. E., and Kupfer, D. J. (eds.) *Psychopharmacology: The Fourth Generation of Progress.* New York: Raven Press, 1995.
19. Cooper, J. R., Bloom, F. E., and Roth, R. H. *The Biochemical Basis of Neuropharmacology.* New York: Oxford University Press, 1996.

20. Schatzberg, A. F., and Nemeroff, C. B. (eds.) *Textbook of Psychopharmacology*. Washington, D.C.: American Psychiatric Press, 1995.

21. Nestler, E. J., and Hyman, S. E. *The Molecular Foundation of Psychiatry*. Washington, D.C.: American Psychiatric Press, 1994.

22. Schildkraut, J. J. The catecholamine hypothesis of affective disorders: A review of supporting evidence. *Am. J. Psychiatry* 122:509–522, 1965.

23. Bunney, W. E., Jr., and Davis, J. M. Norepinephrine in depressive reactions. *Arch. Gen. Psychiatry* 13:483–494, 1965.

24. Heninger, G. R., Delgado, P. L., and Charney, D. S. The revised monoamine theory of depression: A modulatory role for monoamines, based on new findings from monoamine depletion experiments in humans. *Pharmacopsychiatry* 29:2–11, 1996.

25. Mann, J. J., Malone, K. M., Diehl, D. J., Perel, J., Cooper, T. B., and Mintun, M. A. Demonstration *in vivo* of reduced serotonin responsivity in the brain of untreated depressed patients. *Am. J. Psychiatry* 153:174–182, 1996.

26. Mann, J. J., Malone, K. M., Psych, M. R., et al. Attempted suicide characteristics and cerebrospinal fluid amine metabolites in depressed inpatients. *Neuropsychopharmacology* 15:576–586, 1996.

27. Janowsky, D. S., and Overstreet, D. H. The role of acetylcholine mechanisms in mood disorders. In F. E. Bloom and D. J. Kupfer (eds.), *Psychopharmacology: The Fourth Generation of Progress*. New York: Raven Press, 1995, pp. 945–956.

28. Charney, D. S., Menkes, D. B., and Heninger, G. R. Receptor sensitivity and the mechanism of action of antidepressant treatment: Implications for the etiology and therapy of depression. *Arch. Gen. Psychiatry*. 38:1160–1180, 1981.

29. Mann, J. J., Stanley, M., McBride, P. A., and McEwen, B. S. Increased serotonin-2 and β-adrenergic receptor binding in the frontal cortices of suicide victims. *Arch. Gen. Psychiatry* 43:954–959, 1986.

30. Manji, H. K., Potter, W. Z., and Lenox, R. H. Signal transduction pathways: Molecular targets for lithium's actions. *Arch. Gen. Psychiatry* 52: 531–543, 1995.

31. Berridge, M. J., and Irvine, R. F. Inositol phosphates and cell signaling. *Nature* 341:197–204, 1989.

32. Young, E. A., Haskett, R. F., Grunhaus, L., et al. Increased circadian activation of the hypothalamic pituitary adrenal axis in depressed patients in the evening. *Arch. Gen Psychiatry* 51:701–707, 1994.

33. Nemeroff, C. B., Widerlov, E., Bissette, G., et al. Elevated concentrations of corticotropin releasing factor like immunoreactivity in depressed patients. *Science* 226:1342–1344, 1985.

34. Kupfer, D. J. Sleep research in depressive illness: Clinical implications—a tasting menu. *Biol. Psychiatry* 38:391–403, 1995.

35. Oren, D. A., and Rosenthal, N. E. Seasonal affective disorders. In E. S. Paykel (ed.), *Handbook of Affective Disorders*, 2nd ed. New York: Churchill Livingston, 1992, pp. 551–567.

36. Post, R. M. Transduction of psychosocial stress into the neurobiology of recurrent affective disorder. *Am. J. Psychiatry* 149:999–1010, 1992.

37. Zorumski, C. F., and Isenberg, K. E. Insights into the structure and function of GABA-benzodiazepine receptors: Ion channels and psychiatry. *Am. J. Psychiatry* 148:162–173, 1991.

38. Robel, P., and Baulieu, E. E. Neurosteroids: Biosynthesis and function. *Crit. Rev. Neurobiol.* 9:383–394, 1995.

39. Southwick, S., Krystal, J., and Morgan, C. Abnormal noradrenergic function in posttraumatic stress disorder. *Arch. Gen. Psychiatry* 50:266–274, 1993.

40. Bandura, A., Taylor, C. B., Williams, S. L., Mefford, I. N., and Barchas, J. D. Catecholamine secretion as a function of perceived coping self-efficacy. *J. Consult. Clin. Psychol.* 53:406–414, 1985.

41. el Mansari, M., Bouchard, C., and Blier, P. Alteration of serotonin release in the guinea pig orbitofrontal cortex by selective serotonin reuptake inhibitors. Relevance to treatment of obsessive-compulsive disorder. *Neuropsychopharmacology* 13:117–127, 1995.

42. Altemus, M., Pigott, T., Kalogeras, K. T., et al. Abnormalities in the regulation of vasopressin and corticotropin releasing factor secretion in obsessive-compulsive disorder. *Arch. Gen. Psychiatry* 49:9–20, 1992.

43. Wahlestedt, C., Pich, E., Koob, G. F., Yee, F., and Heilig, M. Modulation of anxiety and neuropeptide Y-Y1 receptors by antisense oligodeoxynucleotides. *Science* 259:528–531, 1993.

44. Rapoport, J. L., Ryland, D. H., and Kriete, M. Drug treatment of canine acral lick. *Arch. Gen. Psychiatry* 49:517–521, 1992.

45. Karayiorgou, M., Altemus, M., Galke, B. L., et al. Genotype determining low catechol-O-methyltransferase activity as a risk factor for obsessive-compulsive disorder. *Proc. Natl. Acad. Sci. USA* 94:4572–4575, 1997.

46. Murphy, T., Goodman, W. K., Fudge, M. W., et al. B lymphocyte antigen D8/17: A peripheral

marker for childhood-onset obsessive-compulsive disorder and Tourette's syndrome? *Am. J. Psychiatry* 154:402–407, 1997.

47. Klein, D. F. False suffocation alarms, spontaneous panics, and related conditions: An integrative hypothesis. *Arch. Gen. Psychiatry* 50:306–317, 1993.

48. Insel, T. R. Toward a neuroanatomy of obsessive-compulsive disorder. *Arch. Gen. Psychiatry.* 49:739–744, 1992.

49. Baxter, L. R., Schwartz, J. M., Bergman, K. S., et al. Caudate glucose metabolic rate changes with both drug and behavior therapy for obsessive-compulsive disorder. *Arch. Gen. Psychiatry* 49:681–689, 1992.

50. Rauch, S. L., van der Kolk, B. A., Fisler, R. E., et al. A symptom provocation study of posttraumatic stress disorder using positron emission tomography and script-driven imagery. *Arch. Gen. Psychiatry* 53:380–387, 1996.

51. Duman, R. S., Heninger, G. R., and Nestler, E. J. A molecular and cellular theory of depression. *Arch. Gen. Psychiatry* 54:597–606, 1997.

53

Neurochemical Bases of Drug Abuse

George R. Uhl

Basic Neurochemistry: Molecular, Cellular and Medical Aspects, 6th Ed. edited by G. J. Siegel et al. Published by Lippincott–Raven, Philadelphia, 1999. Correspondence to George R. Uhl, Molecular Neurobiology Branch, Intramural Research Program, National Institute on Drug Abuse, NIH, Box 5180, Baltimore, Maryland 21224 and Departments of Neurology and Neuroscience, The Johns Hopkins University School of Medicine, Baltimore, Maryland 21205.

GENERAL PRINCIPLES

Many individuals try abused substances. By the mid-1990s, more than 23 million Americans had tried cocaine. More than 600,000 frequently were using cocaine and were thus likely to receive a psychiatric diagnosis of drug abuse or dependence. Such drug abuse and dependence is likely to reflect complex interactions between drugs, the brain and environmental and social conditions [1].

Genetic predispositions and a number of environmental and social factors that influence aspects of abuse, including drug availability, may determine which individuals are likely to initiate experimentation with drugs. After initial contact with an abused substance, some of these individuals pursue patterns of escalating drug use that increasingly dominate their lives and interfere with social and job interactions. These hallmarks of drug addiction can also be accompanied by manifestations of physical dependence, depending on the class of drug [2]. The features of physical dependence are often displayed as *dysphoric, aversive* withdrawal symptoms that are manifest when the drug is discontinued. Drug use in some individuals may be sustained, at least in part, by the need to avoid withdrawal symptoms.

Understanding the abuse of addictive substances in humans has been greatly aided by the development of animal behavioral models that predict and reflect human substance abuse behaviors, often with remarkable fidelity. These animal models for pharmacological drug responsiveness are underpinned by studies that have identified brain circuits that underlie reward mechanisms mediated by rewarding drug and non-drug events.

This chapter focuses on the rapidly expanding body of information available concerning the neurochemical bases for the acute brain actions of abused substances, describes approaches to understanding memory-like processes that may underlie drug addictions and introduces the concepts of interindividual differences in vulnerability to drug abuse and possible contributions of genetic differences in brain neurochemistry to differences in acute and chronic drug effects.

MOLECULAR TARGETS FOR DRUG REWARD

A major triumph of drug abuse research over the last several decades has been the identification of primary sites for the rewarding actions of each major class of abused drugs (Fig. 53-1). These studies have also identified a number of other molecular sites that abused substances can bind to in ways that may modulate drug action at primary recognition sites.

The μ opiate receptor is one of the primary sites for opiate reward in the brain

Studies seeking the molecular sites of opiate drug action initially identified opiate receptors as binding sites with properties resembling those of other G protein-linked receptors (see Chaps. 10, 18 and 20) [3,4]. Subsequent studies identified morphine-preferring μ, as well as κ and δ, opiate receptors, each of which displayed distinct affinity patterns for opiate drugs. Cloning of the genes encoding μ, κ and δ opiate receptors revealed that each is a member of the seven-transmembrane-spanning, G protein-linked family of neurotransmitter receptors that largely use the endogenous opioid endomorphin, enkephalin and dynorphin peptides as brain neurotransmitter/neuromodulator ligands (see Chap. 18).

Data supporting the μ receptor as the primary site for morphine reward come from struc-

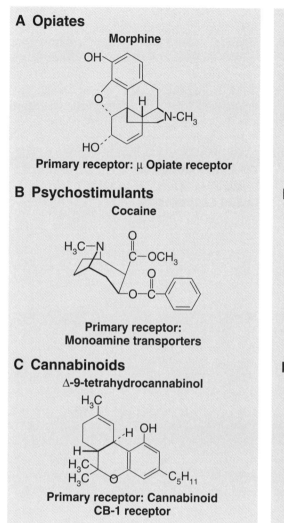

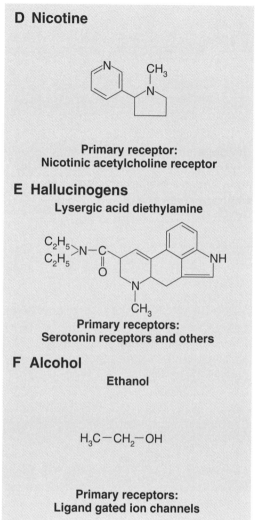

FIGURE 53-1.   Major drug classes, structures of prototypical agonists and "primary receptor" most implicated in drug class reward. See text regarding cocaine and dopamine transporters.

ture-activity studies. μ-Receptor occupancies reasonably parallel the ability of opiate drugs to mediate behavioral reward. Knockout transgenic mice with μ-receptor deletions lose almost all of the rewarding actions of morphine, even though levels of κ and δ receptors are relatively intact [5,6]. These and other convergent lines of evidence point toward seven-transmembrane domain, G protein-linked μ opiate receptors as the primary sites for drug reward mediated by opiate drugs.

Significant features of the μ receptor include its ability to mediate activation of a num-ber of members of the G_i, G_o and even G_q classes of G proteins. These G proteins serve diverse functions in distinct cell types, including effects on G protein-activated K^+ and Ca^{2+} channels and effects on adenylyl cyclase [3]. Consequences of μ-receptor activation in a specific neuronal population can thus depend on the specific complement of G proteins and other effectors that a particular neuron expresses. Studies in transgenic mice that express half the normal concentration of μ receptors reveal an apparent consequence of these sorts of differences: the receptor reductions substantially diminish some morphine effects while failing to reduce others, suggesting varying levels of "receptor reserve" in different circuits that express μ receptors [5,6]. Such studies also reveal that acute morphine actions, morphine tolerance and morphine physical dependence appear to be mediated through these same receptors.

The dopamine transporter is a candidate site for cocaine reward in the brain and is a major contributor to amphetamine reward

Investigators seeking the molecular sites of cocaine action identified high-affinity recognition of cocaine by neurotransmitter transporters for dopamine, serotonin and norepinephrine (see Chaps. 12 and 13). In addition, cocaine blocks voltage-gated Na^+ channels, contributing to its ability to block nerve conduction and local anesthetic properties. Work on cocaine analog structure-activity relationships has been interpreted to reveal that the ability of a compound to block dopamine transporters (DATs) fits best with the ability to mediate behavioral reward [7]. Lesions of the dopaminergic neurons that most intensely express DAT substantially reduce cocaine reward. Cocaine reward is also altered in transgenic mice that express elevated concentrations of DAT [8,9]. However, recent studies in transgenic mice without DATs reveal intact cocaine reward in conditioned place preference and self-administration [10].

These studies have motivated scientists to reconsider the behavioral relevance of cocaine actions at other plasma membrane transporters. Studies in transgenic knockout mice suggest that synaptic vesicles are a second site for amphetamine actions and may contribute significantly to the rewarding properties of this drug [11]. Amphetamine reward is reduced in mice with reduced expression of the vesicular monoamine transporter that pumps monoamines into synaptic vesicles. These results suggest that amphetamine can exert rewarding effects at plasma membrane DATs and by releasing dopamine from synaptic vesicular stores, while cocaine reward is more focused on its actions at plasma membrane transporters.

The function of DAT appears to be modulated through phosphorylation, a feature shared by the μ opiate receptor [12,13]. Addicts relate that the intensity of cocaine and heroin euphoria and reward is closely correlated with the rate at which these substances are administered. This rate dependence of action might be related, in part, to the adaptive actions that phosphorylation can exert at these sites.

Cannabinoids appear to exert their rewarding effects at the G protein-linked CB1 receptor

Another cannabinoid receptor, CB2, is largely expressed in the periphery and could mediate other effects of cannabinoids [14]. The compound anandamide has been proposed as an endogenous neurotransmitter/neuromodulator for these receptors (see Chap. 3).

Interesting features of the CB1 receptor include the density of its expression and its remarkable efficacy in mediating GTPγS binding through G protein subunit activation. Indeed, most neurotransmitter receptors through which abused substances act are present in the brain at levels of expression less than one-tenth that of the CB1 receptor. It is interesting that many of the pharmacological effects of cannabis appear to be much more focal than the multifocal patterns of CB1 receptor expression in the brain would suggest.

Nicotine acts at ligand-gated ion channels that comprise nicotinic acetylcholine receptors

Nicotinic receptors for acetylcholine in the brain are formed by multisubunit structures (see Chap. 11) with compositions that can differ subtly from brain region to region. Salient features of nicotinic receptors include their formation of cation channels that are typically thought of as gating Na^+ [15]. Selective permeation of Ca^{2+} by some nicotinic receptor subtype combinations, however, fits with a role for these often presynaptic receptors in modulating neurotransmitter release, a Ca^{2+}-dependent process. Although most neurotransmitter receptors can be both presynaptic and postsynaptic in different circuits and distinct anatomic contexts, few other receptors may be as dominantly presynaptic as nicotinic receptors in the brain. The nicotine dependence of tobacco users is a major public health problem. A number of pharmacological interventions have been developed in which nicotine is administered orally or subcutaneously to ease withdrawal from chewed or smoked tobacco [16].

Barbiturates and benzodiazepines work at allosteric sites on GABA-gated chloride ion channels

$GABA_A$ receptors modulate inhibitory neurotransmission in many circuits, including those important for behavioral reward (see Chap. 16). Interesting features of the $GABA_A$ receptors include their formation from a pentameric structure of related α, β, γ, δ and even ρ subunits that provide extensive sites for allosteric interactions [17]. Neither barbiturates nor benzodiazepines appear to work directly at the ligand-gated channel or at the GABA recognition sites. Instead, each modulates the functions of GABA receptors at loci that are distant from these primary functional sites. Consequently, the recognition of different classes of these modulators depends more on subunit composition than on the recognition of GABA itself. The homo-oligomeric GABA receptors that are formed from expressed ρ_1 and ρ_2 subunits, for example, are insensitive to both barbiturates and benzodiazepines.

The receptors at which a number of hallucinogens bind have been elucidated

However, the precise sites at which they exert rewarding properties are less well defined. Phencyclidine binds at the N-methyl-D-aspartate (NMDA) class of glutamate-gated ion channels (see Chap. 15). Lysergic acid diethylamide (LSD) binds to monoaminergic receptors of the seven-transmembrane domain class, exerting potent effects on serotonin receptors of several subclasses (see Chaps. 13 and 51) and reasonably potent effects on adrenergic receptor subtypes (see Chap. 12) as well.

Inhalants and ethanol are likely to work at multiple chemical sites

These sites include ligand-gated ion channel receptors for excitatory amino acids, such as glutamate, and inhibitory amino acids, such as GABA. The exact fashion in which actions at these molecular sites contribute to the reward exerted by these substances is less clear. Animals can learn to self-administer these substances, although some strains of mice do so only with some experimental difficulty. It has been proposed that a tyrosine kinase that phosphorylates NMDA receptors plays a role in sensitivity to ethanol, on the basis of knockout mouse experiments [18].

BRAIN CIRCUITS ACTIVATED BY REWARDING DRUGS

Brain circuits that mediate the rewarding actions of abused drugs include a path with cell bodies in the ventral tegmental area of the midbrain

The processes of these neurons widely innervate many structures of the forebrain, including the cerebral cortex, hippocampus, amygdala and other limbic structures (Fig. 53-2).

Behavioral studies of rodents administered electrical current into the brain have found that the ventral tegmental area (VTA) cell body area, its fiber pathways that ascend through the median forebrain bundle and its terminal zones in the nucleus accumbens and frontal cerebral cortex are each reliable sites for electrical self-stimulation in rodents. Lesions of this pathway, or of the associated ventral pallidum, markedly reduce the reward provided by abused drugs of several classes, especially cocaine and amphetamine [19].

Dopamine efflux from ventral tegmental area neuronal terminals increases during treatment with abused drugs

Abused substances of many chemical classes, including opiates, cocaine, amphetamine, ethanol, nicotine and cannabanoids, have this effect [20].

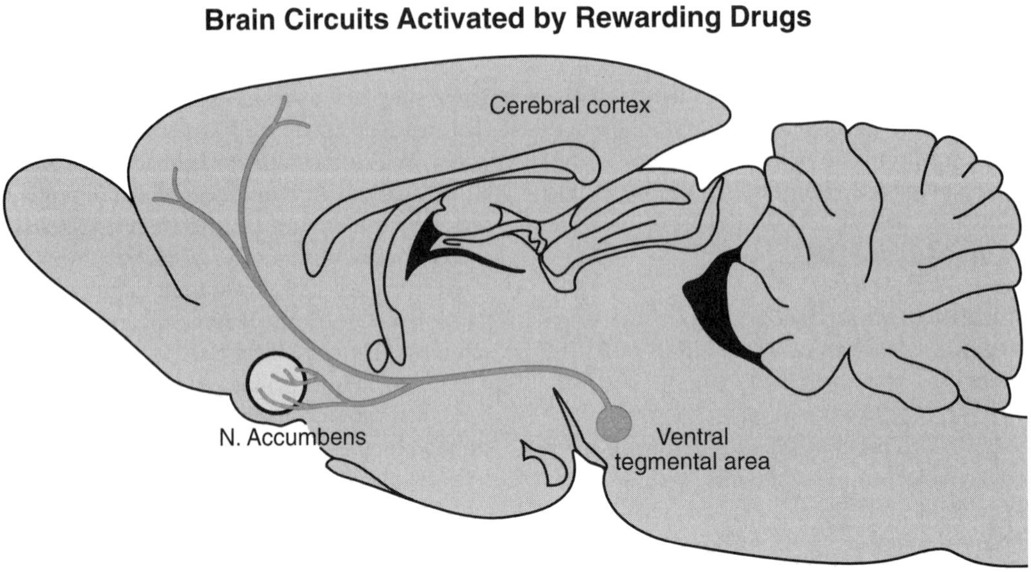

Brain Circuits Activated by Rewarding Drugs

FIGURE 53-2. Schematic depiction of the mesolimbic–mesocortical dopaminergic circuit with cell bodies in the ventral tegmental area and projections to limbic forebrain and frontal cortical structures. Greater distribution of projections in human cerebral cortex is noted in the text. *N. Accumbens*, nucleus accumbens.

This pathway is also activated when a food-deprived animal has access to food and when an animal gains access to a sexually receptive partner. These sorts of data point to ways in which substances of abuse gain access to evolutionarily important brain circuits that have major implications for individual and species survival. These considerations may add to our ability to understand the powerful control that abused substances can gain over complex behaviors.

Several of the primary neurochemical sites for drug action in circuits originating from the VTA have been documented. The DAT at which psychostimulants are active is directly and densely expressed by these dopaminergic neurons. The μ opiate receptor, however, is expressed by afferent terminals that impinge on the dopaminergic cell body areas and on neurons that are poised to receive inputs from these neurons, including those of the nucleus accumbens. Nicotinic, glutamatergic and GABA receptors are expressed by neurons that innervate both the nucleus accumbens and the VTA.

The control of most brain functions often involves a number of different circuits with parallel, series and feedback properties. It seems unlikely that a single brain circuit determines each aspect of biologically crucial reward phenomena. The rewarding functions of many drug classes also seem unlikely to be mediated through a single circuit. Nevertheless, data from the anatomic localization studies noted above, studies with lesions and results of experiments in which locally applied antagonists blocked systemic drug effects suggest that the VTA projection system displays properties of a common reward pathway. The VTA appears to participate, perhaps to varying degrees, in the reward induced by drugs of several different classes.

Brain circuits activated during chronic effects of rewarding drugs are unlikely to be only those that mediate acute drug reward

Studies of brain actions in detecting and processing external inputs have elucidated possible mechanisms for stimulus detection as well as more complex processing, such as those inferred to occur in memory formation (Chap. 50). Analogous brain mechanisms could mediate interoceptive stimuli evoked by substances of abuse.

The brain circuits important for "sensing" acute drug reward might thus be necessary, even if not sufficient, for initiating longer-lasting information storage about abused substance exposure characteristic of addiction.

Circuits implicated in generalized memory processes may play significant roles in long-term consequences of substance abuse

These circuits include those in the hippocampus, amygdala and several related cortical zones. Positron emission tomographic (PET) studies of the brain (see Chap. 54) indicate changes that accompany experimentally induced drug craving. Substantial craving-related metabolic changes are found in brain regions including these limbic and related cerebral cortical structures [21]. Few functionally important neurochemical changes induced by abused drugs in most of these circuits have been clearly eluci-

dated. These circuits extensively use excitatory and inhibitory neurotransmitters. The excitatory neurotransmitters are especially implicated in processes, such as long-term potentiation (see Chap. 50), that provide major model neuroadaptive processes in these regions.

CELLULAR CHANGES EXERTED BY ABUSED SUBSTANCES

By acting at their primary receptor targets, abused substances effect neurochemical changes in cells that express drug "receptor" target molecules

These interactions are shown in Figure 53-3 [22]. Through neuronal connections, they can also alter neurochemical events in cells that receive information from the neurons that express drug receptors.

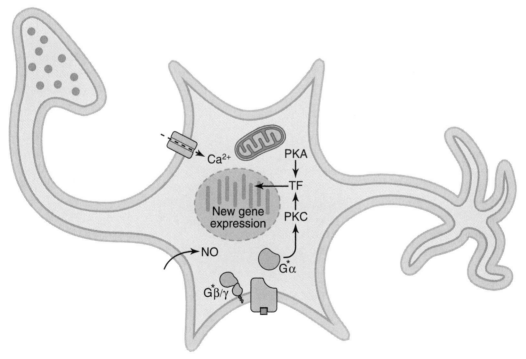

FIGURE 53-3. Representation of a neuron in which receptor occupancies by drugs have consequences for G-protein activation, kinases, transcription factors *(TF)* and channel activities. *PKA,* cAMP-dependent protein kinase; *PKC,* protein kinase C; *NO,* nitric oxide.

Some drug-induced changes occur rapidly, within milliseconds; some occur with time courses of seconds to minutes; and still others with time courses of hours or days. Some of these events display memory-like features that could last for the lifetime of the neuron and of the individual and might be reflected as subtle morphologic changes in neuronal connectivities.

Rapid responses to abused drugs can be induced via ion channel activities

Among the channels affected are those that admit Na^+, Cl^- and Ca^{2+} into neurons when activated by receptors. Entry of Na^+ and Cl^- is especially important for acute control of membrane polarization. Ca^{2+} entry is able to trigger a number of different cellular events. Activation of G proteins through G protein-linked receptors activates G-protein $\beta\gamma$ subunits, which appear to then directly activate cellular components, including K^+ and Ca^{2+} channels. Activated G-protein α subunits also alter the functions of a variety of cellular enzyme systems, including those responsible for phosphorylation of key cellular proteins and changes in phospholipid metabolism that result in the release of important cellular messengers, including inositol $(1, 4, 5)$-trisphosphate (IP_3). Gaseous diffusion from adjacent cells can also affect systems, including nitric oxide effects on cGMP (see Chap. 10).

Cellular Ca^{2+} fluxes might be altered by abused substances in several fashions. Ca^{2+} passes through NMDA-type glutamate receptors, whose activities are modulated by phencyclidine. It is also admitted to cells through voltage-sensitive channels and through putative G protein-gated Ca^{2+} channels. Free intracellular Ca^{2+} stores are also augmented by release from cellular pools maintained in "calciosome" compartments that include mitochondria (see Chap. 23). Each of these processes can be modulated by the consequences of activation of G proteins via G protein-linked receptors directly or indirectly activated by abused substances. Abused substances can alter activities of enzymes, such as phospholipase C, that dramatically change turnover of messengers such as IP_3 (see Chap. 21).

Potassium ion fluxes are altered by several abused substances as well. Opening of G-protein-linked K^+ channels represents a major pathway for opiate receptor activation to be reflected in cells, including those of the locus ceruleus [3]. These channel openings provide hyperpolarizations that are crucial cellular events.

Several abused substances alter levels of cellular second messengers

Drugs can also activate changes in phosphorylation of various membrane, cytoplasmic and nuclear substrates important for information processing [22–24]. Phosphorylation can regulate the functions of neurotransmitter transporters, G protein-linked receptors and ligand-gated ion channels. Functions of DATs, μ opiate receptors, GABA receptors, glutamate receptors and nicotinic acetylcholine receptors can each be significantly altered by phosphorylation. Phosphorylation of DAT by protein kinase C, for example, can reduce the rate of dopamine uptake. μ Opiate receptor phosphorylation by this kinase or through a homologous desensitization mechanism desensitizes its ability to respond to opiate agonists [25]. NMDA and GABA receptor phosphorylation events also alter their properties. The cellular compartmentalization of important regulatory molecules, including products of membrane lipid metabolism and information-carrying ions such as Ca^{2+}, can be altered by phosphorylation, as can the activities of enzymes, including those responsible for synthesis of rapidly diffusing gaseous messengers such as nitric oxide. Phosphorylation changes the expression and activities of transcription factor cascades important for altering expression of numerous genes, as noted below. Major current tasks for drug abuse research are to continue to identify the biochemical changes that occur in the brain after acute and chronic drug administration and which of these are relevant for the behaviorally important phenomena of tolerance, dependence and, ultimately, addiction.

The rates at which abused substances are administered can exert profound influences on their rewarding properties. It is likely that some of the intracellular consequences of abused substance administration, perhaps along with changes in circuitry, could contribute to the rate-dependent effects on drug reward. These same effects might also contribute to the therapeutic effects of drug abuse treatments, such as by the opiate agonist methadone. Studies of methadone now suggest that its robust ability to lead to μ receptor phosphorylation and desensitization could contribute to its therapeutic efficacy in providing agonist blockade of μ receptors [26].

Short-term effects of cellular effectors must also be accompanied by longer-term drug effects

These influences appear likely to display parallels with memory-like brain processes. While the exact biochemical events likely to be involved in memory processes are unknown, studies with inhibitors of protein synthesis have long implicated gene expression in mnemonic processes (see Chap. 50). Blockers of protein synthesis and mRNA synthesis are also able to block several models of longer-term drug effects, including sensitization to psychomotor stimulants [27].

Ca^{2+} concentration and perhaps even cellular oxidative-reductive potentials alter phosphorylation and can therefore change the expression of transcription factor proteins that control the expression of nuclear genes of several different classes [24]. Activation of transcription factors and the resultant altered expression of genes are among the best current biochemical candidates for mediation of the longer-term influences of drug administration (see Chap. 26). The fact that the changes in neuronal gene expression induced during development can persist for the life of the neuron, and thus for the life of the individual, adds confidence that this site of information storage could display the fidelity and long-term storage properties required to explain the long-term, memory-like brain processes that are likely to underlie addiction. Several studies now indicate that a significant fraction of the genes expressed in the brain may be differentially regulated by one or another abused substance. How these gene-regulatory changes contribute to the short- and long-term consequences of drug administration represents an exciting forefront in drug abuse research (see Box 53-1).

INDIVIDUAL DIFFERENCES

Drug abuse vulnerability, like many behavioral disorders, is likely influenced by genetic and environmental factors

Data from family, twin and adoption studies indicate significant genetic contributions to several drug abuse phenotypes [28]. In animal models of substance abuse, genetic influences on drug abuse behaviors can be ascertained by strain comparison, selective breeding, quantitative trait locus, overexpression-transgenic and knockout-transgenic mouse studies [16,29].

Identifying which gene variants contribute to these individual differences in vulnerability to drug abuse provides a major current challenge to drug abuse research. Approaches to studying this problem in humans and in animal models have focused attention on several classes of candidate genes. These include genes that encode for drug receptors and genes expressed in the dopamine brain systems that may play such prominent roles in the reward exerted by abused drugs of a number of different chemical classes. Genes whose expression is altered by administration of abused substances are also candidates for human studies, as are mouse drug abuse vulnerability loci identified by quantitative trait locus approaches.

Studies in transgenic mice in which expression of specific genes is specifically modified can aid in nominating candidate genes for studies in humans. Altered expression of specific dopaminergic genes can substantially influence behavioral responses in principal models of drug abuse vulnerability [9–11]. Studies of the sites for cocaine and amphetamine reward and reinforcement in the brain have focused on actions at the plasma membrane DAT and serotonin transporters (SERT) and on the synaptic vesicles, whose transmitter content is regulated by the synaptic vesicular monoamine transporter, and on dopamine receptors, including D1 and D2 family members [30] (see Chap. 12). Mice overexpressing DAT in catecholaminergic neurons show significantly greater cocaine preference than control mice, although DAT knockout mice retain their reward response to cocaine. Conversely, mice

Box 53-1

A MOLECULAR MECHANISM FOR ADDICTION: cAMP SYSTEMS

Addiction is accompanied by changes that are induced at the molecular level in specific neurons in response to chronic exposure to a drug of abuse. While many chronic adaptations to drug exposure have been observed over the past decade, the major challenge of current research is to relate individual molecular adaptations to specific behavioral features of addiction.

One molecular adaptation that has been associated with chronic drug exposure and, possibly addiction is upregulation of the cAMP pathway, which is known to occur in several neuronal cell types in the CNS as a consequence of chronic drug exposure [1]. A model system for this work is the locus ceruleus, the major noradrenergic nucleus in brain, normally involved in regulating arousal and attentional states. The effects of opiates on locus ceruleus neurons are well established. Acutely, opiates inhibit locus ceruleus firing, whereas after chronic exposure, neuronal firing rates recover toward normal levels, a process termed tolerance. Moreover, upon removal of the opiate, neuronal firing rates increase several-fold above normal levels, termed dependence and withdrawal [1]. This dramatic activation of the locus ceruleus could contribute to somatic signs of opiate withdrawal.

Increasing evidence supports the hypothesis that this withdrawal activation of locus ceruleus neurons occurs, in part, via upregulation of the cAMP pathway induced in the neurons by chronic exposure to opiates. This upregulation includes increased levels of specific subtypes of adenylyl cyclase and specific subunits of protein kinase A (PKA). These adaptations are associated with the higher firing rate of the neurons during withdrawal. Activation of the neurons during withdrawal also occurs from increased glutamatergic transmission to the locus ceruleus, which arises from afferent neurons elsewhere in the brainstem and spinal cord [1].

Part of the mechanism by which chronic opiate exposure causes upregulation of the cAMP pathway involves the transcription factor cAMP response element binding (CREB) protein (Chap. 26). Opiate exposure induces CREB expression and functional activity in locus ceruleus neurons, which then appear to mediate increased expression of certain, although not all, components of the cAMP pathway [2]. Further, indirect support for this scheme comes from analysis of CREB knockout mice, which show an attenuated opiate withdrawal syndrome [3].

The locus ceruleus involvement in somatic opiate withdrawal may be greater than its role in mediating motivational aspects of drug addiction, which comprise the core clinical symptoms of addictive disorders. Nevertheless, upregulation of the cAMP pathway also has been shown to occur in other regions of brain that are implicated in these phenomena. Thus, chronic exposure to several types of drugs of abuse, including opiates, cocaine and alcohol, increases adenylyl cyclase and PKA in the nucleus accumbens, a region critical for mechanisms of drug reward (see text). This upregulation of the cAMP pathway could account for electrophysiological changes observed in nucleus accumbens neurons after chronic drug exposure. According to this scheme, the upregulated cAMP pathway would increase the state of phosphorylation of voltage-gated ion channels in these neurons, thereby altering their conductance [4]. Importantly, recent studies have provided direct support for the hypothesis that upregulation of the cAMP pathway in the nucleus accumbens mediates some of the changes in drug reward, as well as relapse to drug-seeking behavior, that characterize a drug-addicted state [5].

Box 53-1 (Continued)

A major goal of current research is to delineate the molecular mechanisms by which chronic drug exposure leads to upregulation of the cAMP pathway and to altered expression of other signaling proteins in the nucleus accumbens. There is evidence for the involvement of CREB, as found in the locus ceruleus [1,6]. There also is evidence for the involvement of a Fos family member transcription factor called ΔFosB. Whereas acute exposure to any of several drugs of abuse, including opiates, cocaine, amphetamine and nicotine, causes the transient induction of several Fos family proteins, chronic drug exposure results in the gradual accumulation of stable isoforms of ΔFosB. This more stable ΔFosB protein thus persists in nucleus accumbens neurons long after cessation of drug exposure. Thus, ΔFosB can be viewed as a candidate "molecular switch" that could initiate and then maintain relatively long lived adaptations that underlie aspects of drug addiction. Recent studies in FosB knockout mice have provided direct evidence for a role of ΔFosB in behavioral plasticity to drug exposure. Mice that lack ΔFosB show heightened responsiveness to the locomotor-activating and rewarding effects of cocaine [7]. These findings support a scheme wherein induction of ΔFosB represents a "counter-adaptive" compensatory mechanism that serves to dampen responsiveness to further drug exposures.

One of the prominent features of addictive disorders is the persistence of symptoms despite very prolonged periods of abstinence. Drug regulation of transcription factors, such as CREB, ΔFosB and presumably others, clearly represent attractive mechanisms by which relatively stable changes in brain can be induced by repeated drug exposure. It is important to emphasize that components of the cAMP pathway are likely to be among a very large number of proteins that have altered expression as a consequence of these changes. Indeed, drug-induced adaptations have been found for several receptors, transporters and other signaling proteins. Identification and characterization of an increasing number of such molecular adaptations and, increasingly, causally relating them to behavioral features of addiction remain an exciting and challenging area of drug abuse research.

—*Eric J. Nestler*

REFERENCES

1. Nestler, E. J., and Aghajanian, G. K. Molecular and cellular basis of addiction. *Science* 278:58–63, 1997.
2. Lane-Ladd, S. B., Pineda, J., Boundy, V., Pfeuffer, T., Krupinski, J., Aghajanian, G. K., and Nestler, E. J. CREB in the locus coeruleus: Biochemical, physiological, and behavioral evidence for a role in opiate dependence. *J. Neurosci.* 17:7890–7901, 1997.
3. Maldonado, R., Blendy, J. A., Tzavara, E., et al. Reduction of morphine abstinence in mice with a mutation in the gene encoding CREB. *Science* 273:657–659, 1996.
4. Zhang, X.-F., Hu, X.-T., and White, F. J. Whole-cell plasticity in cocaine withdrawal: Reduced sodium currents in nucleus accumbens neurons. *J. Neurosci.* 18:488–498, 1998.
5. Self, D. W., Genova, L. M., Hope, B. T., Barnhart, W. J., Spencer, J. J. and Nestler, E. J. Involvement of cAMP-dependent protein kinase in the nucleus accumbens in cocaine self-administration and relapse of cocaine-seeking behavior. *J. Neurosci.* 18:1848–1859, 1998.
6. Hyman, S. E. Addiction to cocaine and amphetamine. *Neuron* 16:901–904, 1996.
7. Hiroi, N., Brown, J., Haile, C., Ye, H., Greenberg, M. E., and Nestler, E. J. FosB mutant mice: Loss of chronic cocaine induction of Fos-related proteins and heightened sensitivity to cocaine's psychomotor and rewarding effects. *Proc. Natl. Acad. Sci. USA* 94:10397–10402, 1997.

with reduced expression of the synaptic vesicu-lar monoamine transporter gene show no effect on cocaine reward but do manifest reduced amphetamine reward [11]. Mice with dopamine D1 receptor knockouts show slower acquisition of cocaine self-administration but ultimate expression of cocaine reward similar to that of control mice [30].

Human studies of functional allelic differences in the genes expressed in dopamine circuits provide an example of a provisional association of a functional gene variant with substance abuse vulnerability. In initial studies, the proportions of a high activity of the human dopamine-metabolizing gene catechol-*O*-methyltransferase were nearly twice as frequent in polysubstance abusers as in controls free from such use [31]. Replication of this result and identification of genes contributing to complex behavioral disorders will likely permit us to further understand disease nosology, to improve prevention strategies and to better target behavioral and pharmacological treatments (see Box 53-1).

CONCLUSIONS

The complex interactions between drugs, brain, genetic predisposition and environmental factors that result in human drug abuse can now be assigned neurochemical coding at several levels of precision. Knowledge about drug receptors is facilitating increasingly precise hypotheses about the way in which information about drug exposure enters the nervous system. This information in turn is giving fresh impetus to studies elucidating the circuitry and neurochemical bases for longer-term sequelae of drug administration, including development of tolerance, dependence, sensitization and addiction.

ACKNOWLEDGMENTS

The author gratefully acknowledges the contributions to these ideas and work in his laboratory by a number of exceptional students and fellows and support from the NIDA-IRP.

REFERENCES

1. SAMHSA. *National Household Survey on Drug Abuse: Population Estimates, 1994.* Washington, D.C.: U.S. Dept. Health Human Services, 1995.
2. Committee on Opportunities in Drug Abuse Research, Institute of Medicine. *Pathways of Addiction.* Washington, D.C.: National Academy Press, 1966.
3. Uhl, G. R., Childers, S., and Pasternak, G. An opiate receptor gene family reunion. *Trends Neurosci.* 17:89–93, 1994.
4. Wang, J.-B., Imai, Y., Eppler, C. M., Gregor, P., Spivak, and C., Uhl, G. R. μ Opiate receptor/binding protein: cDNA cloning and expression. *Proc. Natl. Acad. Sci. USA* 90:10230–10234, 1993.
5. Sora, I., Takahashi, N., Funada, M., et al. Opiate receptor knockout mice define mu receptor roles in endogenous nociceptive responses and morphine-induced analgesia. *Proc. Natl. Acad. Sci. USA* 94:1544–1549, 1997.
6. Matthes, H. D., Maldonado, R., Simonnin, F., et al. Loss of morphine-induced analgesia, reward effect and withdrawal symptoms in mice lacking the mu opioid receptor gene. *Nature* 383:819–823, 1966.
7. Uhl, G. R., and Hartig, P. R. Transporter explosion: Update on uptake. *Trends Pharmacol. Sci.* 13:421–425, 1992.
8. Donovan, D. M., Miner, L. M., Perry, M., et al. Effects of dopamine transporter overexpression using tyrosine hydroxylase promoter-elements. (*in preparation*).
9. Giros, B., Jaber, M., Jones, S. R., Wightman, R. M., and Caron, M.G. Hyperlocomotion and indifference to cocaine and amphetamine in mice lacking the dopamine transporter. *Nature* 379: 606–612, 1996.
10. Sora, I., Wichems, C., Takahashi, N., et al. Cocaine reward models: Conditioned place preference can be established in dopamine- and serotonin-transporter knockout mice. *Proc. Natl. Acad. Sci. USA* (in press), 1998.
11. Takahashi, N., Miner, L. M., Sora, I., et al. VMAT2 knockout mice: Heterozygotes display reduced amphetamine-conditioned reward, enhanced amphetamine locomotion and enhanced MPTP toxicity. *Proc. Natl. Acad. Sci. USA* (in press), 1998.
12. Zhang, L., Yu, U., Mackin, S., et al. Differential μ opiate receptor phosphorylation and desensitization induced by agonists and phorbol esters. *J. Biol. Chem.* 271:11449–11454, 1996.
13. Vaughan, R. A., Huff, R. A., Uhl, G. R., and Kuhar, M. J. Protein kinase C-mediated phosphorylation and functional regulation of dopamine

transporters in striatal synaptosomes. *J. Biol. Chem.* 272:15541–15546, 1997.

14. Matsuda, L., Lolait, S. J., Brownstein, M. J., Young, A. C., and Bonner, T.I. Structure of a cannabinoid receptor and functional expression of the cloned cDNA. *Nature* 346:561–564, 1990.

15. Colquhoun, L. M., and Patrick, J. W. Pharmacology of neuronal nicotinic acetylcholine receptor subtypes. *Adv. Pharmacol.* 39:191–220, 1997.

16. Hardman, J. G., Limbard, L. E., Molinoff, P. B. and Ruddon, R. W. (eds.) *Goodman and Gilman's The Pharmacologic Basis of Therapeutics* (9th ed.). New York: McGraw-Hill, 1996, pp. 565–566.

17. Gorrie, G. H., Vallis, Y., Stephenson, A., et al. Assembly of GABA$_A$ receptors composed of α1 and β2 subunits in both cultured neurons and fibroblasts. *J. Neurosci.* 17:6587–6596, 1997.

18. Miyakawa, T., Yagi, T., Kitazawa, H., et al. Fyn-kinase as a determinant of ethanol sensitivity: Relation to NMDA-receptor function. *Science* 278:698–701, 1997.

19. Koob, G. F. Drugs of abuse: Anatomy, pharmacology and function of reward pathways. *Trends Pharmacol. Sci.* 13:177–184, 1992.

20. Di Chiara, G., and Imperato, A. Drugs abused by humans preferentially increase synaptic dopamine concentrations in the mesolimbic system of freely moving rats. *Proc. Natl. Acad. Sci. USA* 85:5274–5278, 1988.

21. Grant, S., London, E. D., Newlin, D. B., et al. Activation of memory circuits during drug-elicited cocaine craving. *Proc. Natl. Acad. Sci. USA* 93:12040–12045, 1996.

22. Nestler, E. J. Molecular mechanisms of drug addiction. *J. Neurosci.* 12:2439–2450, 1992.

23. Nestler, E. J., Hope, B. T., and Widnell, K. L. Drug addiction: A model for the molecular basis of neural plasticity. *Neuron* 11:995–1006, 1993.

24. Persico, A. M., and Uhl, G. R. Transcription factors: Potential roles in drug-induced plasticity. *Rev. Neurosci.* 7:233–275, 1997.

25. Huff, R. A., Vaughan, R. A., Kuhar, M. J., and Uhl, G. R. Dopamine transporter: Phorbol esters increase phosphorylation and decrease V_{max}. *J. Neurochem.* 68:225–232, 1997.

26. Yu, Y., Zhang, L., Sun, H., Uhl, G. R., and Wang, J. B. μ Opiate receptor phosphorylation, desensitization and ligand efficacy. *J. Biol. Chem.* (*in press*), 1998.

27. Robinson, T. E., and Berridge, K. C. The neural basis of drug craving: An incentive-sensitization theory of addiction. *Brain Res. Rev.* 18:247–291, 1993.

28. Uhl, G. R., Elmer, G. I., Labuda, M. C., and Pickens, R. W. Genetic influences in drug abuse. In F. E. Bloom and D. J. Kupfer (eds.), *Psychopharmacology: The Fourth Generation of Progress*. New York: Raven Press, 1995, pp. 1793–1806.

29. Crabbe, J. C., Belknap, J. K., and Buck, K. J. Genetic animal models of alcohol and drug abuse. *Science* 264:1715–1723, 1994.

30. Uhl, G. R., Gold, L. H., and Risch, N. Genetic analyses of complex behavioral disorders. *Proc. Natl. Acad. Sci. USA* 94:2785–2786, 1997.

31. Vandenbergh, D. J., Rodriguez, L. A., Miller, I. T., Uhl, G. R., Lachman, H. M. A high-activity catechol-*O*-methyltransferase allele is more prevalent in polysubstance abusers. *Psychiatr. Genet.* 74: 439–442, 1998.

54

Positron Emission Tomography

Kirk A. Frey

Basic Neurochemistry: Molecular, Cellular and Medical Aspects, 6th Ed., edited by G. J. Siegel et al. Published by Lippincott–Raven Publishers, Philadelphia, 1999. Correspondence to Kirk A. Frey, Departments of Internal Medicine (Division of Nuclear Medicine) and Neurology and The Mental Health Research Institute, The University of Michigan Hospitals, B1G 412/0028 AGH, 1500 East Medical Center Drive, Ann Arbor, Michigan 48109-0028.

In vivo determinations of biochemical and physiological processes have provided unique insight into the integrated functioning of the CNS. Approaches to the study of brain function that rely on the use of intact experimental subjects are of particular value for several reasons. First, the metabolic relationships between the brain and its vascular supply represent highly regulated and dynamic processes (Chap. 31). Interruption of the supply of metabolic fuels to the brain results in rapid alteration of both behavior and cerebral metabolism. Second, the blood–brain barrier, acting as a filter, regulates the entry and exit of metabolites and other substances (Chap. 32). In many instances, compounds that could be utilized by the brain as sources of energy are excluded from entry. Other substances with neurotransmitter and neuromodulatory activity in the brain are also excluded; thus, the barrier contributes to regulation of the neuronal microenvironment. Finally, there exists a regional heterogeneity in the populations of neurons, with regard to both their transmitter specificities and their anatomical interconnections. *In vitro* biochemical methods that utilize tissue slices, homogenates or subcellular fractions are generally unsatisfactory for the study of the human diseases that result from disruption of these metabolic relationships. Positron emission tomography (PET) represents an important bridge between *in vitro* and *in vivo* biochemical measures of cerebral function. It is a noninvasive method in which radiotracers are introduced into the bloodstream and their distribution in the brain is subsequently measured by external detectors. Because of the low doses of radiation usually associated with PET, it can be safely applied in clinical research, allowing the direct study of human neurological and psychiatric disease. This chapter provides an overview of PET methods and their applications (see [1] for review).

METHODS IN POSITRON EMISSION TOMOGRAPHY

Positron-emitting tracers are used to produce maps of radioactivity distribution in brain

Positron-emitting nuclides share unique physical properties that permit great flexibility and sensitivity in the design of tracer distribution experiments. Isotopes used frequently in PET research allow a variety of radiochemical approaches to ligand synthesis. Of particular importance, isotopes of carbon and nitrogen may be directly incorporated, and ^{18}F can be substituted for hydrogen or a hydroxyl substituent in many compounds without loss of bioactivity. Because the isotopes used have short half-lives (Table 54-1), a cyclotron dedicated for nuclide production and facilities and methods for rapid radiochemical synthesis are usually required. Some positron-emitting radionuclides are obtained from generators, which contain a long-lived, reactor-produced parent nuclide that decays, yielding the positron emitter as a daughter radionuclide. Chemical differences between the parent and daughter nuclides permit their separation, usually by column chromatography. For example, a generator containing ^{68}Ge (half-life 287 days) may be used for production of the positron emitter ^{68}Ga (half-life 68 min), which is formed following electron-capture decay of the parent nuclide. Other nuclides obtainable from generator systems include ^{62}Cu (from ^{62}Zn, half-life 9.15 hr) and ^{82}Rb (from ^{82}Sr, half-life 25 days). Thus, while the daughter positron-emit-

| | **TABLE 54-1.** | PHYSICAL PROPERTIES OF SELECTED POSITRON-EMITTING NUCLIDES AND POSITRON ANNIHILATION PHOTONS |

Nuclide	Half-life (min)	Maximum energy (MeV)	Maximum range (mm H$_2$O)
^{11}C	20.4	0.97	4
^{13}N	9.96	1.20	5
^{15}O	2.04	1.74	8
^{18}F	109.8	0.64	2
^{62}Cu	9.73	2.92	14
^{68}Ga	68.1	1.90	9
^{82}Rb	1.3	3.35	17
Annihilation photon	—	0.511	7,000[a]

[a] Half-value distance.

ting nuclide is short-lived, generators offer the possibility of providing positron emitters for PET scanning in the absence of a cyclotron. Unfortunately, the nuclides of greatest utility in neurochemical studies, ^{11}C, ^{15}O and ^{18}F, are not obtainable from generator systems. An important advantage of most short-lived positron nuclides is the limited radiation exposure of subjects undergoing PET studies since much of the administered activity decays during the study, contributing directly to the images.

Positron decay. The mode of positron decay is particularly advantageous for detection and quantification by external measurement. The decay process begins in the nucleus of a neutron-deficient isotope upon the conversion of a proton to a neutron with simultaneous emission of a positron, or β^+-particle, from the nucleus [2]. The positron is similar to an electron in physical properties except that it is positively rather than negatively charged. The emitted positron is slowed by loss of energy to the surrounding matter along its path and ultimately combines with an electron. This final interaction, positron annihilation, results in disintegration of both the positron and the electron, with the simultaneous emission of energy equivalent to their combined mass of 1.022 MeV. The emitted energy is in the form of two photons, or γ-rays, with energies of 511 keV that travel in opposite directions.

Photons, unlike positrons, undergo relatively little interaction with surrounding materials of low density; they are not easily deflected from their course and are readily detected at a distance outside the body. Because of the simultaneous emission of the two photons in exactly opposite directions, coincidence-detection algorithms for quantification of positron decay are employed, resulting in images with a high signal-to-noise ratio.

Detection of positron-emitting tracer and construction of images. Detection of positron decay for imaging purposes utilizes multiple detectors arranged in one or more rings surrounding the head. Each ring consists of individual detectors, each of which is paired with an oppositely placed detector by the scanner electronics. Each pair of detectors identifies positron-annihilation events along the line (ray) connecting them in space. A

transverse section image of the distribution of radioactivity within the head is created from the accumulated coincidence counts from each ring. The pair of detectors registering a coincidence defines the ray along which the positron annihilation occurred. Tomographic techniques analogous to those utilized in X-ray computed tomography, termed CT or CAT scanning, are used to reconstruct the image from the rays. Initial PET scanner designs consisted of a single ring of detectors, producing only one cross-sectional image at a time. Second-generation scanners were equipped with multiple adjacent rings of detectors, separated by septa of high-density absorbing material such as tungsten. These scanners allow simultaneous imaging of adjacent brain slices. Pairs of detectors in the same scanner ring define tissue planes in the same manner as the single-ring design. The absorbing septa reduce detection of very oblique coincidences and improve the ability to scan at high background radioactivity. However, most multi-ring scanners have septa that do permit slightly oblique lines of coincidence, involving opposing detectors in adjacent rings. Images from these oblique acquisitions, termed cross planes, depict tissue radioactivity midway between the detector rings and account for the greater number of tissue slices than detector rings in these scanners.

The latest generation of PET scanners (Fig. 54-1) incorporates two additional modifications [3]. First, individual pairs of crystals and photomultiplier tubes that make up the positron detectors in older designs have been replaced by detector blocks, consisting of larger crystals attached to multiple photodetectors. The positioning of a detected photon in the crystal is "decoded" by comparison of the light intensities among the photomultiplier tubes and interpolation, resulting in more possible locations of photon detection than the number of phototubes and improved spatial resolution. The second important modification is the addition of retractable septa. With the interplane septa removed, very oblique lines of coincidence can be scanned. This increases the overall scanner sensitivity by as much as tenfold and permits three-dimensional imaging of tissue sources located near the center of the scanner (Fig. 54-1). However, this design also permits photons originating outside the scanner field of view to reach

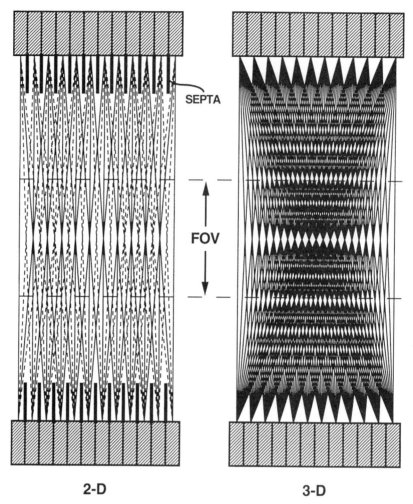

2-D   **3-D**

FIGURE 54-1. Longitudinal cross-sectional views of detector arrangement in positron emission tomography scanners with three-dimensional (*3-D*) imaging capability. In the two-dimensional (*2-D*) mode, annular septa separate detector rings from each other. The septa limit the detection of oblique γ-ray emissions, serving to "focus" the scanner on a limited number of planes for reconstruction. In the three-dimensional mode, the septa are removed, permitting a much greater number of possible tissue planes to be imaged. In each diagram, reconstructed image planes are designated by lines connecting opposing detectors. *FOV,* field of view. (Modified from [3].)

the detectors. While these are not mistaken for coincidences, they may flood the scanner with activity not contributing to the images. In some cases, these scattered events may be so numerous as to "paralyze" the computer software used for coincidence recognition.

Several correction factors are applied to the PET data during reconstruction of the images. The photon counts from each detector are corrected for underestimation errors arising from events missed because of detector and electronic limitations at high counting rates. In addition,

overestimation errors in coincidence detections caused by random coincidence of single events at high count rates are subtracted. Each detector pair is corrected on a regular basis for sensitivity differences by scanning a standard source of known activity. Finally, the coincidence counts from each ray are corrected for attenuation of the emitted 511-keV photons within the body. This correction is based either on direct measurement of attenuation with an external radiation source of known activity or on approximate densities assumed for the tissues within the field of view.

Resolution of PET images. The resulting PET images are spatial maps of radioactivity distribution within tissue slices and are thus analogous to autoradiograms obtained from brain tissue in animal experiments. The PET method, however, has an important distinction: it is noninvasive and may thus be used in clinical research, including longitudinal studies. A second difference between PET methods and tissue autoradiography is in the anatomical resolution. Typical film autoradiographic methods for detection of ^{3}H or ^{14}C provide 50- to 100-μm resolution, allowing clear separation of most brain nuclei from surrounding fiber tracts. The spatial resolution inherent in current PET scans ranges from 3 to 12 mm, resulting from a combination of factors. The number and geometry of detectors in the scanner as well as the number of counts acquired in the image and their statistical imprecision each reduce PET image resolution. These aspects vary between tomographs of different design as well as from study to study, owing to varying image-acquisition times and tissue-radioactivity levels. The ultimate theoretical limit of PET resolution, however, is the distance traveled by the positron in tissue before the annihilation reaction. Maximum tissue ranges vary according to the initial energy of the positron (Table 54-1).

As a consequence of limited spatial resolution, small brain nuclei and thin laminar structures such as the cerebral cortex cannot be completely separated from neighboring tissues and CSF. Reconstructed PET data thus reflect average isotope concentrations in the imaged tissue volume elements. When the actual tracer distribution is heterogeneous but below the resolution of the scan, the data underestimate the highest and overestimate the lowest values owing to this *partial volume averaging* effect.

Positron emission tomography can generate a pictorial representation of a physiological or biochemical process as the process occurs regionally within the brain

Several basic conceptual elements are shared by the variety of PET methods developed and implemented to date. Most significantly, PET mea-

sures generally reflect the functional biochemistry and physiology of the brain, in contrast to other imaging methods, such as CT and magnetic resonance imaging (MRI), which excel in the demonstration of tissue structure. The functional nature of PET imaging confers flexibility in the application of PET to neurochemical analysis, even though it imposes constraints on the experimental design and data analysis.

To achieve functional or parametric images, several conditions must be satisfied by the chosen radiotracer-imaging protocol and the data analysis. First, the process of interest must be precisely specified. Successful PET methods generally rely on a body of basic research experience to characterize the process and to demonstrate the biochemical and physiological significance, regulation and potential pathological alterations that may be encountered. Next, a tracer appropriate for the application must be identified. Tracer properties, including biochemical and physiological specificity, ease of synthesis with a positron-emitting nuclide and metabolic stability, are important factors in the selection of radiotracers. Third, a physiological compartmental model describing tracer distribution and the factors governing the movement of tracer between compartments must be developed [4]. It is the mathematical representation of this model that ultimately permits calculation of a parametric image from PET data.

Finally, the tracer and model must be tested and validated. Studies in experimental animals are utilized to verify the chemical identity of the radioactivity. Kinetic studies are performed under experimental pathological situations, that is, brain lesions and pharmacological treatments, which have predictable effects on the model and the parameter of interest. At any point along this path of development it may be necessary to revise the model or the method. If minimal criteria for quantification cannot be met, a new tracer must be selected.

It must be remembered, in addition, that preliminary work in animal models and in normal human subjects does not guarantee the accuracy of measurements in clinical research applications. Some diseases may cause unforeseen alterations in brain metabolism that invalidate the model and tracer utilized. Thus, understanding the key assumptions, simplifications and metabolic relationships involved in PET tracer methods is essential to data interpretation.

PHYSIOLOGICAL AND BIOCHEMICAL MEASUREMENTS USING POSITRON EMISSION TOMOGRAPHY

The simplest brain parameter to be measured with positron emission tomography is blood volume

The model describing the distribution of blood volume markers consists of a tissue volume element with the intravascular space contained in it representing the only compartment for tracer distribution (Fig. 54-2). It is assumed that the tracer enters and leaves the tissue by blood flow but that it does not enter the extravascular space or undergo metabolism. Carbon monoxide labeled with ^{15}O is inhaled in a single breath. Because of the high specific activity of the $[^{15}O]CO$, the trace chemical amount of gas administered is nontoxic. Following a brief period of mixing to allow the tracer to bind to hemoglobin and distribute evenly within the blood pool, a PET scan is obtained, and a sample of blood is taken simultaneously for measurement of the tracer concentration. The blood volume in tissue is then determined by dividing the tissue tracer concentration by the blood value.

Normal values for cerebral blood volume (CBV) range from 4 to 6% in gray matter and from 2 to 3% in white matter (Fig. 54-2). Regions adjacent to or containing major arteries or venous sinuses have considerably larger values, owing to partial volume averaging with the vessels (see above). Although the intravascular volume itself may occasionally be of interest, the most frequent application is the correction of studies with other tracers for intravascular activity. If the regional intravascular volume and arterial tracer concentrations are known, the measured total tissue activity may be corrected for the intravascular component. This technique is frequently employed in the determination of brain oxygen extraction and metabolism.

Measurement of blood–brain barrier permeability to a test substance is based on a two-compartment model representing the intravascular and extravascular spaces

The movement of tracer into and out of the tissue volume element occurs by flow of blood, whereas capillary blood exchanges tracer with the tissue (see Chap. 32). Two model parameters are estimated following intravenous injection of the tracer [5]: arterial blood samples are used to determine the tracer input curve, and serial PET scans of the brain are obtained to define the regional tracer time–activity curves. The first of the parameters, K_1, represents uptake of the tracer by brain from the blood. It is related to both cerebral blood flow, F, and the regional capillary surface area–permeability product, PS:

$$K_1 = F(1 - e^{-PS/F}).$$

The second parameter, k_2, represents the movement of tracer back to the blood from the brain and is equivalent to K_1 divided by the tracer distribution volume in brain. Selection of tracers with appropriate properties allows direct determination of regional permeability using this model. Specifically, for tracers with very low permeability ($F \gg PS$), $K_1 \sim PS$. In addition, tracers with very large distribution volumes in brain allow k_2 to be neglected early, simplifying estimation of K_1. Tracers satisfying the former condition include $^{82}RbCl$ [5] and $[^{68}Ga]EDTA$ [6]. $[^{11}C]$aminoisobutyric acid, a tracer satisfying both conditions, has been utilized in animal experiments [7]; however, due to the comparative simplicity of $[^{68}Ga]EDTA$ synthesis, it has not gained widespread clinical use.

Determination of regional blood–brain barrier permeability is used primarily when a pathological increase is anticipated. Measurements in brain tumor and in brain infarction, or stroke, have verified the abnormally permeable capillary beds known qualitatively from contrast-enhanced CT scanning and MRI. PET methods, however, allow calculation of the permeability coefficient. This allows quantification of the effects of steroid treatment on

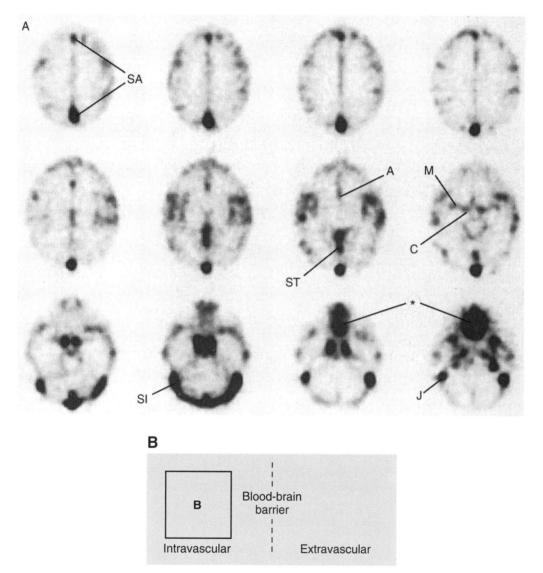

FIGURE 54-2. Positron emission tomographic (PET) measurement of blood volume in normal human subject. **A:** PET images from adjacent transaxial slices extending from the supraventricular level **(upper left)** to the base of the brain **(lower right)** following inhalation of [^{15}O]CO. Blood volume is depicted in gray scale, with increasing image density reflecting higher blood volume. Major cerebral vessels are located on the surface of the brain, and larger volumes are associated with venous sinuses rather than with cerebral arteries. Note that the extracerebral soft tissues (dark gray rim at periphery of images) and nasal sinuses (*) have considerably higher blood volume than does the brain: *A*, anterior cerebral arteries; *C*, carotid artery; *J*, jugular bulb; *M*, middle cerebral artery; *SA*, sagittal sinus; *SI*, sigmoid sinus; *ST*, straight sinus and vein of Galen. **B:** Compartmental model used for calculation of blood volume. Tracer is assumed to remain in the blood pool *(B)* during the study. The PET scanner views a mixture of the intravascular and extravascular compartments, allowing calculation of the intravascular volume. (Images courtesy of Dr. M. E. Phelps, UCLA, Los Angeles, CA.)

blood–brain barrier permeability as well as estimation of regional brain exposure to potential chemotherapeutic agents. Measurement of blood–brain barrier permeability is additionally helpful in excluding potential sources of error from other PET methods, which may be complicated by breakdown of the barrier. Blood–brain barrier permeability to tracers that enter brain readily may be calculated from estimates of their initial uptake combined with independent measurement of regional blood flow according to the relationship given for K_1 above. This may be of benefit in defining the relative flow and permeability contributions to tracer uptake, thereby permitting better understanding of the tracer kinetic model and its sensitivity to pathological blood flow and blood–brain barrier changes.

Determination of regional cerebral blood flow by positron emission tomography is frequently employed to localize "functional" neural activation

The modeling of cerebral blood flow (CBF) tracer distribution is identical with that presented for blood–brain barrier permeability measurements discussed previously. The tissue volume element consists of two tracer-distribution compartments, the intravascular and extravascular spaces (Fig. 54-3). The influx rate constant, K_1, is directly proportional to blood flow when the tracer has a very high blood–brain barrier permeability, that is, $PS \gg F$. Under these conditions, two parameters, K_1 and k_2, are estimated for each tissue volume element: K_1 represents regional CBF, whereas K_1/k_2 is the regional tracer distribution volume. The CBF tracer may be introduced into the circulation either by inhalation or by intravenous injection. Data collected consist of serial PET scans of the brain and the arterial input curve to the brain, approximated from measurement of tracer activity in arterial blood samples [8,9].

Several tracers have been employed for CBF measurement, each of which has relative advantages and disadvantages. Initial CBF measurements were made with [^{13}N]NH$_3$ because of its ease of synthesis; however, NH$_3$ is not inert in cerebral tissue, it is restricted from complete equilibration with brain at high normal CBF

rates and its uptake and distribution are affected by tissue and plasma pH and cerebral NH$_3$ metabolism. Thus, newer agents, including [^{15}O]H$_2$O and [^{11}C]butanol, have replaced [^{13}N]NH$_3$. Water as a CBF tracer is attractive from the standpoint of easy synthesis, formulation and injection; but like ammonia, it is limited by blood–brain barrier permeability at the upper extremes of physiological flow rates [10]. Butanol, by comparison, is not diffusion-limited but is more difficult to synthesize, and the longer half-life of ^{11}C compared to ^{15}O results in greater radiation exposure for an equivalent injected dose. Butanol may be synthesized and labeled with ^{15}O, but the radiochemical synthetic demands are severe, owing to the very short half-life of the nuclide. Preliminary studies suggest the feasibility of CBF measurements using [^{62}Cu]PTSM [pyruvaldehyde bis-(N_4-methylthiosemicarbazone)], a lipophilic, organometallic compound readily synthesized from generator-produced ^{62}Cu. This tracer may permit CBF studies without the need for a local cyclotron, although, as with NH$_3$, it is incompletely extracted and trapped at physiological CBF.

PET-determined values for CBF in normal individuals average approximately 50 ml per minute per 100 g brain, in agreement with the results of global measures by the Kety-Schmidt arteriovenous difference method (see Chap. 31). Regional CBF values range from 40 to 100 in gray matter and from 15 to 30 in white-matter structures (Fig. 54-3). The average ratio of gray to white matter for CBF in the resting state is approximately 3:1 with current PET techniques. This is somewhat less than the ratios of 5:1 or 6:1 obtained in autoradiographic animal experiments, as a result of partial volume averaging in the PET measurements. Global CBF varies substantially with respiration owing to the effect of arterial pCO_2 or pH on the cerebral vasculature (Fig. 54-3C) (see also Chap. 31). Near the physiological pCO_2 of 40 mm Hg, CBF increases approximately 1 to 2% for each 1 mm Hg increase in pCO_2.

In addition to the above global effects, regional CBF changes have been determined both as a result of physiological activation of the brain, in cerebral pathology, and in their interactions. Close regional couplings of CBF to oxida-

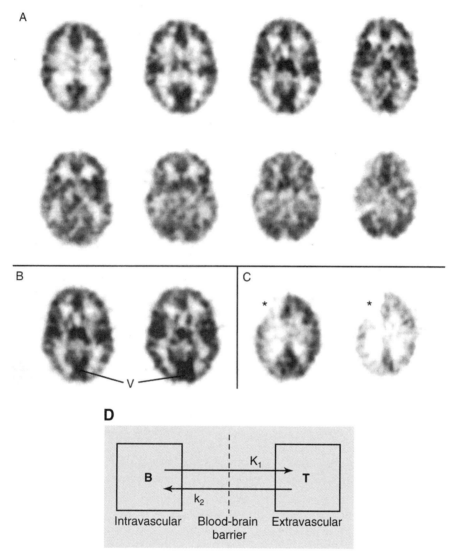

FIGURE 54-3. Positron emission tomographic measurement of cerebral blood flow (CBF). **A:** CBF determined in a normal subject following injection of $[^{15}O]H_2O$. Transaxial images extend from the supraventricular level **(upper left)** to the base of the brain **(lower right). B:** CBF images at the mid-thalamic level from a normal subject during visual deprivation (eyes closed, **left**) and again during audiovisual stimulation (watching a videotape, **right**). Note the focal increase in CBF in the visual cortex *(V)* during stimulation. **C:** CBF at the supraventricular level in a patient at rest **(left)** and again during hyperventilation **(right).** Note the global reduction of CBF due to reduced arterial CO_2 during hyperventilation, without alteration in regional pattern. The patient has undergone prior surgery for removal of a tumor in the frontal lobe (*). **D:** Compartmental model for CBF measurement. Two tracer compartments representing arterial blood *(B)* and brain tissue *(T)* are represented. Blood flow is estimated by the rate of tissue tracer uptake (K_1) from blood. (Images courtesy of Dr. L. Junck, Department of Neurology, The University of Michigan, Ann Arbor, MI.)

tive metabolism and of metabolism to synaptic activity are observed in normal brain, although the exact mechanism(s) underlying these relationships are not yet fully known. Nevertheless, the ability to measure repeatedly the pattern of CBF in human brain permits experimental determinations of altered activity corresponding to different externally imposed stimuli, task performances or internal "states." Powerful statistical methods are employed to detect significant changes within subjects [11] and, in summed studies, across subjects after "warping" individual brains to a common anatomical format [12,13]. The experimental design of within-subject, state-dependent comparisons has provided the means for directly testing the functional involvement of various brain regions in complex cognitive tasks and behaviors, often detecting very subtle, as little as 3 to 5% in some studies, yet significant regional brain activations [14]. This approach provides an *in vivo* complement to the traditional neurological method of correlating behavioral deficits with the locations of brain lesions.

Functional MRI. Functional brain-activation mapping has also been demonstrated with the use of MRI (see also Chap. 50). State- or task-related changes in the proton MRI signal are detected in similar brain regions, as are the PET CBF changes discussed previously. The biophysical explanation for this phenomenon, termed the "BOLD" effect, is that the magnetic field used for MRI is modified locally by the presence of magnetic substances. While only weakly paramagnetic, deoxygenated hemoglobin is able to influence the MR field. Oxygenated hemoglobin is not magnetic. Thus, experimental conditions that alter the concentration of deoxyhemoglobin in MRI will create small signal changes due to its paramagnetic effect. In cerebral "activation" studies, the increased synaptic activity gives rise to increased CBF (see above) and to increased local blood volume. Combined, these effects permit imaging of "functional" changes in proton MRI, termed functional MRI (fMRI), which are analyzed and interpreted in a similar fashion to the PET CBF methods. Advantages of the fMRI technique are that it does not require ionizing radiation and it may be able to image sta-

tistically significant changes in single subjects without the need for group-averaging and summation techniques [15]. If different individual subjects employ unique strategies and brain regions in accomplishing cognitive tasks, this single-subject approach may prove invaluable.

Regional cerebral glucose metabolism is imaged for the study of brain activity *in vivo*

Development of the method for determining the regional cerebral metabolic rate for glucose ($rCMR_{glc}$) and its validation in experimental animals [16] are discussed in detail in Chapter 31. The tracer kinetic model for glucose metabolism is more complex than the previously discussed examples because of an additional tissue compartment representing metabolized tracer (Fig. 54-4). The model consists of intravascular tracer, a tissue precursor pool in exchange with blood and a metabolic pool representing tracer that has been chemically transformed. The compartments are interrelated by the rate constants K_1 and k_2, representing the exchange of tracer across the blood–brain barrier, and by k_3 and k_4, representing the rate of tracer phosphorylation by hexokinase and dephosphorylation by glucose-6-phosphatase, respectively. The tracers employed for measurement of $rCMR_{glc}$ are the 2-deoxy-D-glucoses (2DG), glucose analogs that share transport and phosphorylation processes with the endogenous substrate but that are not appreciably further metabolized following formation of the 6-phosphate derivative. Thus, the 2DG tracers are useful in the determination of the rate of glucose phosphorylation by hexokinase but do not measure subsequent steps in glycolysis or in oxidative metabolism.

At present, two positron-emitting 2DG derivatives are in use: $[^{18}F]$2-fluoro-2-deoxy-D-glucose ($[^{18}F]$FDG) and $[^{11}C]$2DG. The former tracer has the advantage of a longer half-life and is useful in situations in which PET scans of high anatomical resolution and statistical precision at long times following injection are desired. The shorter half-life of $[^{11}C]$2DG, conversely, is useful when multiple sequential studies on the same experimental subject are planned, such as test–retest or baseline and stimulation protocols,

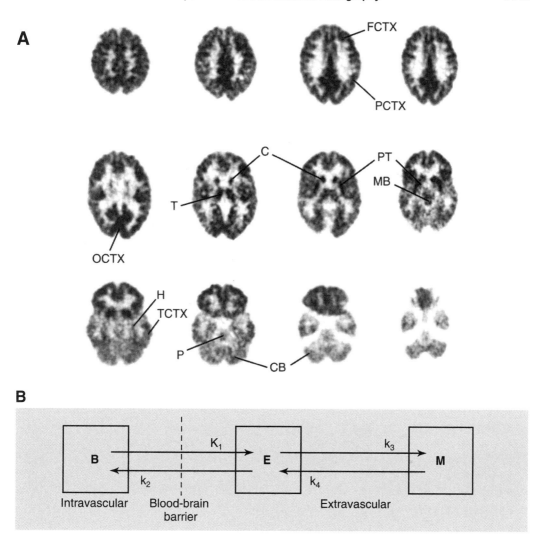

FIGURE 54-4.   Regional cerebral glucose metabolism. **A:** Positron emission tomographic scans obtained 30 to 90 min following injection of [^{18}F]Fluoro-2-deoxy-D-glucose (FDG) in a normal subject. Transaxial slices from the supraventricular level **(upper left)** to the base of the brain **(lower right)** are displayed on a gray scale, with the highest metabolic rates depicted by the darker areas. Anatomical structure is well delineated in the images on the basis of higher glucose metabolism in gray- than in white-matter regions: *C*, caudate nucleus; *CB*, cerebellum; *FCTX*, frontal cortex; *H*, hippocampal formation; *MB*, midbrain; *OCTX*, occipital cortex; *P*, pons; *PCTX*, parietal cortex; *PT*, putamen; *T*, thalamus; *TCTX*, temporal cortex. **B:** Compartmental model for regional cerebral metabolic rate of glucose determination. Tracer compartments include FDG in arterial blood *(B)* and in the extravascular precursor pool *(E)*, as well as FDG-6-phosphate in the metabolic product pool *(M)*. The rate of FDG metabolism is the product of tissue uptake from blood (K_1) and the fraction of tissue precursor metabolized ($k_3/[k_2 + k_3]$).

since the activity decays quickly enough to allow repeat tracer injections on the same day within 3- to 4-hr intervals.

Measurement of rCMR$_{glc}$ is initiated by intravenous injection of labeled DG, followed by collection of timed arterial blood samples for measurement of the tracer input curve [17,18]. The most commonly employed procedure is to obtain PET brain images beginning 30 to 45 min after the injection, at which time the bulk of the activity represents metabolized tracer. These data, combined with the arterial input function, are analyzed according to a modified version of the operational equation of Sokoloff (see Chap. 31). Calculation of rCMR$_{glc}$ by this procedure relies on the use of population average values of the individual rate constants and the lumped constant. The single-scan protocol is thus analogous to the autoradiographic method employed in the determination of rCMR$_{glc}$ using a β^{-}-particle-emitting 2DG tracer in experimental animals.

Under a variety of pathological conditions, some or all of the assumptions about the rate and lumped constants may be invalidated either globally or regionally, leading to inaccuracies in the estimates of rCMR$_{glc}$ provided by the single-scan approach [10,19]. In particular, disruption of the normal relationship and coupling between blood flow and energy metabolism may occur in ischemic states. Wide fluctuations from the normal range of blood glucose concentrations have additionally been demonstrated to produce such alterations. In these circumstances, an alternative experimental protocol involving repeated measurements of tracer distribution may be applied [20]. Serial PET scans are obtained beginning immediately after the injection and ending 45 to 90 min later. The tissue and blood time–activity curves are then fitted to the compartmental model by nonlinear least-squares approximation, defining optimal values for the rate constants. The rate of 2DG "metabolism" (rCMR$_{dg}$) is given by

$$rCMR_{dg} = K_1 \cdot k_3 / (k_2 + k_3)$$

and the glucose metabolic rate by

$$rCMR_{glc} = C_p \cdot rCMR_{dg} / LC$$

where C_p represents the arterial plasma glucose concentration and LC is a lumped constant relating deoxyglucose to glucose metabolism. Using this kinetic approach, the calculated rCMR$_{glc}$ continues to be influenced by the value of the lumped constant but is independent of errors introduced by the application of inappropriate rate constants for 2DG transport and metabolism.

Measurements of CMR$_{glc}$ in normal individuals at rest yield average rates for whole brain of approximately 6 mg per 100 g brain per minute, or 33 μmol per 100 g brain per minute (Fig. 54-4). This is well within the range of values reported using arteriovenous differences, which is between 4.5 and 6.5 mg per 100 g brain per minute. The rCMR$_{glc}$ in normal brain varies between 5 and 11 mg per 100 g brain per minute in gray matter and between 2 and 5 mg per 100 g brain per minute in white matter. These values demonstrate less range than autoradiographic animal studies, in which seven- to eightfold differences between gray- and white-matter regions are seen. This, again, is a result of inherent volume averaging at the PET level of anatomic resolution.

The measurement of rCMR$_{glc}$ has gained wide application in the study of both normal physiological activity and pathological processes, based on the observed relationship between functional neuronal activity and energy metabolism [21]. This relationship has been demonstrated elegantly through a variety of physiological activation and suppression procedures in both experimental animals and normal human volunteers. Results of animal studies suggest that the coupling of metabolism to neuronal activity is due to the increased transmembrane ionic flux associated with synaptic transmission (see Chaps. 5 and 31). In general, areas of dense synaptic content within neuropil show the highest regional rates of metabolism and respond most dramatically to alterations in neuronal activity. White matter is less active or reactive when studied at high anatomic resolution by autoradiography in animals. It should be kept in mind that both pre- and postsynaptic terminals participate in functional metabolic responses and that in some instances the effect of increased neuronal firing may be detected only in distant terminal fields of the activated neurons rather than in the regions of the cell bodies themselves [22]. Thus, the metabolic response to a change in activity within a particular brain region is often detected in remote brain regions receiving its efferent projections.

Applications of PET rCMR$_{glc}$ measurements include primary investigation of cerebral metabolism and the relationships between glucose and oxygen metabolism. In addition, primary disturbances in substrate delivery, as in ischemia, and in metabolic activity, as in metabolic coma, may be directly investigated. Regional glucose metabolism has most frequently been utilized as a tool for localizing alterations in neuronal activity as a consequence of physiological stimulation. Here, changes in metabolism reveal the locations of altered neuronal activity resulting from changes in behavioral states or from pathological processes.

Inhalation of [^{15}O]oxygen allows measurement of regional cerebral oxygen metabolic rate

The regional rate of cerebral oxygen metabolism (rCMRO$_2$) represents one of two PET methods discussed here that cannot be determined in experimental animals by alternative techniques. The known radioisotopes of oxygen are all extremely short-lived and, thus, of little use in conventional biochemical research since the activity decays too rapidly to allow measurement in dissected tissue samples. The longest-lived oxygen isotope, ^{15}O (half-life 2.04 min), administered as [^{15}O]O$_2$, has been successfully employed in the measurement of oxygen metabolism by means of PET. Two methods of administration of the agent by inhalation have been described. They rely on a simple two-compartment model of O$_2$ distribution in which intravascular and extravascular spaces are represented. It is assumed that ^{15}O$_2$ in arterial blood is predominantly bound to hemoglobin with a smaller dissolved fraction. During capillary transit, ^{15}O$_2$ enters the tissue, where it is rapidly metabolized to [^{15}O]H$_2$O. The labeled water then exchanges with the intravascular compartment. Peripheral metabolism also results in production of [^{15}O]H$_2$O, which recirculates in arterial blood to the brain and must be taken into account. Oxygen metabolism is thus defined as the product of regional oxygen extraction and arterial oxygen delivery:

$$rCMRO_2 = E \cdot C_a \cdot rCBF$$

where C_a represents arterial oxygen content, rCBF is regional cerebral blood flow and E is the fraction of available oxygen extracted during a single capillary transit.

The methods employed involve a continuous inhalation protocol with a single-scan determination of regional ^{15}O$_2$ extraction [23] or a kinetic multiple-scan approach following single-breath inhalation of ^{15}O$_2$ [24]. Both methods require arterial blood sampling for determination of O$_2$ content, ^{15}O$_2$ and [^{15}O]H$_2$O. In addition, independent measurement of rCBF, usually with [^{15}O]H$_2$O, is required. Finally, because of the substantial contribution of intravascular activity to the total tissue activity, correction for intravascular volume using [^{15}O]CO is frequently employed.

Results of measurements in normal volunteers indicate resting CMRO$_2$ of 1.8 to 5.8 ml O$_2$ per 100 g brain per minute, or 70 to 230 μmol O$_2$ per 100 g brain per minute, in white and gray matter, respectively. Applications of PET CMRO$_2$ measurements are similar to those discussed above for CMR$_{glc}$.

The metabolism of specific neurotransmitters may be evaluated with the use of labeled precursors

In addition to oxidative energy metabolism, specific processes subserving the synthesis and subsequent disposition of neurotransmitters may be evaluated with PET methods. Measurement of dopamine (DA) synthesis in monoaminergic neurons may be estimated following the injection of [^{18}F]6-fluoro-DOPA (FDOPA). The tracer, an analog of DOPA, is transported across the blood–brain barrier by the large neutral amino acid carrier system. Within nerve terminals, [^{18}F]FDOPA is metabolized by DOPA decarboxylase to the false transmitter [^{18}F]fluorodopamine (FDA), which subsequently undergoes vesicular storage, release on nerve depolarization, presynaptic reuptake and degradative metabolism in parallel with authentic DA. Prominent peripheral metabolism of the tracer by DOPA and aromatic amino acid decarboxylases and by catechol-*O*-methyltransferase (COMT) results in labeled metabolites (see Chap. 12). When the former pathways are inhibited by pre-administration of the peripheral decarboxylase inhibitor carbidopa, brain tracer uptake is enhanced and analysis of blood activity is simplified. Under these conditions, the predominant labeled blood constituents are authentic FDOPA and its COMT metabolite 3-*O*-methyl-FDOPA (MeDOPA). The rate of cerebral FDA synthesis is estimated with a physiological model analogous to that used for FDG metabolism, after correction of both blood and cerebral activities for the estimated contribution of [^{18}F]MeDOPA [25]. A similar method has been proposed for the study of serotonin synthesis, based on uptake and metabolism of [^{11}C]α-methyl-L-tryptophan [26].

Application of FDOPA imaging has been extensive in the evaluation of neurological movement disorders, particularly in Parkinson's disease and other disorders attributed to dopaminergic pathology. The method permits evaluation of presynaptic capacity for DA synthesis, which is known to be impaired in Parkinson's disease and related disorders on the basis of postmortem observations (see Chap. 45).

The *in vivo* quantification of regional ligand-binding sites has been a long anticipated development

The general kinetic ligand-binding model consists of four tracer compartments [27] (Fig. 54-5). The intravascular compartment communicates with the free ligand pool in the tissue by the rate constants K_1 and K_2, which represent exchange across the blood–brain barrier. The extravascular space contains three tracer compartments: free ligand, nonspecifically bound ligand and receptor, or specifically bound ligand. The rate constant k_3 describes specific binding of the ligand to free receptors, and k_4 represents the dissociation of specifically bound ligand. Exchange of free ligand with nonspecific binding

sites that are assumed to be nonsaturable in tissue is represented by k_5 and k_6.

The relationships between the kinetic rate constants and the receptor pharmacological terms k_{on}, k_{off}, K_d and B_{max} are as follows:

$$k_3 = k_{on} \cdot R = k_{on}(B_{max} - RL)$$

$$k_4 = k_{off}$$

where $B_{max} = R + RL$, $K_d = k_{off}/k_{on}$, k_{on} and k_{off} are rate constants for ligand binding to and dissociation from the receptor, B_{max} is the total number of receptor sites, R represents free receptors available for binding and RL represents receptors occupied by ligand (see also Chap. 10). Even under true tracer conditions in PET studies in which radioligand occupies an insignificant number of the total receptor sites, B_{max} and R may be nonidentical, owing to receptor occupancy by endogenous neurotransmitter. Thus, kinetic binding methods estimate the free receptor density (R) rather than the total receptor number (B_{max}) measured by *in vitro* methods. Finally, as is evident from the above equations, B_{max}, or R, is not uniquely specified under *in vivo* binding conditions. Receptor concentration and ligand affinity may be estimated from sequential PET studies, resulting in minimal and substantial occupancy of receptors, respectively, since k_3 is reduced in proportion to receptor availability at pharmacological doses of administered ligand, while k_{on} and k_{off} are unaffected. As an alternative, many investigators choose to determine the $k_{on} \cdot B_{max}$ product (k_3) or the B_{max}/K_d ratio (k_3/k_4) from a single high-specific-activity tracer injection.

In practice, a ligand is injected intravenously and arterial blood samples are withdrawn for determination of the arterial input function. Unlike most of the previously described PET methods, blood radioactivity measurements must be corrected for the presence of labeled metabolites produced *in vivo* in order to define the input curves properly [28]. Sequential PET scans of the brain are obtained, and the resulting tracer time courses in tissue and the arterial blood curve are analyzed by nonlinear least-squares fitting to provide estimates of the model

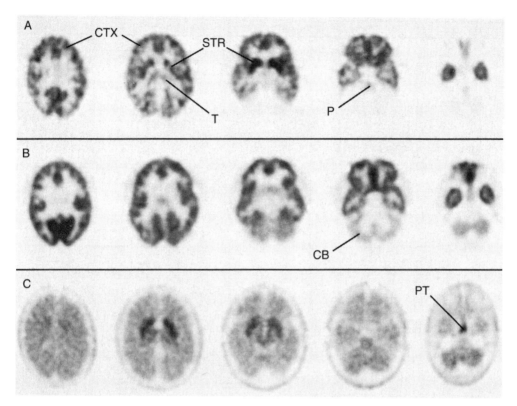

FIGURE 54-5.   Radioligand binding to neurochemical markers in normal human brain. **A:** Distribution of muscarinic acetylcholine receptors as depicted by the tissue distribution volume (DV) for the muscarinic antagonist ligand [^{11}C]*N*-methylpiperidylbenzilate. **B:** Distribution of central-type benzodiazepine-binding sites as depicted by the distribution volume for the benzodiazepine antagonist [^{11}C]flumazenil. **C:** Distribution of monoamine presynaptic terminals as depicted by the accumulation of [^{11}C]tetrabenazine. Comparable images from the supraventricular level **(left)** to the base of the brain **(right)** are shown for the individual binding site ligands. Note the distinction between brain regions according to differential levels of each binding site. Cerebral cortical *(CTX)* areas have high concentrations of muscarinic receptors and benzodiazepine-binding sites; the striatum (caudate and putamen, *STR*) has high concentrations of both muscarinic receptors and monoamine (dopamine) terminals; the thalamus *(T)* has low levels of all three markers (monoaminergic vesicles are predominantly noradrenergic in the diencephalon); the pons *(P)* has low concentrations of muscarinic receptors and monoamine vesicles with virtually no benzodiazepine-binding sites; and the cerebellum *(CB)* has very low muscarinic receptor binding but a modest number of benzodiazepine-binding sites; and monoamine vesicles. The pituitary *(PT)* is distinguished by monoamine vesicles in the terminals of arcuate hypothalamic neurons projecting to its posterior division. (*Figure continues on next page.*)

parameters. Typically, the entire set of six or more parameters in the ligand-binding model cannot be simultaneously estimated from a single PET tracer study. Simplifications of the model, including collapsing of the nonsaturable tissue compartments, and of all three tissue compartments have been applied with success to analyses of specific ligands (Fig. 54-5) [28,29]. Some of these simplifying assumptions permit the calculation of receptor maps, displaying the binding parameter(s) on a pixel-by-pixel basis.

The range of ligand-binding sites that may be studied in this way is potentially as varied as the tracers for their study (Fig. 54-5). It is feasible to measure cerebral DA, opiate, serotonin, benzodiazepine and muscarinic and nicotinic cholinergic receptors. Enzyme concentrations may be determined by using similar modeling assumptions, as demonstrated by the imaging of brain monoamine oxidases [30]. In addition, presynaptic membrane and vesicle transporters may be quantified with appropriately selected

D

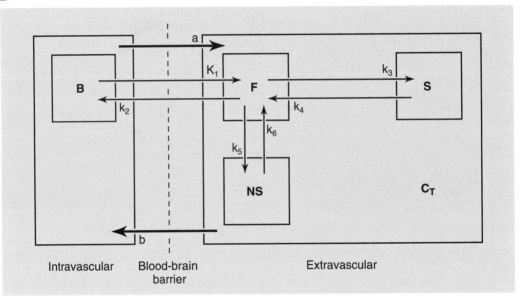

E

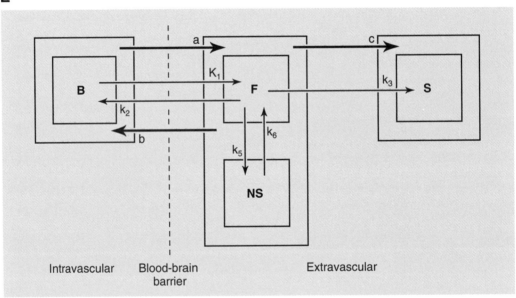

FIGURE 54-5. *(Continued)* **D** and **E:** Two alternative compartmental models depicting simplified algorithms for estimation of ligand binding-site density. In both cases, ligand compartments representing arterial blood *(B)*, free tissue ligand *(F)*, nonspecifically bound ligand *(NS)* and specifically bound ligand *(S)* are considered. These four compartments and six associated rate constants *(inner boxes* in each model) are not independently estimable in most *in vivo* experiments, necessitating introduction of simplified models. In the case of ligands that interact rapidly and reversibly with binding sites ("equilibrium" binding ligands, **D**), the three tissue compartments are kinetically condensed to a single compartment *(outer boxes)* and new rate constants (a and b) are estimated. The degree of specific binding, under appropriate conditions, is proportional to the combined tissue distribution volume, as estimated from the ratio of a/b. This model was applied in calculation of the binding depicted in A and B. Alternatively, modeling of ligands that dissociate very slowly from specific binding sites ("irreversible" binding ligands, **E**) may be simplified by condensing the free and nonspecific binding tissue components and estimating the three remaining rate constants, a, b and c *(outer boxes)*. In this case, the binding-site density is estimated by the magnitude of parameter c.

radioligands [31,32]. The selection of ligands for receptor measurement is a key step in the successful development of *in vivo* binding techniques, and the selection entails greater restrictions on the properties of an acceptable tracer than for *in vitro* binding situations. First, the selected ligand should have specificity for a single receptor type or subtype. The use of antagonist drugs is preferred since antagonist binding is more closely described by the simple association and dissociation reactions assumed in the model than is the binding of agonists. Finally, the labeled ligand must not be metabolized within the brain or converted outside of the brain to labeled metabolites that enter the brain and complicate interpretation of the tissue activity curves.

Applications of *in vivo* ligand-binding methods are potentially diverse, ranging from studies of disease- or therapy-related alterations in the numbers of binding sites to dynamic tests of synaptic function. The latter possibility is based on measurement of changes in free binding sites caused by altered concentrations of endogenous neurotransmitter or substrate. Thus, either physiological or pharmacological challenges that alter presynaptic activity or binding of the endogenous transmitter may produce changes indirectly in the radioligand binding to the receptor sites. A baseline receptor scan followed by a repeat study with such an activation procedure may thus identify the integrity of presynaptic terminals. In addition, the regional receptor occupancies accompanying the use of therapeutic doses of direct receptor agonist or antagonist drugs may be determined by repeat ligand-binding scans before and after a dose of the unlabeled agent.

CLINICAL APPLICATIONS OF CEREBRAL POSITRON EMISSION TOMOGRAPHY

The initial clinical use of cerebral PET techniques was limited largely to research protocols because of its relative expense and limited availability. However, in recent years PET has become widely available in tertiary medical centers throughout the world. The radiosynthesis of many commonly used tracers, such as $[^{15}O]H_2O$, $[^{13}N]NH_3$ and $[^{18}F]2FDG$, has been automated, and the existence of compact medical cyclotrons controlled by personal computers allows PET radiotracer production with reduced personnel. In addition, in many geographic areas, regional cyclotron and radiopharmacy facilities are under development to supply longer-lived PET radiopharmaceuticals, particularly $[^{18}F]2FDG$, to networks of surrounding hospitals. Clinical diagnostic uses of PET in individual patients have been introduced for the management of epilepsy, brain tumor, dementia and cerebrovascular disease. However, the majority of PET research continues to focus on fundamental aspects of neurological and psychiatric disease pathophysiology, rather than on its clinical diagnostic uses. The results of these research directions have broad implications for diagnosis and therapy of all patients with the studied disorders, often applicable without the need for PET in each individual patient. In addition, research applications may uncover unrecognized physiological and biochemical abnormalities, serving to redirect subsequent studies using more conventional methods.

Many degenerative neurological disorders have chronic progressive courses, yet they may respond symptomatically to pharmacological treatment. Thus, postmortem biochemical analyses of the brain may be influenced by the primary disease, medications and nonspecific effects of chronic illness. PET is of particular value in these instances, providing a noninvasive alternative to brain biopsy or other less direct approaches, such as CSF analysis. PET can be applied early in the course of degenerative diseases, often in advance of exposure to medications or other confounding factors. Examples of diseases under study in this manner include Alzheimer's disease, Huntington's disease and Parkinson's disease.

Another alternative goal in PET research is the identification of clinical disease markers or therapeutic responses that might be extrapolated to the subsequent diagnosis or treatment of an entire patient population. In these instances, we seek predictive correlation between PET measurements and results of routinely available and less costly diagnostic tests. Examples of such applications include studies of drug distribution and action, brain tumor response to therapy and the biochemistry and physiology of cerebrovascular disease.

Studies of Alzheimer's disease assist in diagnosis and test pathophysiological hypotheses

A variety of neurochemical and functional PET-imaging approaches have been applied to the study of progressive dementias, particularly Alzheimer's disease (AD) and related disorders. The most reproducible neurochemical imaging abnormality in patients with dementia is cortical glucose hypometabolism, initially reported by Kuhl and co-workers [33]. The typical AD pattern includes reduced 2FDG metabolism in parietal and temporal lobe association and posterior cingulate cortices. Reductions are usually bilateral, yet there often is an asymmetry in the severity or the extent of hypometabolism. Patients with advanced clinical symptoms often demonstrate reduced metabolism in the prefrontal association cortices as well. Metabolism is relatively spared in primary sensory and motor cortical regions, including the somatomotor, auditory and visual cortices. Subcortical structures, including the basal ganglia, thalamus, brainstem and cerebellum, are also preserved in typical AD. The overall distribution of metabolism in AD reflects in part the known regional losses of neurons and synapses but likely also includes effects of cortical disconnection resulting in reduced afferent input to the association areas. The "typical" AD pattern in 2FDG PET is sufficiently specific and sensitive that it may become an important research and clinical diagnostic tool, particularly in patients with memory loss or complaints but without obvious impairment in other areas of cognition.

Specifically designed neurochemical PET-imaging procedures have permitted the testing of pathophysiological hypotheses of the etiology and progression of AD [34]. PET and single-photon emission CT have been applied to imaging the severity and distribution of the cholinergic lesions found at autopsy in the basal forebrain-to-cerebral cortex projection systems in AD. Predominantly postsynaptic in location, muscarinic cholinergic receptors are largely intact in normal aging and in AD by PET studies (see also Chap. 30). Defects in presynaptic markers of cholinergic projections, including concentrations of the vesicular acetylcholine transporter and the activity of acetylcholinesterase, have been identified *in vivo*. However, the severity of these lesions in living patients is less than that reported in autopsy studies, raising questions as to the relationship between cholinergic deficits and the memory impairment characteristic of early AD. Future studies of acetylcholinesterase activity and its response to symptomatic therapies targeting the enzyme may provide important information on the actions of cholinesterase inhibitors in demented patients.

Studies of epilepsy assist in characterizing seizure foci

Although idiopathic epilepsy is one of the most frequently encountered neurological disorders, the underlying pharmacological, metabolic and electrophysiological abnormalities are largely unknown. Medically intractable seizures are frequently associated with epileptogenic foci in the temporal lobes (see Chap. 37).

The first results of PET in partial epilepsy revealed an unanticipated abnormality in the *interictal,* or between seizure, metabolic pattern [35]. The seizure focus showed decreased, rather than increased, blood flow and glucose metabolic rate. In over two-thirds of patients, a well-lateralized zone of hypometabolism is identified on interictal scans. When present, the hypometabolic zone correlates with the location of the seizure focus as determined by *ictal,* or during seizure, depth EEG recordings in greater than 90% of cases. During ictal discharge, the zone of hypometabolism is replaced by a relatively hypermetabolic area that frequently extends beyond the limits of the interictal abnormality.

The etiology of interictal hypometabolism has yet to be conclusively established; however, several hypotheses have been proposed that may account for the phenomenon. Hypometabolism may result from active inhibition of neuronal activity, from loss of neurons or simplification of synaptic architecture or from gross structural atrophy. The frequent finding of mesial temporal

sclerosis, consisting of loss of neurons and gliosis affecting the hippocampus, in surgically re-
sected epileptogenic temporal lobes lends support to the proposed structural mechanisms
[36]. Measurements by PET suggest that the lateral temporal neocortex ipsilateral to the seizure
focus displays a greater degree of metabolic depression, although histological abnormalities in
these areas are not recognized. Thus, metabolic
abnormalities extend beyond known structural
pathology, supporting involvement of functional connections between the seizure focus and
neocortical regions [37].

The coexistence of both PET hypometabolism and ictal-depth EEG localization
is a reliable predictor of good surgical response
in seizure control. Placement of depth electrodes
is an invasive procedure with an associated morbidity. Hence, development of the noninvasive
scheme for localization of a unilateral seizure focus is clinically important. MRI is preferable
when a structural lesion other than mesial temporal sclerosis is present, whereas PET appears
to be more sensitive at detecting sclerotic lesions.
The combination of MRI and PET is routine in
the preoperative evaluation of intractable
seizures at some centers, eliminating the need
for invasive monitoring in most cases.

Ligand-binding sites in the temporal lobe
are altered in temporal lobe epilepsy. Binding of
[^{11}C]carfentanyl, an agonist at μ opiate receptors (see Chap. 18), is increased in the temporal
neocortex ipsilateral to the seizure focus [38];
and binding of [^{11}C]flumazenil, an antagonist of
the central benzodiazepine receptor, is focally
decreased in the hippocampal formation [39].
The former observation suggests a biochemical
disturbance of neurotransmission at a distance
from the presumed focus, as is found metabolically; however, the pathological correlate of altered opiate binding has yet to be established.
The reduction in hippocampal benzodiazepine
receptors appears to be a marker of their loss in
mesial temporal sclerosis, thus enhancing the
anatomical specificity of presurgical imaging.

Several aspects of the underlying pharmacology and physiology of the epileptogenic focus
remain to be examined by PET. The studies reported to date have described patients with well-
established epilepsy who are generally taking at

least one anticonvulsant medication at the time
of study. Some of the observed metabolic
changes may thus relate to effects of either repeated seizures, medications or both. The observation of benzodiazepine receptor loss in the
hippocampal formation may reflect local damage caused by repeated seizures in an area of selective vulnerability, or it may constitute the
necessary substrate for medically refractory
seizures. Future investigations focusing on new-
onset seizures in unmedicated patients may allow
distinctions among pathogenic mechanisms,
therapeutic effects and secondary changes resulting from repeated seizures.

Studies of cerebrovascular disease show the evolution of metabolic and blood flow changes in ischemic brain

The diagnosis and management of patients with
cerebrovascular insufficiency is problematic in
the clinical neurosciences. The factors that lead
to cerebral ischemia are numerous, and there are
a variety of methods proposed for its diagnosis
and management. Potential therapeutic modalities for ischemic cerebrovascular disease include
vascular surgery, anticoagulation or inhibition
of platelet aggregation, thrombolysis and cerebral protection with antioxidant or metabolic
inhibiting agents. Prior to the use of PET, the
pathophysiological evolution from ischemic to
infarcted brain in human stroke was unknown.
Although animal models of stroke have permitted biochemical and physiological measurement
of ischemic brain, the relevance to human cerebrovascular disease is controversial (see also
Chap. 31).

Several PET studies of stroke have examined the evolution of changes in infarcted regions as well as in the surrounding brain (see
also Chap. 34). It was demonstrated by using
[^{18}F]2FDG and [^{13}N]NH$_3$ that glucose
metabolism and blood flow become uncoupled
in the course of ischemic infarction [40]. Very
early after onset of symptoms, within days, regions of reduced blood flow and relatively preserved metabolic activity are observed. Within
the first 2 weeks, these regions become relatively
hyperemic with sustained glucose metabolism.
In chronic lesions that appear atrophic on CT

scans, a relatively matched metabolic and perfusion deficit is observed. A subsequent study of stroke using measures of oxygen metabolism and blood flow [41] revealed an early rise in regional oxygen extraction in the ischemic area that resolves over the first week, becoming hypometabolic, as originally observed with [^{18}F]2FDG. Serial determinations of both oxygen and glucose metabolism in the same patients identified an abnormal relationship in the infarcted regions. The usual coupling ratio of 6 mol of O_2 per mole of glucose oxidized is reduced to 2 mol of O_2, indicating that anaerobic glycolysis or oxidation of alternative substrates occurs in recent cerebral infarction [42]. Studies in experimental animals reveal that the appearance of phagocytic cells in infarcted brain is associated with non-neuronal metabolic activity [22]. Thus, the clinical observation of altered oxygen-to-glucose stoichiometry in early cerebral infarction may reflect that of inflammatory cells rather than viable brain tissue.

Other PET studies in cerebrovascular disease have focused on the pathophysiological changes in ischemic but uninfarcted brain [43]. Patients with occlusive disease of the major cerebral arteries have varied blood flow and metabolic abnormalities. Thus, some patients with adequate collateral circulation may demonstrate no abnormalities of CBF, CBV or oxygen extraction. Patients with compensated disease generally show increased CBV but normal flow on the basis of vasodilation distal to the stenotic lesion. Patients with recurrent ischemic symptoms who have an inadequate compensatory reserve demonstrate normal oxygen metabolism but decreased CBF and increased CBV and oxygen extraction. The latter parameter appears to be the most sensitive and specific marker for inadequate perfusion to meet metabolic demands.

The findings in stroke as well as those in noninfarct cerebrovascular insufficiency suggest a continuum of pathological alterations with physiological compensation by vasodilation and collateral circulation. When the metabolic demands of the tissue can no longer be met by increasing the extractions of oxygen and glucose, infarction results. PET studies suggest that cerebral damage occurs rapidly and that possible interventional therapies must therefore be at-

tempted before or soon after the onset of symptoms to be of benefit. The application of PET to future studies of cerebrovascular disease will focus on prospective monitoring to find changes occurring before or soon after onset of symptoms. Diagnostic probes that will distinguish reversible from irreversible ischemic changes remain to be clinically validated. However, encouraging preliminary results have been obtained in studies employing benzodiazepine receptor binding to distinguish infarcted brain from viable tissue, in which flow and metabolism are reversibly reduced as a result of diaschesis but receptor binding is largely maintained.

Studies of Parkinson's disease reveal distinct subgroups of patients and permit assessment of medication effects

Patients with the clinical syndrome of parkinsonism, including bradykinesia, resting tremor and postural instability, represent a heterogeneous group with a variety of underlying pathologies and distinct therapeutic medication responses. The main postmortem pathological abnormality recognized in Parkinson's disease (PD) is a reduction of striatal dopaminergic nerve terminals attributed to cell loss in the substantia nigra pars compacta (see Chap. 45). In this case, and in other situations where the presynaptic DA system is depleted with relative preservation of postsynaptic striatal elements, patients respond symptomatically to administration of the DA precursor L-DOPA and to DA receptor agonist drugs. However, a subset of parkinsonian patients do not benefit from these medications. It may be difficult to discriminate the presence or absence of initial therapeutic benefit since early symptoms of the disease may be mild, and the possibility of placebo responses cannot be discounted in consideration of subjective effects. In life, the neuropathological bases of drug-resistant parkinsonian syndromes are assumed to be intrinsic striatal pathology or other nondopaminergic lesions.

The availability of several PET ligands for evaluation of the dopaminergic synapse now permits definitive classification of patients early in the course of illness with regard to the site(s) of neurochemical pathology. Presynaptic dopaminergic markers, including presynaptic DA-reuptake sites, termed the DA transporter (DAT) [31]; synaptic vesicular monoamine transporters (VMAT2) [32]; and DOPA decarboxylase activity [25], may be determined with the tracers [^{11}C]cocaine, [^{11}C]dihydrotetrabenazine and [^{18}F]FDOPA, respectively (see Chaps. 5 and 12). The D2-DA receptor, predominantly a postsynaptic striatal marker, may be measured with a variety of radioligands, including [^{11}C]raclopride [44]. Studies with these tracers afford important verifications of postmortem measures since symptomatic therapeutic trials are known to alter many of the biochemical markers of DA synapses.

Patients with typical PD have reduced DOPA decarboxylase activity in the putamen [45,46] and reduced DAT sites [47] with preserved D2 receptors in PET studies. Presynaptic markers are asymmetrically reduced in many early cases, in concordance with individual side-to-side asymmetries in clinical signs. Of particular interest, relatives of patients with a history of familial PD may have reduced decarboxylase activity in the absence of clinical signs or symptoms [46]. This observation supports the hypothesis that PD pathology is present and progressive well in advance of its clinical diagnosis and that PD may reflect a lifelong accelerated loss of neurons due to an initial defect in substantia nigra neurons.

Other parkinsonian syndromes that fail to respond fully to medications include progressive supranuclear palsy (PSP) and multiple system atrophy (MSA). In these instances, there are distinct patterns of dopaminergic marker losses that differ from each other and from PD [47]. Patients with PSP demonstrate loss of striatal D2 receptors, indicating a postsynaptic striatal lesion. Patients with MSA or with PSP demonstrate loss of presynaptic DA terminals in the caudate nucleus as well as in the putamen, again, in distinction to the pattern seen in typical PD. These measurements permit separation of patients early in the course of disease and may assist in determining the causes and pathophysiologies in these disorders.

An additional area of interest in PD is the possible role of differing treatment strategies on the progression of the disease. There has been an intensive search for treatments that might slow or halt progressive losses of dopaminergic neurons, and concern that DA metabolism and, thus, L-DOPA treatment might pose metabolic "stress" on surviving neurons and hasten their deterioration. PET is well suited to the study of problems such as these with longitudinal experimental designs. However, a marker for DA synapses which is not affected by counter-regulatory change or medications is required. Of the previously described markers, only the VMAT2-binding site density has been demonstrated to reflect pathological losses of DA terminals without regulation in response to dopaminergic drug treatments (see discussion in [32]). Future VMAT2 PET studies may thus aid in evaluating potential disease-modifying aspects of existing or of novel treatments for PD.

ACKNOWLEDGMENTS

The author was supported in part by grants MH49748 and NS15655 from the USPHS, National Institutes of Health, during the preparation of this chapter.

REFERENCES

1. Phelps, M. E., Mazziotta, J. C., and Schelbert, H. R. (eds.) *Positron Emission Tomography and Autoradiography. Principles and Applications for the Brain and Heart.* New York: Raven Press, 1986.
2. Sorenson, J. A., and Phelps, M. E. *Physics in Nuclear Medicine,* 2nd ed. New York: Grune and Stratton, 1987.
3. Koeppe, R. A., and Hutchins, G. D. Instrumentation for positron emission tomography: Tomographs and data processing and display systems. *Semin. Nucl. Med.* 22:162–181, 1992.
4. Jacquez, J. A. *Compartmental Analysis in Biology and Medicine,* 2nd ed. Ann Arbor: University of Michigan, 1985.
5. Brooks, D. J., Beaney, R. P., Lammertsma, A. A., et al. Quantitative measurement of blood–brain barrier permeability using rubidium-82 and positron emission tomography. *J. Cereb. Blood Flow Metab.* 4:535–545, 1984.

6. Hawkins, R. A., Phelps, M. E., Huang, S.-C., et al. A kinetic evaluation of blood–brain barrier permeability in human brain tumors with [^{68}Ga]EDTA and positron computed tomography. *J. Cereb. Blood Flow Metab.* 4:507–515, 1984.

7. Washburn, L. C., Blair, L. D., Byrd, B. L., and Sun, T. T. Comparison of 68Ga-EDTA, [1–11C]alpha-aminoisobutyric acid, and [99mTc]sodium pertechnetate in an experimental blood–brain barrier lesion. *Int. J. Nucl. Med. Biol.* 12:267–269, 1985.

8. Huang, S.-C., Carson, R. E., Hoffman, E. J., et al. Quantitative measurement of local cerebral blood flow in humans by positron computed tomography and ^{15}O-water. *J. Cereb. Blood Flow Metab.* 3:141–153, 1983.

9. Herscovitch, P., Markham, J., and Raichle, M. E. Brain blood flow measured with intravenous H$_2$^{15}O. I. Theory and error analysis. *J. Nucl. Med.* 24:782–789, 1983.

10. Hawkins, R. A., Phelps, M. E., Huang, S.-C., and Kuhl, D. E. Effect of ischemia on quantification of local cerebral glucose metabolic rate in man. *J. Cereb. Blood Flow Metab.* 1:37–51, 1981.

11. Worsley, K. J., Marrett, S., Neelin, P., et al. A unified statistical approach for determining significant signals in images of cerebral activation. *Hum. Brain Map.* 4:58–73, 1996.

12. Bookstein, F. L. Principal warps: Thin-plate splines and the decomposition of deformations. *IEEE Trans. Pattern Anal. Mach. Intell.* 11:567–585, 1989.

13. Collins, D. L., Neelin, P., Peters, T. M., and Evans, A. C. Automatic 3D intersubject registration of MR volumetric data in standardized Talairach space. *J. Comput. Assist. Tomogr.* 18:192–205, 1994.

14. Raichle, M. E. Images of the mind: Studies with modern imaging techniques. *Annu. Rev. Psychol.* 45:333–356, 1994.

15. Buckner, R. L., Bandettini, P. A., O'Craven, K. M., et al. Detection of cortical activation during averaged single trials of a cognitive task using functional magnetic resonance imaging. *Proc. Natl. Acad. Sci. USA* 93:14878–14883, 1996.

16. Sokoloff, L., Reivich, M., Kennedy, C., et al. The [^{14}C]deoxyglucose method for the measurement of local cerebral glucose utilization: Theory, procedure, and normal values in the conscious and anesthetized albino rat. *J. Neurochem.* 28:897–916, 1977.

17. Reivich, M., Kuhl, D., Wolf, A., et al. The [^{18}F]fluorodeoxyglucose method for the measurement of local cerebral glucose utilization in man. *Circ. Res.* 44:127–137, 1979.

18. Phelps, M. E., Huang, S.-C., Hoffman, E. J., et al. Tomographic measurement of local cerebral glucose metabolic rate in humans with (F-18)2-fluoro-2-deoxy-D-glucose: Validation of method. *Ann. Neurol.* 6:371–388, 1979.

19. Crane, P. D., Pardridge, W. M., Braun, L. D., and Oldendorf, W. H. Kinetics of transport and phosphorylation of 2-fluoro-2-deoxy-D-glucose in rat brain. *J. Neurochem.* 40:160–167, 1983.

20. Heiss, W.-D., Pawlik, G., Herholz, K., et al. Regional kinetic constants and cerebral metabolic rate for glucose in normal human volunteers determined by dynamic positron emission tomography of [^{18}F]2-fluoro-2-deoxy-D-glucose. *J. Cereb. Blood Flow Metab.* 4:212–223, 1984.

21. Sokoloff, L. Localization of functional activity in the central nervous system by measurement of glucose utilization with radioactive deoxyglucose. *J. Cereb. Blood Flow Metab.* 1:7–36, 1981.

22. Agranoff, B. W., and Frey, K. A. A regional metabolic contrast method for the study of brain pathology. *Ann. Neurol.* 15:S93–S97, 1984.

23. Frackowiack, R. S., Lenzi, G.-L., Jones, T., and Heather, J. D. Quantitative measurement of regional cerebral blood flow and oxygen metabolism in man using ^{15}O and positron emission tomography: Theory, procedure, and normal values. *J. Comput. Assist. Tomogr.* 4:727–736, 1980.

24. Mintun, M. A., Raichle, M. E., Martin, W. R. W., and Herscovitch, P. Brain oxygen utilization measured with O-15 radiotracers and positron emission tomography. *J. Nucl. Med.* 25:177–187, 1984.

25. Gjedde, A., Reith, J., Dyve, S., et al. DOPA decarboxylase activity of the living human brain. *Proc. Natl. Acad. Sci. USA* 88:2721–2725, 1991.

26. Diksic, M., Nagahiro, S., Chaly, T., Sourkes, T. L., Yamamoto, L., and Feindel, W. Serotonin synthesis rate measured in living dog brain by positron tomography. *J. Neurochem.* 56:153–162, 1991.

27. Frey, K. A., Hichwa, R. D., Ehrenkaufer, R. L. E., and Agranoff, B. W. Quantitative *in vivo* receptor binding III: Tracer kinetic modeling of muscarinic cholinergic receptor binding. *Proc. Natl. Acad. Sci. USA* 82:6711–6715, 1985.

28. Frey, K. A., Koeppe, R. A., Mulholland, G. K., et al. *In vivo* muscarinic cholinergic receptor imaging with [^{11}C]scopolamine and positron emission tomography. *J. Cereb. Blood Flow Metab.* 12:147–154, 1992.

29. Frey, K. A., Holthoff, V. A., Koeppe, R. A., et al. Parametric *in vivo* imaging of benzodiazepine receptor distribution in human brain. *Ann. Neurol.* 30:663–672, 1991.

30. Fowler, J. S., MacGregor, R. R., Wolf, A. P., et al. Mapping human brain monoamine oxidase A and B with ^{11}C-labeled suicide inactivators and PET. *Science* 235:481–485, 1987.

31. Volkow, N. D., Fowler, J. S., Wang, G. J., et al. Decreased dopamine transporters with age in healthy human subjects. *Ann. Neurol.* 36:237–239, 1994.

32. Frey, K. A., Koeppe, R. A., Kilbourn, M. R., et al. Presynaptic monoaminergic vesicles in Parkinson's disease and normal aging. *Ann. Neurol.* 40:873–884, 1996.

33. Benson, D. F., Kuhl, D. E., Hawkins, R. A., et al. The fluorodeoxyglucose-18F scan in Alzheimer's disease and multi-infarct dementia. *Arch. Neurol.* 40:711–714, 1983.

34. Frey, K. A., Minoshima, S., and Kuhl, D. E. Neurochemical imaging of Alzheimer's disease and other degenerative dementias. *Q. J. Nucl. Med.* (in press), 1998.

35. Kuhl, D. E., Engel, J., Jr., Phelps, M. E., and Selin, C. Epileptic patterns of cerebral metabolism and perfusion in humans determined by emission computed tomography of 18FDG and 13 NH3. *Ann. Neurol.* 8:348–360, 1980.

36. Engel, J., Jr., Brown, W. J., Kuhl, D. E., et al. Pathological findings underlying focal temporal lobe hypometabolism in partial epilepsy. *Ann. Neurol.* 12:518–528, 1982.

37. Abou-Khalil, B. W., Siegel, G. J., Hichwa, R. D., Sackellares, J. C., and Gilman, S. Topography of glucose metabolism in epilepsy of mesial temporal origin. *Ann. Neurol.* 18:151, 1985.

38. Frost, J. J., Mayberg, H. S., Fisher, R. S., et al. Mu-opiate receptors measured by positron emission tomography are increased in temporal lobe epilepsy. *Ann. Neurol.* 23:231–237, 1988.

39. Henry, T. R., Frey, K. A., Sackellares, J. C., et al. *In vivo* cerebral metabolism and central benzodiazepine receptor binding in temporal lobe epilepsy. *Neurology* 43:1998–2006, 1993.

40. Kuhl, D. E., Phelps, M. E., Kowll, A. P., et al. Effects of stroke on local cerebral metabolism and perfusion: Mapping by emission computed tomography of 18FDG and 13NH$_3$. *Ann. Neurol.* 8:47–60, 1980.

41. Wise, R. J. S., Bernardi, S., Frackowizk, R. S. J., et al. Serial observations on the pathophysiology of acute stroke. The transition from ischaemia to infarction as reflected in regional oxygen extraction. *Brain* 106:197–222, 1983.

42. Wise, R. J. S., Rhodes, C. G., Gibbs, J. M., et al. Disturbance of oxidative metabolism of glucose in recent human cerebral infarcts. *Ann. Neurol.* 14:627–637, 1983.

43. Powers, W. J., Press, G. A., Grubb, R. L., et al. The effect of hemodynamically significant carotid artery disease on the hemodynamic status of the cerebral circulation. *Ann. Intern. Med.* 106:27–35, 1987.

44. Farde, L., Eriksson, L., Blomquist, G., and Halldin, C. Kinetic analysis of central [^{11}C]raclopride binding to D2-dopamine receptors studied by PET: A comparison to the equilibrium analysis. *J. Cereb. Blood Flow Metab.* 9:696–708, 1989.

45. Brooks, D. J., Ibanez, V., Swale, G., et al. Differing patterns of striatal 18F-dopa uptake in Parkinson's disease, multiple system atrophy, and progressive supranuclear palsy. *Ann. Neurol.* 28:547–555, 1990.

46. Swale, G. V., Wroe, S. J., Lees, A. J., et al. The identification of presymptomatic Parkinsonism: Clinical and [^{18}F]dopa positron emission tomography studies in an Irish kindred. *Ann. Neurol.* 32:609–617, 1992.

47. Brooks, D. J. Positron emission tomographic studies of subcortical degenerations and dystonia. *Semin. Neurol.* 9:351–359, 1989.

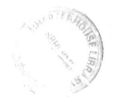

Glossary

AA	arachidonic acid	BAPTA	1,2-*bis*(o-aminophenoxy)ethane-*N*-*N*-*N′*-*N′*-tetraacetic acid
AADC	aromatic L-amino acid decarboxylase	BBB	blood-brain barrier
AANAT	aryl alkylamine *N*-acetyltransferase	BCAA	branched chain amino acids
AAV	adeno-associated virus	BCP	bag cell peptides
ABC	ATP-binding cassette	BCDHC	branched chain dehydrogenase complex
Aβ	amyloid β-peptide		
AC	adenylyl cyclase	BCH	2-aminonorbornane-2-carboxylic acid
ACh	acetylcholine		
AChE	acetylcholinesterase	BDNF	brain-derived neurotrophic factor
AChR	acetylcholine receptor	BH$_4$	tetrahydrobiopterin
ACTH	adrenocorticotrophic hormone	BMAA	β-*N*-methylamino-L-alanine
AD	Alzheimer's disease	BMP	bone morphogenetic proteins
ADP	adenosine 5′-diphosphate	BNP	brain natriuretic peptide
AIDS	acquired immunodeficiency syndrome	BOLD	blood oxygenation level dependent
AIP	acute intermittent porphyria	BPB	*p*-bromophenacyl bromide
AKAP	protein kinase A anchoring protein	BSE	bovine spongiform encephalopathy
AL	argininosuccinate lyase	BTX	batrachotoxin
ALD	adrenoleukodystrophy	BuChE	butyryl (or pseudo) cholinesterases
ALS	amyotrophic lateral sclerosis	CA	catecholamines
AMD	(i) age-related macular degeneration; (ii) acid maltase deficiency	cADPr	cyclic adenosine diphosphate ribose
		CAK	CDK-activating kinase
AMN	adrenomyeloneuropathy	CAKAK	CAK-activating kinase
AMOG	adhesion molecule on glia	CAM	cell adhesion molecule
AMP	adenosine 5′-monophosphate	CaMK	Ca^{2+}-calmodulin-dependent protein kinases
AMP-PNP	adenylylimidodiphosphate		
AMPA	α-amino-3-hydroxy-5-methyl-4-isoxazole propionic acid	cAMP	cyclic AMP; adenosine 3′,5′-monophosphate
AMPT	α-methyl-*p*-tyrosine	CBF	cerebral blood flow
ANP	atrial natriuretic peptide	CBP	CREB-binding protein
L-AP4	L-amino-4-phosphonobutyrate	CBV	cerebral blood volume
ApCAM	*Aplysia* cell adhesion molecule	CCK	cholecystokinin
APDC	2R,4R-4-aminopyrrolidine-2-4-dicarboxylate	cdc	cell division cycle (protein)
		cDNA	complementary DNA
ApoE	apolipoprotein E	CDF	cholinergic differentiation factor
APP	amyloid precursor protein	CDK	cyclin-dependent kinase
APPL	β-amyloid precursor like protein	CDP	cytidine diphosphate
ARAS	ascending reticular activating system	CDP·DAG	cytidine diphosphate diacylglycerol
ARF	ADP-ribosylation factor	Cer-Glc	glucocerebroside
ARIA	ACh receptor-inducing activity	CF	climbing fiber
Arp1	actin related protein 1	CFTR	cystic fibrosis transmembrane conductance regulator
AS	argininosuccinate synthetase		
ATF	activating transcription factor	CG	complementation groups
ATP	adenosine 5′-triphosphate	cGMP	cyclic GMP; guanosine 3′,5′-cyclic monophosphate
βAPP	β-amyloid precursor protein		
βARK	β-adrenergic receptor kinase		
βLPH	β-lipotropin	CGRP	calcitonin gene-related peptide

ChAT	choline acetyltransferase	DARPP-32	dopamine- and cAMP-regulated phosphoprotein of 32 kDa
CICR	Ca^{2+}-induced Ca^{2+} release		
CIDP	chronic inflammatory demyelinating polyneuropathy	DAT	dopamine transporter
		DBH	dopamine β-hydroxylase
CIF	Ca^{2+} influx factor	DBI	diazepam-binding inhibitor
CIRL	Ca^{2+} independent receptor for latrotoxin	DBM	dopamine β-monooxygenase
		5,7-DCK	5,7-dichlorokynurenic acid
CJD	Creutzfeldt-Jakob disease	DDC	dopa decarboxylase
CK	creatine kinase	2DG	2-deoxy-D-glucose
CMR	cerebral metabolic rate	DHA	docosahexaenoic acid
CMR_{glc}	cerebral metabolic rate for glucose	DHAP	dihydroxyacetone phosphate
CMRA	cerebral metabolic rate for ammonia	DHAP-AT	dihydroxyacetone phosphate acyl transferase
$CMRO_2$	cerebral metabolic rate for O_2	DHEA	dihydroepiandrosterone
CMT	Charcot-Marie-Tooth disease	DHT	5α-dihydrotestosterone
cNG	cyclic nucleotide-gated channel	DHPR	dihydropteridine reductase
CNP	2′,3′-cyclic nucleotide 3′-phosphodiesterase	5,7-DHT	5,7-dihydroxytryptamine
		DMD	Duchenne muscular dystrophy
CNS	central nervous system	L-DOPA	3,4-dihydroxyphenylalanine
CNTF	ciliary neurotrophic factor	DOPAC	3,4-dihydroxyphenylacetic acid
rCNT	nucleoside cotransporter	DRG	dorsal root ganglia
CoA	coenzyme A	DS	Down's syndrome
COMT	catechol-O-methyltransferase	DSS	Derjerine-Sottas syndrome
Con A	concanavalin A	EAAC	excitatory amino acid carrier; see EAAT
COP-1	copolymer-1		
CORT	corticosterone	EAAT	excitatory amino acid transporter; see EAAC
COX	(i) cytochrome oxidase; (ii) cyclooxygenase	EAE	experimental allergic encephalomyelitis
CPE	carboxypeptidase E		
CPK	creatine phosphokinase	EAN	experimental allergic neuritis
mCPP	m-chlorophenylpiperazine	ECM	extracellular matrix
2R-CPPene	3-(2-carboxypiperazin-4-yl) 1-propenyl-1-phosphonic acid	ECT	electroconvulsive therapy
		EDRF	endothelium-derived relaxing factor
CPS	carbamyl phosphate synthetase	EEG	electroencephalogram
CPT	carnitine palmitoyltransferase	EGF	epidermal growth factor
CRE	cAMP responsive element	EGFR	epidermal growth factor receptor
CREB	CRE-binding (protein)	ELISA	enzyme-linked immunoabsorbant assay
CREM	CRE-modulatory (protein)		
CRH	corticotropin releasing hormone	ELH	egg laying hormone
CRM	(immunological) cross-reacting material	EM	electron microscopy
		EMG	electromyogram
CRP	creatine phosphate	ENS	enteric nervous system
CS	conditioned stimulus	EPA	eicosapentaenoic acid
CSF	cerebrospinal fluid	Eph	erythropoietin producing hepatocellular receptor
Csk	C-terminal Src kinase		
CSP	cysteine string protein	EPP	evoked end plate potential
CT	computed tomography	EPS	extrapyramidal syndrome
CT-1	cardiotrophin 1	EPSC	excitatory postsynaptic current
CTP	cytidine 5′-triphosphate	EPSP	excitatory postsynaptic potential
CTX	cortex	ER	endoplasmic reticulum
DA	dopamine	ERG	early response genes
DAG	diacylglycerol	ERK	extracellularly regulated kinase
DAO	diamine oxidase	ES	embryonic stem cells
D-AP5	D-2-amino-5-phosphonopentanoic acid	ETF	electron-transferring flavoprotein

FAD	flavin adenine dinucleotide	Gpx	glutathione peroxidase
FAK	focal adhesion kinase	Grb	growth factor receptor binding protein
FDA	[^{18}F]fluorodopamine		
FDOPA	[^{18}F]6-fluoro-DOPA	GRE	glucocorticoid response element
FFA	free fatty acid	GRK	G protein receptor kinase
FFI	fatal familial insomnia	GS	glycogen synthetase
FGF	fibroblast growth factor	GSH	glutathione
FGFR	fibroblast growth factor receptor	GSS	Gerstmann-Straussler-Scheinker syndrome
FMN	flavin mononucleotide		
FMRF-NH$_2$	Phe-Met-Arg-Phe-amide, a molluscan excitatory neuropeptide	GTP	guanosine 5′-triphosphate
		HC	hippocampus; see also HpC
fMRI	functional magnetic resonance imaging	HCHWA-D	hereditary cerebral hemorrhage with amyloidosis of the Dutch type
FSH	follicle stimulating hormone	HDC	L-histidine decarboxylase
G$_{\alpha gust}$	gustducin G$_\alpha$ protein	HE	hepatic encephalopathy
G6P	glucose 6-phosphate	HETE	hydroxyeicosatetraenoic acid
GABA	γ-aminobutyric acid	HGPRT	hypoxanthine-guanine phosphoribosyltransferase
GABA-T	GABA transaminase		
GAD	glutamic acid decarboxylase	5-HIAA	5-hydroxyindoleacetic acid
GAG	glycosaminoglycans	HIOMT	5-hydroxyindole-*O*-methyltransferase
Gal	galactose		
galC	galactocerebroside	HIV	human immunodeficiency virus
GalNAc	*N*-acetylgalactosamine	HLA	human leukocyte antigen
GAP	GTPase-activating protein	HLH	helix-loop-helix transcriptional regulator
GAP-43	growth-associated protein of 43 kDa		
GBS	Guillain-Barré syndrome	HMG	β-hydroxy-β-methylglutaryl
GC	glucocorticoid	HMM	heavy meromyosin
GCS	glycine cleavage system	HMT	histamine *N*-methyltransferase
GDI	GDP-dissociation inhibitor	HNPP	hereditary neuropathy with predisposition to pressure palsies
GDNF	glial-derived neurotrophic factor		
GDP	guanosine 5′-diphosphate	HpC	hippocampus; see also HC
GEF	guanine nucleotide exchange factor	HPETE	hydroperoxyeicosatetraenoic acid
GEMSA	guanidinoethylmercaptosuccinic acid	HPLC	high-performance liquid chromatography
GFAP	glial fibrillary acidic protein	HPRT	hypoxanthine phosphoribosyltransferase
GGF	glial growth factor		
GI	gastrointestinal (tract)	HPTLC	high-performance thin layer chromatography
GIP	GTPase inhibitory protein		
GIRK	G-protein-coupled inwardly rectifying K$^+$ channel	5-HT	5-hydroxytryptamine; serotonin
		5-HTP	5-hydroxytryptophan
GL	granular layer	HVA	homovanillic acid
GLAST	glutamate-aspartate transporter	I$_{CRAC}$	Ca^{2+}-release-activated Ca^{2+} current
Glc	glucose	IAA	imidazoleacetic acid
GLC	gas-liquid chromatography	ICAM	intercellular adhesion molecule
GlcNAc	*N*-acetylglucosamine	IF	intermediate filaments
GluR	glutamate receptor	Ig	immunoglobulin
GLUT	glucose transporter	IGF	insulin-like growth factor
GLT	glutamate transporter	IL	interleukin
GMP	guanosine 5′-monophosphate	INSR	insulin receptor
GnRH	gonadotropin releasing hormone	IP$_1$	inositol 1-phosphate
GPCR	G-protein-coupled receptor	IP$_2$	inositol 1,4-*bis*phosphate
GPI	glycosylphosphatidylinositol	IP$_3$	inositol 1,4,5-*tris*phosphate
Gpl	lateral globus pallidus	IP$_4$	inositol 1,3,4,5-*tetrakis*phosphate
Gpm	medial globus pallidus	IRD	infantile Refsum disease

IPSP	inhibitory postsynaptic potential	MBP	myelin basic protein
IRS	insulin receptor substrate	MCAD	medium chain acyl CoA dehydrogenase
ITP	inosine phosphate		
ITR	inverted repeated sequence	MCHAD	medium chain 3-hydroxyacyl CoA dehydrogenase
IVG	isovalerylglycine		
JP	joining peptide	MDMA	3,4-methylenedioxymethamphetamine
K_{ca}	Ca^{2+}-activated K^+ channels		
K_{erg}	ether-a-go-go-related K^+ channels	MDR	multidrug resistance protein
K_{ir}	inwardly rectifying K^+ channels	MeAIB	2-methylamino-isobutyric acid
K_v	voltage-gated K^+ channels	MeDOPA	3-O-methyl-DOPA
KA	kainic acid	MEK	MAPK/ERK activating kinase
α-KG	α-ketoglutarate	MEKK	MEK kinase
αKGDH	α-ketoglutarate dehydrogenase	MELAS	mitochondrial myopathy, enceph-
KGDHC	α-ketoglutarate dehydrogenase complex		alopathy, lactic acidosis, and stroke-like episodes
KPI	Kunitz-type serine protease inhibitor	MEPP	miniature end plate potential
KRP	kinesin related protein	MERRF	myoclonus epilepsy with ragged red fibers
KSS	Kearns-Sayre syndrome		
LC	locus ceruleus	MF	microfilament
LCAD	long chain acyl-CoA dehydrogenase	MG	myasthenia gravis
LCHAD	long chain-3-hydroxyacyl-CoA dehydrogenase	mGluR	metabotropic glutamate receptor
		MH	malignant hyperthermia
LDCV	large dense-core vesicle	t-MH	*tele*-methylhistamine
LDH	lactate dehydrogenase	MHC	major histocompatibility complex
LDL	low density lipoprotein	MHPG	3-methoxy-4-hydroxyphenylglycol
LEMS	Lambert-Eaton myasthenic syndrome	t-MIAA	*tele*-methylimidazole acetic acid
		MKP	MAP-kinase phosphatases
LH	luteinizing hormone	ML	molecular layer
LHON	Leber's hereditary optic neuropathy	MLD	metachromatic leukodystrophy
LHRH	luteinizing hormone-releasing hormone	MMA	methylmalonic acid
		MMN	multifocal motor neuropathy
LIF	leukemia inhibitory factor	MOG	myelin-oligodendrocyte glycoprotein
LIFR	leukemia inhibitory factor receptor		
LMM	light meromyosin	MPP^+	1-methyl-4-phenylpyridinium
LNAA	large neutral amino acid	MPTP	1-methyl-4-phenyl-1,2,3,6-tetrahydropyridine
LPS	lipopolysaccharide		
LSD	lysergic acid diethylamide	MRP	multidrug resistant proteins
LTD	long-term depression	MRI	magnetic resonance imaging
LTP	long-term potentiation	mRNA	messenger RNA
mAChR	muscarinic acetylcholine receptor	MS	multiple sclerosis
MAG	myelin-associated glycoprotein	MSA	multiple system atrophy
MAGUK	membrane-associated guanylyl kinase homolog	MSD	multiple sulfatase deficiency
		MSUD	maple syrup urine disease
MAO	monoamine oxidase	MT	microtubule
MAOI	monoamine oxidase inhibitors	3-MT	3-methoxytyramine
MAP	microtubule-associated protein	mtDNA	mitochondrial DNA
MAPK	mitogen-activated protein kinase	MTOC	microtubule-organizing center
MAPKAP	MAP-kinase-activated protein kinase	MuSK	muscle specific kinase
MARCKS	myristoylated alanine-rich protein kinase C substrate	Na,K-ATPase	$(Na^+ + K^+)$-stimulated adenosine triphosphatase
MAS	malate-aspartate shuttle	NAAG	N-acetylaspartyl glutamate
MASC	myotube-associated specificity component	NAALADase	N-acetyl alpha-linked acidic dipeptidase
MBO	membrane-bounded organelle	nAChR	nicotinic ACh receptor

NAD$^+$	nicotinamide adenine dinucleotide (oxidized)	PAH	phenylalanine hydroxylase
NADH	nicotinamide adenine dinucleotide (reduced)	PAL	peptidyl-α-hydroxyglycine α-amidating lyase
NADP$^+$	nicotinamide adenine dinucleotide phosphate (oxidized)	PAM	peptidylglycine α-amidating mono-oxygenase
NADPH	nicotinamide adenine dinucleotide phosphate (reduced)	PaO$_2$	partial pressure of ambient arterial oxygen
NAG	*N*-acetylglutamate	PARP	polyADP-ribose polymerase
NALD	neonatal adrenoleukodystrophy	PAS	periodic acid Schiff base
NANA	*N*-acetylneuraminic acid	PBN	*N-tert*-butyl-alpha-phenylnitrone
NBQX	6-nitro 7-sulphamobenzo[f]quin-oxaline-2,3-dione	PC	(i) phosphatidylcholine; (ii) prohormone convertase
NC	neural crest	PCA	*para*chloroamphetamine
NCAM	neural cell adhesion molecule	PCL	Purkinje cell layers
NDF	neu differentiation factor	PCP	phencyclidine
nDNA	nuclear DNA	PCPA	*para*chlorophenylalanine
NE	norepinephrine	PCR	polymerase chain reaction
NET	norepinephrine transporter	PCr	phosphocreatine
NF	(i) neurofilament; (ii) neurofibro-matosis	PD	Parkinson's disease
		PDE	phosphodiesterase
NFT	neurofibrillary tangle	PDGF	platelet-derived growth factor
NgCAM	neuronal glial cell adhesion molecule	PDGFR	platelet-derived growth factor receptor
NGF	nerve growth factor		
NGFR	nerve growth factor receptor	PDHC	pyruvate dehydrogenase complex
NHE	Na$^+$/H$^+$ antiporters	PEPCK	phosphoenolpyruvate carboxykinase
NIPP	nuclear inhibitor of protein phos-phatase	PET	positron emission tomography
		PFC	prefrontal cortex
NKH	nonketotic hyperglycinemia	PFK	phosphofructokinase
NMDA	*N*-methyl-D-aspartate	PG	prostaglandin
NMJ	neuromuscular junction	PGK	phosphoglycerate kinase
NMR	nuclear magnetic resonance	PGM	phosphoglycerate mutase
NO	nitric oxide	PGS	prostaglandin G/H synthase
NOS	nitric oxide synthase	PH	pleckstrin-homology
NPY	neuropeptide Y	PHAL	*Phaseolus vulgaris* leukoagglutinin
NRD	*N*-arginine dibasic	PHF	paired, helically wound, ~10 nm fil-ament
NRPTK	nonreceptor protein tyrosine kinase		
NSAID	nonsteroidal anti-inflammatory drug	PHGPx	phospholipid hydroperoxide glu-tathione peroxidase
		PHM	peptidylglycine α-hydroxylating monooxygenase
NSF	*N*-ethylmaleimide-sensitive factor		
NT	neurotrophin	PI	(i) phosphatidylinositol; (ii) phos-phoinositide
OAG	1-oleoyl, 2-acetyl *sn*-glycerol		
OCD	obsessive-compulsive disorder	PI 3-kinase	phosphatidylinositol 3-kinase
OCRL	oculocerebrorenal syndrome	PIP	phosphatidylinositol 4-phosphate
6-OHDA	6-hydroxydopamine	PIP$_2$	phosphatidylinositol 4,5-*bis*phos-phate
Ol	oligodendrocyte		
3-OMD	3-*O*-methyldopa	PI-PLC	phosphoinositide-specific phospho-lipase C
OTC	ornithine transcarbamylase		
~P	high-energy phosphate bond	PKA	protein kinase A; cAMP-dependent protein kinase
P$_i$	inorganic phosphate		
PA	phosphatidic acid	PKC	protein kinase C; Ca^{2+}/diacylgly-cerol-dependent protein kinase
PACAP	pituitary adenylyl cyclase-activating peptide		
		PKG	protein kinase G; cGMP-dependent protein kinase
PAF	platelet-activating factor		

PKU	phenylketonuria
PLA	phospholipase A
PLC	phospholipase C
PLD	phospholipase D
PLP	proteolipid protein
PMCA	plasma-membrane Ca^{2+} pump
PMD	Pelizaeus-Merzbacher disease
PML	progressive multifocal leukoencephalopathy
PMP	peripheral myelin protein
PNMT	phenylethanolamine *N*-methyltransferase
PNS	peripheral nervous system
pO_2	local partial pressure for O_2
POMC	proopiomelanocortin
POU	a conserved region in pit-1, oct-1, oct-2 and unc-86 proteins
PP1 or PP2	protein phosphatase 1 or 2
PPADS	pyridoxal phosphate-6-azophenyl-2′,4′-disulfonic acid
PRL	prolactin
proANF	proatrial natriuretic factor
PrP	prion protein
PrP^Sc	scrapie prion protein
PS	(i) pregnenolone sulfate; (ii) phosphatidylserine—see PtdSer; (iii) presenilin
PSA	polysialic acid
PSE	portal-systemic encephalopathy
PSEP	postsynaptic excitatory potential; see EPSP
PsmR	presynaptic membrane receptor
PSP	progressive supranuclear palsy
PT	pars tuberalis
PTB	phosphotyrosine binding domain
PTBR	peripheral-type benzodiazepine receptor
PtdCho	phosphatidylcholine
PtdEtn	phosphatidylethanolamine
PtdIns	phosphatidylinositol
PtdIns 4P	phosphatidylinositol 4-phosphate
PtdIns 4,5P_2	phosphatidylinositol 4,5-*bis*phosphate
PtdOH	phosphatidic acid
PtdSer	phosphatidylserine
PTH	parathyroid hormone
PTK	protein tyrosine kinase
PTP	protein tyrosine phosphatase
PTS-1	peroxisomal targeting signals (C-terminal)
PTS-2	peroxisomal targeting signals (N-terminal)
PTSD	post-traumatic stress disorder
PVN	paraventricular nucleus
PYK	proline-rich tyrosine kinase
PZ	pirenzepine
R^*	photoactivated rhodopsin
RACK	receptors for activated protein kinase C
RAGS	repulsive axon guidance signal
RAK	delayed rectifier potassium channel
RCDP	rhizomelic chondrodysplasia punctata
rCMR_{glc}	regional cerebral metabolic rate for glucose
REM	rapid eye movement
RER	rough endoplasmic reticulum
RFLP	restriction fragment length polymorphism
RGS	regulators of G protein signaling
ROS	reactive oxygen species
RP	retinitis pigmentosa
RPTK	receptor protein tyrosine kinase; see also RTK
RQ	respiratory quotient
RR	ryanodine receptor calcium ion channel
Rsk	ribosomal protein S6 kinase
RTK	receptor tyrosine kinase; see also RPTK
RT-PCR	reverse transcriptase-polymerase chain reaction
RVD	regulatory volume decrease
RVI	regulatory volume increase
SAG	Schwann cell membrane associated glycoprotein
SAH	*S*-adenosylhomocysteine
SAM	*S*-adenosylmethionine
SAPK	stress activated protein kinase
SBP	serotonin binding protein
Sca	slow component a (of axonal transport)
SCAD	short chain acyl-CoA dehydrogenase
SCAMP	secretory carrier membrane protein
Scb	slow component b (of axonal transport)
SCG	superior cervical ganglion
SCHAD	short chain 3-hydroxyacyl-CoA dehydrogenase
SCIP	suppressed cyclic AMP-inducible POU domain protein
SCN	suprachiasmatic nuclei
ScTX	scorpion toxin
SDS	sodium dodecylsulfate
SDS-PAGE	sodium dodecylsulfate-polyacrylamide gel electrophoresis
SE	status epilepticus
SEK	SAPK kinase
SER	smooth endoplasmic reticulum

SERCA	smooth endoplasmic reticulum Ca^{2+} antiporter	TGFβ	transforming growth factor β
SERT	serotonin transporter	TH	tyrosine hydroxylase
SGPG	sulfate-3-glucuronyl paragloboside	THIP	4,5,6,7-tetrahydroisoxazolo-[5,4-*c*]-pyridine-3-ol
SH	src homology domain	THPROG	3α, 5α-pregnan-3α-ol-20-one
SHC	src homology collagen-like protein	TK	transketolase
SHP	SH2 domain containing protein tyrosine phosphatase	TLC	thin-layer chromatography
SHIP	src homology inositol phosphatase	TM; TMD	transmembrane spanning domain
SHMT	serine hydroxymethyltransferase	TNF	tumor necrosis factor
SIF	small, intensely fluorescent (cells)	TP	trifunctional protein
SMDF	sensory and motor neuron-derived growth factor	TPA	(i) tissue plasminogen activator; (ii) 12-D-tetradecanoyl phorbol-13-acetate
SMP	Schwann cell myelin protein	TRE	12-D-tetradecanoyl phorbol-13-acetate response element
SNAP	soluble NSF attachment protein		
SNc	substantia nigra pars compacta	TRH	thyrotropin-releasing hormone
SNE	subacute necrotizing encephalo-myelopathy	TSE	transmissible spongiform encephalopathy
SNr	substantia nigra pars reticulata	TSH	thyroid stimulating hormone
SNT	suc-associated neurotrophic factor-induced tyrosine-phosphorylated target	TTP	thiamine triphosphate
		TTX	tetrodotoxin
		Ub	ubiquitin
SOD	superoxide dismutase	UDP	uridine 5′-diphosphate
SOS	son of sevenless (a G protein)	UDP-glucose	uridine diphosphoglucose
SPECT	single photon emission computerized tomography	US	unconditioned stimulus
		UTP	uridine 5′-triphosphate
SR	sarcoplasmic reticulum	VAChT	vesicular acetylcholine transporter
SRF	serum responsive factor	VAMP	vesicle associated membrane protein; synaptobrevin
SRP	signal recognition particle		
SSADH	succinic semialdehyde dehydrogenase	VBR	ventricular:brain ratio
		VGCC	voltage-gated Ca^{2+} channel
SSRI	selective serotonin reuptake inhibitor	VIP	vasoactive intestinal peptide
		VLCAD	very long chain acyl-CoA dehydrogenase
SSPE	subacute sclerosing panencephalomyelitis		
		VLCFA	very long chain fatty acids
SSV	small secretory vesicles	VMAT	vesicular membrane amine transporters
ST	striatum		
STN	subthalamic nucleus	VMH	ventromedial hypothalamus
Str	striatum	VNO	vomeronasal organ
SVZ	subventricular zones	VPM	ventral posterior medial nucleus
SWD	spike and wave discharges	VT	ventral tegmentum
TBPS	*t*-butyl bicyclophosphorothionate	WIPTIDE	Walsh inhibitor protein peptide
TC	transcobalamin	WM	white matter
TCA	(i) tricyclic antidepressant; (ii) tricarboxylic acid (cycle)	YAC	yeast artificial chromosome
		YAP	yeast aspartyl protease
TCR	T cell receptor	ZS	Zellweger syndrome
TEXAN	toxin extruding antiporter		

AMINO ACIDS IN PROTEINS

Symbol		Name	Codons					
One letter	Three letter							
A	Ala	Alanine	GCA	GCC	GCG	GCU		
C	Cys	Cysteine	UGC	UGU				
D	Asp	Aspartate	GAC	GAU				
E	Glu	Glutamate	GAA	GAG				
F	Phe	Phenylalanine	UUC	UUU				
G	Gly	Glycine	GGA	GGC	GGG	GGU		
H	His	Histidine	CAC	CAU				
I	Ile	Isoleucine	AUA	AUC	AUU			
K	Lys	Lysine	AAA	AAG				
L	Leu	Leucine	UUA	UUG	CUA	CUC	CUG	CUU
M	Met	Methionine	AUG					
N	Asn	Asparagine	AAC	AAU				
P	Pro	Proline	CCA	CCC	CCG	CCU		
Q	Gln	Glutamine	CAA	CAG				
R	Arg	Arginine	AGA	AGG	CGA	CGC	CGG	CGU
S	Ser	Serine	AGC	AGU	UCA	UCC	UCG	UCU
T	Thr	Threonine	ACA	ACC	ACG	ACU		
V	Val	Valine	GUA	GUC	GUG	GUU		
W	Trp	Trytophan	UGG					
Y	Tyr	Tyrosine	UAC	UAU				

Subject Index

Note: Page numbers in *italics* indicate figures; page numbers followed by t are tables.

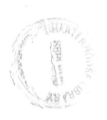